Essential
Clinical Anatomy FOURTH EDITION

Essential
Clinical Anatomy FOURTH EDITION

Keith L. Moore, PhD, FIAC, FRSM, FAAA
Professor Emeritus, Division of Anatomy
Department of Surgery
Former Chair of Anatomy and Associate
Dean for Basic Medical Sciences
Faculty of Medicine, University of Toronto
Toronto, Ontario, Canada

Anne M.R. Agur, BSc(OT), MSc, PhD
Professor, Division of Anatomy
Department of Surgery, Faculty of Medicine
Department of Physical Therapy
Department of Occupational Science & Occupational Therapy
Division of Biomedical Communications
Institute of Medical Science
Graduate Department of Rehabilitation Science
Graduate Department of Dentistry
University of Toronto
Toronto, Ontario, Canada

Arthur F. Dalley II, PhD
Professor, Department of Cell and Developmental Biology
Adjunct Professor, Department of Orthopaedics and Rehabilitation
Director, Structure, Function and
    Development and Anatomical Donations Program
Vanderbilt University School of Medicine
Adjunct Professor for Anatomy
Belmont University School of Physical Therapy
Nashville, Tennessee, U.S.A.

Wolters Kluwer | Lippincott Williams & Wilkins
Health

Philadelphia · Baltimore · New York · London
Buenos Aires · Hong Kong · Sydney · Tokyo

Acquisitions Editor: Crystal Taylor
Product Manager: Julie Montalbano
Marketing Manager: Brian Moody
Design and Art Direction: Jennifer Clements and Doug Smock
Compositor: MPS Content Services

4th Edition

Copyright © 2011, 2007, 2002, 1995 Lippincott Williams & Wilkins, a Wolters Kluwer business.

351 West Camden Street   530 Walnut Street
Baltimore, MD 21201   Philadelphia, PA 19106

Printed in China

9 8 7 6 5 4

ISBN: 978-1-60913-112-8

DISCLAIMER

Care has been taken to confirm the accuracy of the information present and to describe generally accepted practices. However, the authors, editors, and publisher are not responsible for errors or omissions or for any consequences from application of the information in this book and make no warranty, expressed or implied, with respect to the currency, completeness, or accuracy of the contents of the publication. Application of this information in a particular situation remains the professional responsibility of the practitioner; the clinical treatments described and recommended may not be considered absolute and universal recommendations.

The authors, editors, and publisher have exerted every effort to ensure that drug selection and dosage set forth in this text are in accordance with the current recommendations and practice at the time of publication. However, in view of ongoing research, changes in government regulations, and the constant flow of information relating to drug therapy and drug reactions, the reader is urged to check the package insert for each drug for any change in indications and dosage and for added warnings and precautions. This is particularly important when the recommended agent is a new or infrequently employed drug.

Some drugs and medical devices presented in this publication have Food and Drug Administration (FDA) clearance for limited use in restricted research settings. It is the responsibility of the health care provider to ascertain the FDA status of each drug or device planned for use in their clinical practice.

To purchase additional copies of this book, call our customer service department at **(800) 638-3030** or fax orders to **(301) 223-2320**. International customers should call **(301) 223-2300**.

Visit Lippincott Williams & Wilkins on the Internet: http://www.lww.com. Lippincott Williams & Wilkins customer service representatives are available from 8:30 am to 6:00 pm, EST.

Preface

KEITH L. MOORE
PHD, FIAC, FRSM, FAAA

Fifteen years have passed since the first edition of *Essential Clinical Anatomy* was published. As in the previous three editions, the main aim of the fourth edition is to provide a compact yet thorough textbook of clinical anatomy for students and practitioners in the health care professions and related disciplines. We have made the book even more student friendly. The presentations:

- Provide a basic text of human clinical anatomy for use in current health sciences curricula;
- Present an appropriate amount of clinically relevant anatomical material in a readable and interesting form;
- Place emphasis on clinical anatomy that is important for practice;
- Provide a concise clinically oriented anatomical overview for clinical courses in subsequent years;
- Serve as a rapid review when preparing for examinations, particularly those prepared by the National Board of Medical Examiners; and
- Offer enough information for those wishing to refresh their knowledge of clinical anatomy.

This edition has been thoroughly revised keeping in mind the many invaluable comments received from students, colleagues, and reviewers. The key features include:

- Revised text with a stronger clinical orientation.
- A number of new illustrations have been created, and many existing illustrations have been revised, re-colored, and resized. Most illustrations are in full color and designed to highlight important facts and show their relationship to clinical medicine and surgery. A great effort has been made to further improve clarity of labeling, to place illustrations on the pages being viewed as the illustrations are cited in the text, and to eliminate disruptions in the continuity of the running text.
- More illustrated clinical correlations, known as "blue boxes," have been included to help with the understanding of the practical value of anatomy. In response to our readers' suggestions, the blue boxes have been grouped. They are also classified by the following icons to indicate the type of clinical information covered:

 Anatomical variations icon. These blue boxes feature anatomical variations that may be encountered in the dissection lab or in practice, emphasizing the clinical importance of awareness of such variations.

 Life cycle icon. These blue boxes emphasize prenatal developmental factors that affect postnatal anatomy and anatomical phenomena specifically associated with stages of life—childhood, adolescence, adult, and advanced age.

 Trauma icon. The effect of traumatic events—such as fractures of bones or dislocations of joints—on normal anatomy and the clinical manifestations and dysfunction resulting from such injuries are featured in these blue boxes.

 Diagnostic procedures icon. Anatomical features and observations that play a role in physical diagnosis are targeted in these blue boxes.

 Surgical procedures icon. These blue boxes address such topics as the anatomical basis of surgical procedures, such as the planning of incisions and the anatomical basis of regional anesthesia.

 Pathology icon. The effect of disease on normal anatomy, such as cancer of the breast, and anatomical structures or principles involved in the confinement or dissemination of disease within the body are the types of topics covered in these blue boxes.

- Surface anatomy is integrated into the chapter at the time each region is being discussed to demonstrate the relationship between anatomy and physical examination, diagnosis, and clinical procedures.

- Medical images (radiographic, CT, MRI, and ultrasonography studies) have been included, often with correlative illustrations. Current diagnostic imaging techniques demonstrate anatomy as it is often viewed clinically.
- Case studies accompanied by clinico-anatomical problems and USMLE-style multiple-choice questions. Interactive case studies and multiple-choice questions are available to our readers online at http://thePoint.lww.com/ECA4e, providing a convenient and comprehensive means of selftesting and review.
- Instructor's resources and supplemental materials, including images exportable for *Power Point* presentation, are available through http://thePoint.lww.com/ECA4e.

The terminology adheres to the *Terminologica Anatomica* (1998) approved by the International Federation of Anatomists (IFAA). The official English-equivalent terms are used throughout the present edition. When new terms are introduced, however, the Latin forms as used in Europe, Asia and other parts of the world appear in parentheses. The roots and derivation of terms are included to help students understand the meaning of the terminology. Eponyms, although not endorsed by the IFAA, appear in parentheses to assist students during their clinical studies.

The parent of this book, *Clinically Oriented Anatomy* (COA), is recommended as a resource for more detailed descriptions of human anatomy and its relationship and importance to medicine and surgery. It is a pleasure to welcome Arthur F. Dalley II to our team of authors. *Essential Clinical Anatomy*, in addition to its own unique illustrations and manuscript, has utilized from the outset materials from *Clinically Oriented Anatomy* and *Grant's Atlas*. Arthur's expertise, extensive knowledge of clinical anatomy, and innovative eaching methods have enhanced this, the fourth edition of *Essential Clinical Anatomy*.

We again welcome your comments and suggestions for improvements in future editions.

Keith L. Moore
University of Toronto
Faculty of Medicine

Anne M.R. Agur
University of Toronto
Faculty of Medicine

Arthur F. Dalley II
Vanderbilt University
School of Medicine

Acknowledgments

We wish to thank the following colleagues who were invited by the publisher to assist with the development of this fourth edition.

List of Reviewers

Saad Al-Ali
Department of Anatomy with Radiology
University of Auckland
Auckland, New Zealand

Claire Aland
School of Biomedical Sciences
The University of Queensland
Brisbane, Queensland, Australia

Dr. Roscoe Bowen
Human Performance & Natural Science
Campbellsville University
Campbellsville, Kentucky

Richard Boyd
Physiology, Anatomy and Genetics
University of Oxford
Oxford, United Kingdom

Peter Clark
National Heart and Lung Institute
Imperial College London
London, United Kingdom

Anjanette Clifford, MS, DC
Instructor, Gross Anatomy and Neuroanatomy
Logan College of Chiropractic
Chesterfield, Missouri

Jason Cox
School of Medicine
University of Missouri Columbia
Columbia, Missouri

William C. Forbes, DDS
Associate Professor, Anatomy
University of Detroit Mercy School of Dentistry
Detroit, Michigan

Janene H. Fuerch, BS
Medical Student
SUNY Buffalo School of Medicine and Biomedical Sciences
Buffalo, New York

Geraldine Gaik
Anatomical Sciences
Parker College of Chiropractic
Dallas, Texas

Gene Giggleman
Parker College of Chiropractic
Dallas, Texas

Thomas H. Gillingwater, PhD
Senior Lecturer in Anatomy
University of Edinburgh
College of Medicine & Veterinary Medicine
Edinburgh, Scotland, United Kingdom

Roland A. Giolli, PhD
Professor (Recalled)
Department of Anatomy and Neurobiology
University of California School of Medicine
Irvine, California

Seth Goldstein
Johns Hopkins University
Baltimore, Maryland

Lisa Grossman, MD
Resident Physician in Obstetrics and Gynecology
Columbia University Medical Center
New York—Presbyterian Hospital
New York, New York

David Hepworth
Department of Nursing and Midwifery
Saint Martins College
Lancaster, United Kingdom

Edward E. Hurwitz, MD
Department of Internal Medicine
Boston Medical Center
Boston, Massachusetts

George J. R. Maat
Professor, Department of Anatomy
Leiden University Medical Center
Leiden, Netherlands

Charles Marshall
Department of Natural Science
Spalding University
Louisville, Kentucky

Elizabeth A. Martin, DO, MPH
Resident Physician
Jersey Shore University Medical Center
Neptune, New Jersey

Lisa McElroy, MD
General Surgery Resident

Medical College of Wisconsin and Affiliated Hospitals
Milwaukee, Wisconsin

Ruth Morgan
Albany Medical College
Albany, New York

Arash Mozayan Isfahani, MD
Surgery Resident
St. Joseph's Hospital
Phoenix Arizona

Nina Nandy, MD, MS, PGY-1
Internal Medicine
Beth Israel Deaconess Medical Center
Boston, Massachusetts

Tara Neubrand
School of Medicine
University of Texas
Galveston, Texas

Sonja Parisek
Department of Medicine
University of Miami
School of Medicine
Miami, Florida

Kirtan Patel
University of Medicine and Dentistry
New Jersey—New Jersey Medical School
Newark, New Jersey

Shalu Patel
University of Miami
School of Medicine
Miami, Florida

Rebecca L Pratt, PhD
Assistant Professor of Histology/Anatomy
Structural Biology Department
West Virginia School of Osteopathic Medicine
Lewisburg, West Virginia

Logan Schneider
Medical Student
University of Florida College of Medicine
Jacksonville, Florida

Mark Schuenke, PhD
Assistant Professor of Anatomy
University of New England
College of Osteopathic Medicine
Biddeford, Maine

Scott W. Simpson, PhD
Department of Anatomy
Case Western Reserve University School of Medicine
Cleveland, Ohio

Rayapati Sreenathan, PhD
Chairman and Professor of Anatomical Sciences
St. Matthew's University School of Medicine
Grand Cayman, British West Indies

Jason Ting
Oklahoma State University Center for Health Sciences
Tulsa, Oklahoma

Asha Venkatesh
Teaching Fellow in Anatomy
School of Medicine and Dentistry
University of Aberdeen
Aberdeen, United Kingdom

Lawrence M. Witmer, PhD
Professor of Anatomy
Ohio University College of Osteopathic Medicine
Athens, Ohio

Kimberly Yang, MD
University of Michigan
Ann Arbor, Michigan

In addition to reviewers, many people, some of them unknowingly, helped us by discussing parts of the manuscript and/or providing constructive criticism of the text and illustrations in the present and previous editions:

- Dr. Peter Abrahams, Consultant Clinical Anatomist, University of Cambridge and examiner to the Royal College of Surgeons of Edinburgh, Cambridge, UK
- Dr. Robert D. Acland, Professor of Surgery/Microsurgery, Division of Plastic and Reconstructive Surgery, University of Louisville, Louisville, Kentucky
- Dr. Edna Becker, Associate Professor of Medical Imaging, University of Toronto Faculty of Medicine, Toronto, Ontario
- Dr. Donald R. Cahill, Professor of Anatomy (retired; former Chair), Mayo Medical School; former Editor-in-Chief of Clinical Anatomy, Rochester, Minnesota
- Dr. Joan Campbell, Assistant Professor of Medical Imaging, University of Toronto Faculty of Medicine, Toronto, Ontario
- Dr. Stephen W. Carmichael, Professor Emeritus, Mayo Medical School, Editor-in-Chief of Clinical Anatomy, Rochester, Minnesota
- Dr. Carmine D. Clemente, Professor of Anatomy and Cell Biology and Professor of Neurobiology, Emeritus (Recalled), University of California Los Angeles School of Medicine, Los Angeles, California
- Dr. James D. Collins, Distinguished Professor of Radiological Sciences, University of California Los Angeles School of Medicine/Center for Health Sciences, Los Angeles, California

- Dr. Raymond F. Gasser, Emeritus Professor of Cell Biology and Anatomy and Adjunct Professor of Obstetrics and Gynecology, Louisiana State University School of Medicine, New Orleans, Louisiana
- Dr. Ralph Ger, Professor of Anatomy and Structural Biology, Albert Einstein College of Medicine, Bronx, New York
- Dr. Douglas J. Gould, Associate Professor, The Ohio State University, Columbus, Ohio
- Dr. Daniel O. Graney, Professor of Biological Structure, University of Washington School of Medicine, Seattle, Washington
- Dr. David G. Greathouse, former Professor and Chair, Belmont University School of Physical Therapy, Nashville, Tennessee
- Dr. Masoom Haider, Associate Professor of Medical Imaging, University of Toronto Faculty of Medicine, Toronto, Ontario
- Dr. John S. Halle, Professor and Chair, Belmont University School of Physical Therapy, Nashville, Tennessee
- Dr. Jennifer L. Halpern, Associate Professor, Department of Orthopaedic Surgery and Rehabilitation, Vanderbilt University, Nashville, Tennessee
- Dr. Walter Kuchareczyk, Professor, Department of Medical Imaging, Faculty of Medicine, University of Toronto, Toronto, Ontario
- Dr. Nirusha Lachman, Professor of Anatomy, Mayo Medical School, Rochester, Minnesota
- Dr. H. Wayne Lambert, Associate Professor, Department of Neurobiology and Anatomy, West Virginia University School of Medicine, Morgantown, West Virginia
- Dr. Michael von Lüdinghausen, University Professor, Anatomy Institute, University of Würzburg, Würzburg, Germany
- Dr. Shirley McCarthy, Director of MRI, Department of Diagnostic Radiology, Yale University School of Medicine, New Haven, Connecticut
- Dr. Lillian Nanney, Professor of Plastic Surgery and Cell and Developmental Biology, Vanderbilt University School of Medicine, Nashville, Tennessee
- Dr. Todd R. Olson, Professor of Anatomy and Structural Biology, Albert Einstein College of Medicine, Bronx, New York
- Dr. Wojciech Pawlina, Professor and Chair of Anatomy, Mayo Medical School, Rochester, Minnesota
- Dr. T. V. N. Persaud, Professor Emeritus of Human Anatomy and Cell Science, Faculties of Medicine and Dentistry, University of Manitoba, Winnipeg, Manitoba, Canada; Professor of Anatomy and Embryology, St. George's University, Granada, West Indies
- Dr. Cathleen C. Pettepher, Professor of Cancer Biology and Cell and Developmental Biology, Vanderbilt University School of Medicine, Nashville, Tennessee
- Dr. Thomas H. Quinn, Professor of Biomedical Sciences, Creighton University School of Medicine, Omaha, Nebraska
- Dr. George E. Salter, Professor of Anatomy, Department of Cell Biology, University of Alabama, Birmingham, Alabama
- Dr. Tatsuo Sato, Professor and Head (retired), Second Department of Anatomy, Tokyo Medical and Dental University Faculty of Medicine, Tokyo
- Ryckie Wade, MB BS, MClinEd; Yr4, President; UEA Surgical Society, University of East Anglia, School of Medicine, Norwich, United Kingdom
- Professor Colin P. Wendell-Smith, Department of Anatomy and Physiology, University of Tasmania, Hobart, Tasmania, Australia
- Dr. Andreas H. Weiglein, Associate Professor, Institut fur Anatomie, Medical University Graz, Graz, Austria
- Dr. David G. Whitlock, Professor of Anatomy, University of Colorado Medical School, Denver, Colorado

All the new illustrations and changes to the existing artwork were done by Paulette Dennis and Valerie Oxorn, both talented medical illustrators. Their meticulous work and insight into anatomy is invaluable. We also thank Kam Yu, who prepared the illustrations for the first edition. Other illustrations from the sixth edition of *Clinically Oriented Anatomy* and the twelfth edition of *Grant's Atlas* were prepared by Angela Cluer, Nina Kilpatrick, Stephen Mader, David Mazierski, Sari O'Sullivan, Bart Vallecoccia, Valerie Oxorn, J/B Woolsey Associates, and Dragonfly Media Group. We continue to benefit from the extensive surface anatomy project photographed by E. Anne Raynor, Senior Photographer, Vanderbilt Medical Art Group, under the direction of authors Art Dalley and Anne Agur, with the support of Lippincott Williams and Wilkins.

Our appreciation and thanks are extended to the editorial and production team at Lippincott Williams & Wilkins who provided their expertise in the development of this edition: Crystal Taylor, Acquisitions Editor; Julie Montalbano, Product Manager; Jennifer Clements and Doug Smock, Art Directors; and Catherine Noonan, Editorial Assistant. We also wish to acknowledge Kathleen Scogna, former Senior Developmental Editor, for her work on the early part of this edition. Finally thanks to the Sales Division at LWW, which has played a key role in the success of this book.

Keith L. Moore
Anne M.R. Agur
Arthur F. Dalley II

Contents

Preface / vii
Acknowledgments / ix
Figure Credits / xxi

Introduction to Clinical Anatomy / 1

Approaches to Studying Anatomy / 2
Anatomicomedical Terminology / 3
  Anatomical Position / 3
  Anatomical Planes / 3
  Terms of Relationship and Comparison / 4
  Terms of Laterality / 5
  Terms of Movement / 5
  Anatomical Variations / 7
Integumentary System / 7
Skeletal System / 9
  Bones / 11
  Joints / 14
Muscular System / 17
  Skeletal Muscles / 17
  Cardiac Striated Muscle / 20
  Smooth Muscle / 20
Cardiovascular System / 23
  Arteries / 23
  Veins / 25
  Capoid / 28
Lymphoid System / 28
Nervous System / 31
  Central Nervous System / 31
  Peripheral Nervous System / 31
  Somatic Nervous System / 34
  Structure and Components of a Typical Spinal Nerve / 34
  Autonomic Nervous System / 36
  Sympathetic Visceral Motor Innervation / 38
  Parasympathetic Visceral Motor Innervation / 42
  Visceral Afferent Sensation / 42
Imaging of Body Systems / 42
  Conventional Radiography / 42
  Computerized Tomography / 44
  Ultrasonography / 44
  Magnetic Resonance Imaging / 44
  Positron Emission Tomography / 46

1 Thorax / 47

Thoracic Wall / 48
  Skeleton of Thoracic Wall / 48
  Thoracic Apertures / 48
  Joints of Thoracic Wall / 51
  Movements of Thoracic Wall / 51
  Breasts / 53
  Muscles of Thoracic Wall / 60
  Nerves of Thoracic Wall / 61
  Vasculature of Thoracic Wall / 62
Surface Anatomy of Thoracic Wall / 65
Thoracic Cavity and Viscera / 68
  Endothoracic Fascia / 68
  Pleurae and Lungs / 68
Surface Anatomy of Pleurae and Lungs / 70
  Mediastinum / 80
  Anterior Mediastinum / 80
  Middle Mediastinum / 80
  Heart and Great Vessels / 84
Surface Anatomy of Heart / 92
  Superior Mediastinum / 102
  Posterior Mediastinum / 108
Medical Imaging of Thorax / 114

2 Abdomen / 116

Abdominal Cavity / 117
Anterolateral Abdominal Wall / 117
  Fascia of Anterolateral Abdominal Wall / 118
  Muscles of Anterolateral Abdominal Wall / 119
  Internal Surface of Anterolateral Abdominal Wall / 121
Surface Anatomy of Anterolateral Abdominal Wall / 124
  Nerves of Anterolateral Abdominal Wall / 125
  Vessels of Anterolateral Abdominal Wall / 126
  Inguinal Region / 127
Peritoneum and Peritoneal Cavity / 135
  Peritoneal Vessels and Nerves / 136
  Peritoneal Formations / 136
  Subdivisions of Peritoneal Cavity / 138
Abdominal Viscera / 140
  Esophagus / 143
  Stomach / 143
  Small Intestine / 146
Surface Anatomy of Stomach / 148

Large Intestine / 154
Surface Anatomy of Spleen and Pancreas / 161
Spleen / 161
Pancreas / 162
Liver / 165
Surface Anatomy of Liver / 167
Biliary Ducts and Gallbladder / 171
Hepatic Portal Vein and Portal–Systemic Anastomoses / 173
Kidneys, Ureters, and Suprarenal Glands / 174
Summary of Innervation of Abdominal Viscera / 180
Surface Anatomy of Kidneys and Ureters / 180
Diaphragm / 185
Diaphragmatic Apertures / 189
Vasculature and Nerves of Diaphragm / 189
Posterior Abdominal Wall / 192
Fascia of Posterior Abdominal Wall / 192
Muscles of Posterior Abdominal Wall / 193
Nerves of Posterior Abdominal Wall / 193
Vasculature of Posterior Abdominal Wall / 195
Lymphatics of Posterior Abdominal Wall / 196
Medical Imaging of Abdomen / 199

3   Pelvis and Perineum / 204

Pelvis / 205
Pelvic Girdle / 205
Joints and Ligaments of Pelvic Girdle / 209
Peritoneum and Peritoneal Cavity of Pelvis / 211
Walls and Floor of Pelvic Cavity / 211
Pelvic Fascia / 215
Pelvic Nerves / 217
Pelvic Arteries and Veins / 220
Lymph Nodes of Pelvis / 223
Pelvic Viscera / 223
Urinary Organs / 223
Male Internal Genital Organs / 233
Female Internal Genital Organs / 236
Rectum / 245
Perineum / 250
Fascias and Pouches of Urogenital Triangle / 253
Features of Anal Triangle / 257
Male Perineum / 261
Female Perineum / 268
Medical Imaging of Pelvis and Perineum / 271

4   Back / 274

Vertebral Column / 275
Curvatures of Vertebral Column / 276
Surface Anatomy of Curvatures of Vertebral Column / 276
Structure and Function of Vertebrae / 277
Regional Characteristics of Vertebrae / 278
Surface Anatomy of Vertebral Column / 284
Joints of Vertebral Column / 288
Movements of Vertebral Column / 292
Vasculature of Vertebral Column / 294
Innervation of Vertebral Column / 294
Spinal Cord and Meninges / 296
Structure of Spinal Nerves / 297
Spinal Meninges and Cerebrospinal Fluid / 297
Vasculature of Spinal Cord and Spinal Nerve Roots / 301
Muscles of Back / 301
Extrinsic Back Muscles / 303
Intrinsic Back Muscles / 303
Surface Anatomy of Back Muscles / 304
Suboccipital and Deep Neck Muscles / 311
Medical Imaging of Back / 314

5   Lower Limb / 316

Bones of Lower Limb / 318
Hip Bone / 318
Femur / 318
Patella / 322
Tibia / 322
Fibula / 322
Tarsus, Metatarsus, and Phalanges / 323
Surface Anatomy of Lower Limb Bones / 327
Fascia, Vessels, and Cutaneous Nerves of Lower Limb / 329
Subcutaneous Tissue and Fascia / 329
Venous Drainage of Lower Limb / 331
Lymphatic Drainage of Lower Limb / 332
Cutaneous Innervation of Lower Limb / 333
Thigh and Gluteal Region / 336
Anterior Thigh Muscles / 336
Medial Thigh Muscles / 337
Neurovascular Structures and Relationships in Anteromedial Thigh / 341
Femoral Triangle and Adductor Canal / 341
Femoral Nerve / 342
Femoral Sheath / 342
Femoral Artery /343
Femoral Vein / 346
Obturator Artery and Nerve /346
Gluteal Region and Posterior Thigh / 346
Gluteal Muscles / 347
Gluteal Bursae / 348

Posterior Thigh Muscles / 349
Nerves of Gluteal Region and Posterior Thigh / 349
Vasculature of Gluteal and Posterior
  Thigh Regions / 352
Popliteal Fossa / 356
Fascia of Popliteal Fossa / 356
Vessels in Popliteal Fossa / 356
Nerves in Popliteal Fossa / 357
Leg / 357
Anterior Compartment of Leg / 357
Lateral Compartment of Leg / 360
Posterior Compartment of Leg / 363
Foot / 371
Deep Fascia of Foot / 371
Muscles of Foot / 372
Nerves of Foot / 376
Arteries of Foot / 376
Venous Drainage of Foot / 377
Lymphatic Drainage of Foot / 377
Walking: The Gait Cycle / 377
Joints of Lower Limb / 379
Hip Joint / 379
Knee Joint / 385
Tibiofibular Joints / 389
Ankle Joint / 395
Joints of Foot / 398
Arches of Foot / 400
Medical Imaging of Lower Limb / 403

6 Upper Limb / 405

Bones of Upper Limb / 406
Clavicle / 407
Scapula / 407
Humerus / 410
Ulna and Radius / 410
Bones of Hand / 411
Surface Anatomy of Upper Limb Bones / 415
Superficial Structures of Upper Limb / 417
Fascia of Upper Limb / 417
Cutaneous Nerves of Upper Limb / 419
Venous Drainage of Upper Limb / 421
Lymphatic Drainage of Upper Limb / 422
Anterior Axioappendicular Muscles / 422
Posterior Axioappendicular and Scapulohumeral
  Muscles / 423
Superficial Posterior Axioappendicular Muclses /424
Deep Posterior Axioappendicular Muscles /424
Scapulohumeral Muscles /427
*Surface Anatomy of Pectoral and Scapular
  Regions (Anterior and Posterior
  Axioappendicular and Scapulohumeral
  Muscles)* / 428

Axilla / 427
Axillary Artery and Vein / 429
Axillary Lymph Nodes / 432
Brachial Plexus / 433
Arm / 436
Muscles of Arm / 440
Arteries and Veins of Arm /443
Nerves of Arm / 443
Cubital Fossa / 446
Forearm / 446
Muscles of Forearm / 446
Surface Anatomy of Arm and Cubital Fossa / 447
Nerves of Forearm / 456
Arteries and Veins of Forearm / 456
Hand / 461
Fascia of Palm / 461
Muscles of Hand / 462
Flexor Tendons of Extrinsic Muscles / 466
Arteries and Veins of Hand / 466
Nerves of Hand / 468
Surface Anatomy of Forearm and Hand / 473
Joints of Upper Limb / 475
Sternoclavicular Joint / 475
Acromioclavicular Joint / 476
Glenohumeral Joint / 476
Elbow Joint / 482
Proximal Radio-Ulnar Joint / 483
Distal Radio-Ulnar Joint / 485
Joints of Hand / 488
Medical Imaging of Upper Limb / 492

7 Head / 495

Cranium / 496
Facial Aspect of Cranium / 496
Lateral Aspect of Cranium / 496
Occipital Aspect of Cranium / 498
Superior Aspect of Cranium / 498
External Surface of Cranial Base / 499
Internal Surface of Cranial Base / 502
Scalp / 502
Cranial Meninges / 503
Dura Mater / 504
Arachnoid Mater and Pia Mater / 509
Meningeal Spaces / 511
Brain / 512
Parts of Brain / 512
Ventricular System of Brain / 512
Vasculature of Brain / 517
Face / 519
Muscles of Face / 519
Nerves of Face / 519
Superficial Vasculature of Face and Scalp / 522

Parotid Gland / 526
Orbits / 529
 Eyelids and Lacrimal Apparatus / 530
 Eyeball / 533
 Extra-ocular Muscles of Orbit / 540
 Nerves of Orbit / 544
 Vasculature of Orbit / 545
Temporal Region / 549
 Temporal Fossa / 549
 Infratemporal Fossa / 550
Temporomandibular Joint / 555
Oral Region / 557
 Oral Cavity / 557
 Oral Vestibule / 557
 Teeth and Gingivae / 558
 Palate / 560
 Tongue / 563
 Salivary Glands / 567
Pterygopalatine Fossa / 570
Nose / 573
 External Nose / 573
 Nasal Cavities / 573
 Paranasal Sinuses / 574
Ear / 578
 External Ear / 578
 Middle Ear / 580
 Internal Ear / 583
Medical Imaging of Head / 589

8 Neck / 593

Fascia of Neck / 594
 Cervical Subcutaneous Tissue and Platysma / 594
 Deep Cervical Fascia / 594
Superficial Structures of Neck: Cervical
 Regions / 596
 Sternocleidomastoid Region / 596
 Posterior Cervical Region / 598
 Lateral Cervical Region / 598
 Anterior Cervical Region / 604
*Surface Anatomy of Cervical Regions and
 Triangles of Neck* / 611
Deep Structures of Neck / 613
 Prevertebral Muscles / 613
 Root of Neck / 613
Viscera of Neck / 619
 Endocrine Layer of Cervical Viscera / 619
 Respiratory Layer of Cervical Viscera / 623
Surface Anatomy of Larynx / 624
 Alimentary Layer of Cervical Viscera / 631
Lymphatics in Neck / 638
Medical Imaging of Neck / 641

9 Review of Cranial Nerves / 643

Overview of Cranial Nerves / 644
Olfactory Nerve (CN I) / 650
Optic Nerve (CN II) / 652
Oculomotor Nerve (CN III) / 654
Trochlear Nerve (CN IV) / 655
Abducent Nerve (CN VI) / 656
Trigeminal Nerve (CN V) / 659
Facial Nerve (CN VII) / 660
 Somatic (Branchial) Motor / 660
 Visceral (Parasympathetic) Motor / 660
 Somatic (General) Sensory / 660
 Special Sensory (Taste) / 660
Vestibulocochlear Nerve(CN VIII) / 663
Glossopharyngeal Nerve(CN IX) / 664
 Somatic (Branchial) Motor / 664
 Visceral (Parasympathetic) Motor / 664
 Somatic (General) Sensory / 664
 Special Sensory (Taste) / 665
 Visceral Sensory / 665
Vagus Nerve (CN X) / 665
 Somatic (Branchial) Motor / 666
 Visceral (Parasympathetic) Motor / 666
 Somatic (General) Sensory / 668
 Special Sensory (Taste) / 668
 Visceral Sensory / 669
Spinal Accessory Nerve (CN XI) / 669
Hypoglossal Nerve (CN XII) / 671

References and Suggested Readings / 673
Index / 675

Clinical Correlation Blue Boxes

Introduction to Clinical Anatomy
Skin Incisions and Wounds / 8
Heterotopic Bones / 11
Bone Dynamics / 12
Accessory Bones / 14
Assessment of Bone Age / 14
Displacement and Separation of Epiphyses / 14
Avascular Necrosis / 14
Degenerative Joint Disease / 17
Muscle Testing / 22
Electromyography / 22
Muscular Atrophy / 23
Hypertrophy / 23
*Anastomoses, Collateral Circulation,
 and Terminal (End) Arteries* / 25
Arteriosclerosis: Ischemia and Infarction / 25
Varicose Veins / 28

*Lymphangitis, Lymphadenitis, and
      Lymphedema* / 30
Damage to CNS / 31
Peripheral Nerve Degeneration / 34

Chapter 1 Thorax

Role of Costal Cartilages / 54
Rib Fractures / 54
Flail Chest / 54
Supernumerary Ribs / 54
Sternal Fractures / 54
Median Sternotomy / 54
Sternal Biopsies / 54
Paralysis of Diaphragm / 54
*Thoracotomy, Intercostal Space Incisions, and
      Rib Excision* / 55
Thoracic Outlet Syndrome / 55
Dislocation of Ribs / 55
Breast Quadrants / 58
Changes in Breasts / 58
Supernumerary Breasts and Nipples / 58
Carcinoma of Breast / 58
Mammography / 59
Surgical Incisions of Breast / 59
Herpes Zoster Infection / 64
Dyspnea—Difficult Breathing / 64
Intercostal Nerve Block / 64
Pulmonary Collapse / 77
*Pneumothorax, Hydrothorax, Hemothorax, and
      Chylothorax* / 77
Pleuritis / 77
Variation in Lobes of Lungs / 77
Thoracentesis / 78
Auscultation and Percussion of Lungs / 78
Aspiration of Foreign Bodies / 78
Lung Resections / 78
Injury to Pleurae / 78
Thoracoscopy / 78
Pulmonary Embolism / 79
Inhalation of Carbon Particles / 79
Bronchogenic Carcinoma / 79
Bronchoscopy / 79
*Surgical Significance of Transverse Pericardial
      Sinus* / 82
Pericarditis and Pericardial Effusion / 83
Cardiac Tamponade / 84
Levels of Viscera in Mediastinum / 84
Percussion of Heart / 91
Atrial and Ventricular Septal Defects / 91
Thrombi / 91
Valvular Heart Disease / 91
Coronary Artery Disease / 100
Coronary Bypass Graft / 101
Coronary Angioplasty / 101

Variations of Coronary Arteries / 101
Echocardiography / 101
Cardiac Referred Pain / 102
Injury to Conducting System of Heart / 102
Laceration of Thoracic Duct / 112
Collateral Venous Routes to Heart / 112
Aneurysm of Ascending Aorta / 112
Injury to Recurrent Laryngeal Nerves / 112
Variations of Great Arteries / 112
Coarctation of Aorta / 113
Age Changes in Thymus / 113

Chapter 2 Abdomen

*Clinical Significance of Fascia and Fascial
      Spaces of Abdominal Wall* / 122
Abdominal Surgical Incisions / 123
Endoscopic Surgery / 123
Incisional Hernia / 123
Protuberance of Abdomen / 123
Palpation of Anterolateral Abdominal Wall / 123
Hydrocele and Hematocele / 132
Vasectomy / 132
Varicocele / 132
Testicular Cancer / 132
Cremasteric Reflex / 132
Relocation of Gonads / 133
Inguinal Hernias / 134
Palpation of Superficial Inguinal Ring / 135
Cysts and Hernias of Canal of Nuck / 135
The Peritoneum and Surgical Procedures / 141
Peritonitis and Ascites / 141
Peritoneal Adhesions and Adhesiotomy / 141
Abdominal Paracentesis / 141
Functions of Greater Omentum / 141
Spread of Pathological Fluids / 142
*Overview of Embryological Rotation of
      Midgut* / 155
Hiatal Hernia / 159
Carcinoma of Stomach and Gastrectomy / 159
*Gastric Ulcers, Peptic Ulcers, Helicobacter
      pylori, and Vagotomy* / 159
Duodenal (Peptic) Ulcers / 160
Ileal Diverticulum / 160
Diverticulosis / 160
Appendicitis / 160
Appendectomy / 160
Colitis, Colectomy, and Ileostomy / 160
Colonoscopy / 161
Rupture of Spleen and Splenomegaly / 165
Rupture of Pancreas / 165
Pancreatic Cancer / 165
Subphrenic Abscesses / 167
Liver Biopsy / 173
Rupture of Liver / 173

Cirrhosis of Liver / 173
Hepatic Lobectomies and Segmentectomy / 173
Gallstones / 173
Cholecystectomy / 174
Portal Hypertension / 174
Perinephric Abscess / 181
Renal Transplantation / 181
Accessory Renal Vessels / 181
Renal and Ureteric Calculi / 181
Intraperitoneal Injection and Peritoneal Dialysis / 181
Congenital Anomalies of Kidneys and Ureters / 181
Visceral Referred Pain / 186
Section of a Phrenic Nerve / 191
Referred Pain from Diaphragm / 191
Rupture of Diaphragm and Herniation of Viscera / 191
Congenital Diaphragmatic Hernia / 191
Psoas Abscess / 198
Posterior Abdominal Pain / 198
Collateral Routes for Abdominopelvic Venous Blood / 198
Abdominal Aortic Aneurysm / 198

Chapter 3 Pelvis and Perineum
Sexual Differences in Bony Pelves / 209
Pelvic Fractures / 209
Relaxation of Pelvic Ligaments and Increased Joint Mobility During Pregnancy / 211
Injury to Pelvic Floor / 217
Injury to Pelvic Nerves / 218
Ureteric Calculi / 225
Suprapubic Cystotomy / 228
Rupture of Bladder / 228
Cystoscopy / 229
Sterilization of Males / 233
Prostatic Enlargement, Prostatic Cancer, and Prostatectomy / 235
Distention and Examination of Vagina / 238
Culdocentesis / 238
Hysterectomy / 242
Cervical Examination and Pap Smear / 242
Regional Anesthesia for Childbirth / 243
Manual Examination of Uterus / 243
Infections of Female Genital Tract / 247
Patency of Uterine Tubes / 247
Laparoscopic Examination of Pelvic Viscera / 249
Ligation of Uterine Tubes / 249
Ectopic Tubal Pregnancy / 249
Resection of Rectum / 249
Rectal Examination / 249
Disruption of Perineal Body / 253
Episiotomy / 253
Rupture of Urethra in Males and Extravasation of Urine / 256

Ischio-anal Abscesses / 258
Hemorrhoids / 260
Urethral Catheterization / 261
Impotence and Erectile Dysfunction / 266
Phimosis, Paraphimosis, and Circumcision / 266
Dilation of Female Urethra / 270
Inflammation of Greater Vestibular Glands / 270
Pudendal and Ilio-inguinal Nerve Blocks / 270

Chapter 4 Back
Abnormal Curvatures of Vertebral Column / 276
Laminectomy / 278
Fractures of Vertebrae / 278
Spina Bifida / 285
Dislocation of Vertebrae / 286
Lumbar Spinal Stenosis / 286
Aging of Vertebrae and Intervertebral Discs / 290
Injury and Disease of Zygapophysial Joints / 290
Herniation of Nucleus Pulposus / 293
Rupture of Transverse Ligament of Atlas / 293
Rupture of Alar Ligaments / 293
Back Pain / 295
Lumbar Spinal Puncture / 300
Epidural Anesthesia (Blocks) / 300
Ischemia of Spinal Cord / 303
Alternative Circulation Pathways / 303
Reduced Blood Supply to Brainstem / 312
Back Sprains and Strains / 313

Chapter 5 Lower Limb
Fractures of Hip Bone / 318
Femoral Fractures / 325
Coxa Vara and Coxa Valga / 325
Tibial and Fibular Fractures / 326
Bone Grafts / 326
Fractures Involving Epiphysial Plates / 326
Fractures of Foot Bones / 327
Abnormalities of Sensory Function / 335
Compartment Syndromes in Leg and Fasciotomy / 335
Saphenous Cutdown and Saphenous Nerve Injury / 335
Varicose Veins, Thrombosis, and Thrombophlebitis / 335
Enlarged Inguinal Lymph Nodes / 336
Regional Nerve Blocks of Lower Limbs / 336
Hip and Thigh Contusions / 340
Patellar Tendon Reflex / 340
Paralysis of Quadriceps / 340
Chondromalacia Patellae / 340
Transplantation of Gracilis / 340
Groin Pull / 340
Femoral Hernia / 345
Replaced or Accessory Obturator Artery / 345

Femoral Pulse and Cannulation of Femoral Artery / 345
Cannulation of Femoral Vein / 345
Trochanteric and Ischial Bursitis / 353
Injury to Superior Gluteal Nerve / 354
Hamstring Injuries / 354
Injury to Sciatic Nerve / 354
Intragluteal Injections / 354
Popliteal Pulse / 357
Popliteal Aneurysm / 357
Tibialis Anterior Strain (Shin Splints) / 361
Containment and Spread of Compartmental Infections in Leg / 361
Injury to Common Fibular Nerve and Footdrop / 361
Deep Fibular Nerve Entrapment / 362
Superficial Fibular Nerve Entrapment / 362
Palpation of Dorsalis Pedis Pulse / 362
Gastrocnemius Strain / 367
Posterior Tibial Pulse / 367
Injury to Tibial Nerve / 368
Absence of Plantarflexion / 368
Calcaneal Tendon Reflex / 368
Inflammation and Rupture of Calcaneal Tendon / 368
Calcaneal Bursitis / 368
Plantar Fasciitis / 377
Hemorrhaging Wounds of Sole of Foot / 377
Sural Nerve Grafts / 379
Plantar Reflex / 379
Contusion of Extensor Digitorum Brevis / 379
Medial Plantar Nerve Entrapment / 379
Fractures of Femoral Neck ("Hip Fractures") / 384
Surgical Hip Replacement / 384
Dislocation of Hip Joint / 384
Genu Varum and Genu Valgum / 391
Patellofemoral Syndrome / 392
Patellar Dislocation / 392
Popliteal Cysts / 392
Knee Joint Injuries / 393
Arthroscopy of Knee Joint / 394
Knee Replacement / 394
Bursitis in Knee Region / 394
Tibial Nerve Entrapment / 397
Ankle Sprains / 397
Pott Fracture–Dislocation of Ankle / 398
Hallux Valgus / 402
Pes Planus (Flatfeet) / 402

Chapter 6 Upper Limb
Fracture of Clavicle / 412
Ossification of Clavicle / 413
Fracture of Scapula / 413
Fractures of Humerus / 413

Fractures of Ulna and Radius / 414
Fractures of Hand / 414
Paralysis of Serratus Anterior / 424
Venipuncture / 424
Injury to Axillary Nerve / 427
Rotator Cuff Injuries and Supraspinatus / 427
Compression of Axillary Artery / 431
Arterial Anastomoses Around Scapula / 431
Injury to Axillary Vein / 432
Enlargement of Axillary Lymph Nodes / 433
Variations of Brachial Plexus / 438
Brachial Plexus Injuries / 438
Brachial Plexus Block / 439
Biceps Tendinitis / 444
Rupture of Tendon of Long Head of Biceps / 444
Bicipital Myotatic Reflex / 444
Injury to Radial Nerve / 445
Injury to Musculocutaneous Nerve / 445
Occlusion or Laceration of Brachial Artery / 445
Measuring Blood Pressure / 445
Compression of Brachial Artery / 445
Muscle Testing of FDS and FDP / 460
Elbow Tendinitis or Lateral Epicondylitis / 460
Synovial Cyst of Wrist / 460
Mallet or Baseball Finger / 460
Dupuytren Contracture of Palmar Fascia / 470
Hand Infections / 470
Laceration of Palmar Arches / 470
Palmar Wounds and Surgical Incisions / 470
Ischemia of Digits / 470
Tenosynovitis / 470
Carpal Tunnel Syndrome / 471
Trauma to Median Nerve / 471
Ulnar Nerve Injury / 472
Radial Nerve Injury / 472
Rotator Cuff Injuries / 480
Dislocation of Acromioclavicular Joint / 480
Dislocation of Glenohumeral Joint / 481
Calcific Supraspinatus Tendinitis / 481
Adhesive Capsulitis of Glenohumeral Joint / 481
Bursitis of Elbow / 486
Avulsion of Medial Epicondyle / 486
Dislocation of Elbow Joint / 486
Ulnar Collateral Ligament Reconstruction / 487
Subluxation and Dislocation of the Radial Head / 487
Wrist Fractures and Dislocations / 491

Chapter 7 Head
Fractures of Cranium / 498
Scalp Injuries and Infections / 503
Occlusion of Cerebral Veins and Dural Venous Sinuses / 508
Metastasis of Tumor Cells to Dural Sinuses / 508
Fractures of Cranial Base / 508

Dural Origin of Headaches / 508
Head Injuries and Intracranial Hemorrhage / 511
Cerebral Injuries / 512
Cisternal Puncture / 514
Hydrocephalus / 514
Leakage of Cerebrospinal Fluid / 514
Strokes / 518
Transient Ischemic Attacks / 518
Facial Injuries / 519
Trigeminal Neuralgia / 524
Lesions of Trigeminal Nerve / 524
Bell Palsy / 524
Pulses of Arteries of Face / 525
Compression of Facial Artery / 525
Squamous Cell Carcinoma of Lip / 527
Parotidectomy / 528
Infection of Parotid Gland / 528
Fractures of Orbit / 530
Orbital Tumors / 530
Injury to Nerves Supplying Eyelids / 533
Inflammation of Palpebral Glands / 533
Ophthalmoscopy / 538
Detachment of Retina / 538
Papilledema / 539
Presbyopia and Cataracts / 539
Glaucoma / 539
Corneal Ulcers and Transplants / 539
Development of Retina / 539
Blockage of Central Retinal Artery / 548
Blockage of Central Retinal Vein / 548
Pupillary Light Reflex / 548
Corneal Reflex / 548
*Paralysis of Extra-ocular Muscles/Palsies of
    Orbital Nerves* / 548
Oculomotor Nerve (CN III) Palsy / 548
Abducent Nerve (CN VI) Palsy / 548
Mandibular Nerve Block / 556
Inferior Alveolar Nerve Block / 556
Dislocation of TMJ / 556
Arthritis of TMJ / 557
Dental Caries, Pulpitis, and Toothache / 560
Gingivitis and Periodontitis / 560
Sialography / 569
Gag Reflex / 569
Paralysis of Genioglossus / 569
Injury to Hypoglossal Nerve / 569
Sublingual Absorption of Drugs / 569
Lingual Carcinoma / 569
Nasal Fractures / 577
Deviation of Nasal Septum / 577
Rhinitis / 577
Epistaxis / 577
Sinusitis / 577
Infection of Ethmoidal Cells / 577

Infection of Maxillary Sinuses / 577
Relationship of Teeth to Maxillary Sinus / 578
External Ear Injury / 587
Otoscopic Examination / 587
Acute Otitis Externa / 588
Otitis Media / 588
Perforation of Tympanic Membrane / 588

Chapter 8 Neck
Spread of Infection in Neck / 597
Congenital Torticollis / 598
Lesions of Spinal Accessory Nerve (CN XI) / 603
Subclavian Vein Puncture / 603
Prominence of External Jugular Vein / 603
*Severance of Phrenic Nerve and Phrenic Nerve
    Block* / 604
Nerve Blocks in Lateral Cervical Region / 604
Ligation of External Carotid Artery / 610
Surgical Dissection of Carotid Triangle / 610
Carotid Pulse / 610
Carotid Occlusion and Endarterectomy / 610
Internal Jugular Pulse / 611
Internal Jugular Vein Puncture / 611
Cervicothoracic Ganglion Block / 619
Lesion of Cervical Sympathetic Trunk / 619
Pyramidal Lobe of Thyroid Gland / 620
Thyroidectomy / 620
Accessory Thyroid Tissue / 622
Injury to Laryngeal Nerves / 630
Fractures of Laryngeal Skeleton / 630
Laryngoscopy / 630
Aspiration of Foreign Bodies / 630
Tracheostomy / 631
Radical Neck Dissections / 639
Adenoiditis / 639
Foreign Bodies in Laryngopharynx / 639
Tonsillectomy / 640
Zones of Penetrating Trauma / 640

Chapter 9 Review of Cranial Nerves
Anosmia—Loss of Smell / 650
Visual Field Defects / 653
Demyelinating Diseases and the Optic Nerve / 654
Ocular Palsies / 657
Injury to Trigeminal Nerve / 660
Injury to Facial Nerve / 660
Corneal Reflex / 662
Injuries of Vestibulocochlear Nerve / 664
Deafness / 664
Acoustic Neuroma / 664
Lesions of Glossopharyngeal Nerve / 666
Lesions of Vagus Nerve / 669
Injury to Spinal Accessory Nerve / 670
Injury to Hypoglossal Nerve / 671

Figure Credits

All sources are published by Lippincott Williams & Wilkins unless otherwise noted.

INTRODUCTION

Figure I.3, cross-section Moore KL, Dalley AF. Agur, AMR. *Clinically Oriented Anatomy,* 6th edition, 2009, Fig. I.4, p. 8.

Figure I.4 L Moore KL, Dalley AF. Agur, AMR. *Clinically Oriented Anatomy,* 6th edition, 2009, Fig. I.5I, p. 10.

Figure I.8 A&D. Courtesy of Dr. David Cormack, Professor Emeritus, Division of Anatomy, Department of Surgery, University of Toronto.

Figure I.9 Moore KL, Dalley AF. Agur, AMR. *Clinically Oriented Anatomy,* 6th edition, 2009, Fig. I.15 p. 24.

Figure I.11, detail Moore KL, Dalley AF. Agur, AMR. *Clinically Oriented Anatomy,* 6th edition, 2009, Fig. I.18 p. 31.

Figure I.13 Moore KL, Dalley AF. Agur, AMR. *Clinically Oriented Anatomy,* 6th edition, 2009, Fig. I.22A, p. 38.

Figure I.14 E&F Moore KL, Dalley AF. *Clinically Oriented Anatomy,* 5th edition, 2006, Fig. I.23.

Figure I.16 B Moore KL, Dalley AF. Agur, AMR. *Clinically Oriented Anatomy,* 6th edition, 2009, Fig. I.25, p. 41.

Figure I.17 Moore KL, Dalley AF. Agur, AMR. *Clinically Oriented Anatomy,* 6th edition, 2009, Fig. I.27, p. 44.

Figure I.19 based on Moore KL, Dalley AF. *Clinically Oriented Anatomy,* 5th edition, 2006, Fig. I.41.

Figure I.23B Moore KL, Dalley AF. Agur, AMR. *Clinically Oriented Anatomy,* 6th edition, 2009, Fig. I.36 p. 51.

Figure I.25 Moore KL, Dalley AF. *Clinically Oriented Anatomy,* 5th edition, 2006, Fig. I.38, p. 59.

Figure I.28 Moore KL, Dalley AF. *Clinically Oriented Anatomy,* 5th edition, 2006, Fig. I.40, p. 61.

Figure I.29 Moore KL, Dalley AF. *Clinically Oriented Anatomy,* 5th edition, 2006, Fig. I.41, p. 63.

Figure I.32 Wicke L. *Atlas of Radiologic Anatomy,* 6th English ed. Ed. and Trans.: Taylor AN. 1998. [Wicke L. *Roentgen-Anatomie Normalbefunde,* 5th ed. Munich: Urban & Schwarzenberg, 1995.]

Figure I.33B Courtesy of A.M. Arenson, University of Toronto, Canada.

Figure I.33C Wicke L. *Atlas of Radiologic Anatomy,* 6th English ed. Ed. and Trans.: Taylor AN. 1998. [Wicke L. *Roentgen-Anatomie Normalbefunde,* 5th ed. Munich: Urban & Schwarzenberg, 1995.]

Figure I.34 A. Moore KL, *Clinically Oriented Anatomy,* 3rd ed., 1992, Fig.1.30 B. Dean D, Herbener TE. *Cross-Sectional Human Anatomy,* 2000.

Figure I.35 Posner, MI, Raichle M. *Images of Mind.* New York: Scientific American Library, 1994.

Figure BI.1 Willis MC. *Medical Terminology: The Language of Health Care,* 1995.

Figure BI.2 Rassner G, Steinert U. *Dermatologie.* Urban & Schwarzenberg Verlag, Munchen, 1992.

CHAPTER 1

Figure 1.7D&E Moore KL, Dalley AF. *Clinically Oriented Anatomy,* 5th ed., 2006, Fig.1.9D&E, p. 89.

Figure 1.11 Agur AMR, Dalley AF. *Grant's Atlas of Anatomy,* 12th edition, 2009.

Figure 1.19A Agur AMR, Dalley AF. *Grant's Atlas of Anatomy,* 11th ed., 2005.

Figure 1.20A Courtesy of DE Sanders, University of Toronto, Canada.

Figure 1.21 Moore KL, Dalley AF. *Clinically Oriented Anatomy,* 5th ed., 2006, Fig. 1.30, p. 129.

Figure 1.22 Based on Moore KL, Dalley AF. *Clinically Oriented Anatomy,* 5th ed., 2006, figs.1.62, 1.64; p. 180, 182. Also Agur AMR, Ming JL. *Grant's Atlas of Anatomy,* 10th ed., 1999.

Figure 1.25 Moore KL, Dalley AF. *Clinically Oriented Anatomy,* 5th ed., 2006, Fig. 1.36, p. 138.

Figure 1.27C Moore KL et al. *Clinically Oriented Anatomy,* 6th ed., 2009, Fig. 1.59, p. 146.

Figure 1.28 Moore KL, Dalley AF. *Clinically Oriented Anatomy,* 5th ed., 2006, Fig. 1.38, p. 139.

Figure 1.30 Agur AMR. *Grant's Atlas of Anatomy,* 9th ed., 1991.

Figure 1.37 Agur AMR, Dalley AF. *Grant's Atlas of Anatomy,* 11th ed., 2005, Fig. 1.45 A&B, p. 52.

Figure 1.38 Agur AMR, Dalley AF. *Grant's Atlas of Anatomy,* 11th ed., 2005, Fig. 1.46 A&B, p. 53.

Figure 1.40 Moore KL, Dalley AF. *Clinically Oriented Anatomy,* 5th ed., 2006, Fig. 1.39, p. 142.

Figure 1.41D Torrent-Guasp F, Buckberg GD, Clemente C, et al. The structure and function of the helical heart and its buttress wrapping. I. The normal macroscopic structure of the heart. Semin Thoracic Cardiovasc Surg 13:30, 2001.

Figure 1.42 Moore KL, Dalley AF. *Clinically Oriented Anatomy,* 5th ed., 2006, Fig. 1.58 A&B(2), p. 172-173.

Figure 1.46 Agur AMR, Dalley AF. *Grant's Atlas of Anatomy,* 11th ed., 2005, Fig. 1.72, p. 75.

Figure 1.48 Moore KL, Dalley AF. *Clinically Oriented Anatomy,* 5th ed., 2006, Fig. 1.62, p. 180.

Figure 1.49A Agur AMR, Dalley AF. *Grant's Atlas of Anatomy,* 12th edition, 2009, Fig. 1.80G, p. 87.

Figure 1.49B Agur AMR, Dalley AF. *Grant's Atlas of Anatomy,* 12th edition, 2009. Fig. 1.79C, p. 85.

Figure 1.50 Agur AMR, Dalley AF. *Grant's Atlas of Anatomy,* 11th ed., 2005, Fig. 1.47, p. 54; photos courtesy of I. Morrow, University of Manitoba, Canada.

Figure 1.51 Agur AMR, Dalley AF. *Grant's Atlas of Anatomy,* 12th edition, 2009, Fig. 1.84BDE, pp. 92-93.

Figure B1.1 Moore KL, Dalley AF. *Clinically Oriented Anatomy,* 5th ed., 2006, Fig. B1.2, p. 90.

Figure B1.2 Moore KL et al. *Clinically Oriented Anatomy,* 6th ed., 2009, Fig. B1.1, p. 84.

Figure B1.4AB Bickley LS, Szilagyi PG. *Bates' Guide to Physical Examination,* 8th ed, 2002.

Figure B1.5 Moore KL, Dalley AF. *Clinically Oriented Anatomy,* 5th ed., 2006, Fig. B1.3, p. 101.

Figure 2.70 Courtesy of AM Arenson, University of Toronto, Canada.

Figure 2.71A Courtesy of M Asch, University of Toronto, Canada.

Figure 2.71B Dean D, Herbener TE. *Cross-Sectional Human Anatomy*, 2000.

Figure 2.71C Courtesy of CS Ho, University of Toronto, Canada.

Figure B2.1 Moore KL et al. *Clinically Oriented Anatomy*, 6th ed., 2009, Fig. 2.15, p. 204.

Figure B2.2 Moore KL, Dalley AF. *Clinically Oriented Anatomy*, 5th ed., 2006, Fig. B2.1, p. 208.

Figure B2.3 Moore KL et al. *Clinically Oriented Anatomy*, 6th ed., 2009, Fig. 2.4ABC, p. 214.

Figure B2.4 Moore KL, Dalley AF. *Clinically Oriented Anatomy*, 5th ed., 2006, Fig. 2.13 and 2.14, p. 218-219.

Figure B2.5 Moore KL et al. *Clinically Oriented Anatomy*, 6th ed., 2009, Table Fig. B2.1, p. 213.

Figure B2.6 Moore KL et al. *Clinically Oriented Anatomy*, 6th ed., 2009, Fig. B2.3AC, p. 214.

Figure B2.7 Moore KL, Dalley AF. *Clinically Oriented Anatomy*, 5th ed., 2006, Fig. B2.14, p. 269.

Figure B2.8 Radiograph from Brant WE, Helms CA. *Fundamentals of Diagnostic Radiology*, 2nd ed., 1999.

Figure B2.9, inset *Stedman's Medical Dictionary*, 28th edition, 2005.

Figure B2.11A Moore KL, Persaud TVN. *Before We Are Born*, 7th ed., Saunders (Elsevier), Philadelphia, 2008, Fig. 9-10, p. 100. Courtesy of Dr. Nathan E. Wiseman, Professor of Surgery, Children's Hospital, University of Manitoba, Winnipeg, Manitoba, Canada.

Figure B2.11B Moore KL, Persaud TVN. *The Developing Human*, 8th ed., Saunders (Elsevier), Philadelphia 2008, Fig. 8-12C, p.156 Courtesy of Dr. Prem S. Sahni, formerly of Department of Radiology, Children's Hospital, Winnipeg, Manitoba, Canada.

Figure B2.12C Eckert P et al, *Fibrinklebung*, Urban and Schwarzenberg Verlag, Munchen, 1986.

Figure SA2.2 Moore KL et al. *Clinically Oriented Anatomy*, 6th ed., 2009, Fig. 2.36, p. 232.

Figure SA2.3 Moore KL et al. *Clinically Oriented Anatomy*, 6th ed., 2009, Fig. 2.5A-C, p. 264.

Figure SA2.5 Moore KL et al. *Clinically Oriented Anatomy*, 6th ed., 2009, Fig. 2.78, p. 292.

CHAPTER 3

Figure 3.1 Moore KL et al. *Clinically Oriented Anatomy*, 6th ed., 2009, Fig. 3.1, p. 328.

Figure 3.2 Modified from Agur AMR, Dalley AF. *Grant's Atlas of Anatomy*, 11th ed., 2005.

Figure 3.4AB Agur AMR, Dalley AF. *Grant's Atlas of Anatomy*, 11th ed., 2005.

Figure 3.5 Moore KL, Dalley AF. *Clinically Oriented Anatomy*, 5th ed., 2006, 4.27 and 4.28, p. 526 and 528.

Figure 3.7AB Moore KL, Dalley AF. *Clinically Oriented Anatomy*, 5th ed., 2006,Table 3.3, p. 374.

Figure 3.8A&C Agur AMR, Dalley AF. *Grant's Atlas of Anatomy*, 12th edition, 2009, figs.3.49D and Figure 3.39A, p. 259 and 258.

Figure 3.8BD&E Moore KL et al. *Clinically Oriented Anatomy*, 6th ed., 2009, figs 3.13 B&D, 3.14B, p. 346-247.

Figure 3.10 Moore KL, Dalley AF. *Clinically Oriented Anatomy*, 5th ed., 2006, Fig. 3.10B, p. 380.

Figure 3.20B Modified from Tank, PW. *Grant's Dissector*, 13th ed., 2005, fig5.31, p. 117.

Figure 3.24 Modified from Agur AMR, Dalley AF. *Grant's Atlas of Anatomy*, 11th ed., 2005.

Figure 3.27A, left Dauber W. *Pocket Atlas of Human Anatomy*. Rev. 5th ed., New York: Thieme, 2007, p. 195.

Figure 3.27A, right Agur AMR, Dalley AF. *Grant's Atlas of Anatomy*, 12th edition, 2009, Fig. 3.21A, p. 217.

Figure 3.36B&D Courtesy of AM Arenson, University of Toronto, Canada.

Figure 3.37 Agur AMR, Dalley AF. *Grant's Atlas of Anatomy*, 12th edition, 2009, Fig. 3.15A, p. 211; Agur AMR, Dalley AF. *Grant's Atlas of Anatomy*, 11th ed., 2005, p. 199.

Figure 3.41 Modified from Agur AMR, Dalley AF. *Grant's Atlas of Anatomy*, 11th ed., 2005.

Figure 3.42A Moore KL et al. *Clinically Oriented Anatomy*, 6th ed., 2009, 3.51A.

Figure 3.42B Modified from Clemente CD. *Anatomy: A Regional Atlas of the Human Body*, 5th ed. 2006, Fig. 272.I.

Figure 3.44 Moore KL et al. *Clinically Oriented Anatomy*, 6th ed., 2009, Fig. 3.53A-F, p. 407.

Figure 3.45 Moore KL et al. *Clinically Oriented Anatomy*, 6th ed., 2009, Fig. 3.54BC, p. 408.

Figure 3.46 Agur AMR. *Grant's Atlas of Anatomy*, 9th ed. 1991, Fig. 3.60B&C.

Figure 3.47 Agur AMR, Dalley AF. *Grant's Atlas of Anatomy*, 12th edition, 2009, Fig. 3.55, p. 265.

Figure 3.49 Agur AMR, Dalley AF. *Grant's Atlas of Anatomy*, 12th edition, 2009, Fig. 3.55B, p. 264.

Figure 3.51 Modified from Agur AMR, Dalley AF. *Grant's Atlas of Anatomy*, 11th ed., 2005.

Figure 3.52 Agur AMR, Dalley AF. *Grant's Atlas of Anatomy*, 11th ed., 2005.

Figure 3.55 Agur AMR, Dalley AF. *Grant's Atlas of Anatomy*, 11th ed., 2005.

Figure 3.56 Courtesy of MA Haider, University of Toronto, Canada.

Figure 3.58A Beckmann CRB et al., *Obstetrics and Gynecology*, 5th ed, 2006.

Figure 3.58B Courtesy of Dr. A. M. Arenson, Assistant Professor of Medical Imaging, University of Toronto, Ontario, Canada.

Figure 3.58C. Moore KL et al. *Clinically Oriented Anatomy*, 6th ed., 2009, 3.40, p. 384.

Figure 3.58D&F Daffner RH, *Clinical Radiology: The Essentials*, 2nd ed., 1998.

Figure 3.58E Erkonen WE, Smith WL, *Radiology 101: Basics and Fundamentals of Imaging*, 1998.

Figure B3.1 Moore KL, Dalley AF. *Clinically Oriented Anatomy*, 5th ed., 2006, Fig. B3.24B, p. 436.

Figure B3.2 Moore KL, Dalley AF. *Clinically Oriented Anatomy*, 5th ed., 2006, Fig. B3.7, p. 401.

Figure B3.3 Moore KL, Dalley AF. *Clinically Oriented Anatomy*, 5th ed., 2006, Fig. B3.9, p. 409.

Figure B3.4 Moore KL, Dalley AF. *Clinically Oriented Anatomy*, 5th ed., 2006, Fig. B3.14B, p. 418.

Figure B3.5 Moore KL, Dalley AF. *Clinically Oriented Anatomy*, 5th ed., 2006, Fig. B3.18, p. 421.

Figure B3.6 *Stedman's Medical Dictionary*, 27th ed., 2000.

Figure B3.8 Fuller J, Schaller-Ayers J. *A Nursing Approach*, 2nd ed. Philadelphia: Lippincott, 1994. B3.11 (artist: Larry Ward, Salt Lake City, UT).

Figure B3.9 Agur AMR, Dalley AF. *Grant's Atlas of Anatomy*, 11th ed., 2005.

Figure B3.10 Photo courtesy of RE Bristow, John Hopkins School of Medicine, Baltimore, MD.

Figure B3.11 Moore KL, Dalley AF. *Clinically Oriented Anatomy,* 5th ed., 2006, Fig. B3.25., p. 442.

Figure B3.12 Moore KL, Dalley AF. *Clinically Oriented Anatomy,* 5th ed., 2006, Fig. B3.26A, p. 450.

Figure B3.13 Moore KL, Dalley AF. *Clinically Oriented Anatomy,* 5th ed., 2006, Fig. B3.26B, p. 450.

Figure B3.14 Moore KL, Dalley AF. *Clinically Oriented Anatomy,* 5th ed., 2006, Fig. B3.29, p. 466.

CHAPTER 4

Figure 4.1 AB&D Moore KL et al. *Clinically Oriented Anatomy,* 6th ed., 2009, Fig. 4.1, p. 444.

Figure 4.1C Olson TR. *Student Atlas of Anatomy.* 1996.

Figure 4.2 Modified from Agur AMR, Dalley AF. *Grant's Atlas of Anatomy,* 11th ed., 2005.

Figure 4.3A&B Agur AMR, Dalley AF. *Grant's Atlas of Anatomy,* 12th edition, 2009, fig,4.10, p. 295.

Figure 4.3C Agur AMR, Dalley AF. *Grant's Atlas of Anatomy,* 11th ed., 2005.

Figure 4.3D&E Modified from Agur AMR. *Grant's Atlas of Anatomy,* 9th ed. 1991, p. 211.

Figure 4.4 AB&D Agur AMR, Dalley AF. *Grant's Atlas of Anatomy,* 12th edition, 2009, fig,4.12ABD, p. 297.

Figure 4.4C Courtesy of D. Salonen, University of Toronto, Canada.

Figure 4.4E Agur AMR, Dalley AF. *Grant's Atlas of Anatomy,* 12th edition, 2009, fig,4.12E, p. 297.

Figure 4.5A-C Agur AMR, Dalley AF. *Grant's Atlas of Anatomy,* 11th ed., 2005.

Figure 4.5D Becker RF et al. Anatomical Basis of Medical Practice. Williams & Wilkins, 1974.

Figure 4.6A-C Moore KL, Dalley AF. *Clinically Oriented Anatomy,* 5th ed., 2006, Table 4.3, p. 491.

Figure 4.6D Agur AMR, Dalley AF. *Grant's Atlas of Anatomy,* 12th edition, 2009, fig,4.16B, p. 302.

Figure 4.7A&C Agur AMR, Dalley AF. *Grant's Atlas of Anatomy,* 12th edition, 2009, fig,4.24AB, p. 313.

Figure 4.7B&D Olson TR. *Student Atlas of Anatomy.* 1996.

Figure 4.8D-F modified from Moore KL, Dalley AF. *Clinically Oriented Anatomy,* 5th ed., 2006, Fig. 4.9B-D, p. 500.

Figure 4.11 Moore KL et al. *Clinically Oriented Anatomy,* 6th ed., 2009, Fig. 4.19, p. 470.

Figure 4.13 Moore KL et al. *Clinically Oriented Anatomy,* 6th ed., 2009, Fig. 4.22A-C, p. 473.

Figure 4.15 Agur AMR, Dalley AF. *Grant's Atlas of Anatomy,* 11th ed., 2005.

Figure 4.22C-E Olson TR. *Student Atlas of Anatomy.* 1996.

Figure 4.23 D&E Modified from Moore KL, Dalley AF. *Clinically Oriented Anatomy,* 5th ed., 2006, T4.7, p. 539.

Figure 4.25 A Courtesy of D. Salonen, University of Toronto, Canada; B. *Grant's Atlas of Anatomy,* 12th edition, 2009, T7.2, p. 631.

Figure 4.26C Moore KL, Dalley AF. *Clinically Oriented Anatomy,* 5th ed., 2006, Fig. 4.39, p. 551.

Figure 4.27A&B Courtesy of the Visible Human Project; National Library of Medicine; Visible Man 1715.

Figure 4.27C Courtesy of D. Armstrong, University of Toronto, Canada.

Figure B4.1 Moore KL, Dalley AF. *Clinically Oriented Anatomy,* 5th ed., 2006, Fig. B4.16, p. 515.

Figure B4.2 Agur AMR, Dalley AF. *Grant's Atlas of Anatomy,* 11th ed., 2005.

Figure B4.3 van de Graaff K, Human Anatomy, 4th ed. Dubuque, IA: WC Brown, 1995, p. 163.

Figure B4.4 Moore KL, Dalley AF. *Clinically Oriented Anatomy,* 5th ed., 2006, Fig. B4.15, p. 513.

Figure B4.5 Clark,CR et al. *The Cervical Spine,* 1998.

Figure B4.6 Moore KL et al. *Clinically Oriented Anatomy,* 6th ed., 2009, Fig. B4.6, p. 464.

Figure B4.7 Atlas, SW, MD. *Magnetic Resonance Imaging of the Brain and Spinal Cord,* 3rd ed., 2001, Fig. 28.44 B&C.

Figure SA4.2A Moore KL et al. *Clinically Oriented Anatomy,* 6th ed., 2009, Fig. 4.6A, p. 452.

Figure T4.6 Moore KL, Dalley AF. *Clinically Oriented Anatomy,* 5th ed., 2006, Fig. T4.8A-D, p. 541.

Figure T4.7 Moore KL et al. *Clinically Oriented Anatomy,* 6th ed., 2009, Fig. 4.35, p. 491.

Figure T4.10 Moore KL, Dalley AF. *Clinically Oriented Anatomy,* 5th ed., 2006, Fig. T4.11, 546.

Figure T4.11 Moore KL et al. *Clinically Oriented Anatomy,* 6th ed., 2009, Fig. T4.11, p. 494.

CHAPTER 5

Figure 5.1B Agur AMR, Dalley AF. *Grant's Atlas of Anatomy,* 11th ed., 2005 and Moore KL, Dalley AF. *Clinically Oriented Anatomy,* 5th ed., figs. 5.14 and 5.3, p. 588 and 558.

Figure 5.3A Moore KL, Dalley AF. *Clinically Oriented Anatomy,* 5th ed., 2006, Fig. 5.6 A&B, p. 561.

Figure 5.3B Agur AMR, Dalley AF. *Grant's Atlas of Anatomy,* 12th edition, 2009, Fig. 4.23B, p. 312.

Figure 5.3C Agur AMR, Dalley AF. *Grant's Atlas of Anatomy,* 12th edition, 2009, fig,4.23A, p. 312.

Figure 5.7 Agur AMR, Dalley AF. *Grant's Atlas of Anatomy,* 11th ed., 2005

Figure 5.9A Agur AMR, Dalley AF. *Grant's Atlas of Anatomy,* 12th edition, 2009, fig,5.11C, p. 365.

Figure 5.9C Moore KL et al. *Clinically Oriented Anatomy,* 6th ed., 2009, Fig. 5.14D, p. 534.

Figure 5.10 Moore KL et al. *Clinically Oriented Anatomy,* 6th ed., 2009, Fig. 5.14C&E, p. 534.

Figure 5.12F Rose J, Gamble JG. *Human Walking,* 2nd ed. Baltimore: Williams & Wilkins, 1994.

Figure 5.12G Clay JH, Pounds DM. *Basic Clinical Massage Therapy: Integrating Anatomy and Treatment,* 2002.

Figure 5.13C Agur AMR, Ming JL. *Grant's Atlas of Anatomy,* 10th ed.

Figure 5.14B Moore KL, Dalley AF. *Clinically Oriented Anatomy,* 5th ed., 2006, Fig. 5.20A, p. 602.

Figure 5.19D&E Clay JH, Pounds DM. *Basic Clinical Massage Therapy: Integrating Anatomy and Treatment,* 2002.

Figure 5.23E Agur AMR. *Grant's Atlas of Anatomy,* 9th ed and Moore KL et al. *Clinically Oriented Anatomy,* 6th ed., 2009, Fig. 5.43C, P. 575.

Figure 5.26A Moore KL et al. *Clinically Oriented Anatomy,* 6th ed., 2009, Fig. 5.14E, p. 534.

Figure 5.28B Agur AMR, Dalley AF. *Grant's Atlas of Anatomy,* 12th edition, 2009, p. 423.

Figure 5.28C Agur AMR, Dalley AF. *Grant's Atlas of Anatomy,* 12th edition, 2009, Fig. 5.91B, p. 472.

Figure 5.31B Agur AMR, Dalley AF. *Grant's Atlas of Anatomy,* 12th edition, 2009, Fig. 5.59B, p. 433.

Figure 5.31C Agur AMR, Dalley AF. *Grant's Atlas of Anatomy,* 12th edition, 2009, Fig. 5.91B, p. 472.

Figure 5.34 Moore KL, Dalley AF. *Clinically Oriented Anatomy,* 5th ed., 2006, Table 5.11, p. 643.

Figure 5.35 Clay JH, Pounds DM. *Basic Clinical Massage Therapy: Integrating Anatomy and Treatment,* 2002.

Figure 5.38 Moore KL, Dalley AF. *Clinically Oriented Anatomy,* 5th ed., 2006, Fig. 5.43C, p. 662.

Figure 5.40 Moore KL, Dalley AF. *Clinically Oriented Anatomy,* 5th ed., 2006, Table 5.14-IIA, p. 659.

Figure 5.41 Moore KL et al. *Clinically Oriented Anatomy,* 6th ed., 2009, Fig. 5.72, p. 618.

Figure 5.43 Agur AMR, Dalley AF. *Grant's Atlas of Anatomy,* 11th ed., 2005, Fig. 5.32A, p. 380.

Figure 5.45 Moore KL, Dalley AF. *Clinically Oriented Anatomy,* 5th ed., 2006, Fig. 5.52B, p. 677.

Figure 5.47 Moore KL et al. *Clinically Oriented Anatomy,* 6th ed., 2009, Fig. 5.82, p. 632.

Figure 5.48B&D Courtesy of P. Bobechko, University of Toronto, Canada.

Figure 5.51D Agur AMR, Dalley AF. *Grant's Atlas of Anatomy,* 11th ed., 2005, Fig. 5.50B, p. 401.

Figure 5.55A Clay JH, Pounds DM. *Basic Clinical Massage Therapy: Integrating Anatomy and Treatment,* 2002, plate 10-1.

Figure 5.55B Moore KL et al. *Clinically Oriented Anatomy,* 6th ed., 2009, Fig. 5.95B, p. 647.

Figure 5.55C Courtesy of P. Bobechko and E. Becker, Department of Medical Imaging, University of Toronto, Toronto, Ontario, Canada.

Figure 5.59 Clay JH, Pounds DM. *Basic Clinical Massage Therapy: Integrating Anatomy and Treatment,* 2002, plate 10-1.

Figure 5.61C Courtesy of the Visible Human Project: National Library of Medicine; Visible Man 2105.

Figure 5.61D MRI courtesy of D. Salonen, University of Toronto, Canada.

Figure 5.62D-F *Grant's Atlas of Anatomy,* 12th edition, 2009, Fig. 5.91D-E, p. 472-473.

Figure B5.4 ©eMedicine.com, 2008. Available at: http://emedicine.medscape.com/article/411842-overview.

Figure B5.7 Moore KL et al. *Clinically Oriented Anatomy,* 6th ed., 2009, Fig. B5.16B, p. 561.

Figure B5.8 Moore KL et al. *Clinically Oriented Anatomy,* 6th ed., 2009, Fig. B5.15, p. 560.

Figure B5.9 Moore KL et al. *Clinically Oriented Anatomy,* 6th ed., 2009, Fig. B5.18BC, p. 562.

Figure B5.11 Moore KL et al. *Clinically Oriented Anatomy,* 6th ed., 2009, Fig. B5.20, p. 606.

Figure B5.12 Moore KL et al. *Clinically Oriented Anatomy,* 6th ed., 2009, Fig. B5.27, p. 625.

Figure B5.13 Moore KL et al. *Clinically Oriented Anatomy,* 6th ed., 2009, Fig. B5.25, p. 632.

Figure B5.14, drawings Willis MC. *Medical Terminology: A Programmed Learning Approach to the Language of Health Care.* Lippincott Williams & Wilkins: Baltimore, 2002.

Figure B5.14, radiograph Daffner RH: *Clinical Radiology—The Essentials.* Lippincott Williams & Wilkins: Baltimore, 1993.

Figure B5.15 Modified from Palastanga NP, et al. Anatomy and Human Movement, 4th ed. Oxford, UK: Butterworth-Heinemann, 2002.

Figure B5.16D Stedman's Medical Dictionary, 27th ed.

Figure B5.16E Moore KL, Dalley AF. *Clinically Oriented Anatomy,* 5th ed., 2006, Fig. B5.31, p. 701.

Figure B5.16F Moore KL, Dalley AF. *Clinically Oriented Anatomy,* 5th ed., 2006, Fig. B5.29, p. 700.

CHAPTER 6

Figure 6.1 Moore KL et al. *Clinically Oriented Anatomy,* 6th ed., 2009, Fig. 6.1, p. 672.

Figure 6.2 Moore KL et al. *Clinically Oriented Anatomy,* 6th ed., 2009, Fig. 6.2, p. 672.

Figure 6.6 Moore KL et al. *Clinically Oriented Anatomy,* 6th ed., 2009, Fig. 6.7BC, p. 677.

Figure 6.9 Moore KL et al. *Clinically Oriented Anatomy,* 6th ed., 2009, Fig. 6.9C, p. 679.

Figure 6.10 Moore KL, Dalley AF. *Clinically Oriented Anatomy,* 5th ed., 2006, Fig. 6.10A, p. 744.

Figure 6.15A-D Clay JH, Pounds DM. *Basic Clinical Massage Therapy: Integrating Anatomy and Treatment,* 2002.

Figure 6.15E Agur AMR, Dalley AF. *Grant's Atlas of Anatomy,* 11th ed., 2005.

Figure 6.38 Moore KL, Dalley AF. *Clinically Oriented Anatomy,* 5th ed., 2006, Table 6.10, p. 820.

Figure 6.39, left Modified from Agur AMR, Dalley AF. *Grant's Atlas of Anatomy,* 11th ed., 2005.

Figure 6.39, right Agur AMR, Dalley AF. *Grant's Atlas of Anatomy,* 11th ed., 2005.

Figure 6.43 Agur AMR, Dalley AF. *Grant's Atlas of Anatomy,* 11th ed., 2005.

Figure 6.44 Agur AMR, Dalley AF. *Grant's Atlas of Anatomy,* 11th ed., 2005.

Figure 6.45 Moore KL et al. *Clinically Oriented Anatomy,* 6th ed., 2009, Fig. 6.76, p. 774.

Figure 6.47 Agur AMR, Dalley AF. *Grant's Atlas of Anatomy,* 11th ed., 2005.

Figure 6.48B Courtesy of D. Armstrong, University of Toronto, Canada.

Figure 6.50 Moore KL et al. *Clinically Oriented Anatomy,* 6th ed., 2009, Fig. 6.86AB, p. 785.

Figure 6.54A Courtesy of E. L. Landsdown, University of Toronto, Canada.

Figure 6.55A Courtesy of E. Becker, University of Toronto, Canada.

Figure 6.55B Agur AMR, Dalley AF. *Grant's Atlas of Anatomy,* 11th ed., 2005.

Figure 6.58C Courtesy of J. Helsin, University of Toronto, Canada.

Figure 6.61A Dean D, Herbener TE. *Cross-Sectional Anatomy.* 2000, plate 7.2, p. 140-141.

Figure 6.61B Dean D, Herbener TE. *Cross-Sectional Anatomy.* 2000, plate 7.5, p. 140-141.

Figure 6.61C Dean D, Herbener TE. *Cross-Sectional Anatomy.* 2000, plate 7.8.

Figure 6.62A Courtesy of Walter Kucharczyk, University of Toronto, Canada.

Figure 6.62B&C Lee JKT et al, Computed Body Tomography with MRI Correlation, 2003, p. 1491, Fig. 22-13 AC.

Figure B6.4 Moore KL, Dalley AF. *Clinically Oriented Anatomy*, 5th ed., 2006, Fig. B6.4, p. 738.

Figure B6.5 Rowland LF, *Merritt's Textbook of Neurology*, 9th ed., 1995.

Figure B6.7 Moore KL, Dalley AF. *Clinically Oriented Anatomy*, 5th ed., 2006, Fig. B6.15, p. 793.

Figure B6.8 Hall-Craggs, *Anatomy as a Basis of Clinical Medicine*, 3rd ed., 1995.

Figure B6.10 Anderson MK, et al, *Foundations of Athletic Training*, 3rd ed., 1995.

Figure B6.12 Moore KL, Dalley AF. *Clinically Oriented Anatomy*, 5th ed., 2006, Fig. B6.19A, p. 813.

Figure B6.13 Moore KL, Dalley AF. *Clinically Oriented Anatomy*, 5th ed., 2006, Fig. B6.21, p. 814.

Figure B6.16C Agur AMR, Dalley AF. *Grant's Atlas of Anatomy*, 11th ed., 2005.

Figure B6.18 Moore KL et al. *Clinically Oriented Anatomy*, 6th ed., 2009, Fig. 6.10, p. 712.

Figure B6.21 Moore KL, Dalley AF. *Clinically Oriented Anatomy*, 5th ed., 2006, Fig. B6.33, p. 862.

Figure B6.22 MCT/Landov.

Figure B6.23 Moore KL, Dalley AF. *Clinically Oriented Anatomy*, 5th ed., 2006, Fig. B6.36, p. 866.

Figure SA6.1A Moore KL, Dalley AF. *Clinically Oriented Anatomy*, 5th ed., 2006, Fig. SA6.1, p. 739.

Figure SA6.1B Moore KL et al. *Clinically Oriented Anatomy*, 6th ed., 2009, Fig. 6.11, p. 682.

Figure SA6.3 Moore KL, Dalley AF. *Clinically Oriented Anatomy*, 5th ed., 2006, Fig. SA6.8 and 6.9, p. 800.

Figure SA6.4 Moore KL, Dalley AF. *Clinically Oriented Anatomy*, 5th ed., 2006, Fig. SA6.15, p. 845.

CHAPTER 7

Figure 7.1 Agur AMR, Dalley AF. *Grant's Atlas of Anatomy*, 12th ed., 2009, Fig. 7.3B, p. 613.

Figure 7.2 Agur AMR, Dalley AF. *Grant's Atlas of Anatomy*, 12th ed., 2009, Fig. 7.4, p. 614.

Figure 7.3A&C Agur AMR, Dalley AF. *Grant's Atlas of Anatomy*, 12th ed., 2009, Fig. 7.6B, p. 619.

Figure 7.4 Agur AMR, Dalley AF. *Grant's Atlas of Anatomy*, 12th ed., 2009, Fig. 7.16, p. 634.

Figure 7.7B Agur AMR, Dalley AF. *Grant's Atlas of Anatomy*, 12th ed., 2009, Fig. 7.21A, p. 639.

Figure 7.9A Agur AMR, Dalley AF. *Grant's Atlas of Anatomy*, 12th ed., 2009, Fig. 7,17A, p. 635

Figure 7.9B Agur AMR, Dalley AF. *Grant's Atlas of Anatomy*, 12th ed., 2009, Fig. 7.20B, p. 638.

Figure 7.11ABC Agur AMR, Dalley AF. *Grant's Atlas of Anatomy*, 11th ed., 2005, Fig. 7.26C, B, F, p. 626-627.

Figure 7.14 Moore KL, Dalley AF. *Clinically Oriented Anatomy*, 5th ed., 2006, Table 7.3, p. 929.

Figure 7.16A Agur AMR, Dalley AF. *Grant's Atlas of Anatomy*, 12th ed., 2009, Table 7.1 (left), p. 629.

Figure 7.16B Agur AMR, Dalley AF. *Grant's Atlas of Anatomy*, 12th ed., 2009, Table 7.2 (right), p. 631.

Figure 7.17 Moore KL, Dalley AF. *Clinically Oriented Anatomy*, 5th ed., 2006, Table 7.6, p. 948.

Figure 7.24A Courtesy of W. Kucharczyk, University of Toronto, Canada.

Figure 7.24B Agur AMR, Dalley AF. *Grant's Atlas of Anatomy*, 11th ed., 2005, Fig. 7.39B, p. 645.

Figure 7.24C Moore KL, Dalley AF. *Clinically Oriented Anatomy*, 5th ed., 2006, fig 7.23A, p. 938.

Figure 7.26 Moore KL et al. *Clinically Oriented Anatomy*, 6th ed., 2009, Fig. 7.49, p. 894.

Figure 7.27 Moore KL et al. *Clinically Oriented Anatomy*, 6th ed., 2009, Fig. 7.50, p. 895.

Figure 7.28A Melloni, JL, *Melloni's Illustrated Review of Human Anatomy: By Structures–Arteries, Bones, Muscles, Nerves, Veins*, 1988, p. 149.

Figure 7.28B van de Graaf K, *Human Anatomy*, 4th ed., Dubuque, IA: WC Brown, 1995, Fig. 15.18, p. 479.

Figure 7.29 Welch Allyn, Inc., Skaneateles Falls, NY.

Figure 7.30 van de Graaf K, *Human Anatomy*, 4th ed., Dubuque, IA: WC Brown, 1995, Fig. 15.17, p. 479.

Figure 7.31 Moore KL et al. *Clinically Oriented Anatomy*, 6th ed., 2009, Fig. 7.54A, p. 900.

Figure 7.32 Moore KL et al. *Clinically Oriented Anatomy*, 6th ed., 2009, Fig. 7.55B, p. 902.

Figure 7.33A Melloni, JL, *Melloni's Illustrated Review of Human Anatomy: By Structures – Arteries, Bones, Muscles, Nerves, Veins*, 1988, p. 143.

Figure 7.33B Melloni, JL, *Melloni's Illustrated Review of Human Anatomy: By Structures – Arteries, Bones, Muscles, Nerves, Veins*, 1988, p. 141.

Figure 7.33C Moore KL et al. *Clinically Oriented Anatomy*, 6th ed., 2009, Fig. 7.54D, p. 901.

Figure 7.33D Hall-Craggs, ECB, *Anatomy as the Basis of Clinical Medicine*, 3rd ed., 1995.

Figure 7.34A-D Modified from Girard, Louis: Anatomy of the Human Eye. II. The Extra-ocular Muscles. Teaching Films, Inc. Houston, TX.

Figure 7.35 Moore KL et al. *Clinically Oriented Anatomy*, 6th ed., 2009, Fig. 7.59, p. 904.

Figure 7.37A Melloni, JL, *Melloni's Illustrated Review of Human Anatomy: By Structures–Arteries, Bones, Muscles, Nerves, Veins*, 1988, p. 189.

Figure 7.37B Moore KL et al. *Clinically Oriented Anatomy*, 6th ed., 2009, Fig. 7.55A, p. 902.

Figure 7.37C Moore KL et al. *Clinically Oriented Anatomy*, 6th ed., 2009, Fig. 7.58, p. 904.

Figure 7.38A Agur AMR, Dalley AF. *Grant's Atlas of Anatomy*, 11th ed., 2005, Table 7.6, p. 647.

Figure 7.38B Moore KL et al. *Clinically Oriented Anatomy*, 6th ed., 2009, Fig. 7.62, p. 907.

Figure 7.40C Courtesy of D. Armstrong, University of Toronto, Canada.

Figure 7.43 Moore KL et al. *Clinically Oriented Anatomy*, 6th ed., 2009, Fig. 7.73, p. 923.

Figure 7.45A Moore KL et al. *Clinically Oriented Anatomy*, 6th ed., 2009, Fig.7.75, p. 926

Figure 7.45B A. Agur AMR, Dalley AF. *Grant's Atlas of Anatomy*, 11th ed., 2005, Fig. 7.49A, p. 661.

Figure 7.46A Agur AMR, Dalley AF. *Grant's Atlas of Anatomy*, 12th ed., 2009, Fig. 7.46A, p. 675.

Figure 7.46B Agur AMR, Dalley AF. *Grant's Atlas of Anatomy*, 12th ed., 2009, Fig. 7.46C (left), p. 675.

Figure 7.46C & D Agur AMR, Dalley AF. *Grant's Atlas of Anatomy*, 12th ed.,

2009, Fig. 7.46B (middle) and 7.46C (middle), p. 675.

Figure 7.49 Moore KL, Dalley AF. *Clinically Oriented Anatomy*, 5th ed., 2006, Fig. 7.45, p. 990.

Figure 7.51B Courtesy of M. J. Pharaoah, University of Toronto, Canada.

Figure 7.52 Agur AMR, Dalley AF. *Grant's Atlas of Anatomy*, 12th ed., 2009, Fig. 7.79, p. 687.

Figure 7.56 Agur AMR, Dalley AF. *Grant's Atlas of Anatomy*, 11th ed., 2005.

Figure 7.62A Agur AMR, Dalley AF. *Grant's Atlas of Anatomy*, 11th ed., 2005.

Figure 7.62B Modified from Paff, GH. *Anatomy of the Head & Neck*, Philadelphia: WB Sanders Co., 1973, figs. 238-240, p. 142-143.

Figure 7.64AB Modified from Paff, GH. *Anatomy of the Head & Neck*, Philadelphia: WB Sanders Co., 1973, figs. 238-240, p. 142-143.

Figure 7.64D&E Modified from Hall-Craggs ECB. *Anatomy as the Basis of Clinical Medicine*, 2nd ed. Baltimore: Williams & Wilkins, 1990. Fig. 9-100, p. 536.

Figure 7.67B Agur AMR, Dalley AF. *Grant's Atlas of Anatomy*, 11th ed., 2005, table 9.7, p. 809.

Figure 7.68B Agur AMR, Dalley AF. *Grant's Atlas of Anatomy*, 12th ed., 2009, Fig. 7.65C, p. 698.

Figure 7.69C&D Agur AMR, Dalley AF. *Grant's Atlas of Anatomy*, 12th ed., 2009, Fig. 7.68CD, p. 703.

Figure 7.70A Agur AMR, Dalley AF. *Grant's Atlas of Anatomy*, 12th ed., 2009, Fig. 7.71C, p. 706.

Figure 7.70B Courtesy of Welch Allyn, Inc., Skaneateles Falls, NY.

Figure 7.72 Moore KL et al. *Clinically Oriented Anatomy*, 6th ed., 2009, Fig. 7.11B, p. 968.

Figure 7.73A Agur AMR, Dalley AF. *Grant's Atlas of Anatomy*, 11th ed., 2005.

Figure 7.77A Agur AMR, Ming JL. *Grant's Atlas of Anatomy*, 10th ed., 1999.

Figure 7.77B Agur AMR, Dalley AF. *Grant's Atlas of Anatomy*, 11th ed., 2005.

Figure 7.77C&D Moore KL et al. *Clinically Oriented Anatomy*, 6th ed., 2009, Fig. 7.17C&D, p. 974.

Figure 7.78 Moore KL et al. *Clinically Oriented Anatomy*, 6th ed., 2009, Fig. 7.118, p. 976.

Figure 7.79 Agur AMR, Dalley AF. *Grant's Atlas of Anatomy*, 12th ed., 2009, Fig. 7.78A, p. 715.

Figure 7.80 Seeley RR, Stephens TR, and Tate P. *Anatomy & Physiology 6th ed*, New York: McGraw-Hill, 2003. Fig. 15.28, p. 532.

Figure 7.81A&B Courtesy of E. Becker, University of Toronto, Canada.

Figure 7.81C Courtesy of D. Armstrong, University of Toronto, Canada.

Figure 7.82C-F Photos courtesy of The Visible Human Project: National Library of Medicine; Visible Man 1107 and 1168.

Figure B7.3 Visuals Unlimited, Hollis, New Hampshire.

Figure B7.4, bottom Moore KL, Dalley AF. *Clinically Oriented Anatomy*, 5th ed., 2006, Fig. 7.15, p. 931.

Figure B7.6 Skin Cancer Foundation.

Figure B7.7 Welch Allyn, Skaneateles Falls, NY.

Figure B7.8 Cohen BJ. *Medical Terminology*, 4th ed. 2003.

Figure B7.9 Mann IC. *The Development of the Human Eye*. New York: Grune & Stratton. 1974.

Figure B7.10 Moore KL et al. *Clinically Oriented Anatomy*, 6th ed., 2009, Fig. 7.30, p. 913.

Figure B7.11 Moore KL et al. *Clinically Oriented Anatomy*, 6th ed., 2009, Fig. 7.31 (inset), p. 927.

Figure B7.12 Courtesy of Dr. Joseph B. Jacobs, NYU Medical Center, New York, NY.

Figure B7.13 Hall-Craggs ECB, *Anatomy as the Basis of Clinical Medicine, 3rd ed, 1995.*

Figure B7.14 Reprinted with permission of Bechara Y. Ghorayeb MD, Houston, TX.

CHAPTER 8

Figure 8.1 Modified from Moore KL, Dalley AF. *Clinically Oriented Anatomy*, 5th ed., 2006, Fig. 8.3, p. 1048.

Figure 8.2 Moore KL, Dalley AF. *Clinically Oriented Anatomy*, 5th ed., 2006, Fig. 8.4, p. 1050 and Agur AMR, Dalley AF. *Grant's Atlas of Anatomy*, 12th edition, 2009, Fig. 8.1, p. 747.

Figure 8.4A Agur AMR, Dalley AF. *Grant's Atlas of Anatomy*, 12th edition, 2009, Fig. 8.2A, p. 748.

Figure 8.4C Agur AMR, Dalley AF. *Grant's Atlas of Anatomy*, 12th edition, 2009, Fig. 8.5C, p. 755.

Figure 8.5C Modified from Moore KL, Dalley AF. *Clinically Oriented Anatomy*, 5th ed., 2006, Fig. 8.18, p. 1070.

Figure 8.7 Modified from Moore KL, Dalley AF. *Clinically Oriented Anatomy*, 5th ed., 2006, Table 8.5, p. 1094.

Figure 8.10B Modified from Moore KL, Dalley AF. *Clinically Oriented Anatomy*, 5th ed., 2006, Fig. 8.41C, p. 1108.

Figure 8.17A-C Liebgott B, The Anatomical Basis of Dentistry. Philadelphia: Saunders, 1982, Fig. 9.22.

Figure 8.19A&B Modified from Moore KL, Dalley AF. *Clinically Oriented Anatomy*, 5th ed., 2006, Fig. 8. 41A&B, p. 1108.

Figure 8.21A Courtesy of M. Keller, University of Toronto, Canada.

Figure 8.21B&C Courtesy of Walter Kucharczyk, University of Toronto, Canada.

Figure 8.22 Siemens Medical Solutions USA, Inc.

Figure B8.4 Moore KL, Dalley AF. *Clinically Oriented Anatomy*, 5th ed., 2006, Figure B8.4, p. 1073.

Figure B8.5 Agur AMR. *Grant's Atlas of Anatomy*, 9th ed., 1991.

Figure B8.6 Rohen JW et al. *Color Atlas of Anatomy: A Photographic Study of the Human Body*, 5th ed., 2002.

Figure B8.9,left Agur AMR, Dalley AF. *Grant's Atlas of Anatomy*, 12th edition, 2009, Fig. 8.26C, P. 793.

Table 8.1C Moore KL, Dalley AF. *Clinically Oriented Anatomy*, 5th ed., 2006, Table 8.1F, p. 1052.

Table 8.2 Moore KL, Dalley AF. *Clinically Oriented Anatomy*, 5th ed., 2006, Table 8.3, p. 1069.

Table 8.5 Moore KL, Dalley AF. *Clinically Oriented Anatomy*, 5th ed., 2006, Table 8.5, p. 1094.

Figure SA 8.1 Moore KL, Dalley AF. *Clinically Oriented Anatomy*, 5th ed., 2006, Figure SA 8.1A-D&F, p. 1074.

CHAPTER 9

Figure 9.2, inset Agur AMR, Dalley AF. *Grant's Atlas of Anatomy*, 12th edition, 2009, Fig. 4.50C, p. 345.

Figure 9.3B Agur AMR, Dalley AF. *Grant's Atlas of Anatomy,* 12th edition, 2009, Fig.7.6B, p. 619.

Figure 9.4 Modified from Agur AMR, Dalley AF. *Grant's Atlas of Anatomy,* 11th ed., 2005, Fig. 9.3A&B, p. 798-799.

Figure 9.6A Modified from Agur AMR, Dalley AF. *Grant's Atlas of Anatomy,* 11th ed., 2005, Fig. 9.4A, p. 802.

Figure 9.10 Modified from Moore KL, Dalley AF. *Clinically Oriented Anatomy,* 5th ed., 2006, Fig. 9.6, p. 1140.

Figure 9.13A Modified from Agur AMR, Dalley AF. *Grant's Atlas of Anatomy,* 11th ed., 2005.

Figure 9.13B Agur AMR, Dalley AF. *Grant's Atlas of Anatomy,* 12th edition, 2009, Fig. 7.78A, p. 715.

Figure 9.14 Agur AMR, Dalley AF. *Grant's Atlas of Anatomy,* 12th edition, 2009, Table 9.11, p. 834.

Figure 9.15 Agur AMR, Dalley AF. *Grant's Atlas of Anatomy,* 12th edition, 2009, Table 9.11, p. 835.

Figure 9.16 Moore KL, Dalley AF. *Clinically Oriented Anatomy,* 5th ed., 2006, Fig. 9.11, p. 1149.

Figure 9.19 Agur AMR, Dalley AF. *Grant's Atlas of Anatomy,* 11th ed., 2005.

Table 9.1 Agur AMR, Dalley AF. *Grant's Atlas of Anatomy,* 12th edition, 2009, Table Fig. 9.1, p. 814.

Figure B9.7 Agur AMR, Dalley AF. *Grant's Atlas of Anatomy,* 12th edition, 2009, Table Fig. 9.1, p. 841.

Introduction to Clinical Anatomy

APPROACHES TO STUDYING ANATOMY / 2

ANATOMICOMEDICAL TERMINOLOGY / 3
Anatomical Position / 3
Anatomical Planes / 3
Terms of Relationship and Comparison / 4
Terms of Laterality / 5
Terms of Movement / 5
Anatomical Variations / 7

INTEGUMENTARY SYSTEM / 7

SKELETAL SYSTEM / 9
Bones / 11
Joints / 14

MUSCULAR SYSTEM / 17
Skeletal Muscles / 17
Cardiac Striated Muscle / 20
Smooth Muscle / 20

CARDIOVASCULAR SYSTEM / 23
Arteries / 23
Veins / 25
Capillaries / 28

LYMPHOID SYSTEM / 28

NERVOUS SYSTEM / 31
Central Nervous System / 31
Peripheral Nervous System / 31
Somatic Nervous System / 34
Structure and Components of a Typical Spinal Nerve / 34
Autonomic Nervous System / 36
Sympathetic Visceral Motor Innervation / 38
Parasympathetic Visceral Motor Innervation / 42
Visceral Afferent Sensation / 42

IMAGING OF BODY SYSTEMS / 42
Conventional Radiography / 42
Computerized Tomography / 44
Ultrasonography / 44
Magnetic Resonance Imaging / 44
Positron Emission Tomography / 46

1

Essential Clinical Anatomy relates the structure and function of the body to what is commonly required in the general practice of medicine, dentistry, and the allied health sciences. Because the number of details in anatomy overwhelms many beginning students, *Essential Clinical Anatomy* simplifies, correlates, and integrates the information so that it is easier to understand. The *clinical correlation boxes* (blue boxes) and *clinical case studies* (accompanying Web site) illustrate the clinical applications of anatomy. The *surface anatomy boxes* (orange boxes) provide an understanding of what lies under the skin and the *medical imaging techniques* (green boxes), included throughout and at the end of each chapter, illustrate how anatomy is visualized clinically.

APPROACHES TO STUDYING ANATOMY

There are three main approaches to studying human gross anatomy: regional, systemic, and clinical (applied). In this introductory chapter, the systemic approach is used; in subsequent chapters, the clinical and regional approaches are used.

Regional anatomy is based on the organization of the body into parts: head, neck, trunk (further subdivided into thorax, abdomen, pelvis/perineum, back) and paired upper and lower limbs. Emphasis is placed on the relationships of various systemic structures (e.g., muscles, nerves, and arteries) within the region (Fig. I.1). Each region is not an isolated

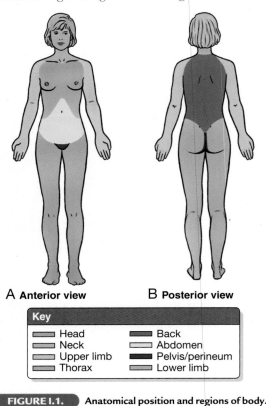

A Anterior view   **B Posterior view**

Key	
Head	Back
Neck	Abdomen
Upper limb	Pelvis/perineum
Thorax	Lower limb

FIGURE I.1.   Anatomical position and regions of body.

part and must be put into the context of adjacent regions and of the body as a whole. Surface anatomy is an essential part of the regional approach, providing a knowledge of what structures are visible and/or palpable (perceptible to touch) in the living body at rest and in action. The physical examination of patients is the clinical extension of surface anatomy. In people with stab wounds, for example, the healthcare worker must be able to visualize the deep structures that might be injured.

Systemic anatomy is an approach to anatomical study organized by *organ systems* that work together to carry out complex functions. None of the organ systems functions in isolation. For example, much of the skeletal, articular, and muscular systems constitute the *locomotor system.* And although the structures directly responsible for locomotion are the muscles, bones, joints, and ligaments, other systems are involved as well. The arteries and veins of the circulatory system supply oxygen to them and remove waste from them, and the nerves of the nervous system stimulate them to act. Brief descriptions of the systems of the body and their fields of study (in parentheses) follow:

- *Integumentary system* (dermatology): consists of the skin (integument) and its appendages, such as the hair and nails. The skin, an extensive sensory organ, forms a protective covering for the body.
- *Skeletal system* (osteology; orthopedics): consists of bones and cartilage. It provides support for the body and protects vital organs. The muscular system acts on the skeletal system to produce movements.
- *Articular system* (arthrology): consists of joints and their associated ligaments. It connects the bony parts of the skeletal system and provides the sites at which movements occur.
- *Muscular system* (myology): consists of muscles that act (contract) to move or position parts of the body (e.g., the bones that articulate at joints).
- *Nervous system* (neurology): consists of the *central nervous system* (brain and spinal cord) and the *peripheral nervous system* (nerves and ganglia, together with their motor and sensory endings). The nervous system controls and coordinates the functions of the organ systems.
- *Circulatory system* (angiology): consists of the cardiovascular and lymphatic systems, which function in parallel to distribute fluids within the body.
  - *Cardiovascular system* (cardiology): consists of the heart and blood vessels that propel and conduct blood through the body.
  - *Lymphoid system:* consists of a network of lymphatic vessels that withdraws excess tissue fluid (lymph) from the body's interstitial (intercellular) fluid compartment, filters it through lymph nodes, and returns it to the bloodstream.
- *Digestive* or *alimentary system* (gastroenterology): consists of the organs and glands associated with the ingestion,

mastication (chewing), deglutition (swallowing), digestion, and absorption of food and the elimination of feces (solid wastes) after the nutrients have been absorbed.

- *Respiratory system* (pulmonology): consists of the air passages and lungs that supply oxygen and eliminate carbon dioxide. The control of airflow through the system produces tone, which is further modified into speech.
- *Urinary system* (urology): consists of the kidneys, ureters, urinary bladder, and urethra, which filter blood and subsequently produce, transport, store, and intermittently excrete liquid waste (urine).
- *Reproductive system* (obstetrics and gynecology for females; andrology for males): consists of the gonads (ovaries and testes) that produce oocytes (eggs) and sperms and the other genital organs concerned with reproduction.
- *Endocrine system* (endocrinology): consists of discrete ductless glands (e.g., thyroid gland) as well as cells of the intestine and blood vessel walls and specialized nerve endings that secrete hormones. Hormones are distributed by the cardiovascular system to reach receptor organs in all parts of the body. These glands influence metabolism and coordinate and regulate other processes (e.g., the menstrual cycle).

Clinical (applied) anatomy emphasizes aspects of the structure and function of the body important in the practice of medicine, dentistry, and the allied health sciences. It encompasses both the regional and the systemic approaches to studying anatomy and stresses clinical application.

ANATOMICOMEDICAL TERMINOLOGY

Anatomy has an international vocabulary that is the foundation of medical terminology. This nomenclature enables precise communication among health professionals worldwide as well as among scholars in basic and applied health sciences. Although *eponyms* (names of structures derived from the names of people) are not used in official anatomical terminology, those commonly used by clinicians appear in parentheses throughout this book to reduce ambiguity and misunderstanding. Similarly, formerly used terms appear in parentheses on first mention—for example, internal thoracic artery (internal mammary artery). The terminology in this book conforms with the *Terminologia Anatomica: International Anatomical Terminology* (Federative Committee on Anatomical Terminology, 1998).

Anatomical Position

All anatomical descriptions are expressed in relation to the anatomical position (Fig. I.1) to ensure that the descriptions are not ambiguous. The anatomical position refers to

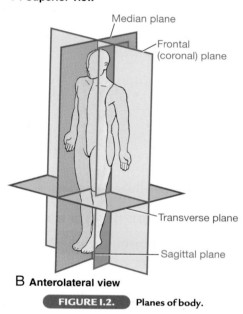

FIGURE I.2. Planes of body.

people—regardless of the actual position they may be in—as if they were standing erect, with their:

- Head, eyes (gaze), and toes directed anteriorly (forward).
- Upper limbs by the sides with the palms facing anteriorly.
- Lower limbs close together with the feet parallel and the toes directed anteriorly.

Anatomical Planes

Anatomical descriptions are based on four imaginary planes that intersect the body in the anatomical position (Fig. I.2). There are many sagittal, frontal, and transverse planes, but there is only one median plane.

- **Median (median sagittal) plane** is the vertical plane passing longitudinally through the center of the body, dividing it into right and left halves.
- **Sagittal planes** are vertical planes passing through the body *parallel to the median plane*. It is helpful to give a point of reference to indicate the position of a specific plane—for example, a sagittal plane through the midpoint of the clavicle. A plane parallel to and near the median plane may be referred to as a *paramedian plane.*
- **Frontal (coronal) planes** are vertical planes passing through the body *at right angles to the median plane*, dividing it into anterior (front) and posterior (back)

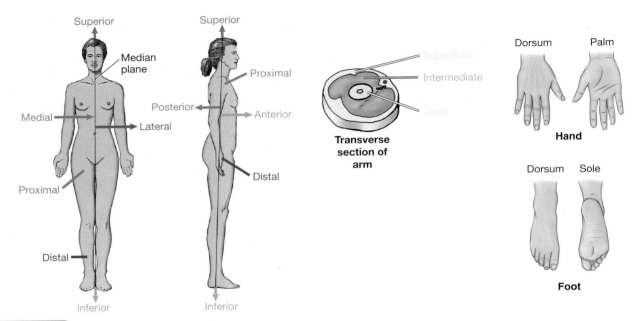

Terms of relationship and comparison.

TABLE I.1 COMMONLY USED TERMS OF RELATIONSHIP AND COMPARISON

Term	Meaning	Example
Superior (cranial)	Nearer to head	Heart is superior to stomach.
Inferior (caudal)	Nearer to feet	Stomach is inferior to heart.
Anterior (ventral)	Nearer to front	Sternum is anterior to heart.
Posterior (dorsal)	Nearer to back	Kidneys are posterior to intestine.
Medial	Nearer to median plane	Fifth digit (little finger) is on medial side of hand.
Lateral	Farther from median plane	First digit (thumb) is on lateral side of hand.
Proximal	Nearer to trunk or point of origin (e.g., of a limb)	Elbow is proximal to wrist; proximal part of artery is its beginning.
Distal	Farther from trunk or point of origin (e.g., of a limb)	Wrist is distal to elbow; distal part of lower limb is foot.
Superficial	Nearer to or on surface	Muscles of arm are superficial to its bone (humerus).
Deep	Farther from surface	Humerus is deep to arm muscles.
Intermediate	Between opposite pairs of terms above	Muscles are intermediate between skin and bones.
Dorsum	Surface of hand, foot, nose, or penis toward back in quadrupedal position	Veins are visible in dorsum of hand.
Palm	Anterior surface of hand	Skin creases are visible on palm.
Sole (plantar)	Inferior surface of foot	Skin is thick on sole of foot.

portions—for example, a frontal plane through the heads of the mandible.

- **Transverse planes** are planes passing through the body *at right angles to the median and frontal planes.* A transverse plane divides the body into superior (upper) and inferior (lower) parts—for example, a transverse plane through the umbilicus. Radiologists refer to transverse planes as *transaxial planes* or simply *axial planes.*

Terms of Relationship and Comparison

Various adjectives, arranged as pairs of opposites, describe the relationship of parts of the body in the anatomical position and compare the position of two structures relative to each other. These pairs of adjectives are explained in Table I.1 and illustrated in Fig. I.3. For example, the eyes are superior to the nose, whereas the nose is inferior to the eyes.

Combined terms describe intermediate positional arrangements:

- **Inferomedial** means nearer to the feet and closer to the median plane—for example, the anterior parts of the ribs run inferomedially.
- **Superolateral** means nearer to the head and farther from the median plane.

Proximal and **distal** are directional terms used when describing positions—for example, whether structures are nearer to the trunk or point of origin (i.e., proximal). **Dorsum** refers to the superior or dorsal (back) surface of any part that protrudes anteriorly from the body, such as the *dorsum of the foot, hand, penis, or tongue*. It is easier to understand why these surfaces are considered dorsal if one thinks of a quadrupedal plantigrade animal that walks on its soles, such as a dog. The **sole** indicates the inferior aspect or bottom of the foot, much of which is in contact with the ground when standing barefoot. The **palm** refers to the flat anterior aspect of the hand, excluding the five digits, and is the opposite of the dorsum of the hand.

Terms of Laterality

Paired structures having right and left members (e.g., the kidneys) are **bilateral,** whereas those occurring on one side only (e.g., the spleen) are **unilateral. Ipsilateral** means occurring on the same side of the body; the right thumb and right great toe are ipsilateral, for example. **Contralateral** means occurring on the opposite side of the body; the right hand is contralateral to the left hand.

Terms of Movement

Various terms describe movements of the limbs and other parts of the body (Fig. I.4). Although most movements take place at joints where two or more bones or cartilages articulate with one another, several non-skeletal structures exhibit movement (e.g., tongue, lips, and eyelids). Movements taking place at joints are described relative to the axes around which the part of the body moves and the plane in which the movement takes place—for example, flexion and extension of the shoulder take place in the sagittal plane around a frontal (coronal) axis.

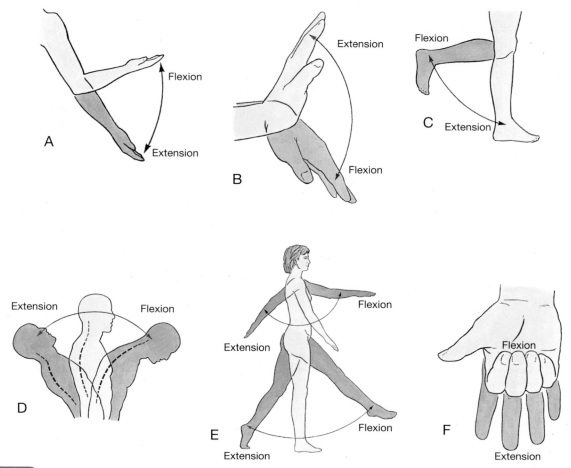

FIGURE I.4.   **Terms of movement. A–G. Flexion** means bending of a part or decreasing the angle between body parts. **Extension** means straightening a part or increasing the angle between body parts. Except for the thumb, flexion and extension movements are in the sagittal plane.

FIGURE I.4. **Terms of movement** (*continued*). **H and I. Abduction** means moving away from the median plane of the body in the frontal plane. **Adduction** means moving toward the median plane of the body in the frontal (coronal) plane. When referring to the digits (fingers and toes), abduction means spreading them, and adduction means drawing them together. **I. Rotation** means moving a part of the body around its long axis. Medial rotation turns the anterior surface medially, and lateral rotation turns this surface laterally. **J. Circumduction** is the circular movement of the limbs, or parts of them, combining in sequence the movements of flexion, extension, abduction, and adduction. **K. Pronation** is a medial rotation of the forearm and hand so that the palm faces posteriorly. **Supination** is a lateral rotation of the forearm and hand so that the palm faces anteriorly, as in the anatomical position. **L. Dorsiflexion** is elevation of the dorsum of the foot at the ankle. **Plantarflexion** is depression of the sole of the foot at the ankle. **Eversion** means turning the sole of the foot outward. **Inversion** means turning the sole of the foot inward. **M. Protrusion** (protraction) means to move the jaw anteriorly. **Retrusion** (retraction) means to move the jaw posteriorly. **N. Elevation** raises or moves a part superiorly. **Depression** lowers or moves a part inferiorly.

Anatomical Variations

Although anatomy books describe the structure of the body observed in most people (i.e., the most common pattern), the structure of individuals varies considerably in the details. Students are often frustrated because the bodies they are examining or dissecting do not conform to the atlas or text-book they are using. Students should expect anatomical variations when dissecting or studying prosected specimens. The bones of the skeleton vary among themselves not only in their basic shape but also in the details of surface structure. There is also a wide variation in the size, shape, and form of the attachment of muscles. Similarly, there is variation in the method of division of vessels and nerves, and the greatest variation occurs in veins. Apart from racial and sexual differences, humans exhibit considerable genetic variation. Approximately 3% of newborns show one or more significant congenital anomalies (Moore & Persaud, 2008).

INTEGUMENTARY SYSTEM

The skin, the largest organ of the body, is readily accessible, and is one of the best indicators of general health (Swartz, 2005). *The skin provides:*

- *Protection* for the body from environmental effects, such as abrasions and harmful substances.
- *Containment* of the tissues, organs, and vital substances of the body, preventing dehydration.
- *Heat regulation* through sweat glands, blood vessels, and fat deposits.
- *Sensation* (e.g., pain) by way of superficial nerves and their sensory endings.
- *Synthesis and storage* of vitamin D.

The skin consists of a superficial cellular layer, the epidermis, which creates a tough protective outer surface, and a basal (deep) regenerative and pigmented connective tissue layer, the dermis (Fig. I.5).

The **epidermis** is a keratinized stratified (layered) epithelium with a tough outer surface composed of keratin (a fibrous protein). The outer layer of the epidermis is continuously "shed" or rubbed away with replacement of new cells from the basal layer. This process renews the epidermis of the entire body every 25 to 45 days. The epidermis is avascular (no blood vessels or lymphatics) and is nourished by the vessels in the underlying dermis. The skin is supplied by afferent nerve endings that are sensitive to touch, irritation (pain), and temperature. Most nerve terminals are in the dermis, but a few penetrate the epidermis.

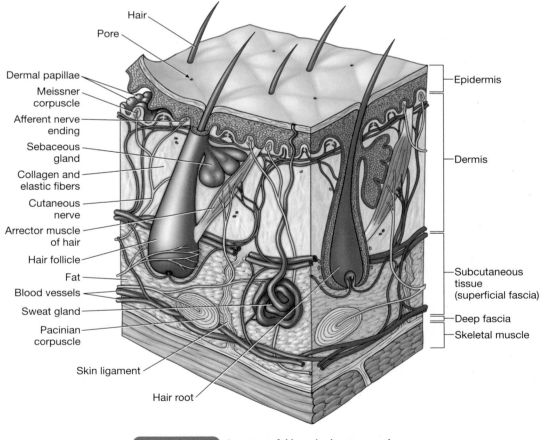

FIGURE I.5. Structure of skin and subcutaneous tissue.

The **dermis** is formed by a dense layer of interlacing *collagen* and *elastic fibers*. These fibers provide skin tone and account for the strength and toughness of the skin. The primary direction of collagen fibers in a particular region determines the characteristic tension lines (cleavage lines) and wrinkle lines in the skin. The deep layer of the dermis contains hair follicles, with their associated smooth arrector (L. *arrector pili*) muscles and sebaceous glands. Contraction of the **arrector muscles** erects the hairs (causing goose bumps), thereby compressing the sebaceous glands and helping them secrete their oily product onto the skin. Other integumentary structures include the hair, nails, mammary glands, and the enamel of teeth.

The **subcutaneous tissue** (superficial fascia) is composed of loose connective tissue and fat. Located between the dermis and underlying deep fascia, the subcutaneous tissue contains the deepest parts of the sweat glands, the blood and lymphatic vessels, and cutaneous nerves. The subcutaneous tissue provides for most of the body's fat storage, so its thickness varies greatly, depending on the person's nutritional state. **Skin ligaments** (L. *retinacula cutis*), consisting of numerous small fibrous bands, extend through the subcutaneous tissue and attach the deep surface of the dermis to the underlying deep fascia. The length and density of these ligaments determine the mobility of the skin over deep structures.

The **deep fascia** is a dense, organized connective tissue layer, devoid of fat, that envelops most of the body deep to the skin and subcutaneous tissue. Extensions from its internal surface:

- Invest deeper structures, such as individual muscles and neurovascular bundles (**investing fascia**).
- Divide muscles into groups or compartments (**intermuscular septa**).
- Lie between the musculoskeletal walls and the serous membranes lining body cavities (**subserous fascia**).

The deep fascia also forms **retinacula,** which hold tendons in place during joint movement.

Bursae (closed sacs containing fluid) prevent friction and enable structures to move freely over another.

In living people, **fascial planes** (interfascial and intrafascial) are potential spaces between adjacent fascias or fascia-lined structures. During operations, surgeons take advantage of these planes, separating structures to create actual spaces that allow access to deeply placed structures. These planes are often fused in embalmed cadavers.

Skin Incisions and Wounds

Tension Lines

 Tension lines (cleavage lines) keep the skin taut, yet allow for creasing with movement. Stab wounds in the skin by an ice pick, for example, are usually slit-like rather than rounded because the pick splits the dermis in the predominant direction of the collagen fibers, which determines the tension lines. Lacerations or surgical incisions that parallel the tension lines usually heal well with little scarring because there is minimal disruption of the collagen fibers. An incision or laceration across tension lines disrupts a greater number of collagen fibers, causing the wound to gape and possibly heal with excessive (keloid) scarring. Surgeons make their incisions parallel with the tension lines when other considerations (e.g., adequate exposure, avoiding nerves) are not of greater importance.

Stretch Marks in Skin

The collagen and elastic fibers in the dermis form a tough, flexible meshwork of tissue. The skin can distend considerably when the abdomen enlarges, as during pregnancy, for example. However, if stretched too far, it can result in damage to the collagen fibers in the dermis. Bands of thin wrinkled skin, initially red, become purple and later white. Stretch marks appear on the abdomen, buttocks, thighs, and breasts during pregnancy. These marks also form in obese individuals. Stretch marks generally fade (but never disappear completely) after pregnancy and weight loss.

Burns

Burns are tissue injuries caused by thermal, electrical, radioactive, or chemical agents.

- In *first-degree burns,* the damage is limited to the superficial part of the epidermis.
- In *second-degree burns,* the damage extends through the epidermis into the superficial part of the dermis. However, except for their most superficial parts, the sweat glands and hair follicles are not damaged and can provide the source of replacement cells for the basal layer of the epidermis.
- In *third-degree burns,* the entire epidermis, dermis, and perhaps underlying muscle are damaged. A minor degree of healing may occur at the edges, but the open ulcerated portions require skin grafting.

The extent of the burn (percent of total body surface affected) is generally more significant than the degree (severity of depth) in estimating its effect on the well-being of the victim.

SKELETAL SYSTEM

The skeleton of the body is composed of bones and cartilages and has two main parts (Fig. I.6):

- The **axial skeleton** consists of the bones of the head (cranium or skull), neck (cervical vertebrae), and trunk (ribs, sternum, vertebrae, and sacrum).

- The **appendicular skeleton** consists of the bones of the limbs, including those forming the pectoral (shoulder) and pelvic girdles.

Bone, a living tissue, is a highly specialized, hard form of connective tissue that makes up most of the skeleton and is the chief supporting tissue of the body. *Bones provide:*

- Protection for vital structures.

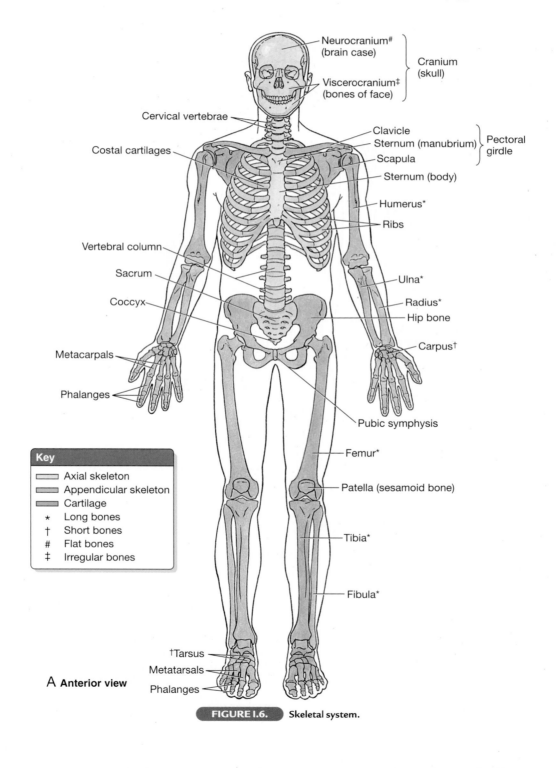

Key
▭	Axial skeleton
▭	Appendicular skeleton
▬	Cartilage
*	Long bones
†	Short bones
#	Flat bones
‡	Irregular bones

Labels in figure:
Neurocranium# (brain case)
Viscerocranium‡ (bones of face)
Cranium (skull)
Cervical vertebrae
Clavicle
Sternum (manubrium)
Pectoral girdle
Scapula
Sternum (body)
Humerus*
Ribs
Costal cartilages
Vertebral column
Sacrum
Coccyx
Ulna*
Radius*
Hip bone
Metacarpals
Carpus†
Phalanges
Pubic symphysis
Femur*
Patella (sesamoid bone)
Tibia*
Fibula*
†Tarsus
Metatarsals
Phalanges

A **Anterior view**

FIGURE I.6. Skeletal system.

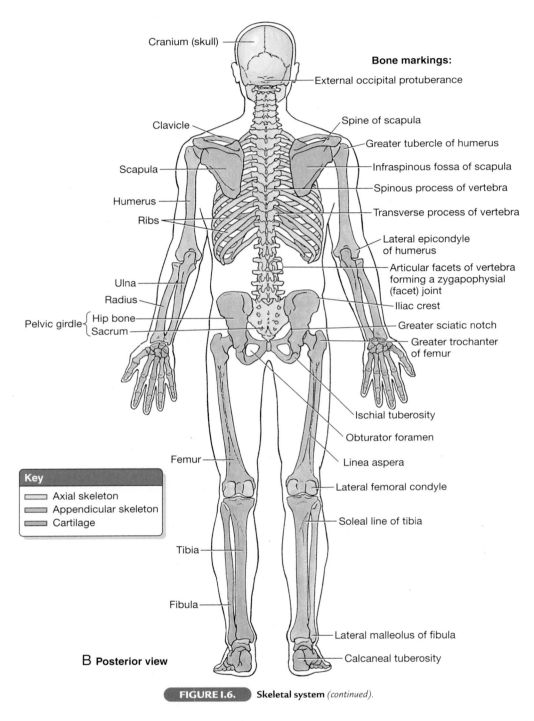

Bone markings:

Cranium (skull)
External occipital protuberance
Spine of scapula
Clavicle
Greater tubercle of humerus
Scapula
Infraspinous fossa of scapula
Humerus
Spinous process of vertebra
Ribs
Transverse process of vertebra
Lateral epicondyle of humerus
Articular facets of vertebra forming a zygapophysial (facet) joint
Ulna
Iliac crest
Radius
Greater sciatic notch
Pelvic girdle { Hip bone
Sacrum
Greater trochanter of femur
Ischial tuberosity
Obturator foramen
Femur
Linea aspera
Lateral femoral condyle
Soleal line of tibia
Tibia
Fibula
Lateral malleolus of fibula
B Posterior view
Calcaneal tuberosity

Key
Axial skeleton
Appendicular skeleton
Cartilage

FIGURE I.6.   Skeletal system *(continued).*

- Support for the body and its vital cavities.
- The mechanical basis for movement.
- Storage for salts (e.g., calcium).
- A continuous supply of new blood cells (produced by the marrow in the medullary cavity of many bones).

Cartilage is a resilient, semirigid, avascular type of connective tissue that forms parts of the skeleton where more flexibility is necessary (e.g., the costal cartilages that attach the ribs to the sternum). The articulating surfaces of bones participating in a synovial joint are capped with **articular cartilage,** which provides smooth, low-friction gliding surfaces for free movement of the articulating bones (e.g., blue areas of the humerus in Fig. I.6A). Cartilage is avascular and therefore its cells obtain oxygen and nutrients by diffusion. The proportion of bone and cartilage in the skeleton changes as the body grows; the younger a person is, the greater the contribution of cartilage. The bones of a newborn infant are soft and flexible because they are mostly composed of cartilage.

The fibrous connective tissue covering that surrounds bone is **periosteum** (Fig. I.9); that surrounding cartilage elements, excluding articular cartilage, is **perichondrium**. The periosteum and perichondrium help nourish the tissue, are capable of laying down more cartilage or bone (particularly during fracture healing), and provide an interface for attachment of tendons and ligaments.

Bones

There are two types of bone: **compact bone** and **spongy** (trabecular or cancellous) **bone**. The differences between these types of bone depend on the relative amount of solid matter and the number and size of the spaces they contain (Fig. I.7). All bones have a superficial thin layer of compact bone around a central mass of spongy bone, except where the latter is replaced by a **medullary (marrow) cavity**. Within this cavity of adult bones, and between the spicules of spongy bone, blood cells and platelets are formed. The architecture of spongy and compact bone varies according to function.

Compact bone provides strength for weight bearing. In long bones, designed for rigidity and attachment of muscles and ligaments, the amount of compact bone is greatest near

the middle of the shaft (body) of the bone, where it is liable to buckle. Living bones have some elasticity (flexibility) and great rigidity (hardness).

CLASSIFICATION OF BONES

Bones are classified according to their shape (Fig. I.6A):

- **Long bones** are tubular structures (e.g., humerus in the arm; phalanges in the fingers).
- **Short bones** are cuboidal and are found only in the ankle (tarsus) and wrist (carpus).
- **Flat bones** usually serve protective functions (e.g., those of the cranium protect the brain).
- **Irregular bones,** such as those in the face, have various shapes other than long, short, or flat.
- **Sesamoid bones** (e.g., patella, or kneecap) develop in certain tendons. These bones protect the tendons from excessive wear and often change the angle of the tendons as they pass to their attachments.

BONE MARKINGS

Bone markings appear wherever tendons, ligaments, and fascia are attached or where arteries lie adjacent to or enter bones. Other formations occur in relation to the passage of a tendon (often to direct the tendon or improve its leverage) or to control the type of movement occurring at a joint. *Some markings and features of bones are as follows* (Fig. I.6B):

- **Condyle:** rounded articular area (e.g., condyles of the femur).
- **Crest:** ridge of bone (e.g., iliac crest).
- **Epicondyle:** eminence superior to a condyle (e.g., epicondyles of the humerus).
- **Facet:** smooth flat area, usually covered with cartilage, where a bone articulates with another bone (e.g., articular facets of a vertebra).
- **Foramen:** passage through a bone (e.g., obturator foramen).
- **Fossa:** hollow or depressed area (e.g., infraspinous fossa of the scapula).
- **Line (linea):** linear elevation (e.g., soleal line of the tibia).

Trabeculae of spongy bone

Spongy bone

Compact bone

Medullary cavity

Shaft (body)

Compact bone

Compact bone
Spongy bone

FIGURE I.7. **Transverse sections of femur (thigh bone).** Observe the trabeculae (tension and pressure lines) related to the weight-bearing function of this bone.

Heterotopic Bones

Bones sometimes form in soft tissues where they are not normally present. Horse riders often develop heterotopic bones in their thighs or buttocks (*rider's bones*), probably because of chronic muscle strain resulting in small hemorrhagic (bloody) areas that undergo calcification and eventual ossification.

- **Malleolus:** rounded prominence (e.g., lateral malleolus of the fibula).
- **Notch:** indentation at the edge of a bone (e.g., greater sciatic notch in the posterior border of the hip bone).
- **Process:** projecting spine-like part (e.g., spinous process of a vertebra).
- **Protuberance:** projection of bone (e.g., external occipital protuberance of the cranium).
- **Spine:** thorn-like process (e.g., spine of the scapula).
- **Trochanter:** large blunt elevation (e.g., greater trochanter of the femur).
- **Tubercle:** small raised eminence (e.g., greater tubercle of the humerus).
- **Tuberosity:** large, rounded elevation (e.g., ischial tuberosity, calcaneal tuberosity).

Bone Dynamics

Bone Adaptation

 Bones are living organs that hurt when injured, bleed when fractured, remodel in relationship to stress placed on them, and change with age. Like other organs, bones have blood vessels, lymphatic vessels, and nerves, and they may become diseased. Unused bones, such as in a paralyzed or immobilized limb, *atrophy* (decrease in size). Bone may be absorbed, which occurs in the mandible after teeth are extracted. Bones *hypertrophy* (enlarge) when they have increased weight to support for a long period.

Bone Trauma and Repair

 Trauma to a bone may *fracture* (break) it. For a fracture to heal properly, the broken ends must be brought together, approximating their normal position (*reduction of fracture*). During bone healing, the surrounding *fibroblasts* (connective tissue cells) proliferate and secrete collagen that forms a *collar of callus* to hold the bones together. Remodeling of bone occurs in the fracture area, and the callus calcifies. Eventually, the callus is resorbed and replaced by bone.

Bone Degeneration—Osteoporosis

As people age, both the organic and inorganic components of bone decrease, often resulting in *osteoporosis,* a reduction in the quantity of bone, or atrophy of skeletal tissue. The bones become brittle, lose their elasticity, and fracture easily.

BONE DEVELOPMENT

All bones are derived from **mesenchyme** (embryonic connective tissue) by one of two different processes: intramembranous ossification (directly from mesenchyme) and endochondral ossification (from cartilage derived from mesenchyme). The histology of a bone is the same either way.

- In **intramembranous ossification** (membranous bone formation), mesenchymal models of bone form during the embryonic period, and direct ossification of the mesenchyme begins in the fetal period.
- In **endochondral ossification** (cartilaginous bone formation), cartilage models of bones form from mesenchyme during the fetal period, and bone subsequently replaces most of the cartilage.

The following brief description of endochondral ossification explains how long bones grow. The mesenchymal cells condense and differentiate into *chondroblasts*, dividing cells in growing cartilage tissue, thereby forming a *cartilaginous bone model* (Fig. I.8A). In the midregion of the bone model, the cartilage *calcifies* (becomes impregnated with calcium salts), and *periosteal capillaries* (capillaries from the fibrous sheath surrounding the model) grow into the calcified cartilage of the bone model and supply its interior. These blood vessels, together with associated *osteogenic* (bone-forming) cells, form a **periosteal bud.**

The capillaries initiate the **primary ossification center,** so named because the bone tissue it forms replaces most of the cartilage in the shaft of the bone model. The shaft of a bone ossified from a primary ossification center is the **diaphysis,** which grows as the bone develops.

Most **secondary ossification centers** appear in other parts of the developing bone after birth; the parts ossified from these centers are **epiphyses.** Epiphysial arteries grow into the developing cavities with associated osteogenic cells. The flared part of the diaphysis nearest to the epiphysis is the **metaphysis** (Fig. I.8C). For growth to continue, the bone formed from the primary center in the diaphysis does not fuse with that formed from the secondary centers in the epiphyses until the bone reaches its adult size. Thus, during growth of a long bone, cartilaginous **epiphysial plates** intervene between the diaphysis and the epiphyses. These growth plates are eventually replaced by bone at each of its two sides, diaphysial and epiphysial. When this occurs, bone growth ceases, and the diaphysis fuses with the epiphyses. The seam formed during this process (*synostosis*) is dense and appears in radiographs as an **epiphysial line** (Fig. I.9). The epiphysial fusion of bones occurs progressively from puberty to maturity.

VASCULATURE AND INNERVATION OF BONES

Bones are richly supplied with blood vessels (Fig. I.9). The arterial supply is from:

- **Nutrient arteries** (one or more per bone) that arise outside the periosteum, pass through the shaft of a long bone

A

B

Secondary (epiphysial) center of ossification

Epiphysial plate

Diaphysis

Nutrient artery

Epiphysial plate

Epiphysial artery

Secondary (epiphysial) center of ossification

Primary center of ossification

Periosteal bud

Cartilage model

Epiphysis

Epiphysial plate

Diaphysis

Metaphysis

Epiphysis

C

Metaphysis

Epiphysial plate

Epiphysis

Cancellous bone

Secondary center of ossificiation

Uncalcified cartilage

Articular cartilage

D

FIGURE I.8. **Development and growth of long bone. A.** Micrograph of primary center of ossification. **B.** Formation of primary and secondary centers of ossification. **C.** Growth in the length of the bone occurs on both sides of the epiphysial plates (*arrowheads*). **D.** Micrograph of secondary ossification center.

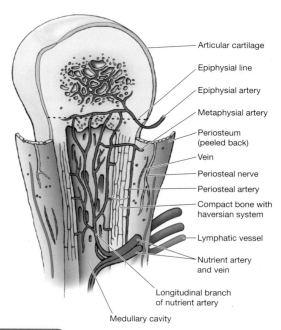

Articular cartilage

Epiphysial line

Epiphysial artery

Metaphysial artery

Periosteum (peeled back)

Vein

Periosteal nerve

Periosteal artery

Compact bone with haversian system

Lymphatic vessel

Nutrient artery and vein

Longitudinal branch of nutrient artery

Medullary cavity

FIGURE I.9. **Vasculature and innervation of long bone.** The bulk of compact bone is composed of haversian systems (osteons). The haversian canal in the system houses one or two small blood vessels for nourishing the osteocytes (bone cells).

via **nutrient foramina,** and split in the medullary cavity into longitudinal branches. These vessels supply the bone marrow, spongy bone, and deeper portions of the compact bone.

- Small branches from the **periosteal arteries** of the periosteum supply most of the compact bone. Consequently, if the periosteum is removed, the bone will die.
- **Metaphysial** and **epiphysial arteries** supply the ends of the bones. These vessels arise mainly from the arteries that supply the joints.

Veins accompany arteries through the *nutrient foramina.* Many large veins leave through foramina near the articular ends of the bones. **Lymphatic vessels** are abundant in the periosteum.

Nerves accompany the blood vessels supplying bones. The **periosteum** is richly supplied with sensory nerves—**periosteal nerves**—that carry pain fibers. The periosteum is especially sensitive to tearing or tension, which explains the acute pain from bone fractures. Bone itself is relatively sparsely supplied with sensory endings. Within bones, *vasomotor nerves* cause constriction or dilation of blood vessels, regulating blood flow through the bone marrow.

Accessory Bones

Accessory (supernumerary) bones develop when additional ossification centers appear and form extra bones. Many bones develop from several centers of ossification, and the separate parts normally fuse. Sometimes one of these centers fails to fuse with the main bone, giving the appearance of an extra bone; however, careful study shows that the apparent extra bone is a missing part of the main bone. Circumscribed areas of bone called *sutural* (*wormian*) *bones* are often seen along the sutures of the cranium where the flat bones come together. It is important to know that accessory bones are common in the foot to avoid mistaking them for bone fragments in medical images (e.g., radiographs).

Assessment of Bone Age

Knowledge of the sites where ossification centers occur, the times of their appearance, the rate at which they grow, and the times of fusion (*synostosis*) of the sites is used to determine the age of a person in clinical medicine, forensic science, and anthropology. The main criteria for determining bone age are (1) the appearance of calcified material in the diaphysis and/or epiphyses and (2) the disappearance of the dark line representing the epiphysial plate (absence of this line indicates epiphysial fusion has occurred; fusion occurs at specific times for each epiphysis). The fusion of epiphyses with the diaphysis occurs 1 to 2 years earlier in girls than in boys. Determination of bone age can be helpful in predicting adult height in early- or late-maturing adolescents and in establishing the approximate age of human skeletal remains in medicolegal cases.

Displacement and Separation of Epiphyses

An injury that causes a fracture in an adult usually causes the displacement of an epiphysis in a child. Without knowledge of bone growth and the appearance of bones in radiographic and other diagnostic images at various ages, a displaced epiphysial plate could be mistaken for a fracture, and separation of an epiphysis could be interpreted as a displaced piece of fractured bone. Bone is smoothly curved on each side of the epiphysial plate, while fractures leave sharp, often uneven edges of bone.

Avascular Necrosis

Loss of blood supply to an epiphysis or other parts of a bone results in death of bone tissue, or *avascular necrosis* (G. *nekrosis,* deadness). After every fracture, small areas of adjacent bone undergo necrosis. In some fractures, avascular necrosis of a large fragment of bone may occur.

Joints

A **joint** is an articulation, or the place of union or junction between two or more rigid components (bones, cartilages, or even parts of the same bone). Joints exhibit a variety of forms and functions. Some joints have no movement; others allow only slight movement, and some are freely movable, such as the glenohumeral (shoulder) joint.

CLASSIFICATION OF JOINTS

The three types of joints (fibrous, cartilaginous, and synovial) are classified according to the manner or type of material by which the articulating bones are united (Table I.2):

- The articulating bones of **fibrous joints** are united by fibrous tissue. The amount of movement occurring at a fibrous joint depends in most cases on the length of the fibers uniting the articular bones. A **syndesmosis** type of fibrous joint unites the bones with a sheet of fibrous tissue, either a ligament or fibrous membrane. Consequently, this type of joint is partially movable. A **gomphosis** (*dentoalveolar syndesmosis*) is a type of fibrous joint in which a peg-like fibrous process stabilizes a tooth and provides proprioceptive information (e.g., about how hard we are chewing or clenching our teeth).
- The articulating structures of **cartilaginous joints** are united by hyaline cartilage or fibrocartilage. *Primary cartilaginous joints (synchondroses)* are united by hyaline cartilage. These joints permit growth of the length of the bone and allow slight bending during early life, until the epiphysial plate converts to bone and the epiphyses fuse with the diaphysis. *Secondary cartilaginous joints (symphyses)* are strong, slightly mobile joints, united by fibrocartilage.
- The articular cavity of **synovial joints** is a potential space that contains a small amount of synovial fluid. Synovial fluid serves the dual function of nourishing the articular cartilage and lubricating the joint surfaces. The distinguishing features of a synovial joint are illustrated and described in Table I.2. Synovial joints, the most common type of joint, are usually reinforced by accessory ligaments that either are separate (extrinsic) or are a thickened part of the joint capsule (intrinsic). Some synovial

TABLE I.2 TYPES OF JOINTS

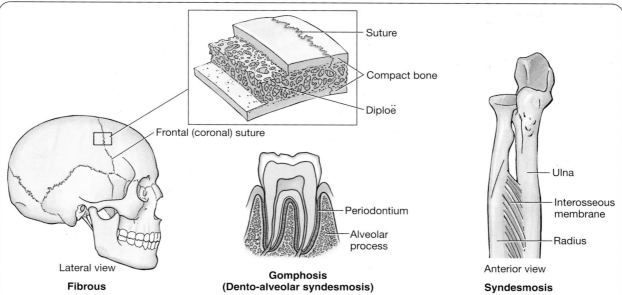

Lateral view
Fibrous

**Gomphosis
(Dento-alveolar syndesmosis)**

Anterior view
Syndesmosis

In **fibrous joints,** articulating bones are joined by fibrous tissue. Sutures of the cranium are fibrous joints in which bones are close together and united by fibrous tissue, often interlocking along a wavy line. Flat bones consist of two plates of compact bone separated by spongy bone and marrow (diploë). In a **syndesmosis joint,** the bones are joined by an interosseous ligament or a sheet of fibrous tissue (e.g., the interosseous membrane joining the forearm bones). In a **gomphosis joint,** a peg-like process fits into a socket (e.g., the articulation between the root of the tooth and the alveolar process). Fibrous tissue, the periodontium, anchors the tooth in the socket.

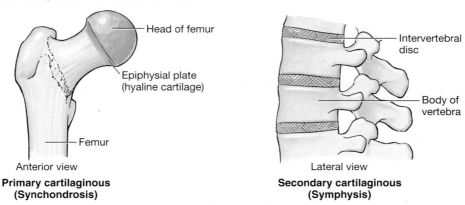

Anterior view
**Primary cartilaginous
(Synchondrosis)**

Lateral view
**Secondary cartilaginous
(Symphysis)**

In **cartilaginous joints,** articulating bones are united by fibrocartilage or hyaline cartilage. In a **synchondrosis,** such as that in a developing long bone, the bony epiphysis and body are joined by an epiphysial plate (hyaline cartilage). In a **symphysis,** the binding tissue is a fibrocartilaginous disc (e.g., between two vertebrae).

In a **synovial joint** (articulation), the two bones are separated by the characteristic joint cavity (containing synovial fluid) but are joined by an articular capsule (fibrous capsule lined with synovial membrane). The bearing surfaces of the bones are covered with articular cartilage. Synovial joints are functionally the most common and important type of joint. They provide free movement between the bones they join and are typical of nearly all joints of the limbs.

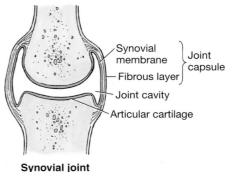

Synovial joint

TABLE I.3 TYPES OF SYNOVIAL JOINTS

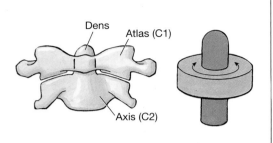

Hinge joints (uniaxial) permit flexion and extension only (e.g., the elbow joint).

Pivot joints (uniaxial) allow rotation. A round process of bone fits into a bony ligamentous socket (e.g., the atlantoaxial joint between the atlas [C1] and axis [C2]).

Saddle joints (biaxial) are shaped like a saddle—that is, they are concave and convex where the bones articulate (e.g., the joint between the first metacarpal and the trapezium).

Condylar (ellipsoid) joints (biaxial) permit a wider range of flexion and extension, and a narrower range of abduction and adduction, and circumduction (e.g., the metacarpophalangeal [knuckle] joints of fingers).

Plane joints permit gliding or sliding movements (e.g., the acromioclavicular joint).

Ball and socket joints (multiaxial) permit movement in several axes (e.g., flexion–extension, abduction–adduction, medial and lateral rotation, and circumduction). A rounded head fits into a concavity (e.g., the hip joint).

joints have other distinguishing features, such as fibrocartilaginous *articular discs* or *menisci,* which are present when the articulating surfaces of the bones are incongruous. The six major types of synovial joints are classified according to the shape of the articulating surfaces and/or the type of movement they permit (Table I.3).

VASCULATURE AND INNERVATION OF JOINTS

Joints receive blood from *articular arteries* that arise from vessels around the joint. The arteries often *anastomose* (communicate) to form networks (*periarticular arterial anastomoses*), which ensure a continuous blood supply to a joint throughout its range of movement. *Articular veins* are communicating veins that accompany the arteries (L. *venae comitantes*) and, like the arteries, are located in the joint capsule, mostly in the synovial membrane.

Joints have a rich nerve supply; the nerve endings are numerous in the joint capsule. In the distal parts of limbs, the *articular nerves* are branches of the cutaneous nerves supplying the overlying skin. Otherwise, most articular nerves are branches of nerves that supply the muscles that cross and therefore move the joint. Hilton's Law states that the nerves supplying a joint also supply the muscles moving the joint and the skin covering their attachments.

Pain fibers are numerous in the fibrous layer of the joint capsule and associated ligaments; the synovial membrane is relatively insensitive. Joints transmit a sensation called *proprioception,* information that provides an awareness of movement and position of the parts of the body.

Degenerative Joint Disease

Synovial joints are well designed to withstand wear, but heavy use over several years can cause degenerative changes. Beginning early in adult life and progressing slowly thereafter, aging of articular cartilage occurs on the ends of the articulating bones, particularly those of the hip, knee, vertebral column, and hands. These irreversible degenerative changes in joints result in the articular cartilage becoming less effective as a shock absorber and a lubricated surface. As a result, the articulation becomes vulnerable to the repeated friction that occurs during joint movements (e.g., during running). In some people these changes cause considerable pain. *Degenerative joint disease,* osteoarthritis (osteoarthrosis), is often accompanied by stiffness, discomfort, and pain. *Osteoarthritis* is common in older people and usually affects joints that support the weight of their bodies (e.g., hips and knees).

MUSCULAR SYSTEM

Muscle cells, often called *muscle fibers* because they are long and narrow when relaxed, are specialized contractile cells, organized into tissues that move body parts or temporarily alter the shape of internal organs. The associated connective tissue conveys nerve fibers and capillaries to the muscle fibers as it binds them into bundles or fascicles. Muscles also give form to the body and provide heat.

There are three types of muscle (Table I.4): (1) **skeletal muscle,** which moves bones and other structures (e.g., the eyes); (2) **cardiac striated muscle,** which forms most of the walls of the heart and adjacent parts of the great vessels; and (3) **smooth muscle,** which forms part of the walls of most vessels and hollow organs, moves substances through viscera such as the intestine, and controls movement through blood vessels.

Skeletal Muscles

All skeletal muscles have a fleshy contractile portion (one or more *heads* or *bellies*) composed of skeletal striated muscle and a white noncontractile portion composed mainly of collagen bundles: *tendons (rounded)* and *aponeuroses (flat sheets).*

When referring to the length of a muscle, both the belly and the tendons are included. Most skeletal muscles are attached directly or indirectly through tendons and aponeuroses to bones, cartilages, ligaments, or fascia or to some combination of these structures; however, some muscles are attached to organs (e.g., the eyeball), to skin (e.g., facial muscles), and to mucous membranes (intrinsic tongue muscles). Muscles are organs of movement but they also provide static support and give form to the body and provide heat. Figure I.10 identifies some of the superficial muscles; the deep muscles are identified when each region is studied.

Most muscles are named on the basis of their function or the bones to which they are attached. The abductor digiti minimi, for example, abducts the little finger. The sternocleidomastoid (L. *kleidos,* bolt) attaches inferiorly to the sternum and clavicle and superiorly to the mastoid process of the temporal bone of the cranium. Other muscles are named on the basis of their shape (G. *deltoid,* triangle), position (medial, lateral, anterior, or posterior), length (brevis, short; longus, long), size (maximus, minimus), or number of attachments (biceps, triceps). Muscles may be described according to their shape and architecture (Fig. I.11). For example:

- **Pennate muscles** are feather-like in the arrangement of their fascicles (fiber bundles): unipennate, bipennate, or multipennate (L. *pennatus,* feather).
- **Fusiform muscles** are spindle-shaped (round, thick belly, and tapered ends).

TABLE I.4 TYPES OF MUSCLE

Skeletal ("striated" or "voluntary") muscle

Striation
Muscle fiber
Nucleus

Location	Appearance	Type of Activity	Stimulation
Composes gross named muscles (e.g., the biceps of the arm) attached to the skeleton and/or fascia of limbs, body wall, and head/neck	Large, long, unbranched, cylindrical fibers with transverse striations (stripes) arranged in parallel bundles; multiple, peripherally located nuclei	Strong, quick intermittent (phasic) contraction above a baseline tonus; acts primarily to produce movement or resist gravity	Voluntary (or reflexive) by the somatic nervous system (SNS, p.34)

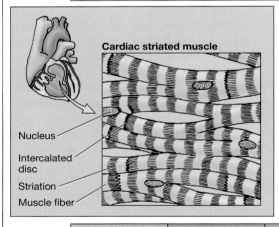

Cardiac striated muscle

Nucleus
Intercalated disc
Striation
Muscle fiber

Location	Appearance	Type of Activity	Stimulation
Muscle of heart (myocardium) and adjacent portions of the great vessels (aorta, vena cava)	Branching and anastomosing shorter fibers with transverse striations (stripes) running parallel and connected end-to-end by complex junctions (intercalated discs); single, central nucleus	Strong, quick, continuous rhythmic contraction; acts to pump blood from heart	Involuntary; intrinsically (myogenically) stimulated and propagated; rate and strength of contraction modified by autonomic nervous system (ANS, p. 36)

TABLE I.4 TYPES OF MUSCLE *(continued)*

Location	Appearance	Type of Activity	Stimulation
Walls of hollow viscera and blood vessels, iris, and ciliary body of eye; attached to hair follicles of skin (arrector muscle of hair)	Single or agglomerated small, spindle-shaped fibers without striations; single, central nucleus	Weak, slow, rhythmic, or sustained tonic contraction; acts mainly to propel substances (peristalsis) and to restrict flow (vasoconstriction and sphincteric activity)	Involuntary by autonomic nervous system (ANS)

- In **parallel muscles**, the fascicles lie parallel to the long axis of the muscle; flat muscles with parallel fibers often have aponeuroses.
- **Convergent muscles** have a broad attachment from which the fascicles converge to a single tendon.
- **Circular muscles** surround a body opening or orifice, constricting it when contracted.
- **Digastric muscles** feature two bellies in series, sharing a common intermediate tendon.

CONTRACTION OF MUSCLES

When muscles contract, the fibers shorten to about 70% of their resting length. Muscles with a long parallel fascicle arrangement shorten the most, providing considerable range of movement at a joint, but are not powerful. Muscle power increases as the total number of muscle cells increases. Therefore, the shorter, wide pennate muscles that "pack in" the most fiber bundles shorten less, but are most powerful.

When a muscle contracts and shortens, one of its attachments usually remains fixed and the other one moves. Attachments of muscles are commonly described as the origin and insertion; the *origin* is usually the proximal end of the muscle, which remains fixed during muscular contraction, and the *insertion* is usually the distal end of the muscle, which is movable. However, some muscles can act in both directions under different circumstances. Therefore, the terms *proximal* and *distal* or *medial* and *lateral* are used in this book when describing most muscle attachments.

Skeletal muscle can undergo contraction in three ways:

1. **Reflexive contraction** is automatic and not voluntarily controlled—for example, respiratory movements of the diaphragm. Muscle stretch is produced by tapping a tendon with a reflex hammer.
2. **Tonic contraction** is a slight contraction (**muscle tone**) that does not produce movement or active resistance but gives the muscle firmness, assisting the stability of joints and the maintenance of posture.
3. There are two principal types of **phasic contraction**. In **isometric contractions,** the muscle length remains the same—no movement occurs but muscle tension is increased above tonic levels (e.g., the deltoid holds the arm in abduction). In **isotonic contractions,** the muscle changes length to produce movement. There are two forms of isotonic contraction: **concentric contraction,** in which movement occurs owing to muscle shortening (e.g., the deltoid muscle shortens to raise the arm into abduction), and **eccentric contraction,** in which the contracting muscle lengthens (e.g., the deltoid lengthens to lower arm in adduction).

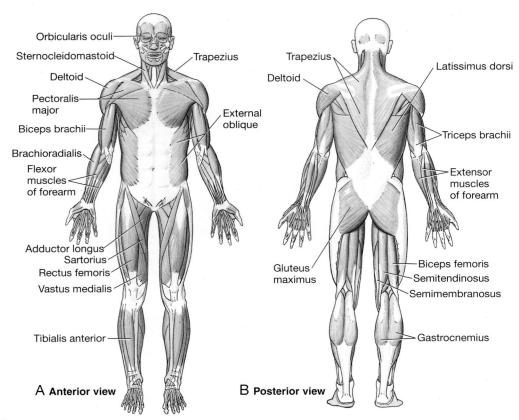

Orbicularis oculi
Sternocleidomastoid
Deltoid
Pectoralis major
Biceps brachii
Brachioradialis
Flexor muscles of forearm
Trapezius
External oblique
Adductor longus
Sartorius
Rectus femoris
Vastus medialis
Tibialis anterior

A Anterior view

Trapezius
Deltoid
Latissimus dorsi
Triceps brachii
Extensor muscles of forearm
Gluteus maximus
Biceps femoris
Semitendinosus
Semimembranosus
Gastrocnemius

B Posterior view

FIGURE I.10.   **Skeletal muscles.** Some larger muscles are labeled.

The *structural unit* of a muscle is a **muscle fiber** (Fig. I.12). Connective tissue covering individual muscle fibers is called **endomysium,** a group of fibers (fiber bundles) is invested by **perimysium,** and the entire muscle is surrounded by **epimysium.** The *functional unit* of a muscle, consisting of a motor neuron and the muscle fibers it controls, is a **motor unit.** When a motor neuron in the spinal cord is stimulated, it initiates an impulse that causes all the muscle fibers supplied by that motor unit to contract simultaneously. The number of muscle fibers in a motor unit varies from one to several hundred, according to the size and function of the muscle. Large motor units, in which one neuron supplies several hundred muscle fibers, are found in the large trunk and thigh muscles. In the small eye and hand muscles, where precision movements are required, the motor units contain only a few muscle fibers.

Muscles serve specific functions in moving and positioning the body. The same muscle may act as a prime mover, antagonist, synergist, or fixator under specific conditions. The functions include:

- A **prime mover** or **agonist** is the main muscle responsible for producing a specific movement of the body (e.g., concentric contraction).
- **Fixators** steady the proximal parts of a limb while movements are occurring in distal parts.

- A **synergist** complements the action of prime movers—for example, by preventing movement of the intervening joint when a prime mover passes over more than one joint.
- An **antagonist** is a muscle that opposes the action of a prime mover. As a prime mover contracts, the antagonist progressively relaxes, producing a smooth movement.

Cardiac Striated Muscle

Cardiac striated muscle forms the muscular wall of the heart—the **myocardium** (Table I.4). Some cardiac muscle is also present in the walls of the aorta, pulmonary vein, and superior vena cava (Fig. I.13). Cardiac muscle contractions are not under voluntary control. Heart rate is regulated intrinsically by a *pacemaker,* composed of special cardiac muscle fibers that are influenced by the autonomic nervous system (discussed later in this chapter).

Smooth Muscle

Smooth muscle, named for the absence of microscopic striations, forms a large part of the middle coat or layer (tunica media) of the walls of most blood vessels and the muscular part of the wall of the digestive tract and ducts (Fig. I.14A; Table I.4). Smooth muscle is also found in skin (*arrector*

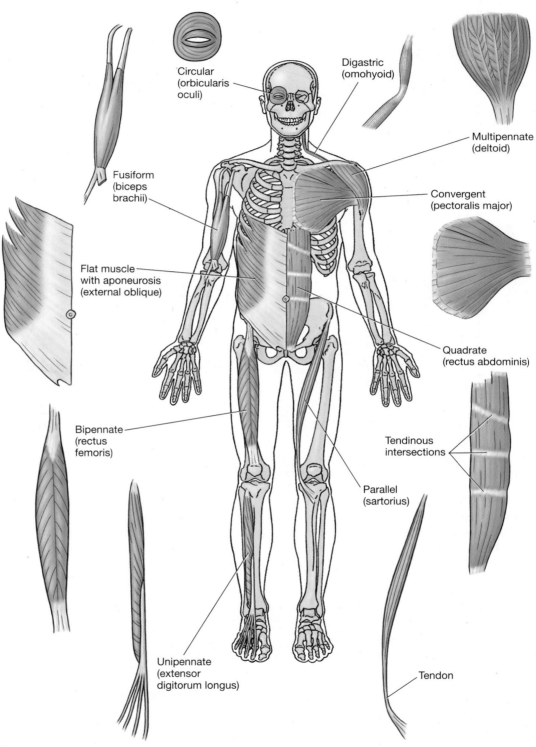

FIGURE I.11. **Architecture and shape of skeletal muscles.** Various types of muscles are shown whose shapes depend on the arrangement of fibers.

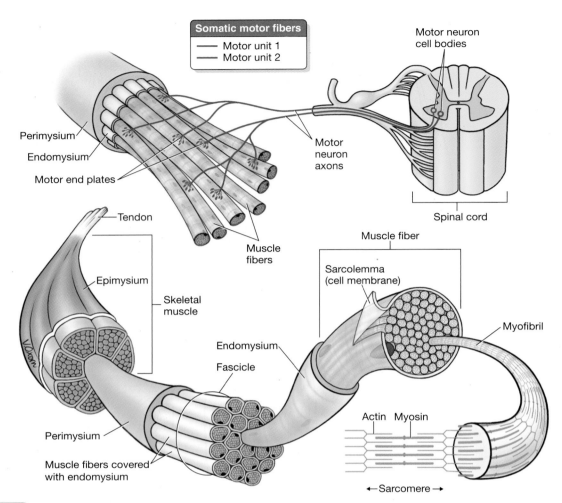

Somatic motor fibers
— Motor unit 1
— Motor unit 2

Motor neuron cell bodies

Perimysium

Endomysium

Motor end plates

Motor neuron axons

Spinal cord

Tendon

Muscle fibers

Muscle fiber

Epimysium

Skeletal muscle

Sarcolemma (cell membrane)

Endomysium

Myofibril

Fascicle

Actin   Myosin

Perimysium

Muscle fibers covered with endomysium

← Sarcomere →

FIGURE I.12. **Structure of skeletal muscle and motor unit.** A motor unit consists of a single motor neuron and all the muscle fibers innervated by it. Actin (thin) and myosin (thick) filaments are contractile elements in the muscle fibers.

muscles associated with hair follicles [Fig. I.5]) and in the eyeball (to controls lens thickness and pupil size). Like cardiac muscle, smooth muscle is innervated by the autonomic nervous system (Table I.4); hence it is an *involuntary muscle* that can undergo partial contraction for long periods. This is important in regulating the size of the lumen of tubular structures; in the walls of the digestive tract, uterine tubes, and ureters, the smooth muscle cells undergo rhythmic contractions (peristaltic waves). This process (**peristalsis**) propels the contents along these tubular structures.

Muscle Testing

Muscle testing helps an examiner diagnose nerve injuries. This technique enables the examiner to gauge the power of the person's movement. Usually muscles are tested in bilateral pairs for comparison. There are two common testing methods:

1. The person performs movements that resist those produced by the examiner (active). When testing flexion of the forearm, the examiner asks the person to flex his or her forearm while the examiner resists the effort.

2. The examiner performs movements against resistance produced by the person. For example, the person keeps the forearm flexed while the examiner attempts to extend it.

Electromyography

The electrical stimulation of muscles through electromyography (EMG) is another method for testing muscle action. The examiner places surface electrodes over a muscle and asks the person to perform certain movements. The examiner then amplifies and records the differences in electrical action potentials of the muscles. A normal resting muscle shows only a baseline activity (tonus), which disappears only during sleep, during paralysis, and when under anesthesia. Contracting muscles demonstrate variable peaks of phasic activity. EMG makes it possible to analyze the activity of an individual muscle during different movements. EMG may also be part of the treatment program for restoring the action of muscles.

Muscular Atrophy

 Wasting of the muscular tissue (atrophy) of a limb, for example, may result from a primary disorder of the muscle or from a lesion of a motor unit. Muscle atrophy may also be caused by immobilization of a limb, such as with a cast.

Hypertrophy

 In *compensatory hypertrophy,* the myocardium responds to increasing demands by increasing the size of its fibers (cells). When cardiac muscle fibers are damaged during a heart attack, the tissue becomes necrotic (dies) and fibrous scar tissue that develops forms a *myocardial infarct* (MI), an area of *myocardial necrosis* (death of myocardial tissue). Smooth muscle cells also undergo compensatory hypertrophy in response to increased demands. During pregnancy, the smooth muscle cells in the wall of the uterus increase not only in size (*hypertrophy*) but also in number (*hyperplasia*).

CARDIOVASCULAR SYSTEM

The **circulatory system** transports fluids throughout the body; it consists of the cardiovascular and lymphatic systems. The heart and blood vessels form the blood transportation network, the **cardiovascular system** (Fig. I.13). The heart pumps blood through the body's vast system of vessels. The blood carries nutrients, oxygen, and waste products to and from cells.

The *heart* consists of two muscular pumps that, although adjacently located, act in a series, dividing the cardiovascular system into two circulations. In the *pulmonary circulation,* the right heart propels low-oxygen blood returned to it into the lungs, where carbon dioxide is exchanged for oxygen. In the *systemic circulation,* oxygen-rich blood returned to the left heart is pumped to the remainder of the body, exchanging oxygen and nutrients for carbon dioxide.

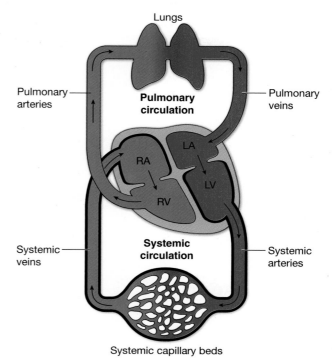

Chambers of heart:
RA = right atrium   LA = left atrium
RV = right ventricle   LV = left ventricle

FIGURE I.13. **Schema of cardiovascular system.** The continuous circuit consists of two loops: the pulmonary and systemic circulations, served by separate halves of the heart.

There are three types of blood vessels: **arteries, veins,** and **capillaries** (Fig. I.14). Blood under high pressure leaves the heart and is distributed to the body by a branching system of thick-walled arteries. The final distributing vessels, **arterioles,** deliver oxygenated blood to capillaries. **Capillaries** form a capillary bed, where the interchange of oxygen, nutrients, waste products, and other substances with the extracellular fluid occurs (Fig. I.14*E*). Blood from the capillary bed passes into thin-walled venules, which resemble wide capillaries. **Venules** drain into small veins that open into larger veins. The largest veins, the superior vena cava (SVC) and inferior vena cava (IVC), return poorly oxygenated blood to the heart.

Most vessels of the circulatory system have three tunics or coats: **tunica intima,** the thin endothelial lining of vessels; **tunica media,** the middle smooth muscle layer; and **tunica adventitia,** the outer connective tissue coat.

Arteries

Arteries carry blood away from the heart and distribute it to the body (Fig. I.15*A*). Blood passes from the heart through arteries of ever-decreasing caliber. The different types of arteries are distinguished from each other on the basis of overall size, relative amounts of elastic tissue or muscle in

FIGURE I.14. **Structures of arteries and veins.** The following structures are shown: **A,** an elastic artery, the aorta (low power); **B,** the inferior vena cava (low power); **C,** a muscular artery and vein (low power); and **D,** an arteriole and venule (high power). **E.** The structure of blood vessels is shown.

the tunica media, and the thickness of the wall relative to the lumen (Fig. I.14). Artery size and type is a continuum—that is, there is a gradual change in morphological characteristics from one type to another. There are three types of arteries:

- **Large elastic arteries** (conducting arteries) have many elastic layers in their walls; examples are the aorta and its branches from the arch of the aorta (Fig. I.14*A*). The maintenance of blood pressure in the arterial system between contractions of the heart results from the elasticity of these arteries. This quality allows them to expand when the heart contracts and to return to normal between cardiac contractions.
- **Medium muscular arteries** (distributing arteries) have walls that consist mainly of smooth muscle, circularly arranged; one example is the femoral artery (Fig. I.14*C*). The ability of these arteries to decrease their diameter (vasoconstrict) regulates the flow of blood to different parts of the body as required.

- **Small arteries and arterioles** have relatively narrow lumina and thick muscular walls (Fig. I.14*D*). The degree of arterial pressure within the vascular system is mainly regulated by the degree of tonus (firmness) in the smooth muscle of the arteriolar walls. If the tonus of muscle in the anterior wall is above normal, *hypertension* (high blood pressure) results.

Veins

Veins return poorly oxygenated blood to the heart from the capillary beds. The large pulmonary veins are atypical in that they carry well-oxygenated blood from the lungs to the heart (Fig. I.15*A*). Because of the lower blood pressure in the venous system, the walls of veins are thinner than those of their companion arteries (Fig. I.14). The smallest veins, **venules,** unite to form larger veins that usually form *venous plexuses*, such as the **dorsal venous arch** of the foot (Fig. I.15*B*). *Medium veins* in the limbs and other locations where

Anastomoses, Collateral Circulation, and Terminal (End) Arteries

Anastomoses (communications) between the multiple branches of an artery provide numerous potential detours for blood flow in case the usual pathway is obstructed by compression, the position of a joint, pathology, or surgical ligation. If a main channel is occluded, the smaller alternate channels can usually increase in size, providing a *collateral circulation* that ensures the blood supply to structures distal to the blockage. However, collateral pathways require time to develop; they are usually insufficient to compensate for sudden occlusion or ligation. There are areas where collateral circulation does not exist or is inadequate to replace the main vessel. Arteries that do not anastomose with adjacent arteries are true *terminal (end) arteries*. Occlusion of a terminal artery disrupts the blood supply to the structure or segment of an organ it supplies. For example, occlusion of the terminal arteries of the retina will result in blindness. Although not true terminal arteries, *functional terminal arteries* (arteries with ineffectual anastomoses) supply segments of the brain, liver, kidney, spleen, and intestines.

Arteriosclerosis: Ischemia and Infarction

The most common acquired disease of arteries is *arteriosclerosis* (hardening of arteries), a group of diseases characterized by thickening

and loss of elasticity of arterial walls. *Atherosclerosis,* a common form of arteriosclerosis, is associated with the buildup of fat (mainly cholesterol) in the arterial walls. Calcium deposits then form an *atheromatous plaque,* resulting in arterial narrowing and irregularity. This may result in thrombosis (local clotting), which may occlude the artery or be flushed into the bloodstream, resulting in ischemia (reduction of blood supply to an organ or region) and infarction (local death of an organ or tissue). Among the consequences of a thrombus are myocardial infarction (heart attack), stroke, and gangrene (necrosis in parts of the limbs) (Fig. BI.1).

Atheromatous plaque

Thrombus

FIGURE BI.1

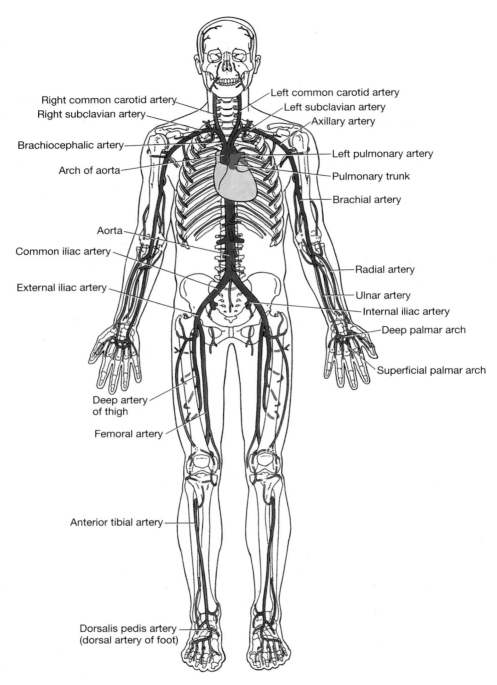

Right common carotid artery
Right subclavian artery
Brachiocephalic artery
Arch of aorta
Aorta
Common iliac artery
External iliac artery
Deep artery of thigh
Femoral artery
Anterior tibial artery
Dorsalis pedis artery (dorsal artery of foot)

Left common carotid artery
Left subclavian artery
Axillary artery
Left pulmonary artery
Pulmonary trunk
Brachial artery
Radial artery
Ulnar artery
Internal iliac artery
Deep palmar arch
Superficial palmar arch

A Anterior view

FIGURE I.15.   **Cardiovascular system. A.** Principal arteries.

the flow of blood is opposed by the pull of gravity have **valves** that permit blood to flow toward the heart but not in the reverse direction (Figs. I.14 and I.16A). **Large veins,** such as the SVC and IVC, are characterized by wide bundles of longitudinal smooth muscle and a well-developed tunica adventitia (Fig. I.14B). Systemic veins are more variable than the arteries and more frequently form anastomoses.

Although often depicted as single vessels, veins tend to be double or multiple. The veins that accompany deep arteries (accompanying veins) surround them in a branching network (Fig. I.16B) and occupy a relatively unyielding *vascular sheath* with the artery they accompany. As a result, they are stretched and flattened as the artery expands during contraction of the heart, which assists in driving the venous

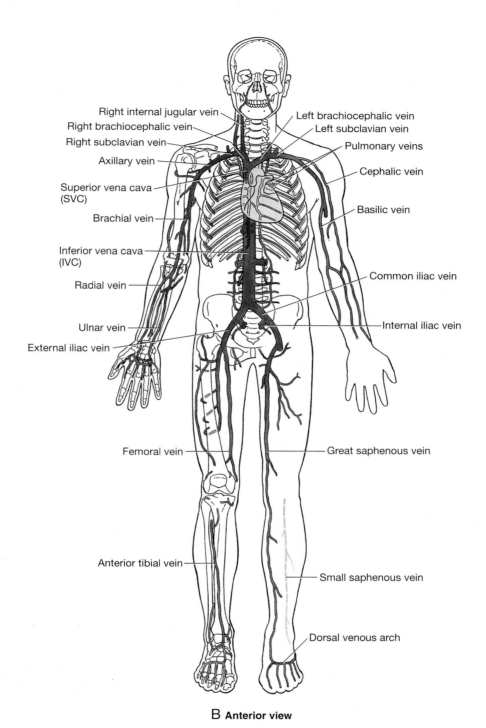

Right internal jugular vein

Right brachiocephalic vein

Right subclavian vein

Axillary vein

Superior vena cava
(SVC)

Brachial vein

Inferior vena cava
(IVC)

Radial vein

Ulnar vein

External iliac vein

Left brachiocephalic vein

Left subclavian vein

Pulmonary veins

Cephalic vein

Basilic vein

Common iliac vein

Internal iliac vein

Femoral vein

Great saphenous vein

Anterior tibial vein

Small saphenous vein

Dorsal venous arch

B Anterior view

FIGURE I.15. **Cardiovascular system** (*continued*). **B.** Principal veins. Superficial veins are shown in the left limbs; deep veins are shown in the right limbs. Most arteries carry oxygenated blood away from the heart, and most veins carry deoxygenated blood to the heart; however, the pulmonary arteries arising from the pulmonary trunk carry deoxygenated blood (*blue*) to the lungs, and the pulmonary veins carry oxygenated blood (*red*) from the lungs to the heart.

blood toward the heart. The outward expansion of the bellies of contracting skeletal muscles in the legs, for example, compresses the veins, "milking" the blood superiorly toward the heart; this is known as the *musculovenous pump* (Fig. I.16A).

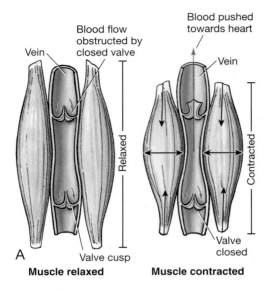

Blood flow obstructed by closed valve

Blood pushed towards heart

Vein

Vein

Relaxed

Contracted

A

Valve cusp

Valve closed

Muscle relaxed　　**Muscle contracted**

Accompanying veins (L. *venae comitantes*)

B

Artery

Vascular sheath

FIGURE I.16. **Veins. A.** The musculovenous pump. *Arrows* indicate the direction of blood flow. **B.** Accompanying veins are shown.

Capillaries

Capillaries are simple endothelial tubes connecting the arterial and venous sides of the circulation. They are generally arranged in networks (**capillary beds**) between the arterioles and venules (Fig. I.14E). The blood flowing through the capillaries is brought to them by arterioles and carried away from them by venules. As the hydrostatic pressure in the arterioles forces blood through the capillary bed, oxygen, nutrients, and other cellular materials are exchanged with the surrounding tissue. In some regions, such as in the fingers, there are direct connections between the small arteries and veins proximal to the capillary beds they supply and drain. The sites of such communications—**arteriovenous anastomoses (AV shunts)**—permit blood to pass directly from the arterial to the venous side of the circulation without passing through capillaries. AV shunts are numerous in the skin, where they have an important role in conserving body heat.

LYMPHOID SYSTEM

The lymphatic system provides for the drainage of surplus tissue fluid and leaked plasma proteins to the bloodstream and for the removal of cellular debris and infection (Fig. I.17). This system collects surplus extracellular tissue fluid as **lymph.** Lymph is usually clear and watery and is similar in composition to blood plasma. The lymphoid system consists of:

- **Lymphatic plexuses,** networks of small lymphatic vessels, **lymphatic capillaries,** that originate in the extracellular spaces of most tissues.
- **Lymphatic vessels (lymphatics),** a nearly bodywide network of thin-walled vessels with abundant *valves,*

Varicose Veins

When the walls of veins lose their elasticity, they become weak and dilate under the pressure of supporting a column of blood against gravity. This results in *varicose veins*, abnormally swollen, twisted veins, most often seen in the legs (Fig BI.2).

Varicose veins have a caliber greater than normal and their valve cusps do not meet or have been destroyed by inflammation. These veins have *incompetent valves;* thus the column of blood ascending toward the heart is unbroken, placing increased pressure on the weakened walls of the veins and exacerbating their varicosities.

Varicose veins

FIGURE BI.2

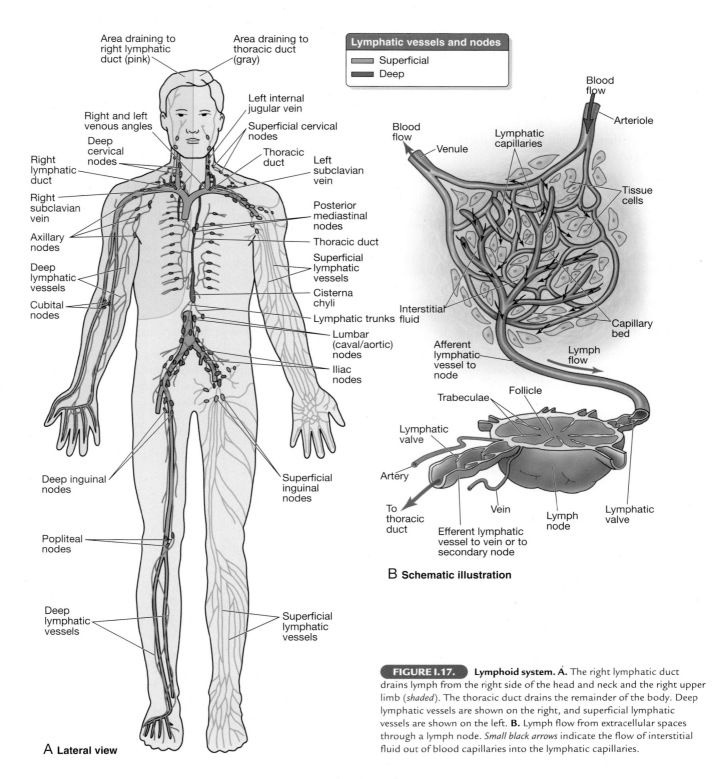

Lymphatic vessels and nodes
- Superficial
- Deep

Area draining to right lymphatic duct (pink)

Area draining to thoracic duct (gray)

Left internal jugular vein

Right and left venous angles

Superficial cervical nodes

Deep cervical nodes

Thoracic duct

Right lymphatic duct

Left subclavian vein

Right subclavian vein

Posterior mediastinal nodes

Axillary nodes

Thoracic duct

Deep lymphatic vessels

Superficial lymphatic vessels

Cubital nodes

Cisterna chyli

Lymphatic trunks

Lumbar (caval/aortic) nodes

Iliac nodes

Deep inguinal nodes

Superficial inguinal nodes

Popliteal nodes

Deep lymphatic vessels

Superficial lymphatic vessels

A **Lateral view**

Blood flow

Arteriole

Blood flow

Venule

Lymphatic capillaries

Tissue cells

Interstitial fluid

Capillary bed

Afferent lymphatic vessel to node

Lymph flow

Follicle

Trabeculae

Lymphatic valve

Artery

Vein

To thoracic duct

Efferent lymphatic vessel to vein or to secondary node

Lymph node

Lymphatic valve

B **Schematic illustration**

FIGURE I.17. **Lymphoid system. A.** The right lymphatic duct drains lymph from the right side of the head and neck and the right upper limb (*shaded*). The thoracic duct drains the remainder of the body. Deep lymphatic vessels are shown on the right, and superficial lymphatic vessels are shown on the left. **B.** Lymph flow from extracellular spaces through a lymph node. *Small black arrows* indicate the flow of interstitial fluid out of blood capillaries into the lymphatic capillaries.

originating from lymphatic plexuses along which lymph nodes are located. Lymphatic vessels occur almost everywhere blood capillaries are found, except, for example, teeth, bone, bone marrow, and the entire central nervous system (excess fluid here drains into the cerebrospinal fluid).

- **Lymph nodes,** small masses of lymphatic tissue through which lymph is filtered on its way to the venous system.
- **Lymphocytes,** circulating cells of the immune system that react against foreign materials.

- **Lymphoid organs**, sites that produce lymphocytes, such as that found in the walls of the digestive tract; in the **spleen, thymus,** and lymph nodes; and in **myeloid tissue** in red bone marrow.

After traversing one or more lymph nodes, lymph enters larger lymphatic vessels, called lymphatic trunks, which unite to form either the right lymphatic duct or the thoracic duct (Fig. I.17A).

- The **right lymphatic duct** drains lymph from the body's right upper quadrant (right side of head, neck, and thorax and the entire right upper limb). The duct ends in the right subclavian vein at its angle of junction with the right internal jugular vein, called the **right venous angle**.
- The **thoracic duct** drains lymph from the remainder of the body. This duct begins in the abdomen as a sac, the **cisterna chyli**, and ascends through the thorax and enters the junction of the left internal jugular and left subclavian veins, called the **left venous angle**.

Superficial lymphatic vessels in the skin and subcutaneous tissue eventually drain into *deep lymphatic vessels* in the deep fascia between the muscles and the subcutaneous tissue; the deep vessels accompany the major blood vessels.

Lymphangitis, Lymphadenitis, and Lymphedema

The terms *lymphangitis* and *lymphadenitis* refer to the secondary inflammation of lymphatic vessels and lymph nodes, respectively. These pathological processes may occur when the lymphatic system is involved in the *metastasis* (spread) of cancer—the lymphogenous dissemination of cancer cells. *Lymphedema* (the accumulation of interstitial fluid) occurs when lymph is not drained from an area of the body. For instance, if *cancerous lymph nodes* are surgically removed from the axilla (armpit), lymphedema of the upper limb may result.

Additional functions of the lymphatic system include:

- *Absorption and transport of dietary fat,* in which special lymphatic capillaries (lacteals) receive all absorbed fat (chyle) from the intestine and convey it through the thoracic duct to the venous system.

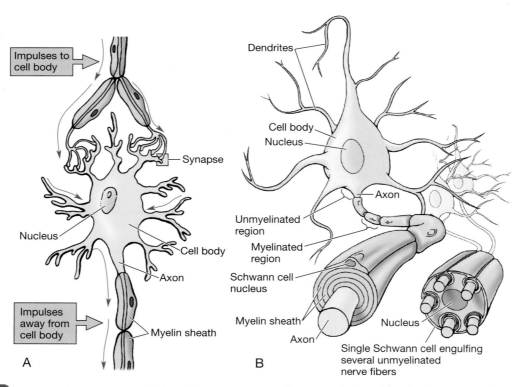

FIGURE I.18.   **Structure of a motor neuron. A.** Parts of a motor neuron are demonstrated. **B.** Myelinated and unmyelinated nerves are shown.

- *Formation of a defense mechanism for the body.* When foreign protein drains from an infected area, antibodies specific to the protein are produced by immunologically competent cells and/or lymphocytes and dispatched to the infected area.

NERVOUS SYSTEM

The nervous system enables the body to react to continuous changes in its external and internal environments. It controls and integrates various activities of the body, such as circulation and respiration. For descriptive purposes, the human nervous system is divided as follows:

- Structurally into the *central nervous system* (CNS), made up of the brain and spinal cord, and the *peripheral nervous system* (PNS), consisting of nerve fibers and cell bodies outside the CNS that conduct impulses to or away from the CNS.
- Functionally into the *somatic nervous system* (SNS), the voluntary nervous system, which carries sensation (e.g., pain) from the skin and joints (e.g., position sense) and supplies skeletal muscle, and the *autonomic nervous system* (ANS), the involuntary/visceral nervous system, which supplies smooth muscle (e.g., in the wall of blood vessels), glands (e.g., sweat glands), and viscera (internal organs) in the body cavities (e.g., heart, stomach, and bladder).

Nervous tissue consists of two main cell types: neurons (nerve cells) and neuroglia (glial cells).

- **Neurons** are the structural and functional units of the nervous system specialized for rapid communication (Fig. I.18). A neuron is composed of a **cell body** with processes (extensions) called **dendrites** and an **axon,** which carry impulses to and away from the cell body, respectively. **Myelin,** layers of lipid and protein substances, forms a **myelin sheath** around some axons, greatly increasing the velocity of impulse conduction. Neurons communicate with each other at **synapses,** points of contact between neurons. The communication occurs by means of *neurotransmitters,* chemical agents released or secreted by one neuron, which may excite or inhibit another neuron, continuing or terminating the relay of impulses or the response to them.
- **Neuroglia** (glial cells or glia) are approximately five times as abundant as neurons, are nonneuronal, nonexcitable cells that form a major component (scaffolding) of nervous tissue. Neuroglia support, insulate, and nourish the neurons.

Central Nervous System

The **central nervous system** (CNS) consists of the **brain** and **spinal cord** (Fig. I.19). The principal roles of the CNS are to integrate and coordinate incoming and outgoing neural signals and to carry out higher mental functions, such as thinking and learning.

A collection of nerve cell bodies in the CNS is a **nucleus** (Fig. I.19*B*). A bundle of nerve fibers (axons) connecting neighboring or distant nuclei of the CNS is a **tract.** The nerve cell bodies lie within and constitute the **gray matter;** the interconnecting fiber tract systems form the **white matter** (Fig. I.20). In transverse sections of the spinal cord, the gray matter appears roughly as an H-shaped area embedded in a matrix of white matter. The struts (supports) of the H are **horns;** therefore, there are right and left **posterior (dorsal)** and **anterior (ventral) gray horns.**

Three membranous layers—pia mater, arachnoid mater, and dura mater—collectively constitute the **meninges** (Fig. I.20). The meninges and the **cerebrospinal fluid** (CSF) surround and protect the CNS. The brain and spinal cord are intimately covered on their outer surface by the innermost meningeal layer, a delicate, transparent covering, the **pia mater** (pia). The CSF is located between the pia and the **arachnoid mater** (arachnoid) in the subarachnoid space. External to the pia and arachnoid is the thick, tough **dura mater** (dura), which is intimately related to the internal aspect of the bone of the surrounding neurocranium (braincase). The dura of the spinal cord is separated from the vertebral column by a fat-filled space, the *epidural space.*

Damage to CNS

When the CNS is damaged, the injured axons do not recover in most circumstances. Their proximal stumps begin to regenerate, sending sprouts into the area of the lesion; however, growth is blocked by astrocyte (a type of glial cell) proliferation at the site of injury. As a result, permanent disability follows destruction of a tract in the CNS.

Peripheral Nervous System

The **peripheral nervous system** (PNS) consists of *nerve fibers* and *nerve cell bodies* that connect the CNS with peripheral structures (Fig. I.19). **Peripheral nerves** consist of bundles of nerve fibers, their connective tissue coverings, and blood vessels (vasa nervorum). A *nerve fiber* consists of an **axon,** the single process of a neuron; its **neurolemma,** the cell membranes of Schwann cells that immediately surround the axon, separating it from other axons; and its **endoneurium,** a connective tissue sheath.

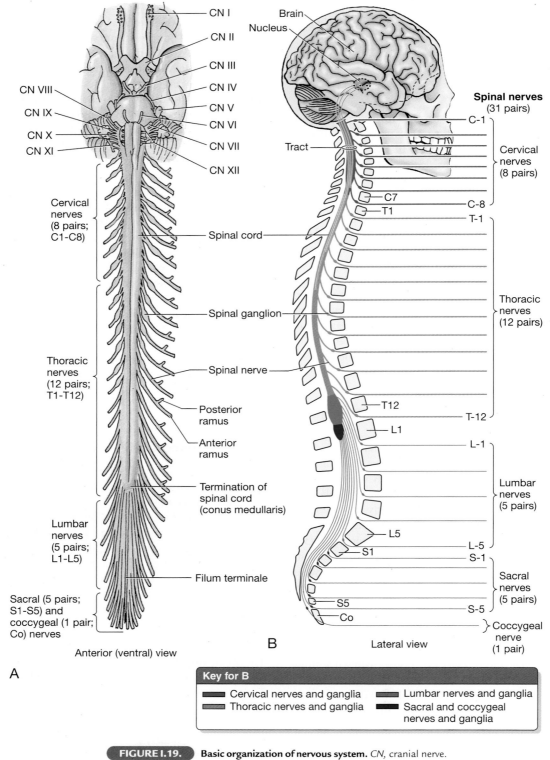

CN I
CN II
CN III
CN IV
CN V
CN VI
CN VII
CN XII

CN VIII
CN IX
CN X
CN XI

Brain
Nucleus

Tract

Spinal nerves
(31 pairs)

C-1

Cervical
nerves
(8 pairs)

C7
T1

C-8

T-1

Cervical
nerves
(8 pairs;
C1-C8)

Spinal cord

Thoracic
nerves
(12 pairs)

Spinal ganglion

Thoracic
nerves
(12 pairs;
T1-T12)

Spinal nerve

Posterior
ramus

Anterior
ramus

T12

T-12

L1

L-1

Termination of
spinal cord
(conus medullaris)

Lumbar
nerves
(5 pairs;
L1-L5)

Lumbar
nerves
(5 pairs)

L5

L-5

S1

S-1

Filum terminale

Sacral (5 pairs;
S1-S5) and
coccygeal (1 pair;
Co) nerves

S5
Co

S-5

Sacral
nerves
(5 pairs)

Coccygeal
nerve
(1 pair)

B

Lateral view

Anterior (ventral) view

A

Key for B	
▬ Cervical nerves and ganglia	▬ Lumbar nerves and ganglia
▬ Thoracic nerves and ganglia	▬ Sacral and coccygeal nerves and ganglia

FIGURE I.19.   **Basic organization of nervous system.** *CN,* cranial nerve.

Posterior horn of gray matter
White matter
Arachnoid mater
Dura mater
Denticulate ligament
Anterior horn of gray matter
Subarachnoid space
Pia mater
A **Transverse section**

Dura mater
Pia mater
Posterior rootlets
Arachnoid mater
Denticulate ligament
Posterior (sensory) root
Posterior ramus
Anterior ramus
Spinal nerve
Spinal ganglion
Anterior (motor) root
B

FIGURE I.20.   Spinal cord and meninges.

In the PNS, the neurolemma may take two forms, creating two classes of nerve fibers (Fig. I.21):

1. The neurolemma of **myelinated nerve fibers** have a myelin sheath that consists of a continuous series of Schwann cells enwrapping an *individual axon*, forming myelin.

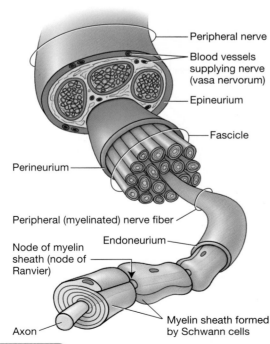

Peripheral nerve
Blood vessels supplying nerve (vasa nervorum)
Epineurium
Fascicle
Perineurium
Peripheral (myelinated) nerve fiber
Endoneurium
Node of myelin sheath (node of Ranvier)
Axon
Myelin sheath formed by Schwann cells

FIGURE I.21.   **Arrangement and ensheathment of peripheral nerve fibers.** The nodes of the myelin sheath are intervals in the myelin sheath (i.e., where short lengths of the axon are not covered by myelin).

2. The neurolemma of **unmyelinated nerve fibers** consist of *multiple axons* separately embedded within the cytoplasm of each Schwann cell. These Schwann cells do not produce myelin. Most fibers in cutaneous nerves (nerves that supply sensation to the skin) are unmyelinated.

Peripheral nerves are fairly strong and resilient because the nerve fibers are supported and protected by three connective tissue coverings (Fig. I.21):

1. **Endoneurium,** a delicate connective tissue sheath that surrounds the neurolemma cells and axons.
2. **Perineurium,** a layer of dense connective tissue that encloses a fascicle (bundle) of peripheral nerve fibers, providing an effective barrier against penetration of the nerve fibers by foreign substances.
3. **Epineurium,** a thick connective tissue sheath that surrounds and encloses a bundle of fascicles, forming the outermost covering of the nerve; it includes fatty tissues, blood vessels, and lymphatics.

A peripheral nerve is much like a telephone cable: the axons are the individual wires insulated by the neurolemma and endoneurium, the insulated wires are bundled by the perineurium, and the bundles are surrounded in turn by the epineurium, forming the outer wrapping of the "cable."

A collection of nerve cell bodies outside the CNS is a **ganglion.** There are both motor (autonomic) and sensory ganglia.

Peripheral nerves are either cranial or spinal nerves. Of the 12 pairs of **cranial nerves (CN),** 11 pairs arise from the brain; one pair (CN XI) arises mostly from the superior part of the spinal cord. All cranial nerves exit the cranial cavity through foramina in the cranium (G. *kranion,* skull). All 31 pairs of **spinal nerves**—8 cervical (C), 12 thoracic (T), 5 lumbar (L), 5 sacral (S), and 1 coccygeal (Co)—arise from the spinal cord and exit through intervertebral foramina in the vertebral column (Fig I.19*B*).

Somatic Nervous System

The **somatic nervous system,** or voluntary nervous system, composed of somatic parts of the CNS and PNS, provides general sensory and motor innervation to all parts of the body (G. *soma*), except the viscera in the body cavities, smooth muscle, and glands. The *somatic (general) sensory fibers* transmit sensations of touch, pain, temperature, and position from sensory receptors (Fig. I.22). The *somatic motor fibers* stimulate skeletal (voluntary) muscle exclusively, evoking voluntary and reflexive movement by causing its contraction, such as occurs when one reaches toward and reflexively withdraws from a candle flame.

Structure and Components of a Typical Spinal Nerve

A typical spinal nerve arises from the spinal cord by **nerve rootlets,** which converge to form two **nerve roots** (Fig. I.22).

Peripheral Nerve Degeneration

When peripheral nerves are crushed or severed, their axons degenerate distal to the lesion because they depend on their cell bodies for survival. A *crushing nerve injury* damages or kills the axons distal to the injury site; however, the nerve cell bodies usually survive and the connective tissue coverings of the nerve are intact. No surgical repair is needed for this type of nerve injury because the intact connective tissue sheaths guide the growing axons to their destinations. Surgical intervention is necessary if the nerve is cut because the regeneration of axons requires apposition of the cut ends by sutures through the epineurium. The individual fascicles (bundles of nerve fibers) are realigned as accurately as possible. Compromising a nerve's blood supply for a long period produces *ischemia* by compression of the vasa nervorum (Fig. I.21), which can also cause nerve degeneration. Prolonged ischemia of a nerve may result in damage no less severe than that produced by crushing or even cutting the nerve.

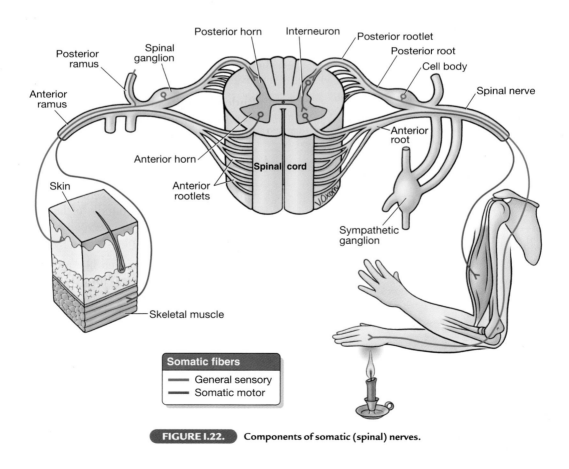

FIGURE I.22. Components of somatic (spinal) nerves.

The **anterior (ventral) root** consists of motor (efferent) fibers passing from nerve cell bodies in the anterior horn of the spinal cord gray matter to effector organs located peripherally. The **posterior (dorsal) root** consists of sensory (afferent) fibers that convey neural impulses to the CNS from sensory receptors in various parts of the body (e.g., in the skin). The posterior root carries general sensory fibers to the posterior horn of the spinal cord. The anterior and posterior roots unite at the intervertebral foramen to form a **spinal nerve,** which immediately divides into two **rami** (branches): a posterior ramus and an anterior ramus. As branches of a mixed spinal nerve, the anterior and posterior rami also carry both motor and sensory nerves, as do all their branches.

- The **posterior rami** supply nerve fibers to synovial joints of the vertebral column, deep muscles of the back, and the overlying skin.
- The **anterior rami** supply nerve fibers to the much larger remaining area, consisting of anterior and lateral regions of the trunk and the upper and lower limbs arising from them.

The components of a typical spinal nerve include:

- **Somatic sensory fibers and motor fibers.**
  - *General sensory (general somatic afferent) fibers* transmit sensations from the body to the CNS; they may be *exteroceptive sensations* (pain, temperature, touch, and pressure) from the skin or pain and *proprioceptive sensations* from muscles, tendons, and joints. Proprioceptive sensations are subconscious sensations that convey information on joint position and the tension of tendons and muscles, providing information on how the body and limbs are oriented in space, independent of visual input. The unilateral area of skin innervated by the general sensory fibers of a single spinal nerve is called a **dermatome.** From

clinical studies of lesions of the posterior roots or spinal nerves, *dermatome maps* have been devised that indicate the typical pattern of innervation of the skin by specific spinal nerves (Fig. I.23). However, a lesion of a single posterior root or spinal nerve would rarely result in numbness over the area demarcated for that nerve in these maps because the general sensory fibers conveyed by adjacent spinal nerves overlap almost completely as they are distributed to the skin, providing a type of double coverage. Clinicians need to understand the dermatomal innervation of the skin so they can determine, using sensory testing (e.g., with a pin) whether a particular spinal nerve/spinal cord segment is functioning normally.

- *Somatic motor (general somatic efferent)* fibers transmit impulses to skeletal (voluntary) muscles (Fig. I.22). The unilateral muscle mass receiving innervation from the somatic motor fibers conveyed by a single spinal nerve is a **myotome** (Fig. I.23). Each skeletal muscle is usually innervated by the somatic motor fibers of several spinal nerves; therefore, the muscle myotome will

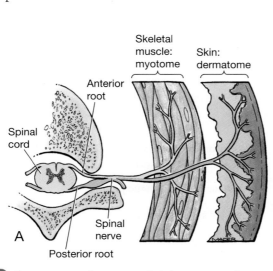

FIGURE I.23. **Dermatomes and myotomes. A.** A dermatome and myotome are shown. **B.** An example of a dermatome map.

consist of several segments. The muscle myotomes have been grouped by joint movement to facilitate clinical testing—for example, muscles that flex the glenohumeral (shoulder) joint are innervated primarily by the C5 spinal nerve, and muscles that extend the knee joint are innervated by the L3 and L4 spinal nerves.

- *Visceral motor fibers* of the sympathetic part of the autonomic nervous system (explained below) are conveyed by all branches of all spinal nerves to the smooth muscle of blood vessels and to sweat glands and arrector pili muscles of the skin. (Visceral motor fibers of the parasympathetic part of the autonomic nervous system and visceral afferent fibers have very limited association with spinal nerves.)
- **Connective tissue coverings** (Fig. I.21).
- **Vasa nervorum,** blood vessels supplying the nerves.

Autonomic Nervous System

The autonomic nervous system (ANS), classically described as the *visceral nervous system* or *visceral motor system,* consists of **visceral efferent (motor) fibers** that stimulate smooth (involuntary) muscle, in the walls of blood vessels and organs, modified cardiac muscle (the intrinsic stimulating and conducting tissue of the heart), and glands. However, the visceral efferent fibers of the ANS serving viscera of the body cavities are accompanied by **visceral afferent (sensory) fibers.** As the afferent component of autonomic reflexes and in conducting pain impulses from internal organs, these visceral afferent fibers also regulate visceral functions (Fig. I.24).

VISCERAL MOTOR INNERVATION

The efferent nerve fibers and ganglia of the ANS are organized into two systems or divisions:

1. **Sympathetic (thoracolumbar) division.** In general, the effects of sympathetic stimulation are *catabolic* (preparing the body for "flight or fight").
2. **Parasympathetic (craniosacral) division.** In general, the effects of parasympathetic stimulation are *anabolic* (promoting normal function and conserving energy).

Visceral fibers

———	Sensory
▪▪▪▪	Presynaptic sympathetic motor
———	Postsynaptic sympathetic motor
▪▪▪▪	Presynaptic parasympathetic motor
———	Postsynaptic parasympathetic motor

Vagus (CN X) nerve

Visceral parasympathetic pathway

Spinal ganglion

Posterior ramus of spinal nerve

Visceral afferent (reflex) fiber

Gray ramus communicans

Sympathetic ganglion

White ramus communicans

Anterior ramus of spinal nerve

Visceral sympathetic pathway

Parasympathetic ganglion

Visceral afferent (pain) fiber

FIGURE I.24. Sympathetic and parasympathetic innervation of the heart.

Although both sympathetic and parasympathetic systems innervate the same structures, they have different (usually contrasting) but coordinated effects (Table I.5).

Conduction of impulses from the CNS to the effector organ involves a series of two neurons in both sympathetic and parasympathetic systems. The cell body of the **presynaptic (preganglionic) neuron** (*first neuron*) is located in the gray matter of the CNS. Its fiber (axon) synapses on the cell body of a **postsynaptic (postganglionic) neuron,** the *second neuron* in the series (Fig. I.24). The cell bodies of such second neurons are located in autonomic ganglia outside the CNS, and the postsynaptic fibers terminate on the effector organ (smooth muscle, modified cardiac muscle, or glands). A functional distinction of pharmacological importance in medical practice is that the postsynaptic neurons of the two systems generally liberate different neurotransmitter substances: *norepinephrine by the sympathetic division* (except in the case of sweat glands) and *acetylcholine by the parasympathetic division.* The anatomical distinction between the sympathetic and the parasympathetic motor divisions of the ANS is based primarily on (1) the location of the presynaptic cell bodies and (2) which nerves conduct the presynaptic fibers from the CNS. These differences are discussed in more detail later in this chapter.

TABLE I.5 FUNCTIONS OF AUTONOMIC NERVOUS SYSTEM

Organ, Tract, or System		Effect of Sympathetic Stimulation[a]	Effect of Parasympathetic Stimulation[b]
Eyes	Pupil	Dilates pupil (admits more light for increased acuity at a distance)	Constricts pupil (protects pupil from excessively bright light)
	Ciliary body		Contracts ciliary muscle, allowing lens to thicken for near vision (accommodation)
Skin	Arrector muscle of hair	Causes hairs to stand on end (gooseflesh or goose bumps)	No effect (does not reach)[c]
	Peripheral blood vessels	Vasoconstricts (blanching of skin and lips; turning fingertips blue)	No effect (does not reach)[c]
	Sweat glands	Promotes sweating[d]	No effect (does not reach)[c]
Other glands	Lacrimal glands	Slightly decreases secretion[e]	Promotes secretion
	Salivary glands	Secretion decreases, becomes thicker, more viscous[e]	Promotes abundant, watery secretion
Heart		Increases rate and strength of contraction; inhibits effect of parasympathetic system on coronary vessels, allowing them to dilate[e]	Decreases rate and strength of contraction (conserving energy); constricts coronary vessels in relation to reduced demand
Lungs		Inhibits effect of parasympathetic system, resulting in bronchodilation and reduced secretion, allowing for maximum air exchange.	Constricts bronchi (conserving energy) and promotes bronchial secretion
Digestive tract		Inhibits peristalsis and constricts blood vessels to digestive tract so blood is available to skeletal muscle; contracts internal anal sphincter to aid fecal continence.	Stimulates peristalsis and secretion of digestive juices; contracts rectum and inhibits internal anal sphincter to cause defecation
Liver and gallbladder		Promotes breakdown of glycogen to glucose (for increased energy)	Promotes building/conservation of glycogen; increases secretion of bile
Urinary tract		Vasoconstriction of renal vessels slows urine formation; internal sphincter of bladder contracted to maintain urinary continence	Inhibits contraction of internal sphincter of bladder, contracts detrusor muscle of bladder wall, causing urination
Genital system		Causes ejaculation and vasoconstriction, resulting in remission of erection.	Produces engorgement (erection) of erectile tissues of external genitals
Suprarenal medulla		Release of adrenaline into blood	No effect (does not innervate)

[a] In general, the effects of sympathetic stimulation are catabolic, preparing body for the flight-or-fight response.

[b] In general, the effects of parasympathetic stimulation are anabolic, promoting normal function and conserving energy.

[c] The parasympathetic system is restricted in its distribution to the head, neck, and body cavities (except for erectile tissues of genitalia); otherwise, parasympathetic fibers are never found in the body wall and limbs. Sympathetic fibers, by comparison, are distributed to all vascularized portions of the body.

[d] With the exception of the sweat glands, glandular secretion is parasympathetically stimulated.

[e] With the exception of the coronary arteries, vasoconstriction is sympathetically stimulated; the effects of sympathetic stimulation on glands (other than sweat glands) are the indirect effects of vasoconstriction.

Sympathetic Visceral Motor Innervation

The cell bodies of *presynaptic* neurons of the sympathetic division of the ANS are located in the **intermediolateral cell columns** (IMLs) or nuclei of the spinal cord (Fig. I.25). The paired (right and left) IMLs are a part of the gray matter, extending between the first thoracic (T1) and the second or third lumbar (L2 or L3) segments of the spinal cord. In horizontal sections of this part of the spinal cord, the IMLs appear as small **lateral horns** of the H-shaped gray matter, looking somewhat like an extension of the cross-bar of the H between the posterior and the anterior horns of matter. The cell bodies of *postsynaptic* neurons of the sympathetic nervous system occur in two locations, the paravertebral and prevertebral ganglia (Fig. I.26):

- **Paravertebral ganglia** are linked to form right and left *sympathetic trunks* (*chains*) on each side of the vertebral column that extend essentially the length of this column. The superior paravertebral ganglion—the **superior cervical ganglion** of each sympathetic trunk—lies at the base of the cranium. The **ganglion impar** forms inferiorly, where the two trunks unite at the level of the coccyx (Fig. I.26).
- **Prevertebral ganglia** are in the plexuses that surround the origins of the main branches of the abdominal aorta (for which they are named), such as the large **celiac ganglia** that surround the origin of the celiac trunk (a major vessel arising from the aorta).

Because they are motor fibers, the axons of presynaptic neurons leave the spinal cord through anterior roots and enter the anterior rami of spinal nerves T1 through L2 or L3 (Fig. I.25). Almost immediately after entering the rami, all the presynaptic sympathetic fibers leave the anterior rami of these spinal nerves and pass to the *sympathetic trunks* through **white rami communicantes.** Within the sympathetic trunks, presynaptic fibers follow one of four possible courses: (1) ascend or (2) descend in the sympathetic trunk to synapse with a postsynaptic neuron of a higher or lower paravertebral ganglion; or (3) enter and synapse immediately with a postsynaptic neuron of the paravertebral ganglion at that level; or (4) pass through the sympathetic trunk without synapsing, continuing on through an abdominopelvic splanchnic nerve (innervates abdominopelvic viscera) to reach the prevertebral ganglia (Fig. I.27).

Presynaptic sympathetic fibers that provide autonomic innervation within the head, neck, body wall, limbs, and thoracic cavity follow one of the first three courses, synapsing within the paravertebral ganglia. Presynaptic sympathetic fibers innervating viscera within the abdominopelvic cavity follow the fourth course.

Postsynaptic sympathetic fibers greatly outnumber the presynaptic fibers; they are destined for distribution within the neck, body wall, and limbs, passing from the paravertebral ganglia of the sympathetic trunks to adjacent anterior rami of spinal nerves through **gray rami communicantes.** By this means, they enter all branches of all 31 pairs of spinal nerves, including the posterior rami, to stimulate contraction of blood vessels (*vasomotion*) and the arrector muscles of hair (*pilomotion,* resulting in goose bumps) and to cause sweating (*sudomotion*). Postsynaptic sympathetic fibers that perform these functions in the head (plus innervation of the dilator

FIGURE I.25. **Intermediolateral cell columns.** The paired intermediolateral cell columns or nuclei constitute the lateral horn of gray matter, seen in the section of spinal cord segments T1 through L2 or L3, and consist of the cell bodies of presynaptic neurons of the sympathetic nervous system. Distribution of the postsynaptic fibers is also shown.

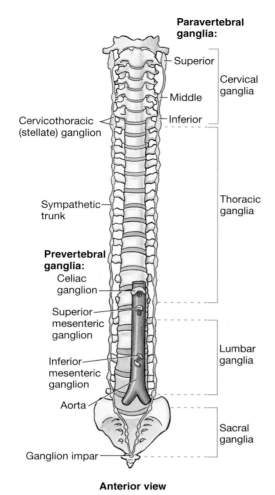

Paravertebral ganglia:
- Superior
- Middle
- Inferior

Cervical ganglia

Cervicothoracic (stellate) ganglion

Sympathetic trunk

Prevertebral ganglia:
- Celiac ganglion
- Superior mesenteric ganglion
- Inferior mesenteric ganglion

Aorta

Ganglion impar

Thoracic ganglia

Lumbar ganglia

Sacral ganglia

Anterior view

FIGURE I.26. **Sympathetic ganglia.** *Paravertebral ganglia* are associated with all spinal nerves, although at the cervical level, eight spinal nerves share three ganglia. *Prevertebral (preaortic) ganglia* occur in the plexuses that surround the origins of the main branches of the abdominal aorta, such as the celiac artery.

Paravertebral ganglion

Abdominopelvic splanchnic nerve

Prevertebral (preaortic) ganglion

Via periarterial plexus

Cells of suprarenal medulla

Cortex of suprarenal (adrenal) gland

Abdominopelvic viscera

Sympathetic motor fibers
- ▪▪▪▪ Presynaptic
- —— Postsynaptic

FIGURE I.27. **Sympathetic supply to medulla of suprarenal gland.**

muscle of the iris) all have their cell bodies in the **superior cervical ganglion** at the superior end of the sympathetic trunk. They pass from the ganglion by means of a **cephalic arterial branch** to form **periarterial plexuses** of nerves (Fig. I.28), which follow branches of the carotid arteries, or they may pass directly to nearby cranial nerves to reach their destination in the head.

Splanchnic nerves convey visceral efferent (autonomic) and afferent fibers to and from viscera of the body cavities (Figs. I.27–I.29). Postsynaptic sympathetic fibers destined for viscera of the thoracic cavity (e.g., heart, lungs, and esophagus) pass through *cardiopulmonary splanchnic nerves* to enter the cardiac, pulmonary, and esophageal plexuses. The presynaptic sympathetic fibers involved in innervation of viscera of the abdominopelvic cavity (e.g., the stomach and intestines) pass to the prevertebral ganglia through *abdominopelvic splanchnic nerves* (the greater,

lesser, least, and lumbar splanchnic nerves). All presynaptic sympathetic fibers of the abdominopelvic splanchnic nerves, except those involved in innervating the suprarenal (adrenal) glands, synapse in the prevertebral ganglia. The postsynaptic fibers from the prevertebral ganglia form periarterial plexuses, which follow branches of the abdominal aorta to reach their destination.

Some presynaptic sympathetic fibers that pass through the prevertebral (celiac) ganglia without synapsing terminate directly on cells in the medulla of the **suprarenal gland** (Fig. I.27). The suprarenal medullary cells function as a special type of postsynaptic neuron that, instead of releasing their neurotransmitter substance onto the cells of a specific effector organ, release it into the bloodstream to circulate throughout the body, producing a widespread sympathetic response. Thus the sympathetic innervation of this gland is exceptional.

As described earlier, postsynaptic sympathetic fibers are components of virtually all branches of all spinal nerves. By this means and via periarterial plexuses, they extend to and innervate all the body's blood vessels (the sympathetic system's primary function) as well as sweat glands, arrector muscles of hairs, and visceral structures. Thus the sympathetic nervous system reaches virtually all parts of the body, with the rare exception of avascular tissues, such as cartilage and nails. The presynaptic fibers are relatively short, whereas the postsynaptic fibers are relatively long, having to extend to all parts of the body.

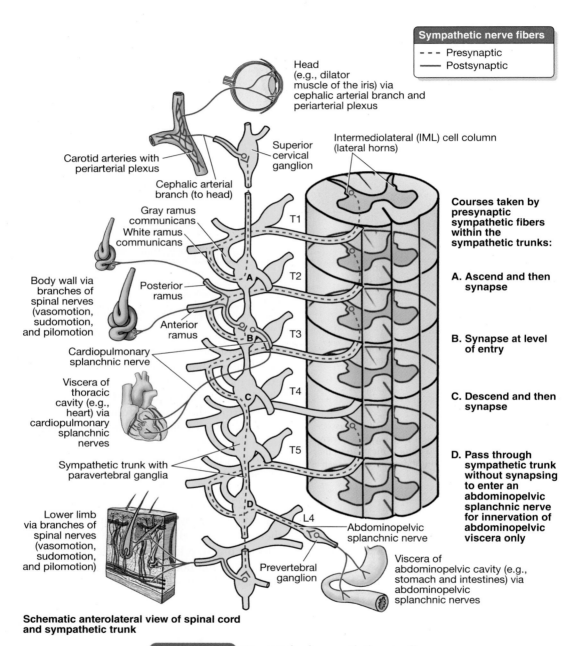

Head
(e.g., dilator
muscle of the iris) via
cephalic arterial branch and
periarterial plexus

Sympathetic nerve fibers
- - - Presynaptic
——— Postsynaptic

Intermediolateral (IML) cell column
(lateral horns)

Carotid arteries with
periarterial plexus

Superior
cervical
ganglion

Cephalic arterial
branch (to head)

Gray ramus
communicans

White ramus
communicans

**Courses taken by
presynaptic
sympathetic fibers
within the
sympathetic trunks:**

T1

Body wall via
branches of
spinal nerves
(vasomotion,
sudomotion,
and pilomotion

Posterior
ramus

A

T2

**A. Ascend and then
synapse**

Anterior
ramus

B

T3

**B. Synapse at level
of entry**

Cardiopulmonary
splanchnic nerve

Viscera of
thoracic
cavity (e.g.,
heart) via
cardiopulmonary
splanchnic
nerves

C

T4

**C. Descend and then
synapse**

Sympathetic trunk with
paravertebral ganglia

T5

Lower limb
via branches of
spinal nerves
(vasomotion,
sudomotion,
and pilomotion)

D

L4

**D. Pass through
sympathetic trunk
without synapsing
to enter an
abdominopelvic
splanchnic nerve
for innervation of
abdominopelvic
viscera only**

Abdominopelvic
splanchnic nerve

Prevertebral
ganglion

Viscera of
abdominopelvic cavity (e.g.,
stomach and intestines) via
abdominopelvic
splanchnic nerves

**Schematic anterolateral view of spinal cord
and sympathetic trunk**

FIGURE I.28.   Courses taken by sympathetic motor fibers.

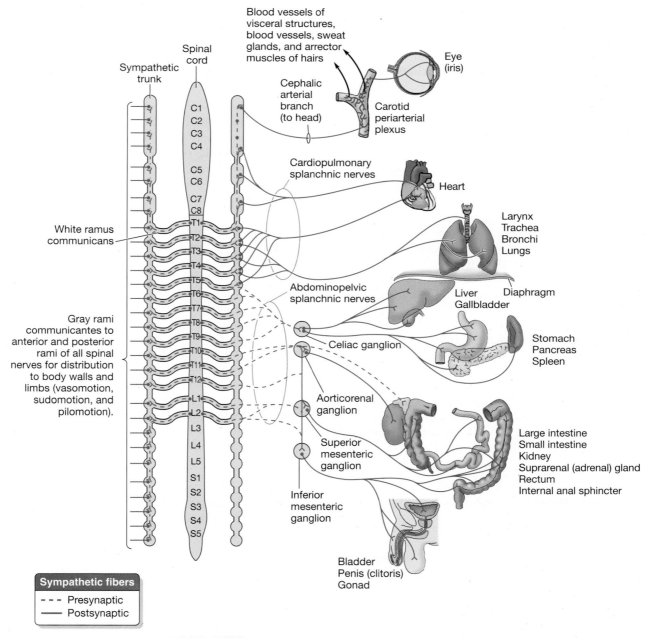

Blood vessels of visceral structures, blood vessels, sweat glands, and arrector muscles of hairs

Eye (iris)

Cephalic arterial branch (to head)

Carotid periarterial plexus

Sympathetic trunk

Spinal cord

C1
C2
C3
C4
C5
C6
C7
C8

Cardiopulmonary splanchnic nerves

Heart

White ramus communicans

T1
T2
T3
T4
T5
T6
T7
T8
T9
T10
T11
T12

Larynx
Trachea
Bronchi
Lungs

Abdominopelvic splanchnic nerves

Liver
Gallbladder

Diaphragm

Celiac ganglion

Stomach
Pancreas
Spleen

Gray rami communicantes to anterior and posterior rami of all spinal nerves for distribution to body walls and limbs (vasomotion, sudomotion, and pilomotion).

L1
L2
L3
L4
L5

Aorticorenal ganglion

S1
S2
S3
S4
S5

Superior mesenteric ganglion

Large intestine
Small intestine
Kidney
Suprarenal (adrenal) gland
Rectum
Internal anal sphincter

Inferior mesenteric ganglion

Bladder
Penis (clitoris)
Gonad

Sympathetic fibers
- - - Presynaptic
——— Postsynaptic

FIGURE I.29.   Distribution of postsynaptic sympathetic nerve fibers.

Parasympathetic Visceral Motor Innervation

Presynaptic parasympathetic neuron cell bodies are located in two sites within the CNS (craniosacral); their fibers exit by two routes (Fig. I.30). This accounts for the alternate name of the parasympathetic (craniosacral) division of the ANS.

- In the gray matter of the brainstem, the fibers exit the CNS within CN III, CN VII, CN IX, and CN X; these fibers constitute the **cranial parasympathetic outflow.**
- In the gray matter of the sacral segments of the spinal cord (S2–S4), the fibers exit the CNS through the anterior roots of spinal nerves S2–S4 and the pelvic splanchnic nerves that arise from their anterior rami; these fibers constitute the **sacral parasympathetic outflow.**

Not surprisingly, the cranial outflow provides parasympathetic innervation of the head, and the sacral outflow provides parasympathetic innervation of the pelvic viscera. However, in terms of the innervation of thoracic and abdominal viscera, the cranial outflow through the vagus nerve (CN X) is dominant. It provides innervation to all the thoracic viscera and most of the gastrointestinal (GI) tract from the esophagus through most of the large intestine (to its left colic flexure). The sacral outflow supplies only the descending and sigmoid colon and rectum.

Regardless of the extensive influence of its cranial outflow, the parasympathetic system is much more restricted than is the sympathetic system in its distribution. The parasympathetic system distributes only to the head, visceral cavities of the trunk, and erectile tissues of the external genitalia. With the exception of the latter, it does not reach the body wall or limbs, and except for initial parts of the anterior rami of spinal nerves S2–S4, its fibers are not components of spinal nerves or their branches.

Four discrete pairs of parasympathetic ganglia occur in the head (see Chapters 7 and 9). Elsewhere, presynaptic parasympathetic fibers synapse with postsynaptic cell bodies, which occur singly in or on the wall of the target organ (*intrinsic* or *enteric ganglia*). Most presynaptic parasympathetic fibers are long, extending from the CNS to the effector organ, whereas the postsynaptic fibers are short, running from a ganglion located near or embedded in the effector organ.

Visceral Afferent Sensation

Visceral afferent fibers have important relationships to the ANS, both anatomically and functionally. We are usually unaware of the sensory input of these fibers, which provides information about the condition of the body's internal environment. This information is integrated in the CNS, often triggering visceral or somatic reflexes or both. Visceral reflexes regulate blood pressure and chemistry by altering such functions as heart and respiratory rates and vascular resistance. Visceral sensation that reaches a conscious level is generally categorized as pain that is usually poorly localized and may be perceived as hunger or nausea. However, adequate stimulation, such as the following, may elicit true pain: sudden distention, spasms or strong contractions, chemical irritants, mechanical stimulation (especially when the organ is active), and pathological conditions (especially *ischemia*—inadequate blood supply) that lower the normal thresholds of stimulation. Normal activity usually produces no sensation but may do so when there is ischemia. Most visceral reflex (unconscious) sensation and some pain travel in visceral afferent fibers that accompany the parasympathetic fibers retrograde. Most visceral pain impulses (from the heart and most organs of the peritoneal cavity) travel centrally along visceral afferent fibers accompanying sympathetic fibers.

Imaging of Body Systems

Familiarity with imaging techniques commonly used in clinical settings enables one to recognize abnormalities such as congenital anomalies, tumors, and fractures. The introduction of contrast media allows the study of various luminal or vascular organs and potential or actual spaces, such as the digestive or alimentary system, blood vessels, kidneys, synovial cavities, and subarachnoid space. This section consists of short descriptions of the principles of some of the commonly used diagnostic imaging techniques:

- Conventional radiography (ordinary X-ray images)
- Computerized tomography (CT)
- Ultrasonography (US)
- Magnetic resonance imaging (MRI)
- Positron emission tomography (PET)

CONVENTIONAL RADIOGRAPHY

The essence of a radiological examination is that a highly penetrating beam of X-rays transilluminates the patient, showing tissues of differing densities of mass within the body as images of differing densities of light and dark on the X-ray film (Fig. I.31). A tissue or organ that is relatively dense in mass, such as compact bone in a rib, absorbs more X-rays than does a less dense tissue, such as spongy (cancellous) bone (Table I.6). Consequently, a dense tissue or organ produces a relatively transparent area on the X-ray film because relatively fewer X-rays reach the emulsion in the film. Therefore, relatively fewer grains of silver are developed at this area when the film is processed. A very dense substance is *radiopaque,* whereas a substance of less density is *radiolucent.*

Many of the same principles that apply to making a shadow apply to conventional radiography. Radiographs are

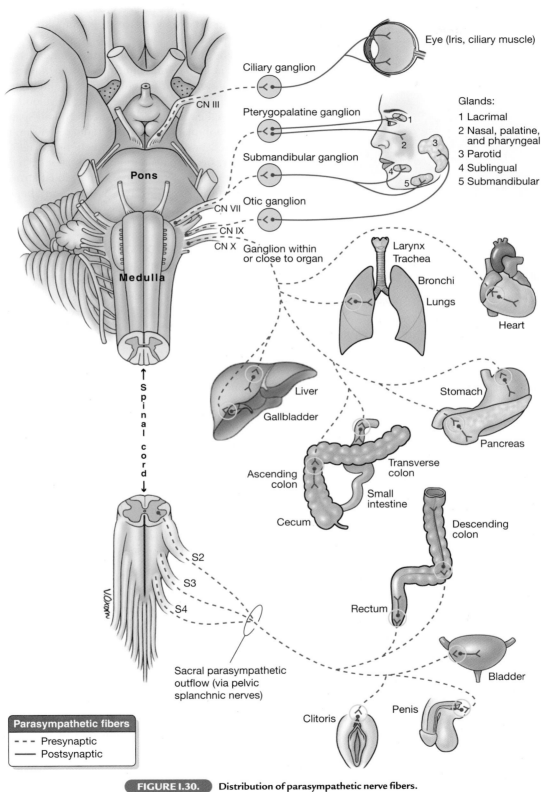

FIGURE I.30. Distribution of parasympathetic nerve fibers.

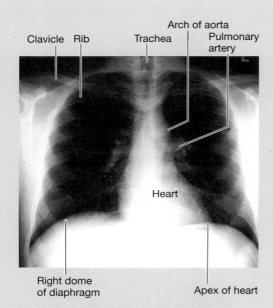

Clavicle Rib   Trachea   Arch of aorta
                             Pulmonary artery

Heart

Right dome
of diaphragm   Apex of heart

Postero-anterior (PA) projection

FIGURE I.31.   **Radiograph of thorax (chest).** (Courtesy of Dr. E. L. Landsdown, Professor of Medical Imaging, University of Toronto, Toronto, Ontario, Canada.)

TABLE I.6 BASIC PRINCIPLES OF X-RAY IMAGE FORMATION

Most radiolucent	Air	Least radiodense
↑	Fat	↑
	Water and most tissues	
	Spongy bone	
↓ Least radiolucent	Compact bone	Most radiodense ↓

made with the part of the patient's body being studied close to the X-ray film or detector to maximize the clarity of the image and minimize magnification artifacts. In basic radiologic nomenclature, *posteroanterior (PA) projection* refers to a radiograph in which the X-rays traversed the patient from posterior (P) to anterior (A); the X-ray tube was posterior to the patient and the X-ray film or detector was anterior. A radiograph using *anteroposterior (AP) projection* radiography is the opposite. Both PA and AP projection radiographs are viewed as if you and the patient were facing each other (the patient's right side is opposite your left); this is referred to as an *anteroposterior (AP) view.* (Thus the standard chest X-ray, taken to examine the heart and lungs, is an AP view of a PA projection.) For lateral radiographs, radiopaque letters (R or L) are used to indicate the side placed closest to the film or detector, and the image is viewed from the same direction that the beam was projected.

The introduction of contrast media (radiopaque fluids such as iodine compounds or barium) allows the study of various luminal or vascular organs and potential or actual spaces—such as the digestive tract, blood vessels, kidneys, synovial cavities, and the subarachnoid space—that are not visible in plain films. Most radiologic examinations are performed in at least two projections at right angles to each other. Because each radiograph presents a two-dimensional representation of a three-dimensional structure, structures sequentially penetrated by the X-ray beam overlap each other. Thus more than one view is usually necessary to detect and localize an abnormality accurately.

COMPUTERIZED TOMOGRAPHY

Computerized tomography (CT) shows images of the body that resemble transverse anatomical sections (Fig. I.32). A beam of X-rays is passed through the body as the X-ray tube and detector rotate around the axis of the body. The amount of radiation absorbed by each different type of tissue of the chosen body plane varies with the amount of fat, bone, and water in each element. A computer compiles and generates images as two-dimensional (2D) slices and total three-dimensional (3D) reconstructions.

ULTRASONOGRAPHY

Ultrasonography is a technique that allows visualization of superficial or deep structures in the body by recording pulses of ultrasonic waves reflecting off the tissues (Fig. I.33). The images can be viewed in real time to demonstrate the motion of structures and flow within blood vessels (Doppler US) and then recorded as single images or as a movie. Because ultrasonography is noninvasive and does not use radiation, it is the standard method of evaluating the growth and development of the embryo and fetus.

MAGNETIC RESONANCE IMAGING

Magnetic resonance imaging (MRI) shows images of the body similar to those produced by CT, but they are better for tissue differentiation (Fig. I.34). Using MRI, the clinician is able to reconstruct the tissues in *any plane,* even arbitrary oblique planes. The person is placed in a scanner with a strong magnetic field, and the body is pulsed with radio waves. Signals subsequently emitted from the patient's tissues are stored in a computer and may be reconstructed in 2D or 3D images. The appearance of tissues on the generated images can be varied by controlling how radiofrequency pulses are sent and received. Scanners can be gated or paced to visualize moving structures, such as the heart and blood flow, in real time.

X-ray tube

Detectors

A

Right   Left

Rib

Pancreas

Liver

Aorta

Vertebra

Left kidney

B **CT image of upper abdomen**

C **Three-dimensional CT reconstruction of bones of wrist and hand**

FIGURE I.32. **CT scanning. A.** The X-ray tube rotates around the person in the CT scanner and sends a fan-shaped beam of X-rays through the person's body from a variety of angles. X-ray detectors on the opposite side of the person's body measure the amount of radiation that passes through a transverse section of the person. **B and C.** A computer reconstructs the CT images. The scan is oriented, so it appears the way an examiner would view it when standing at the foot of the bed and looking toward a supine person's head.

Transducer
Acoustic gel coupling agent
Body wall
Ultrasound waves
Echo
Kidney (K)

A

RK

RK

B

LK

LRV

LRA

C **Doppler ultrasound**

FIGURE I.33. **Ultrasonography. A.** The image results from the echo of ultrasound waves from structures of different densities. **B.** The image of a right kidney (*RK*) is displayed. **C.** Doppler US shows blood flow to and away from the kidney. *LRV,* left renal vein; *LRA,* left renal artery; *LK,* left kidney.

FIGURE I.34. **MRI studies. A.** Sagittal MRI study of the head and upper neck. **B.** MR angiogram of heart and great vessels.

POSITRON EMISSION TOMOGRAPHY

Positron emission tomography (PET) scanning uses cyclotron-produced isotopes of extremely short half-life that emit positrons. PET scanning is used to evaluate the physiological functions of organs such as the brain on a dynamic basis. Areas of increased brain activity will show selective uptake of the injected isotope (Fig. I.35).

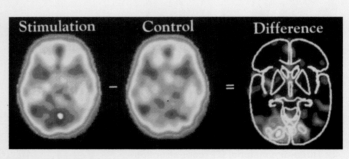

FIGURE I.35. **PET scan.** Observe the differences in brain activity associated with the planning and execution of a specific task in contrast to a control brain.

Go to http://thePoint.lww.com/ECA4e for helpful study tools, including USMLE-style questions, case studies, images, and more!

Thorax

THORACIC WALL / 48

Skeleton of Thoracic Wall / 48

Thoracic Apertures / 48

Joints of Thoracic Wall / 51

Movements of Thoracic Wall / 51

Breasts / 53

Muscles of Thoracic Wall / 60

Nerves of Thoracic Wall / 61

Vasculature of Thoracic Wall / 62

■ Surface Anatomy of Thoracic Wall / 65

THORACIC CAVITY AND VISCERA / 68

Endothoracic Fascia / 68

Pleurae and Lungs / 68

■ Surface Anatomy of Pleurae and Lungs / 70

Mediastinum / 80

Anterior Mediastinum / 80

Middle Mediastinum / 80

Heart and Great Vessels / 84

■ Surface Anatomy of Heart / 92

Superior Mediastinum / 102

Posterior Mediastinum / 108

MEDICAL IMAGING OF THORAX / 114

The thorax is the superior part of the trunk between the neck and abdomen. The thoracic cavity, surrounded by the thoracic wall, contains the heart, lungs, thymus, distal part of the trachea, and most of the esophagus. To perform a physical examination of the thorax, a working knowledge of its structure and vital organs is required.

THORACIC WALL

The thoracic wall consists of skin, fascia, nerves, vessels, muscles, cartilages, and bones. The functions of the thoracic wall include protecting the thoracic and abdominal internal organs; resisting the negative internal pressures generated by the elastic recoil of the lungs and inspiratory movements; providing attachment for and supporting the weight of the upper limbs; and providing attachment for many of the muscles of the upper limbs, neck, abdomen, and back and the muscles of respiration. The mammary glands of the breasts are in the subcutaneous tissue overlying the pectoral muscles covering the anterolateral thoracic wall.

Skeleton of Thoracic Wall

The **thoracic skeleton** forms the osteocartilaginous *thoracic cage* (Fig. 1.1). The thoracic skeleton includes 12 pairs of ribs and costal cartilages, 12 thoracic vertebrae and intervertebral (IV) discs, and the sternum. Costal cartilages form the anterior continuation of the ribs, providing a flexible attachment at their articulation with the sternum (Fig. 1.1A). The ribs and their cartilages are separated by **intercostal spaces,** which are occupied by intercostal muscles, vessels, and nerves.

Thoracic Apertures

The thoracic cavity communicates with the neck and upper limb through the **superior thoracic aperture,** the anatomical *thoracic inlet* (Fig. 1.1A). Structures entering and leaving the thoracic cavity through this aperture include the trachea, esophagus, vessels, and nerves. The adult superior thoracic aperture measures approximately 6.5 cm anteroposteriorly and 11 cm transversely. Because of the obliquity of the first pair of ribs, the superior thoracic aperture slopes anteroinferiorly. The superior thoracic aperture is bounded:

- Posteriorly by the T1 vertebra.
- Laterally by the first pair of ribs and their costal cartilages.
- Anteriorly by the superior border of the manubrium.

The thoracic cavity communicates with the abdomen through the **inferior thoracic aperture,** the anatomical *thoracic outlet* (Fig. 1.1A). In closing the inferior thoracic aperture, the diaphragm separates the thoracic and abdominal cavities almost completely. The inferior thoracic aperture is more spacious than the superior thoracic aperture.

Structures passing to or from the thorax to the abdomen pass through openings in the diaphragm (e.g., the inferior vena cava and esophagus) or posterior to it (e.g., aorta).

The inferior thoracic aperture is bounded:

- Posteriorly by the T12 vertebra.
- Posterolaterally by the eleventh and twelfth pairs of ribs.
- Anterolaterally by the joined costal cartilages of ribs 7–10, forming the costal margin.
- Anteriorly, by the xiphisternal joint.

RIBS AND COSTAL CARTILAGES

The ribs are curved, flat bones that form most of the thoracic cage (Fig. 1.1). They are remarkably light in weight yet highly resilient. Each rib has a spongy interior containing *bone marrow* (Fig. 1.2), which forms blood cells (hematopoietic tissue). There are three types of ribs:

- **True (vertebrocostal) ribs** (first through seventh ribs) attach directly to the sternum through their own costal cartilages.
- **False (vertebrochondral) ribs** (eighth through tenth ribs) have cartilages that are joined to the cartilage of the rib just superior to them; thus, their connection with the sternum is indirect.
- **Floating (free) ribs** (eleventh and twelfth ribs; sometimes the tenth rib) have rudimentary cartilages that do not connect even indirectly with the sternum; instead, they end in the posterior abdominal musculature.

Typical ribs (third through ninth) have a:

- **Head** that is wedge-shaped and two facets that are separated by the **crest of the head** (Fig. 1.2A). One facet is for articulation with the numerically corresponding vertebra, and one facet is for the vertebra superior to it.
- **Neck** that connects the head with the body (shaft) at the level of the tubercle.
- **Tubercle** at the junction of the neck and body. The tubercle has a smooth *articular part* for articulating with the corresponding transverse process of the vertebra and a rough *nonarticular part* for the attachment of the costotransverse ligament.
- **Body** (shaft) that is thin, flat, and curved, most markedly at the **angle** where the rib turns anterolaterally. The concave internal surface has a **costal groove** that protects the intercostal nerve and vessels (Fig. 1.2).

Atypical ribs (first, second, and tenth through twelfth) are dissimilar (Figs. 1.1 and 1.3):

- The first rib is the broadest (i.e., its body is widest and is nearly horizontal), shortest, and most sharply curved of the seven true ribs; it has two grooves crossing its superior surface for the subclavian vessels; the grooves are separated by a **scalene tubercle** and ridge.

A **Anterior view**

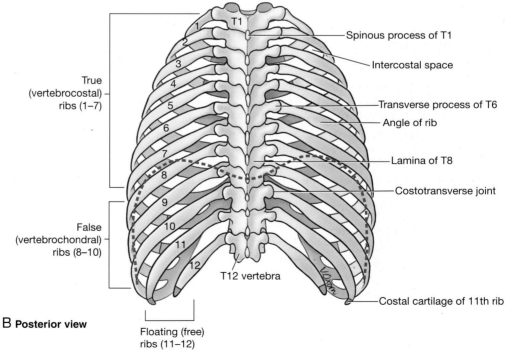

B **Posterior view**

FIGURE 1.1.   **Thoracic skeleton.** The superior and inferior thoracic apertures are outlined in *pink*. Ribs are numbered *1–12. T1,* body of first thoracic vertebra; *T12,* body of twelfth thoracic vertebra. The *dotted lines* indicate the position of the diaphragm, which separates the thoracic and abdominal cavities.

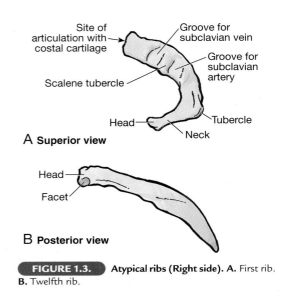

FIGURE 1.3. Atypical ribs (Right side). **A.** First rib. **B.** Twelfth rib.

FIGURE 1.2. Typical rib (Right side). **A.** Features. **B.** Cross section through the middle of body.

rib and the anterior ramus of spinal nerve T12 is the subcostal nerve.

THORACIC VERTEBRAE

Thoracic vertebrae are typical vertebrae in that they are independent and have bodies, vertebral arches, and seven processes for muscular and articular connections (see Chapter 4). Characteristic features of thoracic vertebrae include:

- Bilateral costal facets (demifacets) on their bodies for articulation with the heads of ribs (Fig. 1.4); atypical thoracic vertebrae have one whole costal facet in place of the demifacets.
- Costal facets on their transverse processes for articulation with the tubercles of ribs, except for the inferior two or three thoracic vertebrae.
- Long inferiorly slanting spinous processes.

- The second rib is thinner, less curved, and much longer than the first rib; it has two facets on its head for articulation with the bodies of the T1 and T2 vertebrae.
- The tenth through twelfth ribs, like the first rib, have only one facet on their heads.
- The eleventh and twelfth ribs are short and have no necks or tubercles.

Costal cartilages prolong the ribs anteriorly and contribute to the elasticity of the thoracic wall. *Intercostal spaces* separate the ribs and their costal cartilages from one another. The spaces and neurovascular structures are named according to the rib forming the superior border of the space—that is, there are 11 intercostal spaces and 11 intercostal nerves. The *subcostal space* is below the twelfth

FIGURE 1.4. Costovertebral joints.

FIGURE 1.5. Sternum. **A.** Features. **B.** Relationship of sternum to vertebral column.

STERNUM

The sternum is the flat, vertically elongated bone that forms the middle of the anterior part of the thoracic cage. The sternum consists of three parts: manubrium, body, and xiphoid process (Figs. 1.1A and 1.5).

The **manubrium,** the superior part of the sternum, is a roughly trapezoidal bone that lies at the level of the bodies of the T3 and T4 vertebrae. Its thick superior border is indented by the **jugular notch** (suprasternal notch). On each side of this notch, a **clavicular notch** articulates with the sternal (medial) end of the clavicle. Just inferior to this notch, the costal cartilage of the first rib fuses with the lateral border of the manubrium. The manubrium and body of the sternum lie in slightly different planes, forming a projecting **sternal angle** (of Louis). This readily palpable *clinical landmark* is located opposite the second pair of costal cartilages at the level of the IV disc between the T4 and T5 vertebrae (Fig. 1.5B).

The **body** of the sternum (T5–T9 vertebral level) is longer, narrower, and thinner than the manubrium. Its width varies because of the scalloping of its lateral borders by the **costal notches** for articulation with the costal cartilages.

The **xiphoid process** (T10 vertebral level) is the smallest and most variable part of the sternum. It is relatively thin and elongated but varies considerably in form. The process is cartilaginous in young people but more or less ossified in adults older than 40 years. In elderly people, the xiphoid process may fuse with the sternal body. It is a midline marker for the superior level of the liver, the central tendon of the diaphragm, and the inferior border of the heart.

Joints of Thoracic Wall

Although movements of the joints of the thoracic wall are frequent (e.g., during respiration), the range of movement at the individual joints is small. Any disturbance that reduces the mobility of these joints interferes with respiration. *Joints of the thoracic wall* occur between the (Fig. 1.6 and Table 1.1):

- Vertebrae (intervertebral joints).
- Ribs and vertebrae (costovertebral joints: joints of the heads of ribs and the costotransverse joints).
- Sternum and costal cartilages (sternocostal joints).
- Sternum and clavicle (sternoclavicular joints).
- Ribs and costal cartilages (costochondral joints).
- Costal cartilages (interchondral joints).
- Parts of the sternum (manubriosternal and xiphisternal joints) in young people; usually the manubriosternal joint and sometimes the xiphisternal joint are fused in elderly people.

The *intervertebral joints* between the bodies of adjacent vertebrae are joined together by longitudinal ligaments and *intervertebral discs* (see Chapter 4).

Movements of Thoracic Wall

Movements of the thoracic wall and diaphragm during inspiration increase the intrathoracic volume and diameters of the thorax. Consequent pressure changes result in air being drawn into the lungs (inspiration) through the nose, mouth, larynx, and trachea. During passive expiration, the

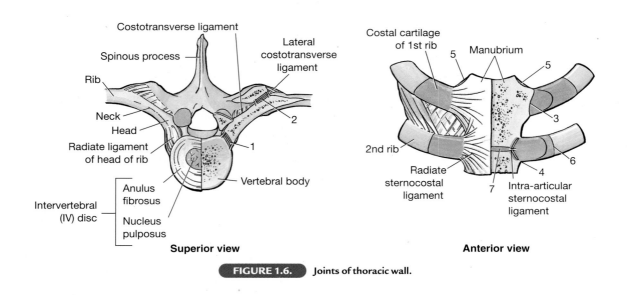

FIGURE 1.6. Joints of thoracic wall.

TABLE 1.1 JOINTS OF THORACIC WALL

Joint[a]	Type	Articulations	Ligaments	Comments
Intervertebral	Symphysis (secondary cartilaginous joint)	Adjacent vertebral bodies bound together by intervertebral disc	Anterior and posterior longitudinal	
Costovertebral joints of head of ribs (*1*)	Synovial plane of joint	Head of each rib with superior demifacet or costal facet of corresponding vertebral body and inferior demifacet or costal facet of vertebral body superior to it	Radiate and intra-articular ligaments of head of rib	Heads of 1st, 11th, and 12th ribs (sometimes 10th) articulate only with corresponding vertebral body
Costotransverse (*2*)		Articulation of tubercle of rib with transverse process of corresponding vertebra	Lateral and superior costotransverse	11th and 12th ribs do not articulate with transverse process of corresponding vertebrae
Sternocostal (*3, 4*)	1st: primary cartilaginous joint	Articulation of 1st costal cartilages with manubrium of sternum		
	2nd–7th: synovial plane joints	Articulation of 2nd–7th pairs of costal cartilages with sternum	Anterior and posterior radiate sternocostal	
Sternoclavicular (*5*)	Saddle type of synovial joint	Sternal end of clavicle with manubrium and 1st costal cartilage	Anterior and posterior sternoclavicular ligaments; costoclavicular ligament	Joint is divided into two compartments by articular disc
Costochondral (*6*)	Primary cartilaginous joint	Articulation of lateral end of costal cartilage with sternal end of rib	Cartilage and bone; bound together by periosteum	Normally, no movement occurs
Interchondral (Fig. 1.1A)	Synovial plane joint	Articulation between costal cartilages of 6th–7th, 7th–8th, and 8th–9th ribs	Interchondral ligaments	Articulation between costal cartilages of 9th–10th ribs is fibrous
Manubriosternal (*7*)	Secondary cartilaginous joint (symphysis)	Articulation between manubrium and body of sternum		Often fuse and become synostosis in older people
Xiphisternal (Fig. 1.1A)	Primary cartilaginous joint (synchondrosis)	Articulation between xiphoid process and body of sternum		

[a]Numbers in parentheses refer to the figures.

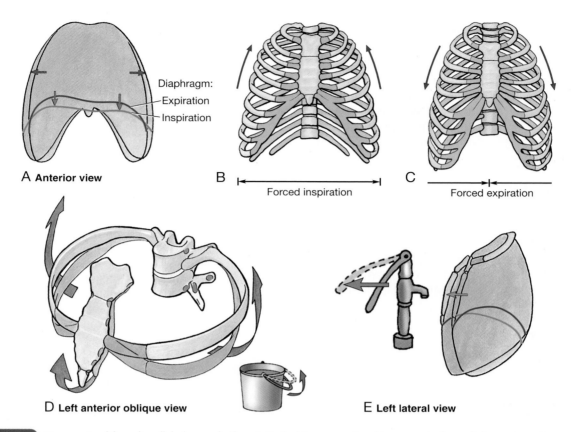

Diaphragm:
Expiration
Inspiration

A **Anterior view**

B Forced inspiration

C Forced expiration

D **Left anterior oblique view**

E **Left lateral view**

FIGURE 1.7. Movements of thoracic wall during respiration. **A.** Vertical (*green arrows*) and transverse (*red arrows*) diameters are increased during inspiration. **B.** Thoracic cage widens during forced inspiration as the ribs are elevated (*arrows*). **C.** Thoracic cage narrows during expiration as the ribs are depressed (*arrows*). **D.** Observe the increased AP (*blue arrow*) and transverse (*red arrows*) diameters. The middle parts of the lower ribs move laterally when they are elevated (bucket-handle movement). **E.** The AP diameter of the thorax is increased (pump-handle movement); a greater excursion (increase) occurs inferiorly.

diaphragm, intercostal muscles, and other muscles relax, decreasing *intrathoracic volume* and increasing *intrathoracic pressure,* expelling air from the lungs (expiration) through the same passages. The stretched elastic tissue of the lungs recoils, expelling most of the air. Concurrently, *intra-abdominal pressure* decreases and the abdominal viscera are decompressed.

The *vertical dimension* (height) of the central part of the thoracic cavity increases during inspiration as the contracting diaphragm descends, compressing the abdominal viscera (Fig. 1.7A,B). During expiration (Fig. 1.7A,C), the vertical diameter returns to the neutral position as the elastic recoil of the lungs produces subatmospheric pressure in the pleural cavities, between the lungs and the thoracic wall. As a result of this and the absence of resistance to the previously compressed viscera, the domes of the diaphragm ascend, diminishing the vertical dimension. The *anteroposterior* (AP) *dimension* of the thorax increases considerably when the intercostal muscles contract (Fig. 1.7D,E). Movement of the upper ribs at the costovertebral joints, about an axis passing through the neck of the ribs, causes the anterior ends of the ribs and sternum, especially its inferior end, to rise like a pump handle, the "pump-handle movement" (Fig. 1.7E). In addition, the *transverse dimension* of the thorax increases

slightly when the intercostal muscles contract, raising the most lateral parts of the ribs, especially the most inferior ones, the "bucket-handle movement" (Fig. 1.7B,D).

Breasts

Both males and females have breasts (L. *mammae*), but normally, the mammary glands are well developed only in women. **Mammary glands** in women are accessory to reproduction, but in men they are functionless, consisting of only a few small ducts or cords. The mammary glands are modified sweat glands and therefore have no special capsule or sheath. The contour and volume of the breasts are produced by subcutaneous fat, except during pregnancy, when the mammary glands enlarge and new glandular tissue forms. During puberty (8 to 15 years of age), the female breasts normally grow because of glandular development and increased fat deposition. Breast size and shape result from genetic, racial, and dietary factors.

The roughly circular base of the female breast extends transversely from the lateral border of the sternum to the midaxillary line and vertically from the second to sixth ribs. A small part of the breast may extend along the inferolateral

Role of Costal Cartilages

 Costal cartilages prolong the ribs anteriorly and contribute to the elasticity of the thoracic wall, preventing many blows from fracturing the sternum and/or ribs. In elderly people, the costal cartilages undergo calcification, making them radiopaque and less resilient.

Rib Fractures

The weakest part of a rib is just anterior to its angle. Rib fractures commonly result from direct blows or indirectly from crushing injuries. The middle ribs are most commonly fractured. Direct violence may fracture a rib anywhere, and its broken ends may injure internal organs such as a lung or the spleen.

Flail Chest

Flail chest occurs when a sizable segment of the anterior and/or lateral thoracic wall moves freely because of *multiple rib fractures*. This condition allows the loose segment of the wall to move paradoxically (inward on inspiration and outward on expiration). Flail chest is an extremely painful injury and impairs ventilation, thereby affecting oxygenation of the blood. During treatment, the loose segment is often fixed by hooks and/or wires so that it cannot move.

Supernumerary Ribs

People usually have 12 ribs on each side, but the number may be increased by the presence of cervical and/or lumbar ribs or decreased by failure of the 12th pair to form. **Cervical ribs** (present in up to 1% of people) articulate with the C7 vertebra and are clinically significant because they may compress spinal nerves C8 and T1 or the inferior trunk of the brachial plexus supplying the upper limb. Tingling and numbness may occur along the medial border of the forearm. They may also compress the subclavian artery, resulting in *ischemic muscle pain* (caused by poor blood supply) in the upper limb. **Lumbar ribs** are less common than cervical ribs, but have clinical significance in that they may confuse the identification of vertebral levels in diagnostic images.

Sternal Fractures

Sternal fractures are not common, but crush injuries can occur during traumatic compression of the thoracic wall (e.g., in automobile accidents when the driver's chest is driven into the steering column). When the body of the sternum is fractured, it is usually a *comminuted fracture* (broken into several pieces). The most common site of sternal fractures is the sternal angle, resulting in dislocation of the manubriosternal joint. In sternal injuries the concern is for the likelihood of heart and pulmonary injury.

Median Sternotomy

 To gain access to the thoracic cavity for surgical procedures—on the heart and great vessels, for example—the sternum is divided ("split") in the median plane and retracted (spread apart). After surgery, the halves of the sternum are reunited and held together with wire sutures.

Sternal Biopsies

 The sternal body is often used for *bone marrow needle biopsy* because of its breadth and subcutaneous position. The needle pierces the thin cortical bone and enters the vascular trabecular (spongy) bone. Sternal biopsy is commonly used to obtain specimens of bone marrow for transplantation and for detection of metastatic cancer.

Paralysis of Diaphragm

 One can detect paralysis of the diaphragm radiographically by noting its paradoxical movement. Paralysis of half of the diaphragm because of *injury to its motor supply from the phrenic nerve* does not affect the other half because each dome has a separate nerve supply. Instead of descending on inspiration, the paralyzed dome is pushed superiorly by the abdominal viscera that are being compressed by the active side. The paralyzed dome descends during expiration as it is pushed down by the positive pressure in the lungs (Fig. B1.1).

FIGURE B1.1.

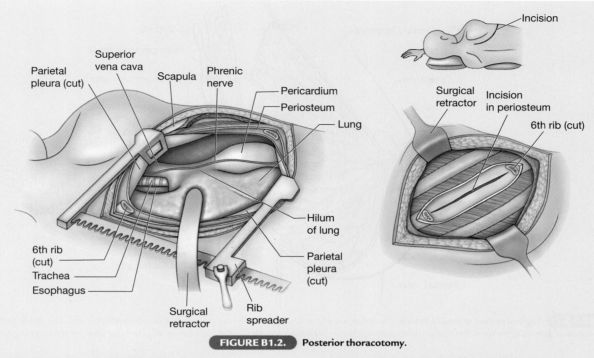

FIGURE B1.2. Posterior thoracotomy.

Thoracotomy, Intercostal Space Incisions, and Rib Excision

The surgical creation of an opening through the thoracic wall to enter a pleural cavity is called a *thoracotomy* (Fig. B1.2). An *anterior thoracotomy* may involve making H-shaped cuts through the perichondrium of one or more costal cartilages and then shelling out segments of costal cartilage to gain entrance to the thoracic cavity.

The posterolateral aspects of the fifth to seventh intercostal spaces are important sites for *posterior thoracotomy* incisions. In general, a lateral approach is most satisfactory for entry through the thoracic cage (Fig. B1.2). With the patient lying on the contralateral side, the upper limb is fully abducted, placing the forearm beside the patient's head. This elevates and laterally rotates the inferior angle of scapula, allowing access as high as the fourth intercostal space.

Surgeons use an H-shaped incision to incise the superficial aspect of the periosteum that ensheaths the rib, strip the periosteum from the rib, and then remove a wide segment of the rib to gain better access, as might be required to enter the thoracic cavity and remove a lung (*pneumonectomy*), for example. In the rib's absence, entry into the thoracic cavity can be made through the deep aspect of the periosteal sheath, sparing the adjacent intercostal muscles. After the operation, the missing pieces of ribs regenerate from the intact periosteum, although imperfectly.

Thoracic Outlet Syndrome

When clinicians refer to the superior thoracic aperture as the thoracic "outlet," they are emphasizing the important nerves and arteries that pass through this aperture into the lower neck and upper limb. Hence various types of thoracic outlet syndromes exist, such as the *costoclavicular syndrome*—pallor and coldness of the skin of the upper limb and diminished radial pulse resulting from compression of the subclavian artery between the clavicle and the first rib, particularly when the angle between the neck and the shoulder is increased.

Dislocation of Ribs

A rib dislocation (*slipping rib syndrome*) or *dislocation of a sternocostal joint* is the displacement of a costal cartilage from the sternum. This causes severe pain, particularly during deep respiratory movements. The injury produces a lump-like deformity at the dislocation site. Rib dislocations are common in body contact sports, and possible complications are pressure on or damage to nearby nerves, vessels, and muscles.

A rib separation refers to *dislocation of a costochondral junction* between the rib and its costal cartilage. In separations of the third through tenth ribs, tearing of the perichondrium and periosteum usually occurs. As a result, the rib may move superiorly, overriding the rib above and causing pain.

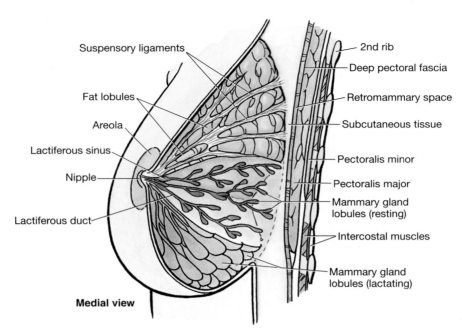

Suspensory ligaments
Fat lobules
Areola
Lactiferous sinus
Nipple
Lactiferous duct
Medial view

2nd rib
Deep pectoral fascia
Retromammary space
Subcutaneous tissue
Pectoralis minor
Pectoralis major
Mammary gland lobules (resting)
Intercostal muscles
Mammary gland lobules (lactating)

FIGURE 1.8.   **Sagittal section of female breast.** The *upper part* of the figure shows the fat lobules and suspensory ligaments. The *middle part* shows the appearance of glandular tissue in the nonlactating (resting) breast. The *lower part* shows the appearance of glandular tissue in the lactating breast.

edge of the pectoralis major muscle toward the axillary fossa, forming an **axillary process** or **tail** (of Spence). Two thirds of the breast rests on the **pectoral fascia** covering the pectoralis major; the other third rests on the fascia covering the serratus anterior muscle (Figs. 1.8 and 1.9). Between the breast and the deep pectoral fascia is a loose connective tissue plane or potential space—the **retromammary space** (bursa). This plane, containing a small amount of fat, allows the breast some degree of movement on the deep pectoral fascia. The mammary glands are firmly attached to the dermis of the overlying skin by the **suspensory ligaments** (of Cooper). These ligaments, particularly well developed in the superior part of the breast (Fig. 1.8), help support the **mammary gland lobules.**

At the greatest prominence of the breast is the **nipple,** surrounded by a circular pigmented area (the **areola**). The breast contains 15 to 20 **lobules** of glandular tissue, which constitute the parenchyma of the mammary gland. Each lobule is drained by a **lactiferous duct,** which opens independently on the nipple. Just deep to the areola, each duct has a dilated portion, the **lactiferous sinus** (Fig. 1.8).

VASCULATURE OF BREAST

The arterial supply of the breast is derived from (Fig. 1.9A):

- **Medial mammary branches of perforating branches** and *anterior intercostal branches of the internal thoracic artery,* originating from the subclavian artery

- **Lateral thoracic** and **thoraco-acromial arteries,** branches of the axillary artery
- *Posterior intercostal arteries,* branches of the thoracic aorta in the intercostal spaces

The **venous drainage of the breast** (Fig. 1.9B) is mainly to the **axillary vein,** but there is some drainage to the *internal thoracic vein.*

The **lymphatic drainage of the breast** is important because of its role in the metastasis (spread) of cancer cells. Lymph passes from the nipple, areola, and lobules of the gland to the **subareolar lymphatic plexus** (Fig. 1.9C), and from it:

- Most lymph (>75%), especially from the lateral quadrants of the breasts, drains to the **axillary lymph nodes** (pectoral, humeral, subscapular, central, and apical).
- Most of the lymph first drains to the *pectoral (anterior) nodes.* However, some lymph may drain directly to other axillary nodes, or to interpectoral, deltopectoral, supraclavicular, or inferior deep cervical nodes.
- Lymph from the medial breast quadrants drains to the **parasternal lymph nodes** or to the opposite breast.
- Lymph from the inferior breast quadrants may pass deeply to **abdominal lymph nodes** (inferior phrenic nodes).

Lymph from the axillary nodes drains to infraclavicular and supraclavicular nodes and from them to the **subclavian lymphatic trunk.** Lymph from the parasternal nodes

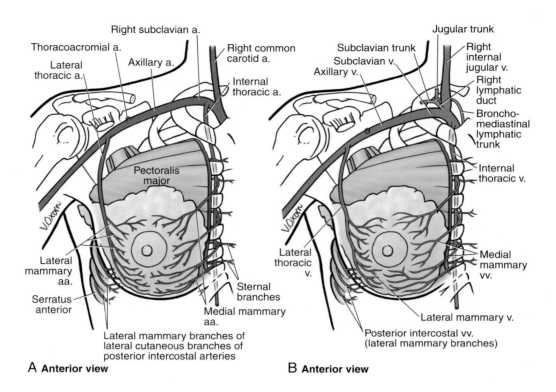

A **Anterior view**

Right subclavian a.
Thoracoacromial a.
Lateral thoracic a.
Axillary a.
Right common carotid a.
Internal thoracic a.
Pectoralis major
Lateral mammary aa.
Serratus anterior
Lateral mammary branches of lateral cutaneous branches of posterior intercostal arteries
Medial mammary aa.
Sternal branches

B **Anterior view**

Subclavian trunk
Subclavian v.
Axillary v.
Jugular trunk
Right internal jugular v.
Right lymphatic duct
Broncho-mediastinal lymphatic trunk
Internal thoracic v.
Lateral thoracic v.
Medial mammary vv.
Lateral mammary v.
Posterior intercostal vv. (lateral mammary branches)

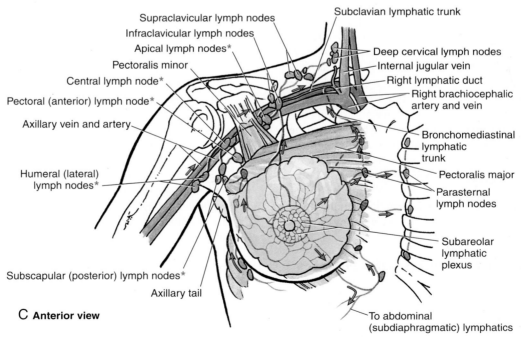

Supraclavicular lymph nodes
Infraclavicular lymph nodes
Apical lymph nodes*
Pectoralis minor
Central lymph node*
Pectoral (anterior) lymph node*
Axillary vein and artery
Humeral (lateral) lymph nodes*
Subscapular (posterior) lymph nodes*
Axillary tail
Subclavian lymphatic trunk
Deep cervical lymph nodes
Internal jugular vein
Right lymphatic duct
Right brachiocephalic artery and vein
Bronchomediastinal lymphatic trunk
Pectoralis major
Parasternal lymph nodes
Subareolar lymphatic plexus
To abdominal (subdiaphragmatic) lymphatics

C **Anterior view**

FIGURE 1.9. **Lymphatic drainage and vasculature of breast. A.** Arteries. **B.** Veins. **C.** Lymphatic drainage. Axillary lymph nodes are indicated by asterisks.

Breast Quadrants

For the anatomical location and description of pathology (e.g., cysts and tumors), the breast is divided into four quadrants. The *axillary tail* is an extension of the mammary gland of the superolateral quadrant (Fig. B1.3).

FIGURE B1.3.   Breast quadrants.

Changes in Breasts

Changes, such as branching of the lactiferous ducts, occur in the breast tissues during the menstrual cycle and pregnancy. Although mammary glands are prepared for secretion by mid-pregnancy, they do not produce milk until shortly after the baby is born. *Colostrum,* a creamy white to yellowish premilk fluid, may secrete from the nipples during the last trimester of pregnancy and during initial episodes of nursing. Colostrum is believed to be especially rich in protein, immune agents, and a growth factor affecting the infant's intestines. In multiparous women (those who have given birth two or more times), the breasts often become large and pendulous. The breasts in elderly women are usually small because of the decrease in fat and the atrophy of glandular tissue.

Supernumerary Breasts and Nipples

Supernumerary (exceeding two) *breasts* (*polymastia*) or nipples (*polythelia*) may occur superior or inferior to the normal breasts. Usually supernumerary breasts consist of only a rudimentary nipple and areola. A supernumerary breast may appear anywhere along a line extending from the axilla to the groin, the location of the embryonic mammary crest (ridge).

Carcinoma of Breast

Understanding the lymphatic drainage of the breasts is of practical importance in predicting the metastasis (dispersal) of cancer cells from a *carcinoma of the breast* (breast cancer). Carcinomas of the breast are malignant tumors, usually adenocarcinomas arising from the epithelial cells of the lactiferous ducts in the mammary gland lobules (Fig. B1.4). Metastatic cancer cells that enter a lymphatic vessel usually pass through two or three groups of lymph nodes before entering the venous system. Breast cancer can spread via lymphatics and veins and as well as by direct invasion.

Interference with the lymphatic drainage by cancer may cause *lymphedema* (edema, excess fluid in the subcutaneous tissue), which in turn may result in deviation of the nipple and a thickened, leather-like appearance of the skin (Fig. B1.4A). Prominent or "puffy" skin between dimpled pores gives it an orange-peel appearance (*peau d'orange* sign). Larger dimples (fingertip size or bigger) result from cancerous invasion of the glandular tissue and fibrosis (fibrous degeneration), which causes shortening or places traction on the suspensory ligaments. *Subareolar breast cancer* may cause inversion of the nipple by a similar mechanism involving the lactiferous ducts.

Breast cancer typically spreads by means of lymphatic vessels (*lymphogenic metastasis*), which carry cancer cells from the breast to the lymph nodes, chiefly those in the axilla. The cells lodge in the nodes, producing nests of tumor cells (*metastases*). Abundant communications among lymphatic pathways and among axillary, cervical, and parasternal nodes may also cause metastases from the breast to develop in the supraclavicular lymph nodes, the opposite breast, or the abdomen. Because most of the lymphatic drainage of the breast is to the *axillary lymph nodes,* they are the most common site of metastasis from a breast cancer. Enlargement of these palpable nodes suggests the possibility of breast cancer and may be key to early detection. However, the absence of enlarged axillary lymph nodes is no guarantee that metastasis from a breast cancer has not occurred because the malignant cells may have passed to other nodes, such as the infraclavicular and supraclavicular lymph nodes. Nodal metastatic breast cancer can be difficult to manage because of the complex system of lymphatic drainage.

The posterior intercostal veins drain into the *azygos/hemiazygos system of veins* alongside the bodies of

Skin dimpling

Abnormal contours

Edema of skin
(Peau d'orange sign)

Nipple retraction
and deviation

A **Signs of carcinoma of breast**

FIGURE B1.4.   Carcinoma of breast.

Cancer

Nipple

B **Mammogram**

C **Carcinoma of breast**

the vertebrae and communicate with the internal vertebral venous plexus surrounding the spinal cord. Cancer cells can also spread from the breast by these venous routes to the vertebrae and from there to the cranium and brain. Cancer also spreads by contiguity (invasion of adjacent tissue). When breast cancer cells invade the retromammary space, attach to or invade the pectoral fascia overlying the pectoralis major, or metastasize to the interpectoral nodes, the breast elevates when the muscle contracts. This movement is a clinical sign of advanced cancer of the breast.

Mammography

Radiographic examination of the breasts, *mammography,* is one of the techniques used to detect breast masses. A carcinoma appears as a large, jagged density in the *mammogram.* The skin is thickened over the tumor (*upper two white arrows* in Fig. B1.4B). The *lower leader* points to the nipple, which is depressed in the mammogram. Surgeons use mammography as a guide when removing breast tumors, cysts, and abscesses.

Surgical Incisions of Breast

Incisions are placed in the inferior breast quadrants when possible because these quadrants are less vascular than the superior ones. The transition between the thoracic wall and breast is most abrupt inferiorly, producing a line, crease, or deep skin fold—the *inferior cutaneous crease.* Incisions made along this crease will be least evident and may actually be hidden by overlap of the breast. Incisions that must be made near the areola or on the breast itself are usually directed radially to either side of the nipple (Langer tension lines run transversely here) or circumferentially.

Mastectomy (breast excision) is not as common as it once was as a treatment for breast cancer. In *simple mastectomy,* the breast is removed down to the retromammary space. *Radical mastectomy,* a more extensive surgical procedure, involves removal of the breast, pectoral muscles, fat, fascia, and as many lymph nodes as possible in the axilla and pectoral region. In current practice, often only the tumor and surrounding tissues are removed—a *lumpectomy* or *quadrantectomy* (known as *breast-conserving surgery,* a wide local excision)—followed by radiation therapy (Goroll, 2005).

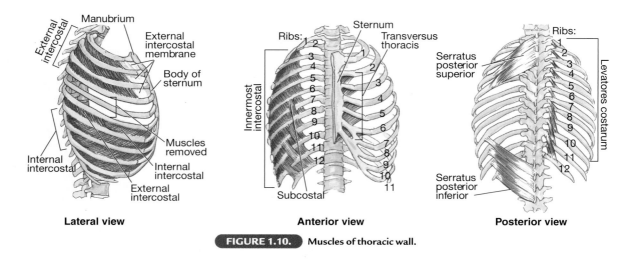

Lateral view   **Anterior view**   **Posterior view**

FIGURE 1.10. Muscles of thoracic wall.

TABLE 1.2 MUSCLES OF THORACIC WALL

Muscles	Superior Attachment	Inferior Attachment	Innervation	Main Action[a]
External intercostal	Inferior border of ribs	Superior border of ribs below	Intercostal nerve	During forced inspiration: elevate ribs
Internal intercostal				During forced inspiration: interosseous part depresses ribs; interchondral part elevates ribs
Innermost intercostal				
Transversus thoracis	Posterior surface of lower sternum	Internal surface of costal cartilages 2–6		Weakly depresses ribs
Subcostal	Internal surface of lower ribs near their angles	Superior borders of 2nd or 3rd ribs below		Probably act in same manner as internal intercostal muscles
Levatores costarum	Transverse processes of T7–T11	Subjacent ribs between tubercle and angle	Posterior rami of C8–T11 nerves	Elevate ribs
Serratus posterior superior	Nuchal ligament, spinous processes of C7–T3 vertebrae	Superior borders of 2nd–4th ribs	2nd–5th intercostal nerves	Elevate ribs[b]
Serratus posterior inferior	Spinous processes of T11–L2 vertebrae	Inferior borders of 8th–12th ribs near their angles	9th–11th intercostal nerves, subcostal (T12) nerve	Depress ribs[b]

[a]All intercostal muscles keep the intercostal spaces rigid, thereby preventing them from bulging out during expiration and from being drawn in during inspiration. The role of individual intercostal muscles and accessory muscles of respiration in moving the ribs is difficult to interpret, despite many electromyographic studies.

[b]Action traditionally assigned on the basis of attachments; these muscles appear to be largely proprioceptive in function.

enters the **bronchomediastinal trunks,** which ultimately drain into the thoracic or right lymphatic duct.

NERVES OF BREAST

The *nerves of the breasts* derive from the anterior and lateral cutaneous branches of the fourth to sixth intercostal nerves (see Fig. 1.11). These branches of the intercostal nerves pass through the deep pectoral fascia covering the pectoralis major to reach the skin. The branches thus convey sensory fibers to the skin of the breast and sympathetic fibers to the blood vessels in the breasts and smooth muscle in the overlying skin and nipple.

Muscles of Thoracic Wall

Several upper limb (axioappendicular) muscles attach to the thoracic cage: pectoralis major, pectoralis minor, serratus anterior anteriorly, and latissimus dorsi posteriorly. In addition, the anterolateral abdominal muscles and some neck and back muscles attach to the thoracic cage. The pectoralis major, the pectoralis minor, and the inferior part of the serratus anterior may also function as accessory muscles of respiration, helping expand the thoracic cavity when inspiration is deep and forceful. The scalene muscles, passing from the neck to the first and second ribs (see Chapter 8),

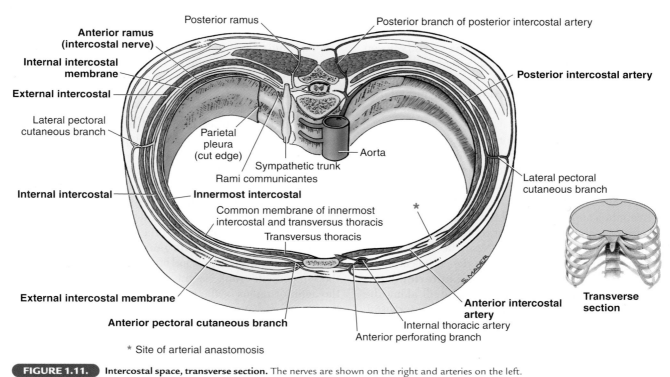

FIGURE 1.11. Intercostal space, transverse section. The nerves are shown on the right and arteries on the left.

also function as accessory respiratory muscles by fixing these ribs and enabling the muscles connecting the ribs below to be more effective in elevating the lower ribs during forced inspiration. The intercostal, transversus thoracis (continuous with the transversus abdominis), subcostal, levatores costarum, and serratus posterior are muscles of the thoracic wall (Fig. 1.10 and Table 1.2).

Typical intercostal spaces contain three layers of intercostal muscles (Figs. 1.11 and 1.12). The superficial layer is formed by the **external intercostal muscles** (fiber bundles oriented inferoanteriorly), the middle layer is formed by the **internal intercostal muscles** (fiber bundles oriented inferoposteriorly), and the deepest layer is formed by the **innermost intercostal muscles** (similar to internal intercostals). Anteriorly, the fleshy external intercostal muscles are replaced by **external intercostal membranes;** posteriorly, the fleshy internal intercostal muscles are replaced by **internal intercostal membranes.** The innermost intercostal muscles are found only at the most lateral parts of the intercostal spaces.

Nerves of Thoracic Wall

The thoracic wall has 12 pairs of thoracic spinal nerves. As they leave the IV foramina, they divide into anterior and posterior rami (Fig. 1.11). The anterior rami of T1–T11 form the **intercostal nerves** that run along the extent of the inter-

costal spaces. The anterior rami of the T12 nerves, inferior to the 12th ribs, form the **subcostal nerves** (see Chapter 3). The posterior rami of the thoracic spinal nerves pass posteriorly immediately lateral to the articular processes of the vertebrae to supply the bones, joints, deep back muscles, and skin of the back in the thoracic region.

Typical intercostal nerves (third through sixth) run initially along the posterior aspects of the intercostal spaces, between the parietal pleura (serous lining of the thoracic cavity) and the internal intercostal membrane. At first they

FIGURE 1.12. Contents of typical intercostal space. Remember the structures in the costal groove, from superior to inferior, as *VAN*, for vein, artery, and nerve.

run across the internal surface of the internal intercostal membrane and muscle near the middle of the intercostal space. Near the angles of the ribs, the nerves pass between the internal intercostal and innermost intercostal muscles (Figs. 1.12 and 1.13). Here the nerves pass to and then continue to course within the **costal grooves,** lying just inferior to the intercostal arteries, which in turn lie inferior to the intercostal veins.

Collateral branches of these nerves arise near the angles of the ribs and run along the superior border of the rib below. The nerves continue anteriorly between the internal and the innermost intercostal muscles, giving branches to these and other muscles and giving rise to **lateral cutaneous branches** approximately at the midaxillary line (Fig. 1.11). Anteriorly, the nerves appear on the internal surface of the internal intercostal muscle. Near the sternum, the nerves turn anteriorly, passing between the costal cartilages and entering the subcutaneous tissue as **anterior cutaneous branches.** *Muscular branches* arise all along the course of the intercostal nerves to supply the intercostal, subcostal, transversus thoracis, levatores costarum, and serratus posterior muscles (Table 1.2).

Atypical intercostal nerves are the first and second and seventh through eleventh. Intercostal nerves 1 and 2 pass on the internal surfaces of the first and second ribs instead of along the inferior margins of the costal grooves. After giving rise to the lateral cutaneous branches, the seventh through eleventh intercostal nerves continue to supply the abdominal skin and muscles.

Through the posterior ramus and the lateral and anterior cutaneous branches of the anterior ramus, each spinal nerve supplies a stripe-like area of skin extending from the posterior median line to the anterior median line. These band-like skin areas (**dermatomes**) are each supplied by the *sensory fibers* of a single posterior root through the posterior and anterior rami of its spinal nerve (Fig. 1.14). Because any particular area of skin usually receives innervation from two adjacent nerves, considerable *overlapping of adjacent dermatomes* occurs. Therefore, complete loss of sensation usually does not occur unless two or more intercostal nerves are anesthetized. The muscles supplied by the *motor fibers* of the posterior and anterior rami of each pair of thoracic spinal nerves constitute a **myotome** (Fig. 1.14).

Rami communicantes, or communicating branches, connect each intercostal and subcostal nerve to the ipsilateral **sympathetic trunk** (Fig. 1.13). Presynaptic fibers leave the initial portions of the anterior ramus of each thoracic (and upper lumbar) nerve by means of a white ramus communicans and pass to a **sympathetic ganglion.** Postsynaptic fibers distributed to the body wall and limbs pass from the ganglia of the sympathetic trunk via gray rami communicantes to join the anterior ramus of the nearest spinal nerve, including all the intercostal nerves. Sympathetic nerve fibers are distributed through the branches of all spinal nerves (anterior and posterior rami) to reach the blood vessels, sweat glands, and smooth muscle of the body wall and limbs.

Vasculature of Thoracic Wall

The **arteries of the thoracic wall** are derived from the **thoracic aorta** through the posterior intercostal and subcostal arteries, the **subclavian artery** through the internal thoracic and supreme intercostal arteries, and the **axillary artery** through the superior and lateral thoracic arteries (Figs. 1.11 and 1.15A; Table 1.3). With the exception of the tenth and eleventh intercostal spaces, each intercostal space

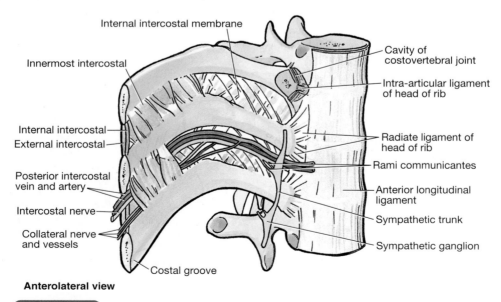

Anterolateral view

FIGURE 1.13. **Vertebral end of intercostal space.** Note the connection of the intercostal nerve to the sympathetic trunk by rami communicantes (communicating branches).

FIGURE 1.14. **Dermatomes and myotomes of the trunk.** Note the relationship between the area of skin (dermatome) and skeletal muscle (myotome) innervated by a spinal nerve or segment of the spinal cord. The dermatomes of the thorax are shown at the right.

is supplied by three arteries: a large posterior intercostal artery (and its collateral branch) and a small pair of anterior intercostal arteries.

The **veins of the thoracic wall** accompany the intercostal arteries and nerves and lie most superior in the costal grooves (Figs. 1.11 and 1.15*B*). There are 11 posterior intercostal veins and one subcostal vein on each side. The posterior intercostal veins anastomose with the anterior intercostal veins, tributaries of the internal thoracic veins. Most posterior intercostal veins end in the *azygos/hemiazygos venous system* (discussed later in this chapter), which conveys venous blood to the superior vena cava.

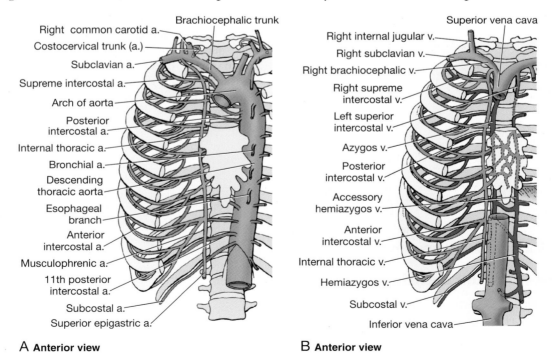

A **Anterior view**

B **Anterior view**

FIGURE 1.15. Arteries and veins of thoracic wall.

TABLE 1.3 ARTERIAL SUPPLY OF THORACIC WALL

Artery	Origin	Course	Distribution
Posterior intercostals	Supreme intercostal arteries (intercostal spaces 1 and 2) and thoracic aorta (remaining intercostal spaces)	Pass between internal and innermost intercostal muscles	Intercostal muscles and overlying skin, parietal pleura
Anterior intercostals	Internal thoracic arteries (intercostal spaces 1–6) and musculophrenic arteries (intercostal spaces 7–9)		
Internal thoracic	Subclavian artery	Passes inferiorly, lateral to sternum, between costal cartilages and internal intercostal muscles to divide into superior epigastric and musculophrenic arteries	By way of anterior intercostal arteries to intercostal spaces 1–6 and musculophrenic arteries to intercostal spaces 7–9
Subcostal	Thoracic aorta	Courses along interior border of 12th rib	Muscles of anterolateral abdominal wall and overlying skin

Herpes Zoster Infection

Herpes zoster **(shingles)**—a viral disease of spinal ganglia—is a *dermatomally distributed skin lesion.* The *herpes virus* invades a spinal ganglion and is transported along the axon to the skin, where it produces an infection that causes a sharp burning pain in the dermatome supplied by the involved nerve. A few days later, the skin of the dermatome becomes red and vesicular eruptions appear (Fig B1.5).

Herpes zoster

FIGURE B1.5. Herpes zoster.

Dyspnea—Difficult Breathing

When people with respiratory problems such as *asthma* or emphysema or with *heart failure* struggle to breathe, they use their accessory respiratory muscles to assist the expansion of their thoracic cavities. They typically lean on a table or their thighs to fix their pectoral girdles (clavicles and scapulae) so the muscles are able to act on their rib attachments and expand the thorax.

Intercostal Nerve Block

Local anesthesia of an intercostal space is produced by injecting a local anesthetic agent around the intercostal nerves. This procedure, an **intercostal nerve block,** involves infiltration of the anesthetic around the intercostal nerve and its collateral branches (Fig. B1.6). Because any particular area of skin usually receives innervation from two adjacent nerves, considerable overlapping of contiguous dermatomes occurs. Therefore, complete loss of sensation usually does not occur unless two or more intercostal nerves in adjacent intercostal spaces are anesthetized.

Lung

Intercostal nerve

Collateral branch

FIGURE B1.6. Intercostal nerve block.

Surface Anatomy of Thoracic Wall

Several bony landmarks and imaginary lines facilitate anatomical descriptions, identification of thoracic areas, and location of lesions such as a bullet wound:

- **Anterior median (midsternal) line** indicates the intersection of the median plane with the anterior thoracic wall (Fig. SA1.1A).

- **Midclavicular lines** pass through the midpoints of the clavicles, parallel to the anterior median line (Fig. SA1.1A).
- **Anterior axillary line** runs vertically along the anterior axillary fold, which is formed by the border of the pectoralis major as it spans from the thorax to the humerus (arm bone) (Fig. SA1.1B).

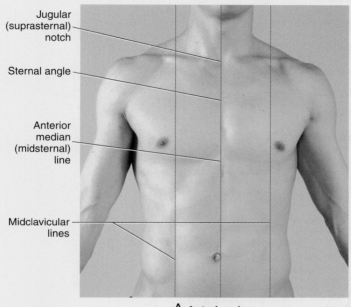

Jugular (suprasternal) notch

Sternal angle

Anterior median (midsternal) line

Midclavicular lines

A Anterior view

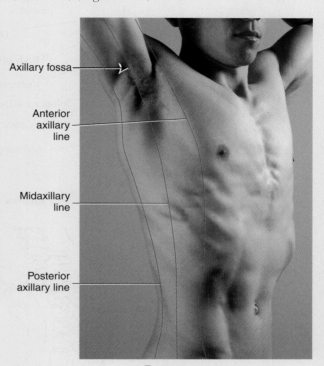

Axillary fossa

Anterior axillary line

Midaxillary line

Posterior axillary line

B Anterolateral view

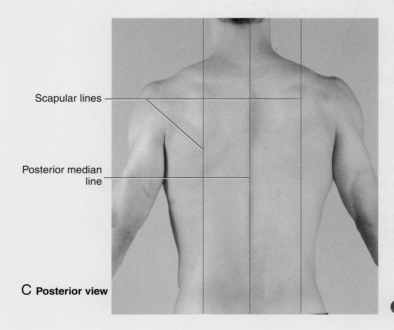

Scapular lines

Posterior median line

C Posterior view

FIGURE SA1.1.

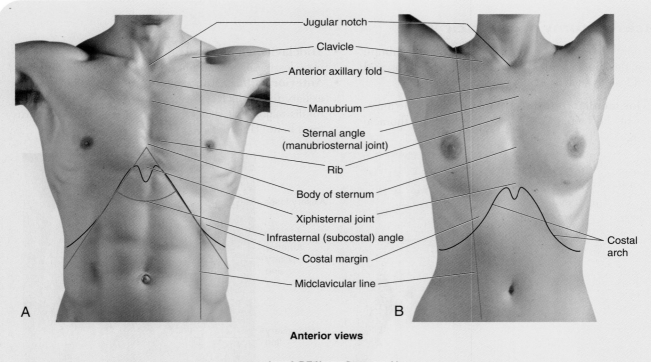

Jugular notch

Clavicle

Anterior axillary fold

Manubrium

Sternal angle
(manubriosternal joint)

Rib

Body of sternum

Xiphisternal joint

Infrasternal (subcostal) angle

Costal margin

Midclavicular line

Costal
arch

A   B

Anterior views

1st rib
Jugular notch
Arch of aorta
Manubrium
Sternal angle
(manubriosternal joint)

Body of sternum
Xiphisternal joint
Epigastric fossa
Xiphoid process
Diaphram
Heart

T2
T3
T4
T5
T6
T7
T8
T9

C   **Lateral view**

* Transverse thoracic plane

FIGURE SA1.2.

- **Midaxillary line** runs from the apex (deepest part) of the axilla, parallel to the anterior axillary line.
- **Posterior axillary line,** also parallel to the anterior axillary line, is drawn vertically along the posterior axillary fold formed by the latissimus dorsi and teres major muscles as they span from the back to the humerus (Fig. SA1.1*B*).

- **Posterior median (midvertebral) line** is a vertical line at the intersection of the median plane with the vertebral column. (Fig. SA1.1*C*).
- **Scapular lines** are parallel to the posterior median line and cross the inferior angles of the scapulae (Fig. SA1.1*C*).

Additional lines (not illustrated) are extrapolated along borders of bony formations—for example, the parasternal line (G. *para*, adjacent to).

The **clavicles** lie subcutaneously, forming bony ridges at the junction of the thorax and neck (Fig. SA1.2). They can be palpated easily throughout their length, especially where their medial ends articulate with the manubrium.

The **sternum** also lies subcutaneously in the anterior median line and is palpable throughout its length. The *manubrium of the sternum:*

- Lies at the level of the bodies of **T3 and T4 vertebrae**
- Is anterior to the **arch of the aorta**
- Has a **jugular notch** that can be palpated between the prominent sternal ends of the clavicles
- Has a **sternal angle** where it articulates with the sternal body at the level of the **T4–T5 IV disc** and the space between the third and fourth spinous processes

The **sternal angle** is a palpable landmark that lies at the level of the second pair of costal cartilages. The main bronchi pass inferolaterally from the bifurcation of the trachea at the level of the sternal angle. The sternal angle also demarcates the division between the superior and inferior mediastina and the beginning of the arch of the aorta. The **superior vena cava** passes inferiorly deep to the manubrium, projecting as much as a fingerbreadth to the right of this bone.

The first rib cannot be palpated because it lies deep to the clavicle; thus **count the ribs and intercostal spaces anteriorly** by sliding the fingers laterally from the sternal angle onto the second costal cartilage. Start counting with rib 2 and count the ribs and spaces by moving the fingers inferolaterally. The first intercostal space is inferior to the first rib; likewise, the other spaces lie inferior to the similarly numbered ribs.

The **body of the sternum** lies anterior to the right border of the heart and vertebrae T5–T9. The **xiphoid process** lies in a slight depression (the **epigastric fossa**) where the converging costal margins form the **infrasternal angle.** The **costal margins,** formed by the medial borders of the seventh through tenth costal cartilages, are easily palpable where they extend inferolaterally from the **xiphisternal**

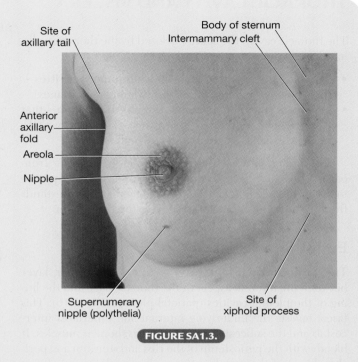

Site of axillary tail

Body of sternum
Intermammary cleft

Anterior axillary fold

Areola

Nipple

Supernumerary nipple (polythelia)

Site of xiphoid process

FIGURE SA1.3.

joint. This articulation, often seen as a ridge, is at the level of the inferior border of the T9 vertebra.

Breasts are the most prominent surface features of the anterior thoracic wall, especially in women. Their flattened superior surfaces show no sharp demarcation from the anterior surface of the thoracic wall; however, laterally and inferiorly their borders are well defined (Fig. SA1.3). The anterior median **intermammary cleft** is the cleavage the between the breasts. The **nipple** in the midclavicular line is surrounded by a slightly raised and circular pigmented area—the **areola.** The color of the areolas varies with the woman's complexion; they darken during pregnancy and retain this color thereafter. The nipple in men lies anterior to the fourth intercostal space, about 10 cm from the anterior median line. The position of the nipple in women is inconstant and so is not reliable as a surface landmark.

THORACIC CAVITY AND VISCERA

The thoracic cavity, the space enclosed by the thoracic walls, has three compartments (Fig. 1.16A):

- Two lateral compartments—the **pulmonary cavities**—that contain the lungs and pleurae (lining membranes).
- One central compartment—the **mediastinum**—that contains all other thoracic structures: heart, great vessels, trachea, esophagus, thymus, and lymph nodes.

The pulmonary cavities are completely separate from each other and, with the lungs and pleurae, occupy the majority of the thoracic cavity. The mediastinum extends from the superior thoracic aperture to the diaphragm.

Endothoracic Fascia

The **endothoracic fascia** is a thin fibroareolar layer between the internal aspect of the thoracic cage and the lining of the pleural cavities (parietal pleura) (Fig. 1.16). This fascia invests the underlying internal and innermost intercostals and the subcostal and transversus thoracis muscles. It blends with the periosteum of the ribs and sternum and perichondrium of the costal cartilages. The endothoracic fascia provides a cleavage plane, allowing the surgeon to separate the parietal pleura from the thoracic wall, providing access to intrathoracic structures.

Pleurae and Lungs

To visualize the relationship of the pleurae and lungs, push your fist into an underinflated balloon (Fig. 1.16A). The part of the balloon wall adjacent to the skin of your fist (which represents the lung) is comparable to the *visceral pleura;* the remainder of the balloon represents the *parietal pleura.* The cavity between the layers of the balloon is analogous to the *pleural cavity.* At your wrist (*root of lung*), the inner and outer walls of the balloon are continuous, as are the visceral and parietal layers of pleura, together forming a *pleural sac.* Note that the lung is outside of but surrounded by the pleural sac, just as your fist is surrounded by but outside of the balloon.

PLEURAE

Each lung is invested by and enclosed in a serous **pleural sac** that consists of two continuous membranes—the pleurae (Fig. 1.16):

- The **visceral pleura** (pulmonary pleura) covers the lungs and is adherent to all its surfaces, including the surfaces within the horizontal and oblique fissures; it cannot be dissected from the lungs.

- The **parietal pleura** lines the pulmonary cavities, adhering to the thoracic wall, the mediastinum, and the diaphragm.

The **root of the lung** is enclosed within the area of continuity between the visceral and parietal layers of pleura, the **pleural sleeve.** Inferior to the root of the lung, this continuity between parietal and visceral pleura forms the **pulmonary ligament** extending between the lung and the mediastinum (Fig. 1.17).

The **pleural cavity**—the potential space between the visceral and the parietal layers of pleura—contains a capillary layer of **serous pleural fluid,** which lubricates the pleural surfaces and allows the layers of pleura to slide smoothly over each other during respiration. Its surface tension also provides the cohesion that keeps the lung surface in contact with the thoracic wall. Consequently, the lung expands and fills with air when the thorax expands while still allowing sliding to occur, much like a layer of water between two glass plates.

The *parietal pleura* consists of four parts (Fig. 1.16):

- **Costal part** covers the internal surfaces of the thoracic wall (sternum, ribs, costal cartilages, intercostal muscles and membranes, and sides of thoracic vertebrae) and is separated from the wall by *endothoracic fascia.*
- **Mediastinal part** covers the lateral aspects of the mediastinum (the central compartment of the thoracic cavity).
- **Diaphragmatic part** covers the superior or thoracic surface of the diaphragm on each side of the mediastinum.
- **Cervical pleura** extends through the superior thoracic aperture into the root of the neck 2 to 3 cm superior to the level of the medial third of the clavicle at the level of the neck of the first rib. It forms a cup-shaped dome over the apex of the lung and is reinforced by a fibrous extension of the endothoracic fascia, the *suprapleural membrane* (Sibson fascia) spanning between the first rib and C7 vertebra.

The relatively abrupt lines along which the parietal pleura changes direction from one wall of the pleural cavity to another are the **lines of pleural reflection.**

- The **sternal line of pleural reflection** is sharp or abrupt and occurs where the costal pleura becomes continuous with the mediastinal pleura anteriorly.
- The **costal line of pleural reflection** is also sharp and occurs where the costal pleura becomes continuous with the diaphragmatic pleura inferiorly.
- The **vertebral line of pleural reflection** is a much rounder, gradual reflection where the costal pleura becomes continuous with the mediastinal pleura posteriorly.

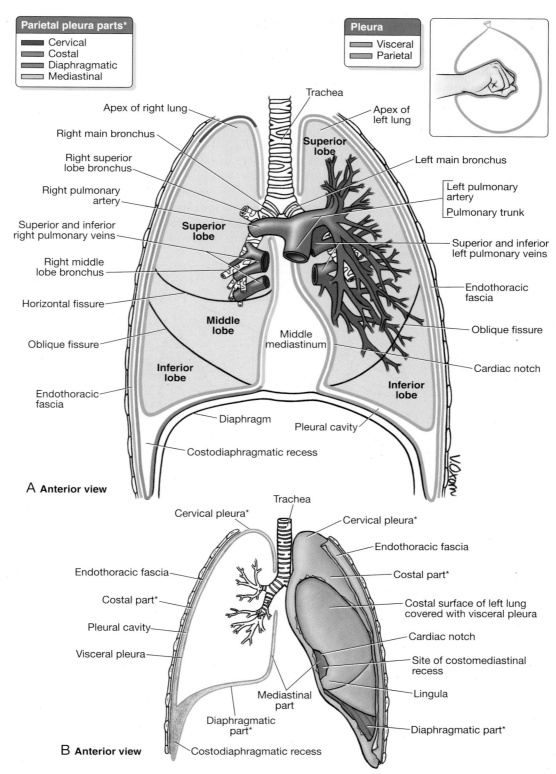

Parietal pleura parts*
- ■ Cervical
- ■ Costal
- ■ Diaphragmatic
- ■ Mediastinal

Pleura
- ■ Visceral
- ■ Parietal

A **Anterior view**

- Trachea
- Apex of right lung
- Apex of left lung
- Right main bronchus
- **Superior lobe**
- Right superior lobe bronchus
- Left main bronchus
- Right pulmonary artery
- Left pulmonary artery
- Pulmonary trunk
- Superior and inferior right pulmonary veins
- **Superior lobe**
- Superior and inferior left pulmonary veins
- Right middle lobe bronchus
- Endothoracic fascia
- Horizontal fissure
- **Middle lobe**
- Oblique fissure
- Oblique fissure
- Middle mediastinum
- Cardiac notch
- **Inferior lobe**
- **Inferior lobe**
- Endothoracic fascia
- Diaphragm
- Pleural cavity
- Costodiaphragmatic recess

B **Anterior view**

- Trachea
- Cervical pleura*
- Cervical pleura*
- Endothoracic fascia
- Endothoracic fascia
- Costal part*
- Costal part*
- Costal surface of left lung covered with visceral pleura
- Pleural cavity
- Cardiac notch
- Visceral pleura
- Site of costomediastinal recess
- Mediastinal part
- Lingula
- Diaphragmatic part*
- Diaphragmatic part*
- Costodiaphragmatic recess

FIGURE 1.16. **Lungs and pleurae. A.** Lungs and pleural cavity. *Inset:* A fist invaginating an underinflated balloon demonstrates the relationship of the lung (represented by fist) to the walls of the pleural sac (parietal and visceral layers of pleura). The cavity of the pleural sac (pleural cavity) is comparable to the cavity of the balloon. **B.** Parts of parietal pleura and recesses of pleural cavities. Asterisks (*) indicate parts of parietal pleura.

Surface Anatomy of Pleurae and Lungs

The cervical pleurae and apices of the lungs pass through the superior thoracic aperture into the root of the neck superior and posterior to the clavicles. The anterior borders of the lungs lie adjacent to the anterior line of reflection of the parietal pleura between the second and fourth costal cartilages (Fig SA1.4). Here the margin of the left pleural reflection moves laterally and then inferiorly at the cardiac notch to reach the level of the sixth costal cartilage. The anterior border of the left lung is more deeply indented by its cardiac notch. On the right side, the pleural reflection continues inferiorly from the fourth to the sixth costal cartilage, paralleled closely by the anterior border of the right lung. Both pleural reflections pass laterally and reach the midclavicular line at the level of the eighth costal cartilage, the tenth rib at the midaxillary line, and the twelfth rib at the scapular line, proceeding toward the spinous process of the T12 vertebra. Thus the parietal pleura extends approximately two ribs inferior to the lung. The *oblique fissure of the lungs* extends from the level of the spinous process of the T2 vertebra posteriorly to the sixth costal cartilage anteriorly, which coincides approximately with the medial border of the scapula when the upper limb is elevated above the head (causing the inferior angle to be rotated laterally). The *horizontal fissure of the right lung* extends from the oblique fissure along the fourth rib and costal cartilage anteriorly.

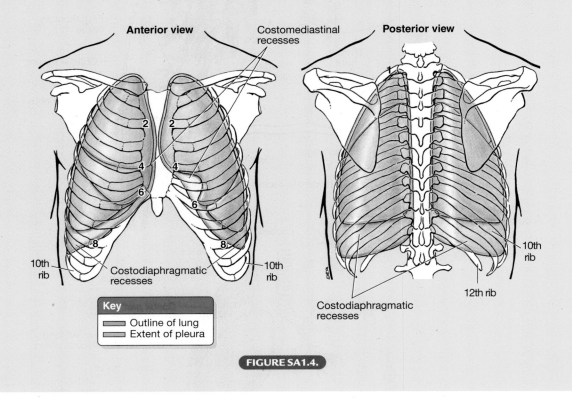

FIGURE SA1.4.

The lungs do not completely occupy the pleural cavities during expiration; thus, the peripheral diaphragmatic pleura is in contact with the lowest part of the costal pleura. The potential pleural spaces here are the **costodiaphragmatic recesses,** the pleural-lined "gutters" that surround the upward convexity of the diaphragm inside the thoracic wall (Fig. 1.16). Similar but smaller pleural recesses are located posterior to the sternum where the costal pleura is in contact with the mediastinal pleura. The potential spaces here are the **costomediastinal recesses** (Fig. 1.16B); the left recess is potentially larger (less occupied) because of the cardiac notch in the left lung. The inferior borders of the lungs move farther into the pleural recesses during deep inspiration and retreat from them during expiration.

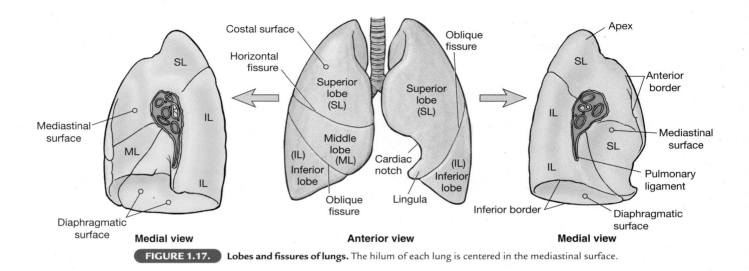

FIGURE 1.17. **Lobes and fissures of lungs.** The hilum of each lung is centered in the mediastinal surface.

LUNGS

The **lungs** are the vital organs of respiration. Their main function is to oxygenate the blood by bringing inspired air into close relation with the venous blood in the pulmonary capillaries. Although cadaveric lungs may be shrunken, firm to the touch, and discolored in appearance, healthy lungs in living people are normally light, soft, and spongy. They are also elastic and recoil to about one-third their size when the thoracic cavity is opened.

The **horizontal and oblique fissures** divide the lungs into lobes (Fig 1.16). *The right lung has three lobes, the left lung has two.* The right lung is larger and heavier than the left, but it is shorter and wider because the right dome of the diaphragm is higher and the heart and pericardium bulge more to the left. The anterior margin of the right lung is relatively straight, whereas this margin of the left lung has a **cardiac notch.** The cardiac notch primarily indents the anteroinferior aspect of the superior lobe of the left lung. This often creates a thin, tongue-like process of the superior lobe—the **lingula** (Fig. 1.17), which extends below the cardiac notch and slides in and out of the costomediastinal recess during inspiration and expiration. Each lung has (Figs. 1.17 and 1.18):

- **An apex:** blunt superior end of the lung ascending above the level of the first rib into the root of the neck; covered by cervical pleura
- **Three surfaces:** *costal surface,* adjacent to the sternum, costal cartilages, and ribs; *mediastinal surface,* including the hilum of the lung and related medially to the mediastinum and posteriorly to the sides of the vertebrae; and *diaphragmatic surface,* resting on the convex dome of the diaphragm
- **Three borders:** *anterior border,* where the costal and mediastinal surfaces meet anteriorly and overlap the heart

(the *cardiac notch* indents this border of the left lung); *inferior border,* which circumscribes the diaphragmatic surface of the lung and separates the diaphragmatic surface from the costal and mediastinal surfaces; and *posterior border,* where the costal and mediastinal surfaces meet posteriorly (it is broad and rounded and lies adjacent to the thoracic region of the vertebral column)

The **root of the lung** is formed by the structures entering and emerging from the lung at its hilum (Figs. 1.17 and 1.18). The root of the lung connects the lung with the heart and trachea. If the root is sectioned before the branching of the main bronchus and pulmonary artery, its general arrangement is:

- Pulmonary artery, superiormost on the left (the superior lobar bronchus may be superiormost on the right)
- Superior and inferior pulmonary veins, anteriormost and inferiormost, respectively
- Bronchus, against and approximately in the middle of the posterior boundary, with bronchial vessels immediately surrounding

The root is enclosed within the area of continuity between the parietal and the visceral layers of pleura—the *pleural sleeve* (Fig. 1.18A) or mesopneumonium (mesentery of the lung). The *hilum of the lung* is the area on the medial surface of each lung at the point at which the structures forming the root—the main bronchus, pulmonary vessels, bronchial vessels, lymphatic vessels, and nerves—enter and leave the lung.

TRACHEA AND BRONCHI

The two **main bronchi** (primary bronchi), one to each lung, pass inferolaterally from the **bifurcation of the trachea,** at the level of the sternal angle, to the hila of the lungs

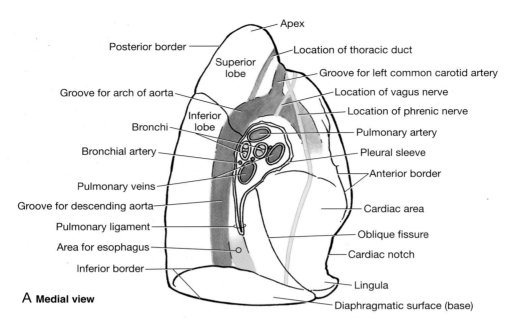

A **Medial view**

Apex
Posterior border
Location of thoracic duct
Superior lobe
Groove for left common carotid artery
Groove for arch of aorta
Location of vagus nerve
Location of phrenic nerve
Inferior lobe
Bronchi
Pulmonary artery
Bronchial artery
Pleural sleeve
Pulmonary veins
Anterior border
Groove for descending aorta
Cardiac area
Pulmonary ligament
Oblique fissure
Area for esophagus
Cardiac notch
Inferior border
Lingula
Diaphragmatic surface (base)

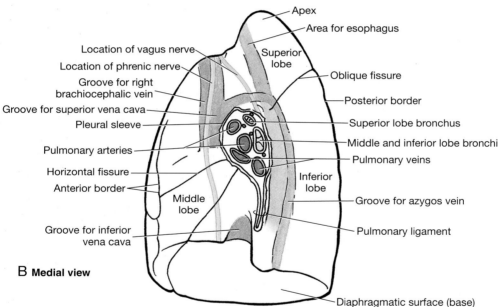

B **Medial view**

Apex
Area for esophagus
Location of vagus nerve
Superior lobe
Location of phrenic nerve
Oblique fissure
Groove for right brachiocephalic vein
Posterior border
Groove for superior vena cava
Superior lobe bronchus
Pleural sleeve
Middle and inferior lobe bronchi
Pulmonary arteries
Pulmonary veins
Horizontal fissure
Anterior border
Inferior lobe
Middle lobe
Groove for azygos vein
Groove for inferior vena cava
Pulmonary ligament
Diaphragmatic surface (base)

FIGURE 1.18. **Mediastinal surfaces of lungs.** Both the left (**A**) and right (**B**) lungs are shown. Observe the somewhat pear-shaped depression, the hilum (doorway) of the lung, near the center of this surface. Embalmed lungs have impressions of the structures in contact with them (e.g., aorta and superior vena cava).

(Figs. 1.19*E* and 1.20*A,B*). The walls of the trachea and bronchi are supported by C-shaped rings of hyaline cartilage.

- The **right main bronchus** is wider and shorter and runs more vertically than the left main bronchus as it passes directly to the hilum of the right lung.
- The **left main bronchus** passes inferolaterally, inferior to the arch of the aorta and anterior to the esophagus and thoracic aorta, to reach the hilum of the left lung.

The main bronchi enter the hila of the lungs and branch in a constant fashion within the lungs to form the **bronchial tree.** Each main bronchus divides into **lobar bronchi** (secondary bronchi), two on the left and three on the right, each of which supplies a lobe of the lung. Each lobar bronchus divides into **segmental bronchi** (tertiary bronchi) that supply the bronchopulmonary segments (Fig. 1.19). Each **bronchopulmonary segment** is pyramidal, with its apex

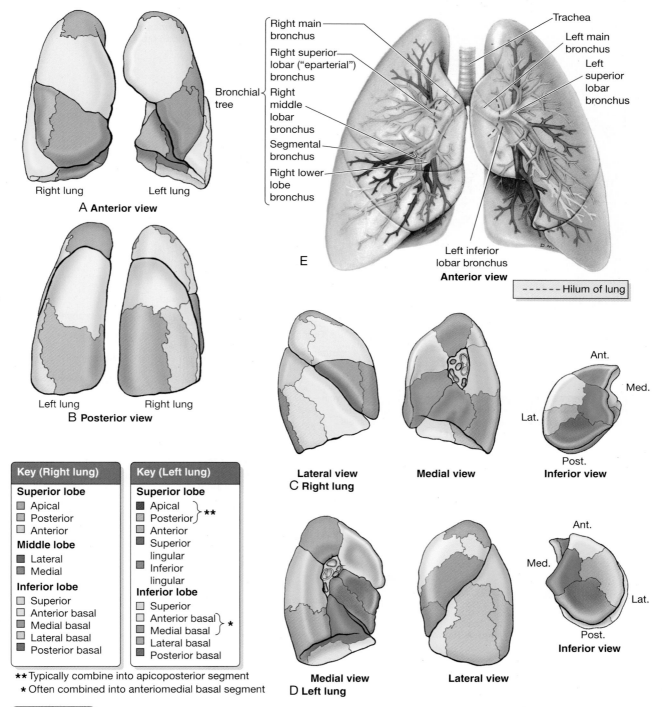

Right lung

Left lung

A **Anterior view**

Bronchial tree

Right main bronchus

Right superior lobar ("eparterial") bronchus

Right middle lobe bronchus

Segmental bronchus

Right lower lobe bronchus

Trachea

Left main bronchus

Left superior lobar bronchus

Left inferior lobar bronchus

E

Anterior view

- - - - - - Hilum of lung

Left lung

Right lung

B **Posterior view**

Lateral view

Medial view

Ant.

Med.

Lat.

Post.

Inferior view

C **Right lung**

Key (Right lung)

Superior lobe
☐ Apical
☐ Posterior
☐ Anterior

Middle lobe
☐ Lateral
☐ Medial

Inferior lobe
☐ Superior
☐ Anterior basal
☐ Medial basal
☐ Lateral basal
☐ Posterior basal

Key (Left lung)

Superior lobe
☐ Apical ⎫
☐ Posterior ⎭ ✶✶
☐ Anterior
☐ Superior lingular
☐ Inferior lingular

Inferior lobe
☐ Superior
☐ Anterior basal ⎫
☐ Medial basal ⎭ ✶
☐ Lateral basal
☐ Posterior basal

✶✶ Typically combine into apicoposterior segment
✶ Often combined into anteriomedial basal segment

Medial view

Lateral view

Ant.

Med.

Lat.

Post.

Inferior view

D **Left lung**

FIGURE 1.19.   **Bronchi and bronchopulmonary segments. A.** The segmental (tertiary) bronchi are indicated by colors (see key). The bronchopulmonary segments of the left (**B**) and right (**C**) lungs are identified.

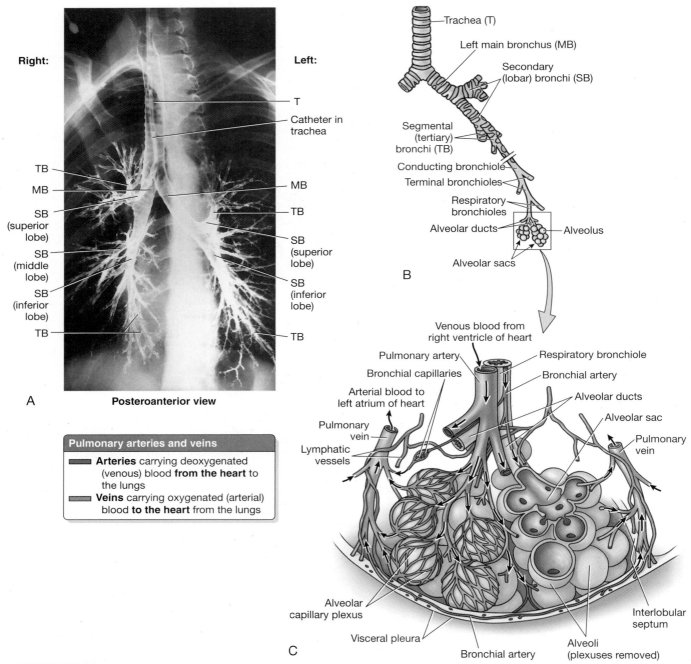

Right:

Left:

T

Catheter in
trachea

TB

MB

SB
(superior
lobe)

SB
(middle
lobe)

SB
(inferior
lobe)

TB

MB

TB

SB
(superior
lobe)

SB
(inferior
lobe)

TB

A

Posteroanterior view

Pulmonary arteries and veins
▬▬ **Arteries** carrying deoxygenated (venous) blood **from the heart** to the lungs
▬▬ **Veins** carrying oxygenated (arterial) blood **to the heart** from the lungs

Trachea (T)

Left main bronchus (MB)

Secondary
(lobar) bronchi (SB)

Segmental
(tertiary)
bronchi (TB)

Conducting bronchiole

Terminal bronchioles

Respiratory
bronchioles

Alveolar ducts

Alveolus

Alveolar sacs

B

Venous blood from
right ventricle of heart

Pulmonary artery

Respiratory bronchiole

Bronchial capillaries

Bronchial artery

Arterial blood to
left atrium of heart

Alveolar ducts

Pulmonary
vein

Alveolar sac

Lymphatic
vessels

Pulmonary
vein

Alveolar
capillary plexus

Interlobular
septum

Visceral pleura

Alveoli
(plexuses removed)

C

Bronchial artery

FIGURE 1.20. **Internal structure of lungs. A.** Bronchogram. Slightly oblique, posteroanterior bronchogram of right and left bronchial tree.
B. Subdivisions of bronchial tree. **C.** Alveoli.

directed toward the root of the lung and its base at the pleural surface, and is named according to the segmental bronchus that supplies it.

Each bronchopulmonary segment is supplied independently by a segmental bronchus and a tertiary branch of the pulmonary artery and is drained by intersegmental parts of the pulmonary veins. Beyond the segmental bronchi, there

are 20 to 25 generations of branches that end in **terminal bronchioles** (Fig. 1.20). Each terminal bronchiole gives rise to several generations of **respiratory bronchioles** and each respiratory bronchiole provides 2 to 11 **alveolar ducts,** each of which gives rise to 5 or 6 **alveolar sacs.** The **pulmonary alveolus** is the basic structural unit of gas exchange in the lung.

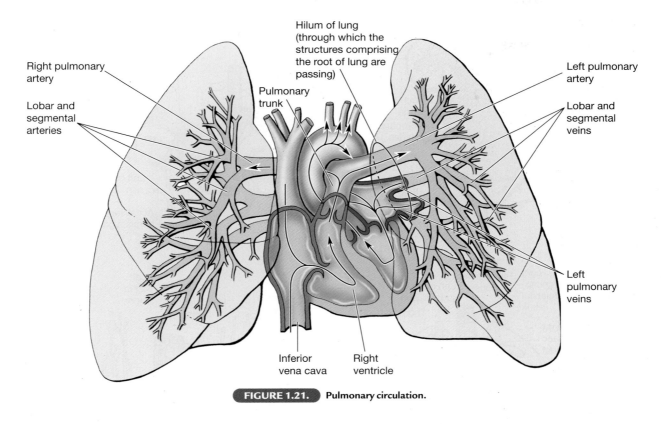

Right pulmonary artery

Lobar and segmental arteries

Hilum of lung (through which the structures comprising the root of lung are passing)

Pulmonary trunk

Left pulmonary artery

Lobar and segmental veins

Left pulmonary veins

Inferior vena cava

Right ventricle

FIGURE 1.21. Pulmonary circulation.

VASCULATURE AND NERVES OF LUNGS AND PLEURAE

Each lung has a large **pulmonary artery** supplying blood to it and two **pulmonary veins** draining blood from it (Fig. 1.21). The right and left pulmonary arteries arise from the **pulmonary trunk** at the level of the sternal angle. The **pulmonary arteries** carry poorly oxygenated ("venous") blood to the lungs for oxygenation. The pulmonary arteries pass to the corresponding root of the lung and give off a branch to the superior lobe before entering the hilum. Within the lung, each artery descends posterolateral to the main bronchus and divides into **lobar** and **segmental arteries.** Consequently, an arterial branch goes to each lobe and bronchopulmonary segment of the lung, usually on the anterior aspect of the corresponding bronchus. The **pulmonary veins,** two on each side, carry well-oxygenated ("arterial") blood from the lungs to the left atrium of the heart. Beginning in the pulmonary capillaries, the veins unite into larger and larger vessels. Intrasegmental veins drain blood from adjacent bronchopulmonary segments into the intersegmental veins in the septa, which separate the segments. A main vein drains each bronchopulmonary segment, usually on the anterior surface of the corresponding bronchus.

The veins from the parietal pleura join the systemic veins in adjacent parts of the thoracic wall. The veins from the visceral pleura drain into the pulmonary veins.

The **bronchial arteries** supply blood to the structures making up the root of the lungs, the supporting tissues of the lung, and the visceral pleura (Figs. 1.18 and 1.22A). The left bronchial arteries arise from the thoracic aorta; however, the right bronchial artery may arise from:

- A superior posterior intercostal artery.
- A common trunk from the thoracic aorta with the right third posterior intercostal artery.
- A left superior bronchial artery.

The small bronchial arteries provide branches to the superior esophagus and then pass along the posterior aspects of the main bronchi, supplying them and their branches as far distally as the respiratory bronchioles. The most distal branches of the bronchial arteries anastomose with branches of the pulmonary arteries in the walls of the bronchioles and in the visceral pleura.

The **bronchial veins** drain only part of the blood supplied to the lungs by the bronchial arteries, primarily that distributed to or near the more proximal part of the root of the lungs (Fig. 1.22B). The remainder of the blood is drained by the pulmonary veins. The right bronchial vein drains into the **azygos vein,** and the left bronchial vein drains into the **accessory hemiazygos vein** or the left superior intercostal vein.

The **lymphatic plexuses in the lungs** communicate freely (Fig. 1.22C).

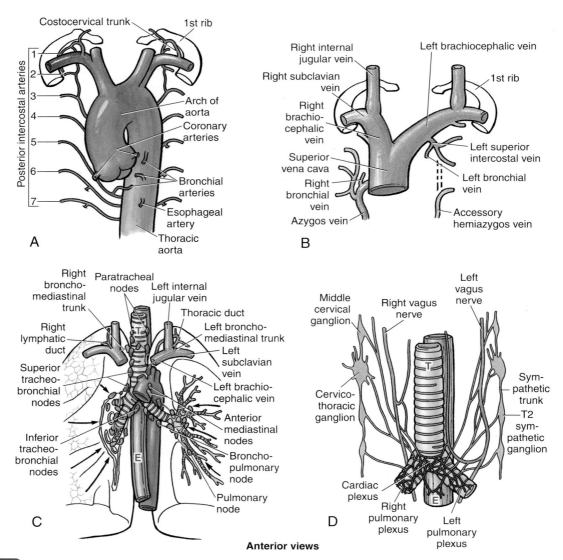

FIGURE 1.22. **Vasculature and nerves of lungs and pleurae. A.** Arteries. **B.** Veins. **C.** Lymphatic drainage. *Arrows* indicate the direction of lymph flow; those on the right show flow from superficial pulmonary lymphatic plexuses, and those on the left indicate flow from deep pulmonary plexuses. **D.** Innervation. *E,* esophagus; *T,* trachea; *orange,* sympathetic; *green,* parasympathetic; *blue,* plexus.

The **superficial lymphatic plexus** lies deep to the visceral pleura and drains the lung parenchyma (tissue) and visceral pleura. Lymphatic vessels from the plexus drain into the **bronchopulmonary (hilar) lymph nodes** in the hilum of the lung.

The **deep lymphatic plexus** is located in the submucosa of the bronchi and in the peribronchial connective tissue. It is largely concerned with draining structures that form the root of the lung. Lymphatic vessels from this plexus drain into the **pulmonary lymph nodes** located along the lobar bronchi. At the hilum of the lung, they drain into bronchopulmonary (hilar) lymph nodes (Fig 1.22C).

Lymph from the superficial and deep plexuses drains from the bronchopulmonary lymph nodes to the superior and inferior **tracheobronchial lymph nodes**, superior and inferior to the bifurcation of the trachea, respectively.

Lymph from the tracheobronchial lymph nodes passes to the **right** and **left bronchomediastinal lymph trunks.** These trunks usually terminate on each side at the *venous angles* (junction of the subclavian and internal jugular veins); however, the right bronchomediastinal trunk may first merge with other lymphatic trunks, converging here to form the **right lymphatic duct.** The left bronchomediastinal trunk may terminate in the **thoracic duct**. The superficial (subpleural) lymphatic plexus drains lymph from the *visceral pleura*. Lymph from the *parietal pleura* drains into the lymph nodes of the thoracic wall (intercostal, parasternal, mediastinal, and phrenic). A few lymphatic vessels from the cervical pleura drain into the axillary lymph nodes.

The **nerves of the lungs and visceral pleura** derive from the pulmonary plexuses located anterior and (mainly) posterior to the roots of the lungs (Fig. 1.22*D*). These nerve networks contain parasympathetic fibers from the **vagus nerves** (CN X) and sympathetic fibers from the sympathetic trunks. *Parasympathetic ganglion cells*—cell bodies of postsynaptic parasympathetic neurons—are in the **pulmonary plexuses** and along the branches of the bronchial tree. The parasympathetic fibers from CN X are motor to the smooth muscle of the bronchial tree (*bronchoconstrictor*), inhibitory to the pulmonary vessels (*vasodilator*), and secretory to the glands of the bronchial tree (*secretomotor*). The visceral afferent fibers of CN X are distributed to the:

- Bronchial mucosa and are probably concerned with tactile sensation for cough reflexes.

- Bronchial muscles, possibly involved in stretch reception.
- Interalveolar connective tissue, in association with Hering–Breuer reflexes (mechanism that tends to limit respiratory excursions).
- Pulmonary arteries serving pressor receptors (blood pressure) and pulmonary veins serving chemoreceptors (blood gas levels).

Sympathetic ganglion cells—cell bodies of postsynaptic sympathetic neurons—are in the **paravertebral sympathetic ganglia** of the sympathetic trunks. The sympathetic fibers are inhibitory to the bronchial muscle (bronchodilator), motor to the pulmonary vessels (vasoconstrictor), and inhibitory to the alveolar glands of the bronchial tree.

Pulmonary Collapse

If a sufficient amount of air enters the pleural cavity, the surface tension adhering visceral to parietal pleura (lung to thoracic wall) is broken, and the lung collapses because of its inherent elasticity (elastic recoil). When a lung collapses, the pleural cavity—normally a potential space (Fig. B1.7, *purple*)—becomes a real space. The pleural cavity is located between the parietal pleura (*blue*) and the visceral pleura (*red*). One lung may be collapsed after surgery, for example, without collapsing the other because the pleural sacs are separate.

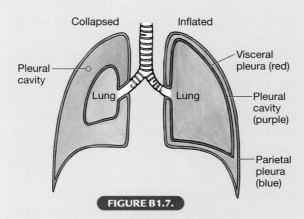

Collapsed   Inflated

Pleural cavity

Lung   Lung

Visceral pleura (red)

Pleural cavity (purple)

Parietal pleura (blue)

FIGURE B1.7.

Pneumothorax, Hydrothorax, Hemothorax, and Chylothorax

Entry of air into the pleural cavity—*pneumothorax*—resulting from a penetrating wound of the parietal pleura or rupture of a lung from a bullet, for example, results in partial collapse of the lung. Fractured ribs may also tear the parietal pleura and produce pneumothorax. This may also occur as a result of leakage from the lung through an opening in the visceral pleura. The accumulation of a significant amount of fluid in the pleural cavity—*hydrothorax*—may result from *pleural effusion* (escape of fluid into the pleural cavity). With a chest wound, blood may also enter the pleural cavity (*hemothorax*); this condition results more often from injury to a major intercostal vessel than from laceration of a lung. Lymph from a torn thoracic duct may also enter the pleural cavity (*chylothorax*). Chyle is a pale white or yellow lymph fluid in the thoracic duct containing fat absorbed by the intestines (see Chapter 2).

Pleuritis

During inspiration and expiration, the normally moist, smooth pleurae make no sound detectable by *auscultation* (listening to breath sounds); however, inflammation of the pleurae—*pleuritis* (pleurisy)—makes the lung surfaces rough. The resulting friction (*pleural rub*) may be heard with a stethoscope. Acute pleuritis is marked by sharp, stabbing pain, especially on exertion, such as climbing stairs, when the rate and depth of respiration may be increased even slightly.

Variation in Lobes of Lungs

Occasionally, an extra fissure divides a lung or a fissure is absent. For example, the left lung sometimes has three lobes and the right lung only two. The most common "accessory" lobe is the *azygos lobe,* which appears in the right lung in approximately 1% of people. In these cases, the azygos vein arches over the apex of the right lung and not over the right hilum, isolating the medial part of the apex as an azygos lobe.

Thoracentesis

 Sometimes it is necessary to insert a hypodermic needle through an intercostal space into the pleural cavity to obtain a sample of pleural fluid or to remove blood or pus. To avoid damage to the intercostal nerve and vessels, the needle is inserted superior to the rib, high enough to avoid the collateral branches (Fig. B1.8).

FIGURE B1.8. Technique for thoracentesis.

Auscultation and Percussion of Lungs

 Auscultation of the lungs (assessing air flow through the tracheobronchial tree into the lung with a stethoscope) and *percussion of the lungs* (tapping the chest over the lungs with the finger) always includes the root of the neck to detect sounds in the apices of the lungs. Percussion helps establish whether the underlying tissues are air-filled (resonant sound), fluid-filled (dull sound), or solid (flat sound). When physicians refer to the base of a lung, they are usually not referring to its diaphragmatic surface (base); rather, they are referring to the inferior part of the posterior costal surface of the inferior lobe. To auscultate this area, physicians apply a stethoscope to the inferoposterior aspect of the thoracic wall at the level of the T10 vertebra.

Aspiration of Foreign Bodies

 Because the right bronchus is wider and shorter and runs more vertically than the left bronchus, aspirated foreign bodies are more likely to enter and lodge in it or one of its branches. A potential hazard encountered by dentists is an aspirated foreign body, such as a piece of tooth or

filling material. Such objects are also most likely to enter the right main bronchus.

Lung Resections

 Knowledge of the anatomy of the bronchopulmonary segments is essential for precise interpretations of diagnostic images of the lungs and for surgical resection (removal) of diseased segments. When resecting a bronchopulmonary segment, surgeons follow the interlobar veins to pass between the segments. Bronchial and pulmonary disorders such as tumors or abscesses (collections of pus) often localize in a bronchopulmonary segment, which may be surgically resected. During the treatment of lung cancer, the surgeon may remove a whole lung (*pneumonectomy*), a lobe (*lobectomy*), or one or more bronchopulmonary segments (*segmentectomy*). Knowledge and understanding of the bronchopulmonary segments and their relationship to the bronchial tree are also essential for planning drainage and clearance techniques used in physical therapy for enhancing drainage from specific areas (e.g., in patients with pneumonia or cystic fibrosis).

Injury to Pleurae

 The *visceral pleura* is insensitive to pain because its innervation is autonomic (motor and visceral afferent). The autonomic nerves reach the visceral pleura in company with the bronchial vessels. The visceral pleura receives no nerves of general sensation.

In contrast, the *parietal pleura* is sensitive to pain, particularly the costal pleura, because it is richly supplied by branches of the somatic intercostal and phrenic nerves. Irritation of the parietal pleura produces local pain and referred pain to the areas sharing innervation by the same segments of the spinal cord. Irritation of the costal and peripheral parts of the diaphragmatic pleura results in local pain and referred pain along the intercostal nerves to the thoracic and abdominal walls. Irritation of the mediastinal and central diaphragmatic areas of the parietal pleura results in pain that is referred to the root of the neck and over the shoulder (C3–C5 dermatomes).

Thoracoscopy

Thoracoscopy is a diagnostic and sometimes therapeutic procedure in which the pleural cavity is examined with a thoracoscope (Fig. B1.9). Small incisions are made into the pleural cavity via an intercostal space. In addition to

Monitor showing excision of pleura (pleurectomy)

FIGURE B1.9. Pleurectomy.

observation, biopsies can be taken and some thoracic conditions can be treated (e.g., disrupting adhesions or removing plaques).

Pulmonary Embolism

 Obstruction of a pulmonary artery by a *blood clot* (*embolus*) is a common cause of morbidity (sickness) and mortality (death). An embolus in a pulmonary artery forms when a blood clot, fat globule, or air bubble travels in the blood to the lungs from a leg vein. The **embolus** passes through the right side of the heart to a lung through a pulmonary artery. The embolus may block a pulmonary artery—*pulmonary embolism*—or one of its branches. The immediate result is partial or complete obstruction of blood flow to the lung. The obstruction results in a sector of lung that is ventilated but not perfused with blood. When a large embolus occludes a pulmonary artery, the person suffers *acute respiratory distress* because of a major decrease in the oxygenation of blood owing to blockage of blood flow through the lung. A medium-size embolus may block an artery supplying a bronchopulmonary segment, producing a *pulmonary infarct,* an area of necrotic (dead) lung tissue.

Inhalation of Carbon Particles

Lymph from the lungs carries *phagocytes,* cells possessing the property of ingesting carbon particles from inspired air. In many people, especially cigarette smokers, these particles color the surface of the lungs and associated lymph nodes a mottled gray to black. *Smokers' cough* results from inhalation of irritants in tobacco.

Bronchogenic Carcinoma

Bronchogenic carcinoma is a common type of lung cancer that arises from the epithelium of the bronchial tree. *Lung cancer* is mainly caused by cigarette smoking. Bronchogenic carcinoma usually metastasizes widely because of the arrangement of the lymphatics. The tumor cells probably enter the systemic circulation by invading the wall of a sinusoid or venule in the lung and are transported through the pulmonary veins, left heart, and aorta to all parts of the body, especially the cranium and brain.

Bronchoscopy

 When examining the bronchi with a *bronchoscope*—an endoscope for inspecting the interior of the tracheobronchial tree for diagnostic purposes—one can observe a ridge, the **carina,** between the orifices of the main bronchi (Fig. B1.10). The carina is a cartilaginous projection of the last tracheal ring. If the tracheobronchial lymph nodes in the angle between the main bronchi are enlarged because cancer cells have metastasized from a bronchogenic carcinoma, for example, the carina is distorted, widened posteriorly, and immobile.

A Bronchoscopic view of trachea

B Bronchoscopic view of carina (C) and main bronchi (MB)

FIGURE B1.10. Bronchoscopy.

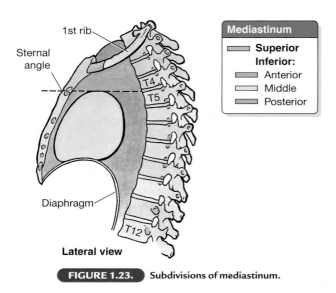

1st rib

Sternal
angle

Diaphragm

T4

T5

T12

Lateral view

Mediastinum
- **Superior**
- **Inferior:**
- Anterior
- Middle
- Posterior

FIGURE 1.23. Subdivisions of mediastinum.

Mediastinum

The mediastinum, occupied by the viscera between the pulmonary cavities, is the central compartment of the thoracic cavity (Fig. 1.23). The mediastinum:

- Is covered on each side by mediastinal pleura and contains all the thoracic viscera and structures, except the lungs.
- Extends from the superior thoracic aperture to the diaphragm inferiorly and from the sternum and costal cartilages anteriorly to the bodies of the thoracic vertebrae posteriorly.
- In living persons is a highly mobile region because it consists primarily of hollow (liquid- or air-filled) visceral structures united only by loose connective tissue, often infiltrated with fat.

The major structures in the mediastinum are also surrounded by blood and lymphatic vessels, lymph nodes, nerves, and fat.

The looseness of the connective tissue and the elasticity of the lungs and parietal pleura on each side of the mediastinum enable it to accommodate movement, as well as volume and pressure changes in the thoracic cavity, such as those resulting from movements of the diaphragm, thoracic wall, and tracheobronchial tree during respiration, contraction (beating) of the heart and pulsations of the great arteries, and passage of ingested substances through the esophagus. The connective tissue here becomes more fibrous and rigid with age; hence, the mediastinal structures become less mobile.

The mediastinum is artificially divided into superior and inferior parts for purposes of description.

- The **superior mediastinum** extends inferiorly from the superior thoracic aperture to the horizontal plane (transverse thoracic plane) passing through the sternal angle and the IV disc of the T4–T5 vertebra (Fig. 1.21). It contains the superior vena cava (SVC), brachiocephalic veins, arch of the aorta, thoracic duct, trachea, esophagus, thymus, vagus nerves, left recurrent laryngeal nerve, and phrenic nerves.
- The **inferior mediastinum,** between the transverse thoracic plane and the diaphragm, is further subdivided by the pericardium into the **anterior mediastinum**, containing remnants of the thymus, lymph nodes, fat, and connective tissue; **middle mediastinum**, containing the pericardium, heart, roots of the great vessels, arch of azygos vein, and main bronchi; and **posterior mediastinum**, containing the esophagus, thoracic aorta, azygos and hemiazygos veins, thoracic duct, vagus nerves, sympathetic trunks, and splanchnic nerves.

The anterior and middle mediastinum are described first, followed by the superior and posterior mediastinum, because many structures (e.g., the esophagus) pass vertically through the superior and posterior mediastinum and, therefore, lie in more than one mediastinal compartment.

Anterior Mediastinum

The anterior mediastinum, the smallest subdivision of the mediastinum, lies between the body of the sternum and the transversus thoracis muscles anteriorly and the pericardium posteriorly (Fig. 1.23). The anterior mediastinum is continuous with the superior mediastinum at the sternal angle and is limited inferiorly by the diaphragm. The anterior mediastinum consists of loose connective tissue (*sternopericardial ligaments*, fibrous bands that pass from the pericardium to the sternum), fat, lymphatic vessels, a few lymph nodes, and branches of the internal thoracic vessels. In infants and children, the anterior mediastinum contains the inferior part of the thymus.

Middle Mediastinum

The middle mediastinum contains the pericardium, heart, ascending aorta, pulmonary trunk, SVC, arch of azygos vein, and main bronchi.

PERICARDIUM

The pericardium is a double-walled fibroserous membrane that encloses the heart and the roots of its great vessels (Fig. 1.24). This conical **pericardial sac** lies posterior to the body of the sternum and the second to sixth costal cartilages at the level of the T5–T8 vertebrae. The tough external fibrous layer of the sac—the **fibrous pericardium**—is continuous with (blends with) the central tendon of the diaphragm (Fig. 1.24A). The internal surface of the fibrous pericardium is lined with a glistening serous

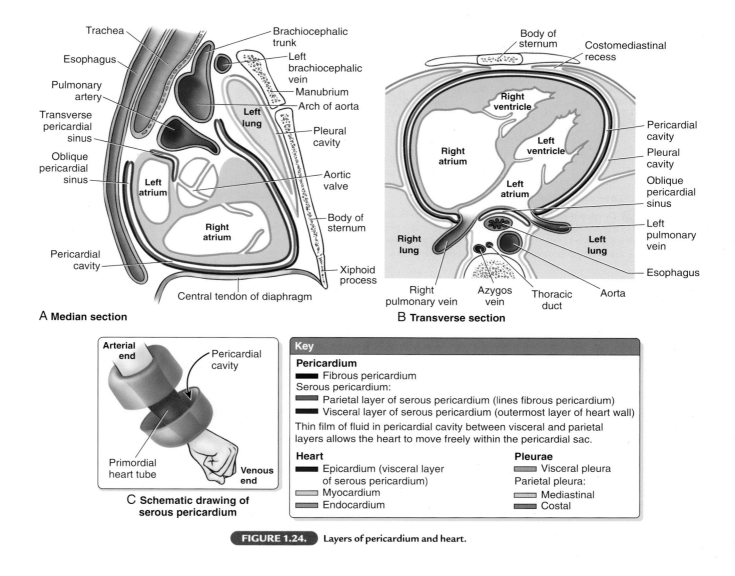

A Median section

B Transverse section

C Schematic drawing of serous pericardium

Key

Pericardium
◼ Fibrous pericardium
Serous pericardium:
◼ Parietal layer of serous pericardium (lines fibrous pericardium)
◼ Visceral layer of serous pericardium (outermost layer of heart wall)
Thin film of fluid in pericardial cavity between visceral and parietal layers allows the heart to move freely within the pericardial sac.

Heart
◼ Epicardium (visceral layer of serous pericardium)
◻ Myocardium
◼ Endocardium

Pleurae
◻ Visceral pleura
Parietal pleura:
◻ Mediastinal
◼ Costal

FIGURE 1.24.   Layers of pericardium and heart.

membrane, the **parietal layer of serous pericardium.** This layer is reflected onto the heart and great vessels as the **visceral layer of serous pericardium.**

The *pericardial sac* is influenced by movements of the heart and great vessels, sternum, and diaphragm because the fibrous pericardium is:

- Fused with the tunica adventitia of the great vessels entering and leaving the heart.
- Attached to the posterior surface of the sternum by sternopericardial ligaments.
- Fused with the central tendon of the diaphragm.

The **fibrous pericardium** protects the heart against sudden overfilling because it is unyielding and closely related to the great vessels that pierce it superiorly and posteriorly (Fig. 1.24B). The ascending aorta carries the pericardium superiorly beyond the heart to the level of the sternal angle.

The **pericardial cavity** is the potential space between the opposing layers of the parietal and visceral layers of serous pericardium (Fig. 1.24C). It normally contains a thin film of serous fluid that enables the heart to move and beat in a frictionless environment.

The visceral layer of serous pericardium forms the **epicardium,** the external layer of the heart wall, and reflects from the heart and great vessels to become continuous with the parietal layer of serous pericardium, where:

- The aorta and pulmonary trunk leave the heart; a finger can be inserted into the **transverse pericardial sinus** located posterior to these large vessels and anterior to the SVC (Figs. 1.24A, 1.25, and B1.11).
- The SVC, inferior vena cava (IVC), and pulmonary veins enter the heart; these vessels are partly covered by serous pericardium, which forms the **oblique pericardial**

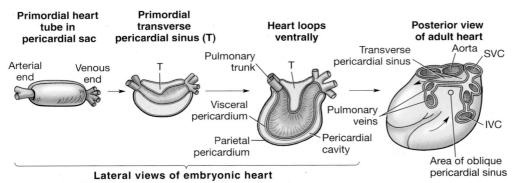

Primordial heart tube in pericardial sac

Primordial transverse pericardial sinus (T)

Heart loops ventrally

Posterior view of adult heart

Arterial end   Venous end

Pulmonary trunk

Visceral pericardium

Parietal pericardium

Pericardial cavity

Transverse pericardial sinus

Pulmonary veins

Aorta SVC

IVC

Area of oblique pericardial sinus

Primordial arterial and venous ends are brought together to form transverse pericardial sinus.

Veins expand and pericardial reflection is carried out around them to form oblique pericardial sinus.

Lateral views of embryonic heart

FIGURE 1.25. **Development of heart and pericardium.** The primordial heart tube invaginates the double-layered pericardial sac (somewhat like placing a hot dog in a bun). The primordial heart then loops ventrally, bringing the primordial arterial and venous ends of the heart together and creating the transverse pericardial sinus between them. The veins expand and move apart. The pericardium is reflected around them to form the boundaries of the oblique pericardial sinus. *IVC,* inferior vena cava; *SVC,* superior vena cava.

sinus (Figs. 1.25 and 1.26), a wide recess posterior to the heart. The oblique sinus can be entered inferiorly and will admit several fingers; however, the fingers cannot pass around any of these vessels because the sinus is a blind recess (cul-de-sac).

These pericardial sinuses form during development of the heart as a consequence of folding of the primordial heart tube (Fig. 1.25). As the heart tube folds, its venous end moves posterosuperiorly so that the venous end of the tube lies adjacent to the arterial end, separated by the transverse pericardial sinus. As these vessels expand and move apart, the pericardium is reflected around them to form the boundaries of the oblique pericardial sinus.

The **arterial supply of the pericardium** is mainly from the **pericardiacophrenic artery** (Fig. 1.26A), a branch of the **internal thoracic artery,** which may accompany or parallel the phrenic nerve to the diaphragm. Smaller contributions of blood to the pericardium come from the *musculophrenic artery,* a terminal branch of the internal thoracic artery; the *bronchial, esophageal,* and *superior phrenic arteries* from the thoracic aorta; and the *coronary arteries,* supplying only the visceral layer of serous pericardium (Fig. 1.15A).

The **venous drainage of the pericardium** is from the (Fig. 1.15B):

- *Pericardiacophrenic veins,* tributaries of the brachiocephalic (or internal thoracic) veins.
- Variable tributaries of the azygos venous system.

The **nerve supply of the pericardium** is from the (Figs. 1.22D and 1.26A):

- *Phrenic nerves* (C3–C5)—a primary source of sensory fibers; pain sensations conveyed by these nerves are commonly referred to the skin (C3–C5 dermatomes) of the top of the shoulder of the same side.

- *Vagus nerves* (CN X)—function uncertain.
- *Sympathetic trunks*—vasomotor.

Surgical Significance of Transverse Pericardial Sinus

The transverse pericardial sinus is especially important to cardiac surgeons. After the pericardial sac has been opened anteriorly, a finger can be passed through the transverse pericardial sinus posterior to the aorta and pulmonary trunk (Fig. B1.11). By passing a surgical clamp or placing a ligature around these vessels, inserting the tubes of a coronary bypass machine, and then tightening the ligature, surgeons can stop or divert the circulation of blood in these large arteries while performing cardiac surgery, such as coronary artery bypass grafting. Cardiac surgery is performed while the patient is on cardiopulmonary bypass.

Superior vena cava

Ascending aorta

Finger passing through transverse pericardial sinus

Pulmonary trunk

FIGURE B1.11. Transverse pericardial sinus.

A **Anterior view**

Key

A	Aorta
AR	Arch of aorta
IVC	Inferior vena cava
LBV	Left brachiocephalic vein
LPA	Left pulmonary artery
LPV	Left pulmonary vein
PT	Pulmonary trunk
RBV	Right brachiocephalic vein
RPV	Right pulmonary vein
SVC	Superior vena cava

Location of

⟷ Transverse pericardial sinus

Oblique pericardial sinus

B **Anterior view**

FIGURE 1.26. **Pericardium. A.** Arterial supply and venous drainage. **B.** Interior of pericardial sac after removal of the heart.

Pericarditis and Pericardial Effusion

Inflammation of the pericardium (*pericarditis*) usually causes chest pain. Normally, the layers of serous pericardium make no detectable sound during auscultation. However, pericarditis makes the surfaces rough and the resulting friction, *pericardial friction rub,* sounds like the rustle of silk when listening with a stethoscope. Certain inflammatory diseases may also produce pericardial effusion (passage of fluid from the pericardial capillaries into the pericardial cavity). As a result, the heart becomes compressed (unable to expand and fill fully) and ineffectual.

Cardiac Tamponade

Cardiac tamponade (heart compression) is a potentially lethal condition because the fibrous pericardium is tough and inelastic. Consequently, heart volume is increasingly compromised by the fluid outside the heart but inside the pericardial cavity. When there is a slow increase in the size of the heart, *cardiomegaly,* the pericardium allows the enlargement of the heart to occur without compression. Stab wounds that pierce the heart, causing blood to enter the pericardial cavity (*hemopericardium*), also risk producing cardiac tamponade. Hemopericardium may also result from perforation of a weakened area of heart muscle after a heart attack. As blood accumulates, the heart is compressed and circulation fails.

Pericardiocentesis (drainage of serous fluid from pericardial cavity) is usually necessary to relieve the cardiac tamponade. To remove the excess fluid, a wide-bore needle may be inserted through the left fifth or sixth intercostal space near the sternum.

Levels of Viscera in Mediastinum

The level of the viscera relative to the mediastinal subdivisions depends on the position of the person. When a person is lying supine, the level of the viscera relative to the subdivisions of the mediastinum is as shown in the figures in this text. Anatomical descriptions traditionally describe the level of the viscera as if the person were supine. However, in the standing position, the levels of the viscera are as shown in Figure B1.12. This occurs because the soft structures in the mediastinum, the heart and great vessels, and the abdominal viscera supporting them sag inferiorly under the influence of gravity. This movement of mediastinal structures must be considered during physical and radiological examinations.

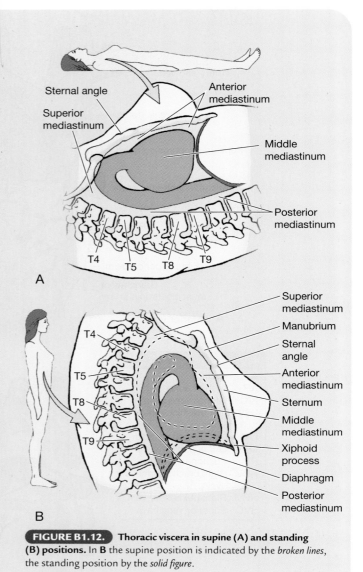

FIGURE B1.12.   **Thoracic viscera in supine (A) and standing (B) positions.** In **B** the supine position is indicated by the *broken lines,* the standing position by the *solid figure.*

Heart and Great Vessels

The heart, slightly larger than a clenched fist, is a double self-adjusting muscular pump, the parts of which work in unison to propel blood to the body. The right side of the heart receives poorly oxygenated blood from the body through the SVC and IVC and pumps it through the pulmonary trunk to the lungs for oxygenation. The left side of the heart receives well-oxygenated blood from the lungs through the pulmonary veins and pumps it into the aorta for distribution to the body.

The wall of the heart consists of three layers; from superficial to deep they are (Fig. 1.24):

- **Epicardium,** a thin external layer (mesothelium) formed by the visceral layer of serous pericardium.
- **Myocardium,** a thick middle layer composed of cardiac muscle.
- **Endocardium,** a thin internal layer (endothelium and subendothelial connective tissue) or lining membrane of the heart that also covers its valves.

ORIENTATION OF HEART

The heart and roots of the great vessels within the pericardial sac are related anteriorly to the sternum, costal cartilages, and the medial ends of the third to fifth ribs on the left

A **Anteroposterior view**

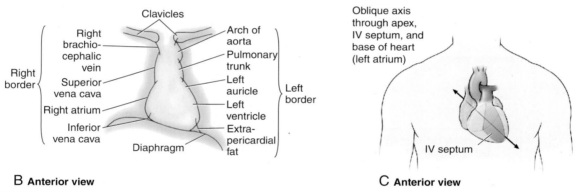

B **Anterior view**

C **Anterior view**

FIGURE 1.27.   **Placement of heart in thorax. A.** Radiograph. **B.** Structures forming the margins of the cardiac silhouette. **C.** Orientation of heart.

side. The heart and pericardial sac are situated obliquely, about two thirds to the left and one third to the right of the median plane. The heart is shaped like a tipped-over, three-sided pyramid with an apex, base, and four surfaces.

The **apex of the heart** (Figs. 1.27*A* and 1.28*A*):

- Is directed anteriorly and to the left and is formed by the inferolateral part of the left ventricle.
- Is located posterior to the left fifth intercostal space in adults, usually 9 cm from the median plane.
- Is where the sounds of mitral valve closure are maximal **(apex beat)**; the apex underlies the site where the heart-beat may be auscultated on the thoracic wall.

The **base of the heart** (Fig. 1.28*B*):

- Is the heart's *posterior aspect*.
- Is formed mainly by the left atrium, with a lesser contri-bution by the right atrium.

- Faces posteriorly toward the bodies of vertebrae T6–T9, and is separated from them by the pericardium, oblique pericardial sinus, esophagus, and aorta.
- Extends superiorly to the bifurcation of the pulmonary trunk and inferiorly to the coronary groove.
- Receives the pulmonary veins on the right and left sides of its left atrial portion and the superior and inferior venae cavae at the superior and inferior ends of its right atrial portion.

The **four surfaces of the heart** are the (Fig. 1.28*A,B*):

- **Anterior (sternocostal) surface,** formed mainly by the right ventricle.
- **Diaphragmatic (inferior) surface,** formed mainly by the left ventricle and partly by the right ventricle; it is related to the central tendon of the diaphragm.
- **Left pulmonary surface,** consists mainly of the left ventricle; it forms the cardiac impression of the left lung.

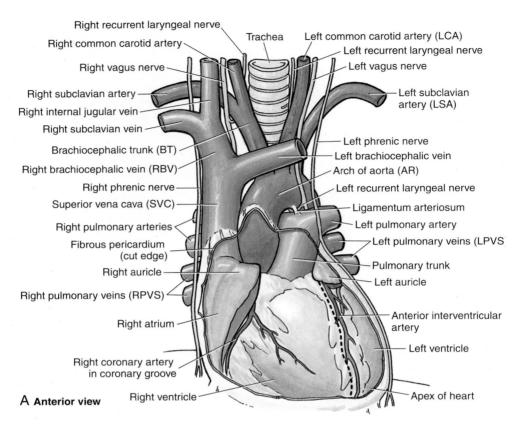

A **Anterior view**

Right recurrent laryngeal nerve
Right common carotid artery
Right vagus nerve
Right subclavian artery
Right internal jugular vein
Right subclavian vein
Brachiocephalic trunk (BT)
Right brachiocephalic vein (RBV)
Right phrenic nerve
Superior vena cava (SVC)
Right pulmonary arteries
Fibrous pericardium (cut edge)
Right auricle
Right pulmonary veins (RPVS)
Right atrium
Right coronary artery in coronary groove
Right ventricle

Trachea

Left common carotid artery (LCA)
Left recurrent laryngeal nerve
Left vagus nerve
Left subclavian artery (LSA)
Left phrenic nerve
Left brachiocephalic vein
Arch of aorta (AR)
Left recurrent laryngeal nerve
Ligamentum arteriosum
Left pulmonary artery
Left pulmonary veins (LPVS)
Pulmonary trunk
Left auricle
Anterior interventricular artery
Left ventricle
Apex of heart

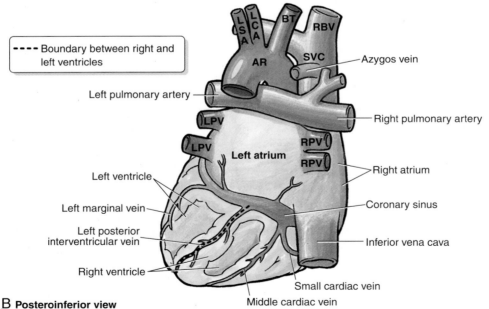

B **Posteroinferior view**

- - - - Boundary between right and left ventricles

LSA LCA BT RBV
AR SVC
Left pulmonary artery
LPV
LPV
Left atrium
Left ventricle
Left marginal vein
Left posterior interventricular vein
Right ventricle
Middle cardiac vein

Azygos vein
Right pulmonary artery
RPV
RPV
Right atrium
Coronary sinus
Inferior vena cava
Small cardiac vein

FIGURE 1.28.   **Exterior of heart. A.** Anterior (sternocostal) and left pulmonary and right pulmonary surfaces. **B.** Diaphragmatic (inferior) surface and base (posterior aspect).

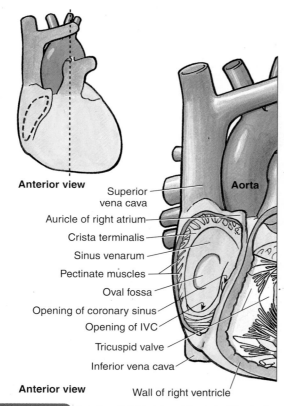

Anterior view

Superior vena cava
Aorta
Auricle of right atrium
Crista terminalis
Sinus venarum
Pectinate muscles
Oval fossa
Opening of coronary sinus
Opening of IVC
Tricuspid valve
Inferior vena cava

Anterior view
Wall of right ventricle

FIGURE 1.29. Interior of right atrium. The *dashed lines* in the orientation figure outline the parts of the heart wall that have been excised to reveal internal structures.

- **Right pulmonary surface,** formed mainly by the right atrium

The heart appears trapezoidal in both anterior and posterior views. The **four borders of the heart** are the (Fig. 1.27):

- **Right border** (slightly convex), formed by the right atrium and extending between the SVC and the IVC
- **Inferior border** (nearly horizontal), formed mainly by the right ventricle and only slightly by the left ventricle
- **Left border** (oblique), formed mainly by the left ventricle and slightly by the left auricle
- **Superior border,** formed by the right and left atria and auricles in an anterior view; the ascending aorta and pulmonary trunk emerge from the superior border, and the SVC enters its right side. Posterior to the aorta and pulmonary trunk and anterior to the SVC, the superior border forms the inferior boundary of the transverse pericardial sinus.

CHAMBERS OF HEART

The heart has four chambers: **right** and **left atria** and **right** and **left ventricles.**

Right Atrium. The right atrium forms the right border of the heart and receives venous blood from the SVC, IVC, and coronary sinus (Figs. 1.28). The ear-like **right auricle** is a small, conical muscular pouch that projects from the **right atrium,** increasing the capacity of the atrium as it overlaps the ascending aorta. The primordial atrium is represented in the adult by the right auricle. The definitive atrium is enlarged by incorporation of most of the embryonic venous sinus (L. *sinus venosus*). The **coronary sinus** lies in the posterior part of the coronary groove and receives blood from the cardiac veins. The coronary sinus is also a derivative of the embryonic venous sinus. The part of the venous sinus incorporated into the primordial atrium becomes the smooth-walled **sinus venarum** of the adult right atrium. The separation between the primordial atrium and the sinus venarum is indicated externally by the **sulcus terminalis** (terminal groove) and internally by the **crista terminalis** (terminal crest). The **interior of the right atrium** has (Figs. 1.29 and 1.30):

- A smooth, thin-walled posterior part (the **sinus venarum**), on which the SVC, IVC, and coronary sinus open, bringing poorly oxygenated blood into the heart
- A rough, muscular wall composed of **pectinate muscles** (L. *musculi pectinati*)
- The **opening of the SVC** into its superior part, at the level of the right third costal cartilage
- The **opening of the IVC** into the inferior part, almost in line with the SVC at approximately the level of the fifth costal cartilage
- The **opening of the coronary sinus** between the right atrioventricular (AV) orifice and the IVC orifice
- A **right AV orifice** through which the right atrium discharges the poorly oxygenated blood into the right ventricle
- The **interatrial septum,** separating the atria, has an oval, thumbprint-size depression, the **oval fossa** (L. *fossa ovalis*), a remnant of the oval foramen and its valve in the fetus (Moore & Persaud, 2008).

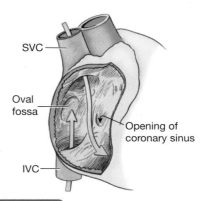

SVC
Oval fossa
Opening of coronary sinus
IVC

FIGURE 1.30. Direction of blood flow in right atrium.

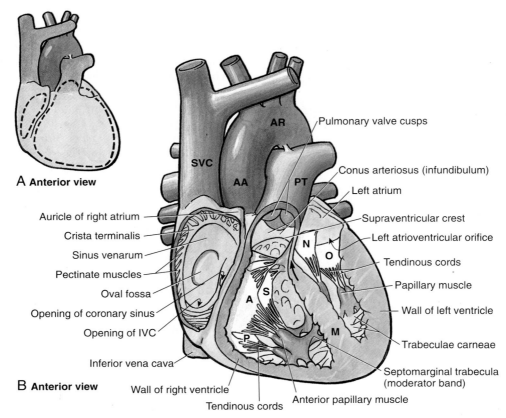

A Anterior view

AR

Pulmonary valve cusps

SVC

Conus arteriosus (infundibulum)

AA   PT

Left atrium

Auricle of right atrium

Supraventricular crest

Crista terminalis

Left atrioventricular orifice

Sinus venarum

N   O

Tendinous cords

Pectinate muscles

Papillary muscle

Oval fossa

A   S

Wall of left ventricle

Opening of coronary sinus

Opening of IVC

P   M

Trabeculae carneae

Inferior vena cava

Septomarginal trabecula
(moderator band)

B Anterior view

Wall of right ventricle

Tendinous cords

Anterior papillary muscle

FIGURE 1.31. **Interior of heart. A.** The *dashed lines* indicate where the heart's wall has been removed in part **B. B.** Observe the features of each chamber. Note the three cusps of the tricuspid valve—*A*, anterior; *P*, posterior; *S*, septal—and the two cusps of the mitral valve—*N*, anterior; *O*, posterior. *AA*, ascending aorta; *AR*, arch of aorta, *IVC*, inferior vena cava; *M*, muscular part of interventricular septum; *PT*, pulmonary trunk; *SVC*, superior vena cava, *arrow*, membranous part of interventricular septum.

Right Ventricle. The right ventricle forms the largest part of the anterior surface of the heart, a small part of the diaphragmatic surface, and almost the entire inferior border of the heart. Superiorly it tapers into an arterial cone, the **conus arteriosus** (infundibulum), which leads into the pulmonary trunk (Fig. 1.31). The interior of the right ventricle has irregular muscular elevations called **trabeculae carneae.** A thick muscular ridge, the **supraventricular crest,** separates the ridged muscular wall of the inflow part of the chamber from the smooth wall of the conus arteriosus or outflow part of the right ventricle. The inflow part of the right ventricle receives blood from the right atrium through the **right AV (tricuspid) orifice,** located posterior to the body of the sternum at the level of the fourth and fifth intercostal spaces. The right AV orifice is surrounded by a fibrous ring (part of the fibrous skeleton of heart) that resists the dilation that might otherwise result from blood being forced through it at varying pressures.

The **tricuspid valve** guards the right AV orifice (Figs. 1.31 and 1.32*A*). The bases of the valve cusps are attached to the fibrous ring around the orifice. **Tendinous cords** (L. *chordae tendineae*) attach to the free edges and ventricular surfaces of the anterior, posterior, and septal cusps—much like the cords attached to a parachute. Because the cords are attached to adjacent sides of two cusps, they prevent separation of the cusps and their inversion when tension is applied to the cords throughout ventricular contraction (systole)—that is, the cusps of the tricuspid valve are prevented from prolapsing (being driven into right atrium) as ventricular pressure rises. Thus regurgitation of blood (backward flow of blood) from the right ventricle into the right atrium is blocked by the valve cusps. The **papillary muscles** form conical projections with their bases attached to the ventricular wall and tendinous cords arising from their apices. There are usually three papillary muscles (anterior, posterior, and septal) in the right ventricle that correspond in name to the cusps of the tricuspid valve. The papillary muscles begin to contract before contraction of the right ventricle, tightening the tendinous cords and drawing the cusps together.

The **interventricular septum,** composed of membranous and muscular parts, is a strong, obliquely placed partition between the right and the left ventricles (Fig. 1.31), forming part of the walls of each. The superoposterior *membranous part of the IV septum* is thin and is continuous with the fibrous skeleton of the heart. The *muscular part of the IV septum* is thick and bulges into the cavity of the right ventricle because of the higher blood pressure in the left ventricle. The **septomarginal trabecula** (moderator band) is a curved muscular bundle that runs from the inferior part of the interventricular septum to the base of the anterior papillary muscle. This trabeculum is important because it carries part of the **right bundle branches of the AV bundle** of the conducting system of the heart to the anterior papillary muscle (discussed later in this chapter). This "shortcut" across the chamber of the ventricle seems to facilitate conduction time, allowing coordinated contraction of the anterior papillary muscle.

When the right atrium contracts, blood is forced through the **right AV orifice** into the right ventricle, pushing the cusps of the tricuspid valve aside like curtains. The inflow of blood into the right ventricle (*inflow tract*) enters posteriorly, and the outflow of blood into the pulmonary trunk (*outflow tract*) leaves superiorly and to the left. Consequently, the blood takes a U-shaped path through the right ventricle. The inflow (AV) orifice and outflow (pulmonary) orifice are approximately 2 cm apart.

The **pulmonary valve** at the apex of the **conus arteriosus** is at the level of the left third costal cartilage (Figs. 1.28 and 1.32*B*). Each of the semilunar **cusps of the pulmonary valve** (anterior, right, and left) is concave when viewed superiorly. The *pulmonary sinuses* are the spaces at the origin of the pulmonary trunk between the dilated wall of the vessel and each cusp of the pulmonary valve. The blood in the pulmonary sinuses prevents the cusps from sticking to the wall of the pulmonary trunk and failing to close.

Left Atrium. The left atrium forms most of the base of the heart (Fig. 1.33). The pairs of valveless right and left **pulmonary veins** enter the left atrium. The left auricle forms the superior part of the left border of the heart and overlaps the pulmonary trunk. The **interior of the left atrium** has:

- A larger smooth-walled part and a smaller muscular auricle containing pectinate muscles.
- Four pulmonary veins (two superior and two inferior) entering its posterior wall.
- A slightly thicker wall than that of the right atrium.
- An interatrial septum that slopes posteriorly and to the right.
- A left AV orifice through which the left atrium discharges the oxygenated blood it receives from the pulmonary veins into the left ventricle.

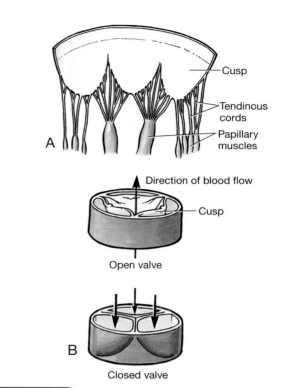

FIGURE 1.32.   **Pulmonary and tricuspid valves. A.** Tricuspid valve spread out. **B.** Blood flow through pulmonary valve.

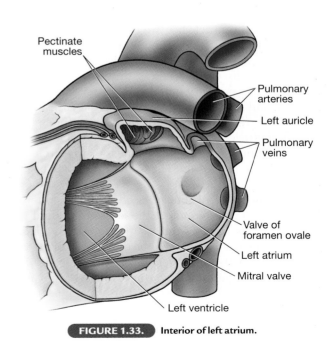

FIGURE 1.33.   Interior of left atrium.

The smooth-walled part of the left atrium is formed by absorption of parts of the embryonic pulmonary veins, whereas the rough-walled part, mainly in the auricle, represents the remains of the left part of the primordial atrium.

Left Ventricle. The left ventricle forms the apex of the heart, nearly all of its left (pulmonary) surface and border, and most of the diaphragmatic surface (Figs. 1.31 and 1.34). Because arterial pressure is much higher in the systemic than in the pulmonary circulation, the **left ventricle** performs more work than the right ventricle.

The **interior of the left ventricle** has (Fig. 1.34):

- A double-leaflet **mitral valve** that guards the left AV orifice.
- Walls that are two to three times as thick as that of the right ventricle.
- A conical cavity that is longer than that of the right ventricle.
- Walls that are covered with thick muscular ridges, **trabeculae carneae,** that are finer and more numerous than those in the right ventricle.
- Anterior and posterior **papillary muscles** that are larger than those in the right ventricle.
- A smooth-walled, nonmuscular, superoanterior outflow part, the **aortic vestibule,** leading to the aortic orifice and aortic valve.
- An **aortic orifice** that lies in its right posterosuperior part and is surrounded by a fibrous ring to which the right, posterior, and left cusps of the **aortic valve** are attached.

The **mitral valve** closing the orifice between the left atrium and left ventricle has two cusps, anterior and posterior (Figs. 1.34 and 1.35). The mitral valve is located posterior to the sternum at the level of the fourth costal cartilage. Each of its cusps receives **tendinous cords** from more than one papillary muscle. These muscles and their cords support the mitral valve, allowing the cusps to resist the pressure developed during contractions (pumping) of the left ventricle. The tendinous cords become taut, just before and during systole, preventing the cusps from being forced into the left atrium. The **ascending aorta** begins at the aortic orifice.

The **aortic valve,** obliquely placed, is located posterior to the left side of the sternum at the level of the third intercostal space. The **aortic sinuses** are the spaces at the origin of the ascending aorta between the dilated wall of the vessel and each cusp of the aortic (semilunar) valve (Fig. 1.36). The mouth of the right coronary artery is in the **right aortic sinus;** the mouth of the left coronary artery is in the **left aortic sinus;** and no artery arises from the **posterior aortic (noncoronary) sinus.**

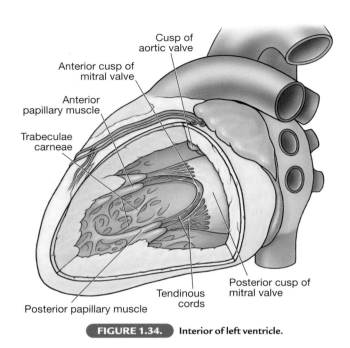

FIGURE 1.34.   Interior of left ventricle.

FIGURE 1.35.   Mitral valve.

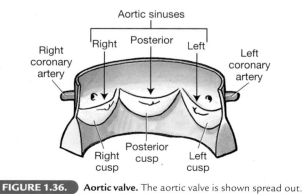

FIGURE 1.36.   **Aortic valve.** The aortic valve is shown spread out.

Percussion of Heart

 Percussion defines the density and size of the heart. The classic percussion technique is to create vibration by tapping the chest with a finger while listening and feeling for differences in sound wave conduction. Percussion is performed at the third, fourth, and fifth intercostal spaces from the left anterior axillary line to the right anterior axillary line. Normally the percussion note changes from resonance to dullness (because of the presence of the heart) approximately 6 cm lateral to the left border of the sternum. The character of the sound changes as different areas of the chest are tapped.

Atrial and Ventricular Septal Defects

 Congenital anomalies of the interatrial septum—usually related to incomplete closure of the oval foramen—are *atrial septal defects* or ASDs (Fig. B1.13*A*). A probe-size patency (defect) appears in the superior part of the oval fossa in 15% to 25% of people. These small ASDs, by themselves, are usually of no clinical significance; however, large ASDs allow oxygenated blood from the lungs to be shunted from the left atrium through the defect into the right atrium, causing enlargement of the right atrium and ventricle and dilation of the pulmonary trunk.

The membranous part of the IV septum develops separately from the muscular part and has a complex embryological origin. Consequently, this part is the common site of *ventricular septal defects* or VSDs (Fig. B1.13*B*). These congenital anomalies rank first on all lists of cardiac defects. Isolated VSDs account for approximately 25% of all forms of congenital heart

A **Atrial septal defect (ASD)**

B **Ventricular septal defect (VSD)**

FIGURE B1.13. Septal defects.

disease (Moore & Persaud, 2008). The size of the defect varies from 1 to 25 mm. A VSD causes a left-to-right shunt of blood through the defect. A large shunt increases pulmonary blood flow, which causes pulmonary disease (*hypertension,* or increased blood pressure) and may cause cardiac failure.

Thrombi

 Thrombi (clots) form on the walls of the left atrium in certain types of heart disease. If these thrombi detach or if pieces break off, they pass into the systemic circulation and occlude peripheral arteries. Occlusion of an artery in the brain results in a stroke or *cerebrovascular accident* (CVA), which may affect, for example, vision, cognition, or sensory or motor function of parts of the body previously controlled by the now-damaged area of the brain.

Valvular Heart Disease

Disorders involving the valves of the heart disturb the pumping efficiency of the heart. *Valvular heart disease* produces either stenosis (narrowing) or insufficiency. **Stenosis** is the failure of a valve to open fully, slowing blood flow from a chamber. **Valvular insufficiency or regurgitation,** on the other hand, is failure of the valve to close completely, usually owing to nodule formation on (or scarring and contraction of) the cusps so that the edges do not meet or align. This allows a variable amount of blood (depending on the severity) to flow back into the chamber it was just ejected from. Both stenosis and insufficiency result in an increased workload for the heart. Restriction of high-pressure blood flow (stenosis) and passage of blood through a narrow opening into a larger vessel or chamber (stenosis and regurgitation) produce turbulence. Turbulence sets up *eddies* (small whirlpools) that produce vibrations that are audible as *murmurs.* Superficial vibratory sensations—*thrills*—may be felt on the skin over an area of turbulence.

Because valvular diseases are mechanical problems, damaged or defective cardiac valves are often replaced surgically in a procedure called *valvuloplasty.* Most commonly, artificial valve prostheses made of synthetic materials are used in these valve replacement procedures, but xenografted valves (valves transplanted from other species, such as pigs) are also used.

A *prolapsed mitral valve* is an insufficient or incompetent valve in which one or both leaflets are enlarged, redundant or "floppy," and extending back into the left atrium during systole. As a result, blood regurgitates into the left atrium when the left ventricle contracts, producing a characteristic murmur.

Aortic valve stenosis is the most frequent valve abnormality and results in *left ventricular hypertrophy.* The great majority of cases of aortic stenosis result from degenerative calcification.

In *pulmonary valve stenosis* (narrowing), the valve cusps are fused, forming a dome with a narrow central opening. In *infundibular pulmonary stenosis,* the conus arteriosus is underdeveloped, producing a restriction of right ventricular outflow. The degree of hypertrophy of the right ventricle is variable.

Surface Anatomy of Heart

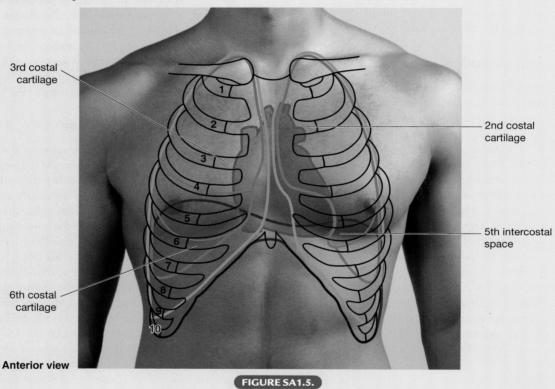

3rd costal cartilage

2nd costal cartilage

5th intercostal space

6th costal cartilage

Anterior view

FIGURE SA1.5.

The heart and great vessels are approximately in the middle of the thorax, surrounded laterally and posteriorly by the lungs and bounded anteriorly by the sternum and the central part of the thoracic cage (Fig. SA1.5). The *outline of the heart* can be traced on the anterior surface of the thorax by using these guidelines:

- The *superior border* corresponds to a line connecting the inferior border of the second left costal cartilage to the superior border of the third right costal cartilage.
- The *right border* corresponds to a line drawn from the third right costal cartilage to the sixth right costal cartilage; this border is slightly convex to the right.
- The *inferior border* corresponds to a line drawn from the inferior end of the right border to a point in the fifth

intercostal space close to the left midclavicular line; the left end of this line corresponds to the location of the apex of the heart and the apex beat.

- The *left border* corresponds to a line connecting the left ends of the lines representing the superior and inferior borders.
- The valves are located posterior to the sternum; however, the sounds produced by them are projected to the **auscultatory areas:** pulmonary, aortic, mitral, and tricuspid (Figs. SA1.6–1.9).

The *apex beat* is an impulse that results from the apex being forced against the anterior thoracic wall when the left ventricle contracts. The *location of the apex beat* (mitral area) varies in position; it may be located in the

FIGURE SA1.6.

FIGURE SA1.7.

FIGURE SA1.8.

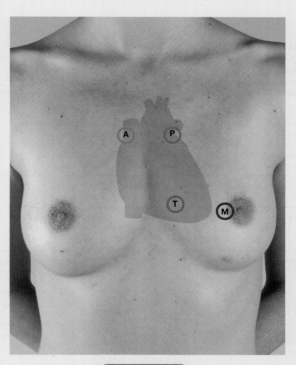

FIGURE SA1.9.

FIGURES SA1.6.–SA1.9. **Location of valves and areas of auscultation.** The location of each valve is indicated by a colored oval and the area of auscultation as a circle of the same color. Tricuspid valve (T) is *green*, mitral valve (M) is *purple*, pulmonary valve (P) is *pink*, and aortic valve (A) is *blue*. The direction of blood flow is indicated by white arrows.

fourth or fifth intercostal spaces, 6 to 10 cm from the midline of the thorax.

Clinicians' interest in the surface anatomy of the heart and cardiac valves results from their need to listen to valve sounds. Because the auscultatory areas are wide apart as possible, the sounds produced at any given valve may be distinguished from those produced at other valves. Blood tends to carry the sound in the direction of its flow. Each area is situated superficial to the chamber or vessel into which the blood has passed and in a direct line with the valve orifice (Figs. SA1.6–1.9).

The **areas of auscultation** are:

- Aortic valve (A): second intercostal space to right of sternal border
- Pulmonary valve (P): second intercostal space to left of sternal border
- Tricuspid valve (T): near left sternal border in fifth or sixth intercostal space
- Mitral valve (M): apex of heart in fifth intercostal space in midclavicular line

ARTERIAL SUPPLY OF HEART

The **coronary arteries** supply the myocardium and epicardium and course just deep to the epicardium, normally embedded in fat. The *right* and *left* coronary arteries arise from the corresponding **aortic sinuses** at the proximal part of the ascending aorta (Figs. 1.36 and 1.37; Table 1.4), just superior to the **aortic valve.** The endocardium receives oxygen and nutrients directly from the chambers of the heart.

The **right coronary artery** (RCA) arises from the *right aortic sinus* and runs in the coronary groove (sulcus). Near its origin, the RCA usually gives off an ascending **sinu-atrial (SA) nodal branch** (Fig. 1.37A) that supplies the *SA node* (part of the cardiac conducting system). The RCA then descends in the coronary groove and gives off the **right marginal branch,** which supplies the right border of the heart as it runs toward (but does not reach) the apex of the

TABLE 1.4 ARTERIAL SUPPLY OF HEART

Artery/Branch	Origin	Course	Distribution	Anastomoses
Right coronary	Right aortic sinus	Follows coronary (AV) groove between atria and ventricles	Right atrium, SA and AV nodes, and posterior part of IV septum	Circumflex and anterior IV branches (left coronary artery)
SA nodal	Right coronary artery near its origin (in 60%)	Ascends to SA node	Pulmonary trunk and SA node	
Right marginal	Right coronary artery	Passes to inferior margin of heart and apex	Right ventricle and apex of heart	IV branches
Posterior IV	Right coronary artery (in 67%)	Runs in posterior IV groove to apex of heart	Right and left ventricles and posterior third of septum	Anterior IV branches of left coronary artery (at apex)
AV nodal	Right coronary artery near origin of posterior IV artery	Passes to AV node	AV node	
Left coronary	Left aortic sinus	Runs in AV groove and gives off anterior IV and circumflex branches	Most of left atrium and ventricle, IV septum, and AV bundles; may supply AV node	Right coronary artery
Anterior IV (LAD)*	Left coronary artery	Passes along anterior IV groove to apex of heart	Right and left ventricles; anterior two thirds of IV septum	Posterior IV branch of left coronary artery
Circumflex	Left coronary artery	Passes to left in AV groove and runs to posterior surface of heart	Left atrium and left ventricle	Right coronary artery
Left marginal	Circumflex branch	Follows left border of heart	Left ventricle	IV branches
Posterior IV	Left coronary artery (in 33%)	Runs in posterior IV groove to apex of heart	Right and left posterior third of IV septum	Anterior IV branch of left coronary artery

AV, atrioventricular; *IV,* interventricular; *LAD,* left anterior descending artery; *SA,* sinu-atrial. *Clinicians continue to use LAD, the abbreviation for the former term "left anterior descending artery."

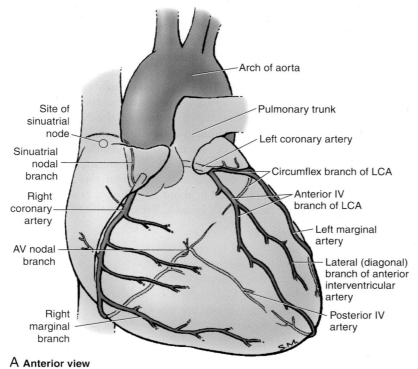

A **Anterior view**

Arch of aorta
Pulmonary trunk
Left coronary artery
Circumflex branch of LCA
Anterior IV branch of LCA
Left marginal artery
Lateral (diagonal) branch of anterior interventricular artery
Posterior IV artery

Site of sinuatrial node
Sinuatrial nodal branch
Right coronary artery
AV nodal branch
Right marginal branch

B **Arteries of isolated interventricular septum (from left side)**

Circumflex branch of LCA
Anterior interventricular branch of LCA
AV bundle
LCA
← 2/3 | 1/3 →
AV node
AV nodal artery
Anterior
Posterior
Septal branches
Posterior IV branch of RCA
AV bundle branches
Apex of heart

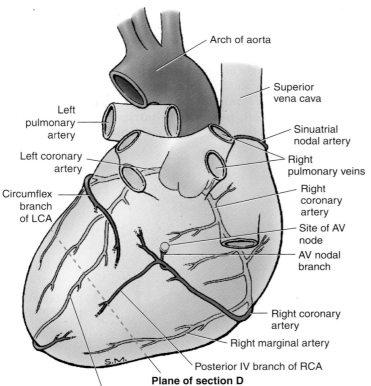

C **Posterior view**

Arch of aorta
Superior vena cava
Sinuatrial nodal artery
Right pulmonary veins
Right coronary artery
Site of AV node
AV nodal branch
Right coronary artery
Right marginal artery
Posterior IV branch of RCA

Left pulmonary artery
Left coronary artery
Circumflex branch of LCA
Plane of section D
Anterior IV branch

Sternocostal surface
AV bundle in IV septum
R
L
Diaphragmatic surface

D **Inferior view of crosssection through ventricles at plane indicated in (C)**

FIGURE 1.37.   **Arterial supply of heart.** *AV,* atrioventricular.

heart. After giving off this branch, the RCA turns to the left and continues in the coronary groove on the posterior aspect of the heart. At the **crux** (cross) of the heart (Fig. 1.39) the junction of the septa and walls of the four heart chambers, the RCA gives rise to the **AV nodal branch,** which supplies the *AV node* (part of the cardiac conducting system). The RCA then gives off the large posterior IV branch that descends in the posterior IV groove toward the apex of the heart (Fig. 1.37). The **posterior IV branch** supplies both ventricles and sends perforating **interventricular septal branches** to the IV septum. The terminal (left ventricular) branch of the RCA then continues for a short distance in the coronary groove. Typically, the RCA supplies:

• The right atrium
• Most of the right ventricle
• Part of the left ventricle (diaphragmatic surface)
• Part of the IV septum (usually the posterior third)
• The SA node (in approximately 60% of people)
• The AV node (in approximately 80% of people)

The **left coronary artery** (LCA) arises from the *left aortic sinus* of the ascending aorta and passes between the left auricle and the left side of the pulmonary trunk in the coronary groove. In approximately 40% of people, the **SA nodal branch** arises from the circumflex branch of the LCA and ascends on the posterior surface of the left atrium to the SA node.

At the left end of the coronary groove, located just left of the pulmonary trunk (Fig. 1.37), the LCA divides into two branches, an **anterior IV branch** (left anterior descending [LAD] branch) and a **circumflex branch.** The anterior IV branch passes along the IV groove to the apex of the heart. Here it turns around the inferior border of the heart and

anastomoses with the posterior IV branch of the right coronary artery. The anterior IV branch supplies both ventricles and the IV septum (Fig. 1.37*C*).

In many people, the anterior IV artery gives rise to a **lateral (diagonal) branch,** which descends on the anterior surface of the heart. The smaller **circumflex branch of the LCA** follows the coronary groove around the left border of the heart to the posterior surface of the heart. The **left marginal artery,** a branch of the circumflex branch, follows the left margin of the heart and supplies the left ventricle. The circumflex branch of the LCA terminates in the coronary groove on the posterior aspect of the heart before reaching the crux, but in about one third of hearts it continues as the posterior IV branch. Typically, the LCA supplies:

• The left atrium.
• Most of the left ventricle.
• Part of the right ventricle.
• Most of the IV septum (usually its anterior two thirds), including the AV bundle of conducting tissue, through its perforating IV septal branches.
• The SA node (in approximately 40% of people).

VENOUS DRAINAGE OF HEART

The heart is drained mainly by veins that empty into the **coronary sinus** and partly by small veins that empty directly into the chambers of the heart. The **coronary sinus,** the main vein of the heart, is a wide venous channel that runs from left to right in the posterior part of the coronary groove. The coronary sinus receives the **great cardiac vein** at its left end and the **middle** and **small cardiac veins** at its right end. The **left posterior ventricular vein** and **left marginal vein** also open into the coronary sinus. The small

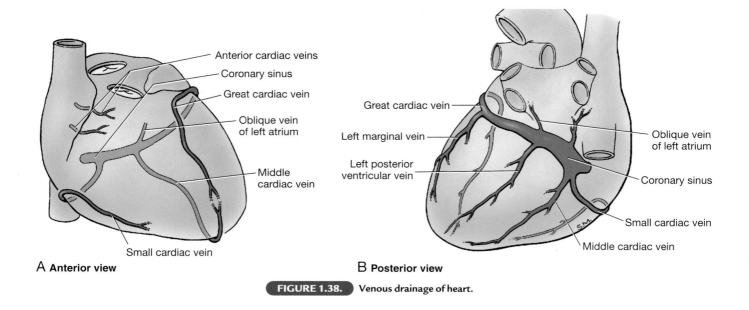

A Anterior view   **B Posterior view**

FIGURE 1.38.   Venous drainage of heart.

anterior cardiac veins empty directly into the right atrium (Fig. 1.38), and the **smallest cardiac veins** (L. *venae cordis minimae*) are minute vessels that begin in the capillary beds of the myocardium and open directly into the chambers of the heart, chiefly the atria. Although called veins, they are valveless communications with the capillary beds of the myocardium and may carry blood from the heart chambers to the myocardium.

LYMPHATIC DRAINAGE OF HEART

Lymphatic vessels in the myocardium and subendocardial connective tissue pass to the *subepicardial lymphatic plexus.* Vessels from this plexus pass to the coronary groove and follow the coronary arteries. A single lymphatic vessel, formed by the union of various vessels from the heart, ascends between the pulmonary trunk and the left atrium and ends in the **inferior tracheobronchial lymph nodes,** usually on the right side (Fig. 1.22C).

CONDUCTING SYSTEM OF HEART

The impulse-conducting system, which coordinates the **cardiac cycle,** consists of cardiac muscle cells and highly specialized conducting fibers for initiating impulses and conducting them rapidly through the heart (Fig. 1.39). Nodal tissue initiates the heartbeat and coordinates the contractions of the four heart chambers. The **SA node** initiates and regulates the impulses for contraction, giving off an impulse about 70 times per minute in most people. The SA node, *the pacemaker of the heart,* is located anterolaterally just deep to the epicardium at the junction of the SVC and right atrium near the superior end of the sulcus terminalis. The **AV node** is a smaller collection of nodal tissue located in the posteroinferior region of the interatrial septum near the opening of the coronary sinus. The signal generated by the SA node passes through the walls of the right atrium propagated by the cardiac muscle (*myogenic conduction*), which transmits the signal rapidly from the SA node to the AV node. The AV node then distributes the signal to the ventricles through the **AV bundle**. Sympathetic stimulation speeds up conduction and parasympathetic stimulation slows it down.

The *AV bundle*, the only bridge of conduction between the atrial and the ventricular myocardium, passes from the AV node through the fibrous skeleton of the heart and along the membranous part of the IV septum. At the junction of the membranous and muscular parts of the septum, the AV bundle divides into **right** and **left bundle branches.** The bundles proceed on each side of the muscular IV septum deep to the endocardium and then ramify into **subendocardial branches** (Purkinje fibers), which extend into the walls of the respective ventricles. The subendocardial branches of the right bundle stimulate the muscle of the IV septum, the anterior papillary muscle (through the **septomarginal trabecula**), and the wall of the right ventricle. The subendocardial branches of the left bundle stimulate the IV septum, the anterior and posterior papillary muscles, and the wall of the left ventricle.

FIGURE 1.39.   **Conducting system of heart.** *Arrows* indicate the flow of impulses initiated at the SA node.

The following is a summary of the conducting system of the heart:

- The SA node initiates an impulse that is conducted to cardiac muscle fibers in the atria, causing them to contract.
- The impulse spreads by myogenic conduction, which transmits the impulse from the SA node to the AV node.
- The signal is distributed from the AV node through the AV bundle and the right and left bundle branches, which pass on each side of the IV septum to supply subendocardial

branches to the papillary muscles and the walls of the ventricles.

INNERVATION OF HEART

The heart is supplied by autonomic nerve fibers from superficial and deep **cardiac plexuses** (Fig. 1.22D). These nerve networks lie anterior to the bifurcation of the trachea and posterior to the ascending aorta. The **sympathetic supply of the heart** is from presynaptic fibers with cell bodies in

Anterior views

FIGURE 1.40. **Cardiac cycle.** Right side of heart (right atrium and right ventricle) is *blue*; left side of heart (left atrium and left ventricle) is *red*.

the intermediolateral cell columns (lateral horns) of the superior five or six thoracic segments of the spinal cord and from postsynaptic sympathetic fibers with cell bodies in the cervical and superior thoracic paravertebral ganglia of the sympathetic trunks. The postsynaptic fibers end in the SA and AV nodes and in relation to the terminations of parasympathetic fibers on the coronary arteries. Sympathetic stimulation of the nodal tissue increases the heart's rate and the force of its contractions. Sympathetic stimulation (indirectly) produces dilation of the coronary arteries by inhibiting their constriction. This supplies more oxygen and nutrients to the myocardium during periods of increased activity.

The **parasympathetic supply of the heart** is from presynaptic fibers of the *vagus nerves* (CN X). Postsynaptic parasympathetic cell bodies (intrinsic ganglia) are located near the SA and AV nodes and along the coronary arteries. Parasympathetic stimulation slows the heart rate, reduces the force of the contraction, and constricts the coronary arteries, saving energy between periods of increased demand.

CARDIAC CYCLE

The cardiac cycle describes the complete movement of the heart or heartbeat and includes the period from the beginning of one heartbeat to the beginning of the next one. The synchronous pumping action of the heart's two AV pumps (right and left chambers) constitutes the cardiac cycle.

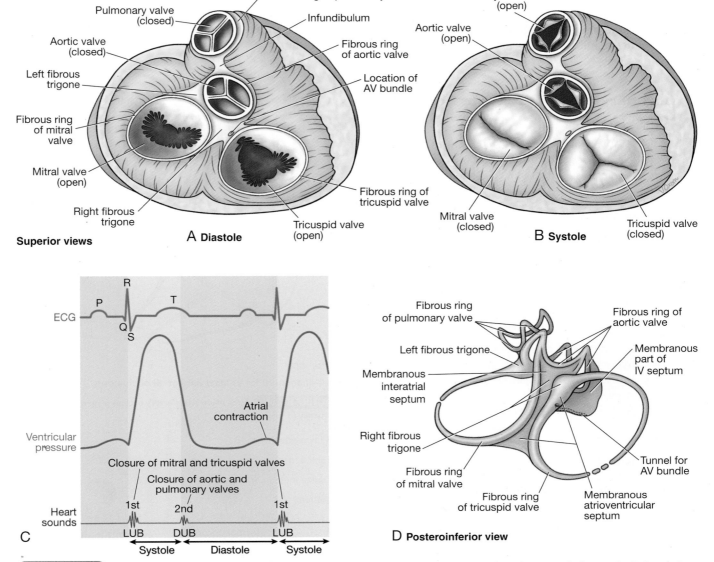

FIGURE 1.41. **Heart valves during diastole and systole and outline of cardiac skeleton. A.** Ventricular diastole. **B.** Ventricular systole. **C.** Correlation of ventricular pressure, electrocardiogram (ECG), and heart sounds. **D.** Cardiac skeleton. *IV,* interventricular; *AV,* atrioventricular.

The atria are receiving chambers that pump blood into the ventricle (the discharging chambers). The right heart (***blue***) is the pump for the pulmonary circuit; the left heart (***red***) is the pump for the systemic circuit (Fig. 1.40). The cycle begins with a period of ventricular elongation and filling (**diastole**) and ends with a period of ventricular shortening and emptying (**systole**). Two *heart sounds*, resulting from valve closures, can be heard with a stethoscope: a *lub* sound as the blood is transferred from the atria to the ventricles and a *dub* sound as the ventricles contract and expel blood from the heart (Fig. 1.41). The heart sounds are produced by the snapping shut of the one-way valves that normally keep blood from flowing backward during contractions of the heart.

When the ventricles contract, they produce a wringing motion. This motion initially ejects the blood from the ventricles, first narrowing and then shortening the heart, reducing the volume of the ventricular chambers. Continued sequential contraction elongates the heart, followed by widening as the myocardium briefly relaxes, increasing the volume of the chambers to draw blood from the atria.

CARDIAC SKELETON

The muscle fibers are anchored to the **fibrous skeleton of the heart** (Fig. 1.41). The fibrous framework of dense collagen forms four **fibrous rings,** which surround the orifices of the valves. The right and left **fibrous trigones** connect the rings, and the membranous parts of the interatrial and interventricular septa. The fibrous skeleton of the heart:

- Keeps the orifices of the AV and semilunar valves patent and prevents them from being overly distended by the volume of blood pumping through them.
- Provides attachments for the leaflets and cusps of the valves.
- Provides attachment for the myocardium.
- Forms an electrical "insulator" by separating the myenterically conducted impulses of the atria and ventricles so that they contract independently and by surrounding and providing passage for the initial part of the AV bundle.

Coronary Artery Disease or Coronary Heart Disease

Coronary artery disease (CAD) is one of the leading causes of death. It has many causes, all of which result in a reduced blood supply to the vital myocardial tissue.

Myocardial Infarction

With sudden occlusion of a major artery by an embolus (G. *embolos,* plug), the region of myocardium supplied by the occluded vessel becomes *infarcted* (rendered virtually bloodless) and undergoes *necrosis* (pathological tissue death). The three most common sites of coronary artery occlusion are (1) the anterior IV (LAD) branch of the LCA (40–50%), (2) the RCA (30–40%), and (3) the circumflex branch of the LCA (15–20%) (Fig. B1.14).

An area of myocardium that has undergone necrosis constitutes a **myocardial infarction** (MI). The most common cause of *ischemic heart disease* is coronary artery insufficiency resulting from atherosclerosis.

Coronary Atherosclerosis

The **atherosclerotic process,** characterized by lipid deposits in the intima (lining layer) of the coronary arteries, begins during early adulthood and slowly results in stenosis of the lumina of the arteries (Fig. B1.15). Insufficiency of blood supply to the heart (**myocardial ischemia**) may result in MI.

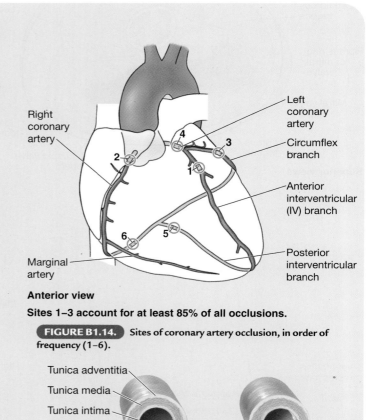

Anterior view

Sites 1–3 account for at least 85% of all occlusions.

FIGURE B1.14.   Sites of coronary artery occlusion, in order of frequency (1–6).

FIGURE B1.15.   Atherosclerosis.

Coronary Bypass Graft

Patients with obstruction of their coronary circulation and severe angina may undergo a **coronary bypass graft** operation. A segment of an artery or vein is connected to the ascending aorta or to the proximal part of a coronary artery and then to the coronary artery distal to the stenosis (Fig. B1.16). The *great saphenous vein* is commonly harvested for coronary bypass surgery because it (1) has a diameter equal to or greater than that of the coronary arteries, (2) can be easily dissected from the lower limb, (3) and offers relatively lengthy portions with a minimum occurrence of valves or branching. Reversal of the implanted segment of vein can negate the effect of a valve if a valved segment must be used. Use of the *radial artery* in bypass surgery has become increasingly more common. A coronary bypass graft shunts blood from the aorta to a stenotic coronary artery to increase the flow distal to the obstruction. Revascularization of the myocardium may also be achieved by surgically anastomosing an internal thoracic artery with a coronary artery.

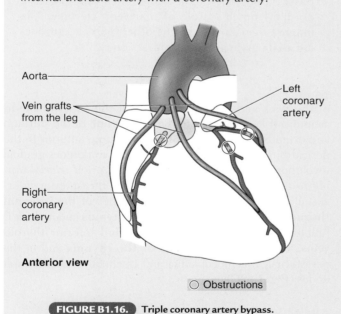

Aorta

Vein grafts from the leg

Left coronary artery

Right coronary artery

Anterior view

○ Obstructions

FIGURE B1.16. Triple coronary artery bypass.

Coronary Angioplasty

In selected patients, surgeons use **percutaneous transluminal coronary angioplasty,** in which they pass a catheter with a small inflatable balloon attached to its tip into the obstructed coronary artery (Fig. B1.17). When the catheter reaches the obstruction, the balloon is inflated, flattening the atherosclerotic plaque against the vessel's wall, and the vessel is stretched to increase the size of the lumen, thus improving blood flow. In other cases, *thrombokinase* is injected through the catheter; this enzyme dissolves the blood clot. After dilation of the vessel, an *intravascular stent* may be introduced to maintain the dilation.

Deflated balloon catheter approaches blockage

Inflated balloon crushes blockage

Circulation reestablished

FIGURE B1.17. Percutaneous transluminal angioplasty.

Variations of Coronary Arteries

Variations in the branching patterns of the coronary arteries are common. In the most common right-dominant pattern, the RCA and LCA share approximately equally in the blood supply to the heart. In approximately 15% of hearts, the LCA is dominant in that the posterior IV branch is a branch of the circumflex artery. There is codominance in about 18% of people, in which branches of both the RCA and LCA reach the crux and give rise to branches that course in or near the posterior IV groove. A few people have only a single coronary artery. In other people, the circumflex artery arises from the right aortic sinus. The branches of coronary arteries are considered to be end arteries—ones that supply regions of the myocardium without functional overlap from other large branches. However, anastomoses exist between small branches of the coronary arteries. The potential for development of collateral circulation likely exists in most hearts.

Echocardiography

Echocardiography (ultrasonic cardiography) is a method of graphically recording the position and motion of the heart by the echo obtained from beams of ultrasonic waves directed through the thorax. This technique may detect as little as 20 mL of fluid in the pericardial cavity, such as that resulting from pericardial effusion. *Doppler echocardiography* is a technique that demonstrates and records the flow of blood through the heart and great vessels by Doppler ultrasonography, making it especially useful in the diagnosis and analysis of problems with blood flow through the heart, such as septal defects, and in delineating valvular stenosis and regurgitation, especially on the left side of the heart.

Cardiac Referred Pain

The heart is insensitive to touch, cutting, cold, and heat; however, ischemia and the accumulation of metabolic products stimulate pain endings in the myocardium. The afferent pain fibers run centrally in the middle and inferior cervical branches and especially in the thoracic cardiac branches of the sympathetic trunk. The axons of these primary sensory neurons enter spinal cord segments T1–T4 or T5, especially on the left side. Cardiac referred pain is a phenomenon whereby noxious stimuli originating in the heart are perceived by the person as pain arising from a superficial part of the body—the skin on the medial aspect of the left upper limb, for example. Visceral pain is transmitted by visceral afferent fibers accompanying sympathetic fibers and is typically referred to somatic structures or areas such as the upper limb having afferent fibers with cell bodies in the same spinal ganglion, and central processes that enter the spinal cord through the same posterior roots.

Injury to Conducting System of Heart

Damage to the conducting system, often resulting from ischemia caused by *coronary artery disease,* produces disturbances of cardiac muscle contraction. Because the anterior IV branch (LAD branch) supplies the AV bundle in most people and because branches of the RCA supply both the SA and the AV nodes, parts of the conducting system of the heart are likely to be affected by their occlusion. Damage to the AV node or bundle results in a *heart block* because the atrial excitation does not reach the ventricles. As a result, the ventricles begin to contract independently at their own rate (25 to 30 times per minute), which is slower than the lowest normal rate of 40 to 45 times per minute. Damage to one of the bundle branches results in a *bundle branch block,* in which excitation passes along the unaffected branch and causes a normally timed systole of that ventricle only. The impulse then spreads to the other ventricle, producing a late asynchronous contraction.

Superior Mediastinum

The superior mediastinum is located superior to the transverse thoracic plane passing through the sternal angle and the junction (IV disc) of vertebrae T4 and T5. From anterior to posterior, **the main contents of the superior mediastinum** are (Fig. 1.42):

- Thymus, a primary lymphoid organ
- Great vessels related to the heart and pericardium:
  - Brachiocephalic veins
  - Superior part of SVC
  - Arch of aorta and roots of its major branches:
    - Brachiocephalic trunk
    - Left common carotid artery
    - Left subclavian artery
- Vagus and phrenic nerves
- Cardiac plexus of nerves
- Left recurrent laryngeal nerve
- Trachea
- Esophagus
- Thoracic duct

THYMUS

The thymus, a lymphoid organ, is located in the lower part of the neck and the anterior part of the superior mediastinum. It lies posterior to the manubrium of the sternum and extends into the anterior mediastinum, anterior to the pericardium. After puberty, the thymus undergoes gradual involution and is largely replaced by fat. A rich *arterial supply to the thymus* derives mainly from the anterior intercostal and anterior mediastinal branches of the **internal thoracic arteries.** The **veins of the thymus** end in the left brachiocephalic, internal thoracic, and inferior thyroid veins. The **lymphatic vessels of the thymus** end in the parasternal, brachiocephalic, and tracheobronchial lymph nodes (Fig. 1.22C).

GREAT VESSELS IN MEDIASTINUM

The *brachiocephalic veins* form posterior to the sternoclavicular joints by the union of the internal jugular and subclavian veins (Figs. 1.42 and 1.43A). At the level of the inferior border of the first right costal cartilage, the brachiocephalic veins unite to form the SVC. The **left brachiocephalic vein** is more than twice as long as the right brachiocephalic vein because it passes from the left to the right side, passing across the anterior aspects of the roots of the three major branches of the arch of the aorta, and shunting blood from the head, neck, and left upper limb to the right atrium. The

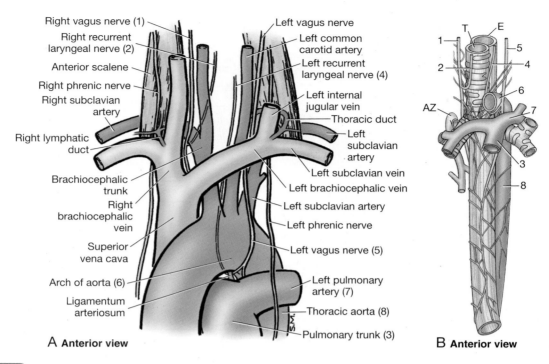

Right vagus nerve (1)
Right recurrent laryngeal nerve (2)
Anterior scalene
Right phrenic nerve
Right subclavian artery
Right lymphatic duct
Brachiocephalic trunk
Right brachiocephalic vein
Superior vena cava
Arch of aorta (6)
Ligamentum arteriosum

Left vagus nerve
Left common carotid artery
Left recurrent laryngeal nerve (4)
Left internal jugular vein
Thoracic duct
Left subclavian artery
Left subclavian vein
Left brachiocephalic vein
Left subclavian artery
Left phrenic nerve
Left vagus nerve (5)
Left pulmonary artery (7)
Thoracic aorta (8)
Pulmonary trunk (3)

A Anterior view

B Anterior view

FIGURE 1.42. **Great vessels and nerves. A.** Vessels in the lower neck and superior mediastinum. **B.** Relationships of trachea (*T*), esophagus (*E*), and azygos vein (*AZ*).

origin of the **right brachiocephalic vein** (by union of the right internal jugular and subclavian veins—the right venous angle) receives lymph from the **right lymphatic duct,** and the origin of the left brachiocephalic vein (by union of the left internal jugular and subclavian veins—the left "venous angle") receives lymph from the **thoracic duct** (Fig. 1.49A).

The **SVC** returns blood from all structures superior to the diaphragm, except the lungs and heart. It passes inferiorly and ends at the level of the third costal cartilage, where it enters the right atrium. The SVC lies in the right side of the superior mediastinum, anterolateral to the trachea and posterolateral to the ascending aorta (Figs. 1.42 and 1.44A). The **right phrenic nerve** lies between the SVC and the mediastinal pleura. The terminal half of the SVC is in the middle mediastinum, where it is adjacent to the ascending aorta and forms the posterior boundary of the transverse pericardial sinus (Fig. 1.26B). The **arch of the aorta,** the curved continuation of the ascending aorta, begins posterior to the second right sternocostal joint at the level of the sternal angle and arches superoposteriorly and to the left (Figs. 1.42 and 1.43). The aortic arch ascends anterior to the right pulmonary artery and the bifurcation of the trachea, reaching its apex at the left side of the trachea and esophagus as it passes over the root of the left lung. The arch descends on the left side of the body of the T4 vertebra and ends by becoming the **thoracic aorta** posterior to the second left sternocostal joint (Fig. 1.44B).

The **ligamentum arteriosum,** the remnant of the fetal ductus arteriosus, passes from the root of the left pulmonary artery to the inferior surface of the arch of the aorta (Fig. 1.42A). The **left recurrent laryngeal nerve** hooks beneath the arch immediately lateral to the ligamentum arteriosum and then ascends between the trachea and esophagus (Fig. 1.42 and Table 1.5). **The branches of the arch of the aorta** are the (Figs. 1.42 and 1.43):

- Brachiocephalic trunk.
- Left common carotid artery.
- Left subclavian artery.

The **brachiocephalic trunk,** the first and largest branch of the arch, arises posterior to the manubrium, where it lies anterior to the trachea and posterior to the left brachiocephalic vein. It ascends superolaterally to reach the right side of the trachea and the right sternoclavicular joint, where it divides into the right common carotid and right subclavian arteries. The **left common carotid artery,** the second branch of the aortic arch, arises posterior to the manubrium, slightly posterior and to the left of the brachiocephalic trunk. It ascends anterior to the left subclavian artery and at first anterior to the trachea and then to its left. It enters the neck by passing posterior to the left sternoclavicular joint. The **left subclavian artery,** the third branch of the aortic arch, arises from the posterior part of the arch, just posterior to the left common carotid artery. It ascends lateral to the trachea

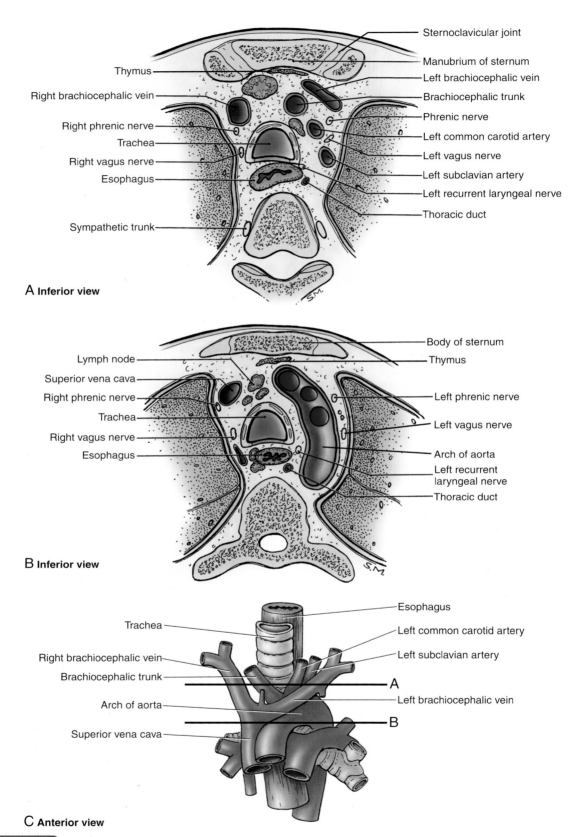

FIGURE 1.43. **Superior mediastinum. A.** Transverse section superior to arch of the aorta. **B.** Transverse section through arch of the aorta. **C.** Level of sections in parts **A** and **B.**

TABLE 1.5 NERVES OF THORAX

Nerve	Origin	Course	Distribution
Vagus (CN X)	8–10 rootlets from medulla of brainstem	Enters superior mediastinum posterior to tracheo-esophageal sternoclavicular joint and brachiocephalic vein; gives rise to recurrent laryngeal nerve; continues into abdomen	Pulmonary plexus, esophageal plexus, and cardiac plexus
Phrenic	Anterior rami of C3–C5 nerves	Passes through superior thoracic aperture and runs between mediastinal pleura and pericardium	Central portion of diaphragm
Intercostals (1–11)	Anterior rami of T1–T11 nerves	Run in intercostal spaces between internal and innermost layers of intercostal muscles	Muscles in and skin over intercostal space; lower nerves supply muscles and skin of anterolateral abdominal wall
Subcostal	Anterior ramus of T12 nerve	Follows inferior border of 12th rib and passes into abdominal wall	Abdominal wall and skin of gluteal region
Recurrent laryngeal	Vagus nerve	On right, loops around subclavian artery; on left, loops around arch of aorta and ascends in tracheo-esophageal groove	Intrinsic muscles of larynx (except cricothyroid); sensory inferior to level of vocal folds
Cardiac plexus	Cervical and cardiac branches of vagus nerve and sympathetic trunk	From arch of aorta and posterior surface of heart, fibers extend along coronary arteries and to sinuatrial node	Impulses pass to sinuatrial node; parasympathetic fibers slow rate; reduce force of heartbeat, and constrict coronary arteries; sympathetic fibers have opposite effect
Pulmonary plexus	Vagus nerve and sympathetic trunk	Forms on root of lung and extends along bronchial subdivisions	Parasympathetic fibers constrict bronchioles; sympathetic fibers dilate them; afferents convey reflexes
Esophageal plexus	Vagus nerve, sympathetic ganglia and greater splanchnic nerve	Distal to tracheal bifurcation, vagus and sympathetic nerves form the plexus around esophagus	Vagal and sympathetic fibers to smooth muscle and glands of inferior two thirds of esophagus

and the left common carotid artery through the superior mediastinum. The left subclavian artery has no branches in the mediastinum. As it leaves the thorax and enters the root of the neck, it passes posterior to the left sternoclavicular joint and lateral to the left common carotid artery.

NERVES IN SUPERIOR MEDIASTINUM

The **vagus nerves** (CN X) arise bilaterally from the medulla of the brain, exit the cranium, and descend through the neck posterolateral to the common carotid arteries. Each nerve enters the superior mediastinum posterior to the respective sternoclavicular joint and brachiocephalic vein (Figs. 1.42, 1.43, and 1.45; Table 1.5). The **right vagus nerve** enters the thorax anterior to the right subclavian artery, where it gives rise to the **right recurrent laryngeal nerve**. This nerve hooks inferior to the right subclavian artery and ascends between the trachea and the esophagus to supply the larynx. The right vagus nerve runs posteroinferiorly through the superior mediastinum on the right side of the trachea. It then passes posterior to the right brachiocephalic vein, SVC, and root of the right lung. Here it breaks up into a number of branches that contribute to the **pulmonary plexus** (Fig. 1.46B). Usually, the right vagus nerve leaves the pulmonary plexus as a single nerve and passes to the esophagus, where it again breaks up and contributes fibers to the **esophageal plexus** (Fig. 1.45A and B). The right vagus nerve also gives rise to nerves that contribute to the **cardiac plexus** (Fig. 1.45C).

The **left vagus nerve** descends in the neck and enters the thorax and mediastinum between the left common carotid and the left subclavian arteries and posterior to the left brachiocephalic vein (Fig. 1.42). When it reaches the left side of the arch of the aorta, the left vagus nerve diverges posteriorly from the left phrenic nerve. It is separated laterally from the phrenic nerve by the left superior intercostal vein. As the left vagus nerve curves medially at the inferior border of the arch of the aorta, it gives off the **left recurrent laryngeal nerve** (Fig. 1.45B). This nerve passes inferior to the arch of the aorta just posterolateral to the **ligamentum arteriosum** and ascends to the larynx in the groove between the trachea and the esophagus (Fig. 1.44 B). The left vagus nerve continues on to pass posterior to the root of the left lung, where it breaks up into many branches, which contribute to the **pulmonary and cardiac plexuses.** The nerve leaves these plexuses as a single trunk and passes to the esophagus, where it joins fibers from the right vagus in the **esophageal plexus** (Fig. 1.45B).

The **phrenic nerves** are the sole motor supply to the diaphragm (Figs. 1.44 and Table 1.5); approximately one third of their fibers are sensory to the diaphragm. Each phrenic nerve enters the superior mediastinum between the subclavian artery and the origin of the brachiocephalic vein. The **right phrenic nerve** passes along the right side of the right brachiocephalic vein, SVC, and pericardium over the right atrium. It also passes anterior to the root of the right lung and descends on the right side of the IVC to the

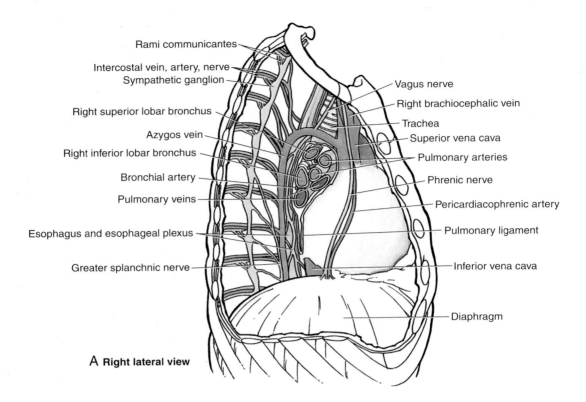

Rami communicantes

Intercostal vein, artery, nerve

Sympathetic ganglion

Right superior lobar bronchus

Azygos vein

Right inferior lobar bronchus

Bronchial artery

Pulmonary veins

Esophagus and esophageal plexus

Greater splanchnic nerve

Vagus nerve

Right brachiocephalic vein

Trachea

Superior vena cava

Pulmonary arteries

Phrenic nerve

Pericardiacophrenic artery

Pulmonary ligament

Inferior vena cava

Diaphragm

A **Right lateral view**

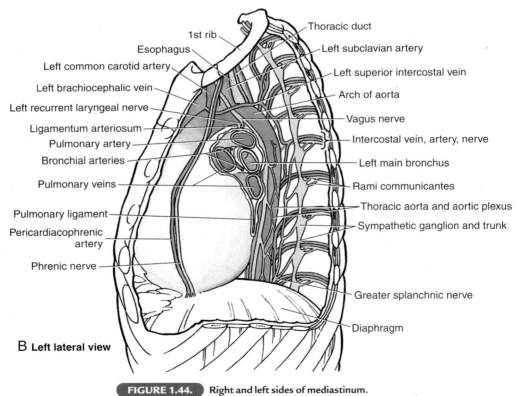

1st rib

Esophagus

Left common carotid artery

Left brachiocephalic vein

Left recurrent laryngeal nerve

Ligamentum arteriosum

Pulmonary artery

Bronchial arteries

Pulmonary veins

Pulmonary ligament

Pericardiacophrenic artery

Phrenic nerve

Thoracic duct

Left subclavian artery

Left superior intercostal vein

Arch of aorta

Vagus nerve

Intercostal vein, artery, nerve

Left main bronchus

Rami communicantes

Thoracic aorta and aortic plexus

Sympathetic ganglion and trunk

Greater splanchnic nerve

Diaphragm

B **Left lateral view**

FIGURE 1.44. Right and left sides of mediastinum.

Cervicothoracic ganglion (stellate ganglion)

Esophagus

Left vagus nerve

Right sympathetic trunk

Cardiac plexus

Left recurrent laryngeal nerve

Rami communicantes

Thoracic aortic plexus

Intercostal nerve

Right vagus nerve (cut end)

Esophageal plexus

Greater splanchnic nerve

Diaphragm

Anterior and posterior vagal trunks

Aortic hiatus

Celiac ganglion
Celiac artery

Splanchnic nerves { Greater / Lesser / Least

Medial arcuate ligament
Left crus of diaphragm

Right sympathetic trunk

A

Right recurrent laryngeal nerve

Left recurrent laryngeal nerve

Right vagus nerve

Left vagus nerve

Cardiac plexus

Right pulmonary plexus

Left pulmonary plexus

Esophageal plexus

B

Middle cervical ganglion

Cervicothoracic ganglion

T1 sympathetic ganglion

Cardiac plexus

Left pulmonary plexus

T3 sympathetic ganglion

Esophageal plexus

C

Innervation
- Sympathetic
- Parasympathetic
- Mixed sympathetic and parasympathetic nerves
- Somatic

FIGURE 1.45. **Nerves in mediastinum. A.** Autonomic nerves in the superior and posterior mediastinum. **B.** Parasympathetic nerves. **C.** Sympathetic nerves. *A,* aorta; *AR,* arch of aorta; *B,* right brachiocephalic artery; *E,* esophagus; *S,* right subclavian artery; *T,* trachea.

diaphragm, which it penetrates or passes through the caval opening (foramen).

The **left phrenic nerve** descends between the left subclavian and the left common carotid arteries (Fig. 1.44*B*). It crosses the left surface of the arch of the aorta anterior to the left vagus nerve and passes over the left superior intercostal vein. It then descends anterior to the root of the left lung and runs along the pericardium, superficial to the left atrium and ventricle of the heart, where it penetrates the diaphragm to the left of the pericardium.

TRACHEA

The trachea descends anterior to the esophagus and enters the superior mediastinum, inclining a little to the right of the median plane (Figs. 1.47*C* and *D*). The posterior surface of the trachea is flat where its cartilaginous "rings" are incomplete and where it is related to the esophagus. The trachea ends at the level of the sternal angle by dividing into the right and left main bronchi.

ESOPHAGUS

The esophagus is a fibromuscular tube that extends from the pharynx to the stomach. It is usually flattened anteroposteriorly (Figs. 1.43 and 1.46). The esophagus enters the superior mediastinum between the trachea and the vertebral column, where it lies anterior to the bodies of vertebrae T1–T4. Initially, the esophagus inclines to the left but is moved by the aortic arch to the median plane opposite the root of the left lung. The **thoracic duct** usually lies on the left side of the esophagus and deep to the aortic arch. Inferior to the arch,

*Areas of constriction where swallowed foreign objects are most likely to lodge and where a stricture may develop, e.g., after drinking caustic liquid.

Labels (top to bottom, right side): Esophagus; Trachea; Arch of aorta*; Left main bronchus*; Left bronchial artery; Thoracic aorta; Esophageal arteries; Esophagus; Diaphragm*; Stomach (cut edge); Left gastric artery; Abdominal aorta

Labels (left side): Esophageal hiatus (opening); Aortic hiatus

Anterior view

FIGURE 1.46. Esophagus.

the esophagus inclines to the left as it approaches and passes through the esophageal hiatus in the diaphragm.

Posterior Mediastinum

The **posterior mediastinum** is located anterior to vertebrae T5–T12, posterior to the pericardium and diaphragm, and between the parietal pleura of the two lungs. The posterior mediastinum contains the (Fig. 1.47):

- Thoracic aorta
- Thoracic duct
- Posterior mediastinal lymph nodes (e.g., tracheobronchial nodes)
- Azygos and hemiazygos veins
- Esophagus
- Esophageal plexus
- Thoracic sympathetic trunks
- Thoracic splanchnic nerves

THORACIC AORTA

The thoracic aorta, the thoracic part of the descending aorta, is the continuation of the **arch of the aorta** (Figs. 1.47, Table 1.6). It begins on the left side of the inferior border of the body of T4 vertebra and descends in the posterior mediastinum on the left sides of T5–T12 vertebrae. As it descends, it approaches the median plane and displaces the esophagus to the right. The **thoracic aortic plexus,** an autonomic nerve network, surrounds it (Fig. 1.45*A*). The thoracic aorta lies posterior to the root of the left lung, the pericardium, and the esophagus. Its name changes to *abdominal aorta* anterior to the inferior border of the T12 vertebra, and it enters the abdomen through the **aortic hiatus** (opening) in the diaphragm (Figs. 1.46 and 1.47). The **thoracic duct** and azygos vein descend on the right side of the thoracic aorta and accompany it through this hiatus (Fig. 1.47*D*).

The **branches of the thoracic aorta** are bronchial, pericardial, posterior intercostals, superior phrenic, esophageal, mediastinal, and subcostal (Fig. 1.48; Table 1.6). The **bronchial arteries** consist of one right and two small left vessels. The bronchial arteries supply the trachea, bronchi, lung tissue, and lymph nodes. The **pericardial arteries** send twigs to the pericardium. The **posterior intercostal arteries** (nine pairs) pass into the third through eleventh intercostal spaces.

The **superior phrenic arteries** pass to the posterior surface of the diaphragm, where they anastomose with the musculophrenic and pericardiacophrenic branches of the internal thoracic artery. Usually, two **esophageal arteries** supply the middle third of the esophagus. The **mediastinal arteries** are small and supply the lymph nodes and other tissues of the posterior mediastinum. The **subcostal arteries** that course on the abdominal side of the origin of the diaphragm are in series with the intercostal arteries.

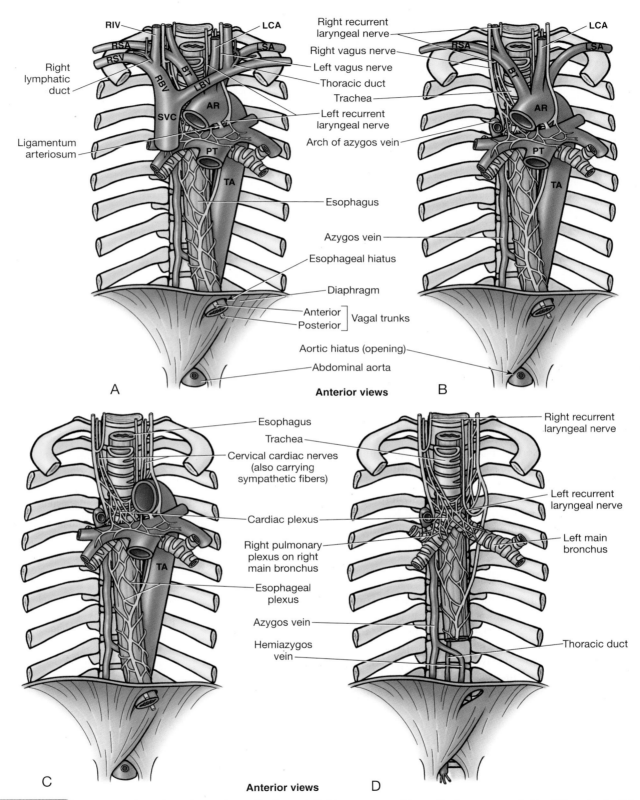

FIGURE 1.47. **Structures of superior and posterior mediastinum. A–D.** The structures of the mediastinum are revealed by different levels of dissection from anterior to posterior. *AR,* aortic arch; *BT,* brachiocephalic trunk; *LBV,* left brachiocephalic vein; *LCA,* left common carotid artery; *LSA,* left subclavian artery; *RBV,* right brachiocephalic vein; *RIV,* right internal jugular vein; *RSA,* right subclavian artery; *RSV,* right subclavian vein; *SVC,* superior vena cava; *TA,* thoracic aorta; *PT,* pulmonary trunk; *T,* trachea.

TABLE 1.6 AORTA AND ITS BRANCHES IN THORAX

Artery	Origin	Course	Branches
Ascending aorta	Aortic orifice of left ventricle	Ascends ~5 cm to sternal angle, where it becomes arch of aorta	Right and left coronary arteries
Arch of aorta	Continuation of ascending aorta	Arches posteriorly on left side of trachea and esophagus and superior to left main bronchus	Brachiocephalic, left common carotid, left subclavian arteries
Thoracic aorta	Continuation of arch of aorta	Descends in posterior mediastinum to left of vertebral column; gradually shifts to right to lie in median plane at aortic hiatus	Posterior intercostal arteries, subcostal, some phrenic arteries, and visceral branches (e.g., esophageal)
Posterior intercostals	Posterior aspect of thoracic aorta	Pass laterally and then anteriorly, parallel to ribs	Lateral and anterior cutaneous branches
Bronchial (1 or 2 branches)	Anterior aspect of aorta or posterior intercostal artery	Run with tracheobronchial tree	Bronchial and peribronchial tissue, visceral pleura
Esophageal (4 or 5 branches)	Anterior aspect of thoracic aorta	Run anteriorly to esophagus	To esophagus
Superior phrenic (vary in number)	Anterior aspect of thoracic aorta	Arise at aortic hiatus and pass to superior aspect of diaphragm	To diaphragm

ESOPHAGUS

The esophagus descends into the posterior mediastinum from the superior mediastinum, passing posterior and to the right of the arch of the aorta and posterior to the pericardium and left atrium. The esophagus constitutes the primary posterior relationship of the base of the heart. It then deviates to the left and passes through the **esophageal hiatus** in the diaphragm at the level of the T10 vertebra, anterior to the aorta (Figs. 1.46 and 1.47). The esophagus may have three impressions, or "constrictions," in its thoracic part. These may be observed as narrowings of the lumen in oblique chest radiographs that are taken as barium is swallowed.

The esophagus is compressed by three structures: the aortic arch, left main bronchus, and diaphragm. No constrictions are visible in the empty esophagus; however, as it expands during filling, these structures compress its walls.

THORACIC DUCT AND LYMPHATIC TRUNKS

In the posterior mediastinum, the **thoracic duct** lies on the bodies of the inferior seven thoracic vertebrae (Fig. 1.49A). The thoracic duct conveys most lymph of the body to the venous system (that from the lower limbs, pelvic cavity, abdominal cavity, left side of thorax, left side of head, neck, and left upper limb). The thoracic duct originates from the **cisterna chyli** in the abdomen and ascends through the aortic hiatus in the diaphragm. The thoracic duct is usually thin-walled and dull white; often, it is beaded because of its numerous valves. It ascends between the thoracic aorta on its left, the azygos vein on its right, the esophagus anteriorly, and the vertebral bodies posteriorly. At the level of the T4–T6 vertebrae, the thoracic duct crosses to the left, posterior to the esophagus, and ascends into the superior mediastinum. The thoracic duct receives branches from the middle and upper intercostal spaces of both sides through

several collecting trunks. It also receives branches from posterior mediastinal structures. Near its termination, it often receives the jugular, subclavian, and bronchomediastinal lymphatic trunks. The thoracic duct usually empties into the venous system near the union of the left internal jugular and

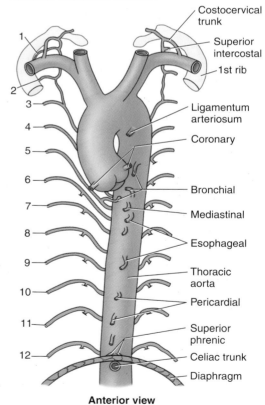

Posterior intercostal arteries:

Costocervical trunk
Superior intercostal
1st rib
Ligamentum arteriosum
Coronary
Bronchial
Mediastinal
Esophageal
Thoracic aorta
Pericardial
Superior phrenic
Celiac trunk
Diaphragm

Anterior view

FIGURE 1.48. **Branches of thoracic aorta.** Superior phrenic arteries arising from the inferior part of the thoracic aorta supply the diaphragm. *1–12,* posterior intercostal arteries.

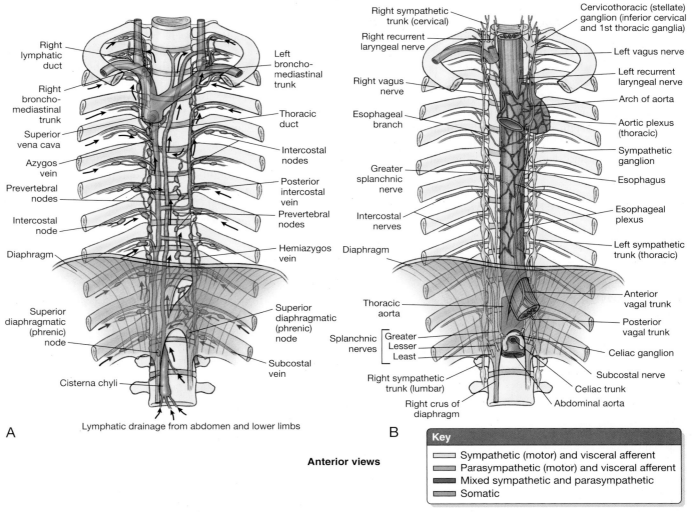

Anterior views

Key
Sympathetic (motor) and visceral afferent
Parasympathetic (motor) and visceral afferent
Mixed sympathetic and parasympathetic
Somatic

FIGURE 1.49. **Posterior mediastinum: lymphatic drainage, azygos system of veins, and nerves. A.** Lymphatic drainage and azygos system of veins. **B.** Nerves.

subclavian veins, the **left venous angle** (Fig. 1.49A), or origin of the left brachiocephalic vein.

VESSELS AND LYMPH NODES OF POSTERIOR MEDIASTINUM

The thoracic aorta and its branches were discussed previously. The **azygos system of veins,** on each side of the vertebral column, drains the back and thoraco-abdominal walls as well as the mediastinal viscera (Fig. 1.49A). The azygos system exhibits much variation, not only in its origin but also in its course, tributaries, anastomoses, and termination. The **azygos vein** and its main tributary, the **hemiazygos vein,** usually arise from "roots" arising from the posterior aspect of the IVC and/or renal vein, respectively, which merge with the ascending lumbar veins. The azygos vein forms a collateral pathway between the SVC and the IVC and drains blood from the posterior walls of the thorax and abdomen. The azygos vein ascends in the posterior mediastinum, passing close to the right sides of the bodies of the inferior eight thoracic vertebrae. It arches over the superior aspect of the root of the right lung to join the SVC (Fig. 1.44A).

In addition to the **posterior intercostal veins,** the azygos vein communicates with the vertebral venous plexuses that drain the back, vertebrae, and structures in the vertebral canal (see Chapter 4). The azygos vein also receives the mediastinal, esophageal, and bronchial veins. The hemiazygos vein ascends on the left side of the vertebral column, posterior to the thoracic aorta as far as T9. Here it crosses to the right, posterior to the aorta, thoracic duct, and esophagus, and joins the azygos vein.

The **accessory hemiazygos vein** descends on the left side of the vertebral column from T5 to T8 and then crosses over the T7–T8 vertebra posterior to the thoracic aorta and thoracic duct to join the azygos vein (Fig. 1.44*B*). Sometimes, the accessory hemiazygos vein joins the hemiazygos vein and drains with it into the azygos vein.

Posterior mediastinal lymph nodes lie posterior to the pericardium, where they are related to the esophagus and thoracic aorta (Fig. 1.49*A*). There are several nodes posterior to the inferior part of the esophagus and more anterior and lateral to it. The posterior mediastinal lymph nodes receive lymph from the esophagus, the posterior aspect of the pericardium and diaphragm, and the middle posterior intercostal spaces.

NERVES OF POSTERIOR MEDIASTINUM

The sympathetic trunks and their associated ganglia form a major portion of the autonomic nervous system (Fig. 1.49*B*, Table 1.5). The **thoracic sympathetic trunks** are in continuity with the cervical and lumbar sympathetic trunks. The thoracic sympathetic trunks lie against the heads of the ribs in the superior part of the thorax, the costovertebral joints in the midthoracic level, and the sides of the vertebral bodies in the inferior part of the thorax. The **lower thoracic splanchnic nerves,** also known as greater, lesser, and least splanchnic nerves, are part of the *abdominopelvic splanchnic nerves* because they supply viscera inferior to the diaphragm. They consist of presynaptic fibers from the fifth to twelfth paravertebral sympathetic ganglia, which pass through the diaphragm and synapse in prevertebral ganglia in the abdomen. They supply sympathetic innervation for most of the abdominal viscera. These splanchnic nerves are discussed further in Chapter 2.

Laceration of Thoracic Duct

 Because the thoracic duct is thin-walled and may be colorless, it may not be easily identified. Consequently, it is vulnerable to inadvertent injury during investigative and/or surgical procedures in the posterior mediastinum. Laceration of the thoracic duct results in chyle escaping into the thoracic cavity. Chyle may also enter the pleural cavity, producing *chylothorax.*

Collateral Venous Routes to Heart

The azygos, hemiazygos, and accessory hemiazygos veins offer alternate means of venous drainage from the thoracic, abdominal, and back regions when *obstruction of the IVC* occurs. In some people, an accessory azygos vein parallels the main azygos vein on the right side. Other people have no hemiazygos system of veins. A clinically important variation, although uncommon, is when the azygos system receives all the blood from the IVC, except that from the liver. In these people, the azygos system drains nearly all the blood inferior to the diaphragm, except from the digestive tract. When *obstruction of the SVC* occurs superior to the entrance of the azygos vein, blood can drain inferiorly into the veins of the abdominal wall and return to the right atrium through the IVC and azygos system of veins.

Aneurysm of Ascending Aorta

The distal part of the ascending aorta receives a strong thrust of blood when the left ventricle contracts. Because its wall is not yet reinforced by fibrous pericardium (the fibrous pericardium blends with the aortic adventitia at the beginning of the arch), an *aneurysm* (localized dilation) may develop. An aortic aneurysm is evident on a chest film (radiograph of the thorax) or a magnetic resonance angiogram as an enlarged area of the ascending aorta silhouette. Individuals with an aneurysm usually complain of chest pain that radiates to the back. The aneurysm may exert pressure on the trachea, esophagus, and recurrent laryngeal nerve, causing difficulty in breathing and swallowing.

Injury to Recurrent Laryngeal Nerves

The recurrent laryngeal nerves supply all the intrinsic muscles of the larynx, except one. Consequently, any investigative procedure or disease process in the superior mediastinum may involve these nerves and affect the voice. Because the left recurrent laryngeal nerve hooks around the arch of the aorta and ascends between the trachea and the esophagus, it may be involved when there is a bronchial or esophageal carcinoma, enlargement of mediastinal lymph nodes, or an aneurysm of the arch of the aorta. In the latter condition, the nerve may be stretched by the dilated arch of the aorta.

Variations of Great Arteries

The most superior part of the arch of the aorta is usually approximately 2.5 cm inferior to the superior border of the manubrium, but it may be more superior or inferior. Sometimes the arch curves over the root of the right lung and passes inferiorly on the right side, forming a **right arch of the aorta.** Less frequently, a **double arch of the aorta** or **retroesophageal right subclavian artery** form a vascular ring around the esophagus and trachea (Fig. B1.18). If the trachea is compressed enough to affect breathing, surgical division of the vascular ring may be needed.

Variations in the origin of the branches of the arch are fairly common. The usual pattern of branches of the arch of the aorta is present in approximately 65% of people. In approximately 27% of people, the left common carotid artery originates from the brachiocephalic trunk. A brachiocephalic trunk fails to form in approximately 2.5% of people; in these cases each of the four arteries (right and left common carotid and subclavian arteries) originate independently from the arch of the aorta (Bergman et al., 1988).

Coarctation of Aorta

In **coarctation of the aorta,** the arch of the aorta or descending aorta has an abnormal narrowing (stenosis) that diminishes the caliber of the aortic lumen, producing an obstruction to blood flow to the inferior part of the body (Fig. B1.19). The most common site for a coarctation is near the ligamentum arteriosum. When the coarctation is inferior to this site (*postductal coarctation*), a good collateral

FIGURE B1.19. Coarctation of aorta.

circulation usually develops between the proximal and distal parts of the aorta through the intercostal and internal thoracic arteries.

Age Changes in Thymus

The thymus is a prominent feature of the superior mediastinum during infancy and childhood. In some infants, the thymus may compress the trachea. The thymus plays an important role in the development and maintenance of the immune system. As puberty is reached, the thymus begins to diminish in relative size. By adulthood, it is usually replaced by adipose tissue and is often scarcely recognizable; however, it continues to produce T lymphocytes.

A Retroesophageal right subclavian artery

B Double arch of aorta

FIGURE B1.18. Aortic arch anomalies.

Medical Imaging of Thorax

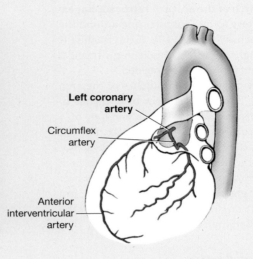

Left coronary artery

Circumflex artery

Anterior interventricular artery

A Left lateral view

Sinu-atrial nodal artery

Right coronary artery

Posterior interventricular branch

B Left anterior oblique view

C Anterior view

Key

1. Superior vena cava	7.	Right ventricle
2. Ascending aorta	8.	Inferior vena cava
3. Right auricle	9.	Left ventricle
4. Right coronary artery	10.	Anterior interventricular artery
5. Right atrium		
6. Coronary (atrioventricular) sulcus	11.	Circumflex branch
	12.	Left auricle
	13	Pulmonary trunk

FIGURE 1.50.   **Imaging of coronary vessels. A and B.** Coronary arteriograms. Radiopaque dye has been injected into the left (**A**) and the right (**B**) coronary arteries. **C.** 3-D volume reconstruction of heart and coronary vessels.

AA	Ascending aorta
AZ	Azygos vein
DA	Descending aorta
E	Esophagus
ILPV	Inferior left pulmonary vein
IRPV	Inferior right pulmonary vein
IS	Interventricular septum
LA	Left atrium
LCA	Left coronary artery
LPA	Left pulmonary artery
LPV	Left pulmonary vein
LV	Left ventricle
MV	Mitral valve
PT	Pulmonary trunk
RA	Right atrium
RCA	Right coronary artery
RPA	Right pulmonary artery
RPV	Right pulmonary vein
RV	Right ventricle
SLPV	Superior left pulmonary vein
SRPV	Superior right pulmonary vein
SVC	Superior vena cava
V	Vertebra
ST	Sternum

FIGURE 1.51. Transverse (axial) 3-D volume reconstructions of thorax (on left side of page) and CT angiograms of thorax (on right side of page).

Go to _http://thePoint.lww.com/ECA4e_ for helpful study tools, including USMLE-style questions, case studies, images, and more!

Page has CHAPTER 2 title page layout

CHAPTER

2 Abdomen

ABDOMINAL CAVITY / 117

ANTEROLATERAL ABDOMINAL WALL / 117

Fascia of Anterolateral Abdominal Wall / 118

Muscles of Anterolateral Abdominal Wall / 119

Internal Surface of Anterolateral Abdominal Wall / 121

Surface Anatomy of Anterolateral Abdominal Wall / 124

Nerves of Anterolateral Abdominal Wall / 125

Vessels of Anterolateral Abdominal Wall / 126

Inguinal Region / 127

PERITONEUM AND PERITONEAL CAVITY / 135

Peritoneal Vessels and Nerves / 136

Peritoneal Formations / 136

Subdivisions of Peritoneal Cavity / 138

ABDOMINAL VISCERA / 140

Esophagus / 143

Stomach / 143

Surface Anatomy of Stomach / 148

Small Intestine / 146

Large Intestine / 154

Surface Anatomy of Spleen and Pancreas / 161

Spleen / 161

Pancreas / 162

Liver / 165

Surface Anatomy of Liver / 167

Biliary Ducts and Gallbladder / 171

Hepatic Portal Vein and Portal–Systemic Anastomoses / 173

Kidneys, Ureters, and Suprarenal Glands / 174

Summary of Innervation of Abdominal Viscera / 180

Surface Anatomy of Kidneys and Ureters / 180

DIAPHRAGM / 185

Diaphragmatic Apertures / 189

Vasculature and Nerves of Diaphragm / 189

POSTERIOR ABDOMINAL WALL / 192

Fascia of Posterior Abdominal Wall / 192

Muscles of Posterior Abdominal Wall / 193

Nerves of Posterior Abdominal Wall / 193

Vasculature of Posterior Abdominal Wall / 195

Lymphatics of Posterior Abdominal Wall / 196

MEDICAL IMAGING OF ABDOMEN / 199

The abdomen is the part of the trunk between the thorax and the pelvis. It has musculotendinous walls, except posteriorly, where the wall includes the lumbar vertebrae and intervertebral (IV) discs. The abdominal wall encloses the abdominal cavity, containing the peritoneal cavity and housing most of the organs (viscera) of the alimentary system and part of the urogenital system.

ABDOMINAL CAVITY

The **abdominal cavity** is the space bounded by the abdominal walls, diaphragm, and pelvis. The abdominal cavity forms the major part of the **abdominopelvic cavity**—the combined and continuous abdominal and pelvic cavities (Fig. 2.1). The abdominal cavity is:

- Enclosed anterolaterally by dynamic musculo-aponeurotic abdominal walls.
- Separated superiorly from the thoracic cavity by the diaphragm.
- Under cover of the thoracic cage superiorly extending to the fourth intercostal space.
- Continuous inferiorly with the pelvic cavity.
- Lined with peritoneum, a serous membrane.
- The location of most of the digestive organs, spleen, kidneys, and ureters for most of their course.

Clinicians subdivide the abdominal cavity into nine regions to locate abdominal organs or pain sites: right and left hypochondriac, right and left lateral (lumbar), right and left inguinal (groin), epigastric, umbilical, and pubic (hypogastric). The nine regions are delineated by four planes (Fig. 2.2A):

- Two horizontal:
  - **Subcostal plane,** passing through the inferior border of the 10th costal cartilage on each side.
  - **Transtubercular plane,** passing through the iliac tubercles and the body of the L5 vertebra.
- Two vertical:
  - **Midclavicular planes,** passing from the midpoints of clavicles to the **midinguinal points,** the midpoints of lines joining the *anterior superior iliac spines* and the superior edge of the *pubic symphysis.*

For general clinical descriptions, clinicians use four quadrants of the abdominal cavity: right upper, right lower, left upper, and left lower. The four quadrants are defined by two planes (Fig. 2.2B):

- **Transumbilical plane,** passing through the umbilicus and IV disc between the L3 and L4 vertebrae.
- **Median plane,** passing longitudinally through the body, dividing it into right and left halves.

ANTEROLATERAL ABDOMINAL WALL

Although the abdominal wall is continuous, it is subdivided for descriptive purposes into the *anterior wall, right and left lateral walls (flanks),* and *posterior wall.* The boundary between the anterior and the lateral walls is indefinite.

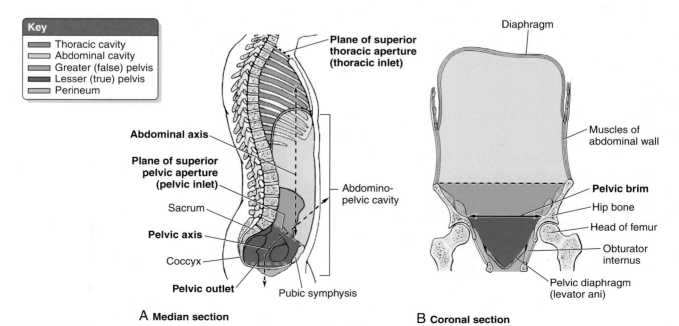

Key
- Thoracic cavity
- Abdominal cavity
- Greater (false) pelvis
- Lesser (true) pelvis
- Perineum

Plane of superior thoracic aperture (thoracic inlet)

Abdominal axis

Plane of superior pelvic aperture (pelvic inlet)

Sacrum

Pelvic axis

Coccyx

Pelvic outlet

Pubic symphysis

Abdomino-pelvic cavity

A Median section

Diaphragm

Muscles of abdominal wall

Pelvic brim

Hip bone

Head of femur

Obturator internus

Pelvic diaphragm (levator ani)

B Coronal section

FIGURE 2.1.   **Thoracic and abdominopelvic cavities. A.** The pelvic inlet (superior pelvic aperture) is the opening into the lesser pelvis. The pelvic outlet (inferior pelvic aperture) is the lower opening of the lesser pelvis. **B.** The plane of the pelvic brim (double-headed arrow) separates the greater pelvis (part of the abdominal cavity) from the lesser pelvis (the pelvic cavity).

Anterior views   **A Nine abdominal regions**

Key
▬ Right hypochondriac (RH)   ▬ Left lateral (lumbar) (LL)
▬ Epigastric (E)   ▬ Right inguinal (groin) (RI)
▬ Left hypochondriac (LH)   ▬ Pubic (hypogastric) (P)
▬ Right lateral (lumbar) (RL)   ▬ Left inguinal (groin) (LI)
▬ Umbilical (U)

B Four abdominal quadrants

Key
▬ Right upper quadrant (RUQ)
▬ Left upper quadrant (LUQ)
▬ Right lower quadrant (RLQ)
▬ Left lower quadrant (LLQ)

FIGURE 2.2.   Subdivisions of abdomen and reference planes.

Consequently, the combined term *anterolateral abdominal wall*, extending from the thoracic cage to the pelvis, is often used. The anterolateral abdominal wall is bounded superiorly by the cartilages of the 7th through 10th ribs and the xiphoid process of the sternum and inferiorly by the inguinal ligament and pelvic bones (Fig. 2.4). The wall consists of skin, subcutaneous tissue (superficial fascia), muscles and their aponeuroses, deep fascia, extraperitoneal fat, and parietal peritoneum (Fig. 2.3). The skin attaches loosely to the subcutaneous tissue except at the umbilicus, where it adheres firmly.

Fascia of Anterolateral Abdominal Wall

The fascial layers from superficial to deep include the **subcutaneous tissue** (superficial fascia), which lies deep to the skin and contains a variable amount of fat (Fig. 2.3). Inferior to the umbilicus, the subcutaneous tissue is composed of two layers: a **superficial fatty layer** (Camper fascia) and a **deep membranous layer** (Scarpa fascia) (see also Fig. B2.1).

The **investing fascia** (epimysium) covers the external aspects of the three muscle layers of the anterolateral abdominal wall and their aponeuroses.

The **endo-abdominal fascia** is a membranous sheet of varying thickness that lines the internal aspect of the abdominal wall. Although continuous, different parts of this

fascia can be named according to the muscle or aponeurosis it is lining—for example, the portion lining the deep surface of the transversus abdominis muscle or aponeurosis is the **transversalis fascia.**

The **parietal peritoneum** lines the abdominal cavity and is located internal to the transversalis fascia. It is separated from the transversalis fascia by a variable amount of **extraperitoneal fat.**

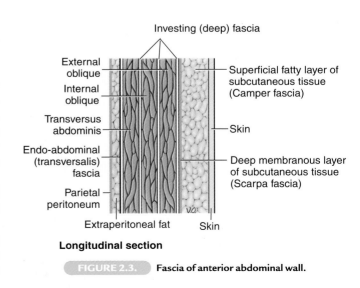

Longitudinal section

FIGURE 2.3.   Fascia of anterior abdominal wall.

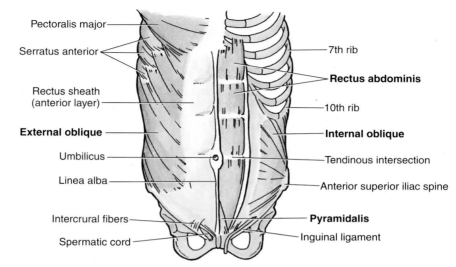

Pectoralis major

Serratus anterior

Rectus sheath (anterior layer)

External oblique

Umbilicus

Linea alba

Intercrural fibers

Spermatic cord

7th rib

Rectus abdominis

10th rib

Internal oblique

Tendinous intersection

Anterior superior iliac spine

Pyramidalis

Inguinal ligament

A **Anterior view**

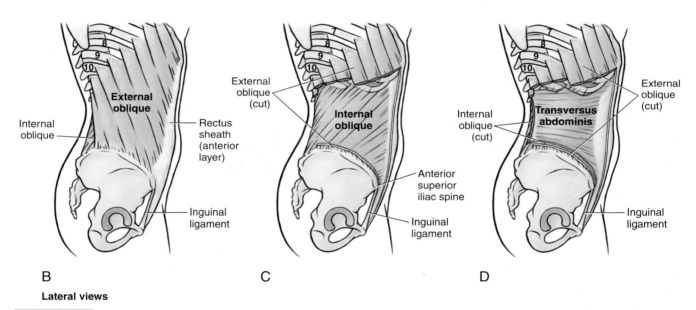

Internal oblique

External oblique

Rectus sheath (anterior layer)

Inguinal ligament

B

External oblique (cut)

Internal oblique

Anterior superior iliac spine

Inguinal ligament

C

Internal oblique (cut)

Transversus abdominis

External oblique (cut)

Inguinal ligament

D

Lateral views

FIGURE 2.4. **Anterolateral abdominal wall. A.** Right side, external oblique and intact rectus sheath; left side, internal oblique and opened rectus sheath, revealing rectus abdominis. **B.** External oblique. **C.** Internal oblique. **D.** Transversus abdominis.

Muscles of Anterolateral Abdominal Wall

There are five (bilaterally paired) muscles in the anterolateral abdominal wall (Fig. 2.4): three flat muscles and two vertical muscles. Their attachments, nerve supply, and main actions are listed in Table 2.1.

The three flat muscles are the:

- **External oblique,** the superficial muscle: Its fibers pass inferomedially and interdigitate with slips of the serratus anterior. The inferior margin is thickened as an under-curving fibrous band that spans between the anterior

superior iliac spine and the pubic tubercle as the **inguinal ligament.**

- **Internal oblique,** the intermediate muscle: Its fibers fan out so that its upper fibers are perpendicular and its lower fibers are parallel to those of the external oblique.
- **Transversus abdominis,** the innermost muscle: Its fibers, except for the most inferior ones, run more or less horizontally.

All three flat muscles end anteriorly in a strong sheet-like **aponeurosis.** Between the midclavicular line and the midline, the aponeuroses form the tough **rectus sheath,** enclosing

TABLE 2.1 PRINCIPAL MUSCLES OF ANTEROLATERAL ABDOMINAL WALL

Muscles[a]	Origin	Insertion	Innervation	Action(s)
External oblique	External surfaces of 5th–12th ribs	Linea alba, pubic tubercle, and anterior half of iliac crest	Thoraco-abdominal nerves (anterior rami of T7–T11) and subcostal nerve	Compress and support abdominal viscera; flex and rotate trunk
Internal oblique	Thoracolumbar fascia, anterior two thirds of iliac crest, and connective tissue deep to inguinal ligament	Inferior borders of 10th–12th ribs, linea alba, and pubis via conjoint tendon	Thoraco-abdominal nerves (anterior rami of T7-T11) and first lumbar nerve	
Transversus abdominis	Internal surfaces of 7th–12th costal cartilages, thoracolumbar fascia, iliac crest, and connective tissue deep to inguinal ligament	Linea alba with aponeurosis of internal oblique, pubic crest, and pectin pubis via conjoint tendon		Compresses and supports abdominal viscera
Rectus abdominis	Pubic symphysis and pubic crest	Xiphoid process and 5th–7th costal cartilages	Thoraco-abdominal nerves (anterior rami of inferior six thoracic nerves)	Flexes trunk (lumbar vertebrae) and compresses abdominal viscera;[b] stabilizes and controls tilt of pelvis (antilordosis)

[a]Approximately 80% of people have a *pyramidalis muscle,* which is located in the rectus sheath anterior to the most inferior part of the rectus abdominis. It extends from the pubic crest of the hip bone to the linea alba. This small muscle tenses on the linea alba.

[b]In so doing, these muscles act as antagonists of the diaphragm to produce expiration.

the rectus abdominis. The aponeuroses interweave, forming a midline raphe (G. *rhaphe,* suture, seam), the **linea alba** (L. white line), which extends from the xiphoid process to the pubic symphysis. The interweaving is not only between right and left sides but also between superficial, intermediate, and deep layers. For example, the tendinous fibers of the external oblique that decussate at the linea alba, for the most part, become continuous with the tendinous fibers of the contralateral internal oblique, forming a two-bellied muscle sharing a common central tendon. These two muscles work together to flex and rotate the trunk (torsional movement of trunk).

The two vertical muscles are the:

- **Rectus abdominis,** a long, broad, strap-like muscle that is mostly enclosed in the *rectus sheath* (Figs. 2.4 and 2.5). The contractile (fleshy) fibers of the rectus do not run the length of the muscle; rather they run between three or more **tendinous intersections** (Fig. 2.4A), which are typically located at the level of the xiphoid process, umbilicus, and a level halfway between these points. Each intersection is firmly attached to the anterior layer of the rectus sheath.
- **Pyramidalis,** a small triangular muscle (absent in about 20% of people), that lies in the rectus sheath anterior to the inferior part of the rectus abdominis (Fig. 2.4A). It ends in the **linea alba** and tenses it.

FUNCTIONS AND ACTIONS OF THE ANTEROLATERAL ABDOMINAL MUSCLES

The muscles of the anterolateral abdominal wall:

- Form a strong expandable support for the anterolateral abdominal wall.
- Protect the abdominal viscera from injury.
- Compress the abdominal viscera to maintain or increase intra-abdominal pressure. Compressing the abdominal viscera and increasing intra-abdominal pressure elevates the relaxed diaphragm to expel air during respiration, coughing, voluntary eructation (burping), yelling, and so on. When the diaphragm contracts during inspiration, the anterolateral abdominal wall expands as the muscles relax to make room for the viscera that are pushed inferiorly.
- Produce the force required for defecation (evacuation of fecal material from the rectum), micturition (urination), vomiting, and parturition (childbirth).
- Produce anterior and lateral flexion of the trunk and torsional (rotatory) movements of the trunk and help maintain posture.

The **rectus sheath** is formed by the interlaced aponeuroses of the flat abdominal muscles (Fig. 2.5). Until about one third of the distance from the umbilicus to the pubic crest, the rectus abdominis is enveloped by the anterior layer of the rectus sheath, formed by the external oblique aponeurosis and the anterior lamina of the internal oblique aponeurosis, and posterior layer of the rectus sheath, formed by the posterior lamina of the internal oblique aponeurosis and the transversus abdominis aponeurosis (Fig. 2.5A). The aponeuroses of all three muscles, the external and internal oblique and the transversus abdominis, pass anterior to the rectus abdominis to form the anterior rectus sheath, leaving only the transversalis fascia to cover the rectus abdominis posteriorly (Fig. 2.5B). An **arcuate line** often demarcates the transition between the posterior rectus sheath covering the superior three quarters of the rectus abdominis proximally and the transversalis fascia covering the inferior quarter (Fig. 2.6).

FIGURE 2.5. Rectus sheath.
A. Transverse section superior to umbilicus.
B. Transverse section inferior to umbilicus.
C. Sagittal section. Planes of sections for A and B are shown in Figure 2.6.

Layers in A, B, & C
- External oblique
- Internal oblique
- Transversus abdominis
- Transversalis fascia
- Parietal peritoneum
- Membranous layer of subcutaneous tissue

The *contents of the rectus sheath* are the rectus abdominis and pyramidalis muscles, the anastomosing superior and inferior epigastric arteries and veins, the lymphatic vessels, and the distal portions of the anterior rami of spinal nerves T7–T12, which supply the muscle and overlying skin (Fig. 2.5C).

Internal Surface of Anterolateral Abdominal Wall

The internal surface of the anterolateral abdominal wall is covered with transversalis fascia, a variable amount of extraperitoneal fat, and parietal peritoneum (Fig. 2.5A,B). The infraumbilical part of this surface of the wall exhibits several peritoneal folds, some of which contain remnants of vessels that carried blood to and from the fetus (Moore and Persaud, 2008).

Five umbilical peritoneal folds—two on each side and one in the median plane—pass toward the umbilicus (Fig. 2.6):

- The **median umbilical fold,** extending from the apex of the urinary bladder to the umbilicus, covers the **median umbilical ligament,** the remnant of the *urachus* that joined the apex of the fetal bladder to the umbilicus.

- Two **medial umbilical folds,** lateral to the median umbilical fold, cover the **medial umbilical ligaments,** formed by the occluded parts of the umbilical arteries.

- Two **lateral umbilical folds,** lateral to the medial umbilical folds, cover the **inferior epigastric vessels** and, therefore, bleed if cut.

The depressions lateral to the umbilical folds are *peritoneal fossae,* some of which are potential sites for a hernia. The location of a hernia in one of these fossae determines how the hernia is classified. The shallow fossae between the umbilical folds are the (Fig. 2.6):

- **Supravesical fossae** between the median and the medial umbilical folds, formed as the peritoneum reflects from the anterior abdominal wall onto the bladder. The level of the supravesical fossae rises and falls with filling and emptying of the bladder.

- **Medial inguinal fossae** between the medial and the lateral umbilical folds, areas also commonly called **inguinal triangles** (Hesselbach triangles). These are potential sites for direct inguinal hernias.

- **Lateral inguinal fossae,** lateral to the lateral umbilical folds; these include the deep inguinal rings and are potential sites for the most common type of inguinal hernia, the indirect inguinal hernia.

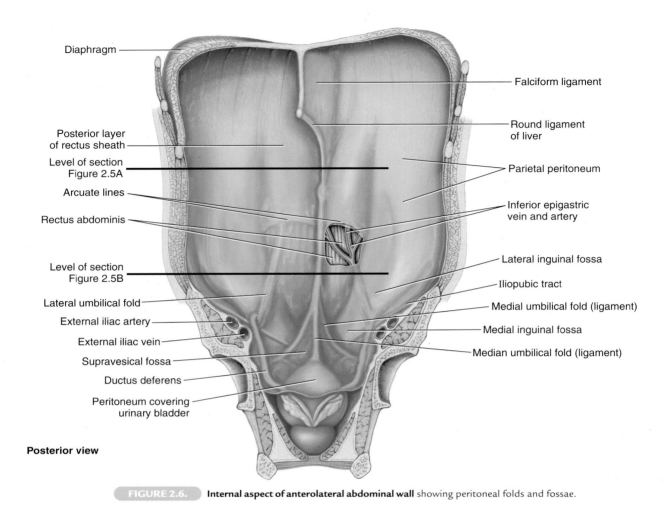

Diaphragm

Posterior layer
of rectus sheath

Level of section
Figure 2.5A

Arcuate lines

Rectus abdominis

Level of section
Figure 2.5B

Lateral umbilical fold

External iliac artery

External iliac vein

Supravesical fossa

Ductus deferens

Peritoneum covering
urinary bladder

Falciform ligament

Round ligament
of liver

Parietal peritoneum

Inferior epigastric
vein and artery

Lateral inguinal fossa

Iliopubic tract

Medial umbilical fold (ligament)

Medial inguinal fossa

Median umbilical fold (ligament)

Posterior view

FIGURE 2.6.   **Internal aspect of anterolateral abdominal wall** showing peritoneal folds and fossae.

Clinical Significance of Fascia and Fascial Spaces of Abdominal Wall

When closing abdominal skin incisions, surgeons include the membranous layer of subcutaneous tissue when suturing because of its strength. Between the membranous layer and the deep fascia covering the rectus abdominis and external oblique muscles is a potential space where fluid may accumulate (e.g., urine from a ruptured urethra). Although no barriers (other than gravity) prevent fluid from spreading superiorly from this space, it cannot spread inferiorly into the thigh because the membranous layer of subcutaneous tissue fuses with the deep fascia of the thigh (fascia lata) along a line inferior and parallel to the inguinal ligament (Fig. B2.1).

Skin

Subcutaneous
tissue:

Fatty layer

Membranous
layer

Anterior wall
of inguinal canal

"Potential space"

Spermatic cord

Fascia lata
of thigh

External oblique aponeurosis

Internal oblique aponeurosis

Transversus abdominis

Transversalis fascia

Retro-inguinal space (of Bogros)

Peritoneum

Inguinal falx (conjoint tendon)
forming posterior wall of
inguinal canal

Iliopubic tract

Inguinal ligament forming
"gutter" (floor of inguinal canal)

Superior ramus of pubis

Sagittal section of anterior abdominal wall

FIGURE B2.1.

Abdominal Surgical Incisions

 Surgeons use various incisions to gain access to the abdominal cavity. The incision that allows adequate exposure and, secondarily, the best possible cosmetic effect is chosen. The location of the incision also depends on the type of operation, the location of the organ(s), bony or cartilaginous boundaries, avoidance of (especially motor) nerves, maintenance of blood supply, and minimizing injury to muscles and fascia of the wall while aiming for favorable healing. Instead of transecting muscles, causing irreversible necrosis (death) of muscle fibers, the surgeon splits them between their fibers. The rectus abdominis is an exception and can be transected because its muscle fibers are short and its nerves entering the lateral part of the rectus sheath can be located and preserved. Cutting a motor nerve paralyzes the muscle fibers supplied by it, thereby weakening the anterolateral abdominal wall. However, because of overlapping areas of innervation between nerves in the abdominal wall, one or two small branches of nerves may be cut without a noticeable loss of motor supply to the muscles or loss of sensation to the skin. Some of the most common surgical incisions are illustrated in Figure B2.2.

Abdominal surgical incisions

- Median or midline incision
- Left paramedian incision
- Gridiron (muscle-splitting) incision
- Transverse (abdominal) incision
- Suprapubic (Pfannenstiel) incision
- Subcostal incision
- ○ McBurney point (usual location of appendix)

Anterior view

FIGURE B2.2.

Endoscopic Surgery

 Many abdominopelvic surgical procedures are now performed using an endoscope, in which tiny perforations into the abdominal wall allow the entry of remotely operated instruments, replacing the larger conventional incisions. Thus the potential for nerve injury, incisional hernia, or contamination through the open wound and the time required for healing are minimized.

Incisional Hernia

 If the muscular and aponeurotic layers of the abdomen do not heal properly, a hernia may occur through the defect. An incisional hernia is a protrusion of omentum (fold of peritoneum) or an organ through a surgical incision or scar.

Protuberance of Abdomen

 The six common causes of abdominal protrusion begin with the letter F: food, fluid, fat, feces, flatus, and fetus. Eversion of the umbilicus may be a sign of increased intra-abdominal pressure, usually resulting from ascites (abnormal accumulation of serous fluid in the peritoneal cavity) or a large mass (e.g., a tumor, a fetus, or an enlarged organ such as the liver).

Excess fat accumulation owing to overnourishment most commonly involves the subcutaneous fatty layer; however, there may also be excessive depositions of extraperitoneal fat in some types of obesity.

Palpation of Anterolateral Abdominal Wall

 Warm hands are important when palpating the abdominal wall because cold hands make the anterolateral abdominal muscles tense, producing involuntary spasms of the muscles, known as **guarding.** Intense guarding, board-like reflexive muscular rigidity that cannot be willfully suppressed, occurs during palpation when an organ (such as the appendix) is inflamed and in itself constitutes a clinically significant sign of *acute abdomen.* The involuntary muscular spasms attempt to protect the viscera from pressure, which is painful when an abdominal infection is present. The common segmental nerve supply of the organ and skin and muscles of the wall explains why these spasms occur.

Palpation of abdominal viscera is performed with the patient in the supine position with thighs and knees semi-flexed to enable adequate relaxation of the anterolateral abdominal wall. Otherwise, the deep fascia of the thighs pulls on the membranous layer of abdominal subcutaneous tissue, tensing the abdominal wall. Some people tend to place their hands behind their heads when lying supine, which also tightens the muscles and makes the examination difficult. Placing the upper limbs at the sides and putting a pillow under the person's knees tends to relax the anterolateral abdominal muscles.

Surface Anatomy of Anterolateral Abdominal Wall

The **umbilicus** is where the umbilical cord entered the fetus and is the reference point for the transumbilical plane (Fig. SA2.1A). It indicates the level of the T10 dermatome and is typically at the level of the IV disc between the L3 and L4 vertebrae; however, its position varies with the amount of fat in the subcutaneous tissue. The **linea alba** is a subcutaneous fibrous band extending from the **xiphoid process** to the **pubic symphysis** that is demarcated by a midline vertical skin groove as far inferiorly as the umbilicus (Fig. SA2.1B). The pubic symphysis can be felt in the median plane at the inferior end of the linea alba. The bony **iliac crest** at the level of the L4 vertebra can be easily palpated as it extends posteriorly from the **anterior superior iliac spine.**

In an individual with good muscle definition, curved skin grooves, the **semilunar lines** (L. *linae semilunares*) demarcate the lateral borders of the rectus abdominis and rectus sheath. The semilunar lines extend from the inferior costal margin near the ninth costal cartilages to the **pubic tubercles.** Three transverse skin grooves overlie the **tendinous intersections** of the rectus abdominis (Fig. SA2.1B). The interdigitating bellies of the **serratus anterior** and **external oblique muscles** are also visible. The site of the **inguinal ligament** is indicated by a skin crease, the inguinal groove, just inferior and parallel to the ligament, marking the division between the anterolateral abdominal wall and the thigh.

Site of xiphoid process

Right costal margin

Iliac crest

Anterior superior iliac spine

Inguinal ligament

Site of pubic tubercle

Epigastric fossa

Semilunar line

Umbilicus

Site of pubic symphysis

A

Location of linea alba

Tendinous intersection

Rectus abdominis

Location of anterior superior iliac spine

Inguinal groove

Location of pubic symphysis

Serratus anterior

External oblique

Rectus abdominis

Semilunar line

Umbilicus

Location of inguinal ligament

B **Anterior views**

FIGURE SA2.1.

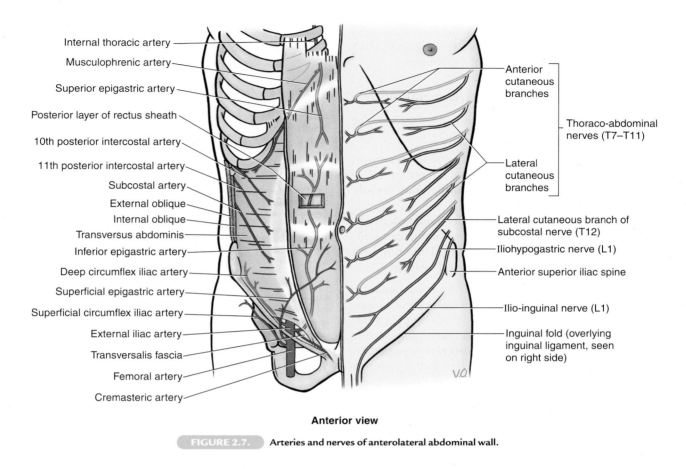

Internal thoracic artery
Musculophrenic artery
Superior epigastric artery
Posterior layer of rectus sheath
10th posterior intercostal artery
11th posterior intercostal artery
Subcostal artery
External oblique
Internal oblique
Transversus abdominis
Inferior epigastric artery
Deep circumflex iliac artery
Superficial epigastric artery
Superficial circumflex iliac artery
External iliac artery
Transversalis fascia
Femoral artery
Cremasteric artery

Anterior cutaneous branches
Thoraco-abdominal nerves (T7–T11)
Lateral cutaneous branches
Lateral cutaneous branch of subcostal nerve (T12)
Iliohypogastric nerve (L1)
Anterior superior iliac spine
Ilio-inguinal nerve (L1)
Inguinal fold (overlying inguinal ligament, seen on right side)

Anterior view

FIGURE 2.7.   Arteries and nerves of anterolateral abdominal wall.

Nerves of Anterolateral Abdominal Wall

The skin and muscles of the anterolateral abdominal wall are supplied mainly by the (Fig. 2.7, Table 2.2):

- **Thoraco-abdominal nerves:** distal, abdominal parts of the anterior rami of the inferior six thoracic spinal nerves (T7–T11), which have muscular branches and **anterior** and **lateral cutaneous branches.** The anterior cutaneous branches pierce the rectus sheath a short distance from the median plane, after the rectus abdominis muscle has been supplied. Spinal nerves T7–T9 supply the skin superior to the umbilicus; T10 innervates the skin around the umbilicus.

- **Subcostal nerve:** large anterior ramus of spinal nerve T12.

- **Iliohypogastric and ilio-inguinal nerves:** terminal branches of the anterior ramus of spinal nerve L1.

TABLE 2.2 NERVES OF ANTEROLATERAL ABDOMINAL WALL

Nerve	Origin	Course	Distribution
Thoraco-abdominal (T7–T11)	Continuation of lower intercostal nerves	Run between second and third layers of abdominal muscles; lateral cutaneous and anterior cutaneous branches enter subcutaneous tissue	Muscles of anterolateral abdominal wall and overlying skin
Subcostal (T12)	Anterior ramus of L1 spinal nerve	Runs along inferior border of 12th rib, then onto subumbilical abdominal wall	Muscles of anterolateral abdominal wall and overlying skin superior to iliac crest and inferior to umbilicus
Iliohypogastric (L1)	Anterior ramus of T12 spinal nerve	Pierces transversus abdominis muscle; branches pierce external oblique aponeurosis of most inferior abdominal wall	Skin overlying iliac crest, upper inguinal and hypogastric regions; internal oblique and transversus abdominis
Ilio-inguinal (L1)	Anterior ramus of L1 spinal nerve	Passes between second and third layers of abdominal muscles, then traverses inguinal canal	Skin of scrotum or labium majus, mons pubis, and adjacent medial aspect of thigh; most inferior internal oblique and transversus abdominis

- Spinal nerve T11, plus the cutaneous branches of the subcostal (T12), iliohypogastric, and ilio-inguinal (L1) nerves: supply the skin inferior to the umbilicus.

Vessels of Anterolateral Abdominal Wall

The blood vessels of the anterolateral abdominal wall are the (Fig. 2.7, Table 2.3):

- **Superior epigastric vessels** and branches of the **musculophrenic vessels** from the internal thoracic vessels.
- **Inferior epigastric** and **deep circumflex iliac vessels** from the external iliac vessels.
- **Superficial circumflex iliac** and **superficial epigastric vessels** from the femoral artery and great saphenous vein.
- **Posterior intercostal vessels** in the 11th intercostal space and anterior branches of **subcostal vessels.**

The **superior epigastric artery,** the direct continuation of the internal thoracic artery, enters the rectus sheath superiorly through its posterior layer (Fig. 2.5C), supplies the upper part of the rectus abdominis, and anastomoses with the inferior epigastric artery. The **inferior epigastric artery** arises from the external iliac artery just superior to the inguinal ligament. It runs superiorly in the transversalis fascia to enter the rectus sheath inferior to the arcuate line. Its branches enter the lower rectus abdominis and anastomose with those of the superior epigastric artery.

The **superficial lymphatic vessels** accompany the subcutaneous veins; those superior to the umbilicus drain mainly to the **axillary lymph nodes,** whereas those inferior to it drain to the **superficial inguinal lymph nodes** (Fig. 2.8). The **deep lymphatic vessels** accompany the deep veins and drain to the external iliac, common iliac, and lumbar (caval and aortic) lymph nodes.

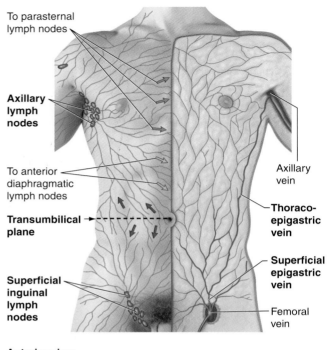

FIGURE 2.8. Lymphatics and superficial veins of anterolateral abdominal wall.

TABLE 2.3 PRINCIPAL ARTERIES OF ANTEROLATERAL ABDOMINAL WALL

Artery	Origin	Course	Distribution
Musculophrenic	Internal thoracic artery	Descends along costal margin	Abdominal wall of hypochondriac region, anterolateral, diaphragm
Superior epigastric		Descends in rectus sheath deep to rectus abdominis	Rectus abdominis and superior part of anterolateral abdominal wall
10th and 11th posterior intercostal	Aorta	Arteries continue beyond ribs to descend in abdominal wall between internal oblique and transversus abdominis	Abdominal wall, lateral region
Subcostal			
Inferior epigastric	External iliac artery	Runs superiorly and enters rectus sheath; runs deep to rectus abdominis	Rectus abdominis and medial part of anterolateral abdominal wall
Deep circumflex iliac		Runs on deep aspect of anterior abdominal wall, parallel to inguinal ligament	Iliacus muscle and inferior part of anterolateral abdominal wall
Superficial circumflex iliac	Femoral artery	Runs in superficial fascia along inguinal ligament	Superficial abdominal wall of inguinal region and adjacent anterior thigh
Superficial epigastric		Runs in superficial fascia toward umbilicus	Subcutaneous tissue and skin over pubic and inferior umbilical region

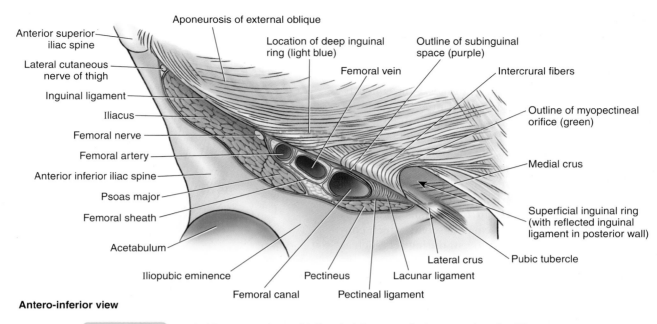

Anterior superior iliac spine

Lateral cutaneous nerve of thigh

Inguinal ligament

Iliacus

Femoral nerve

Femoral artery

Anterior inferior iliac spine

Psoas major

Femoral sheath

Acetabulum

Aponeurosis of external oblique

Location of deep inguinal ring (light blue)

Femoral vein

Outline of subinguinal space (purple)

Intercrural fibers

Outline of myopectineal orifice (green)

Medial crus

Superficial inguinal ring (with reflected inguinal ligament in posterior wall)

Pubic tubercle

Lateral crus

Lacunar ligament

Pectineal ligament

Pectineus

Femoral canal

Iliopubic eminence

Antero-inferior view

FIGURE 2.9. **Inguinal ligament and superficial inguinal ring.** Note the lacunar and pectineal ligaments.

Inguinal Region

The area extends between the anterior superior iliac spine and the pubic tubercle (Fig. 2.9). Anatomically, it is a region where structures exit and enter the abdominal cavity and is, therefore, clinically important because these are potential sites of herniation. Inguinal hernias occur in both sexes, but most (about 86%) occur in males because of the passage of the spermatic cord through the inguinal canal. The migration of the testes from the abdomen into the perineum accounts for many of the structural features of the region. Thus the testis and scrotum are usually studied in relation to the anterior abdominal wall and inguinal region (Fig. 2.10A).

INGUINAL LIGAMENT AND ILIOPUBIC TRACT

The **inguinal ligament,** the most inferior part of the external oblique aponeurosis, and the **iliopubic tract,** the thickened inferior margin of the transversalis fascia, extend from the anterior superior iliac spine to the pubic tubercle. Most of the fibers of the inguinal ligament insert into the pubic tubercle, but some fibers (Fig. 2.9):

1. Attach to the superior ramus of the pubis lateral to the pubic tubercle as the **lacunar ligament** and then continue to run along the pectin pubis as the **pectineal ligament** (of Cooper).
2. Arch superiorly to blend with the contralateral external oblique aponeurosis as the **reflected inguinal ligament.**

The *iliopubic tract* is a fibrous band that runs parallel and posterior (deep) to the inguinal ligament. It is seen in place of

the inguinal ligament when the inguinal region is viewed from its internal (posterior) aspect, as through an endoscope (Figs. 2.6 and 2.10B). The iliopubic tract reinforces the posterior wall and floor of the inguinal canal as it bridges the structures (hip flexors and much of the neurovascular supply of the lower limb) traversing the **subinguinal space** (Fig. 2.9).

INGUINAL CANAL

The inguinal canal is formed in relation to the relocation of the gonad (testes or ovary) during fetal development. The inguinal canal in adults is an approximately 4-cm-long, inferomedially directed oblique passage (between the superficial and deep inguinal rings) that runs through the inferior part of the anterior abdominal wall (Fig. 2.10). The inguinal canal lies parallel and just superior to the medial half of the inguinal ligament. The main occupant of the inguinal canal is the *spermatic cord* in males and the *round ligament of the uterus* in females. The inguinal canal also contains blood and lymphatic vessels and the ilio-inguinal nerve in both sexes. The inguinal canal has an opening at each end.

- The **deep (internal) ring,** the internal entrance to the inguinal canal, is an evagination of the transversalis fascia superior to the middle of the inguinal ligament and lateral to the inferior epigastric vessels (Fig. 2.6).
- The **superficial (external) inguinal ring,** the exit from the inguinal canal, is a slit-like opening between the diagonal fibers of the aponeurosis of the external oblique, superolateral to the pubic tubercle. The lateral and medial margins of the superficial ring formed by the split in the aponeurosis are the **lateral** and **medial crura**

(L. leg-like parts). The **intercrural fibers** help prevent the crura from spreading apart (Fig. 2.9).

The deep and superficial inguinal rings do not overlap because of the oblique path of the inguinal canal through the aponeuroses of the abdominal muscles. Consequently, increases in intra-abdominal pressure force the posterior wall of the canal against the anterior wall, closing this passageway and strengthening this potential defect of the abdominal wall. Simultaneous contraction of the external oblique also approximates the anterior wall of the canal to the posterior wall and increases tension on the crura, resisting dilation of the superficial inguinal ring. Contraction of the internal oblique and transversus abdominis muscles makes the roof of the canal descend, which constricts the canal. All these events occur during acts such as sneezing, coughing, and "bearing down" (Valsalva maneuver) to increase intra-abdominal pressure for elimination (e.g., of feces).

The inguinal canal has two walls (anterior and posterior), a roof, and a floor (Fig. 2.10A).

- **Anterior wall:** formed by external oblique aponeurosis throughout the length of the canal; the anterior wall of the lateral part of the canal is reinforced by fibers of internal oblique.
- **Posterior wall:** formed by transversalis fascia; the posterior wall of the medial part of the canal is reinforced by merging of the pubic attachments of the internal oblique and transversus abdominis aponeuroses into a common tendon—the **inguinal falx (conjoint tendon).**
- **Roof:** formed laterally by transversalis fascia, centrally by the musculo-aponeurotic arches of internal oblique and transversus abdominis muscles, and medially by the medial crus of the external oblique aponeurosis.
- **Floor:** formed laterally by the iliopubic tract, centrally by the superior surface of the inguinal ligament, and medially by the lacunar ligament.

SPERMATIC CORD

The spermatic cord contains structures running to and from the testis and suspends the testis in the scrotum. The spermatic cord begins at the deep inguinal ring lateral to the inferior epigastric vessels, passes through the inguinal canal, exits at the superficial inguinal ring, and ends in the scrotum at the posterior border of the testis (Figs. 2.10A,B and 2.11, and Table 2.4). Fascial coverings derived from the anterolateral abdominal wall during prenatal development include the:

- **Internal spermatic fascia:** derived from the transversalis fascia at the deep inguinal ring.

Peritoneum
Transversalis fascia
Transversus abdominis muscle
Internal oblique muscle
External oblique muscle
Testicular artery and veins
External oblique aponeurosis
Ductus deferens
Ilio-inguinal nerve
Inferior epigastric vessels
Deep inguinal ring
Retroinguinal space (of Bogros)
Internal spermatic fascia
Inguinal ligament
Origin of cremasteric muscle
Inguinal falx (conjoint tendon)
Femoral vessels
Superficial inguinal ring
External spermatic fascia
Reflected inguinal ligament
Cremasteric muscle and fascia
Internal spermatic fascia
Spermatic cord
External spermatic fascia
Testis
* Musculo-aponeurotic arcades of internal oblique & transverse abdominal

A Anterior view

Rectus abdominis
Inferior epigastric artery and vein
Transversus abdominis
Iliopubic tract
Deep inguinal ring
Testicular artery and vein
External iliac artery and vein
Inguinal triangle
Iliopsoas
Ductus deferens
Obturator branch
Pubis
Lacunar ligament

B Posterior view of right anterior abdominal wall

FIGURE 2.10.

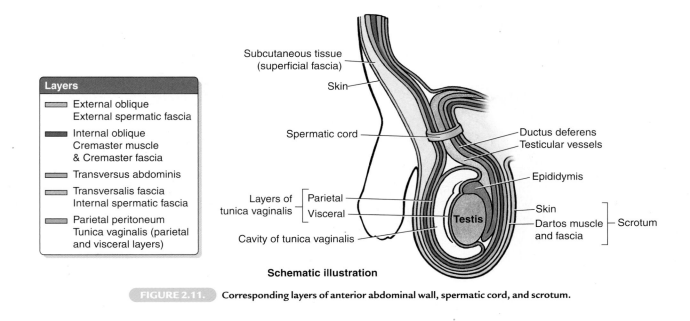

Layers

▭	External oblique External spermatic fascia
▭	Internal oblique Cremaster muscle & Cremaster fascia
▭	Transversus abdominis
▭	Transversalis fascia Internal spermatic fascia
▭	Parietal peritoneum Tunica vaginalis (parietal and visceral layers)

Subcutaneous tissue (superficial fascia)

Skin

Spermatic cord

Ductus deferens

Testicular vessels

Epididymis

Layers of tunica vaginalis — Parietal / Visceral

Cavity of tunica vaginalis

Testis

Skin

Dartos muscle and fascia — Scrotum

Schematic illustration

FIGURE 2.11. Corresponding layers of anterior abdominal wall, spermatic cord, and scrotum.

TABLE 2.4 CORRESPONDING LAYERS OF ANTERIOR ABDOMINAL WALL, SPERMATIC CORD, AND SCROTUM

Layers of the Anterior Abdominal Wall	Scrotum and Covering of the Testis	Coverings of the Spermatic Cord
Skin	Skin	Skin continuous with scrotum (and scrotal septum)
Subcutaneous tissue (superficial fascia)	Subcutaneous tissue (dartos fascia) and dartos muscle	
External oblique aponeurosis or muscle	External spermatic fascia	External spermatic fascia
Internal oblique muscle	Cremaster muscle	Cremaster muscle
Investing fascia of both superficial and deep surfaces of internal oblique muscle	Cremasteric fascia	Cremasteric fascia
Transversus abdominis muscle		
Transversalis fascia	Internal spermatic fascia	Internal spermatic fascia
Extraperitoneal fat		
Peritoneum	Tunica vaginalis (parietal and visceral layers)	Vestige of processus vaginalis

- **Cremasteric fascia:** derived from the fascia of both the superficial and the deep surfaces of the internal oblique muscle.
- **External spermatic fascia:** derived from the external oblique aponeurosis and its investing fascia.

The cremasteric fascia contains loops of the **cremaster muscle,** which is formed by the lowest fascicles of the internal oblique muscle arising from the inguinal ligament. The cremaster reflexively draws the testis superiorly in the scrotum, particularly when it is cold; in a warm environment, the cremaster relaxes and the testis descends deeply in the scrotum. Both responses occur in an attempt to regulate the temperature of the testis for *spermatogenesis* (formation of sperms), which requires a constant temperature of approximately one degree cooler than core temperature. The cremaster acts with the **dartos muscle,** a smooth muscle of the fat-free subcutaneous tissue of the scrotum (dartos fascia), which inserts into the skin. The dartos assists in testicular elevation as it produces contraction of the skin of the scrotum. The cremaster is innervated by the **genital branch of the genitofemoral nerve** (L1, L2), a derivative of the lumbar plexus, whereas the dartos receives autonomic innervation. Although less well developed and usually indistinct, the round ligament of the uterus in the female receives similar contributions from the layers of the abdominal wall as it traverses the canal.

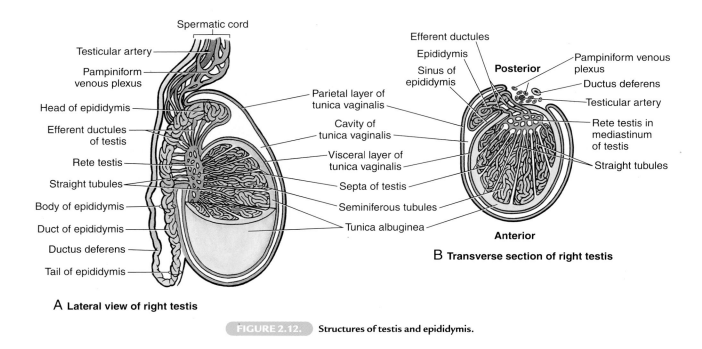

A Lateral view of right testis

B Transverse section of right testis

FIGURE 2.12.   Structures of testis and epididymis.

The **constituents of the spermatic cord** are the (Fig. 2.12A):

- **Ductus deferens** (deferent duct, vas deferens), a muscular tube that conveys sperms from the epididymis to the ejaculatory duct. It courses through the substance of the prostate to open into the prostatic part of the urethra.
- **Testicular artery** arising from the aorta (vertebral level L2) and supplying the testis and epididymis.
- **Artery of ductus deferens** arising from the inferior vesical artery.
- **Cremasteric artery** arising from the inferior epigastric artery.
- **Pampiniform venous plexus,** a network formed by up to 12 veins that converge superiorly as the right or left testicular veins.
- **Sympathetic nerve fibers** on arteries and sympathetic and parasympathetic nerve fibers on the ductus deferens.
- **Genital branch of genitofemoral nerve** supplying the cremaster muscle.
- **Lymphatic vessels** draining the testis and closely associated structures to the lumbar lymph nodes (Fig. 2.13).
- **Vestige of the processus vaginalis,** which may be seen as a fibrous thread in the anterior part of the spermatic cord extending between the abdominal peritoneum and the tunica vaginalis; it may not be detectable.

TESTES

The ovoid testes are suspended in the scrotum by the spermatic cords (Figs. 2.7 and 2.8). The testes produce sperms (spermatozoa) and hormones, principally testosterone. The sperms are formed in the **seminiferous tubules** that are joined by **straight tubules** to the **rete testis.** The testes have a tough outer surface, the **tunica albuginea,** that forms a ridge on its internal, posterior aspect as the **mediastinum of the testis.** The **tunica vaginalis** is a closed peritoneal sac surrounding the testis (Figs. 2.11 and 2.12).

The surface of each testis is covered by the **visceral layer of the tunica vaginalis,** except where the testis attaches to the epididymis and spermatic cord. The visceral layer of the tunica vaginalis, a glistening, transparent serous membrane, is closely applied to the testis, epididymis, and inferior part of the ductus deferens.

The **parietal layer of the tunica vaginalis,** adjacent to the internal spermatic fascia, is more extensive than the visceral layer and extends superiorly for a short distance into the distal part of the spermatic cord. The small amount of fluid in the cavity of the tunica vaginalis separates the visceral and parietal layers, allowing the testis to move freely within its side of the scrotum.

The **testicular arteries** arise from the abdominal aorta (vertebral level L2) just inferior to the renal arteries (Fig. 2.13). The long, slender testicular arteries pass retroperitoneally (posterior to the peritoneum) in an oblique direction, crossing over the ureters and the inferior parts of the external iliac arteries. They traverse the inguinal canals, becoming part of the spermatic cords to supply the testes.

The **testicular veins** emerging from the testis and epididymis form the **pampiniform venous plexus,** consisting of 8 to 12 anastomosing veins lying anterior to the ductus deferens and surrounding the testicular artery in the spermatic cord

Cisterna chyli
Abdominal aorta
Left renal artery
Right renal artery
Right testicular artery
Lumbar plexus
Preaortic lymph nodes
Lymphatic vessels
Lumbar (caval/aortic) lymph nodes
Left testicular artery
Right common iliac artery
Internal iliac artery
External iliac artery
Ilio-inguinal nerve
Sacral plexus
Genital branch of genitofemoral nerve
Pudendal nerve
Posterior scrotal (superficial perineal) nerves
Posterior cutaneous nerve of thigh
Anterior scrotal nerves
Perineal branch of internal pudendal artery
Superficial inguinal lymph node
Cremasteric artery (branch of inferior epigastric artery)
Femoral artery
External pudendal branch of femoral artery
Anterior scrotal arteries
Spermatic cord
Testis   Scrotum

Lymphatic drainage
→ From testis
⇢ From scrotum

Anterior view

FIGURE 2.13.   **Innervation, blood supply, and lymphatic drainage of scrotum, testis, and spermatic cord.** *Arrows,* direction of the flow of lymph to the lymph nodes.

(Fig. 2.12A). The pampiniform plexus is part of the thermoregulatory system of the testis, helping to keep this gland at a constant temperature. The **left testicular vein** originates as the veins of the pampiniform plexus coalesce; it empties into the left renal vein. The **right testicular vein** has a similar origin and course but enters the inferior vena cava (IVC).

The *lymphatic drainage of the testis* follows the testicular artery and vein to the **right and left lumbar (caval/aortic)** and **pre-aortic lymph nodes** (Fig. 2.13). The *autonomic nerves of the testis* arise as the **testicular plexus of nerves** on the testicular artery, which contains vagal parasympathetic and visceral afferent and sympathetic fibers from the T10 (-T11). segment of the spinal cord.

EPIDIDYMIS

The epididymis is an elongated structure on the posterior surface of the testis formed by minute convolutions of the **duct of the epididymis,** so tightly compacted that they appear solid (Fig. 2.12). The **efferent ductules** transport newly formed sperms from the rete testis to the epididymis, where

they are stored until mature. The **rete testis** is a network of canals at the termination of the seminiferous tubules.

The epididymis consists of a:

- **Head:** the superior expanded part composed of lobules formed by the coiled ends of 12 to 14 efferent ductules.
- **Body:** the convoluted duct of the epididymis.
- **Tail:** continuous with the **ductus deferens,** the duct that transports sperms from the epididymis to the ejaculatory duct for expulsion into the prostatic urethra (see Chapter 3).

SCROTUM

The scrotum is a cutaneous sac consisting of two layers: heavily pigmented skin and closely related **dartos fascia,** and a fat-free fascial layer including smooth muscle fibers (dartos muscle) responsible for the rugose (wrinkled) appearance of the scrotum (Fig. 2.11). Because the **dartos muscle** attaches to the skin, its contraction causes the scrotum to wrinkle when cold, which thickens the integumentary layer while reducing the scrotal surface area. This assists the cremaster in holding the testes closer to the body, thus reducing heat loss. *Scrotal veins* accompany the arteries. The *lymphatic vessels* drain into the superficial inguinal lymph nodes.

The *arterial supply of the scrotum* is from the (Fig. 2.13):

- **Posterior scrotal branches of the perineal artery,** a branch of the internal pudendal artery.
- **Anterior scrotal branches of the deep external pudendal artery,** a branch of the femoral artery.
- **Cremasteric artery,** a branch of the inferior epigastric artery.

The *nerves of the scrotum* include the (Fig. 2.13):

- **Genital branch of the genitofemoral nerve** (L1, L2) supplying the anterolateral surface.
- **Anterior scrotal nerves,** branches of the ilio-inguinal nerve (L1) supplying the anterior surface.
- **Posterior scrotal nerves,** branches of the perineal branch of the **pudendal nerve** (S2–S4) supplying the posterior surface.
- **Perineal branches of the posterior cutaneous nerve of the thigh** (S2, S3) supplying the inferior surface.

Hydrocele and Hematocele

 The presence of excess fluid in a persistent processus vaginalis is a *hydrocele of the testis* (Fig. B2.3A). Certain pathological conditions— such as injury or inflammation of the epididymis—may also produce a *hydrocele of the spermatic cord* (Fig. B2.3B). A *hematocele of the testis* is a collection of blood in the cavity of the tunica vaginalis (Fig. B2.3C).

Ductus deferens and spermatic cord

Head of epididymis

Tunica vaginalis

Testis

A Hydrocele (H) of testis   **B** Hydrocele (H) of cord

Injury to the spermatic vessels

C Hematocele of testis

FIGURE B2.3.

Vasectomy

 The *ductus deferens* is ligated bilaterally when sterilizing a man. To perform a vasectomy, also called a *deferentectomy,* the duct is isolated

on each side and transected or a small section of it is removed. Sperms can no longer pass to the urethra; they degenerate in the epididymis and proximal end of the ductus deferens. However, the secretions of the *auxiliary genital glands* (seminal glands, bulbourethral glands, and prostate) can still be ejaculated. The testis continues to function as an endocrine gland for the production of testosterone.

Varicocele

 The pampiniform plexus of veins may become varicose (dilated) and tortuous. These varicose vessels often result from defective valves in the testicular vein. The palpable enlargement, which feels like a bundle of worms, usually drains and thus seems to disappear when the person lies down.

Testicular Cancer

 Because the testes relocate from the dorsal abdominal wall into the scrotum during fetal development, their lymphatic drainage differs from that of the scrotum, which is an outpouching of the anterolateral abdominal skin (Fig. 2.13). Consequently:

- *Cancer of the testis* metastasizes initially to the **lumbar lymph nodes.**
- *Cancer of the scrotum* metastasizes initially to the **superficial inguinal lymph nodes.**

Cremasteric Reflex

 The cremasteric reflex is the rapid elevation of the testis on the same side; this reflex is extremely active in children. Contraction of the cremaster muscle—producing the reflex—can be induced by lightly stroking the skin on the medial aspect of the superior part of the thigh with an applicator stick or tongue depressor. This area is supplied by the *ilio-inguinal nerve.*

Relocation of Gonads

The **fetal testes** relocate from the dorsal abdominal wall in the superior lumbar region to the deep inguinal rings during the 9th to 12th fetal weeks (Fig. B2.4A–C). This movement probably results from growth of the vertebral column and pelvis. The male *gubernaculum,* attached to the caudal pole of the testis and accompanied by an outpouching of peritoneum, the *processus vaginalis,* projects into the scrotum. The testis descends posterior to the processus vaginalis. The inferior remnant of the processus vaginalis forms the *tunica vaginalis* covering the testis. The ductus deferens, testicular vessels, nerves, and lymphatics accompany the testis. The final location of the testis usually occurs before or shortly after birth.

The **fetal ovaries** also relocate from the dorsal abdominal wall in the superior lumbar region during the 12th week but pass into the lesser pelvis (Fig. B2.4D,E). The female gubernaculum also attaches to the caudal pole of the ovary and projects into the labia majora, attaching en route to the uterus; the part passing from the uterus to the ovary forms the *ovarian ligament,* and the remainder of it becomes the *round ligament of the uterus.* For a complete description of the embryology of the inguinal region, see Moore and Persaud (2008).

FIGURE B2.4.

Inguinal Hernias

An inguinal hernia is a protrusion of parietal peritoneum and viscera, such as the small intestine, through a normal or abnormal opening from the abdominal cavity. There are two major categories of inguinal hernia: indirect and direct. More than two thirds are indirect hernias. An indirect inguinal hernia can occur in women, but it is about 20 times more common in males of all ages (Fig. B2.5 and Table B2.1).

Direct (acquired) inguinal hernia

Indirect (congenital) inguinal hernia

Peritoneum

Transversalis fascia

Transversus abdominis muscle

Internal oblique muscle

External oblique muscle

Testicular vessels entering spermatic cord

Ductus deferens

Deep inguinal ring

Lateral umbilical fold

Medial umbilical fold

Median umbilical fold

Inguinal triangle

Herniating bowel passes MEDIAL to inferior epigastric vessels, pushing through peritoneum and transversalis fascia in inguinal triangle to enter inguinal canal.

Femoral artery and vein

Superficial inguinal ring

Hernial sac (parallels spermatic cord)

Spermatic cord

Ductus deferens

Herniating bowel passes LATERAL to inferior epigastric vessels to enter deep inguinal ring.

Inguinal falx (conjoint tendon)

Loop of intestine inside spermatic cord

Hernial sac (within spermatic cord)

FIGURE B2.5. Course of direct and indirect inguinal hernias.

TABLE B2.1 CHARACTERISTICS OF INGUINAL HERNIAS

Characteristics[a]	Direct (Acquired)	Indirect (Congenital)
Predisposing factors	Weakness of anterior abdominal wall in inguinal triangle (e.g., owing to distended superficial ring, narrow inguinal falx, or attenuation of aponeurosis in males > 40 years of age)	Patency of processus vaginalis (complete or at least of superior part) in younger persons, the great majority of whom are males
Frequency	Less common (one third to one quarter of inguinal hernias)	More common (two thirds to three quarters of inguinal hernias)
Coverings at exit from abdominal cavity	Peritoneum plus transversalis fascia (lies outside inner one or two fascial coverings of cord)	Peritoneum of persistent processus vaginalis plus all three fascial coverings of cord/round ligament
Course	Usually traverses only medial third of inguinal canal, external and parallel to vestige of processus vaginalis	Traverses inguinal canal (entire canal if it is sufficient size) within processus vaginalis
Exit from anterior abdominal wall	Via superficial ring, lateral to cord; rarely enters scrotum	Via superficial ring inside cord, commonly passing into scrotum/labium majus

[a]Letters in parentheses refer to the figure parts.

Palpation of Superficial Inguinal Ring

The superficial inguinal ring is palpable supero-lateral to the pubic tubercle by invaginating the skin of the upper scrotum with the index finger. The examiner's finger follows the spermatic cord supero-laterally to the superficial inguinal ring (Fig. B2.6B). If the ring is dilated, it may admit the fingertip without causing pain. With the palmar surface of the finger against the anterior abdominal wall, the deep inguinal ring may be felt as a skin depression superior to the inguinal liga-ment, 2 to 4 cm superolateral to the pubic tubercle. Detection of an impulse against the examining finger, when the person coughs, at the superficial ring and a mass at the site of the deep ring suggests an indirect hernia. Palpation of a direct inguinal hernia is performed by placing the index and/or middle finger over the inguinal triangle and asking the person to cough or strain. If a hernia is present, a forceful impulse is felt against the pad of the finger.

Cysts and Hernias of Canal of Nuck

If the processus vaginalis persists in females, it forms a small peritoneal pouch, the canal of Nuck, in the inguinal canal that may extend to the labium majus. In female infants, such remnants can enlarge and form cysts that have the potential to develop into an indirect inguinal hernia.

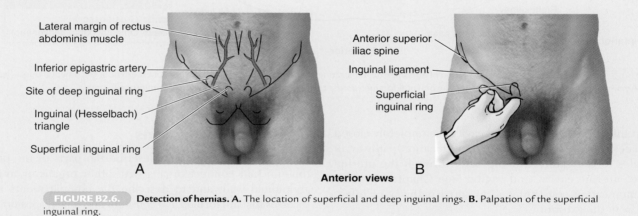

Lateral margin of rectus abdominis muscle
Inferior epigastric artery
Site of deep inguinal ring
Inguinal (Hesselbach) triangle
Superficial inguinal ring

Anterior superior iliac spine
Inguinal ligament
Superficial inguinal ring

A **B**

Anterior views

FIGURE B2.6. **Detection of hernias. A.** The location of superficial and deep inguinal rings. **B.** Palpation of the superficial inguinal ring.

PERITONEUM AND PERITONEAL CAVITY

The **peritoneum** is a glistening, transparent serous membrane that consists of two continuous layers (Fig. 2.14):

- **Parietal peritoneum,** lining the internal surface of the abdominopelvic wall.
- **Visceral peritoneum,** investing viscera (organs) such as the spleen and stomach.

The peritoneum and viscera are in the abdominopelvic cavity. The relationship of the viscera to the peritoneum is as follows:

- **Intraperitoneal organs** are almost completely covered with visceral peritoneum (e.g., the spleen and stomach); intraperitoneal organs have conceptually, if not literally, invaginated into a closed sac, like pressing your fist into an inflated balloon.

- **Extraperitoneal, retroperitoneal, and subperitoneal organs** are outside the peritoneal cavity—external or posterior to the parietal peritoneum—and are only partially covered with peritoneum (usually on one surface). Organs such as the kidneys are between the parietal peritoneum and the posterior abdominal wall and have parietal peritoneum only on their anterior surfaces, often with a considerable amount of intervening fatty tissue (Fig. 2.14).

The **peritoneal cavity** is within the abdominal cavity and continues into the pelvic cavity. It is a potential space of capillary thinness between the parietal and visceral layers of peritoneum. The peritoneal cavity contains a thin layer of **peritoneal fluid** that keeps the peritoneal surfaces moist. *There are no organs in the peritoneal cavity.* Peritoneal fluid lubricates the peritoneal surfaces, enabling the viscera to move over each other without friction and allowing the movements of digestion. In addition, the fluid contains leukocytes and antibodies that

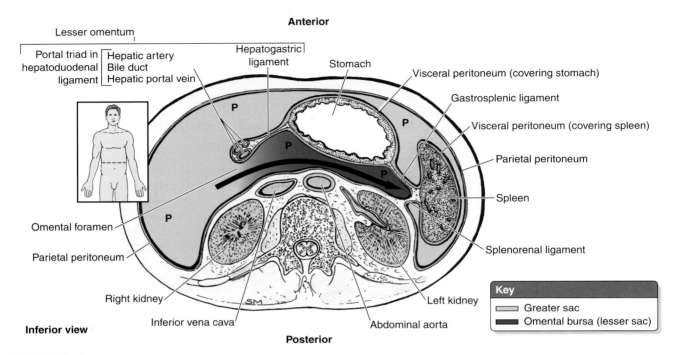

Anterior

Lesser omentum

Portal triad in hepatoduodenal ligament
- Hepatic artery
- Bile duct
- Hepatic portal vein

Hepatogastric ligament

Stomach

Visceral peritoneum (covering stomach)

Gastrosplenic ligament

Visceral peritoneum (covering spleen)

Parietal peritoneum

Spleen

Splenorenal ligament

Omental foramen

Parietal peritoneum

Right kidney

Inferior view

Inferior vena cava

Left kidney

Abdominal aorta

Posterior

Key
	Greater sac
	Omental bursa (lesser sac)

FIGURE 2.14. **Schematic transverse section of abdomen** demonstrating the omental foramen and the horizontal extent of the omental bursa (lesser sac). *Arrow* passes from the greater sac through the omental foramen across the full extent of the omental bursa. *P,* peritoneal cavity.

resist infection. The peritoneal cavity is completely closed in males; however, there is a communication pathway in females to the exterior of the body through the uterine tubes, uterine cavity, and vagina (see Chapter 3). This communication constitutes a potential pathway of infection from the exterior.

Peritoneal Vessels and Nerves

The *parietal peritoneum* is:

- Served by the same blood and lymphatic vasculature and the same somatic nerve supply as the region of the abdominopelvic wall it lines.
- Sensitive to pressure, pain, heat, and cold; pain from the parietal peritoneum is generally well localized.

The *visceral peritoneum* is:

- Served by the same blood and lymphatic vasculature and the same visceral nerve supply as the organs it covers.
- Insensitive to touch, heat, cold, and laceration and is stimulated primarily by stretching and chemical irritation.
- Pain from the visceral peritoneum is poorly localized and is referred to the dermatomes of the spinal ganglia providing the sensory fibers. Pain from the foregut derivatives is usually experienced in the epigastric region; that from the midgut derivatives, in the umbilical region; and that from the hindgut derivatives, in the pubic region.

Peritoneal Formations

Various terms are used to describe the parts of the peritoneum that connect organs with other organs or to the abdominal wall, and to describe the compartments and recesses that are formed as a consequence. The disposition of peritoneum in the adult is easier to understand when developmental changes are considered (for a description of the embryology of the peritoneal cavity and viscera, see Moore and Persaud, 2008, and Moore, Dalley, and Agur, 2009).

A **mesentery** is a double layer of peritoneum that occurs as a result of the invagination of the peritoneum by an organ and constitutes a continuity of the visceral and parietal peritoneum (e.g., *mesentery of small intestine and transverse mesocolon*) (Figs. 2.16B and 2.17; see also Fig. 2.29D). Mesenteries provide a means for neurovascular communication between the organ and the body wall and thus have a core of connective tissue containing blood and lymphatic vessels, nerves, fat, and lymph nodes. Viscera with a mesentery are mobile; the degree of mobility depends on the length of the mesentery.

A **peritoneal ligament** consists of a double layer of peritoneum that connects an organ with another organ or to the abdominal wall. For example, the liver is connected to the anterior abdominal wall by the *falciform ligament* (Fig. 2.15A).

An **omentum** is a double-layered extension of peritoneum passing from the stomach and proximal part of the

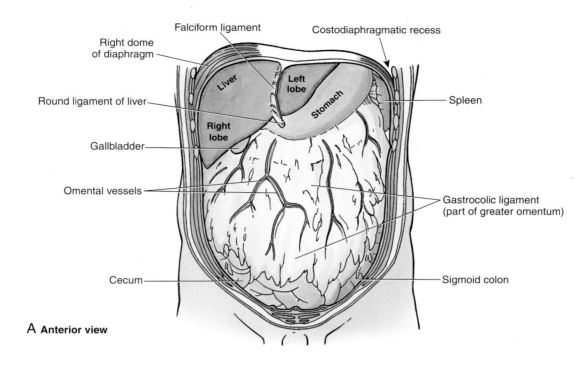

Falciform ligament

Costodiaphragmatic recess

Right dome of diaphragm

Round ligament of liver

Gallbladder

Omental vessels

Cecum

Liver

Left lobe

Stomach

Right lobe

Spleen

Gastrocolic ligament (part of greater omentum)

Sigmoid colon

A Anterior view

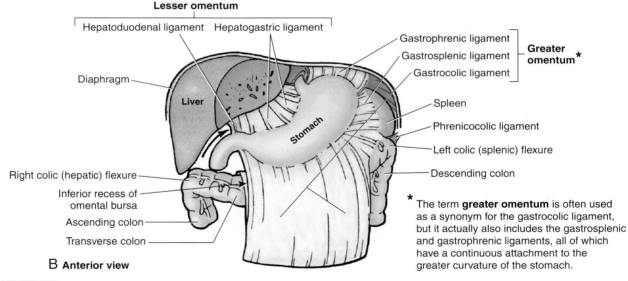

Lesser omentum

Hepatoduodenal ligament   Hepatogastric ligament

Gastrophrenic ligament

Gastrosplenic ligament

Gastrocolic ligament

Greater omentum *

Diaphragm

Liver

Stomach

Spleen

Phrenicocolic ligament

Left colic (splenic) flexure

Descending colon

Right colic (hepatic) flexure

Inferior recess of omental bursa

Ascending colon

Transverse colon

* The term **greater omentum** is often used as a synonym for the gastrocolic ligament, but it actually also includes the gastrosplenic and gastrophrenic ligaments, all of which have a continuous attachment to the greater curvature of the stomach.

B Anterior view

FIGURE 2.15. **Abdominal contents and peritoneum. A.** The anterior thoracic and abdominal walls have been cut away to show the undisturbed contents. **B.** Stomach, lesser and greater omenta, and associated peritoneal ligaments. *Arrow,* site of omental foramen.

duodenum to adjacent organs. The **greater omentum** extends superiorly, laterally to the left, and inferiorly from the greater curvature of the stomach and the proximal part of the duodenum (Fig. 2.15). The greater omentum has three parts:

1. The **gastrophrenic ligament** between the greater curvature of the stomach and the diaphragm.
2. The **gastrosplenic ligament** between the greater curvature of the stomach and the spleen.

3. The **gastrocolic ligament** from the inferior portion of the greater curvature of the stomach. The gastrocolic ligament is the largest part, descending anteriorly and inferiorly beyond the transverse colon and then ascending again posteriorly, fusing with the visceral peritoneum of the transverse colon and the superior layer of its mesentery. The descending and ascending portions of the gastrocolic part of the greater omentum usually fuse together, forming a four-layered fatty "omental apron."

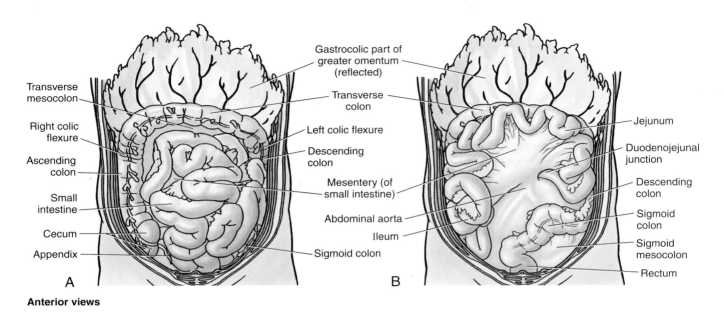

Transverse mesocolon

Right colic flexure

Ascending colon

Small intestine

Cecum

Appendix

Gastrocolic part of greater omentum (reflected)

Transverse colon

Left colic flexure

Descending colon

Mesentery (of small intestine)

Abdominal aorta

Ileum

Sigmoid colon

Jejunum

Duodenojejunal junction

Descending colon

Sigmoid colon

Sigmoid mesocolon

Rectum

A

B

Anterior views

FIGURE 2.16. **Greater omentum and mesentery of small intestine. A.** The gastrocolic ligament, depicted in anatomical position in Fig. 2.15A, has been elevated to reveal the small intestine and ascending and transverse colon. **B.** The small intestine has been elevated to reveal the mesentery, duodeno-jejunal junction, sigmoid colon, and sigmoid mesocolon.

The **lesser omentum** (hepatogastric and hepatoduodenal ligaments) connects the lesser curvature of the stomach and the proximal part of the duodenum to the liver (Fig. 2.15B). The hepatogastric and hepatoduodenal ligaments are continuous parts of the lesser omentum and are separated only for descriptive convenience. The stomach is connected to the liver by the **hepatogastric ligament,** the membranous portion of the lesser omentum. The **hepatoduodenal ligament,** the thickened free edge of the lesser omentum, conducts the *portal triad:* portal vein, hepatic artery, and bile duct.

Every organ must have an area that is not covered with visceral peritoneum to allow the entrance and exit of neurovascular structures. Such areas are called **bare areas** and are formed in relation to the attachments of mesenteries, omenta, and ligaments.

A **peritoneal fold** (e.g., *medial and lateral umbilical folds*) is a reflection of peritoneum that is raised from the body wall by underlying blood vessels, ducts, and obliterated fetal vessels (Fig. 2.6).

A **peritoneal recess,** or fossa, is a pouch or concavity formed by a peritoneal fold (e.g., *inferior recess of the omental bursa* between the layers of the greater omentum [Fig. 2.15B] and the *supravesical* and *umbilical fossae* between the umbilical folds [Fig. 2.6]).

Subdivisions of Peritoneal Cavity

The peritoneal cavity is divided into a greater sac and an omental bursa (Figs. 2.17 and 2.18).

- The **greater sac** is the main and larger part of the peritoneal cavity. A surgical incision through the anterolateral abdominal wall enters the greater sac.
- The **omental bursa** (lesser sac), the smaller part of the peritoneal cavity, lies posterior to the stomach, lesser omentum, and adjacent structures. The omental bursa permits free movement of the stomach on adjacent structures because the anterior and posterior walls of the omental bursa slide smoothly over each other. The omental bursa has two recesses (Fig. 2.17):
  - A **superior recess,** which is limited superiorly by the diaphragm and the posterior layers of the coronary ligament of the liver.
  - An **inferior recess** between the superior part of the layers of the greater omentum.

Most of the inferior recess of the omental bursa is a potential space sealed off from the main part of the omental bursa posterior to the stomach after adhesion of the anterior and posterior layers of the greater omentum (Fig. 2.17A,B). The omental bursa communicates with the greater sac through the **omental foramen** (epiploic foramen), an opening situated posterior to the free edge of the lesser omentum forming the hepatoduodenal ligament (Figs. 2.4 and 2.15B). The boundaries of the omental foramen are:

- *Anteriorly*—the hepatoduodenal ligament (free edge of lesser omentum) containing the portal vein, hepatic artery, and bile duct.
- *Posteriorly*—IVC and right crus of diaphragm, covered with parietal peritoneum. (They are retroperitoneal.)

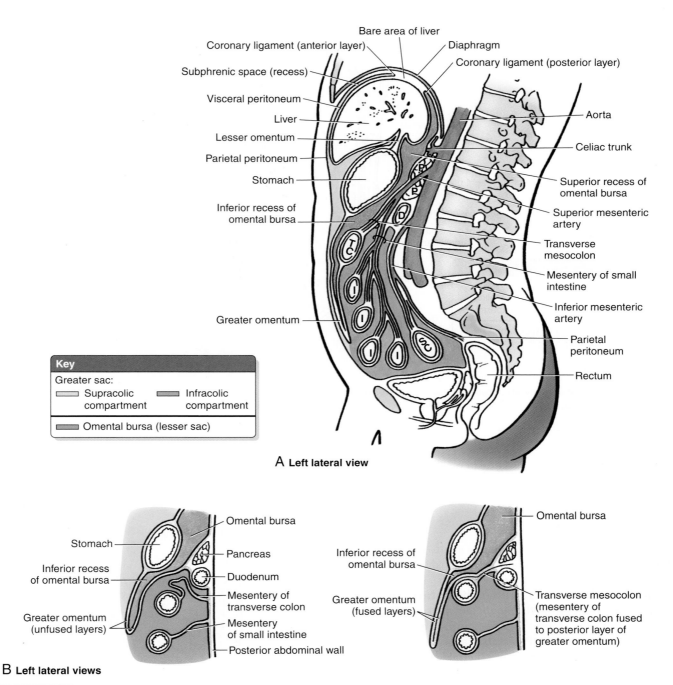

A Left lateral view

Key

Greater sac:
☐ Supracolic compartment   ▨ Infracolic compartment
▨ Omental bursa (lesser sac)

B Left lateral views

FIGURE 2.17. **Mesenteries and blood vessels. A.** Sagittal section of the abdomen and pelvis showing the viscera and the arrangement of the peritoneum. *D,* duodenum; *I,* jejunum and ileum; *P,* pancreas; *SC,* sigmoid colon; *TC,* transverse colon. **B.** Sagittal sections through the inferior recess of the omental bursa showing the formation of the transverse mesocolon and fusion of the layers of the greater omentum in an infant (left) and an adult (right).

- *Superiorly*—the liver, covered with visceral peritoneum.
- *Inferiorly*—superior or first part of the duodenum.

The **transverse mesocolon** (mesentery of transverse colon) divides the abdominal cavity into the following (Fig. 2.19):

- **Supracolic compartment,** containing the stomach, liver, and spleen.

- **Infracolic compartment,** containing the small intestine and ascending and descending colon. The infracolic compartment lies posterior to the greater omentum and is divided into *right* and *left infracolic spaces* by the mesentery of the small intestine.

Free communication occurs between the supracolic and the infracolic compartments through the **paracolic gutters,** the

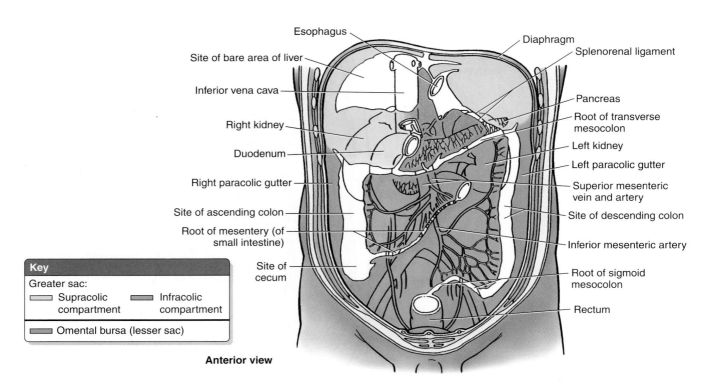

Anterior view

FIGURE 2.18. **Posterior wall of peritoneal cavity and roots of peritoneal reflections.** The liver and the ascending and descending colon have been mobilized and removed, and the transverse and sigmoid mesocolons and the mesentery of the small intestine have been cut at their roots.

grooves between the lateral aspect of the ascending or descending colon and the posterolateral abdominal wall.

ABDOMINAL VISCERA

The principal viscera of the abdomen are the esophagus (terminal part), stomach, intestines, spleen, pancreas, liver, gallbladder, kidneys, and suprarenal glands. The esophagus, stomach, and intestine form the **alimentary (digestive) tract.** Food passes from the *mouth* and *pharynx* through the *esophagus* to the *stomach.* Digestion mostly occurs in the stomach and *duodenum.* **Peristalsis,** a series of ring-like contraction waves that begin around the middle of the stomach and move slowly toward the pylorus, is responsible for mixing of the masticated (chewed) food mass with gastric juices and for emptying the contents of the stomach into the duodenum.

Absorption of chemical compounds occurs principally in the *small intestine,* consisting of the *duodenum, jejunum,* and *ileum* (Fig. 2.20A). The stomach is continuous with the duodenum, which receives the openings of the ducts from the *pancreas* and *liver* (major glands of digestive tract). Peristalsis also occurs in the jejunum and ileum, although it is not forceful unless an obstruction is present. The *large intestine* consists of the *cecum,* which receives the terminal part of the ileum, *appendix, colon* (ascending, transverse, and

descending), *rectum,* and *anal canal* (which ends at the *anus*). Most reabsorption of water occurs in the ascending colon. Feces (stools) are formed in the descending and sigmoid colon and accumulate in the rectum before defecation.

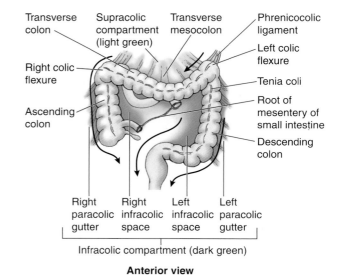

Anterior view

FIGURE 2.19. **Supracolic and infracolic compartments of greater peritoneal sac** after removal of greater omentum. The infracolic spaces and paracolic gutters determine the flow of ascitic fluid (*arrows*) when inclined or upright.

The Peritoneum and Surgical Procedures

 Because the peritoneum is well innervated, patients undergoing abdominal surgery experience more pain with large, invasive, open incisions of the peritoneum (*laparotomy*) than they do with small laparoscopic incisions or vaginal operations. Because of the high incidence of complications such as peritonitis and adhesions after operations in which the peritoneal cavity is opened, efforts are made to remain outside the peritoneal cavity whenever possible (e.g., translumbar or extraperitoneal anterior approach to the kidneys). When opening the peritoneal cavity is necessary, great effort is made to avoid contamination of the cavity.

Peritonitis and Ascites

When bacterial contamination occurs during laparotomy or when the gut is traumatically penetrated or ruptured as the result of infection and inflammation (e.g., appendicitis), allowing gas, fecal matter, and bacteria to enter the peritoneal cavity, the result is infection and inflammation of the peritoneum—**peritonitis.** Exudation of serum, fibrin, cells, and pus into the peritoneal cavity occurs, accompanied by pain in the overlying skin and an increase in the tone of the anterolateral abdominal muscles. Given the extent of the peritoneal surfaces and the rapid absorption of material, including bacterial toxins, from the peritoneal cavity, when peritonitis becomes *generalized* (widespread in the peritoneal cavity), the condition is dangerous and perhaps lethal. In addition to the severe abdominal pain, tenderness, nausea and/or vomiting, fever, and constipation are present.

Excess fluid in the peritoneal cavity is called **ascitic fluid**, clinically called **ascites**. Ascites may also occur as a result of mechanical injury (which may also produce internal bleeding) or other pathological conditions, such as portal hypertension (venous congestion) and widespread metastasis of cancer cells to the abdominal viscera. In all these cases, the peritoneal cavity may be distended with several liters of abnormal fluid, interfering with movements of the viscera.

Rhythmic movements of the anterolateral abdominal wall normally accompany respirations. If the abdomen is drawn in as the chest expands (*paradoxical abdominothoracic rhythm*) and muscle rigidity is present, either peritonitis or pneumonitis (inflammation of the lungs) may be present. Because the intense pain worsens with movement, people with peritonitis commonly lie with their knees flexed to relax their anterolateral abdominal muscles. They also breathe shallowly (and hence more rapidly), reducing the intra-abdominal pressure and pain.

Peritoneal Adhesions and Adhesiotomy

If the peritoneum is damaged, by a stab wound for example, or infected, the peritoneal surfaces become inflamed, making them sticky with *fibrin.* As healing occurs, the fibrin may be replaced with fibrous tissue, forming abnormal attachments between the visceral peritoneum of adjacent viscera, or between the visceral peritoneum of a viscus and the parietal peritoneum of the adjacent abdominal wall. **Adhesions** (scar tissue) may also form after an abdominal operation (e.g., owing to a ruptured appendix) and limit the normal movements of the viscera. This tethering may cause chronic pain or emergency complications such as intestinal obstruction when the gut becomes twisted around an adhesion (*volvulus*).

Adhesiotomy refers to the surgical separation of adhesions. Adhesions are often found during dissection of cadavers (e.g., binding of the spleen to the diaphragm).

Abdominal Paracentesis

Treatment of generalized peritonitis includes removal of the ascitic fluid and, in the presence of infection, administration of large doses of antibiotics. Surgical puncture of the peritoneal cavity for the aspiration or drainage of fluid is called **paracentesis**. After injection of a local anesthetic agent, a needle or trocar and a cannula are inserted through the anterolateral abdominal wall into the peritoneal cavity through the linea alba, for example. The needle is inserted superior to the empty urinary bladder and in a location that avoids the inferior epigastric artery.

Functions of Greater Omentum

The greater omentum, large and fat-laden, prevents the visceral peritoneum from adhering to the parietal peritoneum. It has considerable mobility and moves around the peritoneal cavity with peristaltic movements of the viscera. It often forms adhesions adjacent to an inflamed organ such as the appendix, sometimes walling it off and thereby protecting other viscera from it.

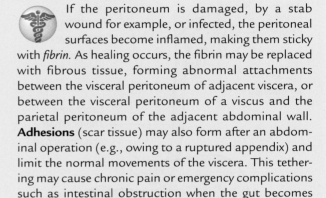

Spread of Pathological Fluids

Peritoneal recesses are of clinical importance in connection with the spread of pathological fluids such as pus, a product of inflammation. The recesses determine the extent and direction of the spread of fluids that may enter the peritoneal cavity when an organ is diseased or injured.

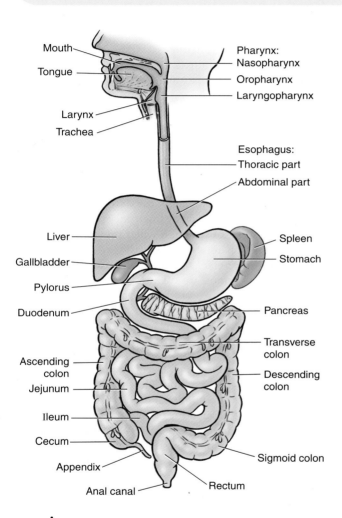

A **Anterior view; medial view of bisected head**

FIGURE 2.20. Schematic overview of alimentary tract and abdominal viscera. **A.** Viscera and parts of alimentary tract. **B.** Overview of arterial supply. **C.** Overview of portal venous drainage.

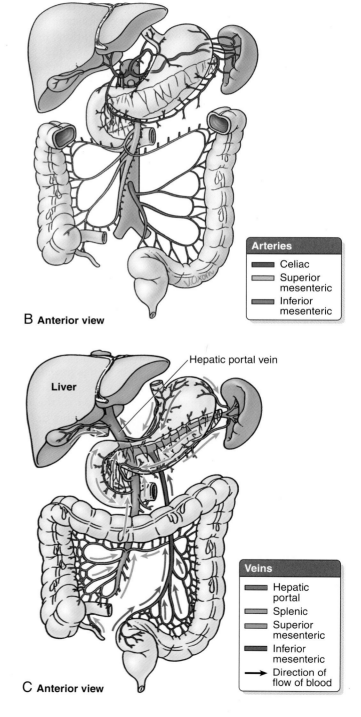

B **Anterior view**

Arteries	
	Celiac
	Superior mesenteric
	Inferior mesenteric

C **Anterior view**

Veins	
	Hepatic portal
	Splenic
	Superior mesenteric
	Inferior mesenteric
→	Direction of flow of blood

The arterial supply to the abdominal part of the alimentary tract, spleen, pancreas, gallbladder, and liver is from the *abdominal aorta* (Fig. 2.20B). The three major branches of the abdominal aorta are the *celiac trunk* and the *superior* and *inferior mesenteric arteries.*

The *hepatic portal vein,* formed by the union of the superior mesenteric and splenic veins (Fig. 2.20C), is the main channel of the *portal venous system*, which collects blood from the abdominal part of the alimentary tract, pancreas, spleen, and most of the gallbladder and carries it to the liver.

Esophagus

The **esophagus** is a muscular tube, approximately 25 cm (10 in) long with an average diameter of 2 cm, that extends from the pharynx to the stomach (Figs. 2.22 and 2.20A). The esophagus:

- Follows the concavity of the vertebral column as it descends through the neck and mediastinum.
- Passes through the elliptical **esophageal hiatus** in the muscular right crus of the diaphragm, just to the left of the median plane at the level of the T10 vertebra (Fig. 2.21A).
- Terminates at the **esophagogastric junction,** where ingested matter enters the cardial orifice of the stomach (Fig. 2.22B). It is located to the left of the midline at the level of the seventh left costal cartilage and the T11 vertebra. The esophagus is retroperitoneal during its short abdominal course.
- Has circular and external longitudinal layers of muscle. In its superior third, the external layer consists of voluntary striated muscle, the inferior third is composed of smooth muscle, and the middle third is made up of both types of muscle.

The esophagogastric junction is marked internally by the abrupt transition from esophageal to gastric mucosa, referred to clinically as the **Z-line** (Fig. 2.21B and 2.23A). Just superior to this junction, the diaphragmatic musculature forming the esophageal hiatus functions as a physiological **inferior esophageal sphincter** that contracts and relaxes. Radiological studies show that food or liquid may be stopped here momentarily and that the sphincter mechanism is normally efficient in preventing reflux of gastric contents into the esophagus.

The abdominal part of the esophagus has its:

- *Arterial supply* from the **esophageal branches of the left gastric artery** (Fig. 2.21B and 2.23A), a branch of the *celiac trunk,* and the **left inferior phrenic artery.**
- *Venous drainage* primarily to the *portal venous system* through the **left gastric vein** (Fig. 2.23), while the proximal thoracic part of the esophagus drains primarily into the *systemic venous system* through the **esophageal veins** entering the *azygos vein* (see Chapter 1). However, the veins of the two parts of the esophagus communicate and provide a clinically important portal–systemic anastomosis.
- *Lymphatic drainage* into the **left gastric lymph nodes,** which in turn drain mainly to the **celiac lymph nodes** (Fig. 2.21A).
- *Innervation* from the **vagal trunks** (becoming anterior and posterior gastric nerves), the **thoracic sympathetic**

Lymphatic drainage
Of thoracic parts:
▭ To jugular trunks
▭ To bronchomediastinal trunks
▭ To superior diaphragmatic nodes
Of abdominal part:
▭ To celiac (abdominal) nodes

Anterior views

⟶ Esophageal hiatus

FIGURE 2.21. Esophagus. **A.** Lymphatic drainage. **B.** Arterial supply.

trunks via the **greater** (abdominopelvic) **splanchnic nerves,** and the **periarterial plexus** around the left gastric artery and left inferior phrenic artery (Fig. 2.24B).

Stomach

The **stomach** acts as a food blender and reservoir; its chief function is enzymatic digestion. The *gastric juice* gradually converts a mass of food into a semiliquid mixture, *chyme* (G. juice), which passes into the duodenum.

PARTS AND CURVATURE OF THE STOMACH

The shape of the stomach is dynamic (changing in shape as it functions) and highly variable from person to person. The stomach has four parts and two curvatures (Fig. 2.22):

- The **cardia** is the part surrounding the **cardial orifice,** the trumpet-shaped opening of the esophagus into the stomach.
- The **fundus** is the dilated superior part of the stomach that is related to the left dome of the diaphragm and is limited inferiorly by the horizontal plane of the cardial orifice. The superior part of the fundus usually reaches the level of the left fifth intercostal space. The **cardial notch** is between the esophagus and the fundus. The fundus may be dilated by gas, fluid, food, or any combination of these.

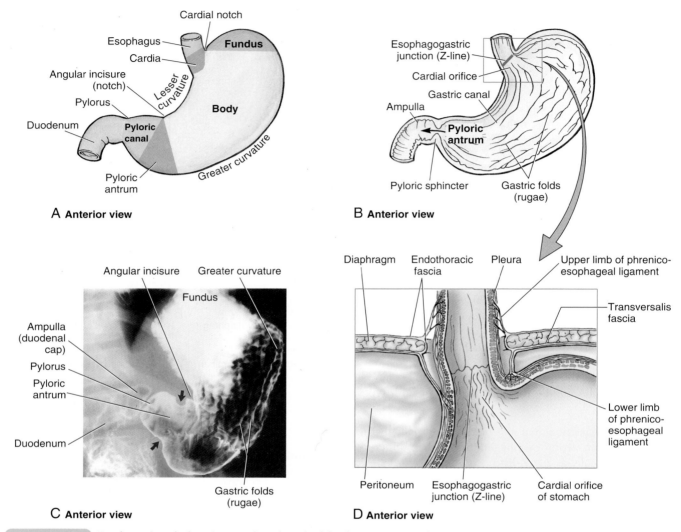

FIGURE 2.22. **Esophagus (terminal part), stomach, and proximal duodenum. A.** Areas of external surface. **B.** Internal surface (mucous membrane). *Arrow* passes from pyloric antrum through pyloric canal. **C.** Radiograph of stomach and duodenum after barium ingestion. *Arrows,* peristaltic wave. **D.** Esophagogastric junction.

- The **body,** the major part of the stomach, lies between the fundus and the pyloric antrum.
- The **pyloric part** of the stomach is the funnel-shaped region; its wide part, the **pyloric antrum,** leads into the **pyloric canal,** its narrow part. The **pylorus,** the distal sphincteric region, is a thickening of the circular layer of smooth muscle, which controls discharge of the stomach contents through the **pyloric orifice** into the duodenum.
- The **lesser curvature** forms the shorter concave border of the stomach; the **angular incisure** (notch) is the sharp indentation approximately two thirds of the distance along the lesser curvature that approximates the junction of the body and pyloric part of the stomach.
- The **greater curvature** forms the longer convex border of the stomach.

INTERIOR OF THE STOMACH

When contracted, the gastric mucosa is thrown into longitudinal **gastric folds** (rugae) (Fig. 2.22B,C). These are most marked toward the pyloric part and along the greater curvature. A **gastric canal** (furrow) forms temporarily during swallowing between the longitudinal gastric folds along the lesser curvature. Saliva and small quantities of masticated food and other fluids pass through the gastric canal to the pyloric canal when the stomach is mostly empty.

VASCULATURE AND NERVES OF STOMACH

The stomach has:

- A rich *arterial supply,* arising from the celiac trunk and its branches (Fig. 2.23A; Table 2.5). Most of the blood is

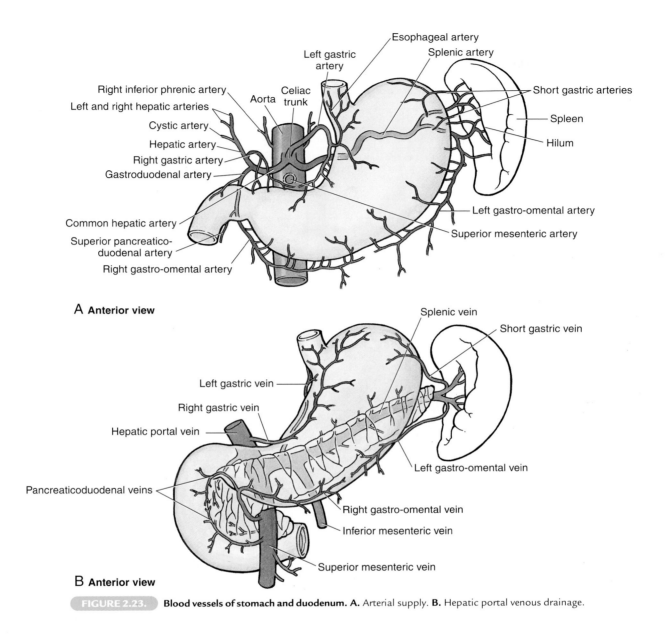

A Anterior view

B Anterior view

FIGURE 2.23. **Blood vessels of stomach and duodenum. A.** Arterial supply. **B.** Hepatic portal venous drainage.

supplied by anastomoses formed along the lesser curvature by the **right** and **left gastric arteries** and, along the greater curvature, by the **right** and **left gastro-omental artery** (gastro-epiploic artery). The fundus and upper body of stomach receive blood from the short and posterior gastric arteries, branches of the splenic artery.

- Gastric *veins* that parallel the arteries in position and course (Fig. 2.23*B*). The **left** and **right gastric veins** drain directly into the *hepatic portal vein.* The **short gastric veins** and the **left gastro-omental veins** drain into the *splenic vein,* which then joins the *superior mesenteric vein* (SMV) to form the hepatic portal vein. The **right gastro-omental vein** usually empties into the SMV.

- *Gastric lymphatic vessels* that accompany the arteries along the greater and lesser curvatures (Fig. 2.24*A*) and drain lymph from its anterior and posterior surfaces toward its curvatures, where the **gastric** and **gastro-omental lymph nodes** are located. The efferent vessels from these nodes via the **pancreaticosplenic, pyloric,** and **pancreaticoduodenal lymph nodes** accompany the large arteries to the *celiac lymph nodes.*

- *Parasympathetic and sympathetic innervation.* The **parasympathetic nerve supply** is from the **anterior vagal trunk** (mainly from the left vagus nerve) and **posterior vagal trunk** (mainly from the right vagus nerve) and their branches, which enter the abdomen through

TABLE 2.5 ARTERIAL SUPPLY TO ESOPHAGUS, STOMACH, DUODENUM, LIVER, GALLBLADDER, PANCREAS, AND SPLEEN

Artery[a]	Origin	Course	Distribution
Celiac trunk	Abdominal aorta (T12) just distal to aortic hiatus of diaphragm	After short anteroinferior course, bifurcates into splenic and common hepatic arteries	Esophagus, stomach, duodenum (proximal to bile duct), liver and biliary apparatus, and pancreas
Left gastric	Celiac trunk	Ascends retroperitoneally to esophageal hiatus, giving rise to an esophageal branch; then descending along lesser curvature to anastomose with right gastric artery	Distal portion of esophagus and left portion of lesser curvature of stomach
Splenic		Runs retroperitoneally along superior border of pancreas, then passes between layers of splenorenal ligament to hilum of spleen	Body of pancreas, spleen, and greater curvature of stomach; posterior gastric branch supplies posterior wall and fundus of stomach
Left gastro-omental (gastro-epiploic)	Splenic artery in hilum of spleen	Passes between layers of gastrosplenic ligament to greater curvature of stomach	Left portion of greater curvature of stomach
Short gastric (n = 4 or 5)		Pass between layers of gastrosplenic ligament to fundus of stomach	Fundus of stomach
Hepatic[b]	Celiac trunk	Passes retroperitoneally to reach hepatoduodenal ligament and passes between its layers to porta hepatis; divides into right and left hepatic arteries	Liver, gallbladder, stomach, pancreas, duodenum, and respective lobes of liver
Cystic	Right hepatic artery	Arises within hepatoduodenal ligament	Gallbladder and cystic duct
Right gastric	Hepatic artery	Runs along lesser curvature of stomach	Right portion of lesser curvature of stomach
Gastroduodenal		Descends retroperitoneally posterior to gastroduodenal junction	Stomach, pancreas, first part of duodenum, and distal part of bile duct
Right gastro-omental (gastro-epiploic)	Gastroduodenal artery	Passes between layers of greater omentum to greater curvature of stomach	Right portion of greater curvature of stomach
Anterior and posterior superior pancreatico-duodenal		Descend on head of pancreas	Proximal portion of duodenum and head of pancreas
Anterior and posterior inferior pancreatico-duodenal	Superior mesenteric artery	Ascend on head of pancreas	Distal portion of duodenum and head of pancreas

[a]For anastomoses, see Figure 2.23.

[b]For descriptive purposes, the hepatic artery is often divided into the common hepatic artery from its origin to the origin of gastroduodenal artery, and the remainder of the vessel is called hepatic artery proper.

the esophageal hiatus (Fig. 2.24B). The **sympathetic nerve supply is** from the T6–T9 segments of the spinal cord, which passes to the **celiac plexus** via the greater splanchnic nerves and is distributed as plexuses around the gastric and gastro-omental arteries.

RELATIONS OF THE STOMACH

The stomach is covered by peritoneum, except where blood vessels run along its curvatures and in a small area posterior to the cardial orifice. The two layers of the lesser omentum separate to extend around the stomach and come together again to leave its greater curvature as the greater omentum.

- *Anteriorly*, the stomach is related to the **diaphragm**, the left lobe of the liver, and the anterior abdominal wall (Fig. SA2.2A).
- *Posteriorly*, the stomach is related to the **omental bursa** and **pancreas**; the posterior surface of the stomach forms most of the anterior wall of the omental bursa (Figs. 2.25 and 2.26).

The **stomach bed** on which the stomach rests when a person is in the supine position is formed by the structures forming the posterior wall of the omental bursa (Table 2.6). From superior to inferior, the stomach bed is formed by the left dome of the diaphragm, spleen, left kidney and suprarenal gland, splenic artery, pancreas, transverse mesocolon, and colon.

Small Intestine

The **small intestine,** consisting of the duodenum, jejunum, and ileum, extends from the pylorus of the stomach to the ileocecal junction, where the ileum joins the cecum, the first part of the large intestine.

DUODENUM

The duodenum, the first and shortest (25 cm) part of the small intestine, is also the widest and most fixed part. The duodenum begins at the pylorus on the right side and ends

Gastric lymph nodes

Celiac lymph nodes

Superior mesenteric lymph nodes

Superior and inferior pyloric lymph nodes

Pancreaticoduodenal lymph nodes

Pancreaticosplenic lymph nodes

Splenic artery

Gastro-omental lymph nodes

Lymph nodes

→ Initial drainage
→ Secondary (subsequent) drainage

Mesenteric lymph nodes

A **Anterior view**

From ileum

From jejunum

Stomach

Anterior and posterior vagal trunks

Thoracic splanchnic nerves (greater, lesser, least)

Celiac ganglion and plexus

Sympathetic trunk and ganglia (lumbar portion)

Lumbar splanchnic nerves

Innervation

☐ Sympathetic nerves and ganglia
☐ Parasympathetic nerves
☐ Plexuses (sympathetic and parasympathetic)

Superior mesenteric ganglion and plexus

Duodenum

Duodenojejunal junction

Jejunum

B **Anterior view**

Ileum

FIGURE 2.24.   Lymphatic drainage (A) and innervation (B) of stomach and duodenum.

Surface Anatomy of Stomach

The surface markings of the stomach vary because its size and position change under various circumstances. The surface markings in the supine position include the (Fig. SA2.2A):

- **Cardial orifice:** usually lies posterior to the *sixth left costal cartilage*, 2 to 4 cm from the median plane at the level of the T10 or T11 vertebra.
- **Fundus:** usually lies posterior to the *fifth left rib* in the midclavicular plane.
- **Greater curvature:** passes inferiorly to the left as far as the *10th left costal cartilage* before turning medially to reach the pyloric antrum.
- **Lesser curvature:** passes from the right side of the cardia to the pyloric antrum. The most inferior part of the curvature is marked by the **angular incisure** (Fig. 2.22A), which lies just to the left of the midline.
- **Pyloric part of the stomach:** usually lies at the level of the ninth costal cartilage at the level of the L1 vertebra. The pyloric orifice is approximately 1.25 cm left of the midline.
- **Pylorus:** usually lies on the right side. Its location varies from the L2 to the L4 vertebra.

A heavily built hypersthenic individual with a short thorax and long abdomen is likely to have a stomach that is placed high and more transversely disposed. In people with a slender, aesthenic physique, the stomach is low and vertical (Fig. SA2.2B).

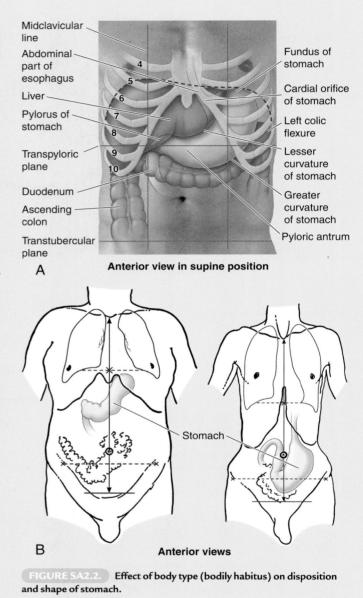

Anterior view in supine position

Anterior views

FIGURE SA2.2.   Effect of body type (bodily habitus) on disposition and shape of stomach.

---

at the **duodenojejunal junction** on the left side. Four parts of the duodenum are (Fig. 2.25 and Table 2.6):

- **Superior (first) part:** short (approximately 5 cm), mostly horizontal, and lies anterolateral to the body of L1 vertebra.
- **Descending (second) part:** longer (7–10 cm) and runs inferiorly along the right sides of the L2 and L3 vertebrae, curving around the head of the pancreas; initially it lies to the right and parallel to the IVC. The *bile duct* and *main*

pancreatic ducts via the hepatopancreatic ampulla enter its posteromedial wall.

- **Inferior (horizontal or third) part:** 6 to 8 cm long and crosses anterior to the IVC and aorta and posterior to the superior mesenteric artery (SMA) and superior mesenteric vein (SMV) at the level of the L3 vertebra.
- **Ascending (fourth) part:** short (approximately 5 cm) and begins at the left of the L3 vertebra and rises superiorly as far as the superior border of the L2 vertebra, 2 to 3 cm to the left of the midline. It passes on the left side of the aorta

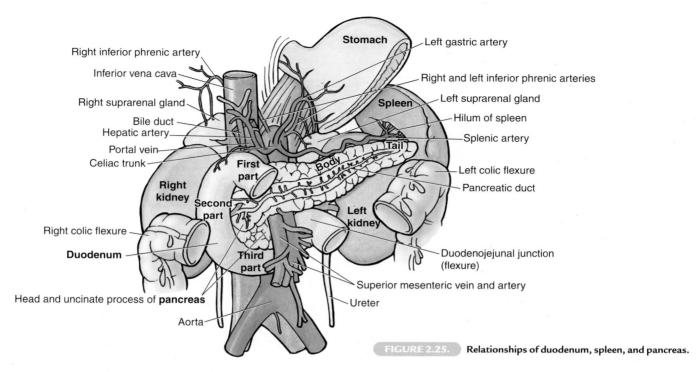

FIGURE 2.25. Relationships of duodenum, spleen, and pancreas.

TABLE 2.6 RELATIONSHIPS OF DUODENUM, SPLEEN, AND PANCREAS

Organ	Anterior	Posterior	Medial	Superior	Inferior	Level
Superior (first) part of duodenum	Peritoneum Gallbladder Quadrate lobe of liver	Bile duct Gastroduodenal artery Hepatic portal vein IVC		Neck of gallbladder	Neck of pancreas	Anterolateral to L1 vertebra
Descending (second) part of duodenum	Transverse colon Transverse mesocolon Coils of small intestine	Hilum of right kidney Renal vessels Ureter Right psoas major	Head of pancreas Pancreatic duct			Right of L2–L3 vertebrae
Inferior (horizontal or third) part of duodenum	SMA SMV coils of small intestine	Right psoas major IVC Aorta Right ureter		Head and uncinate process of pancreas SMV SMA		Anterior to L3 vertebra
Ascending (fourth) part of duodenum	Beginning of root of mesentery Coils of jejunum	Left psoas major Left margin of aorta	Head of pancreas	Body of pancreas		Left of L3 vertebra
Spleen	Stomach	Left part of diaphragm	Left kidney		Left colic flexure	Left upper quadrant between 9th and 11th ribs
Head of pancreas		IVC Right renal artery and vein				
Neck of pancreas	Pylorus of stomach	SMA SMV				
Body of pancreas	Omental bursa	Aorta SMA Left suprarenal gland Left kidney and renal vessels				L2 vertebra
Tail of pancreas		Left kidney				

IVC, inferior vena cava; *SMA*, superior mesenteric artery; *SMV*, superior mesenteric vein.

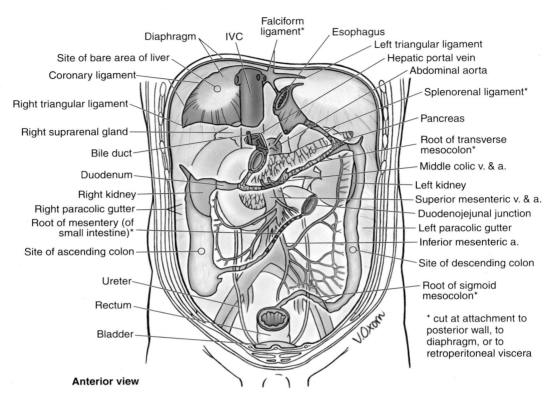

FIGURE 2.26. **Peritoneal relationships of duodenum and pancreas.** The liver, ascending colon, and descending colon have been mobilized and removed, and the transverse and sigmoid mesocolons and the mesentery of the small intestine have been cut at their roots. *IVC,* inferior vena cava.

to reach the inferior border of the body of the pancreas. Here it curves anteriorly to join the jejunum at the **duodenojejunal junction,** which takes the form of an acute angle, the **duodenojejunal flexure.** The flexure is supported by the attachment of the **suspensory muscle of the duodenum** (ligament of Treitz).

The suspensory muscle of the duodenum is commonly composed of a slip of skeletal muscle from the diaphragm and a fibromuscular band of smooth muscle from the third and fouth parts of the duodenum. Contraction of this suspensory muscle widens the angle of the duodenojejunal flexure, facilitating movement of the intestinal contents. The suspensory muscle passes posterior to the pancreas and splenic vein and anterior to the left renal vein.

The first 2 cm of the superior part of the duodenum has a mesentery and is mobile. This free part—relatively dilated and smooth-walled—is called the **ampulla** or duodenal cap (Fig. 2.22*B,C*). The distal 3 cm of the superior part and the other three parts of the duodenum have no mesentery and are immobile because they are retroperitoneal (Fig. 2.26). The principal relations of the duodenum are outlined in Table 2.6.

The duodenum has:

- *An arterial supply* from two different vessels. An important transition in the blood supply of the alimentary tract occurs over the course of the descending (second) part of the duodenum, approximately where the bile duct enters. The basis of this transition is embryological because this is the site of the junction of the foregut and midgut. Consequently, the **duodenal arteries** arise from two different sources (Figs. 2.27 and Table 2.7):
  - Proximally, the abdominal part of the alimentary tract is supplied by the **celiac trunk,** and the first and second parts of the duodenum are supplied via the **gastroduodenal artery** and its branch, the **superior pancreaticoduodenal artery.**
  - Distally, a major part of the alimentary canal (extending as far as the left colic flexure) is supplied by the SMA, and the third and fourth parts of the duodenum are supplied by its branch, the **inferior pancreaticoduodenal artery.** The superior and inferior pancreaticoduodenal arteries form an anastomotic loop between the celiac trunk and the SMA; consequently, there is potential for collateral circulation here.
- *Duodenal veins,* which follow the arteries and drain into the **hepatic portal vein** (Fig. 2.28); some veins drain

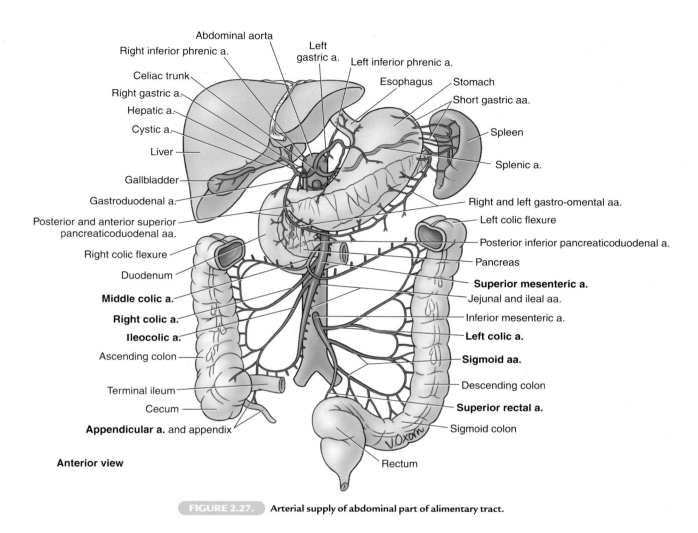

FIGURE 2.27.   Arterial supply of abdominal part of alimentary tract.

TABLE 2.7 ARTERIAL SUPPLY TO INTESTINES

Artery	Origin	Course	Distribution
Superior mesenteric	Abdominal aorta (L1)	Runs in root of mesentery to ileocecal junction	Part of gastrointestinal tract derived from midgut
Intestinal (*n* = 15–18)	Superior mesenteric artery	Passes between two layers of mesentery	Jejunum and ileum
Middle colic		Ascends retroperitoneally and passes between layers of transverse mesocolon	Transverse colon
Right colic		Passes retroperitoneally to reach ascending colon	Ascending colon
Ileocolic	Terminal branch of superior mesenteric artery	Runs along root of mesentery and divides into ileal and colic branches	Ileum, cecum, and ascending colon
Appendicular	Ileocolic artery	Passes between layers of mesoappendix	Appendix
Inferior mesenteric	Abdominal aorta (L3)	Descends retroperitoneally to left of abdominal aorta	Descending colon
Left colic	Inferior mesenteric artery	Passes retroperitoneally toward left to descending colon	
Sigmoid (*n* = 3 or 4)		Passes retroperitoneally toward left to sigmoid colon	Descending and sigmoid colon
Superior rectal	Terminal branch of inferior mesenteric artery	Descends retroperitoneally to rectum	Proximal part of rectum
Middle rectal	Internal iliac artery	Passes retroperitoneally to rectum	Midpart of rectum
Inferior rectal	Internal pudendal artery	Crosses ischio-anal fossa to reach rectum	Distal part of rectum and anal canal

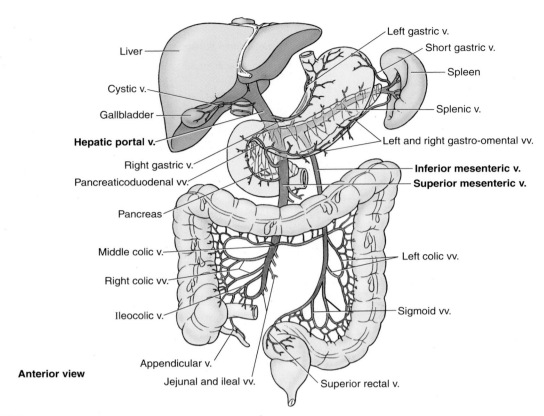

Liver

Cystic v.

Gallbladder

Hepatic portal v.

Right gastric v.

Pancreaticoduodenal vv.

Pancreas

Middle colic v.

Right colic vv.

Ileocolic v.

Appendicular v.

Jejunal and ileal vv.

Anterior view

Left gastric v.

Short gastric v.

Spleen

Splenic v.

Left and right gastro-omental vv.

Inferior mesenteric v.
Superior mesenteric v.

Left colic vv.

Sigmoid vv.

Superior rectal v.

FIGURE 2.28. **Venous drainage of abdominal part of alimentary tract.** The hepatic portal vein drains blood rich in nutrients but reduced in oxygen from the stomach, intestines, spleen, pancreas, and gallbladder to the liver.

directly and others indirectly through the superior mesenteric and splenic veins.

- *Lymphatic vessels,* which follow the arteries in a retrograde direction. The *anterior lymphatic vessels* drain into the **pancreaticoduodenal lymph nodes** located along the superior and inferior pancreaticoduodenal arteries, and into the **pyloric lymph nodes,** which lie along the gastroduodenal artery (Fig. 2.24*A*). The *posterior lymphatic vessels* pass posterior to the head of the pancreas and drain into the **superior mesenteric lymph nodes.** Efferent lymphatic vessels from the duodenal lymph nodes drain into the **celiac lymph nodes.**
- *Parasympathetic innervation* from the **vagus** and *sympathetic innervation* from the **greater** and **lesser splanchnic nerves** by way of the **celiac** and **superior mesenteric plexuses** and then via periarterial plexuses extending to the pancreaticoduodenal arteries (Fig. 2.24*B*).

JEJUNUM AND ILEUM

The jejunum begins at the **duodenojejunal junction** and the ileum ends at the **ileocecal junction,** the union of the terminal ileum and cecum (Fig. 2.29*A*). Together, the jejunum and ileum are 6 to 7 m long in cadavers; however, tonic contraction makes them substantially shorter in living persons. The jejunum constitutes approximately two fifths of the length, and the ileum the remainder. The terminal ileum usually lies in the pelvis, from which it ascends to end in the medial aspect of the cecum. Although no clear line of demarcation between the jejunum and ileum exists, they have distinctive characteristics for most of their lengths (Table 2.8).

The **mesentery,** a fan-shaped fold of peritoneum, attaches the jejunum and ileum to the posterior abdominal wall. The **root (origin) of the mesentery** (approximately 15 cm long) is directed obliquely, inferiorly, and to the right (Fig. 2.26). It extends from the duodenojejunal junction on the left side of the L2 vertebra to the ileocolic junction and the right sacroiliac joint. The root of the mesentery crosses (successively) the ascending and horizontal parts of the duodenum, abdominal aorta, inferior vena cava, right ureter, right psoas major muscle, and right testicular or ovarian vessels.

The jejunum and ileum have:

- *Arterial supply* from the SMA (Fig. 2.27 and Table 2.7). The SMA runs between the layers of the mesentery and sends many branches to the jejunum and ileum. The arteries unite to form loops or arches—**arterial**

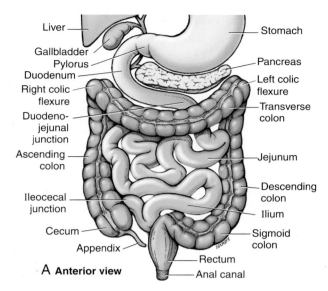

A **Anterior view**

Liver — Stomach
Gallbladder
Pylorus — Pancreas
Duodenum
Right colic flexure — Left colic flexure
Duodeno-jejunal junction — Transverse colon
Ascending colon — Jejunum
Ileocecal junction — Descending colon
Cecum — Ilium
Appendix — Sigmoid colon
— Rectum
— Anal canal

Jejunum

Circular folds
Vasa recta
Arterial arcades

B

Ileum

Circular folds
Vasa recta
Arterial arcades

C

Mesentery

Visceral peritoneum (serosa)
Subserosa
Longitudinal layer — Muscularis externa
Circular layer
Submucosa
Longitudinal layer — Muscularis mucosae
Circular layer
Myenteric plexus (Auerbach plexus)
Submucosal plexus (Meissner plexus)
Lamina propria
Mucous epithelium — Mucosa
Circular folds
D   (L. *plicae circulares*)

FIGURE 2.29.   **Small intestine. A.** Small and large intestine in situ. **B.** Characteristics of jejunum. **C.** Characteristics of ileum. **D.** Layers of wall of small intestine.

TABLE 2.8 DISTINGUISHING CHARACTERISTICS OF JEJUNUM AND ILEUM IN LIVING PERSONS

Characteristic	Jejunum	Ileum
Color	Deeper red	Paler pink
Caliber	2–4 cm	2–3 cm
Wall	Thick and heavy	Thin and light
Vascularity	Greater	Less
Vasas recta	Long	Short
Arcades	A few large loops	Many short loops
Fat in mesentery	Less	More
Circular folds (L. *plicae circulares*)	Large, tall, and closely packed	Low and sparse; absent in distal part

arcades—that give rise to straight arteries—the **vasa recta** (Fig. 2.29*B*,*C*).

- *Venous drainage* from the SMV (Fig. 2.28). The SMV lies anterior and to the right of the SMA in the root of the mesentery. The SMV ends posterior to the neck of the pancreas, where it unites with the splenic vein to form the hepatic portal vein.

- Specialized *lymphatic vessels*, called **lacteals,** in the intestinal villi that absorb fat and drain into the lymphatic plexuses in the walls of the jejunum and ileum. The lymphatic plexuses drain into lymphatic vessels between the layers of the mesentery and then sequentially through three groups of lymph nodes (Fig. 2.24*A*): **juxta-intestinal lymph nodes** (close to the intestinal wall), **mesenteric lymph nodes** (scattered among the arterial arcades), and **central superior nodes** (along the proximal part of the SMA). Efferent lymphatic vessels from these nodes drain into the **superior mesenteric lymph nodes.** Lymphatic vessels from the terminal ileum follow the ileal branch of the ileocolic artery to the **ileocolic lymph nodes.**

- *Sympathetic and parasympathetic innervation.*
  - In general, sympathetic stimulation reduces secretion and motility of the intestine and acts as a vasoconstrictor, reducing or stopping digestion and making blood (and energy) available for "fleeing or fighting." Parasympathetic stimulation increases secretion and motility of the intestine, restoring digestive activity after a sympathetic reaction. The SMA and its branches are surrounded by a dense **perivascular nerve plexus** through which the nerve fibers are conducted to the parts of the intestine supplied by the SMA. The **sympathetic fibers** originate in the T8–T10 segments of the spinal cord and reach the **superior mesenteric nerve plexus** through the *sympathetic trunks* and *thoracic abdominopelvic (greater, lesser, and least) splanchnic nerves* (Figs. 2.24*B* and 2.30). The presynaptic sympathetic fibers synapse on cell bodies of postsynaptic sympathetic neurons in the *celiac and superior mesenteric (prevertebral) ganglia.*
  - The **parasympathetic fibers** derive from the **posterior vagal trunk.** The presynaptic parasympathetic fibers synapse with postsynaptic parasympathetic neurons in the *myenteric and submucous plexuses* in the intestinal wall (Fig. 2.29*D*). The small intestine also has *sensory (visceral afferent) fibers* (Fig. 2.30). The intestine is insensitive to most pain stimuli, including cutting and burning; however, it is sensitive to sudden distention ("gas pains") and transient ischemia from abnormally long contractions that are perceived as **colic** (spasmodic abdominal pains).

FIGURE 2.30. Innervation of small intestine.

Large Intestine

The **large intestine** consists of the *cecum, colon (ascending, transverse, descending,* and *sigmoid), rectum,* and *anal canal* (Fig. 2.29*A* and 2.31*A*). The large intestine can be distinguished from the small intestine by:

- **Teniae coli:** three thickened bands of longitudinal smooth muscle fibers.
- **Haustra:** sacculations or pouches of the colon between the teniae.
- **Omental appendices:** small, fatty appendices (projections) of colon.
- **Caliber:** the internal diameter is much larger.

The three teniae coli make up most of the longitudinal muscle of the large intestine, except in the rectum. Because the teniae are shorter than the large intestine, the colon has the typical sacculated shape formed by the haustra. The teniae begin at the base of the appendix and run the length of the large intestine, merging at the rectosigmoid junction into a continuous layer around the rectum.

CECUM AND APPENDIX

The **cecum,** the first part of the large intestine, which is continuous with the ascending colon, is a blind intestinal pouch in the right lower quadrant, where it lies in the iliac fossa inferior to the junction of the terminal ileum and cecum. The cecum is usually almost entirely enveloped by peritoneum and can be lifted freely; however, the cecum has no

Overview of Embryological Rotation of Midgut

 The primordial gut consists of the *foregut* (esophagus, stomach, pancreas, duodenum, liver, and biliary ducts), *midgut* (small intestine distal to the bile duct, cecum, appendix, ascending colon, and most of the transverse colon), and *hindgut* (distal transverse colon, descending and sigmoid colon, and rectum). For 4 weeks, the rapidly growing midgut, supplied by the SMA, is herniated into the proximal part of the umbilical cord (Fig. B2.7A). It is attached to the

Left anterior oblique views

FIGURE B2.7.

umbilical vesicle (yolk sac) by the omphalo-enteric duct (yolk stalk). As it returns to the abdominal cavity, the midgut rotates 270 degrees around the axis of the SMA (Fig. B2.7B,C). As the parts of the intestine reach their definitive positions, their mesenteric attachments undergo modifications. Some mesenteries shorten and others disappear (Fig. B2.7D,E). Malrotation of the midgut results in several congenital anomalies, such as volvulus (twisting) of the intestine.

mesentery (Fig. 2.26). The ileum enters the cecum obliquely and partly invaginates into it, forming folds superior and inferior to the **ileal orifice** (Fig. 2.31B). These folds form the **ileocecal valve.**

The vermiform (L. worm-like) **appendix,** a blind intestinal diverticulum, extends from the posteromedial aspect of the cecum inferior to the ileocecal junction. The appendix varies in length and has a short triangular mesentery, the **mesoappendix,** which derives from the posterior side of the mesentery of the terminal ileum (Fig. 2.31B). The mesoappendix attaches to the cecum and the proximal part of the appendix. The position of the appendix is variable, but it is usually retrocecal (posterior to the cecum). The base of the appendix most often lies deep to a point that is one third of the way along the oblique line joining the right anterior superior iliac spine to the umbilicus (*spinoumbilical* or *McBurney point*).

The cecum is supplied by the **ileocolic artery,** the terminal branch of the SMA. The appendix is supplied by the **appendicular artery,** a branch of the ileocolic artery (Fig. 2.31B and Table 2.7). A tributary of the SMV, the **ileocolic vein,** drains blood from the cecum and appendix (Fig. 2.28). The **lymphatic vessels** from the cecum and appendix pass to lymph nodes in the mesoappendix and to

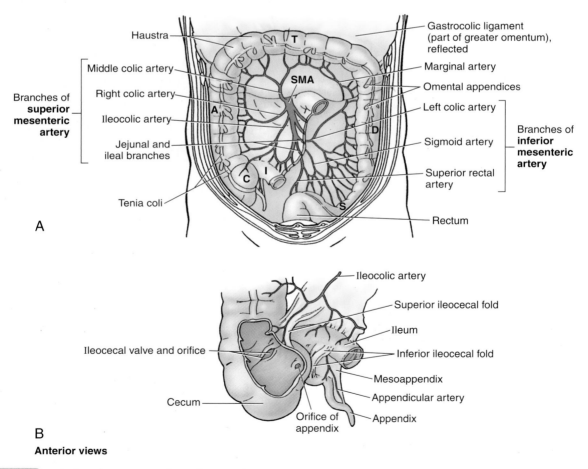

FIGURE 2.31. **Large intestine: parts, arteries, and mesenteries. A.** Most of the small intestine has been removed to show the blood supply of the large intestine. *A*, ascending colon; *C*, cecum; *D*, descending colon; *I*, terminal ileum; *S*, sigmoid colon; *SMA*, superior mesenteric artery; *T*, transverse colon. **B.** Blood supply of cecum and appendix. A window has been cut in the wall of the cecum to expose the ileocecal orifice and the orifice of the appendix.

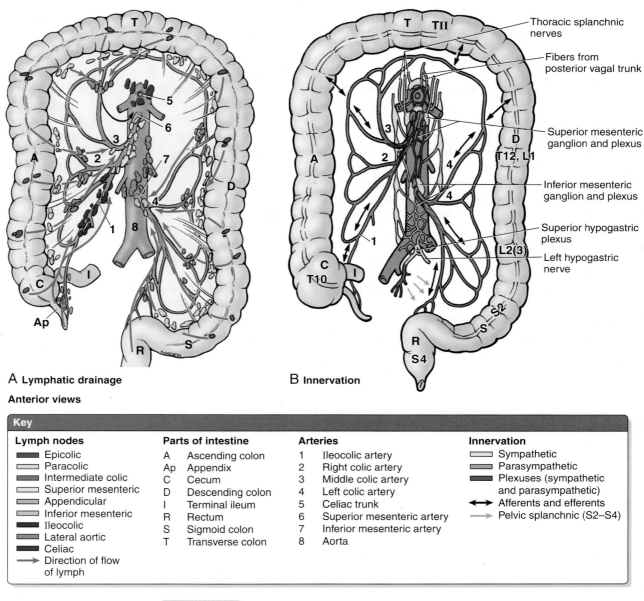

A Lymphatic drainage

B Innervation

Anterior views

Key			
Lymph nodes	**Parts of intestine**	**Arteries**	**Innervation**
Epicolic	A Ascending colon	1 Ileocolic artery	Sympathetic
Paracolic	Ap Appendix	2 Right colic artery	Parasympathetic
Intermediate colic	C Cecum	3 Middle colic artery	Plexuses (sympathetic
Superior mesenteric	D Descending colon	4 Left colic artery	and parasympathetic)
Appendicular	I Terminal ileum	5 Celiac trunk	Afferents and efferents
Inferior mesenteric	R Rectum	6 Superior mesenteric artery	Pelvic splanchnic (S2–S4)
Ileocolic	S Sigmoid colon	7 Inferior mesenteric artery	
Lateral aortic	T Transverse colon	8 Aorta	
Celiac			
Direction of flow of lymph			

FIGURE 2.32.   Lymphatic drainage and innervation of large intestine.

the **ileocolic lymph nodes** that lie along the ileocolic artery (Fig. 2.32*A*). Efferent lymphatic vessels pass to the **superior mesenteric lymph nodes.** The nerve supply to the cecum and appendix derives from sympathetic and parasympathetic nerves from the **superior mesenteric plexus** (Fig. 2.32*B*). The **sympathetic nerve fibers** originate in the lower thoracic part of the spinal cord (T10–T12), and the **parasympathetic nerve fibers** derive from the **vagus nerves.** Afferent nerve fibers from the appendix accompany the sympathetic nerves to the T10 segment of the spinal cord.

COLON

The colon is described as having four parts—ascending, transverse, descending, and sigmoid—that succeed one another in an arch (Fig. 2.31*A*).

The **ascending colon** passes superiorly on the right side of the abdominal cavity from the cecum to the right lobe of the liver, where it turns to the left as the **right colic flexure** (hepatic flexure). The ascending colon, narrower than the cecum, lies retroperitoneally along the right side of the posterior abdominal wall. The ascending colon is covered by peritoneum anteriorly and on its sides; however, in approximately

25% of people, it has a short mesentery. The ascending colon is separated from the anterolateral abdominal wall by the greater omentum. A vertical groove lined with parietal peritoneum (the **right paracolic gutter**) lies lateral to the ascending colon (Fig. 2.26).

The arterial supply to the ascending colon and right colic flexure is from branches of the SMA—the **ileocolic** and **right colic arteries** (Fig. 2.31A; Table 2.7). Tributaries of the SMV, the **ileocolic** and **right colic veins,** drain blood from the ascending colon. The **lymphatic vessels** first pass to the **epicolic and paracolic lymph nodes,** next to the **ileocolic** and intermediate **right colic lymph nodes,** and from them to the **superior mesenteric nodes** (Fig. 2.32A). The **nerves to the ascending colon** derive from the **superior mesenteric plexus** (Fig. 2.32B).

The **transverse colon,** the largest and most mobile part of the large intestine, crosses the abdomen from the right colic flexure to the left colic flexure, where it bends inferiorly to become the descending colon (Fig. 2.29A). The **left colic flexure** (splenic flexure)—usually more superior, more acute, and less mobile than the right colic flexure—lies anterior to the inferior part of the left kidney and attaches to the diaphragm through the **phrenicocolic ligament** (Fig. 2.15B). The mesentery of the transverse colon, the *transverse mesocolon,* loops down, often inferior to the level of the iliac crests, and is adherent to the posterior wall of the omental bursa. The **root of the transverse mesocolon** lies along the inferior border of the pancreas and is continuous with the parietal peritoneum posteriorly (Fig. 2.26).

The arterial supply of the transverse colon is mainly from the **middle colic artery** (Fig. 2.31A; Table 2.7), a branch of the SMA; however, it may also be supplied to variable degrees by the *right* and *left colic arteries* via anastomoses. *Venous drainage of the transverse colon* is through the **SMV.** Lymphatic drainage is to the **middle colic lymph nodes,** which in turn drain to the **superior mesenteric lymph nodes** (Fig. 2.32A). *The nerves of the transverse colon* arise from the **superior mesenteric plexus** and follow the right and middle colic arteries (Fig. 2.32B). These nerves transmit sympathetic and parasympathetic (vagal) nerve fibers. Some nerves derived from the **inferior mesenteric plexus** may follow anastomoses from the left colic artery.

The **descending colon** passes retroperitoneally from the left colic flexure into the left iliac fossa, where it is continuous with the sigmoid colon. Peritoneum covers the colon anteriorly and laterally and binds it to the posterior abdominal wall. Although retroperitoneal, the descending colon, especially in the iliac fossa, has a short mesentery in approximately 33% of people. As it descends, the colon passes anterior to the lateral border of the left kidney (Fig. 2.26). As with the ascending colon, a left **paracolic gutter** lies on the lateral side of the desecending colon.

The **sigmoid colon,** characterized by its S-shaped loop of variable length, links the descending colon and the rectum

(Fig. 2.31A). The sigmoid colon extends from the iliac fossa to the third sacral segment, where it joins the rectum. The termination of the teniae coli indicates the *rectosigmoid junction.* The sigmoid colon usually has a long mesentery (*sigmoid mesocolon*) and, therefore, has considerable freedom of movement, especially its middle part. The **root of the sigmoid mesocolon** has an inverted V-shaped attachment (Fig. 2.26), extending first medially and superiorly along the external iliac vessels and then medially and inferiorly from the bifurcation of the common iliac vessels to the anterior aspect of the sacrum. The left ureter and the division of the left common iliac artery lie retroperitoneally posterior to the apex of the root of the sigmoid mesocolon.

The second important transition in the blood supply to the abdominal portion of the alimentary tract occurs approximately at the left colic flexure. Proximal to this point (back to mid-duodenum), the blood is supplied to the alimentary tract by the **SMA** (embryonic midgut); distal to this point, blood is supplied by the **inferior mesenteric artery** (IMA) (embryonic hindgut). *The arterial supply of the descending and sigmoid colon* is from the **left colic** and **sigmoid arteries,** branches of the IMA (Fig. 2.31A; Table 2.7). The left colic and sigmoid arteries pass to the left, where they divide into ascending and descending branches. Usually all or most of the branches of the arteries supplying blood to the colon (ileocolic; right, middle, and left colic; and sigmoid arteries) anastomose with each other as they approach the colon, thus forming a continuous anastomotic channel, the **marginal artery,** which may provide important collateral circulation (Fig. 2.31A).

The **inferior mesenteric vein (IMV)** returns blood from the descending and sigmoid colon, flowing usually into the splenic vein and then the hepatic portal vein on its way to the liver (Fig. 2.28). The lymphatic vessels from the descending and sigmoid colon pass to the **epicolic** and **paracolic lymph nodes** and then through the **intermediate colic lymph nodes** along the left colic artery (Fig. 2.32A). Lymph from these nodes passes to **inferior mesenteric lymph nodes** that lie around the IMA; however, lymph from the left colic flexure also drains to the *superior mesenteric lymph nodes.*

The **sympathetic nerve supply** of the descending and sigmoid colon is from the lumbar part of the sympathetic trunk via **lumbar (abdominopelvic) splanchnic nerves,** the **inferior mesenteric ganglion,** and the **periarterial plexuses on the IMA** and its branches (Fig. 2.32B). The **parasympathetic nerve supply** is from the **pelvic splanchnic nerves** via the inferior hypogastric (pelvic) plexus and nerves, which ascend retroperitoneally from the plexus, independent of the arterial supply. Proximal to the middle of the sigmoid colon the visceral afferents conveying pain pass retrogradely with sympathetic fibers to thoracolumbar spinal sensory ganglia, whereas those carrying reflex information travel with the parasympathetic fibers to vagal sensory ganglia. Distal to the middle of the sigmoid colon, the visceral afferents follow the parasympathetic fibers retrogradely to the sensory ganglia of spinal nerves S2–S4.

RECTUM AND ANAL CANAL

The rectum, the fixed terminal part of the large intestine, is continuous with the sigmoid colon at the level of the S3 vertebra. The junction is at the lower end of the mesentery of the sigmoid colon (Fig. 2.26). The rectum is continuous inferiorly with the anal canal. These parts of the large intestine are described with the pelvis in Chapter 3.

Hiatal Hernia

 A **hiatal (hiatus) hernia** is a protrusion of part of the stomach into the mediastinum through the esophageal hiatus of the diaphragm. The hernias occur most often in people after middle age, possibly because of weakening of the muscular part of the diaphragm and widening of the esophageal hiatus. Although clinically there are several types of hiatal hernias, the two main types are paraesophageal hiatal hernia and sliding hiatal hernia (Skandalakis et al., 1996).

In the less common **paraesophageal hiatal hernia,** the cardia remains in its normal position (Fig. B2.8A). However, a pouch of peritoneum, often containing part of the fundus, extends through the esophageal hiatus anterior to the esophagus. In these cases, usually no regurgitation of gastric contents occurs because the cardial orifice is in its normal position.

In the common **sliding hiatal hernia,** the abdominal part of the esophagus, the cardia, and parts of the fundus of the stomach slide superiorly through the esophageal hiatus into the thorax, especially when the person lies down or bends over (Fig. B2.8B). Some regurgitation of stomach contents into the esophagus is possible because the clamping action of the right crus of the diaphragm on the inferior end of the esophagus is weak.

Carcinoma of Stomach and Gastrectomy

 When the body or pyloric part of the stomach contains a malignant tumor, the mass may be palpable. Using *gastroscopy,* physicians can inspect the lining of the air-inflated stomach, enabling them to observe gastric lesions and take biopsies. **Partial gastrectomy** (removal of part of the stomach) may be performed to remove the region of the stomach involved by carcinoma. Because of the anastomoses of the arteries supplying the stomach provide good collateral circulation, one or more arteries may be ligated during this procedure without seriously affecting the blood supply of the remaining part of the stomach.

Partial gastrectomy to remove a carcinoma usually also requires removal of all involved regional lymph

Barium swallow radiograph of sliding hiatal hernia

 FIGURE B2.8.   Barium swallow radiograph of sliding hiatal hernia.

nodes. Because cancer frequently occurs in the pyloric region, removal of the *pyloric lymph nodes* as well as the right *gastro-omental lymph nodes* also receiving lymph drainage from this region is especially important. As stomach cancer becomes more advanced, the lymphogenous dissemination of malignant cells involves the *celiac lymph nodes,* to which all gastric nodes drain.

Gastric Ulcers, Peptic Ulcers, *Helicobacter pylori,* and Vagotomy

Gastric ulcers are open lesions of the mucosa of the stomach, whereas *peptic ulcers* are lesions of the mucosa of the pyloric canal or, more often, the duodenum. Most ulcers of the stomach and duodenum are associated with an infection of a specific bacterium, *Helicobacter pylori* (*H. pylori*). People experiencing severe chronic anxiety are most prone to the development of peptic ulcers. They often have gastric acid secretion rates that are markedly higher than normal between meals. It is thought that the high acid level in the stomach and duodenum overwhelms the bicarbonate normally produced by the duodenum and reduces the effectiveness of the mucous lining, leaving it vulnerable to *H. pylori*. The bacteria erode the protective mucous lining of the stomach, inflaming the mucosa and making it vulnerable to the effects of the gastric acid and digestive enzymes (pepsin) produced by the stomach.

If the ulcer erodes into the gastric arteries, it can cause life-threatening bleeding. Because the secretion of acid by parietal cells of the stomach is largely controlled by the vagus nerves, *vagotomy* (surgical section of the vagus nerves) is performed in some people with chronic or recurring ulcers to reduce the production of acid.

A *posterior gastric ulcer* may erode through the stomach wall into the pancreas, resulting in referred pain to the back. In such cases, *erosion of the splenic artery* results in severe hemorrhage into the peritoneal cavity.

Duodenal (Peptic) Ulcers

 Most inflammatory erosions of the duodenal wall, *duodenal ulcers,* are in the posterior wall of the superior part of the duodenum within 3 cm of the pylorus. Occasionally, an ulcer perforates the duodenal wall, permitting its contents to enter the peritoneal cavity and produce *peritonitis*. Because the superior part of the duodenum closely relates to the liver and gallbladder, either of them may adhere to and be ulcerated by a duodenal ulcer. *Erosion of the gastroduodenal artery,* a posterior relation of the superior part of the duodenum, by a duodenal ulcer results in severe hemorrhage into the peritoneal cavity.

Ileal Diverticulum

 An *ileal diverticulum* (of Meckel) is a congenital anomaly that occurs in 1% to 2% of people. A remnant of the proximal part of the embryonic omphalo-enteric duct (yolk stalk), the diverticulum usually appears as a finger-like pouch 3 to 6 cm long. It is always on the antimesenteric border of the ileum—the border of the intestine opposite the mesenteric attachment. An ileal diverticulum may become inflamed and produce pain mimicking appendicitis.

Diverticulosis

Diverticulosis is a disorder in which multiple false *diverticula* (external evaginations or outpocketings of the mucosa of the colon) develop along the intestine. It primarily affects middle-

aged and elderly people. Diverticulosis is commonly found in the sigmoid colon. Diverticula are subject to infection and rupture, leading to diverticulitis.

Appendicitis

Acute inflammation of the appendix is a common cause of an *acute abdomen* (severe abdominal pain arising suddenly). Digital pressure over the McBurney point produces the maximum abdominal tenderness. The pain of appendicitis usually commences as a vague pain in the periumbilical region because afferent pain fibers enter the spinal cord at the T10 level. Later, severe pain in the right lower quadrant results from irritation of the parietal peritoneum lining the posterior abdominal wall.

Appendectomy

Surgical removal of the appendix (**appendectomy**) may be performed through a transverse or gridiron (muscle-splitting) incision centered at the McBurney point in the right lower quadrant.

Laparoscopic appendectomy has become a standard procedure selectively used to remove the appendix. The peritoneal cavity is first inflated with carbon dioxide gas, distending the abdominal wall, to provide viewing and working space. The laparoscope is passed through a small incision in the anterolateral abdominal wall (e.g., near or through the umbilicus). One or two other small incisions ("portals") are required for surgical (instrument) access to the appendix and related vessels.

In unusual cases of *malrotation of the intestine,* or failure of descent of the cecum, the appendix is not in the lower right quadrant (LRQ). When the cecum is high (*subhepatic cecum*), the appendix is in the right hypochondriac region and the pain localizes there, not in the LRQ.

Colitis, Colectomy, and Ileostomy

  Chronic inflammation of the colon (*ulcerative* **colitis**, *Crohn disease*) is characterized by severe inflammation and ulceration of the colon and rectum. In some cases, a **colectomy** is performed, during which the terminal ileum and colon as well as the rectum and anal canal are removed. An **ileostomy** is then constructed to establish an artificial cutaneous opening between the ileum and the skin of the anterolateral abdominal wall. Following a partial colectomy, a **colostomy** or *sigmoidostomy* is performed to create an artificial cutaneous opening for the terminal part of the colon.

Colonoscopy

The interior surface of the colon can be observed and photographed in a procedure called **colonoscopy** or *coloscopy*, using a long fiberoptic endoscope (*colonoscope*) inserted into the colon through the anus and rectum. Small instruments can be passed through the colonoscope to perform minor operative procedures, such as biopsies or removal of polyps. Most tumors of the large intestine occur in the rectum; approximately 12% of them appear near the rectosigmoid junction. The interior of the sigmoid colon is observed with a *sigmoidoscope*, a shorter endoscope, in a procedure called *sigmoidoscopy*.

Surface Anatomy of Spleen and Pancreas

The **spleen** lies superficially in the left upper abdominal quadrant between the 9th and the 11th ribs (Fig. SA2.3). Its convex, costal surface fits the inferior surface of the diaphragm and the curved bodies of the ribs. In the supine position, the long axis of the spleen is roughly parallel to the long axis of the 10th rib. The spleen is seldom palpable through the anterolateral abdominal wall unless it is enlarged. The **neck of the pancreas** overlies the L1 and L2 vertebrae in the transpyloric plane. Its head is to the right and inferior to this plane, and its body and tail are to the left and superior to this level. Because the pancreas is deep in the abdominal cavity, posterior to the stomach and omental bursa, it is usually not palpable.

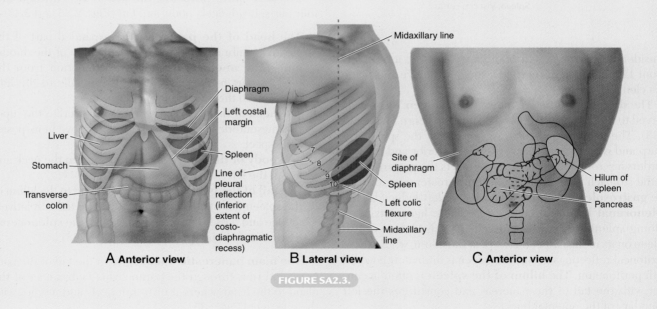

FIGURE SA2.3.

Spleen

The **spleen,** a mobile ovoid lymphatic organ, lies intraperitoneally in the left upper quadrant. The spleen is entirely surrounded by peritoneum except at the **hilum** (Fig. 2.33), where the splenic branches of the splenic artery and vein enter and leave. It is associated posteriorly with the left 9th through 11th ribs and separated from them by the diaphragm and the **costodiaphragmatic recess,** the cleft-like extension of the pleural cavity between the diaphragm and the lower part of the thoracic cage (Fig. SA2.3B). The spleen normally does not descend inferior to the costal region; it rests on the left colic flexure. The spleen varies

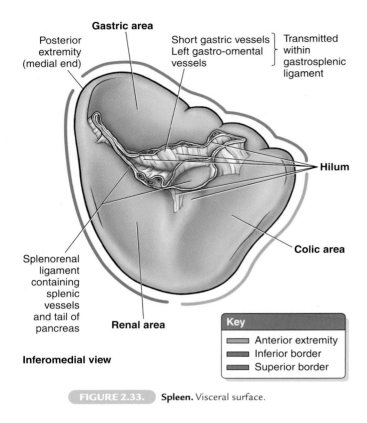

Gastric area

Posterior extremity (medial end)

Short gastric vessels
Left gastro-omental vessels
] Transmitted within gastrosplenic ligament

Hilum

Colic area

Splenorenal ligament containing splenic vessels and tail of pancreas

Renal area

Inferomedial view

Key
- Anterior extremity
- Inferior border
- Superior border

FIGURE 2.33. **Spleen.** Visceral surface.

considerably in size, weight, and shape; however, it is usually about 12 cm long and 7 cm wide, roughly the size and shape of a clenched fist.

The **diaphragmatic surface of the spleen** is convexly curved to fit the concavity of the diaphragm (Figs. SA2.3 and 2.33). The anterior and superior borders of the spleen are sharp and often notched, whereas its posterior and inferior borders are rounded. The spleen contacts the posterior wall of the stomach and is connected to its greater curvature by the **gastrosplenic ligament** and to the left kidney by the **splenorenal ligament** (Fig. 2.14). These ligaments, containing splenic vessels, are attached to the hilum of the spleen on its medial aspect. Except at the hilum, where these peritoneal reflections occur, the spleen is intimately covered with peritoneum. The **hilum of the spleen** is often in contact with the tail of the pancreas and constitutes the left boundary of the omental bursa.

The **splenic artery,** the largest branch of the celiac trunk, follows a tortuous course posterior to the omental bursa, anterior to the left kidney, and along the superior border of the pancreas (Fig. 2.34A). Between the layers of the splenorenal ligament, the splenic artery divides into five or more branches that enter the hilum of the spleen, dividing it into two to three vascular segments. The **splenic vein** is formed by several tributaries that emerge from the hilum (Fig. 2.34B). It is joined by the IMV and runs posterior to the

body and tail of the pancreas throughout most of its course. The splenic vein unites with the SMV posterior to the neck of the pancreas to form the **hepatic portal vein.**

The *splenic lymphatic vessels* leave the lymph nodes in the hilum and pass along the splenic vessels to the **pancreaticosplenic lymph nodes** (Fig. 2.34C). These nodes relate to the posterior surface and superior border of the pancreas. The **nerves of the spleen** derive from the **celiac plexus** (Fig. 2.34D). They are distributed mainly along branches of the splenic artery and are vasomotor in function.

Pancreas

The **pancreas,** an elongated accessory digestive gland, lies retroperitoneally and transversely across the posterior abdominal wall, posterior to the stomach between the duodenum on the right and the spleen on the left (Fig. 2.25). The root of the transverse mesocolon lies along its anterior margin. The pancreas produces an exocrine secretion (*pancreatic juice* from the acinar cells) that enters the duodenum and endocrine secretions (*glucagon* and *insulin* from the pancreatic islets [of Langerhans]) that enter the blood.

For descriptive purposes, the pancreas is divided into four parts: head, neck, body, and tail (Figs. 2.25 and 2.35).

- The **head of the pancreas,** the expanded part of the gland, is embraced by the C-shaped curve of the duodenum. The **uncinate process,** a projection from the inferior part of the head, extends medially to the left, posterior to the SMA.
- The **neck of the pancreas** is short and overlies the superior mesenteric vessels, which form a groove in its posterior aspect.
- The **body of the pancreas** continues from the neck and lies to the left of the SMA and SMV.
- The **tail of the pancreas** is closely related to the hilum of the spleen and the left colic flexure. The tail is relatively mobile and passes between the layers of the **splenorenal ligament** with the splenic vessels (Fig. 2.33).

The **main pancreatic duct** begins in the tail of the pancreas and runs through the parenchyma (substance) of the gland to the head, where it turns inferiorly and merges with the bile duct (Fig. 2.35).

The **bile duct** (common bile duct) crosses the posterosuperior surface of the head of the pancreas or is embedded in its substance. The pancreatic and bile ducts unite to form a short, dilated **hepatopancreatic ampulla** (Fig. 2.35B), which opens into the descending part of the duodenum at the summit of the **major duodenal papilla.** Several smooth-muscle sphincters occur in this area. The **sphincter of the bile duct** (around the termination of the bile duct) controls the flow of bile. The **sphincter of the pancreatic**

A Arteries

Aorta
Celiac artery
Common hepatic artery
Gastroduodenal artery
Right gastro-omental artery
Dorsal pancreatic artery
Greater pancreatic artery
Splenic artery
Inferior pancreatico-duodenal artery (dividing into anterior and posterior branches)
Anterior and posterior superior pancreatico-duodenal arteries
Uncinate process of pancreas (posterior to superior mesenteric artery)
Superior mesenteric artery (SMA)

B Veins

Short gastric vein
Superior pancreatico-duodenal vein
Hepatic portal vein
Pancreatic veins
Splenic vein
Inferior mesenteric vein (IMV)
Inferior pancreatico-duodenal vein
Superior mesenteric vein (SMV)

Anterior views

C Lymphatic drainage

Splenic artery

Key
	Pancreaticosplenic
	Celiac
	Superior mesenteric
	Pyloric
	Hepatic
→	Direction of flow of lymph

D Innervation

Vagus nerve (CN X)
Abdominopelvic (greater, lesser, least) splanchnic nerves
Celiac ganglion, trunk, and plexus
Sympathetic trunk and ganglion
Superior mesenteric ganglion, plexus, and artery
Esophagus
Spleen
Pancreas
Aorta

Key
	Sympathetic nerves and ganglia
	Parasympathetic nerves
	Plexuses (sympathetic and parasympathetic)

Anterior views

FIGURE 2.34.   Neurovasculature of spleen and pancreas.

duct (around the terminal part of the pancreatic duct) prevents reflux of bile into the duct, and the **hepatopancreatic sphincter** (sphincter of Oddi) around the hepatopancreatic ampulla prevents duodenal content from entering the ampulla. The **accessory pancreatic duct** drains the uncinate process and the inferior part of the head of the pancreas and opens into the duodenum at the **minor duodenal papilla** (Fig. 2.35B). Usually, the accessory duct communicates with the main pancreatic duct but in some people it is a separate duct.

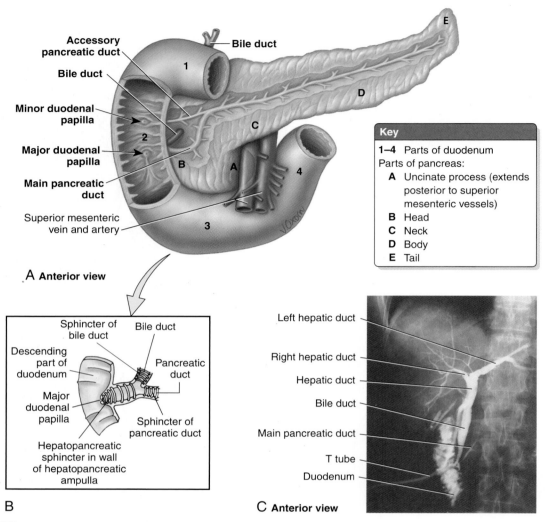

Accessory
pancreatic duct

Bile duct

Bile duct

Minor duodenal
papilla

Major duodenal
papilla

Main pancreatic
duct

Superior mesenteric
vein and artery

A Anterior view

Key

1–4	Parts of duodenum
	Parts of pancreas:
A	Uncinate process (extends posterior to superior mesenteric vessels)
B	Head
C	Neck
D	Body
E	Tail

Sphincter of
bile duct

Bile duct

Descending
part of
duodenum

Pancreatic
duct

Major
duodenal
papilla

Sphincter of
pancreatic duct

Hepatopancreatic
sphincter in wall
of hepatopancreatic
ampulla

B

Left hepatic duct

Right hepatic duct

Hepatic duct

Bile duct

Main pancreatic duct

T tube

Duodenum

C Anterior view

FIGURE 2.35. **Pancreas and biliary system. A.** Extrahepatic bile passages and pancreatic ducts. **B.** *Inset,* Sphincters. **C.** Endoscopic retrograde cholangiography and pancreatography reveals the bile and pancreatic ducts. The T tube delivers radiopaque dye into ducts.

The **pancreatic arteries** derive mainly from the branches of the splenic artery (Fig. 2.34A and Table 2.5). The anterior and posterior **superior pancreaticoduodenal arteries,** branches of the gastroduodenal artery, and the anterior and posterior **inferior pancreaticoduodenal arteries,** branches of the SMA, supply the head of the pancreas. The **pancreatic veins** are tributaries of the splenic and superior mesenteric parts of the hepatic portal vein; however, most of them empty into the **splenic vein** (Fig. 2.34B). The *pancreatic lymphatic vessels* follow the blood vessels (Fig. 2.34C). Most of them end in the **pancreaticosplenic nodes** that lie along the splenic artery, but some vessels end in the **pyloric lymph nodes.** Efferent vessels from these nodes drain to the **superior mesenteric**

lymph nodes or to the **celiac lymph nodes** via the **hepatic lymph nodes.**

The *nerves of the pancreas* are derived from the **vagus** and **abdominopelvic splanchnic nerves** passing through the diaphragm (Fig. 2.34D). The **parasympathetic** and **sympathetic nerve fibers** reach the pancreas by passing along the arteries from the **celiac plexus** and **superior mesenteric plexus.** In addition to the sympathetic fibers that pass to blood vessels, sympathetic and parasympathetic fibers are distributed to pancreatic acinar cells and islets. The parasympathetic fibers are secretomotor, but pancreatic secretion is primarily mediated by hormones, secretin and cholecystokinin formed in the duodenum and proximal intestine.

Rupture of Spleen and Splenomegaly

Although well protected by the 9th through 12th ribs, the spleen is the most frequently injured organ in the abdomen. Severe blows on the left side may fracture one or more ribs, resulting in sharp bone fragments that can lacerate the spleen. Blunt trauma to other regions of the abdomen that cause a sudden, marked increase in intra-abdominal pressure (e.g., by impalement on the steering wheel of a car) can also rupture the spleen because its capsule is thin and its parenchyma (essential substance) is soft and pulpy. If ruptured, the spleen bleeds profusely. Rupture of the spleen causes severe intraperitoneal hemorrhage and shock. Repair of a ruptured spleen is difficult; consequently, *splenectomy* (removal of the spleen) or *subtotal (partial) splenectomy* (removal of one or more segments of the spleen) is often performed to prevent the patient from bleeding to death. Even total splenectomy usually does not produce serious side effects, especially in adults, because most of its functions are assumed by other reticuloendothelial organs (e.g., liver and bone marrow), but the person will be more susceptible to certain bacterial infections.

When the spleen is diseased, resulting from, for example, granulocytic leukemia (high leukocyte and white blood cell count), it may enlarge to 10 or more times its normal size and weight (**splenomegaly**). Spleen engorgement sometimes accompanies hypertension (high blood pressure). The spleen is not usually palpable in the adult.

Rupture of Pancreas

Pancreatic injury can result from sudden, severe, forceful compression of the abdomen such as the force of impalement on steering wheel in an automobile accident. Because the pancreas lies transversely, the vertebral column acts like an anvil and the traumatic force may rupture the pancreas. Rupture of the pancreas frequently tears its duct system, allowing pancreatic juice to enter the parenchyma of the gland and to invade adjacent tissues. Digestion of pancreatic and other tissues by pancreatic juice is very painful.

Pancreatic Cancer

Cancer involving the pancreatic head accounts for most cases of extrahepatic obstruction of the biliary ducts. Because of the posterior relationships of the pancreas, cancer of the head often compresses and obstructs the bile duct and/or the hepatopancreatic ampulla. This causes obstruction, resulting in the retention of bile pigments, enlargement of the gallbladder, and jaundice (obstructive jaundice). *Jaundice* (Fr. *jaune*, yellow) is the yellow staining of most body tissues, skin, mucous membranes, and conjunctiva by circulating bile pigments.

Most people with pancreatic cancer have *ductular adenocarcinoma*. Severe pain in the back is frequently present. Cancer of the neck and body of the pancreas may cause portal or inferior vena caval obstruction because the pancreas overlies these large veins. The pancreas's extensive drainage to relatively inaccessible lymph nodes and the fact that pancreatic cancer typically metastasizes to the liver early, via the hepatic portal vein, make surgical resection of the cancerous pancreas nearly futile.

Liver

The **liver,** the largest internal organ and largest gland in the body, weighs about 1500 g. The diaphragm separates the liver from the pleura, lungs, pericardium, and heart. With the exception of lipids, every substance absorbed by the alimentary tract is received first by the liver. In addition to its many metabolic activities, the liver stores glycogen and secretes bile.

SURFACES OF LIVER

The liver has a convex **diaphragmatic surface** (anterior, superior, and some posterior) and a relatively flat, concave **visceral surface** (posteroinferior), which are separated anteriorly by the sharp **inferior border** (Fig. 2.36A,B). The diaphragmatic surface is smooth and dome-shaped where it is related to the concavity of the inferior surface of the diaphragm. **Subphrenic recesses**, superior extensions of the peritoneal cavity, are located between the anterior and the superior aspects of the liver and the diaphragm (Fig. 2.36C). The subphrenic spaces are separated by the **falciform ligament,** which extends between the liver and the anterior abdominal wall, into right and left recesses. The **hepatorenal recess** (Morrison pouch) of the subhepatic space is a deep recess of the peritoneal cavity on the right side inferior to the liver and anterior to the kidney and suprarenal gland.

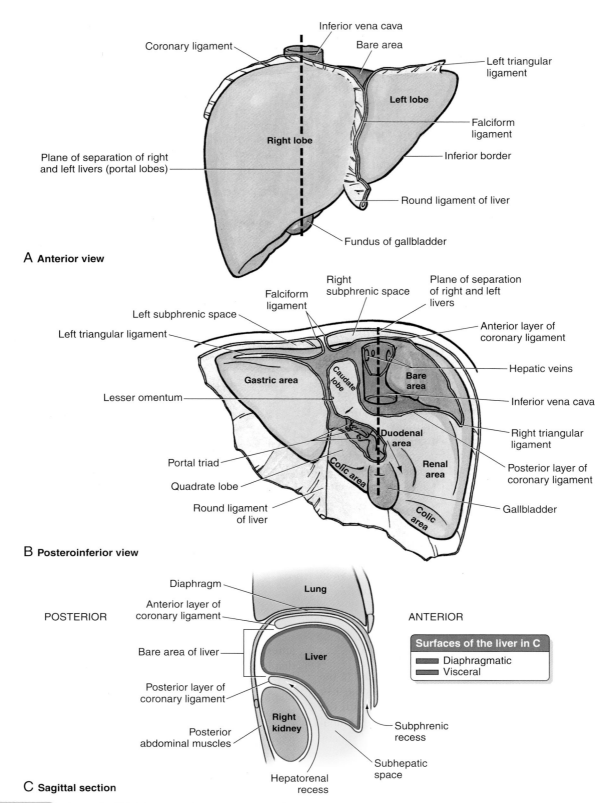

A Anterior view

B Posteroinferior view

C Sagittal section

FIGURE 2.36. **Liver and gallbladder. A.** Diaphragmatic surface of liver. **B.** Visceral surface of liver. The bare area is demarcated by the reflection of peritoneum from the diaphragm to the liver as the anterior (upper) and posterior (lower) layers of the coronary ligament. These layers meet at the right to form the right triangular ligament and diverge toward the left to enclose the bare area. The anterior layer of the coronary ligament is continuous on the left with the right layer of the falciform ligament, and the posterior layer is continuous with the right layer of the lesser omentum. The left layers of the falciform ligament and lesser omentum meet to form the left triangular ligament. **C.** Surfaces and recesses.

Surface Anatomy of Liver

The liver lies mainly in the right upper quadrant, where it is hidden and protected by the thoracic cage and diaphragm (Fig. SA2.4). The normal liver lies deep to ribs 7 to 11 on the right side and crosses the midline toward the left nipple. The liver is located more inferiorly when one is erect because of gravity. Its sharp inferior border follows the right costal margin. When the person is asked to inspire deeply, the liver may be palpated because of the inferior movement of the diaphragm and liver.

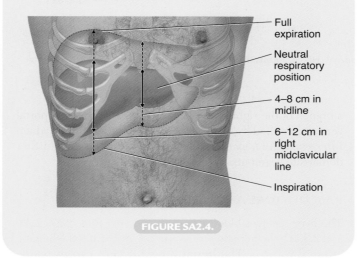

- Full expiration
- Neutral respiratory position
- 4–8 cm in midline
- 6–12 cm in right midclavicular line
- Inspiration

FIGURE SA2.4.

The *hepatorenal recess* is a gravity-dependent part of the peritoneal cavity when a person is in the supine position; fluid draining from the omental bursa flows into this recess. The hepatorenal recess communicates anteriorly with the right subphrenic space. The diaphragmatic surface is covered with peritoneum, except posteriorly in the **bare area of the liver,** where it lies in direct contact with the diaphragm (Fig. 2.36B,C). The **visceral surface of the liver** is covered with peritoneum, except at the *bed of the gallbladder* and the *porta hepatis.* The **porta hepatis** is a transverse fissure in the middle visceral surface of the liver that gives passage to the hepatic portal vein, hepatic artery, hepatic nerve plexus, hepatic ducts, and lymphatic vessels (Fig. 2.38B). The visceral surface of the liver is related to the:

- Right side of the anterior aspect of the stomach—*gastric* and *pyloric areas.*
- Superior part of the duodenum—*duodenal area.*
- Lesser omentum.
- Gallbladder—fossa for gallbladder.
- Right colic flexure and right transverse colon—*colic area.*
- Right kidney and suprarenal gland—*renal* and *suprarenal areas.*

Subphrenic Abscesses

Peritonitis may result in the formation of abscesses (localized collections of pus) in various parts of the peritoneal cavity. A common site for an abscess is in the subphrenic recesses. Subphrenic abscesses occur much more frequently on the right side because of the frequency of ruptured appendices and perforated duodenal ulcers. Because the right and left subphrenic recesses are continuous with the hepatorenal recess (Fig. 2.36C), pus from a subphrenic abscess may drain into one of the hepatorenal recesses, especially when the individual is bedridden. A subphrenic abscess is often drained by an incision inferior to, or through, the bed of the 12th rib.

The **lesser omentum,** enclosing the **portal triad** (portal vein, hepatic artery, and bile duct), passes from the liver to the lesser curvature of the stomach and the first 2 cm of the superior part of the duodenum (Fig. 2.37A). The thickened free edge of the lesser omentum extending between the porta hepatis and the duodenum is the **hepatoduodenal ligament** (Fig. 2.37B); it encloses the structures that pass through the porta hepatis (Fig. 2.38B).

LOBES AND SEGMENTS OF LIVER

Anatomically, based only on external features, the liver is described as having four "lobes": right, left, caudate, and quadrate; however, functionally, in terms of blood supply and glandular secretion, the liver is divided into independent right and left livers—portal lobes (Fig. 2.38A). The anatomical large **right lobe** is separated from the smaller **left lobe** by the falciform ligament and the left sagittal fissure. On the visceral surface, the right and left sagittal fissures and porta hepatis demarcate the **caudate lobe** (posterior and superior) and **quadrate lobe** (anterior and inferior)—both are parts of the right lobe. The **right sagittal fissure** is the continuous groove formed by the fossa for the gallbladder anteriorly and the groove for the inferior vena cava posteriorly. The **left sagittal fissure** is the continuous groove formed anteriorly by the **fissure for the round ligament** (L. *ligamentum teres*) and posteriorly by the **fissure for the ligamentum venosum** (Fig. 2.38B). The **round ligament of the liver** is the obliterated remains of the umbilical vein, which carried well-oxygenated blood from the placenta to the fetus. The **ligamentum venosum** is the fibrous remnant of the fetal ductus venosus, which shunted blood from the umbilical vein to the IVC, short-circuiting the liver (Moore and Persaud, 2008).

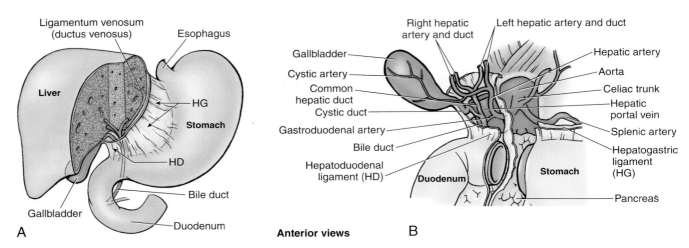

FIGURE 2.37. **Lesser omentum. A.** Hepatogastric (HG) and hepatoduodenal (HD) ligaments. **B.** Portal triad (bile duct, hepatic artery, and portal vein) within the hepatoduodenal ligament.

The division between **right** and **left livers** (parts or portal lobes) is approximated by the sagittal plane passing through the gallbladder fossa and the fossa for the IVC on the visceral surface of the liver and an imaginary line over the diaphragmatic surface that runs from the fundus of the gallbladder to the IVC (Fig. 2.38*B*). The left liver includes the anatomical caudate lobe and most of the quadrate lobe. The right and left livers are closer in mass than the anatomical lobes, but the right lobe is still somewhat larger. Each portal lobe has its own blood supply from the hepatic artery and hepatic portal vein and its own venous and biliary drainage. The portal lobes of the liver are further subdivided into eight **segments** (Fig. 2.39). The segmentation is based on the principal branches of the right and left hepatic arteries, hepatic portal veins, and hepatic ducts. Each segment is supplied by

a branch of the right or left hepatic artery and hepatic portal vein and drained by a branch of the right or left hepatic duct. *Intersegmental hepatic veins* pass between and thus further demarcate segments on their way to the IVC.

VASCULATURE AND NERVES OF LIVER

The liver receives blood from two sources (Figs. 2.27, 2.28, and 2.39*A*): the hepatic portal vein (75–80%) and the hepatic artery (20–25%). The **hepatic portal vein** carries poorly oxygenated blood from the abdominopelvic portion of the gastrointestinal tract. The **hepatic artery,** a branch of the celiac trunk, carries well-oxygenated blood from the aorta. At or close to the porta hepatis, the hepatic artery and hepatic portal vein terminate by dividing into right and left

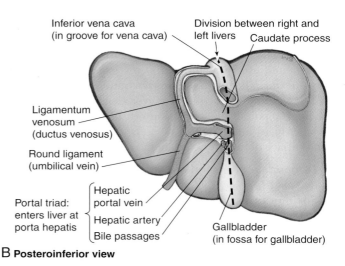

FIGURE 2.38. **Anatomical lobes and fissures of liver, visceral surface. A.** Four anatomical lobes. **B.** Structures forming and occupying fissures.

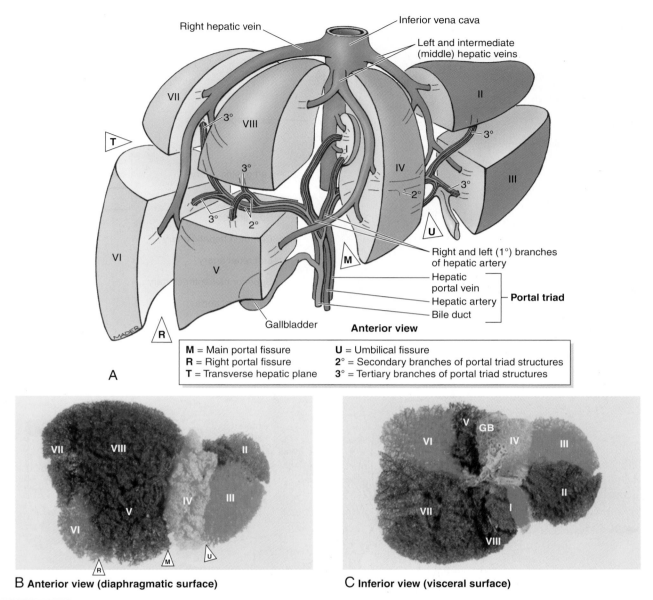

FIGURE 2.39.   **Hepatic segmentation. A.** Each segment (I–VIII) has its own intrasegmental blood supply and biliary drainage. **B and C.** Injection of different colors of latex into the branches of the hepatic portal vein to demonstrate hepatic segments.

branches, which supply the right and left livers, respectively. Within each lobe, the primary branches of the hepatic portal vein and hepatic artery are consistent enough to form **vascular segments** (Fig. 2.39). Between the segments are the **right, intermediate (middle),** and **left hepatic veins,** which drain parts of adjacent segments. The hepatic veins open into the IVC just inferior to the diaphragm (Fig. 2.39A). The attachment of these veins to the IVC helps hold the liver in position.

The liver is a major lymph-producing organ; between one quarter and one half of the lymph received by the thoracic duct comes from the liver. The **lymphatic vessels of the liver** occur as superficial lymphatics in the subperitoneal *fibrous capsule of the liver* (Glisson capsule), which form its outer surface, and as *deep lymphatics* in the connective tissue that accompany the ramifications of the portal triad and hepatic veins. Superficial lymphatics from the anterior aspects of the diaphragmatic and visceral surfaces and the deep lymphatic vessels accompanying the interlobular portal triads converge toward the porta hepatis and drain to the **hepatic lymph nodes** scattered along the hepatic vessels and ducts in the lesser omentum (Fig. 2.40A). Efferent

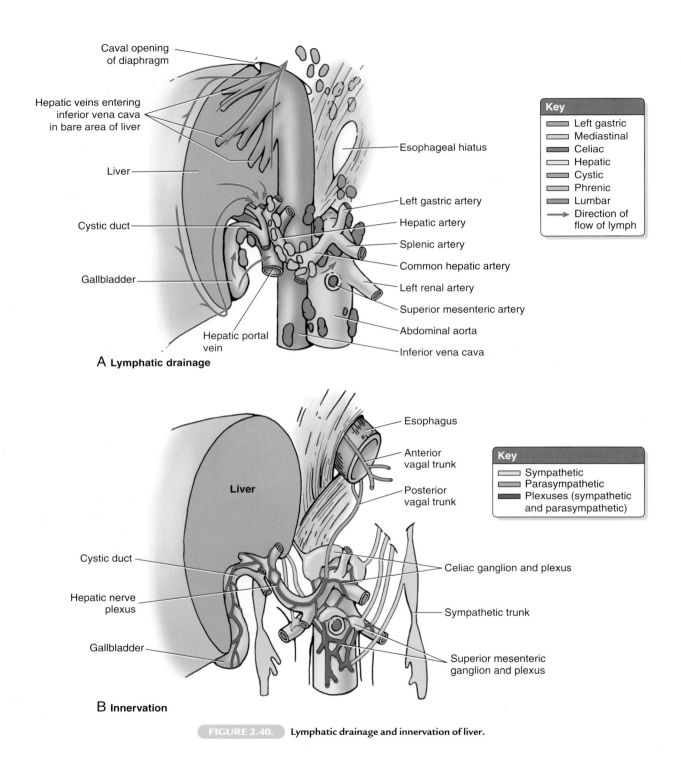

Key
- Left gastric
- Mediastinal
- Celiac
- Hepatic
- Cystic
- Phrenic
- Lumbar
- → Direction of flow of lymph

Caval opening of diaphragm

Hepatic veins entering inferior vena cava in bare area of liver

Liver

Cystic duct

Gallbladder

Hepatic portal vein

Esophageal hiatus

Left gastric artery

Hepatic artery

Splenic artery

Common hepatic artery

Left renal artery

Superior mesenteric artery

Abdominal aorta

Inferior vena cava

A Lymphatic drainage

Key
- Sympathetic
- Parasympathetic
- Plexuses (sympathetic and parasympathetic)

Liver

Esophagus

Anterior vagal trunk

Posterior vagal trunk

Cystic duct

Hepatic nerve plexus

Gallbladder

Celiac ganglion and plexus

Sympathetic trunk

Superior mesenteric ganglion and plexus

B Innervation

FIGURE 2.40. Lymphatic drainage and innervation of liver.

lymphatic vessels from these lymph nodes drain into the **celiac lymph nodes,** which in turn drain into the **cisterna chyli** at the inferior end of the thoracic duct. Superficial lymphatics from the posterior aspects of the diaphragmatic and visceral surfaces of the liver drain toward the bare area of the liver. Here, they drain into **phrenic lymph nodes** or

join deep lymphatics that have accompanied the hepatic veins converging on the IVC and then pass with this large vein through the diaphragm to drain into the **posterior mediastinal lymph nodes.** Efferent vessels from these nodes join the right lymphatic and thoracic ducts. A few lymphatic vessels also drain to the left gastric nodes, along

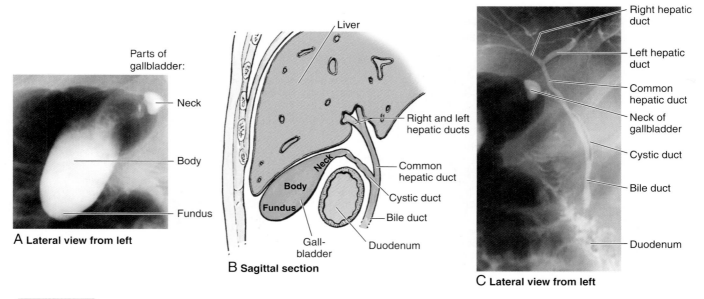

Parts of gallbladder:

- Neck
- Body
- Fundus

A Lateral view from left

Liver

Right and left hepatic ducts

Neck

Body

Fundus

Common hepatic duct

Cystic duct

Bile duct

Duodenum

Gall-bladder

B Sagittal section

Right hepatic duct

Left hepatic duct

Common hepatic duct

Neck of gallbladder

Cystic duct

Bile duct

Duodenum

C Lateral view from left

FIGURE 2.41. Normal disposition of gallbladder and extrahepatic biliary ducts. **A.** Gallbladder demonstrated by endoscopic retrograde cholangiography. **B.** Schematic sagittal section showing relationships to superior part of duodenum. **C.** Endoscopic retrograde cholangiogram of bile passages. Most often the cystic duct lies anterior to the common hepatic duct. (**A** and **C** courtesy of Dr. G.B. Haber, University of Toronto, Canada.)

the falciform ligament to the parasternal lymph nodes and along the round ligament of the liver to the lymphatics of the anterior abdominal wall. The **nerves of the liver** derive from the **hepatic nerve plexus** (Fig. 2.40B), the largest derivative of the celiac plexus. The hepatic plexus accompanies the branches of the hepatic artery and hepatic portal vein to the liver. It consists of *sympathetic fibers* from the **celiac plexus** and *parasympathetic fibers* from the anterior and posterior **vagal trunks.**

Biliary Ducts and Gallbladder

Bile is produced continuously in the liver and stored in the gallbladder (Fig. 2.41). In addition to storing bile, the gallbladder concentrates it by absorbing water and salts. When fat enters the duodenum, the gallbladder sends concentrated bile through the cystic and bile ducts to the duodenum. Bile emulsifies the fat so it can be absorbed in the distal intestine. The *hepatocytes* (liver cells) secrete bile into the **bile canaliculi** formed between them (Fig. 2.42). The canaliculi drain into the small *interlobular biliary ducts* and then into large collecting bile ducts of the intrahepatic portal triad, which merge to form the right and left hepatic ducts. The **right** and **left hepatic ducts** drain the right and left livers (portal lobes), respectively. Shortly after leaving the porta hepatis, the right and left hepatic ducts unite to form the **common hepatic duct,** which is joined on the right side by the **cystic duct** to form the **bile duct** (Fig. 2.41).

BILE DUCT

The bile duct (formerly called the common bile duct) is formed in the free edge of the lesser omentum by the union of the *cystic duct* and *common hepatic duct*. The bile duct descends posterior to the superior part of the duodenum and lies in a groove on the posterior surface of the head of the pancreas. On the left side of the descending part of the duodenum, the bile duct comes into contact with the **main pancreatic duct** (Fig. 2.43). The two ducts run obliquely through the wall of this part of the duodenum, where they unite to form the **hepatopancreatic ampulla** (ampulla of Vater). The distal end of the ampulla opens into the duodenum through the **major duodenal papilla.** The muscle around the distal end of the bile duct is thickened to form the **sphincter of the bile duct.** When this sphincter contracts, bile cannot enter the ampulla and/or the duodenum; hence bile backs up and passes along the cystic duct to the *gallbladder* for concentration and storage.

The arteries supplying the bile duct include the (Figs. 2.37B and 2.44):

- **Posterior superior pancreaticoduodenal artery** and **gastroduodenal artery,** supplying the retroduodenal part of the duct.
- **Cystic artery,** supplying the proximal part of the duct.
- **Right hepatic artery,** supplying the middle part of the duct.

The veins from the proximal part of the bile duct and the hepatic ducts generally enter the liver directly. The **posterior**

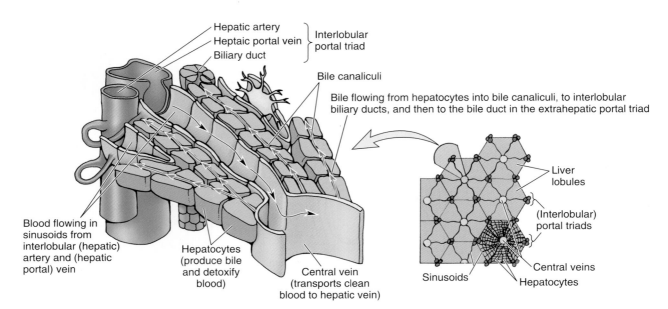

FIGURE 2.42. **Flow of blood and bile in the liver.** This small part of a liver lobule shows the components of the interlobular portal triad and the positioning of the sinusoids and bile canaliculi. At right, the cut surface of the liver shows the hexagonal pattern of the lobules.

superior pancreaticoduodenal vein drains the distal part of the bile duct and empties into the **hepatic portal vein** or one of its tributaries (Fig. 2.28). The lymphatic vessels from the bile duct pass to the **cystic lymph node** near the neck of the gallbladder, the **node of the omental foramen** and the **hepatic lymph nodes** (Fig. 2.40A). Efferent lymphatic vessels from the bile duct pass to the **celiac lymph nodes.**

GALLBLADDER

The pear-shaped **gallbladder** (7–10 cm long) lies in the **gallbladder fossa** on the visceral surface of the liver (Figs. 2.38B and 2.41). Peritoneum completely surrounds the fundus of the gallbladder and binds its body and neck to the liver. The hepatic surface of the gallbladder attaches to the liver by connective tissue of the fibrous capsule of the liver. The gallbladder has three parts (Figs. 2.41 and 2.43):

- The **fundus,** the wide end, projects from the inferior border of the liver and is usually located at the tip of the right ninth costal cartilage in the midclavicular line.
- The **body** contacts the visceral surface of the liver, the transverse colon, and the superior part of the duodenum.
- The **neck** is narrow, tapered, and directed toward the porta hepatis.

The neck makes an S-shaped bend and joins the **cystic duct.** Internally, the mucosa of the neck spirals into a **spiral fold** (spiral valve), which keeps the cystic duct open so that bile can easily divert into the gallbladder when the distal end of the bile duct is closed by the sphincter of the bile duct and/or the hepatopancreatic sphincter, or when bile passes to the duodenum as the gallbladder contracts. The **cystic**

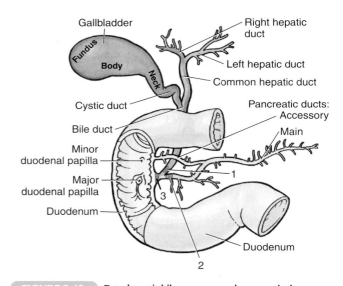

FIGURE 2.43. **Extrahepatic bile passages and pancreatic ducts.** 1. Sphincter of bile duct. 2. Sphincter of pancreatic duct. 3. Hepatopancreatic sphincter.

duct (approximately 4 cm long) connects the *neck of the gallbladder* to the common hepatic duct. The cystic duct passes between the layers of the lesser omentum, usually parallel to the **common hepatic duct,** which it joins to form the bile duct.

The **cystic artery,** which supplies the gallbladder and cystic duct, commonly arises from the **right hepatic artery** in the angle between the common hepatic duct and the cystic duct (Fig. 2.44). Variations in the origin and course of the cystic artery are common. The **cystic veins** draining the biliary ducts and the neck of the gallbladder may pass to the liver directly or drain through the hepatic portal vein to the liver. The veins from the fundus and body pass directly into the visceral surface of the liver and drain into the hepatic sinusoids. The lymphatic drainage of the gallbladder is to the **hepatic lymph nodes** (Fig. 2.40A), often by way of the **cystic lymph node** located near the neck of the gallbladder. Efferent lymphatic vessels from these nodes pass to the **celiac lymph nodes.** The nerves to the gallbladder and cystic duct pass along the cystic artery from the **celiac nerve plexus** (sympathetic and visceral [pain] afferents), the **vagus nerve** (parasympathetic), and the **right phrenic nerve** (somatic afferent fibers) (Fig. 2.40B).

Hepatic Portal Vein and Portal–Systemic Anastomoses

The **hepatic portal vein** is the main channel of the **portal venous system** (Fig. 2.45). It collects poorly oxygenated but nutrient-rich blood from the abdominal part of the alimentary tract, including the gallbladder, pancreas, and spleen, and carries it to the liver. Within the liver, its branches are distributed in a segmental pattern and end in expanded capillaries, the **venous sinusoids of the liver** (Fig. 2.42).

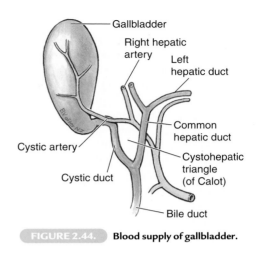

FIGURE 2.44.   **Blood supply of gallbladder.**

Portal–systemic anastomoses, in which the portal venous system communicates with the systemic venous system, are in the following locations (Fig. 2.45B):

- Between the **esophageal veins** draining into either the **azygos vein** (systemic system) or the **left gastric vein**

Liver Biopsy

Hepatic tissue may be obtained for diagnostic purposes by liver biopsy. The *needle puncture* is commonly made through the right 10th intercostal space in the midaxillary line. Before the physician takes the biopsy, the person is asked to hold his or her breath in full expiration to reduce the *costodiaphragmatic recess* and to lessen the possibility of damaging the lung and contaminating the pleural cavity.

Rupture of Liver

Although less so than the spleen, the liver is vulnerable to rupture because it is large, fixed in position, and friable. Often the liver is torn by a fractured rib that perforates the diaphragm. Because of the liver's great vascularity and friability, liver lacerations often cause considerable hemorrhage and right upper quadrant pain.

Cirrhosis of Liver

In cirrhosis of the liver, hepatocytes are destroyed and replaced by fibrous tissue. This tissue surrounds the intrahepatic blood vessels and biliary ducts, making the liver firm and impeding

circulation of blood through it. Cirrhosis, the most common of many causes of *portal hypertension,* frequently develops in chronic alcoholics.

Hepatic Lobectomies and Segmentectomy

When it was discovered that the right and left hepatic arteries and ducts, as well as branches of the right and left hepatic portal veins, do not communicate significantly, it became possible to perform *hepatic lobectomies*—removal of the right or left part of the liver—with minimal bleeding. If a severe injury or tumor involves one segment or adjacent segments, it may be possible to resect (remove) only the affected segment(s): *segmentectomy.* The intersegmental hepatic veins serve as guides to the interlobular planes.

Gallstones

Gallstones are concretions (L. *calculi,* pebbles) in the gallbladder cystic duct, hepatic ducts, or bile duct. The distal end of the hepatopancreatic ampulla is the narrowest part of the biliary passages and is the common site for impaction of a gallstone. Gallstones may produce **biliary colic** (pain in the epigastric region). When the gallbladder relaxes, the stone in the cystic duct may pass back into the gallbladder. If a stone blocks the cystic duct, *cholecystitis* (inflammation of the gallbladder) occurs because of bile accumulation, causing enlargement of the gallbladder. Pain develops in the epigastric region and later shifts to the right hypochondriac region at the junction of the ninth costal cartilage and the lateral border of the rectus sheath. Inflammation of the gallbladder may cause pain in the posterior thoracic wall or right shoulder as a result of irritation of the diaphragm. If bile cannot leave the gallbladder, it enters the blood and causes *obstructive jaundice* (see the clinical correlation box "Pancreatic Cancer" in this chapter).

Cholecystectomy

 People with severe *biliary colic* usually have their gallbladders removed. *Laparoscopic cholecystectomy* often replaces the open-incision surgical method. The cystic artery most commonly arises from the right hepatic artery in the **cystohepatic triangle** (Calot triangle). In current clinical use, the cystohepatic triangle is defined inferiorly by the cystic duct, medially by the common hepatic duct, and superiorly by the inferior surface of the liver (Fig. 2.44). Careful dissection of the cystohepatic triangle early during cholecystectomy safeguards these important structures should there be anatomical variations.

Portal Hypertension

When scarring and fibrosis from cirrhosis of the liver obstruct the hepatic portal vein, pressure rises in the hepatic portal vein and

its tributaries, producing **portal hypertension.** At the sites of anastomoses between portal and systemic veins, portal hypertension produces enlarged varicose veins and blood flow from the portal to the systemic system of veins. The veins may become so dilated that their walls rupture, resulting in hemorrhage. Bleeding from *esophageal varices* (dilated esophageal veins) at the distal end of the esophagus is often severe and may be fatal. A common method for reducing portal hypertension is to divert blood from the portal venous system to the systemic venous system by creating a communication between the portal vein and the IVC or by joining the splenic and left renal veins—a **portacaval anastomosis** or **portosystemic shunt** (Fig. B2.9).

"Hobnail" appearance of cirrhotic liver

Side to side

End to side

Central splenorenal

Hepatic portal vein

IVC

Splenic vein

L. renal v.

FIGURE B2.9. Portosystemic shunts *(red arrows)*.

(portal system); when dilated these are *esophageal varices.*

• Between the **rectal veins,** the inferior and middle veins draining into the IVC (systemic system) and the superior rectal vein continuing as the inferior mesenteric vein (portal system); when abnormally dilated these are *hemorrhoids.*

• **Paraumbilical veins** of the anterior abdominal wall (portal system) anastomosing with **superficial epigastric veins** (systemic system); when dilated these veins produce *caput medusae*—varicose veins radiating from the umbilicus. These dilated veins were called caput medusae because of their resemblance to the

serpents on the head of Medusa, a character in Greek mythology.

• Twigs of **colic veins** (portal system) anastomosing with retroperitoneal veins (systemic system).

Kidneys, Ureters, and Suprarenal Glands

The **kidneys** lie retroperitoneally on the posterior abdominal wall, one on each side of the vertebral column (Fig. 2.46). These urinary organs remove excess water, salts, and wastes of protein metabolism from the blood while returning nutrients and chemicals to the blood. The kidneys convey the waste products from the blood into the urine, which drains

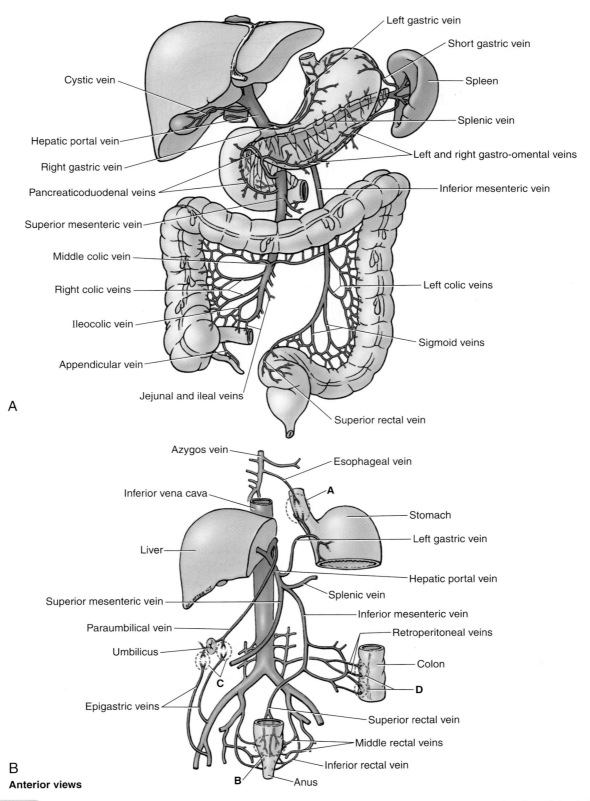

FIGURE 2.45. **Hepatic portal venous system. A.** Overview. **B.** Portal–systemic anastomoses. These anastomoses provide collateral circulation in cases of obstruction in the liver or hepatic portal vein. *Darker blue,* portal tributaries; *lighter blue,* systemic tributaries; *A,* anastomoses between esophageal veins; *B,* anastomoses between rectal veins; *C,* anastomoses between paraumbilical veins (portal) and small epigastric veins of the anterior abdominal wall; *D,* anastomoses between the twigs of colic veins (portal) and the retroperitoneal veins.

Hepatic veins
IVC
Right superior suprarenal arteries
Right suprarenal vein
Right suprarenal gland
Celiac trunk
Right kidney
Superior mesenteric artery
Right renal artery
Quadratus lumborum
Aorta
Right testicular vein and artery
Right external iliac artery and vein

Left inferior phrenic artery
Diaphragm
Spleen
Left suprarenal gland
Left middle suprarenal artery
Inferior suprarenal vein and artery
Left renal vein
Left kidney
Ureter
Inferior mesenteric artery
Left testicular artery and vein
Urinary bladder

Anterior view

FIGURE 2.46. Retroperitoneal viscera and vessels of posterior abdominal wall. *IVC,* inferior vena cava.

through the ureters to the urinary bladder. The *ureters* run inferiorly from the kidneys, passing over the pelvic brim at the bifurcation of the common iliac arteries. They then run along the lateral wall of the pelvis and enter the *urinary bladder.* The superomedial aspect of each kidney normally contacts a suprarenal gland. A weak fascial septum separates these glands from the kidneys. The *suprarenal glands* function as part of the endocrine system, completely separate in function from the kidneys so they are not attached to each other. They secrete corticosteroids and androgens and make epinephrine and norepinephrine hormones.

RENAL FASCIA AND FAT

Perinephric fat (**perirenal fat capsule**) surrounds the kidneys and suprarenal glands and is continuous with the fat in the renal sinus (Fig. 2.47). The kidneys, suprarenal glands, and perinephric fat surrounding them are enclosed (except inferiorly) by a membranous layer of **renal fascia.** Inferomedially, the renal fascia is prolonged along the ureters as **periureteric fascia.** External to the renal fascia is the **paranephric fat (pararenal fat body),** the extraperitoneal fat of the lumbar region that is most obvious posterior to the kidney. The renal fascia sends collagen bundles through the paranephric fat. Movement of the kidneys occurs during respiration and when changing from supine to erect positions;

normal renal mobility is about 3 cm. Superiorly, the renal fascia is continuous with the diaphragmatic fascia on the inferior surface of the diaphragm. Inferiorly, the anterior and posterior layers of renal fascia are loosely united, if attached at all.

KIDNEYS

The **kidneys** lie on the posterior abdominal wall at the level of the T12–L3 vertebrae. The *right kidney* lies at a slightly lower level than the *left kidney*, probably owing to its relationship to the liver. Each kidney has anterior and posterior surfaces, medial and lateral margins, and superior and inferior poles (Fig. 2.48). The lateral margin is convex, and the medial margin is concave where the renal sinus and renal pelvis are located, giving the kidney a somewhat kidney bean–shaped appearance. At the concave medial margin of each kidney is a vertical cleft, the **renal hilum.** The hilum is the entrance to the space within the kidney, the **renal sinus,** which is occupied mostly by fat in which the renal pelvis, calices, vessels, and nerves are embedded. At the hilum, the **renal vein** is anterior to the **renal artery,** which is anterior to the **renal pelvis.**

Superiorly, the kidneys are related to the diaphragm, which separates them from the pleural cavities and the 12th pair of ribs. More inferiorly, the posterior surface of the kidney is related to the quadratus lumborum muscle (Fig. 2.46).

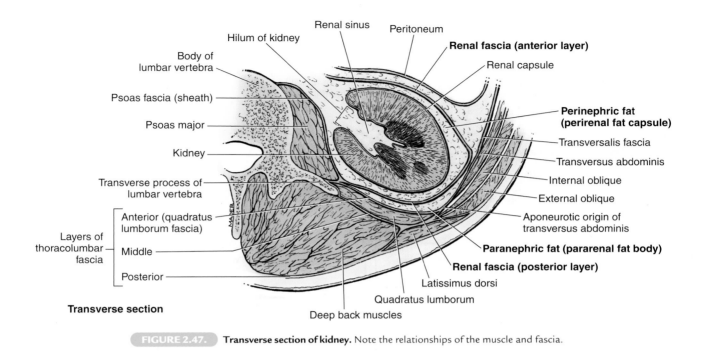

Hilum of kidney
Body of
lumbar vertebra
Psoas fascia (sheath)
Psoas major
Kidney
Transverse process of
lumbar vertebra
Anterior (quadratus
lumborum fascia)
Middle
Posterior
Layers of
thoracolumbar
fascia

Renal sinus Peritoneum
Renal fascia (anterior layer)
Renal capsule
**Perinephric fat
(perirenal fat capsule)**
Transversalis fascia
Transversus abdominis
Internal oblique
External oblique
Aponeurotic origin of
transversus abdominis
Paranephric fat (pararenal fat body)
Renal fascia (posterior layer)
Latissimus dorsi
Quadratus lumborum
Deep back muscles

Transverse section

FIGURE 2.47. **Transverse section of kidney.** Note the relationships of the muscle and fascia.

The subcostal nerve and vessels and the iliohypogastric and ilio-inguinal nerves descend diagonally across the posterior surfaces of the kidneys (see Fig. SA2.3B). The liver, duodenum, and ascending colon are anterior to the right kidney. The left kidney is related to the stomach, spleen, pancreas, jejunum, and descending colon (Fig. 2.25; Table 2.6).

URETERS

The **ureters** are muscular ducts with narrow lumina that carry urine from the kidneys to the urinary bladder. The superior expanded end of the ureter, the **renal pelvis,** is formed through the merging of two or three **major calices**

(calyces), each of which was formed by the merging of two or three **minor calices** (Figs. 2.49 and 2.50). Each minor calyx is indented by the apex of the **renal pyramid—the renal papilla.** The abdominal parts of the ureters adhere closely to the parietal peritoneum and are retroperitoneal throughout their course. The ureters run inferomedially along the transverse processes of the lumbar vertebrae and cross the external iliac artery just beyond the bifurcation of the common iliac artery. They then run along the lateral wall of the pelvis to enter the urinary bladder (Fig. 2.51). The ureters are normally constricted to a variable degree in three places: (1) at the junction of the ureters and renal pelves, (2) where the ureters cross the brim of the pelvic inlet, and (3) during their passage through the wall of the urinary bladder. These constricted areas are potential sites of obstruction by ureteric (kidney) stones.

SUPRARENAL GLANDS

The **suprarenal (adrenal) glands** are located between the superomedial aspects of the kidneys and the diaphragmatic crura (Fig. 2.46), where they are surrounded by connective tissue containing considerable perinephric fat. The glands are enclosed by renal fascia by which they are attached to the *crura of the diaphragm;* however, they are separated from the kidneys by fibrous tissue. The shape and relations of the suprarenal glands differ on the two sides.

- The pyramid-shaped right gland lies anterior to the diaphragm and makes contact with the IVC anteromedially and the liver anterolaterally.

Suprarenal gland
Renal artery
Renal vein
Renal pelvis
Ureter
Superior pole
Lateral margin
Kidney
Anterior surface
Renal hilum
Medial margin
Inferior pole

Anterior view

FIGURE 2.48. **Right kidney and suprarenal gland.**

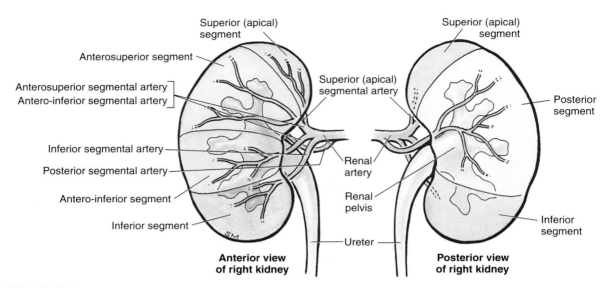

Superior (apical) segment

Anterosuperior segment

Anterosuperior segmental artery
Antero-inferior segmental artery

Superior (apical) segmental artery

Inferior segmental artery

Posterior segmental artery

Antero-inferior segment

Inferior segment

Renal artery

Renal pelvis

Ureter

Anterior view of right kidney

Superior (apical) segment

Posterior segment

Inferior segment

Posterior view of right kidney

FIGURE 2.49. **Segments and segmental arteries of kidneys.** Only the superior and inferior arteries supply the whole thickness of the kidney.

- The crescent-shaped left gland is related to the spleen, stomach, pancreas, and the left crus of the diaphragm.

Each suprarenal gland has two parts: the **suprarenal cortex** and **suprarenal medulla** (Fig. 2.50). These parts have different embryological origins and different functions (Moore and Persaud, 2008). The suprarenal cortex secretes corticosteroids and androgens, and the medulla secretes epinephrine (adrenalin) and norepinephrine (noradrenalin).

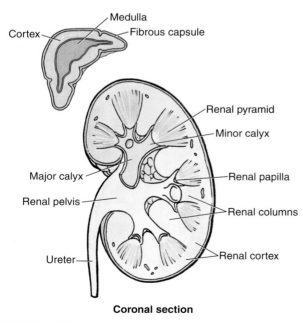

Medulla
Cortex
Fibrous capsule

Renal pyramid
Minor calyx

Major calyx
Renal papilla

Renal pelvis
Renal columns

Ureter
Renal cortex

Coronal section

FIGURE 2.50. **Internal features of kidney and suprarenal gland.**

12th rib
Minor calix
Major calix
Renal pelvis

Ureter

Gas in intestine

Sacrum

Ureter

Catheter (in urinary bladder)

A **Anteroposterior pyelogram**   B

FIGURE 2.51. Normal constrictions of ureters demonstrated by retrograde pyelogram. **A.** Contrast medium was injected into the ureters from a flexible endoscope (urethroscope) in the bladder. *Arrows* represent papillae bulging into minor calyces. **B.** Sites at which relative constrictions in the ureters normally appear: (**1**) ureteropelvic junction, (**2**) crossing external iliac vessels and/or pelvic brim, and (**3**) as ureter traverses bladder wall.

FIGURE 2.52. **Lymphatics of kidneys and suprarenal glands.** The *arrows* indicate the direction of lymph flow to the lymph nodes.

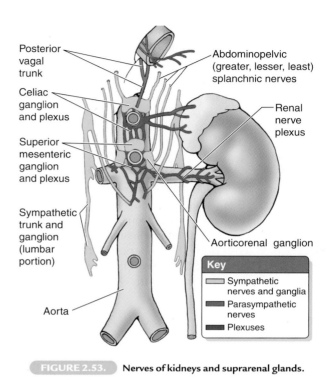

FIGURE 2.53. **Nerves of kidneys and suprarenal glands.**

VASCULATURE OF KIDNEYS, URETERS, AND SUPRARENAL GLANDS

The **renal arteries** arise at the level of the IV disc between the L1 and L2 vertebrae (Fig. 2.46). The longer **right renal artery** passes posterior to the IVC. Typically, each artery divides close to the hilum into five **segmental arteries** that are end arteries—that is, they do not anastomose (Fig. 2.49). Segmental arteries are distributed to the **segments of the kidney.** Several veins drain the kidney and unite in a variable fashion to form the renal vein. The **renal veins** lie anterior to the renal arteries, and the longer left renal vein passes anterior to the aorta (Fig. 2.46). Each renal vein drains into the IVC.

The **arteries to the ureters** arise mainly from three sources: the *renal artery, testicular or ovarian arteries,* and *abdominal aorta.* The **veins of the ureters** drain into the renal and testicular or ovarian veins (Fig. 2.46).

The endocrine function of the suprarenal glands makes their abundant blood supply necessary. The **suprarenal arteries** arise from three sources:

- **Superior suprarenal arteries** (six to eight) from the *inferior phrenic artery.*
- **Middle suprarenal arteries** (one or more) from the *abdominal aorta* near the origin of the SMA.
- **Inferior suprarenal arteries** (one or more) from the *renal artery.*

The venous drainage of the suprarenal gland is into a large **suprarenal vein** (see Fig. 2.58A). The **short right**

suprarenal vein drains into the IVC, whereas the longer **left suprarenal vein,** often joined by the inferior phrenic vein, empties into the left renal vein.

The **renal lymphatic vessels** follow the renal veins and drain into the **lumbar lymph nodes** (Fig. 2.52). Lymphatic vessels from the superior part of the ureter may join those from the kidney or pass directly to the lumbar (caval and aortic) nodes. Lymphatic vessels from the middle part of the ureter usually drain into the **common iliac lymph nodes,** whereas vessels from its inferior part drain into the common, external, or internal **iliac lymph nodes.** The **suprarenal lymphatic vessels** arise from a plexus deep to the capsule of the gland and from one in its medulla. The lymph passes to the **lumbar lymph nodes.**

NERVES OF KIDNEYS, URETERS, AND SUPRARENAL GLANDS

The nerves to the kidneys and ureters arise from the **renal nerve plexus** and consist of sympathetic, parasympathetic, and visceral afferent fibers (Fig. 2.53). The renal nerve plexus is supplied by fibers from the abdominopelvic (especially the least) splanchnic nerves. The nerves to the abdominal part of the ureters derive from the renal, abdominal aortic, and superior hypogastric plexuses. Visceral afferent fibers conveying pain sensations follow the sympathetic fibers retrograde to spinal ganglia and cord segments T11–L2. The **suprarenal glands** have a rich nerve supply from the **celiac plexus** and **abdominopelvic** (greater, lesser, and least) **splanchnic nerves.** The nerves are mainly myelinated presynaptic sympathetic fibers that derive from the lateral horn of the spinal cord and traverse the paravertebral and prevertebral ganglia, without synapse, to be distributed to the chromaffin cells in the suprarenal medulla (Fig. 2.54).

Summary of Innervation of Abdominal Viscera

The autonomic nerves of the abdomen consist of several different splanchnic nerves and one cranial nerve (the vagus, CNX) that deliver presynaptic sympathetic and parasympa-

Surface Anatomy of Kidneys and Ureters

The hilum of the left kidney lies near the transpyloric plane, approximately 5 cm from the median plane (Fig. SA2.5A). The transpyloric plane passes through the superior pole of the right kidney, which is approximately 2.5 cm lower than the left pole. Posteriorly, the superior parts of the kidneys lie deep to the 11th and 12th ribs. The levels of the kidneys change during respiration and with changes in posture by 2

to 3 cm in a vertical direction. The kidneys may be impalpable. In lean adults, the inferior pole of the right kidney is palpable by bimanual examination as a firm, smooth, somewhat rounded mass that descends during inspiration. The left kidney is usually not palpable unless it is enlarged or displaced. The ureters occupy a sagittal plane that intersects the tips of the transverse processes of the lumbar vertebrae.

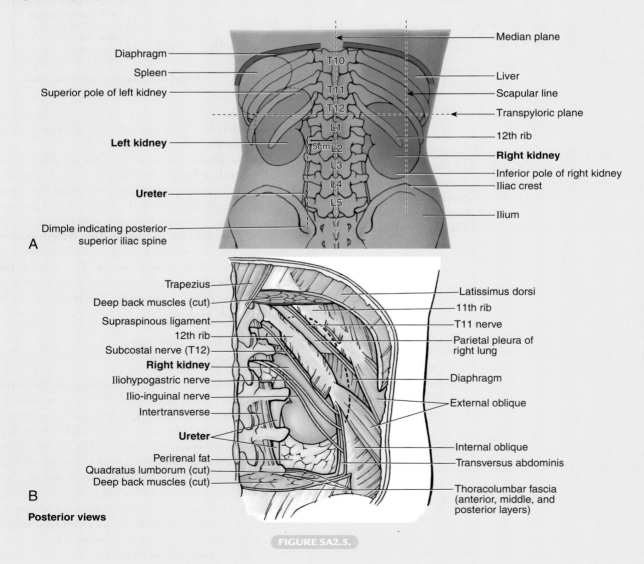

FIGURE SA2.5.

Perinephric Abscess

The attachments of the renal fascia determine the path of extension of a *perinephric abscess*. For example, the fascia at the renal hilum firmly attaches to the renal vessels and ureter, usually preventing spread of pus to the contralateral side. However, pus from an abscess (or blood from an injured kidney) may force its way into the pelvis between the loosely attached anterior and posterior layers of the pelvic fascia.

Renal Transplantation

Renal transplantation is now an established operation for the treatment of selected cases of chronic renal failure. The site for the transplanted kidney is in the iliac fossa of the greater pelvis (see Chapter 3), where it is firmly supported and where only short lengths of renal vessels and ureters are required for transplantation. The renal artery and vein are joined to the adjacent external iliac artery and vein, respectively; and the ureter is sutured into the nearby urinary bladder.

Accessory Renal Vessels

During their "ascent" to their final site, the embryonic kidneys receive their blood supply and venous drainage from successively more superior vessels. Usually, the inferior vessels degenerate as superior ones take over the blood supply and venous drainage. Failure of some of these vessels to degenerate results in *accessory (or polar) renal arteries and veins*. Variations in the number and position of these vessels occur in about 25% of people.

Renal and Ureteric Calculi

Excessive distention of the ureter owing to a **renal calculus** (kidney stone) causes severe intermittent pain, *ureteric colic,* as it is gradually forced down the ureter by waves of contraction. The calculus may cause complete or intermittent obstruction of urinary flow. Depending on the level of obstruction, the pain may be referred to the lumbar (loin) or inguinal regions (groin), the proximal anterior aspect of the thigh, or the external genitalia and/or testis. The pain is referred to the cutaneous areas innervated by the spinal cord segments and sensory ganglia, which supply the ureter—mainly

T11–L2. Ureteric calculi can be observed and removed with a *nephroscope*. Another technique, *lithotripsy*, focuses a shock wave through the body that breaks the stones into fragments, which then pass with the urine.

Intraperitoneal Injection and Peritoneal Dialysis

The peritoneum is a semipermeable membrane with an extensive surface area, much of which (subdiaphragmatic portions in particular) overlies blood and lymphatic capillary beds. Therefore, fluid injected into the peritoneal cavity is absorbed rapidly. For this reason, anesthetic agents, such as solutions of barbiturate compounds, may be injected into the peritoneal cavity by **intraperitoneal injection.**

In *renal failure*, waste products such as urea accumulate in the blood and tissues and ultimately reach fatal levels. *Peritoneal dialysis* may be performed, in which soluble substances and excess water are removed from the system by transfer across the peritoneum, using a dilute sterile solution that is introduced into the peritoneal cavity on one side and then drained from the other side. Diffusible solutes and water are transferred between the blood and the peritoneal cavity as a result of concentration gradients between the two fluid compartments. Peritoneal dialysis is usually employed only temporarily; however, for the long term it is preferable to use direct blood flow through a renal dialysis machine.

Congenital Anomalies of Kidneys and Ureters

Bifid renal pelvis and ureter are fairly common. These anomalies result from division of the *metanephric diverticulum* (ureteric bud), the primordium of the renal pelvis and ureter. The extent of ureteral duplication depends on the completeness of embryonic division of the metanephric diverticulum. The bifid renal pelvis and/or ureter may be unilateral or bilateral; however, separate openings into the bladder are uncommon. Incomplete division of the metanephric diverticulum results in a bifid ureter; complete division results in a *supernumerary kidney*.

The kidneys are close together in the embryonic pelvis. In approximately 1 in 600 fetuses, the inferior poles (rarely, the superior poles) of the kidneys fuse to form a *horseshoe kidney*. This U-shaped kidney usually lies at the level of the L3–L5 vertebrae because the root of the *inferior mesenteric artery* prevented normal relocation of the kidneys. Horseshoe kidney usually produces no symptoms; however, associated abnormalities of the kidney and renal pelvis may be present, obstructing the ureter.

Sometimes the embryonic kidney on one or both sides fails to reach the abdomen and lies anterior to the sacrum. Although uncommon, awareness of the possibility of an *ectopic pelvic kidney* should prevent it from being mistaken for a pelvic tumor and removed.

thetic fibers, respectively, to the abdominal aortic plexus and its associated sympathetic ganglia. The periarterial extensions of these plexuses deliver postsynaptic sympathetic fibers and the continuation of the parasympathetic fibers to the abdominal viscera, where intrinsic parasympathetic ganglia are located (Figs. 2.54 and 2.55; Table 2.9).

The sympathetic part of the autonomic nervous system in the abdomen consists of:

- *Abdominopelvic splanchnic* nerves consisting of *lower thoracic splanchnic nerves* (greater, lesser, and least) from the thoracic part of the sympathetic trunks and *lumbar splanchnic nerves* from the lumbar part of the sympathetic trunks.
- Prevertebral sympathetic ganglia.
- *Abdominal aortic plexus* and its extensions, the periarterial plexuses. The plexuses are mixed, shared with the parasympathetic nervous system and visceral afferent fibers.

The **abdominopelvic splanchnic nerves** convey presynaptic sympathetic fibers to the abdominopelvic cavity (Fig. 2.56). These presynaptic sympathetic fibers originate from cell bodies in the intermediolateral cell column, or lateral horn, of the gray matter of spinal cord segments T7–L2 or L3. The fibers pass successively through the anterior roots, anterior rami, and white communicating branches of thoracic and upper lumbar spinal nerves to reach the sympathetic trunks. They pass through the paravertebral ganglia of the sympathetic trunks without synapsing to enter the abdominopelvic splanchnic nerves, which convey them to the prevertebral ganglia of the abdominal cavity. The abdominopelvic splanchnic nerves include the lower thoracic splanchnic nerves and the lumbar splanchnic nerves.

The **lower thoracic splanchnic nerves** are the main source of presynaptic sympathetic fibers serving abdominal viscera (Figs. 2.55 and 2.56; Table 2.9). The **greater splanchnic nerve** (from the sympathetic trunk from the T5–T9 or T10 vertebral levels), **lesser splanchnic nerve** (from the T10–T11 levels), and **least splanchnic nerve** (from the T12 level) are the specific thoracic splanchnic nerves that arise from the thoracic part of the sympathetic trunks and pierce the corresponding crus of the diaphragm to convey the presynaptic sympathetic fibers to

the celiac, aorticorenal, and superior mesenteric (prevertebral) sympathetic ganglia and plexuses, respectively.

The **lumbar splanchnic nerves** arise from the abdominal part of the sympathetic trunks. Medially, the lumbar sympathetic trunks give off three or four lumbar splanchnic nerves, which pass to the **intermesenteric, inferior mesenteric, and superior hypogastric plexuses,** conveying presynaptic sympathetic fibers to the associated prevertebral ganglia of those plexuses.

The cell bodies of postsynaptic sympathetic neurons constitute the major prevertebral ganglia that cluster around the roots of the major branches of the abdominal aorta—the *celiac, aorticorenal, superior mesenteric,* and *inferior mesenteric ganglia*—and minor, unnamed prevertebral ganglia that occur

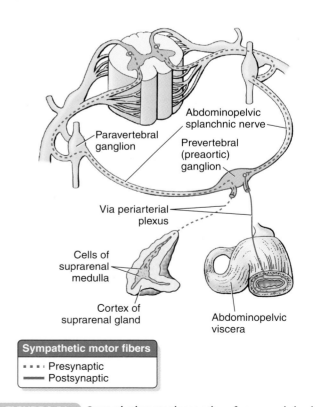

FIGURE 2.54. **Sympathetic motor innervation of suprarenal gland and abdominopelvic viscera.**

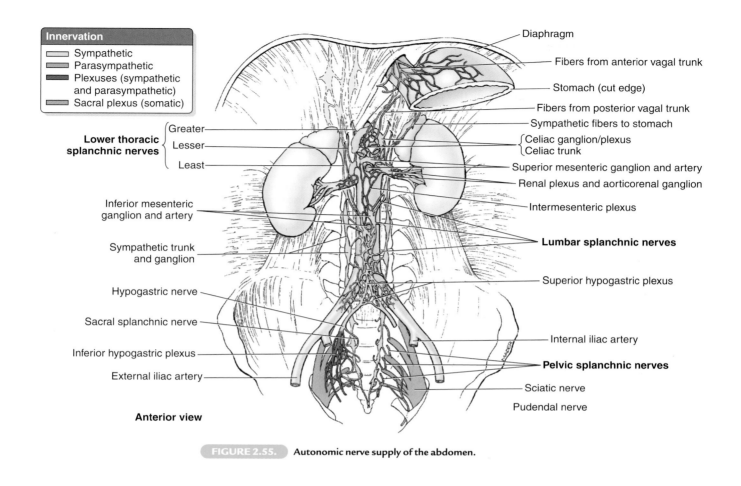

Innervation
- Sympathetic
- Parasympathetic
- Plexuses (sympathetic and parasympathetic)
- Sacral plexus (somatic)

Lower thoracic splanchnic nerves { Greater — Lesser — Least —

Inferior mesenteric ganglion and artery

Sympathetic trunk and ganglion

Hypogastric nerve

Sacral splanchnic nerve

Inferior hypogastric plexus

External iliac artery

Anterior view

Diaphragm
Fibers from anterior vagal trunk
Stomach (cut edge)
Fibers from posterior vagal trunk
Sympathetic fibers to stomach
Celiac ganglion/plexus
Celiac trunk
Superior mesenteric ganglion and artery
Renal plexus and aorticorenal ganglion
Intermesenteric plexus

Lumbar splanchnic nerves

Superior hypogastric plexus

Internal iliac artery

Pelvic splanchnic nerves

Sciatic nerve
Pudendal nerve

FIGURE 2.55. Autonomic nerve supply of the abdomen.

TABLE 2.9 SPLANCHNIC NERVES

Splanchnic Nerves	Autonomic Fiber Type[a]	System	Origin	Destination
A. Cardiopulmonary (cervical and upper thoracic)	Postsynaptic	Cervical and superior thoracic sympathetic trunk	Thoraco-abdominal nerves (anterior rami of T7–T11) and subcostal nerve	Thoracic cavity (viscera superior to level of diaphragm)
B. Abdominopelvic			Lower thoracic and abdominal sympathetic trunk	Abdominopelvic cavity (prevertebral ganglia serving viscera below level of diaphragm)
1. Lower thoracic a. Greater b. Lesser c. Least	Presynaptic	Sympathetic	Thoracic sympathetic trunk T5–T9 (T10) level T10–T11 level T12 level	Abdominal prevertebral ganglia Celiac ganglia Aorticorenal Other abdominal prevertebral ganglia
2. Lumbar	Presynaptic		Abdominal sympathetic trunk	Superior and inferior mesenteric ganglia and intermesenteric hypogastric plexuses
3. Sacral	Presynaptic		Pelvic (sacral) sympathetic trunk	Pelvic prevertebral ganglia
C. Pelvic	Presynaptic	Parasympathetic	Anterior rami of S2–S4 spinal nerves	Intrinsic ganglia of descending and sigmoid colon, rectum, and pelvic viscera

[a]Splanchnic nerves also convey visceral afferent fibers.

within the intermesenteric, abdominal, aortic, and superior hypogastric plexuses. The synapse between presynaptic and postsynaptic neurons occurs in the prevertebral ganglia. Postsynaptic sympathetic nerve fibers pass from the prevertebral ganglia to the abdominal viscera through the periarterial plexuses associated with the branches of the abdominal aorta. Sympathetic innervation in the abdomen, as elsewhere, is primarily involved in producing vasoconstriction. In regard to

the alimentary tract, it acts to inhibit (slow down or stop) peristalsis. The sympathetic supply to the suprarenal gland is an exception. The secretory cells of the medulla are postsynaptic sympathetic neurons that lack axons or dendrites. Consequently, the **suprarenal medulla** is supplied directly by presynaptic sympathetic neurons (Fig. 2.54).

Visceral afferent fibers conveying pain sensations accompany the sympathetic (visceral motor) fibers. The pain

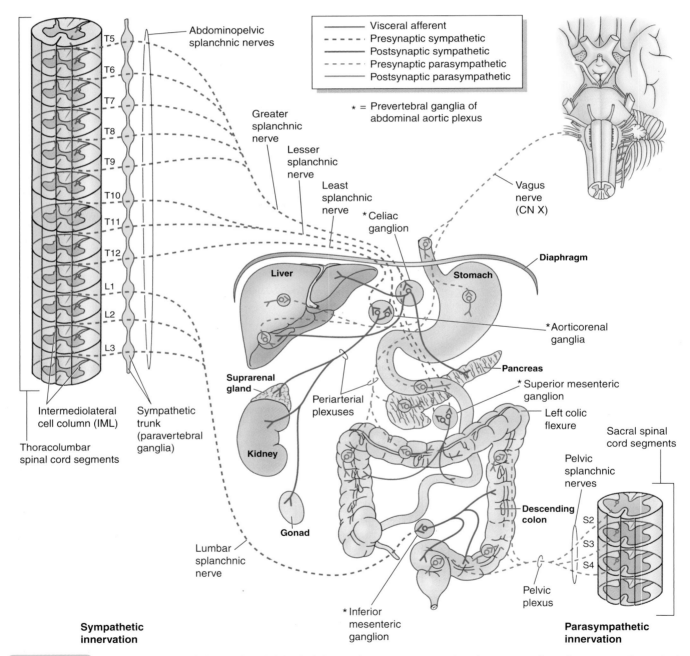

FIGURE 2.56. **Overview of autonomic innervation of abdominal viscera.** The approximate spinal cord segments and spinal sensory ganglia involved in sympathetic and visceral afferent innervation of the abdominal viscera are listed on each organ.

impulses pass retrogradely to those of the motor fibers along the splanchnic nerves to the sympathetic trunk. The fibers then pass through white rami communicantes to the anterior rami of the spinal nerves, and then enter the posterior root to the spinal sensory ganglia and spinal cord. The stomach (foregut) receives information from the T6–T9 levels; the small intestine through the transverse colon (midgut), from the T8–T12 levels; and the descending colon (hindgut), from the T12–L2 levels. Starting from the midpoint of the sigmoid colon, visceral pain fibers run with parasympathetic fibers to the S2–S4 sensory ganglia and spinal cord. These are the same spinal cord segments involved in the sympathetic innervation of those portions of the gastrointestinal tract.

The parasympathetic part of the autonomic nervous system in the abdomen consists of the (Figs. 2.55 and 2.56; Table 2.9):

* *Anterior and posterior vagal trunks.*
* *Pelvic splanchnic nerves.*
* *Abdominal (para-aortic) autonomic nerve plexuses* and their extensions, the periarterial plexuses; the nerve plexuses are mixed—that is, are shared with the sympathetic nervous system and visceral afferent fibers.
* *Intrinsic* (enteric) *parasympathetic ganglia.*

The **anterior and posterior vagal trunks** are the continuation of the left and right vagus nerves, which emerge from the esophageal plexus and pass through the esophageal hiatus on the anterior and posterior aspects of the esophagus and stomach. The vagus nerves convey presynaptic parasympathetic and visceral afferent fibers (mainly for unconscious sensations associated with reflexes) to the abdominal aortic plexuses and the periarterial plexuses.

The **pelvic splanchnic nerves** are distinct from other splanchnic nerves in that they:

* Have nothing to do with the sympathetic trunks.
* Derive directly from anterior rami of spinal nerves S2–S4.
* Convey presynaptic parasympathetic fibers to the inferior hypogastric (pelvic) plexus.

Presynaptic fibers terminate on the isolated and widely scattered cell bodies of the postsynaptic neurons lying on or within the abdominal viscera, constituting intrinsic ganglia. The presynaptic parasympathetic and visceral afferent reflex fibers conveyed by the vagus nerves extend to intrinsic ganglia of the lower esophagus, stomach, small intestine (including the duodenum), ascending and most of the transverse colon; those conveyed by the pelvic splanchnic nerves supply the descending and sigmoid parts of the colon, rectum, and pelvic organs. In terms of the alimentary tract, the vagus nerves provide parasympathetic innervation of the smooth muscle and glands of the gut as far as the left colic flexure; the pelvic splanchnic nerves provide the remainder.

The **abdominal autonomic plexuses** are networks consisting of both sympathetic and parasympathetic fibers that surround the abdominal aorta and its major branches. The celiac, superior mesenteric, and inferior mesenteric plexuses are interconnected. The **prevertebral sympathetic ganglia** are scattered among the celiac and mesenteric plexuses. The **intrinsic parasympathetic ganglia,** such as the *myenteric plexus* (Auerbach plexus) in the muscular coat of the stomach and intestine, are in the walls of the viscera.

The **celiac plexus,** surrounding the root of the celiac trunk, contains right and left *celiac ganglia* (approximately 2 cm long) that may unite superior or inferior to the celiac trunk (Fig. 2.55). The *parasympathetic root of the celiac plexus* is a branch of the *posterior vagal trunk,* which contains fibers from the right and left vagus nerves. The *sympathetic roots of the celiac plexus* are the greater and lesser splanchnic nerves.

The **superior mesenteric plexus** and ganglion or ganglia surround the origin of the SMA. The plexus has one median and two lateral branches. The median branch is from the celiac plexus, and the lateral branches arise from the lesser and least splanchnic nerves, sometimes with a contribution from the first lumbar ganglion of the sympathetic trunk. The **inferior mesenteric plexus** and ganglia surround the inferior mesenteric artery and the plexus gives off shoots to its branches. It receives a medial root from the intermesenteric plexus and lateral roots from the lumbar ganglia of the sympathetic trunks.

The **intermesenteric plexus** is part of the aortic plexus of nerves between the superior and the inferior mesenteric arteries. It gives rise to renal, testicular or ovarian, and ureteric plexuses. The **superior hypogastric plexus** is continuous with the intermesenteric plexus and inferior mesenteric plexus and lies anterior to the inferior part of the abdominal aorta and its bifurcation. Right and left **hypogastric nerves** join the superior hypogastric plexus to the **inferior hypogastric plexus.** The superior hypogastric plexus supplies *ureteric* and *testicular plexuses* and a plexus on each common iliac artery. The right and left **inferior hypogastric plexuses** are formed by hypogastric nerves from the superior hypogastric plexus. The right and left plexuses are situated on the sides of the rectum, uterine cervix, and urinary bladder. The plexuses receive small branches from the superior sacral sympathetic ganglia and the sacral parasympathetic outflow from the S2–S4 spinal nerves (**pelvic parasympathetic splanchnic nerves**). Extensions of the inferior hypogastric plexus send autonomic fibers along the blood vessels, which form visceral plexuses on the walls of the pelvic viscera (e.g., *the rectal and vesical plexuses*).

DIAPHRAGM

The **diaphragm** is a dome-shaped, musculotendinous partition separating the thoracic and abdominal cavities. The diaphragm, the chief muscle of inspiration, forms the convex

Visceral Referred Pain

Pain arising from a viscus such as the stomach varies from dull to severe. The pain is poorly localized; it radiates to the dermatome level that receives visceral sensory fibers from the organ concerned (Fig. B2.10; Table B2.2).

Duodenum, head of pancreas
Gallbladder
Liver
Appendix
Cecum and ascending colon
Liver, gallbladder, and duodenum (resulting from irritation of diaphragm)
Stomach
Spleen
Small intestine (pink)
Sigmoid colon
Kidney and ureter
Gallbladder
Liver

FIGURE B2.10. Areas of referred pain.

TABLE B2.2 VISCERAL REFERRED PAIN

Origin	Nerve Supply	Spinal Cord	Referred Site and Clinical Example
Stomach	Anterior and posterior vagal trunks; presynaptic sympathetic fibers reach celiac and other ganglia through greater splanchnic nerves	T6–T9 or T10	Epigastric and left hypochondriac regions (e.g., gastric peptic ulcer)
Duodenum	Vagus nerves; presynaptic sympathetic fibers reach celiac and superior mesenteric ganglia through greater splanchnic nerves	T5–T9 or T10	Epigastric region (e.g., duodenal peptic ulcer); right shoulder (if ulcer perforates)
Pancreatic head	Vagus and thoracic splanchnic nerves	T8–T9	Inferior part of epigastric region (e.g., pancreatitis)
Small intestine (jejunum and ileum)	Posterior vagal trunks; presynaptic sympathetic fibers reach celiac ganglion through greater splanchnic nerves	T5–T9	Periumbilical region (e.g., acute intestinal obstruction)
Colon	Vagus nerves; presynaptic sympathetic fibers reach celiac, superior mesenteric, and inferior mesenteric ganglia through greater splanchnic nerves; parasympathetic supply to distal colon derived from pelvic splanchnic nerves through hypogastric nerves and inferior hypogastric plexus	T10–T12 (proximal colon) L1–L3 (distal colon)	Hypogastric region (e.g., ulcerative colitis); left lower quadrant (e.g., sigmoiditis)
Spleen	Celiac plexus, especially from greater splanchnic nerve	T6–T8	Left hypochondriac region (e.g., splenic infarct)
Appendix	Sympathetic and parasympathetic nerves from superior mesenteric plexus; afferent nerve fibers accompany sympathetic nerves to T10 segment of spinal cord	T10	Periumbilical region and later to right lower quadrant (e.g., appendicitis)
Gallbladder and liver	Nerves derived from celiac plexus (sympathetic), vagus nerve (parasympathetic), and right phrenic nerve (sensory)	T6–T9	Epigastric region and right hypochondriac region; may cause pain on posterior thoracic wall or right shoulder owing to diaphragmatic irritation
Kidneys and ureters	Nerves arise from renal plexus and consist of sympathetic, parasympathetic, and visceral afferent fibers from thoracic and lumbar splanchnics and vagus nerve	T11–T12	Small of back, flank (lumbar quadrant), extending to groin (inguinal region) and genitals (e.g., renal or ureteric calculi)

Right subclavian artery

Brachiocephalic trunk

Right phrenic nerve

Right pericardiacophrenic artery & vein

Central tendon of diaphragm

Right dome of diaphragm

Right internal thoracic artery & vein

Right superior epigastric artery & vein

Right musculophrenic artery & vein

Left subclavian artery

Right and left brachiocephalic veins

Left pericardiacophrenic vein & artery

Left phrenic nerve

Pericardium

Xiphoid process of sternum

Left dome of diaphragm

Esophageal hiatus

Left intercostal nerves

L1

L2

Left crus

Right crus

A **Anterior view**

Sternal part

Caval opening

Costal part

Central tendon

Vertebral body

Costodiaphragmatic recess

Esophageal hiatus

Aorta passing through aortic hiatus

B **Superior view**

FIGURE 2.57.   **Superior surface of diaphragm. A.** Arteries, veins, and nerves. **B.** Diaphragm as viewed from thorax.

floor of the thoracic cavity and the concave roof of the abdominal cavity (Figs. 2.57 and 2.58). The diaphragm descends during inspiration; however, only its central part moves because its periphery, as the fixed origin of the muscle, attaches to the inferior margin of the thoracic cage and the superior lumbar vertebrae. The diaphragm curves superiorly into **right** and **left domes;** normally, the right dome is higher than the left owing to the presence of the liver (Fig. 2.57). During expiration, the right dome reaches as high as

the fifth rib and the left dome ascends to the fifth intercostal space. The level of the domes of the diaphragm varies according to the phase of respiration (inspiration or expiration), posture (e.g., supine or standing), and size and degree of distention of the abdominal viscera.

The muscular part of the diaphragm is situated peripherally with fibers that converge radially on the trifoliate central aponeurotic part, the **central tendon.** This tendon has no bony attachments and is incompletely divided into three

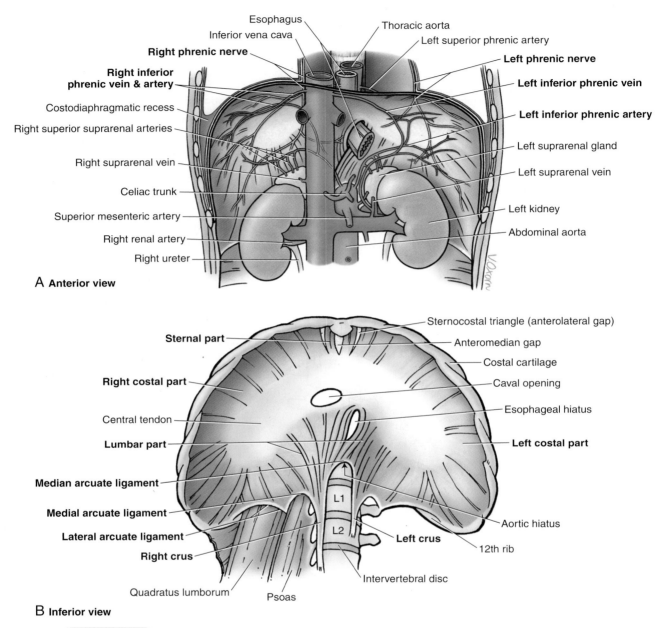

FIGURE 2.58. Inferior surface of diaphragm. **A.** Arteries, veins, and nerves. **B.** Diaphragm as viewed from abdomen.

leaves, resembling a wide cloverleaf. Although it lies near the center of the diaphragm, the central tendon is closer to the anterior part of the thorax. The superior aspect of the central tendon is fused with the inferior surface of the fibrous pericardium. The surrounding muscular part of the diaphragm forms a continuous sheet; however, for descriptive purposes it is divided into three parts, based on the peripheral attachments:

- A **sternal part,** consisting of two muscular slips that attach to the posterior aspect of the xiphoid process of the sternum; this part is not always present.

- A **costal part,** consisting of wide muscular slips that attach to the internal surfaces of the inferior six costal cartilages and their adjoining ribs on each side; this part forms the domes of the diaphragm.

- A **lumbar part,** arising from two aponeurotic arches, the *medial* and *lateral arcuate ligaments,* and the three superior lumbar vertebrae; this part forms right and left muscular crura that ascend to the central tendon.

The **crura of the diaphragm** are musculotendinous bundles that arise from the anterior surfaces of the bodies of the superior three lumbar vertebrae, the anterior longitudinal ligament, and the IV discs (Fig. 2.58*B*). The **right crus,** larger and longer than the left crus, arises from the first three or four lumbar vertebrae, whereas the **left crus** arises from only the first two or three. The crura are united by the **median arcuate ligament,** which passes over the anterior surface of the aorta. The diaphragm is also attached on each side to the **medial** and **lateral arcuate ligaments,** which are thickenings of the fascia covering the psoas and quadratus lumborum muscles, respectively.

Diaphragmatic Apertures

The **diaphragmatic apertures** permit structures (e.g., esophagus, vessels, nerves, and lymphatics) to pass between the thorax and the abdomen (Figs. 2.57, 2.58 and 2.59). The three large apertures for the IVC, esophagus, and aorta are the caval opening, esophageal hiatus, and aortic hiatus, respectively.

CAVAL OPENING

The **caval opening** is an aperture in the central tendon primarily for the IVC. Also passing through the caval opening are terminal branches of the right phrenic nerve and some lymphatic vessels on their way from the liver to the middle phrenic and mediastinal lymph nodes. The caval opening is located to the right of the median plane at the junction of the tendon's right and middle leaves. The most superior of the three diaphragmatic apertures, the caval opening lies at the level of the IV disc between the T8 and the T9 vertebrae. The IVC is adherent to the margin of the opening; consequently, when the diaphragm contracts during inspiration, it widens the opening and dilates the IVC. These changes facilitate blood flow to the heart through this large vein.

ESOPHAGEAL HIATUS

The **esophageal hiatus** is an oval aperture for the esophagus in the muscle of the right crus of the diaphragm at the

FIGURE 2.59. Diaphragmatic apertures.

level of the T10 vertebra. The fibers of the right crus decussate (cross one another) inferior to the hiatus, forming a muscular sphincter for the esophagus that constricts it when the diaphragm contracts. In 30% of individuals, a superficial muscular bundle from the left crus contributes to the formation of the right margin of the hiatus. The esophageal hiatus also transmits the anterior and posterior vagal trunks, esophageal branches of the left gastric vessels, and a few lymphatic vessels.

AORTIC HIATUS

The **aortic hiatus** is an opening posterior to the diaphragm for the aorta. The aortic hiatus transmits the aorta, azygos vein, and the thoracic duct. Because the aorta does not pierce the diaphragm, blood flow through it is not affected by the muscle's movements during respiration. The aorta passes between the crura of the diaphragm posterior to the median arcuate ligament, which is at the level of the T12 vertebra (Fig. 2.58*B*).

OTHER APERTURES IN DIAPHRAGM

There is a small opening, the **sternocostal triangle** (foramen), between the sternal and the costal attachments of the diaphragm. This triangle transmits lymphatic vessels from the diaphragmatic surface of the liver and the superior epigastric vessels. The sympathetic trunks pass deep to the medial arcuate ligament. There are two small apertures in each crus of the diaphragm; one transmits the greater and the other the lesser splanchnic nerve.

Vasculature and Nerves of Diaphragm

The **arteries of the diaphragm** form a branch-like pattern on both its superior and inferior surfaces. The arteries supplying the superior surface of the diaphragm are the **pericardiacophrenic and musculophrenic arteries,** branches of internal thoracic artery, and the **superior phrenic arteries** arising from thoracic aorta (Figs. 2.57*A* and 2.58*A*; Table 2.10). The arteries supplying the inferior surface of the diaphragm are the **inferior phrenic arteries,** which typically are the first branches of the abdominal aorta; however, they may arise from the celiac trunk.

The veins draining the superior surface of the diaphragm are the **pericardiacophrenic** and **musculophrenic veins,** which empty into the *internal thoracic veins,* and on the right side, a *superior phrenic vein,* which drains into the IVC. Posteriorly, some veins drain into the *azygos and hemiazygos veins.* The inferior phrenic veins drain blood from the inferior surface of the diaphragm. The **right inferior phrenic vein** usually opens into the IVC, whereas the **left inferior phrenic vein** is usually double, with one branch passing anterior to the esophageal hiatus to end in the IVC

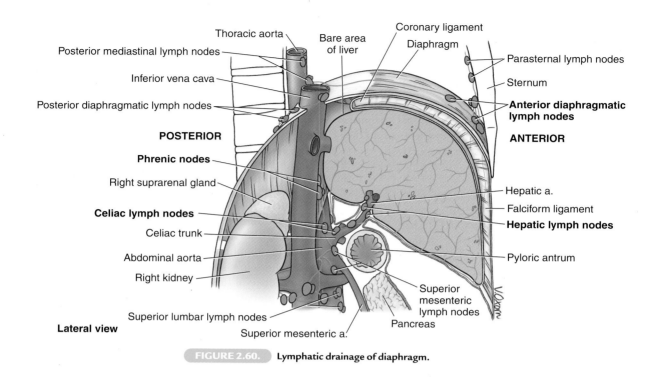

FIGURE 2.60.   Lymphatic drainage of diaphragm.

and the other, more posterior branch usually joining the left suprarenal vein.

The **lymphatic plexuses** on the thoracic and abdominal surfaces of the diaphragm communicate freely (Fig. 2.60). The anterior and posterior **diaphragmatic lymph nodes** are on the thoracic surface of the diaphragm. Lymph from these nodes drains into the *parasternal, posterior mediastinal,* and *phrenic lymph nodes.* Lymph vessels from the abdominal surface of the diaphragm drain into the anterior diaphragmatic, phrenic, and *superior lumbar (caval/aortic) lymph nodes.* Lymphatic vessels are dense on the inferior

surface of the diaphragm, constituting the primary means for absorption of peritoneal fluid and substances introduced by intraperitoneal injection.

The entire motor supply to the diaphragm is from the **right** and **left phrenic nerves,** each of which is distributed to half of the diaphragm and arises from the anterior rami of the C3–C5 segments of the spinal cord. The phrenic nerves also supply sensory fibers (pain and proprioception) to most of the diaphragm. Peripheral parts of the diaphragm receive their sensory nerve supply from the **intercostal nerves** (lower six or seven) and the **subcostal nerves.**

TABLE 2.10 NEUROVASCULATURE OF DIAPHRAGM

Vessels and Nerves	Superior Surface of Diaphragm	Inferior Surface of Diaphragm
Arterial supply	Superior phrenic arteries from thoracic aorta; musculophrenic and pericardiacophrenic arteries from internal thoracic arteries	Inferior phrenic arteries from abdominal aorta
Venous drainage	Musculophrenic and pericardiacophrenic veins drain into internal thoracic veins; superior phrenic vein (right side) drains into IVC	Inferior phrenic veins: right vein drains into IVC; left vein is doubled and drains into IVC and left suprarenal vein
Lymphatic drainage	Diaphragmatic lymph nodes to phrenic nodes, then to parasternal and posterior mediastinal nodes	Superior lumbar lymph nodes; lymphatic plexuses on superior and inferior surfaces communicate freely
Innervation	*Motor supply:* phrenic nerves (C3–C5) *Sensory supply:* centrally by phrenic nerves (C3–C5); peripherally by intercostal nerves (T5–T11) and subcostal nerves (T12)	

IVC, inferior vena cava.

Section of a Phrenic Nerve

Section of a phrenic nerve in the neck results in complete paralysis and eventual atrophy of the muscular part of the corresponding half of the diaphragm, except in persons who have an accessory phrenic nerve. *Paralysis of a hemidiaphragm* can be recognized radiographically by its permanent elevation and paradoxical movement.

Referred Pain from Diaphragm

Pain from the diaphragm radiates to two different areas because of the difference in the sensory nerve supply of the diaphragm. Pain resulting from irritation of the diaphragmatic pleura or the diaphragmatic peritoneum is referred to the shoulder region, the area of skin supplied by the C3–C5 segments of the spinal cord. These segments also contribute anterior rami to the phrenic nerves. Irritation of peripheral regions of the diaphragm, innervated by the inferior intercostal nerves, is more localized, being referred to the skin over the costal margins of the anterolateral abdominal wall.

Rupture of Diaphragm and Herniation of Viscera

Rupture of the diaphragm and herniation of viscera can result from a sudden large increase in either the intrathoracic or intra-abdominal pressure. The common cause of this injury is severe trauma to the thorax or abdomen during a motor vehicle accident. Most diaphragmatic ruptures are on the left side (95%) because the substantial mass of the liver, intimately associated with the diaphragm on the right side, provides a physical barrier.

A nonmuscular area of variable size called the *lumbocostal triangle* usually occurs between the costal and lumbar parts of the diaphragm. This part of the diaphragm is normally formed only by fusion of the superior and inferior fascias of the diaphragm. When a *traumatic diaphragmatic hernia* occurs, the stomach, small intestine and mesentery, transverse colon, and spleen may herniate through this area into the thorax.

Hiatal or hiatus hernia, a protrusion of part of the stomach into the thorax through the esophageal hiatus, was discussed earlier in this chapter. The structures that pass through the esophageal hiatus (vagal trunks, left inferior phrenic vessels, esophageal branches of the left gastric vessels) may be injured in surgical procedures on the esophageal hiatus (e.g., repair of a hiatus hernia).

Congenital Diaphragmatic Hernia

In congenital diaphragmatic hernia (CDH), part of the stomach and intestine herniate through a large posterolateral defect (foramen of Bochdalek) in the region of the lumbocostal trigone of the diaphragm (Fig. B2.11). Herniation almost always occurs on the left owing to the presence of the liver on the right. This type of hernia results from the complex development of the diaphragm.

Posterolateral defect of the diaphragm is the only relatively common congenital anomaly of the diaphragm, occurring approximately once in 2200 newborn infants (Moore and Persaud, 2008). With abdominal viscera in the limited space of the prenatal pulmonary cavity, one lung (usually the left lung) does not have room to develop normally or to inflate after birth. Because of the consequent *pulmonary hypoplasia,* the mortality rate in these infants is high (approximately 76%).

Key
H	Heart
I	Intestine
L	Liver
LL	Location of left lung
H	Heart
RL	Location of right lung
S	Stomach

FIGURE B2.11. **Congenital diaphragmatic hernia (CDH).** As seen radiographically in a newborn.

POSTERIOR ABDOMINAL WALL

The posterior abdominal wall is composed mainly—from deep (posterior) to superficial (anterior)—of the:

- Five lumbar vertebrae and associated IV discs.
- Posterior abdominal wall muscles—psoas, quadratus lumborum, iliacus, transversus abdominis, and oblique muscles.
- Lumbar plexus, composed of the anterior rami of lumbar spinal nerves.
- Fascia, including thoracolumbar fascia.
- Diaphragm, contributing to the superior part of the posterior wall.
- Fat, nerves, vessels, and lymph nodes.

Fascia of Posterior Abdominal Wall

The posterior abdominal wall is covered with a continuous layer of endo-abdominal fascia, which lies between the parietal peritoneum and the muscles. The fascia lining the posterior abdominal wall is continuous with the transversalis fascia that lines the transversus abdominis muscle (Fig. 2.61). It is customary to name the fascia according to the structure it covers. The **psoas fascia** covering the psoas major is attached medially to the lumbar vertebrae and pelvic brim. The psoas fascia is thickened superiorly to form the **medial arcuate ligament** and fuses laterally with the quadratus lumborum and thoracolumbar fascia (Fig. 2.61*B*). Inferior to the iliac crest, the psoas fascia is continuous with the part of the iliac fascia covering the iliacus muscle.

The **thoracolumbar fascia** is an extensive fascial complex that has anterior, middle, and posterior layers with muscles enclosed between them. It is thin and transparent where it covers thoracic parts of the deep muscles but is thick and strong in the lumbar region. The **posterior and middle layers of thoracolumbar fascia** enclose the vertical deep back muscles (erector spinae). The lumbar part of this posterior layer, extending between the 12th rib and the iliac crest, attaches laterally to the internal oblique and transversus abdominis muscles. The **anterior layer of the thoracolumbar fascia** (quadratus lumborum fascia) covering the quadratus lumborum muscle attaches to the anterior surfaces of the transverse processes of the lumbar vertebrae, the iliac crest, and the 12th rib and is continuous laterally with the aponeurotic origin of the transversus abdominis muscle. The anterior layer of the thoracolumbar fascia is thickened superiorly to form the **lateral arcuate ligaments** and is adherent inferiorly to the iliolumbar ligaments.

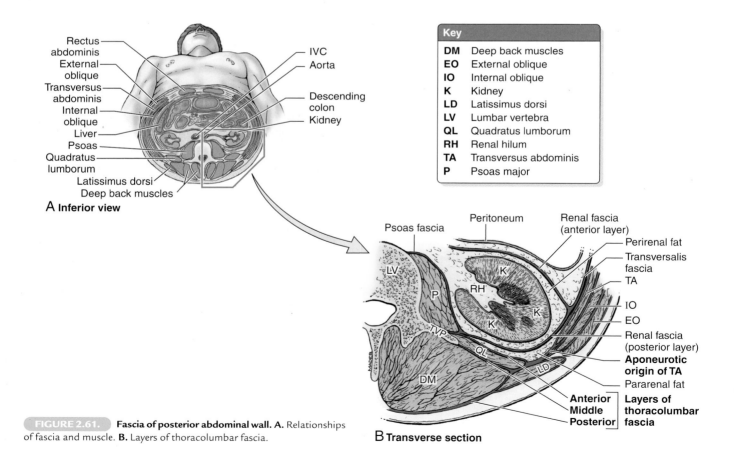

Key

DM	Deep back muscles
EO	External oblique
IO	Internal oblique
K	Kidney
LD	Latissimus dorsi
LV	Lumbar vertebra
QL	Quadratus lumborum
RH	Renal hilum
TA	Transversus abdominis
P	Psoas major

A Inferior view

B Transverse section

FIGURE 2.61. **Fascia of posterior abdominal wall. A.** Relationships of fascia and muscle. **B.** Layers of thoracolumbar fascia.

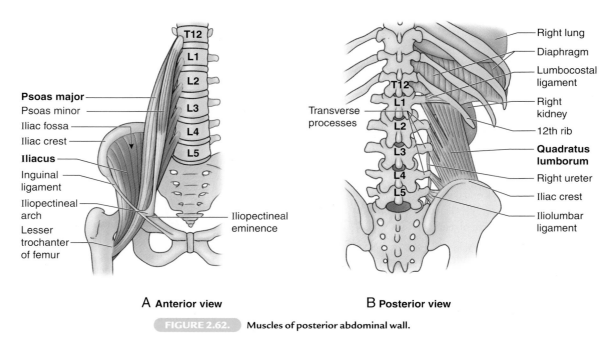

A Anterior view   **B** Posterior view

FIGURE 2.62.   Muscles of posterior abdominal wall.

TABLE 2.11 MAIN MUSCLES OF POSTERIOR ABDOMINAL WALL

Muscle	Superior Attachments	Inferior Attachment(s)	Innervation	Actions
Psoas major[a]	Transverse processes of lumbar vertebrae; sides of bodies of T12–S1 vertebrae and intervening IV discs	By a strong tendon to lesser trochanter of femur	Lumbar plexus via anterior branches of nerves L2–L4	Acting inferiorly with iliacus, flexes thigh. Acting superiorly, flexes vertebral column laterally to balance the trunk. When sitting, acts inferiorly with iliacus to flex trunk.
Iliacus[a]	Superior two thirds of iliac fossa, ala of sacrum, and anterior sacro-iliac ligaments	Lesser trochanter of femur and shaft inferior to it, and to psoas major tendon	Femoral nerve (L2–L4)	Flexes thigh and stabilizes hip joint. Acts with psoas major.
Quadratus lumborum	Medial half of inferior border of 12th rib and tips of lumbar transverse processes	Iliolumbar ligament and internal lip of iliac crest	Anterior branches of T12 and L1–L4 nerves	Extends and laterally flexes vertebral column. Fixes 12th rib during inspiration.

[a]Psoas major and iliacus muscles are often described together as the iliopsoas muscle when flexion of the thigh is discussed (see Chapter 5). The iliopsoas is the chief flexor of the thigh; and when thigh is fixed, it is a strong flexor of the trunk (e.g., during sit-ups). *IV*, intervertebral.

Muscles of Posterior Abdominal Wall

The main paired muscles in the posterior abdominal wall (Fig. 2.62) are the:

- **Psoas major,** passing inferolaterally.
- **Iliacus,** lying along the lateral sides of the inferior part of the psoas major; together the psoas and iliacus form the **iliopsoas.**
- **Quadratus lumborum,** lying adjacent to the transverse processes of the lumbar vertebrae and lateral to the superior parts of the psoas major.

The attachments, nerve supply, and main actions of these muscles are summarized in Table 2.11.

Nerves of Posterior Abdominal Wall

There are somatic and autonomic nerves in the posterior abdominal wall. The somatic nerves will be discussed here.

The **subcostal nerves,** the anterior rami of T12, arise in the thorax, pass posterior to the lateral arcuate ligaments into the abdomen, and run inferolaterally on the anterior surface of the quadratus lumborum muscle (Fig. 2.63). They pass through the transversus abdominis and internal oblique muscles to supply the external oblique and skin of the anterolateral abdominal wall.

The **lumbar spinal nerves** pass from the spinal cord through the IV foramina inferior to the corresponding vertebrae, where they divide into posterior and anterior rami.

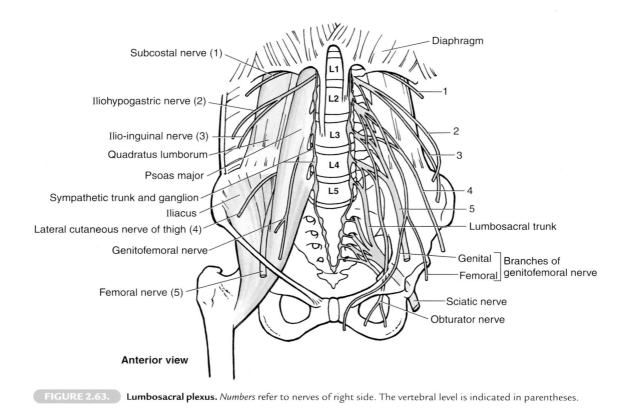

Subcostal nerve (1)
Iliohypogastric nerve (2)
Ilio-inguinal nerve (3)
Quadratus lumborum
Psoas major
Sympathetic trunk and ganglion
Iliacus
Lateral cutaneous nerve of thigh (4)
Genitofemoral nerve
Femoral nerve (5)
Anterior view

Diaphragm
L1
L2
L3
L4
L5
1
2
3
4
5
Lumbosacral trunk
Genital] **Branches of**
Femoral] **genitofemoral nerve**
Sciatic nerve
Obturator nerve

FIGURE 2.63.   **Lumbosacral plexus.** *Numbers* refer to nerves of right side. The vertebral level is indicated in parentheses.

Each ramus contains sensory and motor fibers. The posterior rami pass posteriorly to supply the deep back muscles and skin of the back, whereas the anterior rami pass inferolaterally through the psoas major to supply the skin and muscles of most inferior trunk and lower limb. The proximal parts of the anterior rami of L1–L2 or L3 give rise to *white rami communicantes* that convey presynaptic sympathetic fibers to the lumbar sympathetic trunks. The lumbar sympathetic trunks descend on the anterolateral aspects of the bodies of the lumbar vertebrae in a groove formed by the psoas major (Fig. 2.63).

For the innervation of the abdominal wall and lower limbs, synapses occur in the sympathetic ganglia of the sympathetic trunks. Postsynaptic sympathetic fibers then travel via the *gray communicating branches* to the anterior rami. The anterior rami become the thoraco-abdominal and subcostal nerves, and the lumbar plexus (somatic nerves) and the accompanying postsynaptic sympathetic fibers stimulate vasomotor, sudomotor, and pilomotor action in the distribution of these nerves. The *lumbar splanchnic nerves* that innervate pelvic viscera are described in Chapter 4.

The **lumbar plexus of nerves** is in the posterior part of the psoas major, anterior to the lumbar transverse processes (Fig. 2.63). This nerve network is composed of the anterior rami of L1–L4 nerves. All rami receive *gray communicating branches* from the sympathetic trunks. The following nerves are **branches of the lumbar plexus;** the three largest are listed first:

- The **obturator nerve** (L2–L4) emerges from the medial border of the psoas major and passes through the pelvis to the medial thigh, supplying the adductor muscles.
- The **femoral nerve** (L2–L4) emerges from the lateral border of the psoas major and innervates the iliacus and passes deep to the inguinal ligament to the anterior thigh, supplying the flexors of the hip and extensors of the knee.
- The **lumbosacral trunk** (L4, L5) passes over the ala (wing) of the sacrum and descends into the pelvis to participate in the formation of the sacral plexus along with the anterior rami of the S1–S4 nerves.
- The **ilio-inguinal and iliohypogastric nerves** (L1) arise from the anterior ramus of L1 and enter the abdomen posterior to the medial arcuate ligaments and pass inferolaterally, anterior to the quadratus lumborum. They pierce the transversus abdominis muscles near the anterior superior iliac spines and pass through the internal and external oblique muscles to supply the abdominal muscles and skin of the pubic and inguinal regions.
- The **genitofemoral nerve** (L1, L2) pierces the anterior surface of the psoas major and runs inferiorly on it deep to the psoas fascia; it divides lateral to the common and external iliac arteries into femoral and genital branches.

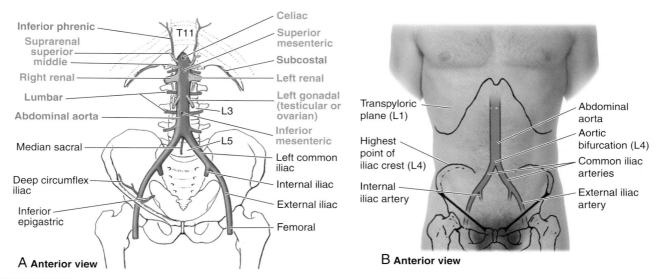

A Anterior view

B Anterior view

FIGURE 2.64. **Branches of abdominal aorta. A.** Paired visceral branches (orange), unpaired visceral branches (green), and parietal branches (purple). **B.** Surface anatomy.

- The **lateral cutaneous nerve of the thigh** (L2, L3) runs inferolaterally on the iliacus muscle and enters the thigh posterior to the inguinal ligament, just medial to the anterior superior iliac spine; it supplies the skin on the anterolateral surface of the thigh.

Vasculature of Posterior Abdominal Wall

Most arteries supplying the posterior abdominal wall arise from the **abdominal aorta** (Fig. 2.64); however, the **subcostal arteries** arise from the thoracic aorta and distribute inferior to the 12th rib. The abdominal aorta, approximately 13 cm in length, begins at the aortic hiatus in the diaphragm at the level of the T12 vertebra and ends at the level of the L4 vertebra by dividing into two common iliac arteries. The **level of the aortic bifurcation** is 2 to 3 cm inferior and to the left of the umbilicus at the level of the iliac crests. Four or five pairs of **lumbar arteries** arise from the abdominal aorta and supply the lumbar vertebrae, back muscles, and posterior abdominal wall.

The **common iliac arteries**, terminal branches of the abdominal aorta, diverge and run inferolaterally, following the medial border of the psoas muscles to the pelvic brim. Here each common iliac artery divides into the **internal** and **external iliac arteries.** The internal iliac artery enters the pelvis; its course and branches are described in Chapter 4. The external iliac artery follows the iliopsoas muscle. Just before leaving the abdomen, the external iliac artery gives rise to the **inferior epigastric** and **deep iliac circumflex arteries,** which supply the anterolateral abdominal wall.

From superior to inferior, the important *anterior relations* of the abdominal aorta are the celiac plexus and ganglion, body of pancreas, splenic and left renal veins, horizontal part of the duodenum, and the coils of small intestine (Table 2.6). The left lumbar veins pass *posterior* to the aorta to reach the IVC. On the *right*, the aorta is related to the azygos vein, cisterna chyli, right crus of diaphragm, and right celiac ganglion. On the *left*, the aorta is related to the left crus of diaphragm and left celiac ganglion. The branches of the abdominal aorta may be described as visceral or parietal and paired or unpaired (Figs. 2.64 and 2.65A).

The **paired visceral branches** (vertebral level of origin) are the:

- Suprarenal arteries (L1).
- Renal arteries (L1).
- Gonadal arteries, the ovarian or testicular arteries (L2).

The **unpaired visceral branches** (vertebral level of origin) are the:

- Celiac trunk (T12).
- Superior mesenteric artery (L1).
- Inferior mesenteric artery (L3).

The **paired parietal branches** are the:

- Inferior phrenic arteries that arise just inferior to the aortic hiatus and supply the inferior surface of the diaphragm and the suprarenal glands.
- Lumbar arteries that pass around the sides of the superior four lumbar vertebrae to supply the posterior abdominal wall.

The **unpaired parietal branch** is the **median sacral artery,** which arises from the aorta at its bifurcation and descends into the lesser pelvis.

FIGURE 2.65. **Aorta and inferior vena cava. A.** Branches of aorta. **B.** Tributaries of inferior vena cava.

The **veins of the posterior abdominal wall** are tributaries of the IVC, except for the **left testicular** or **ovarian vein,** which enters the **left renal vein** instead of entering the IVC (Fig. 2.65*B*). The IVC, the largest vein in the body, has no valves except for a variable, nonfunctional one at its orifice in the right atrium of the heart. The IVC returns poorly oxygenated blood from the lower limbs, most of the back, the abdominal walls, and the abdominopelvic viscera. Blood from the viscera passes through the *portal venous system* and the liver before entering the IVC via the hepatic veins. The IVC begins anterior to the L5 vertebra by the union of the common iliac veins. This union occurs approximately 2.5 cm to the right of the median plane, inferior to the bifurcation of the aorta and posterior to the proximal part of the right *common iliac artery.* The IVC ascends on the right side of the bodies of the L3–L5 vertebrae and on the psoas major muscle to the right of the aorta. The IVC leaves the abdomen by passing through the caval opening in the diaphragm to enter the thorax. The tributaries of the IVC correspond to branches of the aorta:

- Common iliac veins, formed by union of external and internal iliac veins.
- Third (L3) and fourth (L4) lumbar veins.
- Right testicular or ovarian veins (the left testicular or ovarian veins usually drain into the left renal vein).
- Right and left renal veins.

- Ascending lumbar veins (the azygos and hemiazygos veins arise, in part, from ascending lumbar veins (see Chapter 1); the ascending lumbar and azygos veins connect the IVC and superior vena cava, either directly or indirectly.
- Right suprarenal vein (the left suprarenal vein; usually drains into the left renal vein).
- Inferior phrenic veins.
- Hepatic veins.

Lymphatics of Posterior Abdominal Wall

Lymphatic vessels and **lymph nodes** lie along the aorta, IVC, and iliac vessels. The **common iliac lymph nodes** receive lymph from the external and internal iliac lymph nodes. Lymph from the common iliac lymph nodes passes to the **lumbar lymph nodes** (Fig. 2.66). These nodes receive lymph directly from the posterior abdominal wall, kidneys, ureters, testes or ovaries, uterus, and uterine tubes. They also receive lymph from the descending colon, pelvis, and lower limbs through the **inferior mesenteric** and **common iliac lymph nodes.** Efferent lymphatic vessels from the lymph nodes form the right and left **lumbar lymph trunks.** Lymphatic vessels from the intestine, liver, spleen, and pancreas pass along the celiac, superior, and inferior mesenteric arteries to the **preaortic lymph nodes** (celiac and superior and inferior mesenteric nodes)

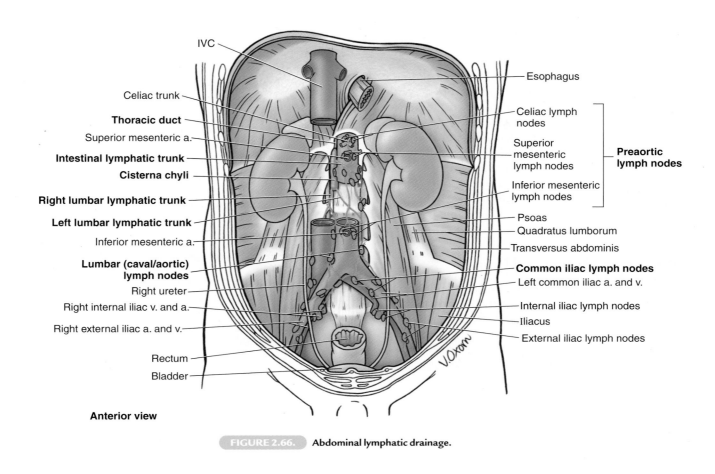

FIGURE 2.66.   Abdominal lymphatic drainage.

scattered around the origins of these arteries from the aorta. Efferent vessels from these nodes form the **intestinal lymphatic trunks,** which may be single or multiple and participate in the confluence of lymphatic trunks that gives rise to the thoracic duct.

The **cisterna chyli** is a thin-walled sac at the inferior end of the **thoracic duct,** variable in size and shape, located anterior to the bodies of the L1 and L2 vertebrae between the right crus of the diaphragm and the aorta (Fig. 2.67). A pair of **descending thoracic lymphatic trunks** carry lymph from the lower six intercostal spaces on each side. More often there is merely a simple or plexiform convergence of the right and left lumbar lymphatic trunks, the intestinal lymph trunk(s), and a pair of **descending thoracic lymphatic trunks.** Consequently, essentially all the lymphatic drainage from the lower half of the body (deep lymphatic drainage inferior to the level of the diaphragm and all superficial drainage inferior to the level of the umbilicus) converges in the abdomen to enter the beginning of the thoracic duct. The thoracic duct ascends through the aortic hiatus in the diaphragm into the posterior mediastinum, where it collects more parietal and visceral drainage, particularly from the left upper

quadrant of the body, and ultimately ends by entering the venous system at the junction of the **left subclavian and internal jugular veins** (the left venous angle).

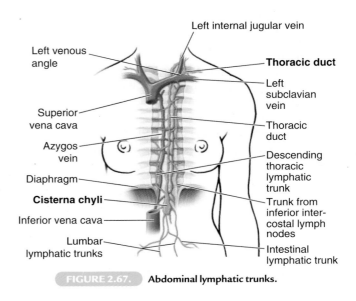

FIGURE 2.67.   Abdominal lymphatic trunks.

Psoas Abscess

An abscess resulting from tuberculosis in the lumbar region tends to spread from the vertebrae into the psoas sheath, where it produces a *psoas abscess*. As a consequence, the psoas fascia thickens to form a strong stocking-like tube. Pus from the psoas abscess passes inferiorly along the psoas within this fascial tube over the pelvic brim and deep to the inguinal ligament. The pus usually surfaces in the superior part of the thigh. Pus can also reach the psoas sheath by passing from the posterior mediastinum when the thoracic vertebrae are diseased.

Posterior Abdominal Pain

The *iliopsoas muscle* has extensive and clinically important relations to the kidneys, ureters, cecum, appendix, sigmoid colon, pancreas, lumbar lymph nodes, and nerves of the posterior abdominal wall. When any of these structures is diseased, movement of the iliopsoas usually causes pain. When intra-abdominal inflammation is suspected, the **iliopsoas test** is performed. The person is asked to lie on the unaffected side and to extend the thigh on the affected side against the resistance of the examiner's hand. Pain resulting from this maneuver is a *positive psoas sign*. An acutely inflamed appendix, for example, will produce a positive sign.

Collateral Routes for Abdominopelvic Venous Blood

Three collateral routes, formed by valveless veins of the trunk, are available for venous blood to return to the heart when the IVC is obstructed or ligated:

- The *inferior epigastric* veins, tributaries of the external iliac veins of the inferior caval system, anastomose in the rectus sheath with the superior epigastric veins, which drain in sequence through the internal thoracic veins of the superior caval system.
- The *superficial epigastric* or superficial circumflex iliac veins, normally tributaries of the great saphenous vein

of the inferior caval system, anastomose in the subcutaneous tissues of the anterolateral body wall with one of the tributaries of the axillary vein, commonly the lateral thoracic vein. When the IVC is obstructed, this subcutaneous collateral pathway—called the *thoraco-epigastric vein*—becomes particularly conspicuous.

- The *epidural venous plexus* inside the vertebral column (see Chapter 4) communicates with the lumbar veins of the inferior caval system, and the tributaries of the azygos system of veins, which is part of the superior caval system.

Abdominal Aortic Aneurysm

Rupture of an aneurysm (localized enlargement) of the abdominal aorta causes severe pain in the abdomen or back (Fig. B2.12). If unrecognized, a ruptured aneurysm has a mortality rate of nearly 90% because of heavy blood loss. Surgeons can repair an aneurysm by opening it, inserting a prosthetic graft (such as one made of Dacron), and sewing the wall of the aneurysmal aorta over the graft to protect it. Aneurysms may also be treated by endovascular catheterization procedures.

FIGURE B2.12. Abdominal aortic aneurysm (A).

Medical Imaging of Abdomen

Examples of some of the modalities used in medical imaging of the abdomen follow. Radiographs of the abdomen demonstrate normal and abnormal anatomical relationships, such as those resulting from tumors. CT (computed tomography) scans (Fig. 2.68), MRI (magnetic resonance imaging) studies (Fig. 2.69), and ultrasound (Fig. 2.70) are also used to examine the abdominal viscera. MRI studies provide better differentiation than CT scans between soft tissues.

FIGURE 2.68.   **CT scans of abdomen at progressively lower levels.** *A,* aorta; *C,* celiac trunk; *D,* duodenum; *DBM,* deep back muscles; *I,* intestine, *IVC;* inferior vena cava; *L,* liver; *LA,* left renal artery; *LC,* left crus of diaphragm; *LK,* left kidney; *LV,* left renal vein; *P,* pancreas; *PS,* psoas major; *RC,* right crus of diaphragm; *RK,* right kidney; *RM,* rectus abdominis; *RV,* right renal vein; *SP,* spleen; *ST,* stomach; *SV,* splenic vessels; *V,* vertebral body; *X,* superior mesenteric artery.

A Transverse section, inferior view

B Transverse section, inferior view

C Median section, right lateral view

FIGURE 2.69. **Ultrasound scans of abdomen. A.** Transverse scan through the celiac trunk. **B.** Transverse scan through the pancreas. **C.** Transverse scan through the aorta. *Ao,* aorta; *BD,* bile duct; *CA,* celiac artery; *D,* duodenum; *FL,* falciform ligament; *GD,* gastroduodenal artery; *GE,* gastroesophageal junction; *HA,* hepatic artery; *IVC,* inferior vena cava; *L,* liver; *LCr,* left crus of diaphragm; *LGA,* left gastric artery; *LR,* left renal vein; *P,* pancreas; *Pu,* uncinate process of pancreas; *PV,* hepatic portal vein; *PVC,* hepatic portal venous confluence; *RCr,* right crus of diaphragm; *SA,* splenic artery; *SMA,* superior mesenteric artery; *SMV,* superior mesenteric vein; *SV,* splenic vein; *V,* vertebra.

Key	
Ac	Ascending colon
AF	Air-fluid level of stomach
Ao	Aorta
Az	Azygos vein
CA	Celiac artery
cc	Costal cartilage
CD	Cystic duct
CHA	Common hepatic artery
CHD	Common hepatic duct
CL	Caudate lobe of liver
DBM	Deep back muscles
Dc	Descending colon
D2	2nd part of duodenum
D3	3rd part of duodenum
E	Esophagus
FL	Falciform ligament
GB	Gallbladder
HA	Hepatic artery
Hz	Hemiazygos vein
IVC	Inferior vena cava
L1	1st lumbar vertebra
L2	2nd lumbar vertebra
L3	3rd lumbar vertebra
LC	Left crus of diaphragm
LG	Left suprarenal gland
LHV	Left hepatic vein
LIL	Left inferior lobe of lung
LK	Left kidney
LL	Left lobe of liver
LRV	Left renal vein
MHV	Middle hepatic vein

FIGURE 2.70.   Transverse MRI studies of the abdomen.

Key (continued)

P	Pancreas
PA	Pyloric antrum of stomach
PB	Body of pancreas
PC	Portal confluence
PF	Perirenal fat
PH	Head of pancreas
PS	Psoas
PT	Tail of pancreas
PU	Uncinate process of pancreas
PV	Hepatic portal vein
QL	Quadratus lumborum
R	Rib
RA	Rectus abdominis
RC	Right crus of diaphragm
RF	Retroperitoneal fat
RG	Right suprarenal gland
RHV	Right hepatic vein
RIL	Right inferior lobe of lung
RK	Right kidney
RL	Right lobe of liver
RP	Renal pelvis
RPV	Right branch of hepatic portal vein
RRA	Right renal artery
RRV	Right renal vein
RU	Right ureter
S	Spinous process
SA	Splenic artery
SC	Spinal cord
SF	Splenic flexure
SI	Small intestine
SMA	Superior mesenteric artery
SMV	Superior mesenteric vein
Sp	Spleen
St	Stomach
SV	Splenic vein
T11	11th thoracic vertebra
T12	12th thoracic vertebra
Tc	Transverse colon
TVP	Transverse process
Xp	Xiphoid process

FIGURE 2.70. *(Continued)*

Abdominal arteriography, radiography after the injection of radiopaque material directly into the bloodstream, detects abnormalities of the abdominal arteries (Fig. 2.71*A,B*).

Angiographic studies may also be performed using MRI. To examine the colon a barium enema is given after the bowel is cleared of fecal material by a cleansing enema (Fig. 2.71*B,C*).

12th rib
Minor calyx
Major calyx
Renal pelvis
L1
L2
Ureter
Gas in intestine
Sacrum
Ureter
Catheter (in urinary bladder)

A **Anteroposterior pyelogram**

ST
Ao
CA
SA
K
RRA
LRA
K
SMA

B **Anterior view**

S
H
U U U
T
A
C
D
G
R

C **Posteroanterior radiograph**

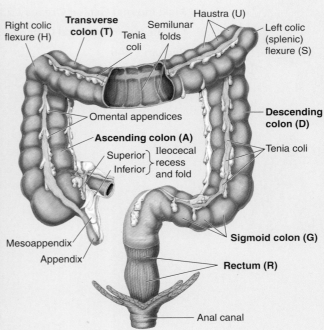

Right colic flexure (H)
Transverse colon (T)
Tenia coli
Semilunar folds
Haustra (U)
Left colic (splenic) flexure (S)
Omental appendices
Descending colon (D)
Tenia coli
Ascending colon (A)
Superior
Inferior
Ileocecal recess and fold
Mesoappendix
Appendix
Sigmoid colon (G)
Rectum (R)
Anal canal

D **Anterior view**

FIGURE 2.71. **Abdominal images after introduction of contrast material. A.** Pyelogram (radiograph of renal pelves and ureters). **B.** MR angiogram (MRA). *Ao,* aorta; *CA,* celiac trunk; *K,* kidney; *LRA,* left renal artery; *RRA,* right renal artery; *SA,* splenic artery; *SMA,* superior mesenteric artery; *ST,* stomach. **C.** Single-contrast radiograph of colon after a barium enema. Letters are identified in D. **D.** Overview of characteristics of the large intestine.

 Go to <u>http://thePoint.lww.com/ECA4e</u> *for helpful study tools, including USMLE-style questions, case studies, images, and more!*

PELVIS / 205

Pelvic Girdle / 205

Joints and Ligaments of Pelvic Girdle / 209

Peritoneum and Peritoneal Cavity of
Pelvis / 211

Walls and Floor of Pelvic Cavity / 211

Pelvic Fascia / 215

Pelvic Nerves / 217

Pelvic Arteries and Veins / 220

Lymph Nodes of Pelvis / 223

PELVIC VISCERA / 223

Urinary Organs / 223

Male Internal Genital Organs / 233

Female Internal Genital Organs / 236

Rectum / 245

PERINEUM / 250

Fascias and Pouches of Urogenital
Triangle / 253

Features of Anal Triangle / 257

Male Perineum / 261

Female Perineum / 268

**MEDICAL IMAGING OF PELVIS AND
PERINEUM / 271**

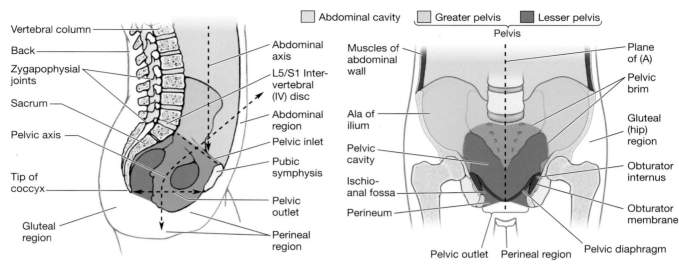

A **Medial view of left half of bisected lower trunk**

B **Anterior view of posterior half of coronally-sectioned lower trunk**

FIGURE 3.1.   **Abdominopelvic cavity. A.** and **B.** The pelvis is the space within the pelvic girdle, overlapped externally by the abdominal and gluteal (lower limb) regions and the perineum. Thus the pelvis has no unique external surface area. *Light green,* greater pelvis; *dark green,* lesser pelvis.

The pelvis (L. *basin*) is the part of the trunk inferoposterior to the abdomen and is the area of transition between the trunk and the lower limbs (Fig. 3.1). The perineal region refers to the area of the trunk between the thighs and the buttocks, extending from the pubis to the coccyx. The perineum is a shallow compartment lying deep to this area and inferior to the pelvic diaphragm.

PELVIS

The superior boundary of the **pelvic cavity** is the **pelvic inlet,** the superior pelvic aperture (Figs. 3.1 and 3.2). The pelvis is limited inferiorly by the **pelvic outlet,** the inferior pelvic aperture, which is bounded anteriorly by the **pubic symphysis** (L. *symphysis pubis*) and posteriorly by the **coccyx.**

The **pelvic inlet** (*superior pelvic aperture*) is bounded by the **linea terminalis** of the pelvis, which is formed by the:

- Superior margin of the pubic symphysis anteriorly.
- Posterior border of the pubic crest.
- Pecten pubis, the continuation of the superior ramus of the pubis, which forms a sharp ridge.
- **Arcuate line** of the ilium.
- Anterior border of the ala (L. *wing*) of the sacrum.
- **Sacral promontory.**

The **pelvic outlet** (*inferior pelvic aperture*) is bounded by the:

- Inferior margin of the pubic symphysis anteriorly.
- Inferior rami of the pubis and ischial tuberosities anterolaterally.

- Sacrotuberous ligaments posterolaterally (Fig. 3.3*B*)
- Tip of the coccyx posteriorly

Pelvic Girdle

The **pelvic girdle** is a basin-shaped ring of bones that connects the vertebral column to the two femurs in the thighs. The main functions of the strong pelvic girdle are to transfer the weight of the upper body from the axial to the lower appendicular skeleton for standing and walking, and to withstand compression and other forces resulting from its support of body weight. The bony pelvis is formed by three bones (Fig. 3.2; Table 3.1):

- Right and left **hip bones:** two large, irregularly shaped bones, each of which forms at puberty by fusion of three bones—*ilium, ischium,* and *pubis.*
- **Sacrum:** formed by the fusion of five, originally separate, sacral vertebrae.

The hip bones are joined at the *pubic symphysis* anteriorly and to the sacrum posteriorly at the **sacro-iliac joints** to form a bony ring, the *pelvic girdle.*

The **ilium** is the superior, flattened, fan-shaped part of the hip bone (Fig. 3.2). The **ala** of the ilium represents the spread of the fan and the **body** of the ilium, the handle of the fan. The body of the ilium forms the superior part of the **acetabulum,** the cup-shaped depression on the external surface of the hip bone with which the head of the femur articulates. The **iliac crest,** the rim of the ilium, has a curve that follows the contour of the ala between the **anterior** and the **posterior superior iliac spines.** The anterior concave part of the ala forms the **iliac fossa.**

A **Anterior view**

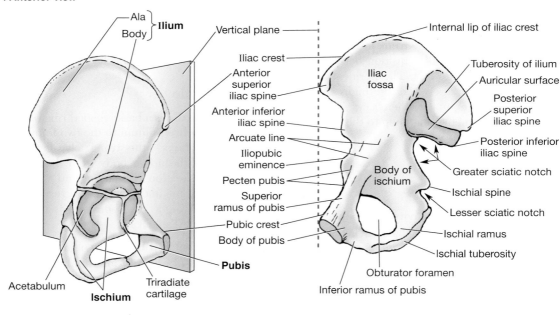

B **Lateral view**   C **Medial view**

FIGURE 3.2.   **Bony pelvis. A.** Articulated pelvis. **B.** Child's right hip bone. **C.** Adult's right hip bone. In the anatomical position the anterior superior iliac spine and the anterior aspect of the pubis lie in the same vertical plane.

The **ischium** has a body and a ramus (L. *branch*). The **body** of the ischium forms the posterior part of the acetabulum, and the **ramus** forms the posterior part of the inferior boundary of the **obturator foramen.** The large posteroinferior protuberance of the ischium is the **ischial tuberosity** (Fig. 3.2). The small pointed posterior projection near the junction of the ramus and body is the **ischial spine.**

The **pubis** is an angulated bone that has the **superior pubic ramus,** which forms the anterior part of the acetabulum, and the **inferior pubic ramus,** which forms the anterior part of the

inferior boundary of the *obturator foramen.* The superior pubic ramus has an oblique ridge, the **pecten pubis** (pectineal line of pubis), on its superior aspect. A thickening on the anterior part of the **body of the pubis** is the **pubic crest,** which ends laterally as a swelling—the **pubic tubercle** (Fig. 3.3A).

The **pubic arch** is formed by the **ischiopubic rami** (conjoined inferior rami of the pubis and ischium) of the two sides. These rami meet at the *pubic symphysis,* and their inferior borders define the **subpubic angle** (the distance between the right and the left ischial tuberosities), which can

Anterior longitudinal ligament

Iliolumbar ligament

Anterior sacro-iliac ligament

Inguinal ligament

Sacrospinous ligament

Superior pubic ligament

Pubic symphysis

Inferior (arcuate) pubic ligament

A Anterior view

Transverse process of L5 vertebra

Iliac crest

L5/S1 intervertebal (IV) disc=lumbosacral joint

Anterior superior iliac spine (ASIS)

Greater sciatic foramen

Sacrotuberous ligament

Anterior sacrococcygeal ligament

Obturator membrane

Pubic tubercle

Iliolumbar ligament

Posterior sacro-iliac ligament

Greater sciatic foramen

Ischial spine

Lesser sciatic foramen

Pubic symphysis

Pelvic outlet (red line)

B Posterior view

Joint capsule of posterior lumbosacral (zygapophysis) joint

Iliac crest

Posterior superior iliac spine (PSIS)

Posterior sacrococcygeal ligament

Sacrospinous ligament

Sacrotuberous ligament

Ischial tuberosity

Obturator membrane

FIGURE 3.3. Ligaments of pelvis.

be approximated by the angle between the abducted middle and index fingers for the male, and the angle between the index finger and extended thumb for the female (Fig. 3.4).

The bony pelvis is divided into *greater (false)* and *lesser (true) pelves* by the oblique plane of the **pelvic inlet** (superior pelvic aperture) (Figs. 3.1 and 3.2). The bony edge (rim) surrounding the pelvic inlet is the **pelvic brim.**

The **greater pelvis** (L. *pelvis major*) is:

- Superior to the pelvic inlet.
- Bounded by the abdominal wall anteriorly, the alea of illun laterally, and the L5 and S1 vertebrae posteriorly.

- The location of some abdominal viscera, such as the sigmoid colon and some loops of ileum.

The **lesser pelvis** (L. *pelvis minor*) is:

- Between the *pelvic inlet* and the *pelvic outlet* (Fig. 3.3B).
- The location of the pelvic viscera—urinary bladder and reproductive organs, such as the uterus and ovaries.
- Bounded by the pelvic surfaces of the hip bones, sacrum, and coccyx.
- Limited inferiorly by the musculomembranous pelvic diaphragm (levator ani) (Table 3.2, Fig. 3.1B).

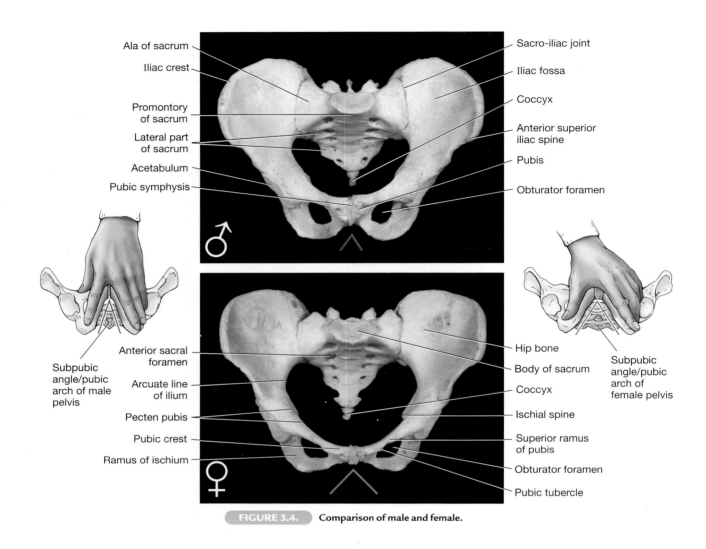

FIGURE 3.4. Comparison of male and female.

TABLE 3.1 COMPARISON OF MALE AND FEMALE BONY PELVES

Bony Pelvis	Male (♂)	Female (♀)	
General structure	Thick and heavy	Thin and light	
Greater pelvis (pelvis major)	Deep	Shallow	
Lesser pelvis (pelvis minor)	Narrow and deep	Wide and shallow	
Pelvic inlet (superior pelvic aperture)	Heart-shaped	Oval or rounded	
Pelvic outlet (inferior pelvic aperture)	Comparatively small	Comparatively large	
Pubic arch and subpubic angle (∧)	Narrow (<70°)	Wide (>80°)	
Obturator foramen	Round	Oval	
Acetabulum	Large	Small	

Sexual Differences in Bony Pelves

The male and female bony pelves differ in several respects (Fig. 3.4 and Table 3.1). These sexual differences are related mainly to the heavier build and larger muscles of men, and to the adaptation of the pelvis, particularly the lesser pelvis, in women for childbearing. Hence, the **male pelvis** is heavier and thicker than the female pelvis and usually has more prominent bone markings. In contrast, the **female pelvis** is wider and shallower and has a larger pelvic inlet and outlet. The shape and size of the pelvic inlet (and the pelvic brim) are significant because it is through this opening that the fetal head enters the lesser pelvis during labor. To determine the capacity of the pelvis for childbirth, the diameters of the lesser pelvis are noted during a pelvic examination. The *ischial spines* face each other and the **interspinous distance** between them is the narrowest part of the pelvic canal (the passageway traversing the pelvic inlet, lesser pelvis, and pelvic outlet through which a baby's head must pass at birth).

Pelvic Fractures

Pelvic fractures can result from direct trauma to the pelvic bones, such as may occur during an automobile accident, or from forces transmitted to these bones from the lower limbs during falls on the feet. Pelvic fractures may cause injury to pelvic soft tissues, blood vessels, nerves, and organs.

Joints and Ligaments of Pelvic Girdle

The primary joints of the pelvis are the *sacro-iliac joints* and the *pubic symphysis*, which link the skeleton of the trunk and the lower limb (Fig. 3.2A). The *lumbosacral* and *sacrococcygeal* joints are directly related to the pelvic girdle. Strong ligaments support and strengthen these joints (Fig. 3.3).

SACRO-ILIAC JOINTS

The sacro-iliac joints are strong, weight-bearing, compound joints, consisting of an anterior synovial joint (between the ear-shaped *auricular surfaces* of the sacrum and ilium covered with articular cartilage) and a posterior syndesmosis (between the tuberosities of the same bones) (Figs. 3.2C and 3.5). The articular (auricular) surfaces of the synovial joint have irregular but congruent elevations and depressions that interlock. The sacro-iliac joints differ from most synovial joints in that they have limited mobility, a consequence of their role in transmitting the weight of most of the body to the hip bones.

The sacrum is suspended between the iliac bones and is firmly attached to them by posterior and interosseous sacro-iliac ligaments. The thin **anterior sacro-iliac ligaments** form the anterior part of the fibrous capsule of the synovial joint. The **interosseous sacro-iliac ligaments** occupy an area of about 10 cm^2 each and are the primary structures involved in transferring the weight of the upper body from the axial skeleton to the two ilia and then to the femurs during standing and to the ischial tuberosities during sitting. The **posterior sacro-iliac ligaments** are posterior external continuations of the interosseous sacro-iliac ligaments.

Usually movement is limited to slight gliding and rotary movements, except when subject to considerable force such as occurs after a high jump (or during late pregnancy—see next Blue Box). Then the weight of the body is transmitted through the sacrum anterior to the rotation axis, tending to push the superior sacrum inferiorly, thereby causing the inferior sacrum to rotate superiorly. This tendency is resisted by the strong **sacrotuberous** and **sacrospinous ligaments** (Fig. 3.3). These ligaments allow only limited upward movement of the inferior end of the sacrum, thus providing resilience to the sacro-iliac region when the vertebral column sustains sudden weight increases (Fig. 3.5C).

PUBIC SYMPHYSIS

The pubic symphysis is a secondary cartilaginous joint that is formed by the union of the bodies of the pubic bones in the median plane (Figs. 3.3 and 3.5D). The fibrocartilaginous **interpubic disc** is generally wider in women than in men. The ligaments joining the pubic bones are thickened superi they orly and inferiorly to form the **superior pubic ligament** and the **inferior** (arcuate) **pubic ligament,** respectively. The decussating fibers of tendinous attachments of the rectus abdominis and external oblique muscles also strengthen the pubic symphysis anteriorly.

LUMBOSACRAL JOINTS

The L5 and S1 vertebrae articulate anteriorly at the anterior **intervertebral joint,** formed by the L5/S1 intervertebral (IV) disc between their bodies posteriorly and (Fig. 3.1A) at two **zygapophysial joints** (facet joints) between the articular processes of these vertebrae (Fig. 3.3B). The facets on the S1 vertebra face posteromedially, interlocking with the anterolaterally facing inferior articular facets of the L5 vertebra, preventing L5 from sliding anteriorly. **Iliolumbar ligaments** unite the transverse processes of L5 to the ilia.

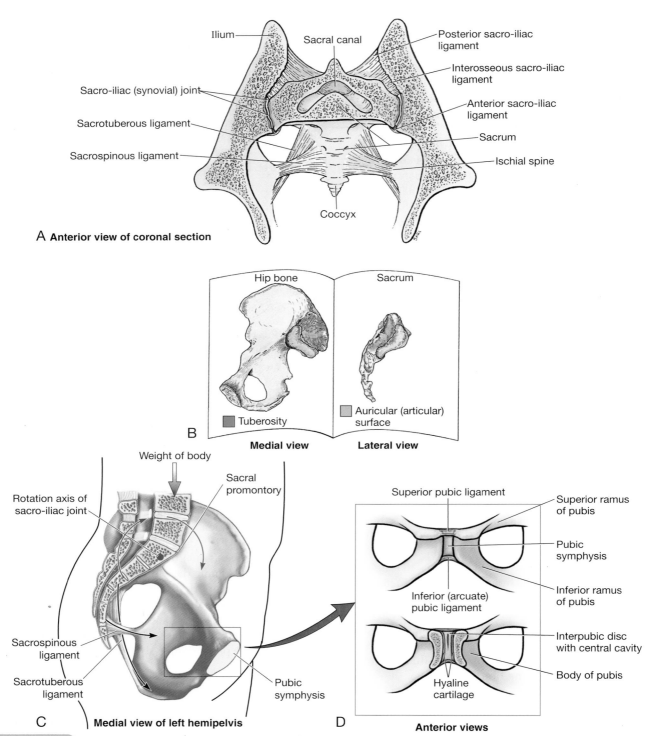

FIGURE 3.5. **Sacro-iliac joints and ligaments. A.** Coronal section of the pelvis. **B.** Articular surfaces of sacro-iliac joint. **C.** Role of sacrotuberous and sacrospinous ligaments in resisting anterior rotation of pelvis. **D.** Structure of the pubic symphysis.

Relaxation of Pelvic Ligaments and Increased Joint Mobility During Pregnancy

During pregnancy, the pelvic joints and ligaments relax and pelvic movements increase. This relaxation during the latter half of pregnancy is caused by the increase in levels of the sex hormones and the presence of the hormone relaxin. The sacro-iliac interlocking mechanism is less effective because the relaxation permits greater rotation of the pelvis and contributes to the lordotic posture often assumed during pregnancy with the change in the center of gravity. Relaxation of the sacro-iliac joints and pubic symphysis permits as much as a 10% to 15% increase in diameters (mostly transverse), facilitating passage of the fetus through the pelvic canal. The coccyx is also allowed to move posteriorly.

SACROCOCCYGEAL JOINT

The sacrococcygeal joint is a secondary cartilaginous joint with an IV disc. Fibrocartilage and ligaments join the apex of the sacrum to the base of the coccyx (Fig. 3.3A).

The anterior and posterior **sacrococcygeal ligaments** are long strands that reinforce the joint, much like the anterior and posterior longitudinal ligaments do for superior vertebrae.

Peritoneum and Peritoneal Cavity of Pelvis

The **peritoneum** lining the abdominal cavity continues into the pelvic cavity, reflecting onto the superior aspects of most pelvic viscera (Fig. 3.6 and Table 3.2). Only the uterine tubes—except for their ostia, which are open—are intraperitoneal and suspended by a mesentery. The ovaries, although suspended in the peritoneal cavity by a mesentery, are not covered with peritoneum. The peritoneum creates a number of folds and fossae as it reflects onto most of the pelvic viscera.

The peritoneum is not firmly bound to the suprapubic crest, allowing the bladder to expand between the peritoneum and the anterior abdominal wall as it fills.

Walls and Floor of Pelvic Cavity

The pelvic cavity has an *anteroinferior wall,* two *lateral walls,* and a *posterior wall.* Muscles of the pelvic walls are summarized in Figure 3.7A–E and Table 3.3.

The **anteroinferior pelvic wall:**

- Is formed primarily by the bodies and rami of the pubic bones and the pubic symphysis.
- Participates in bearing the weight of the urinary bladder.

The **lateral pelvic walls:**

- Have a bony framework formed by the hip bones, including the obturator foramen (Fig. 3.2C); the **obturator foramen** is closed by the **obturator membrane** (Fig. 3.3).
- Are covered and padded by the **obturator internus muscles** (Fig. 3.7A–D). Each obturator internus passes posteriorly from its origin within the lesser pelvis, exits through the lesser sciatic foramen, and turns sharply laterally to attach to the femur (Fig. 3.7E). The medial surfaces of these muscles are covered by **obturator fascia,** thickened centrally as a tendinous arch that provides attachment for the levator ani (pelvic diaphragm) (Fig. 3.7A,C).
- Have the obturator nerves and vessels and other branches of the internal iliac vessels located on their medial aspects (medial to obturator internus muscles).

The *posterior pelvic wall:*

- Consists of a bony wall and roof in the midline (formed by the sacrum and coccyx) and musculoligamentous posterolateral walls (formed by the sacro-iliac joints and their associated ligaments and piriformis muscles). Each **piriformis muscle** leaves the lesser pelvis through the *greater sciatic foramen* to attach to the femur (Fig. 3.7D,E).
- Is the site of the nerves forming the **sacral plexus;** the piriformis muscles form a "muscular bed" for this nerve network (Fig. 3.7A,C,D).

The **pelvic floor** is formed by the bowl- or funnel-shaped **pelvic diaphragm,** which consists of the *levator ani* and *coccygeus* muscles and the fascias (L. *fasciae*) covering the superior and inferior aspects of these muscles (Fig. 3.7B). The **coccygeus muscles** extend from the ischial spines to the inferior sacrum and coccyx. The **levator ani** is attached to the pubic bones anteriorly, to the ischial spines posteriorly, and to a thickening in the obturator fascia (**tendinous arch of levator ani**) on each side (Fig. 3.7A,C). The levator ani consists of three parts, each named according to the attachment of its fibers (Fig. 3.7A,C; Table 3.3). The parts of the levator ani are:

- The **puborectalis,** consisting of the thicker, narrower, medial part of the levator ani, which is continuous between the posterior aspects of the right and left pubic bones. It forms a U-shaped muscular sling (puborectal sling) that passes posterior to the anorectal junction. This part plays a major role in maintaining fecal continence.
- The **pubococcygeus,** the wider but thinner intermediate part of the levator ani, arises from the posterior aspect of the body of the pubis and the anterior part of the tendinous arch and passes posteriorly in a nearly horizontal plane. The lateral fibers attach posteriorly to the coccyx, and the medial fibers merge with those of the contralateral side to form part of the **anococcygeal body** or **ligament.**

A **Anterior view of female**

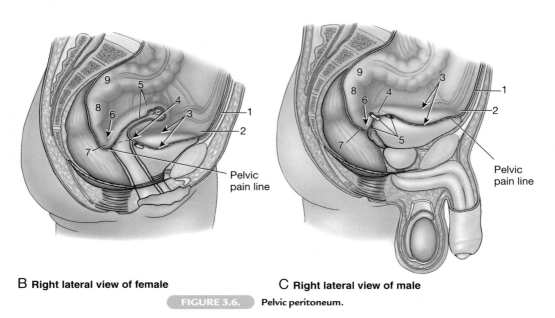

B **Right lateral view of female**   C **Right lateral view of male**

FIGURE 3.6.   Pelvic peritoneum.

TABLE 3.2 PERITONEAL REFLECTIONS IN PELVIS

Female (Parts A & B)[a]	Male (Part C)[a]
1 Descends anterior abdominal wall (loose attachment allows insertion of bladder as it fills)	1 Descends anterior abdominal wall (loose attachment allows insertion of bladder as it fills)
2 Reflects onto superior surface of bladder, creating **supravesical fossa**	2 Reflects onto superior surface of bladder, creating **supravesical fossa**
3 Covers convex superior surface of bladder; slopes down sides of bladder to ascend lateral wall of pelvis, creating **paravesical fossae** on each side	3 Covers convex superior surface (roof) of bladder, sloping down sides of roof to ascend lateral wall of pelvis, creating **paravesical fossae** on each side
4 Reflects from bladder body of uterus, forming **vesico-uterine pouch**	4 Descends posterior surface of bladder as much as 2 cm
5 Covers body and fundus of uterus, posterior fornix of vagina; extends laterally from uterus as double fold of mesentery, the **broad ligament** that engulfs uterine tubes, and round ligaments of uterus, and suspends ovaries	5 Laterally, forms fold over ureters (**ureteric fold**), ductus deferentes, and superior ends of seminal glands
6 Reflects from vagina onto rectum, forming **recto-uterine pouch**[b] (pouch of Douglas)	6 Reflects from bladder and seminal glands onto rectum, forming **rectovesical pouch**[b]
7 Recto-uterine pouch extends laterally and posteriorly to form **pararectal fossae** on each side of rectum	7 Rectovesical pouch extends laterally and posteriorly to form **pararectal fossae** on each side of rectum
8 Ascends rectum; from inferior to superior, rectum is subperitoneal and then retroperitoneal	8 Ascends rectum; from inferior to superior, rectum is subperitoneal and then retroperitoneal
9 Engulfs sigmoid colon beginning at rectosigmoid junction	9 Engulfs sigmoid colon beginning at rectosigmoid junction

[a]Numbers refer to Figure 3.6.
[b]Low point of peritoneal cavity in erect position.

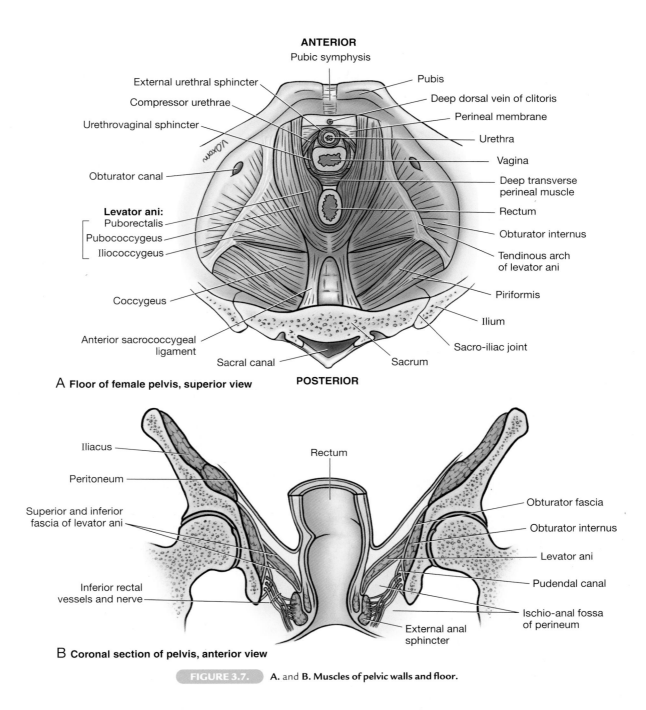

A Floor of female pelvis, superior view

B Coronal section of pelvis, anterior view

FIGURE 3.7. A. and B. Muscles of pelvic walls and floor.

TABLE 3.3 MUSCLES OF PELVIC WALLS AND FLOOR

Muscle	Proximal Attachment	Distal Attachment	Innervation	Main Action
Levator ani (pubococcygeus and iliococcygeus)	Body of pubis, tendinous arch of levator ani, ischial spine	Perineal body, coccyx, anococcygeal ligament, walls of prostate or vagina, rectum, anal canal	Nerve to levator ani (branches of S4), inferior anal (rectal) nerve, coccygeal plexus	Helps support pelvic viscera; resists increases in intra-abdominal pressure
Coccygeus (ischiococcygeus)	Ischial spine	Inferior end of sacrum	Branches of S4 and S5 nerves	Forms small part of pelvic diaphragm that supports pelvic viscera; flexes coccyx

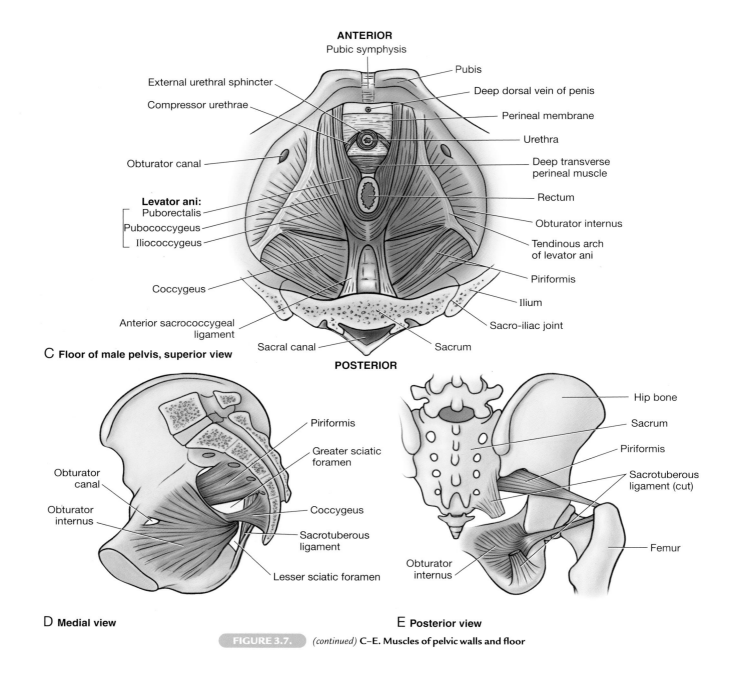

ANTERIOR
Pubic symphysis

External urethral sphincter

Compressor urethrae

Obturator canal

Levator ani:
Puborectalis

Pubococcygeus

Iliococcygeus

Coccygeus

Anterior sacrococcygeal ligament

Sacral canal

Pubis

Deep dorsal vein of penis

Perineal membrane

Urethra

Deep transverse perineal muscle

Rectum

Obturator internus

Tendinous arch of levator ani

Piriformis

Ilium

Sacro-iliac joint

Sacrum

C **Floor of male pelvis, superior view**

POSTERIOR

Piriformis

Greater sciatic foramen

Coccygeus

Sacrotuberous ligament

Lesser sciatic foramen

Obturator canal

Obturator internus

D **Medial view**

Hip bone

Sacrum

Piriformis

Sacrotuberous ligament (cut)

Femur

Obturator internus

E **Posterior view**

FIGURE 3.7. *(continued)* **C–E. Muscles of pelvic walls and floor**

TABLE 3.3 MUSCLES OF PELVIC WALLS AND FLOOR (*continued*)

Muscle	Proximal Attachment	Distal Attachment	Innervation	Main Action
Obturator internus	Pelvic surface of ilium and ischium; obturator membrane	Greater trochanter of femur	Nerve to obturator internus (L5, S1, S2)	Rotates thigh laterally; assists in holding head of femur in acetabulum
Piriformis	Pelvic surface of 2nd–4th sacral segments; superior margin of greater sciatic notch and sacrotuberous ligament		Anterior rami of S1 and S2	Rotates thigh laterally; abducts thigh; assists in holding head of femur in acetabulum

- The **iliococcygeus,** the posterolateral part of the levator ani, arises from the posterior part of the tendinous arch and ischial spine; it is thin and often poorly developed and blends with the anococcygeal body posteriorly.

The levator ani forms a dynamic floor for supporting the abdominopelvic viscera. Acting together, the parts of the levator ani raise the pelvic floor, following its descent when relaxed to allow defecation and urination, restoring its normal position. Further contraction occurs when the thoracic diaphragm and anterolateral abdominal wall muscles contract to compress the abdominal and pelvic contents. Therefore, it can resist the increased intra-abdominal pressure that would otherwise force the abdominopelvic contents (gas, solid and liquid wastes, and the viscera) through the pelvic outlet. This action occurs reflexively during forced expiration, coughing, sneezing, vomiting, and fixation of the trunk during strong movements of the upper limbs, as occurs when lifting a heavy object. The levator ani also has important functions in the voluntary control of urination, fecal continence (via the puborectalis), and support of the uterus.

Pelvic Fascia

The **pelvic fascia** is connective tissue that occupies the space between the membranous peritoneum and the muscular pelvic walls and floor not occupied by pelvic organs (Fig. 3.8). This "layer" is a continuation of the comparatively thin endoabdominal fascia that lies between the muscular abdominal walls and the peritoneum superiorly.

MEMBRANOUS PELVIC FASCIA: PARIETAL AND VISCERAL

The **parietal pelvic fascia** is a membranous layer of variable thickness that lines the internal (deep or pelvic) aspect of the muscles forming the walls and floor of the pelvis. The parietal pelvic fascia covers the pelvic surfaces of the obturator internus, piriformis, coccygeus, levator ani, and part of the urethral sphincter muscles (Fig. 3.8A–D). The name given to the fascia is derived from the muscle it encloses (e.g., obturator fascia). This layer is continuous superiorly with the transversalis and iliopsoas fascias.

The **visceral pelvic fascia** includes the membranous fascia that directly ensheathes the pelvic organs, forming the adventitial layer of each. The membranous parietal and visceral layers become continuous where the organs penetrate the pelvic floor (Fig. 3.8A,C,E). Here the parietal fascia thickens, forming the **tendinous arch of pelvic fascia,** a continuous bilateral band running from the pubis to the sacrum along the pelvic floor adjacent to the viscera.

The most anterior part of this tendinous arch (**puboprostatic ligament** in males; **pubovesical ligament** in females) connects the prostate to the pubis in the male or the fundus (base) of the bladder to the pubis in the female. The most posterior part of the band runs as the sacrogenital ligaments from the sacrum around the side of the rectum to attach to the prostate in the male or the vagina in the female.

ENDOPELVIC FASCIA: LOOSE AND CONDENSED

Usually, the abundant connective tissue remaining between the parietal and visceral membranous layers is considered part of the visceral fascia, but various authors label parts of it as parietal. It is probably more realistic to consider this remaining fascia simply as extraperitoneal or **subperitoneal endopelvic fascia** (Fig. 3.8A–D), which is continuous with both the parietal and the visceral membranous fascias.

Some of this fascia is extremely *loose areolar (fatty) tissue*, relatively devoid of all but minor lymphatics and nutrient vessels. The **retropubic** (or *prevesical*, extended posterolaterally as *paravesical*) and **retrorectal** (or *presacral*) **spaces** are *potential spaces* in the loose fatty tissue that accommodate the expansion of the urinary bladder and rectal ampulla as they fill (Fig. 3.8B,D). Other parts of the endopelvic fascia have a fibrous consistency, the *ligamentous fascia*. These parts are often described as "fascial condensations" or pelvic "ligaments."

The **hypogastric sheath** is a thick band of condensed pelvic fascia that gives passage to essentially all the vessels and nerves passing from the lateral wall of the pelvis to the pelvic viscera, along with the ureters and, in the male, the ductus deferens. As it extends medially from the lateral wall, the hypogastric sheath divides into three laminae ("leaflets" or "wings") that pass to or between the pelvic organs, conveying neurovascular structures and providing support. The three laminae of the hypogastric sheath, from anterior to posterior, are:

- The **lateral ligament of the bladder,** passing to the bladder, conveying the superior vesical arteries and veins.
- The middle lamina in the male, forming the **rectovesical septum** between the posterior surface of the bladder and the prostate anteriorly and the rectum posteriorly (Fig. 3.8D). In the female, the middle lamina is substantial and passes medially to the uterine cervix and vagina as the **cardinal ligament** (transverse cervical), also known clinically as the *lateral cervical* or *Mackenrodt ligament* (Fig. 3.8B,E). In its most superior portion, at the base of the broad ligament, the uterine artery runs transversely toward the cervix while the ureters course immediately inferior to them as they pass on each side of the cervix toward the bladder.
- The most posterior lamina passes to the rectum, conveying the middle rectal artery and vein (Fig. 3.8B,D).

The transverse cervical ligament, and the way in which the uterus normally "rests" on top of the bladder, provides the main passive support for the uterus. The bladder, in

Key

- ☐ Loose areolar fascia ⎱ Endopelvic
- ☐ Ligamentous fascia ⎰ fascia
- ── Visceral ⎱ Membranous fascia
- ── Parietal ⎰
- ── Peritoneum

A Anterior view of coronal section of female pelvis

- Endo-abdominal fascia
- Cervix
- Uterine artery
- Cardinal ligament
- Paracolpium
- Vagina
- Vestibule
- Obturator internus
- Obturator fascia
- Plane of section for **B** & **D**
- Visceral fascia
- Tendinous arch of levator ani
- Superior and inferior fascia of pelvic diaphragm
- Levator ani
- Tendinous arch of pelvic fascia
- External urethral sphincter

C Anterior view of coronal section of male pelvis

- Urinary bladder
- Prostate
- Prostatic urethra

B Superior view of transverse section of female pelvis

- Pubic bone
- Bladder
- Visceral fascia of bladder
- Paravesical space
- Obturator internus
- Obturator fascia
- Plane of (A)
- Cervix
- Recto-uterine space
- Retropubic (prevesical) space
- Obturator membrane
- Lateral ligament of bladder
- Ureter
- Paravesical space
- Rectovesical septum
- Cardinal ligament
- Hypogastric sheath
- Lateral ligament of rectum
- Visceral fascia of rectum
- Piriformis
- Sacrum
- Rectum
- Retrorectal (presacral) space

D Superior view of transverse section of male pelvis

- Pubic symphysis
- Retropubic (prevesical) space
- Visceral fascia of bladder
- Plane of (C)
- Ampulla of ductus deferens
- Seminal gland
- Lateral ligament of bladder
- Pelvirectal spaces

E Left anterolateral view

- *Location of ischial spine
- Uterosacral ligament
- Cervix
- Tendinous arch of levator ani
- Levator ani
- Pubic bones
- Rectum
- Cardinal (transverse cervical) ligament
- Bed of bladder (outlined)
- Paracolpium
- Neck of bladder
- Obturator internus muscle
- Tendinous arch of pelvic fascia
- Pubic symphysis
- Uterus

FIGURE 3.8. Pelvic fascia: endopelvic fascia and fascial ligaments.

turn, rests on the pubic bones and the symphysis uniting them anteriorly, and on the anterior wall of the vagina posteriorly (Fig. 3.8E). The vagina, in turn, is suspended between the tendinous arches of the pelvic fascia by the **paracolpium** (Fig. 3.8A,E). In addition to this *passive support*, the perineal muscles provide *dynamic support* for the uterus, bladder, and rectum by contracting during moments of increased intra-abdominal pressure.

There are surgically important potential **pelvirectal spaces** in the loose extraperitoneal connective tissue superior to the pelvic diaphragm. The spaces are divided into anterior and posterior regions by the **lateral rectal ligaments** (rectal stalks), which are the posterior laminae of the hypogastric sheaths. These ligaments connect the rectum to the parietal pelvic fascia at the S2–S4 levels (Fig. 3.8B,D).

Pelvic Nerves

Pelvic structures are innervated mainly by the **sacral** (S1–S4) and **coccygeal spinal nerves** and the *pelvic part of the autonomic nervous system*. The piriformis and coccygeus muscles form a bed for the sacral and coccygeal nerve plexuses (Fig. 3.9C,D). The anterior rami of the S2 and S3 nerves emerge between the digitations of these muscles. The descending part of the anterior ramus of L4 nerve unites with the anterior ramus of the L5 nerve to form the thick, cord-like **lumbosacral trunk.** It passes inferiorly, anterior to the ala of the sacrum to join the sacral plexus.

SACRAL PLEXUS

The **sacral plexus** is located on the posterolateral wall of the lesser pelvis, where it is closely related to the anterior surface of the piriformis. The two main nerves of the sacral plexus are the *sciatic* and *pudendal.* Most branches of the sacral plexus leave the pelvis through the *greater sciatic foramen* (Fig. 3.9A).

The **sciatic nerve,** the largest nerve in the body, is formed by the anterior rami of spinal nerves L4–S3 (Fig. 3.9; Table 3.4). The anterior rami converge on the anterior surface of the piriformis. Most commonly, the sciatic nerve passes through the *greater sciatic foramen* inferior to the piriformis to enter the gluteal (buttock) region.

The **pudendal nerve** is the main nerve of the perineum and the chief sensory nerve of the external genitalia. It is derived from the anterior rami of spinal nerves S2–S4. It accompanies the internal pudendal artery and leaves the pelvis through the greater sciatic foramen between the piriformis and the coccygeus muscles. The pudendal nerve hooks around the ischial spine and sacrospinous ligament and enters the perineum through the lesser sciatic foramen. It supplies the skin and muscles of the perineum.

The **superior gluteal nerve** arises from the anterior rami of spinal nerves L4–S1 and leaves the pelvis through the greater sciatic foramen, superior to the piriformis. It supplies three muscles in the gluteal region: the gluteus medius and minimus and the tensor fasciae latae (see Chapter 5).

The **inferior gluteal nerve** arises from the anterior rami of spinal nerves L5–S2 and leaves the pelvis through the greater sciatic foramen, inferior to the piriformis and superficial to the sciatic nerve. It accompanies the inferior gluteal artery and breaks up into several branches that supply the overlying gluteus maximus muscle (see Chapter 5).

COCCYGEAL PLEXUS

The **coccygeal plexus** is a small network of nerve fibers formed by the anterior rami of spinal nerves S4 and S5 and the **coccygeal nerves** (Fig. 3.9B). It lies on the pelvic surface of the coccygeus and supplies this muscle, part of the levator ani, and the sacrococcygeal joint. The **anococcygeal nerves** arising from this plexus pierce the sacrotuberous ligament and supply a small area of skin between the tip of the coccyx and the anus (Fig. 3.9D).

Injury to Pelvic Floor

During childbirth, the pelvic floor supports the fetal head while the cervix of the uterus is dilating to permit delivery of the fetus. The perineum, levator ani, and pelvic fascia may be injured during childbirth. It is the pubococcygeus, the main, intermediate part of the levator ani, that is usually torn (Fig. B3.1). This part of the muscle is important because it encircles and supports the urethra, vagina, and anal canal. Weakening of the levator ani and pelvic fascia resulting from stretching or tearing during childbirth may alter the position of the neck of the bladder and urethra. These changes may cause *urinary stress incontinence,* characterized by dribbling of urine when intra-abdominal pressure is raised during coughing and lifting, for instance.

Tear of pubococcygeus

FIGURE B3.1.

OBTURATOR NERVE

Although it passes through the pelvis, the obturator nerve is not a "pelvic nerve," but is rather the primary nerve to the medial thigh. It arises from the lumbar plexus (anterior rami of spinal nerves L2–L4) in the abdomen (greater pelvis) and enters the lesser pelvis (Fig. 3.9C,D). It runs in the extraperitoneal fat along the lateral wall of the pelvis to the obturator canal, the opening in the obturator membrane, where it exits the pelvis and enters the medial thigh.

Injury to Pelvic Nerves

During childbirth, the fetal head may compress the mother's sacral plexus, producing pain in her lower limbs. The obturator nerve is vulnerable to injury during surgery (e.g., during removal of cancerous lymph nodes from the lateral pelvic wall). *Injury to the obturator nerve* may cause painful spasms of the adductor muscles of the thigh and sensory deficits in the medial thigh region (see Chapter 5).

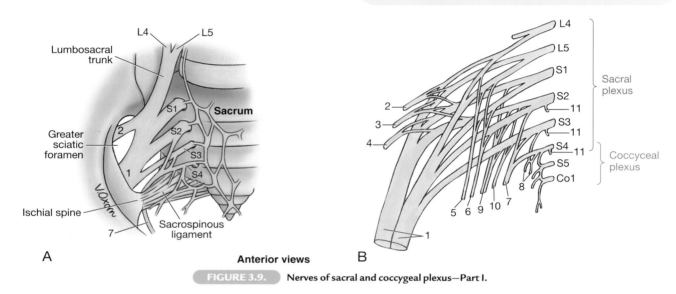

FIGURE 3.9. Nerves of sacral and coccygeal plexus—Part I.

TABLE 3.4 NERVES OF SACRAL AND COCCYGEAL PLEXUSES

Nerve[a]	Segmental Origin (Anterior Rami)	Distribution
1 Sciatic	L4, L5, S1, S2, S3	Articular branches to hip joint and muscular branches to flexors of knee (hamstring muscles), and all muscles in leg and foot
2 Superior gluteal	L4, L5, S1	Gluteus medius, gluteus minimus, and tensor fasciae latae muscles
3 Inferior gluteal	L5, S1, S2	Gluteus maximus muscle
4 Nerve to piriformis	S1, S2	Piriformis muscle
5 Nerve to quadratus femoris and inferior gemellus	L4, L5, S1	Quadratus femoris and inferior gemellus muscles
6 Nerve to obturator internus and superior gemellus	L5, S1, S2	Obturator internus and superior gemellus muscles
7 Pudendal	S2, S3, S4	Structures in perineum: sensory to genitalia, muscular branches to perineal muscles, sphincter urethrae, and external anal sphincter
8 Nerves to levator ani and coccygeus	S3, S4	Levator ani and coccygeus muscles
9 Posterior femoral cutaneous	S2, S3	Cutaneous branches to buttock and uppermost medial and posterior surfaces of thigh
10 Perforating cutaneous	S2, S3	Cutaneous branches to medial part of buttock
11 Pelvic splanchnic	S2, S3, S4	Pelvic viscera via inferior hypogastric and pelvic plexus

[a]Numbers refer to Figure 3.9.

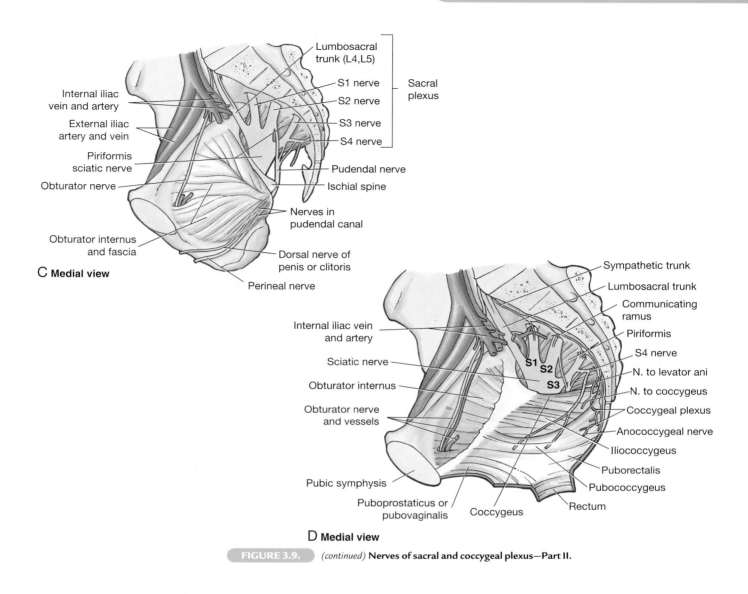

C Medial view

D Medial view

FIGURE 3.9. *(continued)* **Nerves of sacral and coccygeal plexus—Part II.**

PELVIC AUTONOMIC NERVES

Autonomic innervation of the pelvic cavity is via four routes: the *sacral sympathetic trunks, periarterial plexuses, hypogastric plexuses,* and *pelvic splanchnic nerves.*

The **sacral sympathetic trunks** are the inferior continuations of the lumbar sympathetic trunks (Fig. 3.9A,C,D). Each sacral trunk usually has four sympathetic ganglia. The sacral trunks descend on the pelvic surface of the sacrum just medial to the pelvic sacral foramina, and commonly converge to form the small median **ganglion impar** anterior to the coccyx (Fig. 3.10). The sympathetic trunks descend posterior to the rectum in the extraperitoneal connective tissue and send communicating branches, gray rami communicantes, to each of the anterior rami of the sacral and coccygeal nerves. They also send branches to the median sacral artery and the inferior hypogastric plexus. The primary function of the sacral

sympathetic trunks is to provide postsynaptic fibers to the sacral plexus for sympathetic innervation of the lower limb.

The **periarterial plexuses** of the superior rectal, ovarian, and internal iliac arteries provide postsynaptic, sympathetic, vasomotor fibers to each of the arteries and its derivative branches.

The **hypogastric plexuses** (superior and inferior) are networks of sympathetic and visceral afferent nerve fibers. The main part of the **superior hypogastric plexus** lies just inferior to the bifurcation of the aorta and descends into the pelvis. This plexus is the inferior prolongation of the **intermesenteric plexus** (see Chapter 2), which also receives the L3 and L4 splanchnic nerves. The superior hypogastric plexus enter the pelvis, dividing into **left** and **right hypogastric nerves,** which descend anterior to the sacrum. These nerves descend lateral to the rectum within

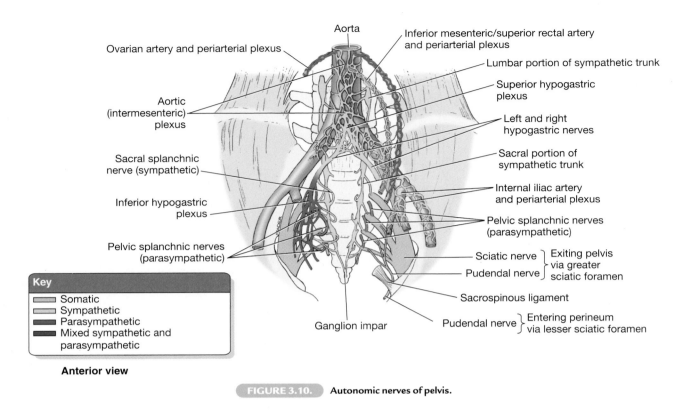

Aorta

Ovarian artery and periarterial plexus

Inferior mesenteric/superior rectal artery and periarterial plexus

Aortic (intermesenteric) plexus

Lumbar portion of sympathetic trunk

Superior hypogastric plexus

Sacral splanchnic nerve (sympathetic)

Left and right hypogastric nerves

Inferior hypogastric plexus

Sacral portion of sympathetic trunk

Internal iliac artery and periarterial plexus

Pelvic splanchnic nerves (parasympathetic)

Pelvic splanchnic nerves (parasympathetic)

Sciatic nerve ⎱ Exiting pelvis
Pudendal nerve ⎰ via greater sciatic foramen

Sacrospinous ligament

Ganglion impar

Pudendal nerve ⎱ Entering perineum
⎰ via lesser sciatic foramen

Key
- Somatic
- Sympathetic
- Parasympathetic
- Mixed sympathetic and parasympathetic

Anterior view

FIGURE 3.10. Autonomic nerves of pelvis.

the *hypogastric sheaths* and then spread as they merge with pelvic splanchnic nerves (parasympathetic) to form the **right** and **left inferior hypogastric plexuses.** Sub-plexuses of the inferior hypogastric plexuses, **pelvic plexuses,** in both sexes pass to the lateral surfaces of the rectum and to the inferolateral surfaces of the urinary bladder, and in males to the prostate and seminal glands (vesicles) and in females to the cervix of the uterus and lateral parts of the fornix of the vagina.

The **pelvic splanchnic nerves** contain presynaptic parasympathetic and visceral afferent fibers derived from the S2–S4 spinal cord segments and visceral afferent fibers from cell bodies in the spinal ganglia of the corresponding spinal nerves (Figs. 3.9B and 3.10; Table 3.4). The pelvic splanchnic nerves merge with the hypogastric nerves to form the inferior hypogastric (and pelvic) plexuses.

The **hypogastric/pelvic system of plexuses,** receiving sympathetic fibers via the lumbar splanchnic nerves and parasympathetic fibers via the pelvic splanchnic nerves, innervates the pelvic viscera. The **sympathetic component** produces vasomotion, inhibits peristaltic contraction of the rectum, and stimulates contraction of the genital organs during orgasm (producing ejaculation in the male). The **parasympathetic fibers** stimulate contraction of the rectum and bladder for defecation and urination, respectively. Parasympathetic fibers in the prostatic plexus penetrate the pelvic floor to supply the erectile bodies of the external genitalia, producing erection.

VISCERAL AFFERENT INNERVATION IN PELVIS

Visceral afferent fibers travel with the autonomic nerve fibers, although the sensory impulses are conducted centrally retrograde to the efferent impulses. In the pelvis, visceral afferent fibers conducting *reflexive sensation* (information that does not reach consciousness) travel with parasympathetic fibers to the spinal sensory ganglia of S2–S4. The route taken by visceral afferent fibers conducting *pain sensation* differs in relationship to an imaginary line, the **pelvic pain line,** that corresponds to the inferior limit of peritoneum (Fig. 3.6B, C), except in the case of the large intenstine, where the pain line occurs midway along the length of the sigmoid colon. Visceral afferent fibers that transmit pain sensations from the viscera *inferior to the pelvic pain line* (structures that do not contact the peritoneum, and the distal sigmoid colon and rectum) also travel with parasympathetic fibers to the spinal ganglia of S2–S4. However, visceral afferent fiber conducting pain from the viscera *superior to the pelvic pain line* (structures in contact with the peritoneum, except for the distal sigmoid colon and rectum) follow the sympathetic fibers retrogradely to inferior thoracic and superior lumbar spinal ganglia.

Pelvic Arteries and Veins

Four main arteries enter the lesser pelvis in females, three in males:

- The paired **internal iliac arteries** deliver the most blood to the lesser pelvis (Fig. 3.11A,D). They bifurcate into an

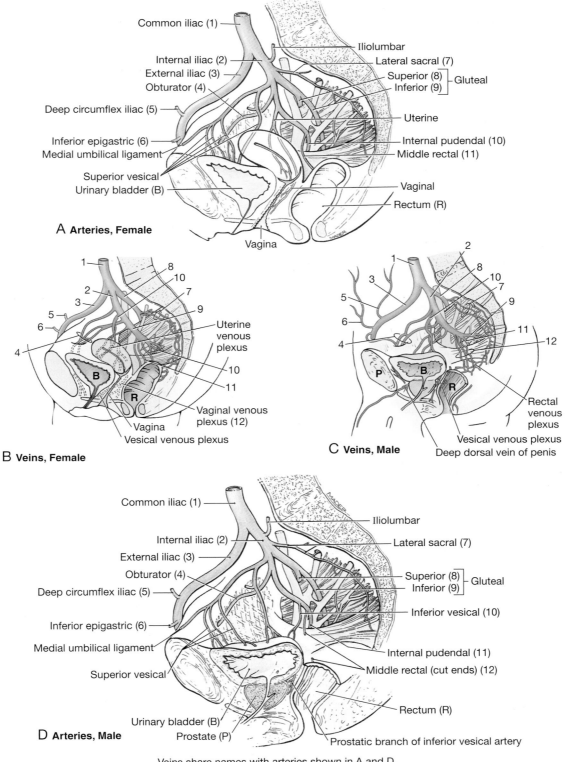

A Arteries, Female

Common iliac (1)
Internal iliac (2)
External iliac (3)
Obturator (4)
Deep circumflex iliac (5)
Inferior epigastric (6)
Medial umbilical ligament
Superior vesical
Urinary bladder (B)

Iliolumbar
Lateral sacral (7)
Superior (8)
Inferior (9) Gluteal
Uterine
Internal pudendal (10)
Middle rectal (11)
Vaginal
Rectum (R)
Vagina

B Veins, Female

1
8
10
2
7
3
9
5
6
4
B
R
Vagina
Vesical venous plexus

Uterine venous plexus
10
11
Vaginal venous plexus (12)

C Veins, Male

1
2
3
8
10
5
7
6
9
4
11
P   B
12
R

Rectal venous plexus
Vesical venous plexus
Deep dorsal vein of penis

D Arteries, Male

Common iliac (1)
Internal iliac (2)
External iliac (3)
Obturator (4)
Deep circumflex iliac (5)
Inferior epigastric (6)
Medial umbilical ligament
Superior vesical
Urinary bladder (B)
Prostate (P)

Iliolumbar
Lateral sacral (7)
Superior (8)
Inferior (9) Gluteal
Inferior vesical (10)
Internal pudendal (11)
Middle rectal (cut ends) (12)
Rectum (R)
Prostatic branch of inferior vesical artery

Veins share names with arteries shown in A and D.

Median section

FIGURE 3.11.   Arteries and veins of pelvis.

TABLE 3.5 ARTERIES OF PELVIS

Artery	Origin	Course	Distribution
Internal iliac	Common iliac artery	Passes over pelvic brim to reach pelvic cavity	Main blood supply to pelvic organs, gluteal muscles, and perineum
Anterior division of internal iliac artery	Internal iliac artery	Passes anteriorly and divides into visceral branches and obturator artery	Pelvic viscera and muscles in medial compartment of thigh
Umbilical	Anterior division of internal iliac artery	Short pelvic course; obliterates after origin of superior vesical artery	Via superior vesical artery
Obturator		Runs anteroinferiorly on lateral pelvic wall	Pelvic muscles, nutrient artery to ilium, and head of femur
Superior vesical artery	Patent part of umbilical artery	Passes to superior aspect of urinary bladder	Superior aspect of urinary bladder; often ductus deferens in male
Artery to ductus deferens	Superior or inferior vesical artery	Runs retroperitoneally to ductus deferens	Ductus deferens
Inferior vesical[a]	Anterior division of internal iliac artery	Passes retroperitoneally to inferior aspect of male urinary bladder	Urinary bladder, pelvic part of ureter, seminal gland, and prostate
Middle rectal		Descends in pelvis to rectum	Seminal gland, prostate, and rectum
Internal pudendal		Leaves pelvis through greater sciatic foramen and enters perineum (ischio-anal fossa) by passing through lesser sciatic foramen	Main artery to perineum, including muscles of anal canal and perineum; skin and urogenital triangle; erectile bodies
Inferior gluteal		Leaves pelvis through greater sciatic foramen inferior to piriformis	Piriformis, coccygeus, levator ani, and gluteal muscles
Uterine		Runs medially on levator ani; crosses ureter to reach base of broad ligament	Pelvic part of ureter, uterus, ligament of uterus, uterine tube, and vagina
Vaginal	Uterine artery	At junction of body and cervix of uterus, it descends to vagina	Vagina and branches to inferior part of urinary bladder
Gonadal (testicular and ovarian)	Abdominal aorta	Descends retroperitoneally; testicular artery passes into deep inguinal ring; ovarian artery crosses brim of pelvis and runs medially in suspensory ligament to ovary	Testis and ovary, respectively
Posterior division of internal iliac artery	Internal iliac artery	Passes posteriorly and gives rise to parietal branches	Pelvic wall and gluteal region
Iliolumbar	Posterior division of internal iliac artery	Ascends anterior to sacro-iliac joint and posterior to common iliac vessels and psoas major	Iliacus, psoas major, quadratus lumborum muscles, and cauda equina in vertebral canal
Lateral sacral (superior and inferior)		Run on superficial aspect of piriformis	Piriformis and vertebral canal
Superior gluteal		Leaves pelvis through greater sciatic foramen, superior to piriformis	Gluteal muscles and tensor fasciae latae

[a]Often arises from posterior division of internal iliac artery

anterior division and a posterior division, providing the visceral branches and parietal branches, respectively.

- The paired **ovarian arteries.**
- The **median sacral artery.**
- The **superior rectal artery.**

The origin, course, and distribution of these arteries and their branches are summarized in Table 3.5.

The pelvis is drained by the following:

- Mainly, the **internal iliac veins** and their tributaries.
- Superior rectal veins (see portal venous system, Chapter 2).
- Median sacral vein.
- Gonadal veins.
- Internal vertebral venous plexus (see Chapter 4).

Pelvic venous plexuses are formed by the interjoining of veins in the pelvis (Fig. 3.11B,C). The various plexuses (rectal, vesical, prostatic, uterine, and vaginal) unite and drain mainly into the **internal iliac vein,** but some drain through the superior rectal vein into the inferior mesenteric vein or through lateral sacral veins into the internal vertebral venous plexus.

Lymph Nodes of Pelvis

The lymph nodes draining pelvic organs are variable in number, size, and location. They are somewhat arbitrarily divided into four primary groups of nodes named for the blood vessels with which they are associated (Fig. 3.12):

- **External iliac lymph nodes** receive lymph mainly from the inguinal lymph nodes; however, they also receive lymph from pelvic viscera, especially the superior parts of the anterior pelvic organs. Whereas most of the lymphatic drainage from the pelvis tends to parallel routes of venous drainage, the lymphatic drainage to the external iliac nodes does not. These nodes drain into the common iliac nodes.
- **Internal iliac lymph nodes** receive drainage from the inferior pelvic viscera, deep perineum, and gluteal region and drain into the common iliac nodes.
- **Sacral lymph nodes,** in the concavity of the sacrum, receive lymph from posteroinferior pelvic viscera and drain either to internal or to common iliac nodes.
- **Common iliac lymph nodes** receive drainage from the three main groups listed above. These nodes begin a common route for drainage from the pelvis that passes next to the lumbar (caval/aortic) nodes.

Additional minor groups of nodes (e.g., the **pararectal nodes**) occupy the connective tissue along the branches of the internal iliac vessels.

Both primary and minor groups of pelvic nodes are highly interconnected, so that many nodes can be removed without disturbing drainage. This also allows cancer to spread in virtually any direction, to any pelvic or abdominal viscus. The drainage pattern is not sufficiently predictable to allow the progress of metastatic cancer from pelvic organs to be reliably staged in a manner comparable to that of breast cancer.

PELVIC VISCERA

The pelvic viscera include the inferior part of the intestinal tract (rectum), the urinary bladder, and parts of the ureters and reproductive system (Figs. 3.13–3.15). Although the sigmoid colon and parts of the small bowel extend into the pelvic cavity, they are mobile at their abdominal attachments; therefore, they are abdominal rather than pelvic viscera.

Urinary Organs

The pelvic urinary organs are the (Fig. 3.13):

- Ureters, which carry urine from the kidneys.
- Urinary bladder, which temporarily stores urine.
- Urethra, which conducts urine from the urinary bladder to the exterior.

URETERS

The **ureters** are retroperitoneal muscular tubes that connect the kidneys to the urinary bladder. Urine is transported down the ureters by peristaltic contractions. The ureters run inferiorly from the kidneys, passing over the pelvic brim at

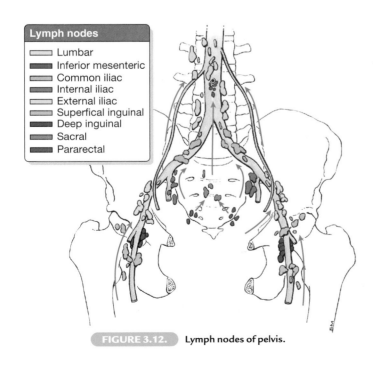

Lymph nodes
- Lumbar
- Inferior mesenteric
- Common iliac
- Internal iliac
- External iliac
- Superfical inguinal
- Deep inguinal
- Sacral
- Pararectal

FIGURE 3.12. Lymph nodes of pelvis.

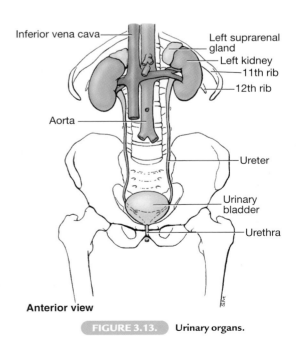

Inferior vena cava
Left suprarenal gland
Left kidney
11th rib
12th rib
Aorta
Ureter
Urinary bladder
Urethra

Anterior view

FIGURE 3.13. Urinary organs.

Common iliac vein and artery

Ureter

External iliac artery and vein

Cut edge of peritoneum

Ductus deferens

Inferior vesical artery

Retropubic space

Puboprostatic ligament

Dorsal vein of penis

Urethra

Corpus cavernosum

Corpus spongiosum

Glans penis

External urethral orifice

Bifurcation of common iliac artery

Internal iliac artery and vein

Sciatic nerve

Ampulla of ductus deferens

Urinary bladder

Rectum

Coccyx

PS

Internal urethral orifice

P P

Ejaculatory duct

Perineal membrane

External anal sphincter

Internal anal sphincter

Bulb of penis

Testis

Scrotum

Median section

FIGURE 3.14.   **Male pelvis.** *P,* prostate; *PS,* pubic symphysis.

Common iliac vein and artery

Ureter

Ovarian vessels

Cut edge of peritoneum

External iliac artery

Round ligament of uterus

Linea alba

Apex of bladder

Retropubic space

Internal urethral orifice

Pubovesical ligament

Urethra

External urethral orifice

Vestibule of vagina

Labium minus

Labium majus

Sacrum

Internal iliac artery

Posterior fornix of vagina

SN

Uterus

O

Urinary bladder

C C

Rectum

Coccyx

Fundus of bladder

Neck of bladder

PS

Levator ani m.

External anal sphincter

Internal anal sphincter

Vagina

Perineal membrane

Median section

FIGURE 3.15.   **Female pelvis.** *C,* cervix of uterus; *O,* ovary; *PS,* pubic symphysis; *SN,* sciatic nerve; *UT,* uterine tube.

the bifurcation of the common iliac arteries (Figs. 3.14 and 3.15). The ureters then run posteroinferiorly on the lateral walls of the pelvis, and anterior to the internal iliac arteries. Opposite the ischial spine, they curve anteromedially, superior to the levator ani, to enter the urinary bladder. The ureters pass inferomedially through the muscular wall of the urinary bladder. This oblique passage through the bladder wall forms a one-way "flap valve"; the internal pressure of the filling bladder causes the intramural passage to collapse. In males, the only structure that passes between the ureter and the peritoneum is the *ductus deferens*. The ureter lies posterolateral to the ductus deferens and enters the posterosuperior angle of the bladder (Fig. 3.14). In females, the ureter passes medial to the origin of the uterine artery and continues to the level of the ischial spine, where it is crossed superiorly by the uterine artery (Fig. 3.15). The ureter then passes close to the lateral part of the fornix of the vagina and enters the posterosuperior angle of the bladder.

Vasculature of Ureters. Branches of the common and internal iliac arteries supply the pelvic part of the ureters (Fig. 3.16). The most constant arteries supplying this part of the ureters in females are branches of the **uterine arteries.** The sources of similar branches in males are the **inferior vesical arteries.** Veins from the ureters accompany the arteries and have corresponding names. **Lymph** drains into the lumbar (caval/aortic), common iliac, external iliac, and internal iliac lymph nodes (Fig. 3.12).

Innervation of Ureters. The nerves to the ureters derive from adjacent autonomic plexuses (renal, aortic, superior and inferior hypogastric). The ureters are superior to the pelvic pain line (Figs. 3.6 and 3.24); therefore, afferent (pain) fibers from the ureters follow sympathetic fibers retrogradely to reach the spinal ganglia and spinal cord segments T11–L1 or L2 (Fig. 3.17).

Ureteric Calculi

Ureteric calculi (stones) may cause complete or intermittent *obstruction of urinary flow*. The obstruction may occur anywhere along the ureter; however, it occurs most often where the ureters are relatively constricted: (1) at the junction of the ureters and renal pelvis, (2) where they cross the external iliac artery and the pelvic brim, and (3) where they pass through the wall of the bladder. The severity of the pain associated with calculi can be extremely intense; it depends on the location, type, size, and texture of the calculus. Ureteric calculi can be removed by open surgery, endoscopy, or **lithotripsy** (shock waves are used to break the stones into small fragments that can be passed in the urine).

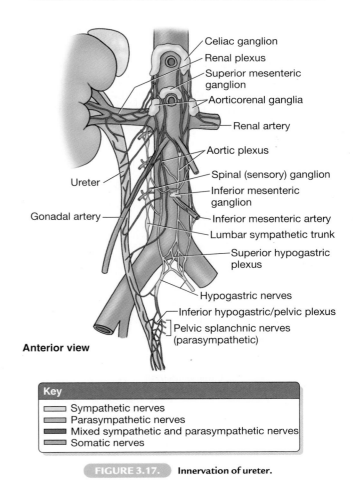

Celiac ganglion
Renal plexus
Superior mesenteric ganglion
Aorticorenal ganglia
Renal artery
Aortic plexus
Spinal (sensory) ganglion
Inferior mesenteric ganglion
Inferior mesenteric artery
Lumbar sympathetic trunk
Superior hypogastric plexus
Hypogastric nerves
Inferior hypogastric/pelvic plexus
Pelvic splanchnic nerves (parasympathetic)

Ureter
Gonadal artery

Anterior view

Key	
▭	Sympathetic nerves
▭	Parasympathetic nerves
▭	Mixed sympathetic and parasympathetic nerves
▭	Somatic nerves

From renal artery
From gonadal artery
From aorta
From common iliac artery
From internal iliac artery
From superior vesical artery
From uterine artery (F)
From middle rectal artery
From vaginal artery (F)
From inferior vesical artery (M)

Anterior view

FIGURE 3.16.   **Arterial supply of ureter.** F = female, M = male.

FIGURE 3.17.   **Innervation of ureter.**

URINARY BLADDER

The **urinary bladder,** a hollow viscus with strong muscular walls, is in the lesser pelvis when empty, posterior and slightly superior to the pubic bones. It is separated from these bones by the *retropubic space* and lies inferior to the peritoneum, where it rests on the pelvic floor (Figs. 3.18–3.20). The bladder is relatively free within the extraperitoneal subcutaneous fatty tissue, except for its neck, which is held firmly by the lateral ligaments of the bladder and the tendinous arch of pelvic fascia, especially the *puboprostatic ligament* in males and the *pubovesical ligament* in females. As the bladder fills, it ascends superiorly into the extraperitoneal fatty tissue of the anterior abdominal wall and enters the greater pelvis. A full bladder may ascend to the level of the umbilicus.

When empty the bladder is somewhat tetrahedral and externally has an apex, body, fundus, and neck. The four surfaces are a superior surface, two inferolateral surfaces, and a posterior surface (Fig. 3.19). The **apex of the bladder** (anterior end) points toward the superior edge of the pubic symphysis. The **fundus of the bladder** is opposite the apex, formed by the somewhat convex posterior wall. The **body of the bladder** is the part between the apex and the fundus. *In females,* the fundus is closely related to the anterior wall of the vagina; *in males,* it is related to the rectum. The **neck of the bladder** is where the fundus and inferolateral surfaces converge inferiorly.

The **bladder bed** is formed on each side by the pubic bones and the fascia covering the obturator internus and levator ani muscles and posteriorly by the rectum or vagina (Figs 3.19 and 3.20). The bladder is enveloped by loose connective tissue, the vesical fascia. Only the superior surface is covered by peritoneum.

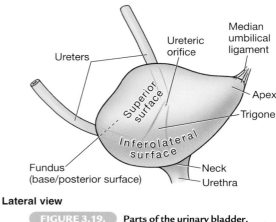

Lateral view

FIGURE 3.19.   Parts of the urinary bladder.

The walls of the bladder are composed chiefly of the **detrusor muscle** (Fig. 3.20A). Toward the neck of the male bladder, its muscle fibers form the involuntary **internal urethral sphincter.** This sphincter contracts during ejaculation to prevent retrograde ejaculation of semen into the bladder. Some fibers run radially and assist in opening the **internal urethral orifice.** In males, the muscle fibers in the neck of the bladder are continuous with the fibromuscular tissue of the prostate, whereas in females, these fibers are continuous with muscle fibers in the wall of the urethra.

The **ureteric orifices** and the internal urethral orifice are at the angles of the **trigone of the bladder.** The ureteric orifices are encircled by loops of detrusor musculature that tighten when the bladder contracts to assist in preventing reflux of urine into the bladder. The **uvula of the bladder** is a slight elevation of the trigone in the internal urethral orifice.

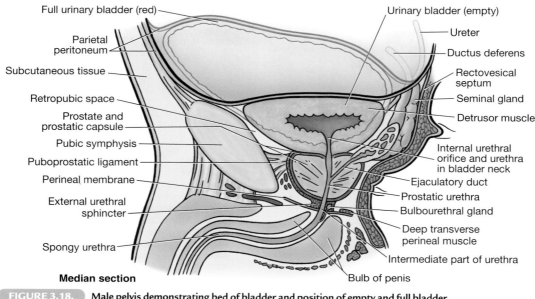

Median section

FIGURE 3.18.   Male pelvis demonstrating bed of bladder and position of empty and full bladder.

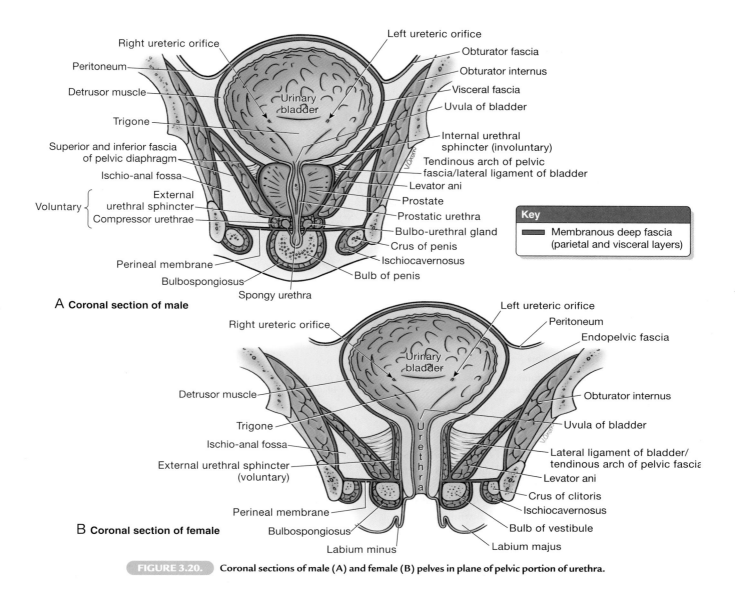

FIGURE 3.20.   Coronal sections of male (A) and female (B) pelves in plane of pelvic portion of urethra.

Vasculature of Bladder. The main arteries supplying the bladder are branches of the **internal iliac arteries** (Fig. 3.11A,D; Table 3.5). The *superior vesical arteries* supply the anterosuperior parts of the bladder. In males, the fundus and neck of the bladder are supplied by the *inferior vesical arteries* (Fig. 3.21). In females, the inferior vesical arteries are replaced by the *vaginal arteries,* which send small branches to the posteroinferior parts of the bladder. The obturator and inferior gluteal arteries also supply small branches to the bladder.

The names of the **veins draining the bladder** correspond to the arteries and are tributaries of the internal iliac veins. In males, the *vesical venous plexus* is continuous with the *prostatic venous plexus* (Fig. 3.21), and the combined plexus envelops the fundus of the bladder and prostate, the

seminal glands, the ductus deferentes (plural of ductus deferens), and the inferior ends of the ureters. The prostatic venous plexus also receives blood from the *deep dorsal vein of the penis.* The *vesical venous plexus* mainly drains through the inferior vesical veins into the internal iliac veins (Fig. 3.11B,C); however, it may drain through the sacral veins into the *internal vertebral venous plexuses* (see Chapter 4).

In females, the vesical venous plexus envelops the pelvic part of the urethra and the neck of the bladder, receives blood from the *dorsal vein of the clitoris,* and communicates with the *vaginal or uterovaginal venous plexus* (Fig. 3.11B).

In both sexes, **lymphatic vessels** leave the superior surface of the bladder and pass to the *external iliac lymph nodes* (Figs. 3.22 and 3.23; Tables 3.6 and 3.7), whereas those from

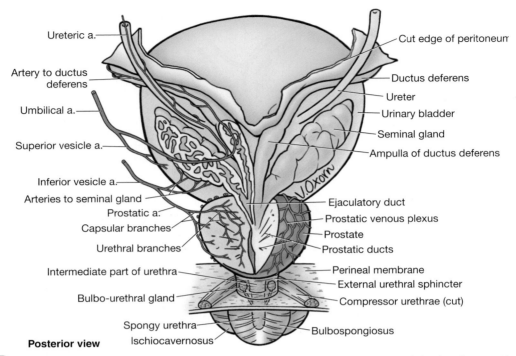

Ureteric a.

Artery to ductus deferens

Umbilical a.

Superior vesicle a.

Inferior vesicle a.
Arteries to seminal gland
Prostatic a.
Capsular branches
Urethral branches

Intermediate part of urethra

Bulbo-urethral gland

Spongy urethra
Ischiocavernosus

Posterior view

Cut edge of peritoneum

Ductus deferens
Ureter
Urinary bladder
Seminal gland
Ampulla of ductus deferens

Ejaculatory duct
Prostatic venous plexus
Prostate
Prostatic ducts
Perineal membrane
External urethral sphincter
Compressor urethrae (cut)

Bulbospongiosus

FIGURE 3.21. **Male pelvic genitourinary organs.** On the left side, the ampulla of ductus deferens, seminal gland, and prostate have been sectioned to the midline in a coronal plane, and the arterial supply to these structures and the bladder is demonstrated.

the fundus pass to the *internal iliac lymph nodes.* Some vessels from the neck of the bladder drain into the sacral or common iliac lymph nodes.

Innervation of Bladder. Sympathetic fibers to the bladder are conveyed from the T11–L2 or L3 spinal cord levels to the vesical (pelvic) plexuses, primarily through the hypogastric plexuses and nerves, whereas parasympathetic fibers from the sacral spinal cord levels are conveyed by the pelvic splanchnic nerves and the inferior hypogastric plexuses (Fig. 3.24). *Parasympathetic fibers* are motor to the detrusor muscle in the bladder wall and inhibitory to the internal sphincter of males. Hence, when the visceral afferent fibers are stimulated by stretching, the bladder contracts, the internal sphincter relaxes in males, and urine flows into the urethra. Adults suppress this reflex until it is convenient to void. The sympathetic innervation that stimulates ejaculation simultaneously causes contraction of the internal urethral sphincter, to prevent reflux of semen into the bladder.

Sensory fibers from the bladder are visceral; reflex afferents and pain afferents (e.g., from overdistention) from the inferior part of the bladder follow the course of the parasympathetic fibers. The superior surface of the bladder is covered with peritoneum and is, therefore, superior to the pain line; thus, pain fibers from the superior part of the bladder follow the sympathetic fibers retrogradely.

Suprapubic Cystotomy

 As the bladder fills, it extends superiorly in the extraperitoneal fatty tissue of the anterior abdominal wall (Fig. 3.18). The bladder then lies adjacent to this wall without the intervention of peritoneum. Consequently, the distended bladder may be punctured (*suprapubic cystostomy*) or approached surgically for the introduction of indwelling catheters or instruments without traversing the peritoneum and entering the peritoneal cavity.

Rupture of Bladder

 Because of the superior position of a distended bladder, it may be ruptured by injuries to the inferior part of the anterior abdominal wall or by fractures of the pelvis. The rupture of the superior part of the bladder frequently tears the peritoneum, resulting in passage (extravasation) of urine into the peritoneal cavity. Posterior rupture of the bladder usually results in passage of urine subperitoneally into the perineum.

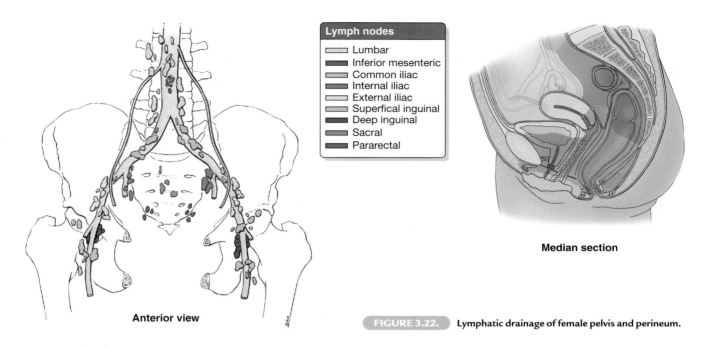

Lymph nodes
- Lumbar
- Inferior mesenteric
- Common iliac
- Internal iliac
- External iliac
- Superficial inguinal
- Deep inguinal
- Sacral
- Pararectal

Anterior view

Median section

FIGURE 3.22. Lymphatic drainage of female pelvis and perineum.

TABLE 3.6 LYMPHATIC DRAINAGE OF FEMALE PELVIS AND PERINEUM

Lymph Node Group	Typically Drains
Lumbar (along ovarian vessels)	Gonads and associated structures, common iliac nodes (ovary, uterine tube except isthmus and intrauterine parts, fundus of uterus)
Inferior mesenteric	Superiormost rectum, sigmoid colon, descending colon, pararectal nodes
Internal iliac	Inferior pelvic structures, deep perineal structures, sacral nodes (base of bladder, inferior pelvic ureter, anal canal above pectinate line, inferior rectum, middle and upper vagina, cervix, body of uterus)
External iliac	Anterosuperior pelvic structures, deep inguinal nodes (superior bladder, superior pelvic ureter, upper vagina, cervix, lower body of uterus)
Superficial inguinal	Lower limb; superficial drainage of inferolateral quadrant of trunk, including anterior abdominal wall inferior to umbilicus, gluteal region, superficial perineal structures (superolateral uterus near attachment of round ligament, skin of perineum including vulva, ostium of vagina inferior to hymen, prepuce of clitoris, perianal skin, anal canal inferior to pectinate line)
Deep inguinal	Glans clitoris, superficial inguinal nodes
Sacral	Posteroinferior pelvic structures, inferior rectum, inferior vagina
Pararectal	Superior rectum

Cystoscopy

The interior of the bladder and its three orifices can be examined with a *cystoscope,* a lighted tubular endoscope that is inserted through the urethra into the bladder. The cystoscope consists of a light; an observing lens; and various attachments for grasping, removing, cutting, and cauterizing (Fig. B3.2).

Urinary bladder

Cytoscope in urethra

Prostate

Rectum

Sagittal section

FIGURE B3.2.

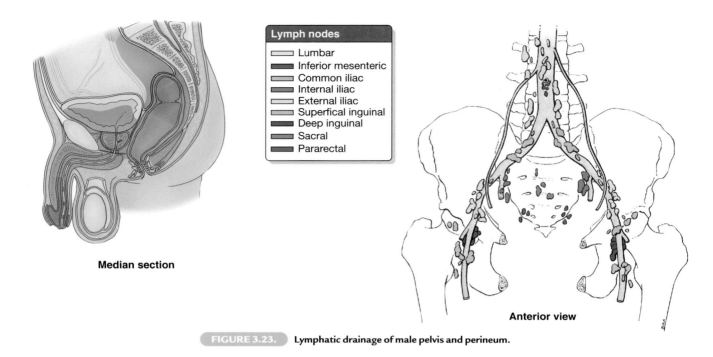

Lymph nodes
- Lumbar
- Inferior mesenteric
- Common iliac
- Internal iliac
- External iliac
- Superfical inguinal
- Deep inguinal
- Sacral
- Pararectal

Median section

Anterior view

FIGURE 3.23.   Lymphatic drainage of male pelvis and perineum.

TABLE 3.7   LYMPHATIC DRAINAGE OF MALE PELVIS AND PERINEUM

Lymph Node Group	Typically Drains
Lumbar along testicular vessels	Urethra, testis, epididymis
Inferior mesenteric	Superiormost rectum, sigmoid colon, descending colon, pararectal nodes
Internal iliac	External and internal iliac lymph nodes
External iliac	Inferior pelvic structures, deep perineal structures, sacral nodes (prostatic urethra, prostate, base of bladder, inferior pelvic ureter, inferior seminal glands, cavernous bodies, anal canal above pectinate line, inferior rectum)
Superficial inguinal	Lower limb; superficial drainage of inferolateral quadrant of trunk, including anterior abdominal wall inferior to umbilicus, gluteal region, superficial perineal structures (skin of perineum including skin and prepuce of penis, scrotum, perianal skin, anal canal inferior to pectinate line)
Deep inguinal	Glans of penis, superficial inguinal nodes, distal spongy urethra
Sacral	Posteroinferior pelvic structures, inferior rectum
Pararectal	Superior rectum

FEMALE URETHRA

The short **female urethra** passes anteroinferiorly from the *internal urethral orifice* of the urinary bladder, posterior, and then inferior to the pubic symphysis to the *external urethral orifice* in the vestibule of the vagina (Fig. 3.20B). The urethra lies anterior to the vagina; its axis is parallel with the vagina. The urethra passes with the vagina through the pelvic diaphragm, external urethral sphincter, and perineal membrane. Urethral glands are present, particularly in its superior part; the **paraurethral glands** are homologs to the prostate. These glands have a common paraurethral duct, which opens (one on each side) near the external urethral orifice. The inferior half of the urethra is in the perineum and is discussed in that section.

Vasculature of Female Urethra. Blood is supplied by the *internal pudendal* and *vaginal arteries* (Fig. 3.11A; Table 3.5). The veins follow the arteries and have similar names. Most lymphatic vessels from the urethra pass to the *sacral* and *internal iliac lymph nodes* (Fig. 3.22; Table 3.6). A few vessels drain into the *inguinal lymph nodes*.

Innervation of Female Urethra. The nerves to the urethra arise from the *vesical (nerve) plexus* and the *pudendal nerve* (Fig. 3.24). The pattern is similar to that in the male, given the absence of a prostatic plexus and an internal urethral sphincter. Visceral afferents from most of the urethra run in the *pelvic splanchnic nerves,* but the termination receives somatic afferents from the pudendal nerve.

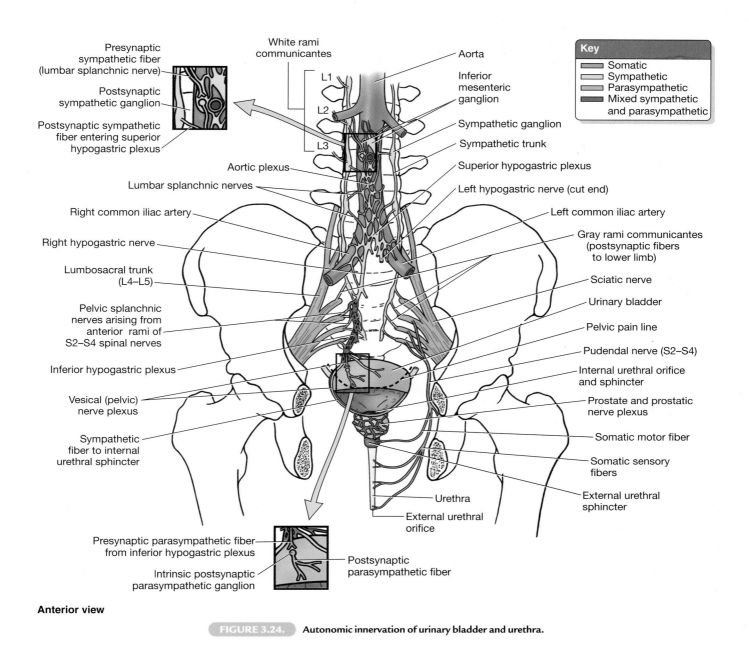

Presynaptic
sympathetic fiber
(lumbar splanchnic nerve)

Postsynaptic
sympathetic ganglion

Postsynaptic sympathetic
fiber entering superior
hypogastric plexus

Aortic plexus

Lumbar splanchnic nerves

Right common iliac artery

Right hypogastric nerve

Lumbosacral trunk
(L4–L5)

Pelvic splanchnic
nerves arising from
anterior rami of
S2–S4 spinal nerves

Inferior hypogastric plexus

Vesical (pelvic)
nerve plexus

Sympathetic
fiber to internal
urethral sphincter

White rami
communicantes

L1

L2

L3

Aorta

Inferior
mesenteric
ganglion

Sympathetic ganglion

Sympathetic trunk

Superior hypogastric plexus

Left hypogastric nerve (cut end)

Left common iliac artery

Gray rami communicantes
(postsynaptic fibers
to lower limb)

Sciatic nerve

Urinary bladder

Pelvic pain line

Pudendal nerve (S2–S4)

Internal urethral orifice
and sphincter

Prostate and prostatic
nerve plexus

Somatic motor fiber

Somatic sensory
fibers

External urethral
sphincter

Urethra

External urethral
orifice

Presynaptic parasympathetic fiber
from inferior hypogastric plexus

Intrinsic postsynaptic
parasympathetic ganglion

Postsynaptic
parasympathetic fiber

Key
Somatic
Sympathetic
Parasympathetic
Mixed sympathetic
and parasympathetic

Anterior view

FIGURE 3.24. Autonomic innervation of urinary bladder and urethra.

MALE URETHRA

The **male urethra** is a muscular tube that conveys urine from the *internal urethral orifice* of the urinary bladder to the exterior through the *external urethral orifice* at the tip of the glans penis (Fig. 3.24). The urethra also provides an exit for semen (sperm and glandular secretions). For descriptive purposes, the urethra is divided into four parts: intramural part of the urethra (preprostatic urethra), prostatic urethra, intermediate (membranous) part of the urethra, and spongy (penile) part of the urethra (Figs. 3.20A and 3.25; Table 3.8).

The *intramural part of the male urethra* is surrounded by an internal urethral sphincter composed of sympathetically innervated smooth muscle (Fig. 3.26). This sphincter prevents semen from entering the bladder during ejaculation (retrograde ejaculation). The prostate surrounds the prostatic urethra. The *intermediate part of the male urethra* is surrounded by the external urethral sphincter, composed of somatically innervated voluntary muscle. The tonic and phasic contraction of this muscle primarily controls urinary continence, but several other muscles may also contribute by compressing the urethra. Stimulation of both sphincters must be inhibited to enable urination.

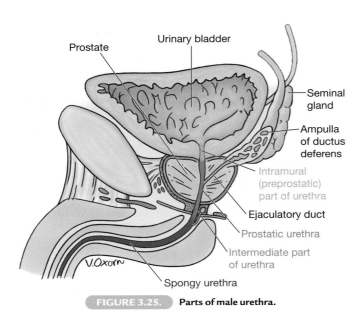

FIGURE 3.25.   Parts of male urethra.

Vasculature of Male Urethra. The intramural part of the urethra and the prostatic urethra are supplied by the *prostatic branches of the inferior vesical and middle rectal arteries* (Fig. 3.11D; Table 3.5). The intermediate and spongy parts of the urethra are supplied by the *internal pudendal artery*. The **veins** accompany the arteries and have similar names. The **lymphatic vessels** drain mainly into the *internal iliac lymph nodes* (Fig. 3.23; Table 3.7), but some lymph passes to the *external iliac lymph nodes*. Lymphatic vessels from the spongy urethra pass to the *deep inguinal lymph nodes*.

Innervation of Male Urethra. The nerves of the male urethra are derived from the **prostatic nerve plexus** (mixed sympathetic, parasympathetic, and visceral afferent fibers) (Fig. 3.24). This plexus is one of the pelvic plexuses (an inferior extension of the vesical plexus) arising as an organ-specific extension of the inferior hypogastric plexus.

TABLE 3.8 PARTS OF MALE URETHRA

Part	Length (cm)	Location/Disposition	Features
Intramural (preprostatic) part	0.5–1.5	Extends almost vertically through neck of bladder	Surrounded by internal urethral sphincter; diameter and length vary, depending on whether bladder is filling or emptying
Prostatic urethra	3.0–4.0	Descends through anterior prostate, forming gentle, anteriorly concave curve; is bounded anteriorly by vertical, trough-like part (rhabdosphincter) of external urethral sphincter	Widest and most dilatable part; features urethral crest with seminal colliculus, flanked by prostatic sinuses into which the prostatic ducts open; ejaculatory ducts open onto colliculus; hence urinary and reproductive tracts merge in this part
Intermediate (membranous) part	1.0–1.5	Passes through deep perineal pouch, surrounded by circular fibers of external urethral sphincter; penetrates perineal membrane	Narrowest and least distensible part (except for external urethral orifice)
Spongy urethra	~15	Courses through corpus spongiosum; initial widening occurs in bulb of penis; widens again distally as navicular fossa (in the glans penis)	Longest and most mobile part; bulbourethral glands open into bulbous part; distally, urethral glands open into small urethral lacunae entering lumen of this part

Key: Male

- Puboprostaticus
- Pubococcygeus
- Puborectalis
- Muscle of uvula
- Rectovesicalis

Muscles compressing urethra:

- Internal urethral sphincter
- Pubovesicalis
- External urethral sphincter
- Compressor urethrae

Male

FIGURE 3.26.   Supporting and compressor muscles of male pelvis.

Male Internal Genital Organs

The male internal genital organs include the testes, epididymides (plural of epididymis), ductus deferentes (plural of ductus deferens), seminal glands, ejaculatory ducts, prostate, and bulbourethral glands (Fig. 3.14). The testes and epididymides are described in Chapter 2.

DUCTUS DEFERENS

The **ductus deferens** (vas deferens) is the continuation of the duct of the epididymis (see Chapter 2). The ductus deferens (Figs. 3.14 and 3.21):

- Begins in the tail of the epididymis at the inferior pole of the testis.
- Ascends in the spermatic cord.
- Passes through the inguinal canal.
- Crosses over the external iliac vessels and enters the pelvis.
- Passes along the lateral wall of the pelvis where it lies external to the parietal peritoneum.
- Ends by joining the duct of the seminal gland to form the *ejaculatory duct*.

During the course of the ductus deferens, no other structure intervenes between it and the peritoneum. The ductus crosses superior to the ureter near the posterolateral angle of the bladder, running between the ureter and the peritoneum to reach the fundus of the urinary bladder. Posterior to the bladder, the ductus deferens at first lies superior to the seminal gland, then it descends medial to the ureter and the gland. Here, the ductus deferens enlarges to form the **ampulla of the ductus deferens** before its termination. The ductus then narrows and joins the duct of the seminal gland to form the **ejaculatory duct.**

Vasculature of Ductus Deferens. The tiny *artery to the ductus deferens* usually arises from a superior (sometimes inferior) vesical artery and accompanies the ductus deferens as far as the testis (Table 3.5). It terminates by anastomosing with the testicular artery, posterior to the testis. The veins accompany the arteries and have similar names. The lymphatic vessels from the ductus deferens drain into the *external iliac lymph nodes* (Fig. 3.23; Table 3.7).

SEMINAL GLANDS

Each **seminal gland** (vesicle) is an elongated structure that lies between the fundus of the bladder and the rectum (Fig. 3.25). The seminal glands are obliquely placed structures superior to the prostate and do not store sperms. They secrete a thick alkaline fluid that mixes with the sperms as they pass into the ejaculatory ducts and urethra. The superior ends of the seminal glands are covered with peritoneum and lie posterior to the ureters, where the peritoneum of the *rectovesical pouch* separates them from the rectum (Fig. 3.6, Table 3.2). The inferior ends of the seminal glands are

Sterilization of Males

The common method of sterilizing males is **deferentectomy,** popularly called a *vasectomy*. During this procedure, part of the ductus deferens is ligated and/or excised through an incision in the superior part of the scrotum. Hence, the ejaculated fluid from the seminal glands, prostate, and bulbourethral glands contains no sperms. The unexpelled sperms degenerate in the epididymis and the proximal part of the ductus deferens.

closely related to the rectum and are separated from it only by the rectovesical septum.

Vasculature of Seminal Glands. The arteries to the seminal glands derive from the *inferior vesical* and *middle rectal arteries* (Table 3.5). The veins accompany the arteries and have similar names. The iliac lymph nodes receive lymph from the seminal glands: the *external iliac nodes* from the superior part, and the *internal iliac lymph nodes* from the inferior part (Table 3.7).

EJACULATORY DUCTS

Each **ejaculatory duct** is a slender tube that arises by the union of the duct of a seminal gland with the ductus deferens (Figs. 3.21 and 3.25). The ejaculatory ducts arise near the neck of the bladder and run close together as they pass anteroinferiorly through the posterior part of the prostate. The ducts converge to open by slit-like apertures on, or just within, the opening of the prostatic utricle (Fig. 3.28). Prostatic secretions join the seminal fluid in the prostatic urethra after the termination of the ejaculatory ducts.

Vasculature of Ejaculatory Ducts. The *arteries to the ductus deferentes,* usually branches of the superior (but frequently inferior) vesical arteries, supply the ejaculatory ducts (Table 3.5). The veins join the *prostatic* and *vesical venous plexuses*. The lymphatic vessels drain into the *external iliac lymph nodes* (Table 3.7).

PROSTATE

The walnut-size **prostate** surrounds the *prostatic urethra* (Figs. 3.25 and 3.27). The glandular part makes up approximately two thirds of the prostate; the other third is fibromuscular. The structure has a dense **fibrous capsule of the prostate** that incorporates the prostatic plexuses of nerves and veins. This is surrounded by the visceral layer of the pelvic fascia, forming a fibrous *prostatic sheath* that is thin anteriorly, continuous anterolaterally with the *puboprostatic* *ligaments,* and dense posteriorly, continuous with the *rectovesical septum.*

The prostate has (Fig. 3.27*B*):

- A **base** (superior aspect) that is closely related to the neck of the bladder.
- An **apex** (inferior aspect) that is in contact with fascia on the superior aspect of the urethral sphincter and deep perineal muscles.
- A muscular **anterior surface** that features mostly transversely oriented muscle fibers forming a vertical trough-like hemisphincter (rhabdosphincter), which is part the urethral sphincter, separated from the pubic symphysis by retroperitoneal fat in the **retropubic space** (Fig. 3.18).
- A **posterior surface** that is related to the ampulla of the rectum.
- **Inferolateral surfaces** that are related to the levator ani.

Although not clearly distinct anatomically, the following **lobes and lobules of the prostate** are described (Fig. 3.27*A*):

- The **isthmus of the prostate** (anterior muscular zone; historically, the anterior lobe) lies anterior to the urethra. It is primarily muscular and represents the superior continuation of the urethral sphincter muscle.
- **Right** and **left lobes** (peripheral zones), each divided in turn into four indistinct *lobules* in two concentric bands, defined by their relationship to the urethra and ejaculatory ducts:
  1. A superfical **inferoposterior lobule**, posterior to the urethra and inferior to the ejaculatory ducts, is readily palpable by digital rectal examination.
  2. A superficial **inferolateral lobule**, lateral to the urethra, forms the major part of the prostate.
  3. A **superomedial lobule** surrounds the ejaculatory duct, deep to the inferoposterior lobule.
  4. An **anteromedial lobule**, deep to the inferolateral lobule, is directly lateral to the proximal prostatic urethra.

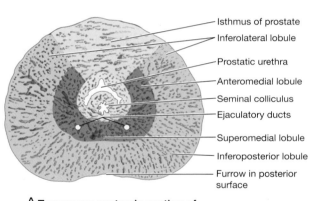

A **Transverse anatomic section of prostate at level of red line in (B)**

Isthmus of prostate
Inferolateral lobule
Prostatic urethra
Anteromedial lobule
Seminal colliculus
Ejaculatory ducts
Superomedial lobule
Inferoposterior lobule
Furrow in posterior surface

B **Median section of prostate**

Internal urethral sphincter
Seminal gland
Base of prostate
Superomedial lobule
Ejaculatory duct
Prostatic urethra
Inferoposterior lobule
Isthmus of prostate
Apex of prostate
Intermediate urethra
External urethral sphincter

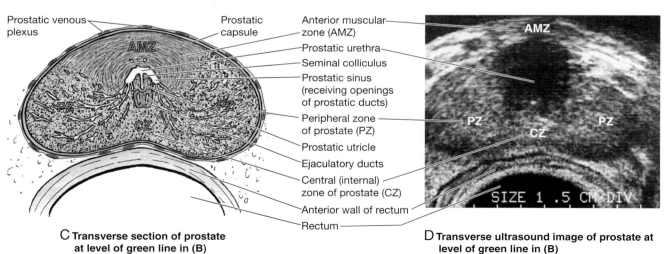

Prostatic venous plexus
Prostatic capsule
AMZ
PZ
PZ
CZ

Anterior muscular zone (AMZ)
Prostatic urethra
Seminal colliculus
Prostatic sinus (receiving openings of prostatic ducts)
Peripheral zone of prostate (PZ)
Prostatic utricle
Ejaculatory ducts
Central (internal) zone of prostate (CZ)
Anterior wall of rectum
Rectum

C **Transverse section of prostate at level of green line in (B)**

AMZ
PZ
CZ
PZ
SIZE 1 .5 CM/DIV

D **Transverse ultrasound image of prostate at level of green line in (B)**

FIGURE 3.27. Lobules and zones of prostate demonstrated by anatomical section and ultrasonographic imaging.

An embryonic middle (median) lobe gives rise to super-omedial and anteromedial lobules. This region tends to undergo hormone-induced hypertrophy in advanced age, forming a **middle lobule** (central zone) believed to be partially responsible for the formation of the *uvula* that may project into the internal urethral orifice (Fig. 3.28).

Urologists and sonographers usually divide the prostate into peripheral and central (internal) zones (Fig. 3.27C,D).

The **prostatic ducts** (20–30) open chiefly into the **prostatic sinuses** that lie on either side of the **seminal colliculus** on the posterior wall of the prostatic urethra (Fig. 3.28). Prostatic fluid provides about 20% of the volume of **semen** (a mixture of secretions).

Vasculature of Prostate. The prostatic **arteries** are mainly branches of the *internal iliac artery* (Table 3.5), especially the *inferior vesical arteries* but also the *internal pudendal* and *middle rectal arteries*. The **veins** join to form the **prostatic venous plexus** around the sides and base of the prostate (Figs. 3.21 and 3.27B). This plexus, between the fibrous capsule of the prostate and the prostatic sheath, drains into the *internal iliac veins*. The plexus is continuous superiorly with the *vesical venous plexus* and communicates posteriorly with the *internal vertebral venous plexus* (see Chapter 4). The lymphatic vessels drain chiefly into the *internal iliac nodes*, but some pass to the *sacral lymph nodes* (Table 3.7).

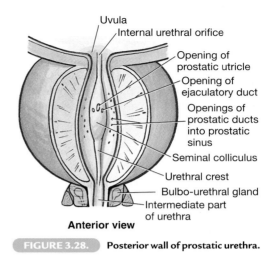

Anterior view

FIGURE 3.28.   Posterior wall of prostatic urethra.

BULBO-URETHRAL GLANDS

The two pea-size **bulbo-urethral glands** (Cowper glands) lie posterolateral to the intermediate part of the urethra, largely embedded within the external urethral sphincter (Figs. 3.20A, 3.21, and 3.28). The **ducts of the bulbo-urethral glands** pass through the perineal membrane with the intermediate urethra and open through minute apertures into the proximal part of the spongy urethra in the bulb of the penis. Their mucus-like secretion enters the urethra during sexual arousal.

Prostatic Enlargement, Prostatic Cancer, and Prostotectomy

The prostate is of medical interest because benign enlargement or **benign hypertrophy of the prostate** (BHP) is common after middle age. An enlarged prostate projects into the urinary bladder and impedes urination by distorting the prostatic urethra. The middle lobule usually enlarges the most and obstructs the internal urethral orifice.

Prostatic cancer is common in men older than 55 years. In most cases, the cancer develops in the posterolateral region. This may be palpated during a digital rectal examination (Fig. B3.3). A malignant prostate feels hard and often irregular. In advanced stages, cancer cells metastasize (spread) to the iliac and sacral lymph nodes and later to distant nodes and bone. The prostatic plexus, closely associated with the prostatic sheath, gives passage to parasympathetic fibers, which give rise to the cavernous nerves that convey the fibers that cause penile erection. A major concern regarding **prostatectomy** is that impotency may

be a consequence. All or part of the prostate, or just the hypertrophied part, is removed (*transurethral resection of the prostate* [TURP]).

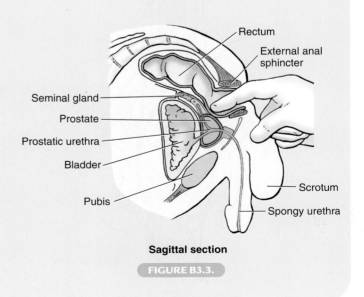

Sagittal section

FIGURE B3.3.

INNERVATION OF INTERNAL GENITAL ORGANS OF MALE PELVIS

The ductus deferens, seminal glands, ejaculatory ducts, and prostate are richly innervated by *sympathetic nerve fibers* originating from cell bodies in the intermediolateral cell column. They traverse the paravertebral ganglia of the sympathetic trunk to become components of the lumbar (abdominopelvic) splanchnic nerves and the hypogastric and pelvic plexuses (Fig. 3.29). *Presynaptic parasympathetic fibers* from the S2–S4 spinal cord segments traverse the pelvic splanchnic nerves, which also join the inferior hypogastric–pelvic plexuses. Synapses with postsynaptic sympathetic and parasympathetic neurons occur with the plexuses, en route to or near the pelvic viscera. As part of an orgasm, the sympathetic system stimulates contractions of the ductus deferens, and the combined contraction of and secretion from the seminal and prostate glands provide the vehicle (semen) and the expulsive force to discharge the sperms during ejaculation. The function of the parasympathetic innervation is unclear. However, the parasympathetic fibers in the prostatic nerve plexus form the cavernous nerves that pass to the erectile bodies of the penis, which are responsible for producing penile erection.

Female Internal Genital Organs

The female internal genital organs include the vagina, uterus, uterine tubes, and ovaries.

Anterior view

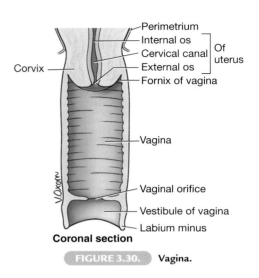

Coronal section

FIGURE 3.30. Vagina.

VAGINA

The **vagina,** a mostly subperitoneal musculomembranous tube, extends from the cervix of the uterus to the **vestibule of the vagina,** the cleft between the labia minora into which the vagina and urethra open (Fig. 3.30). The vestibule contains the vaginal and external urethral orifices and the openings of the two greater vestibular glands. The superior end of the vagina surrounds the *cervix* of the uterus.

The vagina:

- Serves as a canal for menstrual fluid.
- Forms the inferior part of the birth canal.
- Receives the penis and ejaculate during sexual intercourse.
- Communicates superiorly with the **cervical canal,** and inferiorly with the vestibule. The cervical canal extends from the isthmus of the uterus to the external os (opening) of the uterus.

The vagina is usually collapsed, so its anterior and posterior walls are in contact, except at its superior end, where the

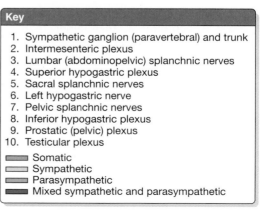

Key

1. Sympathetic ganglion (paravertebral) and trunk
2. Intermesenteric plexus
3. Lumbar (abdominopelvic) splanchnic nerves
4. Superior hypogastric plexus
5. Sacral splanchnic nerves
6. Left hypogastric nerve
7. Pelvic splanchnic nerves
8. Inferior hypogastric plexus
9. Prostatic (pelvic) plexus
10. Testicular plexus

- Somatic
- Sympathetic
- Parasympathetic
- Mixed sympathetic and parasympathetic

FIGURE 3.29. Autonomic innervation of testis, ductus deferens, prostate, and seminal glands.

A Coronal section

B Left lateral view

FIGURE 3.31.   Supporting and compressive muscles of female pelvis.

cervix holds them apart. The **vaginal fornix,** the recess around the protruding cervix, is usually described as having *anterior, posterior,* and *lateral parts.* The **posterior vaginal fornix** is the deepest part and is closely related to the recto-uterine pouch (Fig. 3.32*B*).

Four muscles compress the vagina and act like sphincters: **pubovaginalis, external urethral sphincter, urethrovaginal sphincter,** and **bulbospongiosus** (Fig. 3.31). The relations of the vagina are:

- Anteriorly: the fundus of the urinary bladder and urethra.
- Laterally: the levator ani, visceral pelvic fascia, and ureters.
- Posteriorly (inferior to superior): the anal canal, rectum, and recto-uterine pouch (Fig. 3.4*A*).

Vasculature of Vagina. The **arteries** supplying the superior part of the vagina derive from the *uterine arteries;* the arteries supplying the middle and inferior parts of the vagina derive from the *vaginal arteries* and *internal pudendal arteries* (Fig. 3.32*A*; Table 3.5). The **veins** form the **vaginal venous plexuses** along the sides of the vagina and within the vaginal mucosa (Fig. 3.32*B*). These veins communicate with the *uterine venous plexus* as the **uterovaginal plexus** and drain into the internal iliac veins through the uterine vein.

The lymphatic vessels drain from the vagina as follows (Fig. 3.22; Table 3.6):

- Superior part: to the internal and external iliac lymph nodes.
- Middle part: to the internal iliac lymph nodes.
- Inferior part: to the sacral and common iliac nodes.
- External orifice: to the superficial inguinal lymph nodes.

UTERUS

The uterus (womb) is a thick-walled, pear-shaped, hollow muscular organ. The nongravid (not pregnant) uterus usually lies in the lesser pelvis, with its body lying on the urinary bladder and

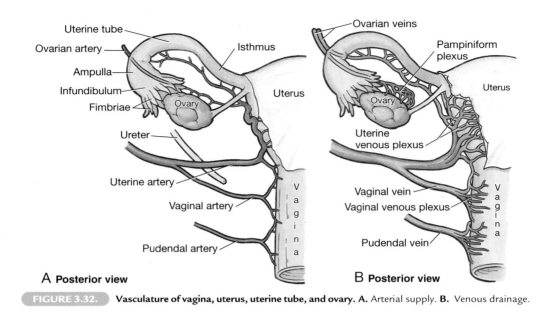

FIGURE 3.32.   **Vasculature of vagina, uterus, uterine tube, and ovary. A.** Arterial supply. **B.** Venous drainage.

Distention and Examination of Vagina

The vagina can be markedly distended by the fetus during childbirth, particularly in an anteroposterior direction. Lateral distention of the vagina is limited by the ischial spines, which project posteromedially, and the sacrospinous ligaments extending from these spines to the lateral margins of the sacrum and coccyx. The interior of the vagina can be distended for examination using a *vaginal speculum* (Fig. B3.4). The cervix, ischial spines, and sacral promontory can be palpated with the gloved digits in the vagina and/or rectum (*manual pelvic examination*).

Culdocentesis

An endoscopic instrument (*culdoscope*) can be inserted through an incision made in the posterior part of the vaginal fornix into the peritoneal cavity to drain a pelvic abscess (collection of pus) in the recto-uterine pouch (*culdocentesis*). Similarly, fluid in this part of the perineal cavity (e.g., blood) can be aspirated at this site.

FIGURE B3.4.

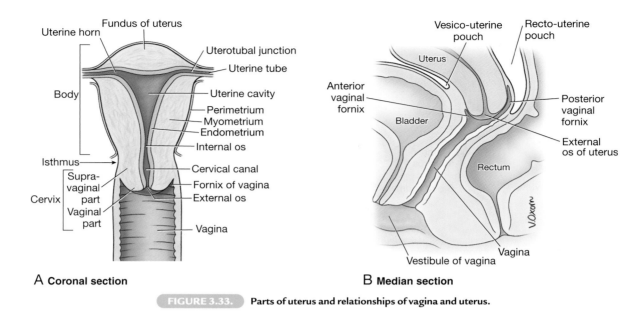

A Coronal section   **B** Median section

FIGURE 3.33.   Parts of uterus and relationships of vagina and uterus.

its cervix between the urinary bladder and the rectum (Fig. 3.33*B*). The adult uterus is usually *anteverted* (tipped anterosuperiorly relative to the axis of the vagina) and *anteflexed* (uterine body is flexed or bent anteriorly relative to the cervix) so that its mass lies over the bladder. The position of the uterus changes with the degree of fullness of the bladder and rectum. The uterus is divisible into two main parts (Fig. 3.33*A*):

- The **body of the uterus,** forming the superior two thirds of the structure, includes the **fundus of the uterus,** the rounded part of the body that lies superior to the orifices of the uterine tubes, and the **isthmus of the uterus,** the relatively constricted region of the body (about 1-cm long) just superior to the cervix. The **uterine horns** (L. *cornua*) are the superolateral regions where the uterine tubes enter. The body of the uterus lies between the layers of the broad ligament and is freely movable (Fig. 3.34*A*).
- The **cervix of the uterus,** the cylindrical, narrow inferior part of the uterus, which has a *supravaginal part* between the isthmus and the vagina and a *vaginal part* that protrudes into the vagina and surrounds the *external os of the uterus.* The *supravaginal part of the cervix* is separated from the bladder anteriorly by loose connective tissue and from the rectum posteriorly by the recto-uterine pouch (Fig. 3.33*B*). The cervix is mostly fibrous, with a small amount of smooth muscle and elastin.

The *wall of the body of the uterus* consists of three layers (Fig. 3.33*A*):

- **Perimetrium:** the outer serous coat, which consists of peritoneum supported by a thin layer of connective tissue.
- **Myometrium:** the middle muscular coat of smooth muscle, which becomes greatly distended during pregnancy; the main branches of the blood vessels and nerves of the uterus are located in this coat.

- **Endometrium:** the inner mucous coat, which firmly adheres to the myometrium and is actively involved in the menstrual cycle, differing in structure with each stage; if conception occurs, the blastocyst becomes implanted in this layer; if conception does not occur, the inner surface of the coat is shed during menstruation.

Ligaments of Uterus. Externally, the **ligament of the ovary** attaches to the uterus posteroinferior to the uterotubal junction (Fig. 3.34*A*). The **round ligament of the uterus** attaches anteroinferiorly to this junction. These two ligaments are vestiges of the *ovarian gubernaculum,* related to the descent of the gonad from its developmental position on the posterior abdominal wall (see Chapter 2).

The **broad ligament of the uterus** is a double layer of peritoneum (mesentery) that extends from the sides of the uterus to the lateral walls and floor of the pelvis. This ligament assists in keeping the uterus relatively centered in the pelvis but mostly contains the ovaries, uterine tubes, and related structures as well as the vasculature that serves them. The two layers of the ligament are continuous with each other at a free edge, which surrounds the uterine tube. Laterally, the ligament is prolonged superiorly over the ovarian vessels as the **suspensory ligament of the ovary** (Fig. 3.34). Between the layers of the broad ligament on each side of the uterus, the *ligament of the ovary* lies posterosuperiorly and the *round ligament of the uterus* lies anteroinferiorly. The part of the broad ligament by which the ovary is suspended is the **mesovarium** (Fig. 3.34*B*). The part of the broad ligament forming the mesentery of the uterine tube is the **mesosalpinx.** The major part of the broad ligament serves as a mesentery for the uterus and is the **mesometrium,** which lies inferior to the mesosalpinx and mesovarium.

The principal supports of the uterus are both dynamic and passive. Dynamic support is provided by the pelvic

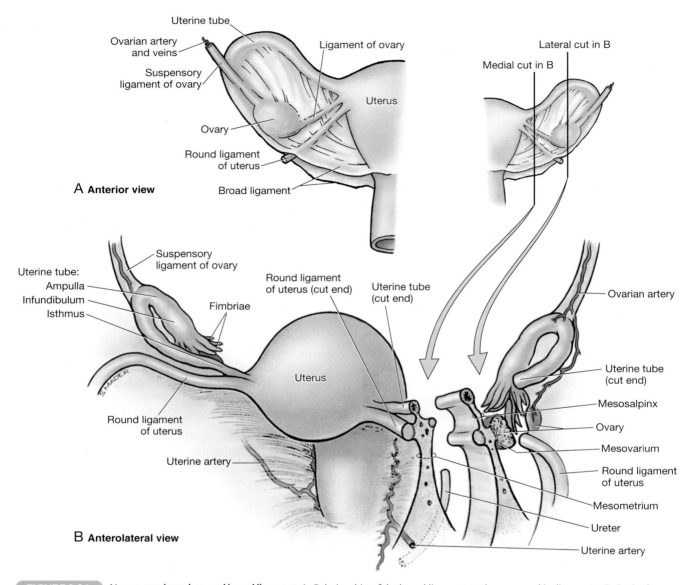

FIGURE 3.34. **Uterus, uterine tubes, and broad ligament. A.** Relationship of the broad ligament to the ovary and its ligaments. **B.** Sagittal sections showing the mesentery of the uterus (mesometrium), ovary (mesovarium), and uterine tube (mesosalpinx).

fascia. Passive support is provided by the way in which the uterus normally rests on top of the bladder. The cervix is the least mobile part of the uterus because of the passive support provided by attached condensations of endopelvic fascia (ligaments), which may also contain smooth muscle (Figs. 3.8A,B,E and 3.31A):

- *Transverse cervical* (cardinal) *ligaments* extend from the cervix and lateral parts of the fornix of the vagina to the lateral walls of the pelvis.
- *Uterosacral ligaments* pass superiorly and slightly posteriorly from the sides of the cervix to the middle of the sacrum (Fig. 3.8E); they are palpable on rectal examination.

Relationships of Uterus. Peritoneum covers the uterus anteriorly and superiorly, except for the cervix (Figs. 3.6A,C and 3.34; Table 3.3). The peritoneum is reflected anteriorly from the uterus onto the bladder and posteriorly over the posterior part of the fornix of the vagina onto the rectum. Anteriorly, the uterine body is separated from the urinary bladder by the **vesico-uterine pouch** where the peritoneum is reflected from the uterus onto the posterior margin of the superior surface of the bladder (Fig. 3.33B); the inferior uterine body (isthmus) and cervix lie in direct contact with the bladder without intervening peritoneum. This allows uterine/cervical cancer to invade the urinary bladder. Posteriorly, the uterine body and the supravaginal part of the cervix are separated from the sigmoid colon by a layer of peritoneum and the peritoneal cavity and from the rectum by the *recto-uterine pouch.* Laterally, the uterine artery crosses the ureter superiorly, near the cervix, in the root of the broad ligament (Fig. 3.34*B*).

Vasculature of Uterus. The *arteries* derive mainly from the **uterine arteries,** with potential collateral supply from the ovarian arteries (Figs. 3.11*A* and 3.32*A*; Table 3.5). The *uterine veins* run in the broad ligament, draining the **uterine venous plexus** formed on each side of the uterus and vagina (Fig. 3.32*B*). Veins from this plexus drain into the internal iliac veins.

The *uterine lymphatic vessels* follow three main routes (Fig. 3.22 and Table 3.6):

- Most vessels from the uterine fundus and superior uterine body pass along the ovarian vessels to the lumbar (caval/aortic) lymph nodes, but some vessels pass along the round ligament of the uterus to the *superficial inguinal lymph nodes.*
- Vessels from most of the uterine body pass within the broad ligament to the *external iliac lymph nodes.*
- Vessels from the uterine cervix pass along the uterine vessels, within the transverse cervical ligaments, to the *internal iliac lymph nodes* and along the uterosacral ligaments to the *sacral lymph nodes.*

Innervation of Vagina and Uterus. The innervation of the inferior part of the vagina is somatic, from the *deep perineal nerve,* a branch of the *pudendal nerve.* The innervation of most of the vagina and the entire uterus, however, is visceral. The nerves are derived from the **uterovaginal nerve plexus,** which travels with the uterine artery at the junction of the base of the peritoneal broad ligament and the superior part of the transverse cervical ligament (Fig. 3.35). The uterovaginal plexus is one of the pelvic plexuses that extend to the pelvic viscera from the inferior hypogastric plexus. Sympathetic, parasympathetic, and visceral afferent fibers pass through this plexus. Sympathetic innervation originates in the inferior thoracic spinal cord segments and passes through *lumbar splanchnic nerves* and the intermesenteric–hypogastric–pelvic series of plexuses. Parasympathetic innervation originates in the S2–S4 spinal cord segments and passes through the *pelvic splanchnic nerves* to the inferior hypogastric–uterovaginal plexus. Visceral afferent fibers, carrying pain sensation from the intraperitoneal uterine fundus and body, travel retrogradely with the sympathetic fibers to the lower thoracic–upper lumbar spinal ganglia; those from the subperitoneal uterine cervix and vagina (inferior to the pelvic pain line) travel with the parasympathetic fibers to the spinal sensory ganglia of S2–S4. All visceral afferent fibers from the uterus and vagina not concerned with pain (those conveying unconscious sensations) also follow the latter route.

UTERINE TUBES

The **uterine tubes** (formerly called fallopian tubes) extend laterally from the *uterine horns* and open into the peritoneal cavity near the ovaries (Figs. 3.33 and 3.34*B*). The uterine tubes lie in the *mesosalpinx* in the free edges of the broad ligament. In the "ideal" disposition, the tubes extend posterolaterally to the lateral pelvic walls, where they ascend and arch over the ovaries; however, ultrasound studies demonstrate that the position of the tubes and ovaries is variable (dynamic) in life, and right and left sides are often asymmetrical.

A **Anterior view**

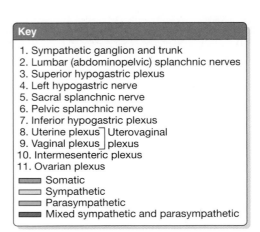

Key
1. Sympathetic ganglion and trunk
2. Lumbar (abdominopelvic) splanchnic nerves
3. Superior hypogastric plexus
4. Left hypogastric nerve
5. Sacral splanchnic nerve
6. Pelvic splanchnic nerve
7. Inferior hypogastric plexus
8. Uterine plexus ⎤ Uterovaginal
9. Vaginal plexus ⎦ plexus
10. Intermesenteric plexus
11. Ovarian plexus

▬▬ Somatic
▭▭ Sympathetic
▬▬ Parasympathetic
▬▬ Mixed sympathetic and parasympathetic

FIGURE 3.35. Autonomic innervation of uterus, vagina, and ovaries.

B Anterior view

FIGURE 3.35. *(continued)* **Autonomic innervation of uterus, vagina, and ovaries.**

Labels on figure: Superior hypogastric plexus; Inferior hypogastric plexuses; Uterine plexus; Ovarian plexus; Pelvic plexus; Uterovaginal plexus; Pelvic intra-peritoneal viscera; Peritoneum (lower limit); Pelvic pain line; Pelvic plexus; Pudendal nerve; Pelvic sub-peritoneal viscera; Perineum

Innervation

——	Postsynaptic sympathetic
····	Presynaptic parasympathetic
——	Postsynaptic parasympathetic
——	Visceral afferents running with sympathetic and parasympathetic fibers
——	Somatic afferent
——	Somatic motor

Hysterectomy

Hysterectomy (excision of the uterus) is performed through the lower anterior abdominal wall or through the vagina (Fig. B3.5). Because the uterine artery crosses anterior to the ureter near the lateral fornix of the vagina, the ureter is in danger of being inadvertently clamped or severed when the uterine artery is tied off during a hysterectomy. The point of crossing of the artery and the ureter is approximately 2 cm superior to the ischial spine.

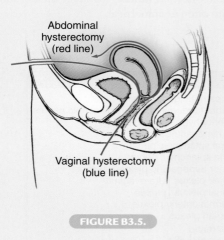

Abdominal hysterectomy (red line)

Vaginal hysterectomy (blue line)

FIGURE B3.5.

Cervical Examination and Pap Smear

The vagina can be distended with a vaginal speculum to enable inspection of the cervix and prepare a Pap smear. A spatula is placed on the external os of the uterus (Fig. B3.6). The spatula is rotated to scrape cellular material from the vaginal surface of the cervix, followed by insertion of a cytobrush into the cervical canal that is used to gather cellular material from the supravaginal cervical mucosa. The cellular material is placed on glass slides for microscopic examination.

A

B

C

Spatula

Speculum

Vagina

Cervix

FIGURE B3.6.

Regional Anesthesia for Childbirth

Several types of regional anesthesia are used to reduce pain during childbirth. Lumbar epidural and low spinal blocks anesthetize somatic and visceral afferent fibers distributed below waist level, anesthetizing the uterus, entire birth canal, and perineum, but also the lower limbs (Fig. B3.7*I*, *J*). A caudal epidural block is a popular choice for participatory childbirth (*K*). It must be administered in advance of childbirth, which is not possible with precipitous birth. The anesthetic agent is administered using an indwelling catheter in the sacral canal (see Chapter 4), enabling administration of more anesthetic agent for a deeper or prolonged anesthesia if necessary. Within the sacral canal, the anesthesia bathes the S2–S4 spinal nerve roots, including visceral pain fibers from the uterine cervix and upper vagina, and somatic pain fibers of the pudendal nerve. Thus, the birth canal is anesthetized but the lower limbs are not usually affected. Because visceral pain fibers to the uterine fundus ascend to lower thoracic and upper lumbar spinal levels, they are also not affected and sensations of uterine contraction are still perceived. Pudendal nerve blocks (*A*) and local infiltration of the perineum (*B*) provide only somatic anesthesia of the perineum.

Manual Examination of Uterus

The size and disposition of the uterus may be examined by *bimanual palpation* (Fig. B3.8). Two gloved fingers of the examiner's dominant hand are passed superiorly in the vagina, while the other hand is pressed inferoposteriorly on the pubic region of the anterior abdominal wall. The size and other characteristics of the uterus can be determined in this way (e.g., whether the uterus is in its normal anteverted position).

─── Visceral and somatic afferents from S2–S4 cord levels
─── Visceral afferents from T12–L2(3) cord levels

Regional anesthesia for childbirth: sites of injection; (A) pudendal block, (B) local infiltration of perineum, (C) pia mater, (D) arachnoid mater, (E) dura mater, (F) spinal cord, (G) subarachnoid space, (H) epidural space, (I) lumbar epidural block, (J) low spinal block, (K) saddle block

FIGURE B3.7.   **Regional anesthesia for childbirth.**

Bimanual palpation; uterus anteverted and anteflexed

— Uterus

Medial view

FIGURE B3.8.

Each uterine tube is divisible into four parts (Fig. 3.34*B*):

- The **infundibulum** is the funnel-shaped distal end that opens into the peritoneal cavity through the **abdominal ostium.** The finger-like processes of the infundibulum, the **fimbriae,** spread over the medial surface of the ovary; one large **ovarian fimbria** is attached to the superior pole of the ovary.

- The **ampulla,** the widest and longest part, begins at the medial end of the infundibulum.
- The **isthmus,** the thick-walled part, enters the uterine horn.
- The **uterine part** is the short intramural segment that passes through the wall of the uterus and opens through the **uterine ostium** into the uterine cavity at the uterine horn (Fig. 3.33*A*).

OVARIES

The almond-shaped **ovaries** are typically located near the attachment of the broad ligament to the lateral pelvic walls, suspended from both by peritoneal folds, the *mesovarium* from the posterosuperior aspect of the broad ligament and the *suspensory ligament of the ovary* from the pelvic wall (Figs. 3.34*A* and 3.36*A,B*). The suspensory ligament conveys the ovarian vessels, lymphatics, and nerves to and from the ovary and constitutes the lateral part of the mesovarium. The ovary also attaches to the uterus by the *ligament of ovary,* which runs within the mesovarium. This ligament is a remnant of the superior part of the ovarian gubernaculum of the fetus and connects the proximal (uterine) end of the ovary to the lateral angle of the uterus, just inferior to the entrance of the uterine tube. Because the ovary is suspended in the peritoneal cavity and its surface is not covered by peritoneum, the oocyte expelled at ovulation passes into the peritoneal cavity but is usually trapped by the fimbriae of the uterine tube and carried to the ampulla.

Vasculature of Ovaries and Uterine Tubes. The ***ovarian arteries*** arise from the abdominal aorta and descend along the posterior abdominal wall. At the pelvic brim, they cross over the external iliac vessels and enter the suspensory ligaments (Figs. 3.32*A* and 3.34*B*). The ovarian artery sends branches through the mesovarium to the ovary and through the mesosalpinx to supply the uterine tube. The ascending branches of the uterine arteries (branches of the internal iliac arteries) course along the lateral aspects of the uterus to approach the medial aspects of the ovaries and tubes. The ovarian and ascending uterine arteries terminate by bifurcating into ovarian and tubal branches and anastomose with each other, providing a collateral circulation from abdominal and pelvic sources.

Ovarian veins draining the ovary form a **pampiniform plexus of veins** in the broad ligament near the ovary and uterine tube (Fig. 3.32*B*). The veins of the plexus merge to form a singular **ovarian vein,** which leaves the lesser pelvis with the ovarian artery. The *right ovarian vein* ascends to

A Transverse section

B

- Distended urinary bladder
- Ovary
- Uterus
- Rectum

C Transverse section

- Pubic symphysis
- Femoral vessels
- Urethra
- Vagina
- Rectovaginal spetum
- Rectum
- Ischium
- Anococcygeal body
- Gluteus maximus

D

FIGURE 3.36.   **Imaging of female pelvis. A.** and **B.** Structures seen on an ultrasound scan. **C.** and **D.** Structures seen via MRI.

enter the *inferior vena cava;* the *left ovarian vein* drains into the *left renal vein.* The tubal veins drain into the *ovarian veins* and *uterine (uterovaginal) venous plexus.* The lymphatic vessels from the ovary join those from the uterine tubes and fundus of the uterus as they ascend to the *right* and *left* (caval/aortic) *lumbar lymph nodes* (Fig. 3.22 and Table 3.6).

Innervation of Ovaries and Uterine Tubes. The nerves descend along the ovarian vessels from the *ovarian plexus,* and from the *uterine (pelvic) plexus* (Fig. 3.35). Because the ovaries and uterine tubes are superior to the *pelvic pain line,* the visceral afferent pain fibers ascend retrogradely with the sympathetic fibers of the ovarian plexus and lumbar splanchnic nerves to the cell bodies in the T11–L1

spinal sensory ganglia. Visceral afferent reflex fibers follow parasympathetic fibers retrogradely through the uterine (pelvic) and inferior hypogastric plexuses and pelvic splanchnic nerves to cell bodies in the S2–S4 spinal sensory ganglia.

Rectum

The **rectum** is the pelvic part of the alimentary tract that is continuous proximally with the sigmoid colon and distally with the anal canal (Fig. 3.37*A*). The **rectosigmoid junction** lies at the level of the S3 vertebra. The rectum follows the curve of the sacrum and coccyx, forming the **sacral flexure**

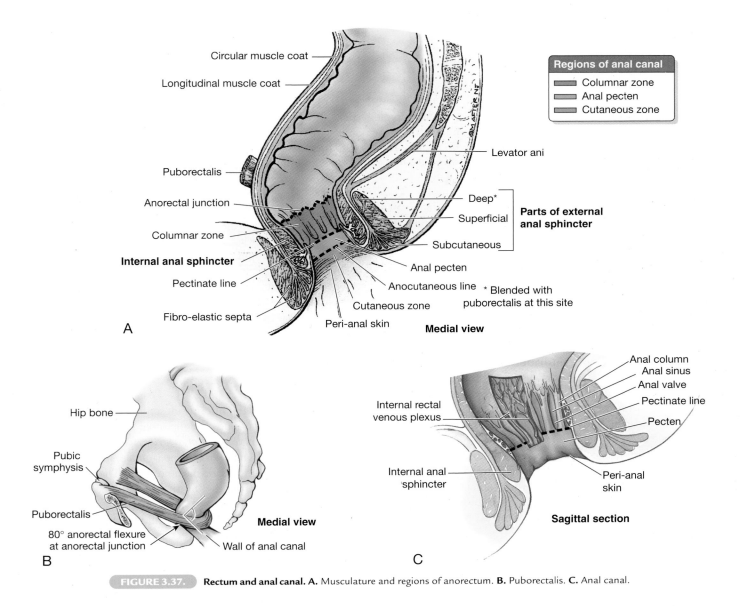

FIGURE 3.37.   **Rectum and anal canal. A.** Musculature and regions of anorectum. **B.** Puborectalis. **C.** Anal canal.

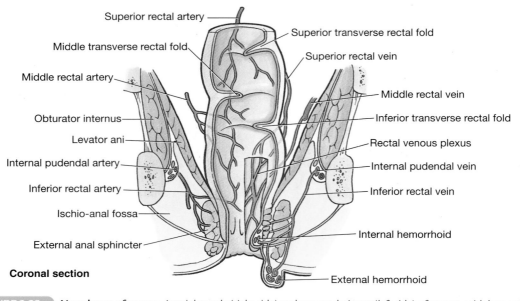

FIGURE 3.38. **Vasculature of rectum.** Arterial supply (right side) and venous drainage (left side) of rectum, with hemorrhoids.

of the rectum. The rectum ends anteroinferior to the tip of the coccyx, where the rectum turns posteroinferiorly and becomes the **anal canal.** The dilated terminal part, the **ampulla of the rectum,** supports and retains the fecal mass before it is expelled during defecation. The rectum is S-shaped and has three flexures as it follows the sacrococcygeal curve (Fig. 3.37*B*). Its terminal part bends sharply in a posterior direction, **anorectal flexure,** as it perforates the pelvic diaphragm to become the anal canal (Fig. 3.37*A*).

The roughly 80-degree anorectal flexure (angle) is an important mechanism for fecal continence and is maintained during the resting state by the tonus of the puborectalis muscle and by its active contraction during peristaltic contractions if defecation is not to occur (Fig. 3.37*B*). The relation of the puborectalis during defecation results in straightening of the anorectal junction. Three sharp **lateral flexures of the rectum** (**superior, intermediate,** and **inferior**) are apparent when the rectum is viewed anteriorly (Fig. 3.38). The flexures are formed in relation to three internal infoldings (**transverse rectal folds**): two on the left and one on the right side. The folds overlie thickened parts of the circular muscle layer of the rectal wall.

Peritoneum covers the anterior and lateral surfaces of the superior third of the rectum (Fig. 3.6 and Table 3.2), only the anterior surface of the middle third, and no surface of the inferior third because it is subperitoneal. In males, the peritoneum reflects from the rectum to the posterior wall of the bladder, where it forms the floor of the *rectovesical pouch.* In females, the peritoneum reflects from the rectum to the posterior fornix of the vagina, where it forms the floor of the *recto-uterine pouch.* In both sexes, lateral reflections of peritoneum from the upper third of the rectum form

pararectal fossae, which permit the rectum to distend as it fills with feces.

The rectum rests posteriorly on the inferior three sacral vertebrae and the coccyx, anococcygeal ligament, median sacral vessels, and inferior ends of the sympathetic trunks and sacral plexuses. In males, the rectum is related anteriorly to the fundus of the urinary bladder, terminal parts of the ureters, ductus deferentes, seminal glands, and prostate (Figs. 3.14 and 3.18). The *rectovesical septum* lies between the fundus of the bladder and the ampulla of the rectum and is closely associated with the seminal glands and prostate. In females, the rectum is related anteriorly to the vagina and is separated from the posterior part of the fornix and cervix by the *recto-uterine pouch* (Figs. 3.15 and 3.33*B*). Inferior to this pouch, the weak rectovaginal septum separates the superior half of the posterior wall of the vagina from the rectum (Fig. 3.36*C,D*).

VASCULATURE OF RECTUM

The continuation of the inferior mesenteric artery, the *superior rectal artery,* supplies the proximal part of the rectum. The right and left *middle rectal arteries,* usually arising from the inferior vesical (male) or uterine (female) arteries, supply the middle and inferior parts of the rectum. The *inferior rectal arteries,* arising from the internal pudendal arteries, supply the anorectal junction and anal canal (Fig. 3.38). Blood from the rectum drains via superior, middle, and inferior rectal veins. Because the superior rectal vein drains into the portal venous system and the middle and inferior rectal veins drain into the systemic system, this communication is an important area of *portacaval anastomosis* (see Chapter 2). The submucosal rectal venous plexus surrounds the rectum

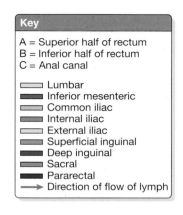

Key

A = Superior half of rectum
B = Inferior half of rectum
C = Anal canal

☐ Lumbar
☐ Inferior mesenteric
☐ Common iliac
☐ Internal iliac
☐ External iliac
☐ Superficial inguinal
☐ Deep inguinal
☐ Sacral
☐ Pararectal
→ Direction of flow of lymph

Anterior view

FIGURE 3.39. Lymphatic drainage of rectum and anal canal.

and communicates with the vesical venous plexus in males and the uterovaginal venous plexus in females. The **rectal venous plexus** consists of two parts, the **internal rectal venous plexus** just deep to the epithelium of the rectum and the external **rectal venous plexus** external to the muscular wall of the rectum.

Lymphatic vessels from the superior half of the rectum pass to the **pararectal lymph nodes,** located directly on the muscle layer of the rectum (Fig. 3.39), and then ascend to the *inferior mesenteric lymph nodes* either via the *sacral lymph nodes* or by passing through the nodes along the superior rectal vessels. Lymphatic vessels from the inferior half of the rectum drain into the *sacral lymph nodes* or, especially from the distal ampulla, follow the middle rectal vessels to drain into the *internal iliac lymph nodes.*

INNERVATION OF RECTUM

The nerve supply to the rectum is from the sympathetic and parasympathetic systems (Fig. 3.40). The *sympathetic supply* is from the lumbar spinal cord, conveyed via the lumbar splanchnic nerves and the hypogastric (pelvic) plexuses and through periarterial plexuses on the branches of the inferior mesenteric artery and superior rectal arteries. The *parasympathetic supply* is from the S2–S4 spinal cord level, passing via the pelvic splanchnic nerves (S2–S4) and inferior hypogastric plexuses to the rectal (pelvic) plexus. Because the rectum is inferior (distal) to the pelvic pain line, all visceral afferent fibers follow the parasympathetic fibers retrogradely to the S2–S4 spinal sensory ganglia.

Infections of Female Genital Tract

Because the female genital tract communicates with the peritoneal cavity through the abdominal ostia of the uterine tubes, infections of the vagina, uterus, and uterine tubes may result in *peritonitis.* Conversely, inflammation of the tubes (*salpingitis*) may result from infections that spread from the peritoneal cavity. A major cause of infertility in women is blockage of the uterine tubes, often the result of infection that causes salpingitis.

Patency of Uterine Tubes

Patency of the uterine tubes may be determined by a radiographic procedure involving injection of a water-soluble radiopaque material or carbon dioxide gas into the uterus,

Hysterosalpingogram. *Arrowheads,* uterine tubes; *c* catheter in the cervical canal; *vs,* vaginal speculum

FIGURE B3.9.

Spinal ganglion

Upper lumbar
sympathetic trunk

T12
L1
L2
L3
L4
L5

Lumbar
splanchnic
nerves

Spinal
ganglion

Pelvic splanchnic
nerves

S1

S2

S3

S4

Pelvic
plexus

Prevertebral ganglia

Para-aortic
plexus

Sacral
plexus

Superior
rectal nerves

Pudendal
nerve

Superior
hypogastric
plexus

Inferior
hypogastric
plexuses

Pelvic
plexus

Innervation

∙∙∙∙ Presynaptic sympathetic
——— Postsynaptic sympathetic
∙∙∙∙ Presynaptic parasympathetic
——— Postsynaptic parasympathetic
——— Visceral afferent running
with sympathetic and
parasympathetic fibers
——— Somatic sensory
——— Somatic motor

Internal anal
sphincter

External anal sphincter

Inferior anal
(rectal) nerve

FIGURE 3.40. **Innervation of rectum and anal canal.** The lumbar and pelvic spinal nerves and hypogastric plexuses have been retracted laterally for clarity.

hysterosalpingography. The material enters the uterine tubes and, if the tubes are patent, passes from the abdominal ostium into the peritoneal cavity (Fig. B3.9). Patency can also be determined by **hysteroscopy,** examination of the interior of the tubes using an endoscopic instrument (*hysteroscope*) introduced through the vagina and uterus.

Laparoscopic Examination of Pelvic Viscera

Laparoscopy involves inserting a *laparoscope* into the peritoneal cavity through a small incision below the umbilicus (Fig. B3.10). Insufflation of inert gas creates a pneumoperitoneum to provide space to visualize the pelvic organs. Additional

Uterine cannula Operating laparoscope Forceps
Pneumoperitoneum

Key

B	Urinary bladder
L	Ligament of ovary
O	Ovary
P	Recto-uterine pouch
R	Round ligament of uterus
T	Uterine tube
U	Fundus of uterus

Laparoscopic view of normal pelvis

FIGURE B3.10.

openings (ports) can be made to introduce other instruments for manipulation or to enable therapeutic procedures (e.g., ligation of the uterine tubes).

Ligation of Uterine Tubes

Ligation of the uterine tubes is a surgical method of birth control. **Abdominal tubal ligation** is usually performed through a short suprapubic incision made just at the pubic hairline. **Laparoscopic tubal ligation** is done with a laparoscope, which is similar to a small telescope with a powerful light. It is inserted through a small incision, usually near the umbilicus.

Ectopic Tubal Pregnancy

Occasionally, a blastocyst fails to reach the uterus and may implant in the mucosa of the uterine tube (most commonly the ampulla), producing an **ectopic tubal pregnancy.** On the right side, the appendix often lies close to the ovary and uterine tube. This close relationship explains why a *ruptured tubal pregnancy* and the resulting peritonitis may be misdiagnosed as acute appendicitis. In both cases, the parietal peritoneum is inflamed in the same general area and the pain is referred to the right lower quadrant of the abdomen. Tubal rupture and the severe hemorrhage constitute a threat to the mother's life and result in death of the embryo.

Resection of Rectum

When resecting the rectum in males (e.g., during cancer treatment), the plane of the rectovesical septum (a fascial septum extending superiorly from the perineal body) is located so that the prostate and urethra can be separated from the rectum. In this way, these organs are not often damaged during surgery.

Rectal Examination

Many structures related to the anteroinferior part of the rectum may be palpated through its walls (e.g., the prostate and seminal glands in males [Fig. B3.4] and the cervix in females). In both sexes, the pelvic surfaces of the sacrum and coccyx may be palpated. The ischial spines and tuberosities may also be palpated. Enlarged internal iliac lymph nodes, pathologic thickening of the ureters, swellings in the ischio-anal fossae (e.g., ischio-anal abscesses and abnormal contents in the rectovesical pouch in the male or the recto-uterine pouch in the female) may also be palpated. Tenderness of an inflamed appendix may also be detected rectally if it descends into the lesser pelvis (pararectal fossa).

PERINEUM

The term "perineum" is frequently used to refer to both an external surface area (perineal region) and a shallow "compartment" of the body (Fig. 3.41). The **perineum** (perineal compartment) lies inferior to the inferior pelvic aperture and is separated from the pelvic cavity by the pelvic diaphragm. In the anatomical position, the surface of the perineum (**perineal region**) is the narrow region between the proximal parts of the thighs. However, when the lower limbs are abducted, the perineal region is a diamond-shaped area extending from the mons pubis anteriorly, the medial surfaces (insides) of the thighs laterally, and the gluteal folds and superior end of the intergluteal (natal) cleft posteriorly (Fig. 3.43A).

The osseofibrous structures marking the boundaries of the perineum (perineal compartment) are the (Fig. 3.42):

* *Pubic symphysis*, anteriorly.
* *Inferior pubic* and *ischial (ischiopubic) rami*, anterolaterally.
* *Ischial tuberosities*, laterally.
* *Sacrotuberous ligaments*, posterolaterally.
* Inferiormost *sacrum* and *coccyx*, posteriorly.

A transverse line joining the anterior ends of the ischial tuberosities divides the perineum into two triangles (Fig. 3.42A):

* The **anal triangle** lies posterior to this line and contains the anal canal and its orifice, the anus.
* The **urogenital (UG) triangle,** containing the root of the scrotum and penis in males and the vulva of females, is anterior to this line.

The UG triangle is "closed" by the **perineal membrane** (Fig. 3.43C), a thin sheet of tough deep fascia, which stretches between the right and the left sides of the pubic arch. The perineal membrane covers the anterior part of the pelvic outlet and is perforated by the urethra in both sexes and by the vagina of the female. The **perineal body** is an irregular fibromuscular mass located in the median plane between the anal canal and the perineal membrane. It lies deep to the skin, with relatively little overlying subcutaneous tissue, posterior to the vestibule of the vagina or bulb of the penis and anterior to the anus and anal canal. Anteriorly, the perineal body blends with the posterior border of the perineal membrane and superiorly with the rectovesical or rectovaginal septum. It contains collagenous and elastic fibers and both skeletal and smooth muscle.

The perineal body is the site of convergence of several muscles (Fig. 3.43B and Table 3.9):

* Bulbospongiosus.
* External anal sphincter.
* Superficial and deep transverse perineal muscles.
* Smooth and voluntary slips of muscle from the external urethral sphincter, levator ani, and muscular coats of the rectum.

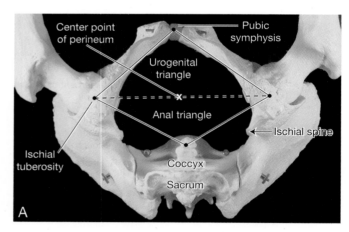

Female pelvis, inferior views (lithotomy position)

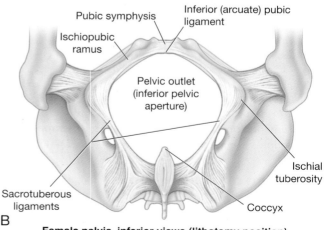

FIGURE 3.42.   Osseoligamentous boundaries of perineum.

Outline of perineum ⋯⋯⋯   Greater pelvis   Lesser pelvis

Pelvis

Ilium

Pelvic brim

Pelvic cavity

Obturator Internus

Obturator membrane

Ischio-anal fossa

Pelvic outlet   Perineal region   Pelvic diaphragm

Anterior view of posterior half of coronallysectioned lower trunk

FIGURE 3.41.   Perineum and perineal region.

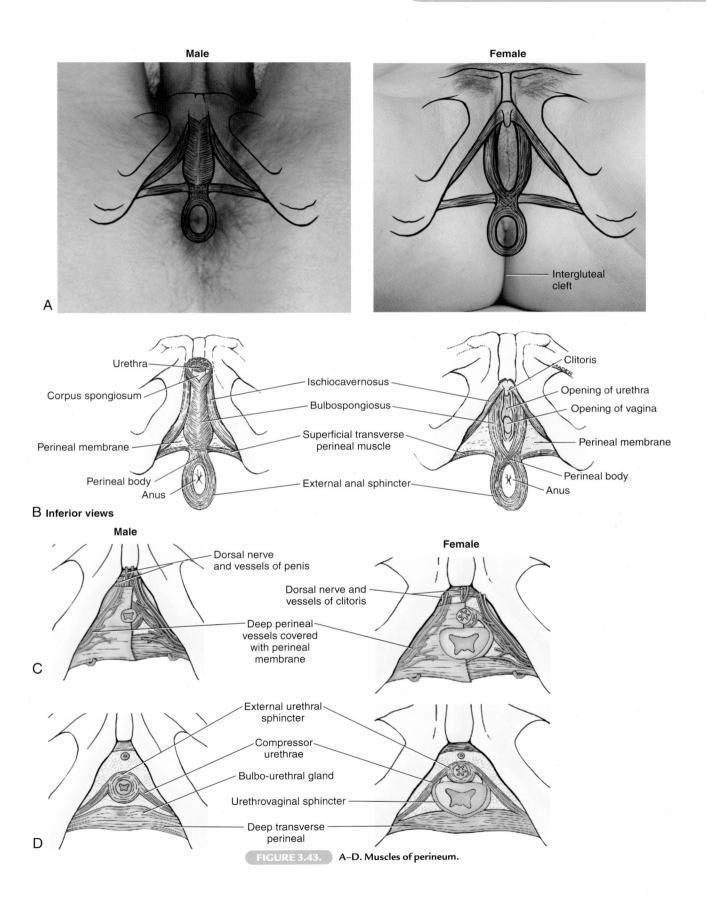

Male

Female

Intergluteal cleft

A

Urethra

Corpus spongiosum

Perineal membrane

Perineal body

Anus

Clitoris

Opening of urethra

Opening of vagina

Perineal membrane

Perineal body

Anus

Ischiocavernosus

Bulbospongiosus

Superficial transverse perineal muscle

External anal sphincter

B **Inferior views**

Male

Female

C

Dorsal nerve and vessels of penis

Dorsal nerve and vessels of clitoris

Deep perineal vessels covered with perineal membrane

D

External urethral sphincter

Compressor urethrae

Bulbo-urethral gland

Urethrovaginal sphincter

Deep transverse perineal

FIGURE 3.43.   A–D. Muscles of perineum.

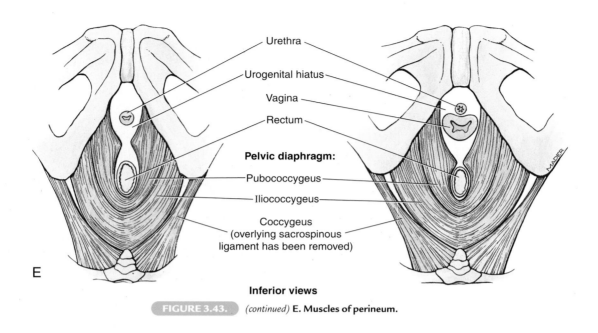

Inferior views

FIGURE 3.43. *(continued)* **E. Muscles of perineum.**

TABLE 3.9 MUSCLES OF PERINEUM

Muscle	Origin	Course and Insertion	Innervation	Main Action(s)
External anal sphincter	Skin and fascia surrounding anus and coccyx via anococcygeal ligament	Passes around lateral aspects of anal canal, inserting into perineal body	Inferior anal nerve, branch of pudendal nerve (S2–S4)	Constricts anal canal during peristalsis, resisting defecation; supports and fixes perineal body/pelvic floor
Bulbospongiosus	*Male:* median raphe on ventral surface of bulb of penis and perineal body *Female:* perineal body	*Male:* surrounds lateral aspects of bulb of penis and most proximal part of body of penis, inserting into perineal membrane, dorsal aspect of corpora spongiosum and cavernosa, and fascia of bulb of penis *Female:* passes on each side of lower vagina, enclosing bulb and greater vestibular gland; inserts onto pubic arch and fascia of corpora cavernosa of clitoris	Muscular (deep) branch of perineal nerve, branch of pudendal nerve (S2–S4)	Supports and fixes perineal body/pelvic floor *Male:* compresses bulb of penis to expel last drops of urine/semen; assists erection by compressing outflow via deep perineal vein and by pushing blood from bulb into body of penis *Female:* "sphincter" of vagina; assists in erection of clitoris (and bulb of vestibule); compresses greater vestibular gland
Ischiocavernosus	Internal surface of ischiopubic ramus and ischial tuberosity	Embraces crus of penis or clitoris, inserting onto inferior and medial aspects of crus and to perineal membrane medial to crus	Muscular (deep) branch of perineal nerve, branch of pudendal nerve	Maintains erection of penis or clitoris by compressing outflow veins and pushing blood from root of penis or clitoris into body
Superficial transverse perineal		Passes along superior posterior border of perineal membrane to perineal body		
Deep transverse perineal	Internal surface of ischiopubic ramus and ischial tuberosity; compressor urethrae portion only	Passes along superior posterior border of perineal membrane to perineal body, and external anal sphincter	Muscular (deep) branch of perineal nerve, branch of pudendal nerve (S2–S4); dorsal nerve of penis or clitoris, terminal branch of pudendal nerve (S2–S4)	Support and fix perineal body (pelvic floor) to support abdominopelvic viscera and resist increased intra-abdominal pressure
External urethral sphincter		Surrounds urethra superior to perineal membrane *Male:* also ascends anterior aspect of prostate *Female:* some fibers also enclose vagina (urethrovaginal sphincter)		Compresses urethra to maintain urinary continence *Female:* urethrovaginal sphincter portion also compresses vagina

Disruption of Perineal Body

The perineal body is an especially important structure in women because it is the final support of the pelvic viscera. Stretching or tearing of this attachment of the perineal muscles from the perineal body can occur during childbirth, removing support provided by the pelvic floor. As a result, *prolapse of pelvic viscera,* including prolapse of the bladder (through the urethra) and prolapse of the uterus and/or vagina (through the vaginal orifice), may occur.

Episiotomy

During vaginal surgery and labor, an *episiotomy* (surgical incision of the perineum and inferoposterior vaginal wall) may be made to enlarge the vaginal orifice with the intention of decreasing excessive tearing of the perineum and perineal muscles. Episiotomies are still performed in a large portion of vaginal deliveries. It is generally agreed that episiotomy is indicated when descent of the fetus is arrested or protracted, when instrumentation is necessary (e.g., obstetrical forceps), or to expedite delivery when there are signs of fetal distress. However, routine prophylactic episiotomy is widely debated and declining in frequency.

Fascias and Pouches of Urogenital Triangle

PERINEAL FASCIAS

The **perineal fascia** consists of superficial and deep layers (Fig. 3.44). The **subcutaneous tissue of the perineum,** or *superficial perineal fascia,* consists of a fatty superficial layer and a deep membranous layer (Colles fascia). In females, the **fatty layer of subcutaneous tissue of the perineum** makes up the substance of the labia majora and mons pubis and is continuous anteriorly and superiorly with the *fatty layer of subcutaneous tissue of the abdomen (Camper fascia)* (Fig. 3.44A,C). In males, the fatty layer is greatly diminished in the urogenital triangle and is replaced altogether in the penis and scrotum with smooth (dartos) muscle. It is continuous between the penis or scrotum and the thighs with the fatty layer of subcutaneous tissue of the abdomen (Fig. 3.44B,F). In both sexes, it is continuous posteriorly with the ischio-anal fat pad in the anal region (Fig. 3.44E).

The **membranous layer of subcutaneous tissue of the perineum** is attached posteriorly to the posterior margin of the perineal membrane and the perineal body (Fig. 3.44A,B). Laterally, it is attached to the fascia lata (deep fascia) of the superiormost medial aspect of the thigh. Anteriorly, in the male, the membranous layer of subcutaneous tissue is continuous with the dartos fascia of the penis and scrotum; however, on each side of and anterior to the scrotum, the membranous layer becomes continuous with the *membranous layer of subcutaneous tissue of the abdomen (Scarpa fascia)* (Fig. 3.44B,F). In females, the membranous layer passes superior to the fatty layer forming the labia majora and becomes continuous with the membranous layer of the subcutaneous tissue of the abdomen (Fig. 3.44A,C).

The **perineal fascia** (deep perineal, investing, or Gallaudet fascia) intimately invests the ischiocavernosus, bulbospongiosus, and superficial transverse perineal muscles (Fig. 3.44C,D). It is also attached laterally to the ischiopubic rami. Anteriorly, it is fused to the suspensory ligament of the penis and is continuous with the deep fascia covering the external oblique muscle of the abdomen and the rectus sheath. The deep perineal fascia is fused with the suspensory ligament of the clitoris in females and with the deep fascia of the abdomen in males.

SUPERFICIAL PERINEAL POUCH

The **superficial perineal pouch** (compartment) is a potential space between the membranous layer of subcutaneous tissue and the perineal membrane, bounded laterally by the ischiopubic rami (Fig. 3.44A–D).

In males, the superficial perineal pouch contains the (Fig. 3.44B,D):

- *Root* (bulb and crura) *of the penis* and associated muscles (*ischiocavernosus* and *bulbospongiosus*).
- Proximal (bulbous) part of the *spongy urethra.*
- *Superficial transverse perineal muscles.*
- *Deep perineal branches* of the internal pudendal vessels and pudendal nerves.

In females, the superficial perineal pouch contains the (Fig. 3.44A,C):

- *Clitoris* and associated muscle (ischiocavernosus).
- *Bulbs of the vestibule* and the surrounding muscle (bulbospongiosus).
- *Greater vestibular glands.*
- *Deep perineal branches* of the internal pudendal vessels and pudendal nerves.
- *Superficial transverse perineal muscles.*

DEEP PERINEAL POUCH

The **deep perineal pouch** (space) is bounded inferiorly by the perineal membrane, superiorly by the inferior fascia of the pelvic diaphragm, and laterally by the inferior portion of the obturator fascia (covering obturator internus muscle). It includes the fat-filled anterior recesses of the ischio-anal fossa (Figs. 3.44C,D and Fig. 3.46). In both sexes, the deep perineal pouch contains part of the urethra centrally, the inferior part of the external urethral sphincter muscle, and the anterior extensions of the ischio-anal fat pads. In males, the deep perineal pouch contains the *intermediate part of the urethra,*

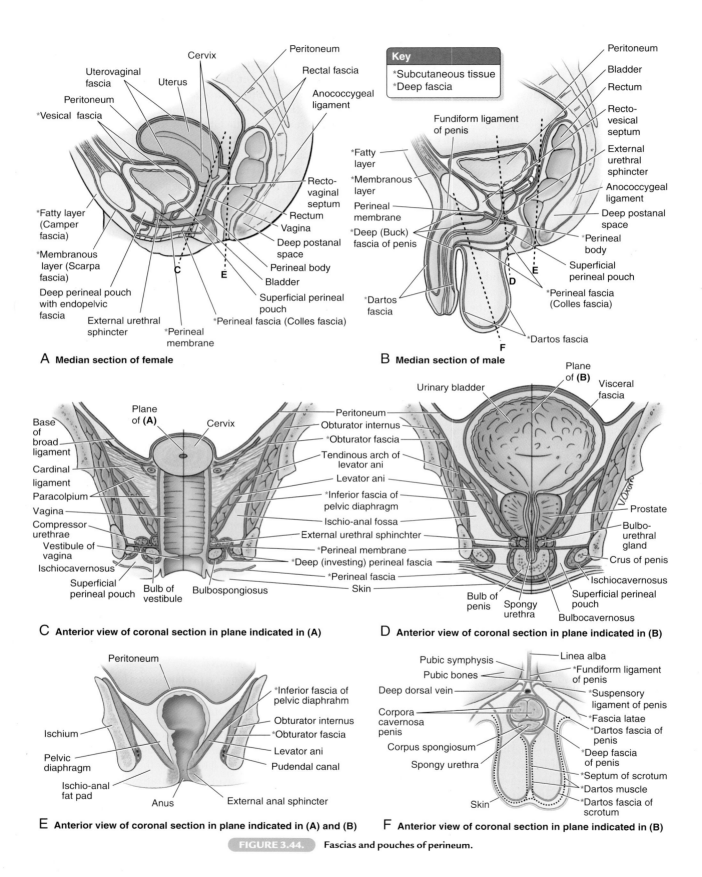

A Median section of female

B Median section of male

Key
*Subcutaneous tissue
*Deep fascia

C Anterior view of coronal section in plane indicated in (A)

D Anterior view of coronal section in plane indicated in (B)

E Anterior view of coronal section in plane indicated in (A) and (B)

F Anterior view of coronal section in plane indicated in (B)

FIGURE 3.44. Fascias and pouches of perineum.

deep transverse perineal muscles, bulbourethral glands, and dorsal neurovascular structures of the penis (Fig. 3.44*D*). In females, it contains the proximal part of the *urethra,* a mass of smooth muscle in place of deep transverse perineal muscles, and the dorsal neurovasculature of the clitoris (Fig. 3.44*C*).

Traditionally, a trilaminar UG diaphragm was described as making up the deep perineal pouch. The long-held concept of a flat, essentially two-dimensional UG diaphragm is erroneous (Wendell-Smith, 1995). According to this concept, the UG diaphragm consisted of the perineal membrane (inferior fascia of UG diaphragm) inferiorly and a superior fascia of the UG diaphragm superiorly, between which was a flat muscular sheet composed of a disc-like sphincter urethra and the transversely oriented deep transverse perineal muscle. The descriptions of only the perineal membrane and of the deep transverse perineal muscles of the male appear to be supported by evidence (Myers et al., 1998*a,b*).

In the female, deep transverse perineal muscles are mainly smooth muscle. Immediately superior to the posterior half of the perineal membrane, the flat, sheet-like deep transverse perineal muscle, when developed (typically only in males), offers dynamic support for the pelvic viscera. As described by Oelrich (1980), however, the urethral sphincter muscle is not a flat, planar structure, and the only "superior fascia" is the fascia of the external urethral sphincter muscle. In both views, the strong perineal membrane is the inferior boundary (floor) of the deep pouch. The perineal membrane, with the perineal body, is the final passive support of the pelvic viscera.

The **external urethral sphincter** is more tube- and trough-like than disc-like, and in the male, only a part of the muscle forms a circular investment (a true sphincter) for the intermediate part of the urethra inferior to the prostate (Fig. 3.45*A*). Its larger, trough-like part extends vertically to the neck of the bladder, displacing the prostate and investing the prostatic urethra anteriorly and anterolaterally only. As the prostate develops from the urethral glands, the posterior and posterolateral muscle atrophies or is displaced by the prostate. Whether this part of the muscle compresses or dilates the prostatic urethra is a matter of some controversy.

In the female, the external urethral sphincter is more properly a "urogenital sphincter," according to Oelrich (1983). Here, too, he described a part forming a true anular sphincter around the urethra, with several additional parts extending from it (Fig. 3.45*B*): a superior part, extending to the neck of the bladder; a subdivision described as extending inferolaterally to the ischial ramus on each side (the **compressor urethrae muscle**); and another band-like part, which encircles both the vagina and the urethra (**urethrovaginal sphincter**). In both males and females, the musculature described is oriented perpendicular to the perineal membrane rather than lying in the plane parallel to it. Some dispute the encircling of the urethra in the female, stating that the muscle is not capable of sphincteric action.

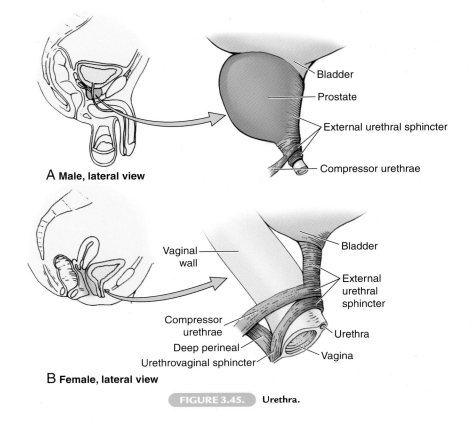

A **Male, lateral view**

- Bladder
- Prostate
- External urethral sphincter
- Compressor urethrae

B **Female, lateral view**

- Vaginal wall
- Compressor urethrae
- Deep perineal
- Urethrovaginal sphincter
- Bladder
- External urethral sphincter
- Urethra
- Vagina

FIGURE 3.45. Urethra.

Rupture of Urethra in Males and Extravasation of Urine

Fractures of the pelvic girdle often cause a *rupture of the intermediate part of the urethra*. This results in extravasation of urine and blood into the deep perineal pouch (Fig. B3.11A). The fluid may pass superiorly through the urogenital hiatus and distribute extraperitoneally around the prostate and bladder.

Rupture of the spongy urethra in the bulb of the penis results in urine passing (extravasating) into the superficial perineal space (Fig. B3.11B). The attachments of the perineal fascia determine the direction of flow of the extravasated urine. Urine and blood may pass into the loose connective tissue in the scrotum, around the penis, and superiorly, deep to the membranous layer of subcutaneous connective tissue of the inferior anterior abdominal wall. The urine cannot pass far into the thighs because the membranous layer of superficial perineal fascia blends with the fascia lata (deep fascia) enveloping the thigh muscles, just distal to the inguinal ligament. In addition, urine cannot pass posteriorly into the anal triangle because the superficial and deep layers of perineal fascia are continuous with each other around the superficial perineal muscles and with the posterior edge of the perineal membrane between them.

A

- Peritoneum
- Bladder
- Prostate
- Bloody extravasation
- Pubic symphysis
- Torn and separated intermediate part of urethra
- External urethral sphincter
- Perineal membrane

B

- Membranous layer of superficial abdominal (Scarpa) fascia
- Bloody extravasation
- Deep (Buck) fascia of penis
- Intercavernous septum
- Dartos fascia
- Perforation of spongy urethra
- Fatty layer of perineal fascia
- Deep (Buck) fascia of penis
- Membranous layer of perineal (Colles) fascia
- Bloody extravasation

Median sections

FIGURE B3.11.

Features of Anal Triangle

ISCHIO-ANAL FOSSAE

The **ischio-anal fossae** (formerly ischiorectal fossae) around the wall of the anal canal are large fascia-lined, wedge-shaped spaces between the skin of the anal region and the pelvic diaphragm (Fig. 3.46). The apex of each fossa lies superiorly where the levator ani muscle arises from the obturator fascia. The ischio-anal fossae, wide inferiorly and narrow superiorly, are filled with fat and loose connective tissue. The two ischio-anal fossae communicate by means of the *deep postanal space* over the *anococcygeal ligament* (body), a fibrous mass located between the anal canal and the tip of the coccyx (Fig. 3.46A).

Each ischio-anal fossa is bounded (Fig. 3.46A,B):

- Laterally by the ischium and the inferior part of the obturator internus, covered with obturator fascia.
- Medially by the external anal sphincter, with a sloping superior medial wall or roof formed by the levator ani as it descends to blend with the sphincter; both structures surround the anal canal.
- Posteriorly by the sacrotuberous ligament and gluteus maximus.
- Anteriorly by the bodies of the pubic bones, inferior to the origin of the puborectalis; these parts of the fossae, extending into the UG triangle superior to the perineal membrane, are known as the **anterior recesses of the ischio-anal fossae.**

The ischio-anal fossae are traversed by tough, fibrous bands and filled with fat, forming the **fat bodies of the ischio-anal fossae.** These fat bodies support the anal canal but are readily displaced to permit expansion of the anal canal during the passage of feces. The fat bodies are traversed by several neurovascular structures, including the inferior anal/rectal vessels and nerves and two other cutaneous nerves: the perforating branch of S2 and S3 and the perineal branch of the S4 nerve.

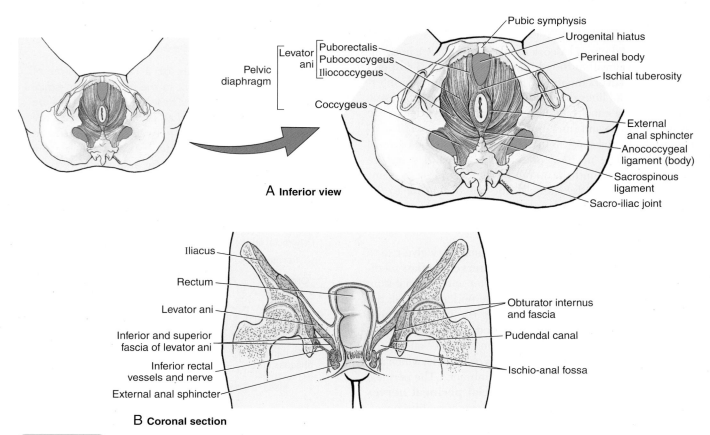

FIGURE 3.46. **Pelvic diaphragm and ischio-anal fossae. A.** Pelvic diaphragm. *Arrow* passes through deep postanal space. **B.** Section of the pelvis through the rectum, anal canal, and ischio-anal fossae.

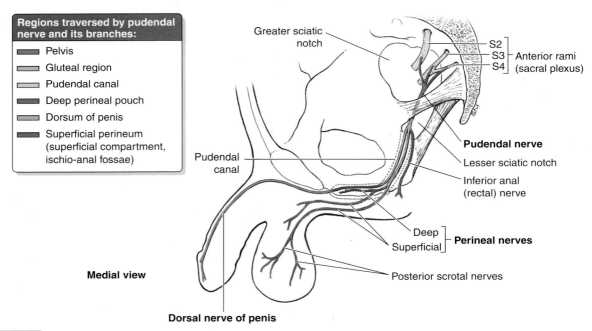

Regions traversed by pudendal nerve and its branches:
- Pelvis
- Gluteal region
- Pudendal canal
- Deep perineal pouch
- Dorsum of penis
- Superficial perineum (superficial compartment, ischio-anal fossae)

Greater sciatic notch

S2
S3 Anterior rami
S4 (sacral plexus)

Pudendal nerve

Lesser sciatic notch

Inferior anal (rectal) nerve

Pudendal canal

Deep ⎱ **Perineal nerves**
Superficial ⎰

Posterior scrotal nerves

Medial view

Dorsal nerve of penis

FIGURE 3.47. **Pudendal nerve.** The five regions in which the nerve runs are color-coded. In females, the superficial perineal nerve gives rise to posterior labial nerves and the terminal branch of the pudendal nerve is the dorsal nerve of the clitoris.

PUDENDAL CANAL

The **pudendal canal** (Alcock canal) is essentially a horizontal passageway within the obturator fascia (Figs. 3.46B and 3.47), which covers the medial aspect of the obturator internus muscle and lines the lateral wall of the ischio-anal fossa. The pudendal canal begins at the posterior border of the ischio-anal fossa and runs from the *lesser sciatic notch* adjacent to the ischial spine to the posterior edge of the perineal membrane. The internal pudendal artery and vein, the pudendal nerve, and the nerve to the obturator internus enter this canal at the lesser sciatic notch, inferior to the ischial spine. The internal pudendal vessels supply and drain blood from the perineum; the pudendal nerve innervates most of the same area.

As the artery and nerve enter the canal, they give rise to the **inferior anal** (rectal) **artery** and **nerve** that pass medially to supply the external anal sphincter and perianal skin. Toward the distal (anterior) end of the pudendal canal, the artery and nerve both bifurcate, giving rise to the **perineal nerve** and **artery**, which are distributed mostly to the superficial pouch (inferior to the perineal membrane) and to the **dorsal artery** and **nerve of the penis** or **clitoris,** which run in the deep pouch (superior to the membrane). The perineal nerve has two branches: the **superficial perineal nerves** give rise to *posterior scrotal* or *labial (cutaneous) branches,* and the **deep perineal nerve** supplies the muscles of the deep and superficial perineal pouches, the skin of the vestibule of the vagina, and the mucosa of the inferiormost

Ischio-anal Abscesses

The ischio-anal fossae are occasionally the sites of infection, which may result in the formation of *ischio-anal abscesses* (Fig. B3.12). These collections of pus are painful. Diagnostic signs of an ischio-anal abscess are fullness and tenderness between the anus and the ischial tuberosity. A perianal abscess may rupture spontaneously, opening into the anal canal, rectum, or perianal skin.

Rectum

Pelvirectal space

Levator ani

Obturator internus

Pudendal canal

Perianal abscess in ischio-anal fossa

Fistula

Pectinate line

External anal sphincter

FIGURE B3.12.

part of the vagina. The **dorsal nerve of the penis** or **clitoris** is the primary sensory nerve serving the male or female organ, especially the glans.

ANAL CANAL

The **anal canal** is the terminal part of the large intestine that extends from the superior aspect of the pelvic diaphragm to the **anus.** The canal begins where the ampulla of the rectum abruptly narrows at the level of the U-shaped sling formed by the puborectalis muscle (Fig. 3.37A,B). The canal ends at the anus, the external outlet of the alimentary tract. The **anal canal,** surrounded by internal and external anal sphincters, descends posteroinferiorly between the **anococcygeal ligament** and the **perineal body.** The anal canal is normally collapsed except during passage of feces. Both sphincters must relax before defecation can occur.

The **external anal sphincter** is a large voluntary sphincter that forms a broad band on each side of the inferior two thirds of the anal canal (Fig. 3.37A). This sphincter blends superiorly with the puborectalis muscle and is described as having subcutaneous, superficial, and deep parts. The external anal sphincter is supplied mainly by S4 through the inferior anal (rectal) nerve (Fig. 3.40).

The **internal anal sphincter** is an involuntary sphincter surrounding the superior two thirds of the anal canal (Fig. 3.37A). It is a thickening of the circular muscle layer. Its contraction (tonus) is stimulated and maintained by the sympathetic fibers from the superior rectal (periarterial) and hypogastric plexuses. It is inhibited (loses its tonic contraction and is allowed to expand passively) by the parasympathetic fibers. This sphincter is tonically contracted most of time to prevent leakage of fluid or flatus; however, it relaxes temporarily in response to distention of the rectal ampulla by feces or gas, requiring voluntary contraction of the puborectalis and the external anal sphincter if defecation or flatulence is not to occur.

Interior of Anal Canal. The superior half of the mucous membrane of the anal canal is characterized by a series of longitudinal ridges called **anal columns** (Fig. 3.37A,C). These columns contain the terminal branches of the superior rectal artery and vein. The **anorectal junction,** indicated by the superior ends of the anal columns, is where the rectum joins the anal canal. The inferior ends of these columns are joined by **anal valves.** Superior to the valves are small recesses called **anal sinuses** (Fig. 3.37C). When compressed by feces, the anal sinuses exude mucus that aids in evacuation of feces from the anal canal. The inferior comb-shaped limit of the anal valves forms an irregular line, the **pectinate line** (Figs. 3.37A,C and 3.48), which indicates the junction of the superior part of the anal canal (visceral; derived from the hindgut) and the inferior part (somatic; derived from the embryonic proctodeum). The anal canal superior to the pectinate line differs from the part inferior to the pectinate line in its arterial supply, innervation, and venous and lymphatic drainage. These differences result from their different embryological origins (Moore & Persaud, 2008).

Vasculature and Lymphatic Drainage of Anal Canal. The *superior rectal artery* supplies the anal canal superior to the pectinate line (Figs. 3.38 and 3.48). The two *inferior rectal arteries* supply the inferior part of the anal canal as well as the surrounding muscles and perianal skin. The *middle rectal arteries* assist with the blood supply to the anal canal

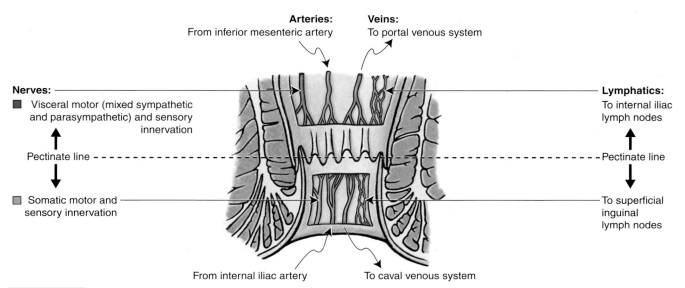

Arteries:
From inferior mesenteric artery

Veins:
To portal venous system

Nerves:
■ Visceral motor (mixed sympathetic and parasympathetic) and sensory innervation

Pectinate line

■ Somatic motor and sensory innervation

Lymphatics:
To internal iliac lymph nodes

Pectinate line

To superficial inguinal lymph nodes

From internal iliac artery

To caval venous system

FIGURE 3.48. **Innervation and vascular supply of anal canal superior and inferior to pectinate line.** The vessels and nerves superior to the pectinate line are visceral; those inferior to the pectinate line are somatic.

by forming anastomoses with the superior and inferior rectal arteries.

The *internal rectal venous plexus* drains in both directions from the level of the pectinate line. Superior to the pectinate line, the internal rectal venous plexus drains chiefly into the *superior rectal vein* (a tributary of the inferior mesenteric vein) and the portal system. Inferior to the pectinate line, the internal rectal venous plexus drains into the *inferior rectal veins* (tributaries of the caval venous system) around the margin of the external anal sphincter. The *middle rectal veins* (tributaries of the internal iliac veins) mainly drain the muscularis externa of the rectal ampulla and form anastomoses with the superior and inferior rectal veins. The rectal venous plexuses receive multiple arteriovenous anastomoses from the superior and middle rectal arteries.

Superior to the pectinate line, the lymphatic vessels drain into the *internal iliac lymph nodes* and through them into the common iliac and lumbar lymph nodes (Fig. 3.39). Inferior to the pectinate line, the lymphatic vessels drain into the *superficial inguinal lymph nodes.*

Innervation of Anal Canal. The nerve supply to the anal canal superior to the pectinate line is visceral innervation from the *inferior hypogastric plexus* (sympathetic, parasympathetic, and visceral afferent fibers) (Figs. 3.40 and 3.48). The superior part of the anal canal is inferior to the pelvic pain line; all visceral afferents travel with the parasympathetic fibers to spinal sensory ganglia S2–S4. Superior to the pectinate line, the anal canal is sensitive only to stretching. The nerve supply of the anal canal inferior to the pectinate line is somatic, derived from the *inferior anal (rectal) nerves,* branches of the pudendal nerve. Therefore, this part of the anal canal is sensitive to pain, touch, and temperature. Somatic efferent fibers stimulate the contraction of the voluntary external anal sphincter.

Hemorrhoids

Internal hemorrhoids ("piles") are prolapses of the rectal mucosa containing the normally dilated veins of the *internal rectal venous plexus* (Fig. B3.13). They are thought to result from a breakdown of the muscularis mucosae, a smooth muscle layer deep to the mucosa. Internal hemorrhoids that prolapse through the anal canal are often compressed by the contracted sphincters, impeding blood flow. As a result, they tend to strangulate and ulcerate. Owing to the presence of abundant arteriovenous anastomoses, bleeding from internal hemorrhoids is usually bright red.

External hemorrhoids are thromboses (blood clots) in the veins of the *external rectal venous plexus* and are covered by skin. Predisposing factors for hemorrhoids include pregnancy, chronic constipation, and any disorder that impedes venous return, including increased intra-abdominal pressure.

The anastomoses among the superior, middle, and inferior rectal veins form clinically important communications between the portal and the systemic venous systems (Fig. 3.48). The superior rectal vein drains into the inferior mesenteric vein, whereas the middle and inferior rectal veins drain through the systemic system into the inferior vena cava. Any abnormal increase in pressure in the valveless portal system or veins of the trunk may cause enlargement of the superior rectal veins, resulting in increase in blood flow or stasis in the internal rectal venous plexus. In *portal hypertension,* as in *hepatic cirrhosis,* the portocaval anastomosis among the superior, middle, and inferior rectal veins, along with portocaval anastomoses elsewhere, may become varicose. It is important to note that the veins of the rectal plexuses *normally* appear varicose (dilated and tortuous) and that internal hemorrhoids occur most commonly in the absence of portal hypertension.

Because visceral afferent nerves supply the anal canal superior to the pectinate line, an incision or a needle insertion in this region is painless. However, the anal canal inferior to the pectinate line is quite sensitive (e.g., to the prick of a hypodermic needle) because it is supplied by the *inferior rectal nerves,* containing somatic sensory fibers.

Anterior view of coronal sections

FIGURE B3.13.

Male Perineum

The male perineum includes the external genitalia (urethra, scrotum, and penis), perineal muscles, and anal canal.

DISTAL MALE URETHRA

The urethra in the bladder neck (intramural part) and the prostatic urethra, the first two parts of the male urethra, are described with the pelvis (Fig. 3.25 and Table 3.8). The **intermediate (membranous) part of the urethra** begins at the apex of the prostate and traverses the deep perineal pouch, surrounded by the external urethral sphincter. It then penetrates the perineal membrane, ending as the urethra enters the bulb of the penis (Fig. 3.18). Posterolateral to this part of the urethra are the small *bulbourethral glands* (Figs. 3.18 and 3.20A) and their slender ducts, which open into the proximal part of the spongy urethra.

The **spongy urethra** begins at the distal end of the intermediate part of the urethra and ends at the **external urethral orifice** (Figs. 3.18 and 3.49B,D). The lumen of the spongy urethra is expanded in the bulb of the penis to form the **intrabulbar fossa** and in the glans of the penis to form the **navicular fossa.** On each side, the ducts of the bulbourethral glands open into the proximal part of the spongy urethra. There are also many minute openings of the ducts of mucus-secreting **urethral glands** (Littré glands) into the spongy urethra.

The arterial supply of the intermediate and spongy parts of the urethra is from branches of the *dorsal artery of the* penis (Fig. 3.50B). The veins accompany the arteries and have similar names. Lymphatic vessels from the intermediate part of the urethra drain mainly into the *internal iliac lymph nodes* (Fig. 3.51), whereas most vessels from the spongy urethra pass to the deep inguinal lymph nodes, but some vessels pass to the external iliac lymph nodes. The innervation of the intermediate part of the urethra is the same as that of the prostatic part (Fig. 3.52). The dorsal nerve of the penis, a branch of the *pudendal nerve,* provides somatic innervation of the spongy part of the urethra.

Urethral Catheterization

Urethral catheterization is done to remove urine from a person who is unable to micturate. It is also performed to irrigate the bladder and to obtain an uncontaminated sample of urine. When inserting the catheters and urethral sounds (slightly conical instruments for exploring and dilating a constricted urethra) the curves of the male urethra must be considered.

SCROTUM

The **scrotum** is a cutaneous fibromuscular sac for the testes and associated structures. It is situated posteroinferior to the penis and inferior to the pubic symphysis (Fig. 3.49). The bilateral embryonic formation of the scrotum is indicated by the midline **scrotal raphe** (Fig. 3.49C), which is continuous on the ventral surface of the penis with the **penile raphe** and posteriorly along the median line of the perineum as the **perineal raphe.** Internally deep to the scrotal raphe, the scrotum is divided into two compartments, one for each testis, by a prolongation of dartos fascia, the **septum of the scrotum.** The contents of the scrotum (testes and epididymides) are described with the abdomen (see Chapter 2).

Vasculature of Scrotum. The anterior aspect of the scrotum is supplied by the **anterior scrotal arteries,** terminal branches of the **external pudendal arteries** (Fig. 3.50B and Table 3.10), and the posterior aspect is supplied by the **posterior scrotal arteries,** terminal branches of the *internal pudendal arteries.* The scrotum also receives branches from the cremasteric arteries, branches of inferior epigastric arteries. The *scrotal veins* accompany the arteries and drain primarily to the *external pudendal veins.* Lymphatic vessels from the scrotum drain into the *superficial inguinal lymph nodes* (Fig. 3.51).

Innervation of Scrotum. The anterior aspect of the scrotum is supplied by the **anterior scrotal nerves** derived from the *ilio-inguinal nerve,* and by the *genital branch of the genitofemoral nerve.* The posterior aspect of the scrotum is supplied by **posterior scrotal nerves,** branches of the superficial perineal branches of the pudendal nerve (Fig. 3.52), and by the *perineal branch of the posterior femoral cutaneous nerve.*

PENIS

The penis is the male organ of copulation and the outlet for urine and semen. The penis consists of a *root, body,* and *glans penis* (Fig. 3.49D). It is composed of three cylindrical bodies of erectile cavernous tissue: the paired **corpora cavernosa** and the single **corpus spongiosum** ventrally. (Note that in the anatomical position, the penis is erect; when the penis is flaccid, its dorsum is directed anteriorly.) Each *cavernous body* has a fibrous outer covering or capsule, the **tunica albuginea** (Fig. 3.49B). Superficial to the outer covering is the **deep fascia of the penis** (Buck fascia), the continuation of the deep perineal fascia that forms a membranous covering for the corpora, binding them together. The corpus spongiosum contains the spongy urethra. The corpora cavernosa are fused with each other in the median plane except posteriorly, where they separate to form the **crura of the penis** (Figs. 3.49A and 3.53).

The **root of the penis** consists of the crura, bulb, and **ischiocavernosus** and **bulbospongiosus muscles**

A Lateral view

Ductus deferens
Fundiform ligment
Suspensory ligament of penis
Deep dorsal vein of penis
Superficial dorsal vein of penis
Corona
Neck of penis
Prepuce (foreskin)
Glans penis

Ureter
Urinary bladder
Seminal gland
Prostate
Dorsal artery and nerve of penis
Crus of penis
Bulb of penis
Testicular vessels
Ductus deferens
Epididymis
Testis
Scrotum
Dartos muscle

B Transverse section

Spongy urethra
Prepuce
Glans penis
Scrotum

Dorsal vein {Superficial, Deep}
Corpora cavernosa
Deep artery
Septum penis
Spongy urethra
Dorsal artery and nerve
Skin
Loose areolar tissue
Deep fascia
Tunica albuginea
Corpus spongiosum

C Ventral view

Glans penis
Corona of glans penis
Scrotum
Anus

Frenulum of prepuce
Penile raphe
Scrotal raphe
Perineal raphe

D Dorsal view

Pubic hairs covering site of pubic symphysis
Root of penis
Body of penis
Corona of glans penis
Glans penis
External urethral orifice

FIGURE 3.49. **Male urogenital organs. A.** Internal structures. **B.** Male external genitalia: uncircumcised penis and scrotum, and section through the body of the penis. **C.** and **D.** Surface anatomy of male external genitalia; penis is circumcised.

(Fig. 3.53; Table 3.9). The root is located in the superficial perineal pouch (Fig. 3.44*B,D*). The **crura** and **bulb of the penis** contain masses of erectile tissue. Each crus is attached to the inferior part of the internal surface of the corresponding ischial ramus, anterior to the ischial tuberosity. The bulb

of the penis is penetrated by the urethra, continuing from its intermediate part.

The **body of the penis** (usually pendulous) is the free part that is suspended from the pubic symphysis. Except for a few fibers of the bulbospongiosus near the root of the penis and the ischiocavernosus that embrace the crura, the penis has no muscles. Distally, the corpus spongiosum of the penis expands to form the **glans penis** (Fig. 3.49). The margin of the glans (head) projects beyond the ends of the corpora cavernosa to form the **corona of the glans.** The corona overhangs the neck of the glans. The **neck of the glans** separates the glans from the body of the penis. The slit-like opening of the spongy urethra, the *external urethral orifice,* is located near the tip of the glans (Fig. 3.49*D*). The thin skin and fascia of the penis are prolonged as a double layer of skin, the **prepuce** (foreskin), which covers the glans to a variable extent (Fig. 3.49*A,B*). The **frenulum of the prepuce** is a median fold that passes from the prepuce to the urethral surface of the glans (Fig. 3.49*C*).

The **suspensory ligament of the penis** is a condensation of the deep fascia that arises from the anterior surface of the pubic symphysis and splits to form a sling that is attached to the deep fascia of the penis at the junction of its root and body (Fig. 3.49*A*). The fibers of the suspensory ligament are short and taut. The **fundiform ligament of the penis** is a band of the subcutaneous tissue that descends in the midline from the linea alba superior to the pubic symphysis (Fig. 3.15*A*). It passes inferiorly and splits to surround the penis and then unites and blends with the dartos fascia forming the scrotal septum.

The **superficial perineal muscles** are the superficial transverse perineal, bulbospongiosus, and ischiocavernosus (Fig. 3.43*B* and Table 3.9). These muscles are in the super-ficial perineal pouch and are supplied by the perineal nerves. Because of their function during erection and the activity of the bulbospongiosus subsequent to urination and ejaculation, to expel the last drops of urine and semen, the perineal muscles are generally more developed in males than in females.

Vasculature of Penis. The penis is supplied by *branches of the internal pudendal arteries* (Fig. 3.50*B* and Table 3.10).

- **Dorsal arteries of the penis** run in the interval between the corpora cavernosa on each side of the deep dorsal vein, supplying the fibrous tissue around the corpora cavernosa and the penile skin.
- **Deep arteries of the penis** pierce the crura and run distally near the center of the corpora cavernosa, supplying the erectile tissue in these structures.
- **Arteries of the bulb of the penis** supply the posterior (bulbous) part of the corpus spongiosum and the bulbourethral gland. They give off numerous branches (**helicine arteries of penis**) that open directly into the cavernous spaces. When the penis is flaccid, these arteries are coiled, restricting blood flow.
- **Superficial** and **deep branches of the external pudendal arteries** supply the penile skin, anastomosing with branches of the internal pudendal arteries.

Blood from the cavernous spaces of the corpora cavernosa is drained by a venous plexus that becomes the **deep**

TABLE 3.10 ARTERIAL SUPPLY OF PERINEUM

Artery	Origin	Course	Distribution
Internal pudendal	Internal iliac artery	Leaves pelvis through greater sciatic foramen; hooks around ischial spine to enter perineum via lesser sciatic foramen; enters pudendal canal	Primary artery of perineum and external genital organs
Inferior rectal	Internal pudendal artery	Arises at entrance to pudendal canal; crosses ischio-anal fossa to anal canal	Anal canal inferior to pectinate line; anal sphincters; perianal skin
Perineal		Arises within pudendal canal; passes to superficial perineal pouch (space) on exit	Supplies superficial perineal muscles and scrotum in male; vestibule in female
Posterior scrotal or labial	Terminal branch of perineal artery	Runs in subcutaneous tissue of posterior scrotum or labia majora	Skin of scrotum or labia majora and minora
Artery of bulb of penis or vestibule		Pierces perineal membrane to reach bulb of penis or vestibule of vagina	Supplies bulb of penis and bulbourethral gland in male; bulb of vestibule and greater vestibular gland in female
Deep artery of penis or clitoris	Terminal branch of internal pudendal artery	Pierces perineal membrane to reach corpora cavernosa of penis or clitoris	Supplies most erectile tissue of penis or clitoris via helicine arteries
Dorsal artery of penis or clitoris		Pierces perineal membrane and passes through suspensory ligament of penis or clitoris to run on dorsum of penis or clitoris	Deep perineal pouch; skin of penis; erectile tissue of penis or clitoris; distal corpus spongiosum of penis, including spongy urethra
External pudendal, superficial and deep branches	Femoral artery	Pass medially across thigh to reach scrotum or labia majora (anterior aspect of urogenital triangle)	Anterior aspect of scrotum and skin at root of penis in male; mons pubis and anterior aspect of labia in female

Abdominal aorta

Inferior mesenteric a.

Left common iliac a.

Superior rectal a.

Left internal iliac a.

Left external iliac a.

Lateral sacral aa.

Umbilical a.

Uterine a.

Left ureter

Ovaries

Uterus

Right ureter

Middle rectal a.

Bladder

Inferior vesical a.

Superior vesical a.

Spine of ischium

Pubic symphysis

Internal pudendal a.

Crus of clitoris

Levator ani

Dorsal artery of clitoris

Inferior rectal aa.

Deep artery of clitoris

Anterior labial a.

Artery of vestibule of vagina

Posterior labial a.

Perineal a.

External pudendal a.

A Female

Femoral a.

Superior rectal a.

Left external iliac a.

Umbilical a.

Rectum

Left ureter

Right ureter

Middle rectal a.

Artery to ductus deferens

Superior vesical a.

Inferior vesical a.

Bladder

Spine of ischium

Pubic symphysis

Internal pudendal a.

Deep artery of penis

Levator ani

Dorsal artery of penis

Inferior rectal aa.

Artery of bulb of penis

Anterior scrotal a.

Perineal a.

Femoral a.

External pudendal a.

B Male

Posterior scrotal a.

FIGURE 3.50. **Arterial supply of perineum.** Superficial and deep dissections of male perineum.

dorsal vein of the penis in the deep fascia (Fig. 3.49A,B). This vein passes deep between the laminae of the suspensory ligament of the penis, anterior to the perineal membrane, to enter the prostatic venous plexus. Blood from the superficial coverings of the penis drains into the **superficial dorsal vein(s),** which ends in the *superficial external pudendal vein.* Some blood also passes to the internal pudendal vein.

Lymph from the skin of the penis drains initially to the *superficial inguinal lymph nodes,* and lymph from the glans and distal spongy urethra drains to the *deep inguinal* and *external iliac nodes.* The cavernous bodies and proximal spongy urethra drain to the *internal iliac nodes* (Fig. 3.51).

Innervation of Penis. The nerves derive from the S2–S4 segments of the spinal cord. Sensory and sympathetic innervation is primarily from the *dorsal nerve of the penis,* a terminal branch of the **pudendal nerve** (Fig. 3.52), which arises in the pudendal canal and passes anteriorly into the deep perineal pouch. It then runs along the dorsum of the penis lateral to the dorsal artery and supplies the skin and glans. The penis is supplied with a variety of sensory nerve endings, especially the glans penis. Branches of the *ilioinguinal nerve* supply the skin at the root of the penis. Cavernous nerves, conveying parasympathetic fibers independently from the prostatic nerve plexus, innervate the helicine arteries.

Erection, Emission, Ejaculation, and Remission. Most of the time, the penis is flaccid. In this state, most arterial blood bypasses the "empty" potential spaces or *sinuses of the corpora cavernosa* by means of arteriovenous anastomoses. Only enough blood to bring oxygen and nutrition to the tissues circulates through the sinuses. When a male is stimulated erotically, parasympathetic stimulation by the *cavernous nerves* (conveying fibers from S2–S4 spinal cord levels via the prostatic nerve plexus) closes the arteriovenous anastomoses.

Simultaneously, the tonic contraction of the smooth muscle in the fibrous trabeculae and coiled *helicine arteries* (terminal branches of the arteries serving the erectile tissue) is inhibited. As a result, the arteries straighten, enlarging their lumina. Blood flow no longer diverted from the cavernous spaces increases in volume, filling the sinuses of the corpora of the penis. The bulbospongiosus and ischiocavernosus muscles reflexively contract, compressing the veins of the corpora cavernosa, impeding the return of venous blood. **Erection** occurs as the corpora cavernosa and corpus spongiosum become engorged with blood at arterial pressure, causing the erectile bodies to become turgid (enlarged and rigid), elevating the penis.

During **emission,** semen (sperms and glandular secretions) is delivered to the prostatic urethra through the ejaculatory ducts after peristalsis of the ductus deferentes and

A = Glans penis
B = Spongy/bulbar urethra
C = Skin of body of penis/ scrotum

Key
◻ Lumbar
◻ Common iliac
◼ Internal iliac
◻ External iliac
◻ Superficial inguinal
◼ Deep inguinal
→ Direction of flow of lymph

Anterior view

FIGURE 3.51. Lymphatic drainage of male perineum.

seminal glands. Prostatic fluid is added to the seminal fluid as the smooth muscle in the prostate contracts. Emission is a sympathetic response (L1–L2 nerves).

During **ejaculation,** semen is expelled from the urethra through the external urethral orifice. Ejaculation results from:

- Closure of the internal urethral sphincter at the neck of the urinary bladder, a sympathetic response (L1–L2 nerves) preventing retrograde ejaculation into the bladder.
- Contraction of the urethral muscle, a parasympathetic response (S2–S4 nerves).
- Contraction of the bulbospongiosus muscles, from the pudendal nerves (S2–S4).

After ejaculation, the penis gradually returns to a flaccid state (**remission**), resulting from sympathetic stimulation that opens the arteriovenous anastomoses and causes contraction of smooth muscle of the helicine arteries, recoiling them. This reduces blood inflow as the bulbospongiosus and ischiocavernosus muscles relax, allowing more blood to be drained from the cavernous spaces into the deep dorsal vein.

Lumbar splanchnic nerves

Superior hypogastric plexus

Sacral splanchnic nerve

Vesical plexus

Pelvic pain line

Dorsal nerve of penis

Sympathetic trunk

Lumbosacral trunk

Left hypogastric nerve

Pelvic splanchnic nerves

Inferior hypogastric plexus

Prostatic plexus

Inferior anal (rectal) nerve

Pudendal nerve

Cavernous nerves

Perineal nerve

Posterior scrotal nerves

Lateral view

Key
- [ ] Sympathetic nerves
- [ ] Parasympathetic nerves
- [ ] Mixed sympathetic and parasympathetic nerves
- [ ] Somatic nerves

FIGURE 3.52. Innervation of male perineum.

Impotence and Erectile Dysfunction

Inability to obtain an erection (**impotence**) may result from several causes. When a lesion of the prostatic plexus or cavernous nerves results in an inability to achieve an erection, a surgically implanted, semirigid or inflatable penile prosthesis may assume the role of the erectile bodies, providing the rigidity necessary to insert and move the penis within the vagina during intercourse.

Erectile dysfunction (ED) may occur in the absence of a nerve insult. Central nervous system (hypothalamic) and endocrine (pituitary or testicular) disorders may result in reduced testosterone (male hormone) secretion. Autonomic nerve fibers may fail to stimulate erectile tissues, or blood vessels may be insufficiently responsive to stimulation. In many such cases erection can be achieved with the assistance of oral medications or injections that increase blood flow into the cavernous sinusoids by causing relaxation of smooth muscle.

Phimosis, Paraphimosis, and Circumcision

An uncircumcised prepuce covers all or most of the glans penis (Fig. 3.49B). The prepuce is usually sufficiently elastic to allow retraction over the glans. In some males, it is tight and cannot be retracted easily (phimosis) if at all. Secretions (smegma) may accumulate in the preputial sac, located between the glans penis and prepuce, causing irritation.

In some cases, retraction of the prepuce constricts the neck of the glans so that there is interference with the drainage of blood and tissue fluid (paraphimosis). The glans may enlarge so much that the prepuce cannot be distracted. Circumcision, surgical excision of the prepuce, must be performed.

Circumcision exposes most, or all, of the glans (Fig. 3.49C,D) and is the most common minor surgical operation performed on male infants. Although it is a religious practice in Islam and Judaism, it is often done routinely for nonreligious reasons.

PERINEAL MUSCLES OF MALES

The *superficial perineal muscles* include the *superficial transverse perineal, ischiocavernosus,* and *bulbospongiosus* (Fig. 3.53). Details of their attachments, innervation, and actions are provided in Table 3.9. The ischiocavernosus and bulbospongiosus muscles both constrict venous outflow from the erectile bodies to assist erection, simultaneously pushing blood from the penile root into the body. The bulbospongiosus muscle constricts around the bulb of the penis to express the final drops of urine or semen.

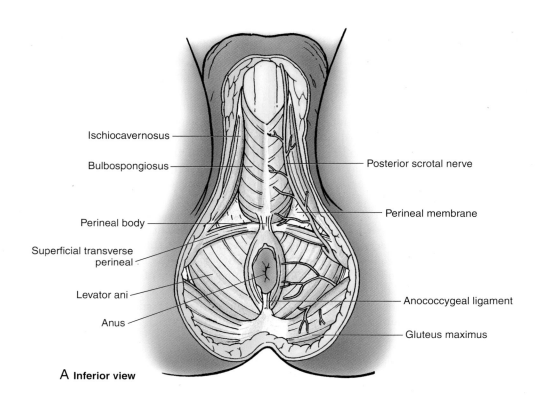

A Inferior view

- Ischiocavernosus
- Bulbospongiosus
- Perineal body
- Superficial transverse perineal
- Levator ani
- Anus
- Posterior scrotal nerve
- Perineal membrane
- Anococcygeal ligament
- Gluteus maximus

B Inferior view

- Corpus spongiosum
- Urethra
- Dorsal vein of penis
- Crus of penis
- Urethra
- Perineal membrane
- Anus
- Corpus cavernosum
- Dorsal artery of penis
- Dorsal nerve of penis
- Bulb of penis (cut)
- Perineal artery
- Internal pudendal artery

FIGURE 3.53.   Superficial and deep dissections of male perineum.

Female Perineum

The female perineum includes the female external genitalia, perineal muscles, and anal canal.

FEMALE EXTERNAL GENITALIA

The **female external genitalia** include the mons pubis, labia majora (enclosing the pudendal cleft), labia minora (enclosing the vestibule), clitoris, bulbs of the vestibule, and greater and lesser vestibular glands. The synonymous terms **pudendum** and **vulva** include all these parts. The term *pudendum* is commonly used clinically (Fig. 3.54). The pudendum vulva serves as sensory and erectile tissue for sexual arousal and intercourse, directs the flow of urine, and prevents entry of foreign material into the urogenital tract.

Mons Pubis.   The **mons pubis** is the rounded fatty eminence anterior to the pubic symphysis, pubic tubercle, and superior pubic rami. The amount of fat in the mons increases at puberty and decreases after menopause. After puberty, the mons pubis is covered with coarse pubic hairs (Fig. 3.54A).

Labia Majora.   The **labia majora** are prominent folds of skin that bound the **pudendal cleft,** the slit between the labia majora, and indirectly provide protection for the urethral and vaginal orifices. Each labium majus—largely filled with subcutaneous fat containing smooth muscle and the termination of the round ligament of the uterus—passes inferoposteriorly from the mons pubis toward the anus. The external aspects of the labia in the adult are covered with pigmented skin containing many sebaceous glands and are covered with crisp pubic hair. The internal aspects of the labia are smooth, pink, and hairless. The labia are thicker anteriorly where they join to form the **anterior commissure.** Posteriorly, they merge to form the **posterior commissure,** which usually disappears after the first vaginal birth.

Labia Minora.   The **labia minora** are folds of fat-free, hairless skin. They have a core of spongy connective tissue containing erectile tissue and many small blood vessels. Although the internal surface of each labium minus consists of thin moist skin, it has the typical pink color of a mucous membrane and contains many sensory nerve endings. The labia minora are enclosed in the pudendal cleft within the labia majora and surround the vestibule into which the external urethral and vaginal orifices open. Anteriorly, the labia minora form two laminae: the medial laminae unite as the **frenulum of the clitoris,** and the lateral laminae unite to form the **prepuce of the clitoris** (Fig 3.54). In young women, especially virgins, the labia minora are connected posteriorly by a small transverse fold, the **frenulum of the labia minora** (fourchette).

Clitoris.   The **clitoris** is an erectile organ located where the labia minora meet anteriorly. The clitoris consists of a **root** and a **body,** which are composed of two crura, two corpora cavernosa, and the **glans of the clitoris.** The glans is covered by the prepuce of the clitoris (Figs. 3.54A and 3.55A). The clitoris is highly sensitive and enlarges on tactile stimulation. The glans is the most highly innervated part of the clitoris.

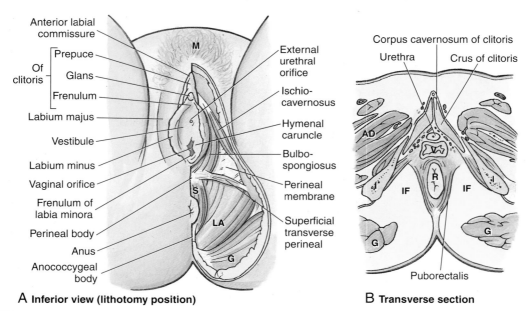

A Inferior view (lithotomy position)   **B** Transverse section

FIGURE 3.54.   **Female perineum. A.** Surface anatomy and perineal muscles. **B.** Structures on section. *AD,* adducter muscles of thigh; *G,* gluteus maximus; *I,* ischium; *IF,* ischio-anal fossa; *LA,* levator ani; *M,* mons pubis; *S,* external anal sphincter; *R,* rectum; *V,* vagina.

Pubic symphysis

Dorsal artery of clitoris

Deep artery of clitoris

Artery of vestibule

Posterior labial arteries

Greater vestibular gland

Perineal membrane

Superficial transverse perineal muscle

Transverse perineal artery

Perineal artery

Internal pudendal artery

Inferior rectal artery

Anus

External anal sphincter

A Inferior view

Dorsal nerve of clitoris

Glans of clitoris

Crus of clitoris

External urethral orifice

Opening of paraurethral gland

Opening of greater vestibular gland

Vaginal orifice

Posterior labial nerves

Bulb of vestibule

Perineal body

Perineal nerve

Pudendal nerve

Ischial tuberosity

Inferior rectal nerves

Levator ani

B Anterior view

Key

A = Vulva
B = Glans clitoris, labia minora
C = Urethra

Lumbar
Common iliac
Internal iliac
External iliac
Superficial inguinal
Deep inguinal
Sacral
→ Direction of flow of lymph

FIGURE 3.55. Blood supply, innervation, and lymphatic drainage of vulva (pudendum).

Vestibule. The **vestibule** is the space surrounded by the labia minora, which contains the openings of the urethra, vagina, and ducts of the greater and lesser vestibular glands. The **external urethral orifice** is located posteroinferior to the glans clitoris and anterior to the vaginal orifice. On each side of the external urethral orifice are the openings of the

ducts of the **paraurethral glands.** The size and appearance of the **vaginal orifice** vary with the condition of the **hymen,** a thin fold of mucous membrane within the vaginal orifice surrounding the lumen. After its rupture, only remnants of the hymen, **hymenal caruncles** (tags), are visible (Fig. 3.54A).

Bulbs of Vestibule. The **bulbs of the vestibule** are paired masses of elongated erectile tissue that lie along the sides of the vaginal orifice under cover of the bulbospongiosus muscles (Fig. 3.55A). The bulbs are homologous with the bulb of the penis and the corpus spongiosum.

Vestibular Glands. The **greater vestibular glands** (Bartholin glands) are located on each side of the vestibule, posterolateral to the vaginal orifice. These glands are round or oval and are partly overlapped posteriorly by the bulbs of the vestibule, and both are partially surrounded by the bulbospongiosus muscles. The slender ducts of these glands pass deep to the bulbs and open into the vestibule on each side of the vaginal orifice. These glands secrete mucus into the vestibule during sexual arousal. The **lesser vestibular**

glands are smaller glands on each side of the vestibule that open into it between the urethral and the vaginal orifices. These glands secrete mucus into the vestibule, which moistens the labia and vestibule (Fig. 3.54A).

Vasculature of Vulva. The *arterial supply* to the vulva is from the *external and internal pudendal arteries* (Fig. 3.50A and Table 3.10). The *internal pudendal artery* supplies most of the skin, external genitalia, and perineal muscles. The labial arteries are branches of the internal pudendal artery, as are those of the clitoris (Fig. 3.55A). The *labial veins* are tributaries of the *internal pudendal veins* and accompanying veins (L. *venae comitantes*). Venous engorgement during the excitement phase of the sexual response causes an increase in the size and consistency of the clitoris and the bulbs of the vestibule. As a result the clitoris becomes turgid.

The vulva contains a rich network of *lymphatic vessels* that pass laterally to the *superficial inguinal lymph nodes* (Fig. 3.55B). The glans of the clitoris and anterior labia minora may also drain to the deep inguinal nodes or internal iliac nodes.

Innervation of Vulva. The anterior aspect of the vulva is supplied by the **anterior labial nerves,** derived from the *ilio-inguinal nerve* and the *genital branch of the genitofemoral nerve.* The posterior aspect is supplied by the *perineal branch of the posterior cutaneous nerve of the thigh* laterally and the *pudendal nerve* centrally. The pudendal nerve is the main nerve of the perineum. Its **posterior labial nerves** supply the labia; *deep* and *muscular branches* supply the orifice of the vagina and superficial perineal muscles; and the *dorsal nerve of the clitoris* supplies deep perineal muscles and sensation to the clitoris (Fig. 3.55A). The bulb of the vestibule and erectile bodies of the clitoris receive parasympathetic fibers via cavernous nerves from the uterovaginal plexus. Parasympathetic stimulation produces increased vaginal secretion, erection of the clitoris, and engorgement of erectile tissue in the bulbs of the vestibule.

PERINEAL MUSCLES OF THE FEMALE

The *superficial perineal muscles* include the *superficial transverse perineal, ischiocavernosus,* and *bulbospongiosus* (Fig. 3.54A). Details of the attachments, innervation, and actions of the muscles are provided in Table 3.9.

Dilation of Female Urethra

The female urethra is distensible because it contains considerable elastic tissue, as well as smooth muscle. It can easily dilate without injury to it. Consequently, the passage of catheters or cystoscopes in females is much easier than it is in males.

Inflammation of Greater Vestibular Glands

The greater vestibular glands (Bartholin glands) are usually not palpable, except when infected. *Bartholinitis,* inflammation of the greater vestibular glands, may result from a number of pathogenic organisms. Infected glands may enlarge to a diameter of 4 to 5 cm and impinge on the wall of the rectum.

Pudendal and Ilio-inguinal Nerve Blocks

To relieve the pain experienced during childbirth, *pudendal nerve block anesthesia* may be performed by injecting a local anesthetic agent into the tissues surrounding the pudendal nerve. The injection may be made where the pudendal nerve crosses the lateral aspect of the sacrospinous ligament, near its attachment to the ischial spine.

Although a pudendal nerve block anesthetizes most of the perineum, it does not abolish sensation from the anterior part of the perineum that is innervated by the ilio-inguinal nerve. To abolish pain from the anterior part of the perineum, an *ilio-inguinal nerve block* is performed (Fig. B3.14).

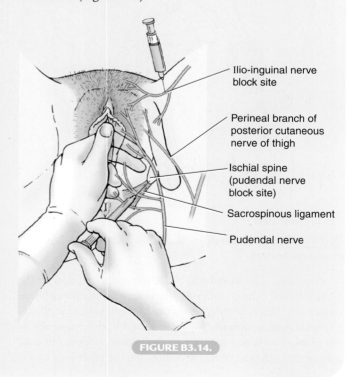

Ilio-inguinal nerve block site

Perineal branch of posterior cutaneous nerve of thigh

Ischial spine (pudendal nerve block site)

Sacrospinous ligament

Pudendal nerve

FIGURE B3.14.

Medical Imaging of Pelvis and Perineum

MRI provides excellent evaluation of male and female pelvic structures (Figs. 3.56 and 3.57). It also permits the identification of tumors and congenital anomalies.

A Median section

B Transverse section

C Transverse section

Key	
A	Anus
Ad	Adductor muscles
B	Bulb of penis
C	Conjoint ramus
Cav	Corpus cavernosum of penis
Cox	Coccyx
Cr	Crus of penis
IAF	Ischio-anal fossa
IL	Iliacus
IT	Ischial tuberosity
LA	Levator ani
Max	Gluteus maximus
OE	Obturator externus
OI	Obturator internus
P	Prostate
PP	Prostatic venous plexus
R	Rectum
RP	Root of penis
RVP	Rectovesical pouch
S	Sacrum
SGI	Seminal gland
Sy	Pubic symphysis
U	Urethra
UB	Urinary bladder

D Coronal section

E Coronal section

FIGURE 3.56.   MRI studies of male pelvis and perineum.

A Median section

B Transverse section

C Transverse section

D Transverse section

Key					
A	Anus	LM	Labium majus	RA	Rectus abdominis
B	Body of uterus	M	Myometrium	Sc	Sacrum
C	Cervix of uterus	Max	Gluteus maximus	SP	Superior ramus of pubis
Cox	Coccyx	OE	Obturator externus	Sy	Pubic symphysis
CJ	Conjoint ramus	OI	Obturator internus	U	Uterus
E	Endometrium	Ov	Ovary	UB	Urinary bladder
F	Fundus of uterus	Pm	Perineal membrane	V	Vagina
IAF	Ischio-anal fossa	PV	Perivaginal veins	Ve	Vestibule of vagina
IT	Ischial tuberosity	R	Rectum	VU	Vesico-uterine pouch
LA	Levator ani				

FIGURE 3.57. MRI studies of female pelvis and perineum.

The female pelvis is commonly examined using ultrasonography. The viscera may be examined by placing a transducer on the lower abdomen, just superior to the pubic symphysis (A in Fig. 3.58A). For the nongravid uterus, the full bladder serves as an acoustical "window," conducting transmitted and reflected sound waves to and from the viscera, the uterus retroverted by the full bladder (Fig. 3.58B,E). Currently, viscera is studied most often by means of a slender transducer passed into the vagina (B in Fig. 3.58A and Fig. 3.58D). Ultrasonography is the procedure of choice for examining the developing embryo and fetus (Fig. 3.58E,F).

A Ultrasound scanning: (A) transabdominal; (B) transvaginal

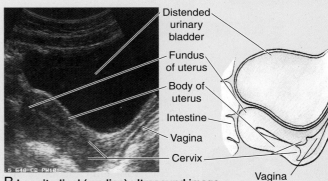

B Longitudinal (median) ultrasound image

- Distended urinary bladder
- Fundus of uterus
- Body of uterus
- Intestine
- Vagina
- Cervix
- Vagina

C Transverse transabdominal ultrasound (US) image

- Ovary
- Distended urinary bladder
- Broad ligament
- Follicle
- Ovary
- Uterus
- Intestine

D Longitudinal transvaginal US image of nongravid uterus

UT

E Longitudinal transvaginal US scan of early gravid uterus

- 9-week fetus
- Amniotic fluid
- Placenta
- Uterine wall

F Progressive growth and development of embryo/fetus

FIGURE 3.58. Ultrasonographic (US) studies of the pelvis. **A.** Placement of the transducer for US scanning of pelvis. **B.** and **C.** Appearance of normal pelvic viscera in transabdominal scans. **D.** Transvaginal US scan of nongravid uterus; *arrows,* endometrium and uterine canal. **E.** Gestational sac in gravid uterus. **F.** US study of embryonic/fetal growth and development. *A,* Only the gestational sac is evident (*arrow*). *B,* Limbs (*solid arrows*) and head (*outlined arrow*) are visible. *C,* Sagittal section of fetal head, neck and thorax (*P, placenta*). *D,* Profile of face and upper limb (*arrow*).

 Go to http://thePoint.lww.com/ECA4e for helpful study tools, including USMLE-style questions, case studies, images, and more!

CHAPTER

4 Back

VERTEBRAL COLUMN / 275

Curvatures of Vertebral Column / 276

Surface Anatomy of Curvatures of Vertebral Column / 276

Structure and Function of Vertebrae / 277

Regional Characteristics of Vertebrae / 278

Surface Anatomy of Vertebral Column / 284

Joints of Vertebral Column / 288

Movements of Vertebral Column / 292

Vasculature of Vertebral Column / 294

Innervation of Vertebral Column / 294

SPINAL CORD AND MENINGES / 296

Structure of Spinal Nerves / 297

Spinal Meninges and Cerebrospinal Fluid / 297

Vasculature of Spinal Cord and Spinal Nerve Roots / 301

MUSCLES OF BACK / 301

Extrinsic Back Muscles / 303

Intrinsic Back Muscles / 303

Surface Anatomy of Back Muscles / 304

Suboccipital and Deep Neck Muscles / 311

MEDICAL IMAGING OF BACK / 314

The back, the posterior aspect of the trunk inferior to the neck and superior to the gluteal region (buttocks), is the region of the body to which the head, neck, and limbs are attached. Because of their close association with the trunk, the back of the neck and the posterior and deep cervical muscles and vertebrae are described in this chapter. The back consists of:

- Skin.
- Subcutaneous tissue.
- Deep fascia.
- Muscles (a superficial layer, concerned with positioning and moving the upper limbs, and deeper layers, concerned with posture, moving or maintaining the position of the axial skeleton).
- Ligaments.
- Vertebral column.
- Ribs (in the thoracic region).
- Spinal cord and meninges (membranes covering the spinal cord).
- Various segmental nerves and vessels.

VERTEBRAL COLUMN

The vertebral column (spine), extending from the cranium (skull) to the apex of the coccyx, forms the skeleton of the neck and back and is the main part of the axial skeleton (articulated bones of the cranium, vertebral column, ribs, and sternum). The vertebral column protects the spinal cord and spinal nerves, supports the weight of the body superior to the level of the pelvis, provides a partly rigid and flexible axis for the body and a pivot for the head, and plays an important role in posture and locomotion.

The adult vertebral column typically consists of 33 vertebrae arranged in five regions: 7 cervical, 12 thoracic, 5 lumbar, 5 sacral, and 4 coccygeal (Fig. 4.1A–D). The **lumbosacral angle** is located at the junction of the lumbar region of the vertebral column and sacrum. Significant motion occurs between only the superior 25 vertebrae. The five sacral vertebrae (segments) are fused in adults to form the **sacrum,** and the four coccygeal vertebrae (segments) are fused to form the **coccyx.** The vertebrae gradually become larger as the vertebral column descends to the sacrum and then become progressively smaller toward the apex of the coccyx. These structural differences are related to the fact that the successive vertebrae bear increasing amounts of the body's weight. The vertebrae reach maximum size immediately superior to the sacrum, which transfers the weight to the pelvic girdle at the sacro-iliac joints. The presacral vertebral column is flexible because it consists of **vertebrae** joined together by semi-rigid **intervertebral (IV) discs.** The 25 cervical, thoracic, lumbar, and first sacral vertebrae also articulate at synovial *zygapophysial joints*, which facilitate and control the vertebral column's flexibility. The vertebral

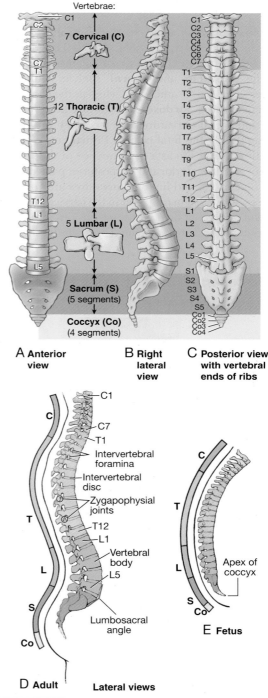

A Anterior view   **B Right lateral view**   **C Posterior view with vertebral ends of ribs**

D Adult   **Lateral views**   **E Fetus**

FIGURE 4.1.   **Vertebral column and curvatures. A–C.** Regions of adult vertebral column. **D.** Curvatures of adult vertebral column. **E.** Curvatures of fetal vertebral column. C + T + L = presacral vertebral column

bodies contribute approximately three quarters of the height of the presacral vertebral column, and the fibrocartilage of IV discs contributes approximately one quarter. The shape and strength of the vertebrae and IV discs, ligaments, and muscles provide stability to the vertebral column.

Curvatures of Vertebral Column

The vertebral column in adults has four curvatures: cervical, thoracic, lumbar, and sacral (Fig. 4.1D). The curvatures provide a flexible support (shock-absorbing resilience) for the body. The **thoracic** and **sacral** (pelvic) **curvatures** (**kyphoses**) are concave anteriorly, whereas the **cervical** and **lumbar curvatures** (**lordoses**) are concave posteriorly. The thoracic and sacral curvatures are **primary curvatures,** developing during the fetal period. Primary curvatures are retained throughout life as a consequence of differences in height between the anterior and the posterior parts of the vertebrae. The cervical and lumbar curvatures are **secondary curvatures,** which begin to appear in the cervical region during the fetal period but do not become obvious until infancy. Secondary curvatures are maintained primarily by differences

Surface Anatomy of Curvatures of Vertebral Column

Cervical lordosis (2° curvature)

Thoracic kyphosis (1° curvature)

Lumbar lordosis (2° curvature)

Sacral kyphosis (1° curvature)

Lateral view of normal curvatures of back

FIGURE SA4.1.

When the posterior surface of the trunk is observed, especially in a lateral view, the normal curvatures of the vertebral column are apparent.

Abnormal Curvatures of Vertebral Column

 Abnormal curvatures in some people result from developmental anomalies and in others from pathological processes such as *osteoporosis*. Osteoporosis is characterized by a net demineralization of bones and results from a disruption of the normal balance of calcium deposition and resorption. The bones become weakened and brittle and are subject to fracture. Vertebral body osteoporosis occurs in all vertebrae but is most common in thoracic vertebrae and is an especially common finding in postmenopausal women.

A Normal

B Excessive kyphosis

C Excessive lordosis

Lateral views

FIGURE B4.1.

Excessive thoracic kyphosis (clinically shortened to **kyphosis**; colloquially called "humpback") is characterized by an abnormal increase in the thoracic curvature; the vertebral column curves posteriorly (Fig. B4.1A,B). This abnormality can result from erosion of the anterior part of one or more vertebrae. Progressive erosion and collapse of vertebrae results in an overall loss of height. *Dowager's hump* is a colloquial name for excess thoracic kyphosis in older women resulting from osteoporosis; however, kyphosis occurs in geriatric people of both sexes.

Excessive lumbar lordosis (clinically shortened to **lordosis**; colloquially called "hollow back") is characterized by an anterior rotation of the pelvis, producing an abnormal increase in the lumbar curvature; the vertebral column becomes more convex anteriorly (Fig. B4.1A,C). This *abnormal extension deformity* may be associated with weakened trunk musculature, especially of the anterolateral abdominal wall. To compensate for alterations to their normal line of gravity, women develop a temporary lordosis during late pregnancy.

(Continued on next page)

FIGURE 4.2. Typical vertebra, represented by second lumbar vertebra. A and B. Bony features. C. Functional components. D. Formation of intervertebral foramen.

Scoliosis (curved back) is characterized by an abnormal lateral curvature that is accompanied by rotation of the vertebrae (Fig. B4.1*D,E*). The spinous processes turn toward the cavity of the abnormal curvature. Scoliosis is the most common deformity of the vertebral column in pubertal girls (aged 12–15 years). Asymmetric weakness of the intrinsic back muscles (*myopathic scoliosis*), failure of half of a vertebra to develop (*hemivertebra*), and a difference in the length of the lower limbs are causes of scoliosis.

D Normal   **E Scoliosis**
Posterior views

FIGURE B4.1.

in thickness between the anterior and the posterior parts of the IV discs (Fig. 4.1*E*). The **cervical curvature** becomes prominent when an infant begins to hold his or her head erect.

The **lumbar curvature** becomes apparent when an infant begins to walk and assumes the upright posture. This curvature, generally more pronounced in females, ends at the **lumbosacral angle,** formed at the junction of the L5 vertebra with the sacrum. The **sacral curvature** of females is reduced so that the coccyx protrudes less into the pelvic outlet (birth canal).

The curvatures provide additional flexibility (shock-absorbing resilience) to the vertebral column, augmenting that provided by the IV discs. Although the flexibility provided by the IV disc is passive and limited primarily by the zygapophysial (facet) joints and longitudinal ligaments, that provided by the curvatures is actively resisted by the contraction of muscle groups antagonistic to the movement.

Structure and Function of Vertebrae

Vertebrae vary in size and other characteristics from one region of the vertebral column to another and to a lesser degree within each region. A *typical vertebra* consists of a vertebral body, vertebral arch, and seven processes (Fig. 4.2*A–C*). The **vertebral body** (the anterior, more massive part of the vertebra) gives strength to the vertebral column and supports body weight. The size of vertebral bodies, especially from T4 inferiorly, increases to bear the progressively greater body weight. In life, most of the superior and inferior surfaces of vertebral bodies are covered with hyaline cartilage, which are remnants of the cartilaginous model from which the bone develops, except at the periphery, where there is a ring of smooth bone, the **epiphysial rim** (Fig. 4.2A). The cartilaginous remnants permit some diffusion of fluid between the IV disc and capillaries in the vertebral body.

The **vertebral arch** lies posterior to the vertebral body and is formed by right and left pedicles and laminae (Fig. 4.2C). The **pedicles** are short, stout processes that join the vertebral arch to the vertebral body. The pedicles project posteriorly to meet two broad, flat plates of bone, called **laminae,** which unite in the midline (Fig. 4.2A–C). The vertebral arch and the posterior surface of the vertebral body form the walls of the **vertebral foramen.** The succession of vertebral foramina in the articulated column forms the **vertebral canal,** which contains the spinal cord, meninges (protective membranes), fat, spinal nerve roots, and vessels. The indentations formed by the projection of the body and articular processes superior and inferior of the pedicles are **vertebral notches** (Fig. 4.2B). The superior and inferior vertebral notches of adjacent vertebrae contribute to the formation of the **IV foramina,** which give passage to spinal nerve roots and accompanying vessels and contain the spinal ganglia (Fig. 4.2D).

Seven processes arise from the vertebral arch of a typical vertebra (Fig. 4.2A–C):

- One median **spinous process** projects posteriorly (and usually inferiorly) from the vertebral arch at the junction of the laminae and typically overlaps the vertebra below.
- Two **transverse processes** project posterolaterally from the junctions of the pedicles and laminae.
- Four **articular processes**—two **superior** and two **inferior**—also arise from the junctions of the pedicles and laminae, each bearing an **articular surface (facet).**

The spinous process and two transverse processes project from the vertebral arch and afford attachments for deep back muscles and serve as levers that help the muscles move the vertebrae (Fig. 4.2C). The four articular processes are in apposition with corresponding processes of vertebrae superior and inferior to them, forming *zygapophysial (facet) joints* (Fig. 4.2D). The direction of the articular facets on the articular processes determines the types of movements permitted and restricted between the adjacent vertebrae of each region. The interlocking of the articular processes also assists in keeping adjacent vertebrae aligned, particularly preventing one vertebra from slipping anteriorly on the vertebra below.

Regional Characteristics of Vertebrae

Each of the 33 vertebrae is unique. However, most of the vertebrae demonstrate characteristic features identifying

Laminectomy

A **laminectomy** is the surgical excision of one or more spinous processes and their supporting laminae in a particular region of the vertebral column (1 in Fig. B4.2) and also commonly denotes the removal of most of the vertebral arch by transecting the pedicles (2 in Fig. B4.2). Laminectomies provide access to the vertebral canal to relieve pressure on the spinal cord or nerve roots, commonly caused by a tumor, herniated IV disc, or bony hypertrophy (excess growth).

Spinous process

Lamina

Vertebral arch

Pedicle

Vertebral foramen (vertebral canal in the articulated vertebral column)

Vertebral body

FIGURE B4.2.

Fractures of Vertebrae

Fractures and fracture-dislocations of the vertebral column usually result from sudden forceful flexion, as in an automobile accident. Typically, the injury is a crush or compression fracture of the body of one or more vertebrae. If violent anterior movement of the vertebra occurs in addition to compression, a vertebra may be displaced anteriorly on the vertebra inferior to it. Usually this dislocates and fractures the articular facets between the two vertebrae and ruptures the interspinous ligaments. Irreparable injuries to the spinal cord accompany most severe flexion injuries of the vertebral column.

them as belonging to one of the five regions of the vertebral column (e.g., cervical vertebrae are characterized by the presence of foramina in their transverse processes). In each region, the articular facets are oriented on the articular processes of the vertebrae in a characteristic direction that determines the type of movement permitted between the adjacent vertebrae and, in aggregate, for the region. Regional variations in the size and shape of the vertebral canal accommodate the varying thickness of the spinal cord. The main regional characteristics of vertebrae are summarized in Tables 4.1 through 4.4 and Figures 4.3 through 4.7.

A **Lateral view**

B **Anterior view**

C **Lateral view (M, mandible)**

D **Superior view**

E **Lateral view**

FIGURE 4.3. **Cervical vertebrae. A and B.** Articulated vertebrae. **C.** Lateral radiograph. **D and E.** Bony features of typical cervical vertebrae,* occurs at C6 only.

TABLE 4.1 CERVICAL VERTEBRAE

Cervical vertebrae (C1–C7) form the skeleton of the neck; the atlas (C1) and the axis (C2) are atypical cervical vertebrae.

Part (Typical Vertebrae)	Distinctive Characteristics
Body	Small and wider from side to side than anteroposteriorly; superior surface is concave between adjacent (uncinate) processes; inferior surface is convex
Vertebral foramen	Large and triangular
Transverse processes	Foramina transversaria; small or absent in C7; vertebral arteries and accompanying venous and sympathetic plexuses pass through foramina (except C7, which transmits only small accessory vertebral veins); anterior and posterior tubercles
Articular processes	Superior facets directed superoposteriorly; inferior facets directed inferoanteriorly
Spinous process	C3–C5 short and bifid (split in two parts); process of C6 is long but that of C7 is longer (C7 is called *vertebra prominens*)

Superior views

A Atlas

B Axis

C Anteroposterior view

D Anterior view

Key for C and D

A	Lateral mass of atlas
D	Dens of axis
C2	Axis

E Posterior view

Key for E

AA	Anterior arch of C1	PA	Posterior arch of C1
AT	Anterior tubercle of C1	PT	Posterior tubercle of C1
C1–C4	Cervical vertebrae	SF	Superior articular facet
D	Dens (odontoid) process		of C1
	of C2	SP	Spinous process
FJ	Zygapophysial (facet) joint	T	Foramen transversarium
La	Lamina	VC	Vertebral canal

FIGURE 4.4. Atlas (C1) and axis (C2). **A** and **B.** Bony features. **C.** Anteroposterior radiograph. **D.** Anterior view. **E.** Three-dimensional reconstructed computed tomographic (CT) image.

TABLE 4.1 CERVICAL VERTEBRAE (*continued*)

Vertebrae (Atypical)	Distinctive Characteristics	
Atlas (C1)	• Ring-like; somewhat kidney-shaped when viewed superiorly or inferiorly • No spinous process or body; consists of two lateral masses connected by anterior and posterior arches • Concave superior articular facets create atlanto-occipital joints with the occipital condyles; flat inferior facets meet with the C2 vertebra to create lateral atlanto-axial joints	
Axis (C2)	• Strongest cervical vertebra • Distinguishing feature is the dens, which projects superiorly from its body and provides a pivot around which the atlas turns and carries the cranium • Articulates anteriorly with the anterior arch of the atlas and posteriorly with the transverse ligament of the atlas	

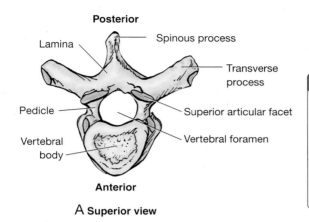

A Superior view

Posterior

Spinous process

Lamina

Transverse process

Pedicle

Superior articular facet

Vertebral body

Vertebral foramen

Anterior

Key

H = Head of rib
P = Pedicle of vertebra
TP = Transverse process of vertebra
SP = Spinous process (tip overlaps inferior IV disc and vertebra)
Arrows = Joints of heads of ribs

B Anteroposterior view

C Lateral view

Superior

Transverse costal facet (for tubercle of rib)

Zygapophysial joint

Superior and inferior costal facets (for head of rib)

Vertebral body

Inferior articular facet

Spinous process

Inferior

D Lateral view

Radiologic "disc space" (intervertebral disc)

Intervertebral foramen

Pedicle

Head of 10th rib (note position of attachment on vertebral body)

Spinous process

Articular processes { inferior / superior }

Head of 11th rib

Body of vertebra T12

FIGURE 4.5. **Thoracic vertebrae. A.** Bony features of typical vertebra. **B.** Anteroposterior radiograph. **C.** Articulated vertebrae. **D.** Lateral radiograph.

TABLE 4.2 THORACIC VERTEBRAE

Thoracic vertebrae (T1–T12) form the posterior part of the skeleton of the thorax and articulate with the ribs. The space between the vertebral bodies is the site of the intervertebral disc.

Part	Distinctive Characteristics
Body	Heart-shaped; bears one or two costal facets for articulation with head of rib (*H*)
Vertebral foramen	Circular and smaller than those in cervical and lumbar regions
Transverse process (*TP*)	Long and strong; extends posterolaterally; length diminishes from T1 to T12; those of T1–T10 have transverse costal facets for articulation with tubercle of rib
Articular processes	Superior articular facets directed posteriorly and slightly laterally; inferior articular facets directed anteriorly and slightly medially
Spinous process (*SP*)	Long; slopes posteroinferiorly; tip extends to level of vertebral body below

FIGURE 4.6.   **Lumbar vertebrae. A and B.** Bony features. **C.** Lateral radiograph of lumbar spine. **D.** Lateral radiograph of L1–L2 region. Letters refer to structures labeled in **C**.

TABLE 4.3 LUMBAR VERTEBRAE

Part	Distinctive Characteristics	
Body	Massive; kidney-shaped when viewed superiorly; larger and heavier than those of other regions	
Vertebral foramen	Triangular; larger than in thoracic vertebrae and smaller than in cervical vertebrae	
Transverse processes	Long and slender; accessory process on posterior surface of base of each process	
Articular processes	Superior articular facets directed posteromedially (or medially); inferior articular facets directed anterolaterally (or laterally); mammillary process on posterior surface of each superior articular process	
Spinous process	Short and sturdy; hatchet-shaped	

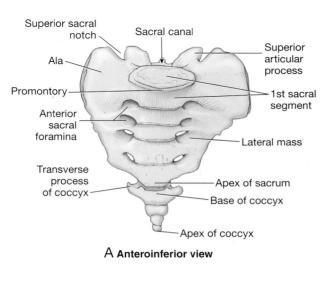

Superior sacral notch
Ala
Promontory
Anterior sacral foramina
Transverse process of coccyx
Sacral canal
Superior articular process
1st sacral segment
Lateral mass
Apex of sacrum
Base of coccyx
Apex of coccyx

A Anteroinferior view

Zygapophysial joint
Sacro-iliac joint
Sacral foramina
Sacrococcygeal joint
Coccyx (partly fused)
Sacrum

B Posteroanterior view

Superior articular facet
Auricular surface
Median crest
Intermediate crest
Lateral crest
Posterior sacral foramina
Sacral hiatus
Cornua of sacrum and coccyx
Apex of coccyx
Sacral canal

C Posterosuperior view

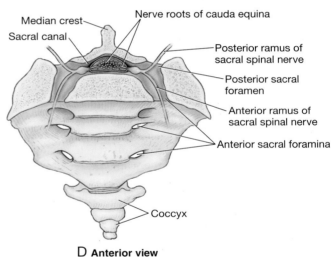

Median crest
Sacral canal
Nerve roots of cauda equina
Posterior ramus of sacral spinal nerve
Posterior sacral foramen
Anterior ramus of sacral spinal nerve
Anterior sacral foramina
Coccyx

D Anterior view

FIGURE 4.7. **Sacrum and coccyx. A.** Base and pelvic surface. **B.** Posteroanterior radiograph. **C.** Dorsal surface. **D.** Coronal section through first sacral foramina.

TABLE 4.4 SACRUM AND COCCYX

The large, wedge-shaped **sacrum** in adults is composed of five fused sacral vertebrae. The sacrum provides strength and stability to the pelvis and transmits body weight to the pelvic girdle through the **sacro-iliac joints.** The base of the sacrum is formed by the superior surface of the S1 vertebra. Its superior articular processes articulate with the inferior articular processes of the L5 vertebra. The projecting anterior edge of the body of the first sacral vertebra is the **sacral promontory.** On the pelvic and dorsal surfaces are four pairs of sacral foramina for the exit of the rami of the first four sacral nerves and the accompanying vessels. The pelvic surface of the sacrum is smooth and concave. The four transverse lines indicate where fusion of the sacral vertebrae occurred. The posterior surface of the sacrum is rough and convex. The fused spinous processes form the **median sacral crest.** The fused articular processes form the **intermediate sacral crests,** and the fused tips of the transverse processes form the **lateral sacral crests.** The inverted U-shaped **sacral hiatus** results from the absence of the laminae and spinous processes of the S4 and S5 vertebrae. The hiatus leads into the sacral canal, the inferior end of the vertebral canal. The **sacral cornua** (L. *horns*), representing the inferior articular processes of the S5 vertebra, project inferiorly on each side of the sacral hiatus and are a helpful guide to its location. The lateral surface of the sacrum has an ear-shaped (auricular) articular surface that participates in the sacro-iliac joint. The four vertebrae of the tapering **coccyx** are remnants of the skeleton of the embryonic tail-like caudal eminence. The distal three vertebrae fuse during middle life to form the coccyx, a beak-like bone that articulates with the sacrum.

Surface Anatomy of Vertebral Column

The spinous processes from the C7 vertebra inferiorly can be observed when the back is flexed (Fig. SA4.2*A,B*), but most of the spinous processes can be palpated, even in an obese individual, because the fat does not normally accumulate in the midline. Although C7 is the most superior process that is visible (*vertebra prominens*), the spinous process of T1 may be the most prominent. The spinous processes of C2–C6 may be palpated in the nuchal groove between the neck muscles; the C3–C5 spinous processes are separated from the surface by the nuchal ligament, making them harder to palpate. C1 has no spinous process. The transverse processes of the C1, C6, and C7 vertebrae are also palpable. Those of C1 can be palpated by deep pressure posteroinferior to the tips of the mastoid processes of the temporal bones (bony prominences posterior to the ears).

The spinous processes of thoracic vertebrae may be observed in thin people and can be palpated from superior to inferior starting at the C7 spinous process. The tips of the thoracic spinous processes do not indicate the level of the corresponding vertebral bodies because they overlap (lie at the level of) the vertebra below. The transverse processes of the thoracic vertebrae can usually be palpated on each side of the spinous processes in the thoracic region; and in thin individuals, the ribs can be palpated from tubercle to angle, at least in the lower back (inferior to the scapula).

The spinous processes of the lumbar vertebrae are large and easy to observe when the trunk is flexed and can be palpated in the **posterior median furrow** (Fig. SA4.2*C*). A horizontal line joining the highest points of the iliac crests passes through the tip of the L4 spinous process and the L4–L5 IV disc. This is a useful landmark when performing lumbar puncture to obtain a sample of cerebrospinal fluid (see the "Lumbar Spinal Puncture" blue box discussed subsequently in this chapter). The transverse processes are covered with thick muscles and may or may not be palpable.

The S2 spinous process lies at the middle of a line drawn between the posterior superior iliac spines, indicated by the skin dimples formed by the attachment of skin and deep fascia to these spines. This level indicates the inferior extent of the subarachnoid space (lumbar cistern). The median crest of the sacrum can be palpated in the midline inferior to the L5 spinous process (Fig. SA4.2*D*). The *sacral hiatus* can be palpated at the inferior end of the sacrum in the superior part of the *intergluteal (natal) cleft* between the buttocks. Clinically the coccyx is examined with a gloved finger in the anal canal and its apex can be palpated approximately 2.5 cm posterosuperior to the anus. The *sacral triangle* is formed by the lines joining the posterior superior iliac spines and the superior part of the intergluteal cleft. The sacral triangle outlining the sacrum is a common area of pain resulting from low back sprains.

Site of external occipital protuberance

Nuchal groove (nuchal ligament deep to skin)

C7 spinous process (vertebra prominens)

T1 spinous process

T2 spinous process

Supraspinous ligament

T4 spinous process

A Posterior view

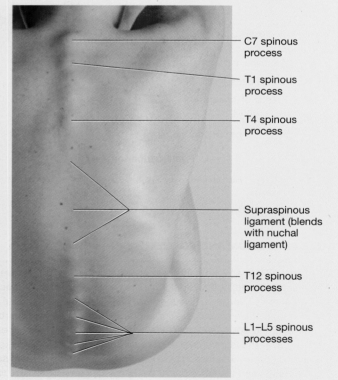

C7 spinous process

T1 spinous process

T4 spinous process

Supraspinous ligament (blends with nuchal ligament)

T12 spinous process

L1–L5 spinous processes

B Posterior view

FIGURE SA4.2. **A and B.** Neck and back flexed with scapulae protracted.

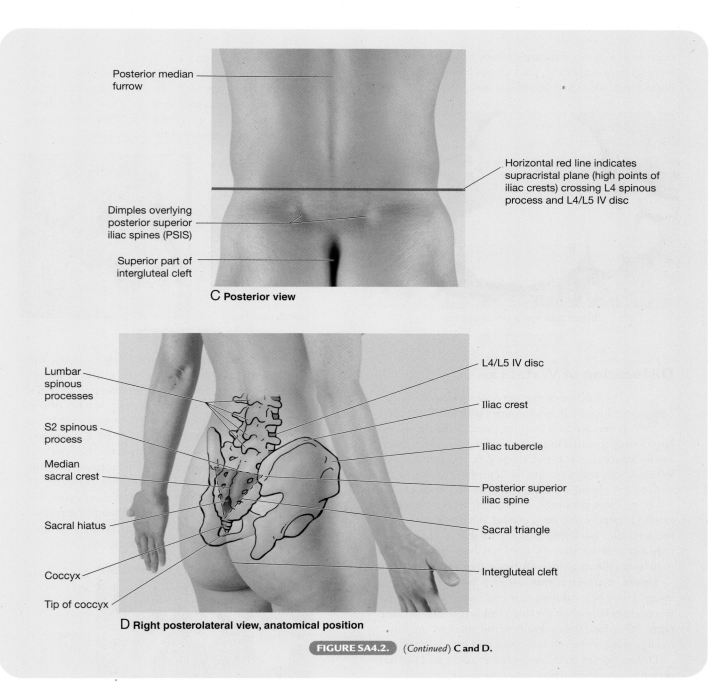

C **Posterior view**

- Posterior median furrow
- Horizontal red line indicates supracristal plane (high points of iliac crests) crossing L4 spinous process and L4/L5 IV disc
- Dimples overlying posterior superior iliac spines (PSIS)
- Superior part of intergluteal cleft

- Lumbar spinous processes
- L4/L5 IV disc
- S2 spinous process
- Iliac crest
- Median sacral crest
- Iliac tubercle
- Sacral hiatus
- Posterior superior iliac spine
- Coccyx
- Sacral triangle
- Tip of coccyx
- Intergluteal cleft

D **Right posterolateral view, anatomical position**

FIGURE SA4.2.   (*Continued*) **C and D.**

Spina Bifida

The most common congenital anomaly of the vertebral column is **spina bifida occulta,** in which the laminae (embryonic neural arches) of L5 and/or S1 fail to develop normally and fuse. This bony defect, present in up to 24% of people, is concealed by skin but its location is often indicated by a tuft of hair. Most people with spina bifida occulta have no back problems. In severe types of the anomaly, such as **spina bifida cystica,** one or more vertebral arches may almost completely fail to develop (Moore & Persaud, 2008) (Fig. B4.3). Spina bifida cystica is associated with herniation of the meninges (*meningocele*) and/or the spinal cord (*meningomyelocele*). Usually, neurological symptoms are present in severe cases of meningomyelocele (e.g., paralysis of limbs and disturbances in bladder and bowel control).

Infant with spina bifida cystica

FIGURE B4.3.

Dislocation of Vertebrae

The bodies of the cervical vertebrae can be dislocated in neck injuries with less force than is required to fracture them. Because of the large vertebral canal in the cervical region, slight dislocation can occur without damaging the spinal cord. When a cervical vertebra is severely dislocated, it injures the spinal cord. If the dislocation does not result in "facet jumping" with locking of the displaced articular processes, the cervical vertebrae may self-reduce ("slip back into place") so that a radiograph may not indicate that the cord has been injured. MRI may reveal the resulting soft tissue damage.

Severe hyperextension of the neck ("whiplash injury") may occur during rear-end motor vehicle collisions, especially when the head rest is too low. In these types of hyperextension injuries, the anterior longitudinal ligament is severely stretched and may be torn.

Dislocation of vertebrae in the thoracic and lumbar regions is uncommon because of the interlocking of their articular processes; however, owing to the abrupt transition from the relatively inflexible thoracic region to the much more mobile lumbar region, T11 and T12 are the most commonly fractured noncervical vertebrae.

Fractures of the interarticular parts of the vertebral laminae of L5 (*spondylolysis of L5*) may result in forward displacement of the L5 vertebral body relative to the sacrum (*spondylolisthesis*). (Fig. B4.4) Spondylolysis of L5, or susceptibility to it, probably results from a failure of the centrum of L5 to unite adequately with the neural arches during development. Spondylolisthesis

at the L5–S1 articulation may (but does not necessarily) result in pressure on the spinal nerves of the cauda equina as they pass into the superior part of the sacrum, causing back and lower limb pain. The intrusion of the L5 body into the pelvic inlet reduces the anteroposterior diameter of the pelvic inlet.

Spondylolisthesis

FIGURE B4.4.

Severe hyperextension is most likely to injure the posterior parts of the vertebrae—the vertebral arches and their processes. Severe hyperextension of the neck (e.g., as occurs in diving injuries) may pinch the posterior arch of C1 vertebra between the occipital bone and the C2 vertebra. In these cases, the C1 vertebra usually breaks at one or both grooves for the vertebral arteries (*white arrows*, Fig. B4.5). The anterior longitudinal ligament and adjacent anulus fibrosus of the C2–C3 IV disc may also rupture. If this occurs, the cranium, C1, and C2 are separated from the rest of the axial skeleton, and the spinal cord is usually severed. Individuals with this injury seldom survive.

Anterior arch

Lateral mass

Posterior arch

FIGURE B4.5.   *Red arrows* indicate fractures.

Lumbar Spinal Stenosis

Lumbar spinal stenosis describes a stenotic (narrow) vertebral foramen in one or more lumbar vertebrae (Fig. B4.6). Stenosis of a lumbar vertebral foramen alone may cause compression of one or more of the spinal nerve roots occupying the vertebral canal. Surgical treatment may consist of decompressive laminectomy. Lumbar spinal stenosis may be a hereditary anomaly that can make a person more vulnerable to age-related degenerative changes such as IV disc protrusion. When IV disc protrusion occurs in a patient with spinal stenosis, it further compromises the size of the vertebral canal, as does arthritic proliferation and ligamentous degeneration. It should also be noted that lumbar spinal nerves increase in size as the vertebral column descends, but the IV foramina decease in size.

A Normal vertebral foramen   **B Stenotic vertebral foramen**
Superior views

FIGURE B4.6.

A Anterior view

B Dissected isolated disc

C Sagittal section

D Lateral view of disc when recumbent

E Lateral view of disc when erect (weight bearing)

F Anterior view during lateral flexion

FIGURE 4.8.   Structure and function of intervertebral (IV) discs.

Joints of Vertebral Column

The joints of the vertebral column include the joints of vertebral bodies, joints of the vertebral arches, craniovertebral joints, costovertebral joints (Chapter 1), and sacro-iliac joints (Chapter 3).

JOINTS OF VERTEBRAL BODIES

The joints of the vertebral bodies are *symphyses* (*secondary cartilaginous joints*) designed for weight bearing and strength. The articulating surfaces of adjacent vertebrae are connected by ***IV discs*** and ligaments (Fig. 4.8). The IV discs, interposed between the bodies of adjacent vertebrae, provide strong attachments between the vertebral bodies. As well as permitting movement between adjacent vertebrae, the discs have resilient deformability, which allows them to serve as shock absorbers. Each IV disc consists of an *anulus fibrosus*, an outer fibrous part, and a gelatinous central mass, the *nucleus pulposus.*

The **anulus fibrosus** is a ring consisting of concentric lamellae of fibrocartilage forming the circumference of the IV disc. The anuli insert into the smooth, rounded *epiphysial rims* on the articular surfaces of the vertebral bodies (Fig. 4.8C). The fibers forming each lamella run obliquely from one vertebra to another; the fibers of one lamella typically run at right angles to those of adjacent ones.

The **nucleus pulposus** is the central core of the IV disc (Fig. 4.8) and, at birth, the nuclei are about 85% water. The pulpy nuclei become broader when compressed and thinner when tensed or stretched. Compression and tension occur simultaneously in the same disc during movement of the _vertebral column (e.g., anterior and lateral flexion, extension, rotation); the turgid nucleus acts as a semifluid fulcrum (Fig. 4.8D–F). With age, the nuclei pulposi dehydrate and lose elastin and proteoglycans while gaining collagen, eventually becoming dry and granular. As a result, the IV discs lose their turgor, becoming stiffer and more resistant to deformation. As this occurs, the anulus assumes a greater share of the vertical load and the associated stresses and strains.

The lamellae of the anulus thicken with age and often develop fissures and cavities. Because the lamellae are thinner and less numerous posteriorly than they are anteriorly or laterally, the nucleus pulposus is not centered in the disc but is more posteriorly placed (Fig. 4.8C). The nucleus pulposus is avascular. It receives its nourishment by diffusion from blood vessels at the periphery of the anulus fibrosus and vertebral body.

There is no IV disc between the C1 (atlas) and C2 (axis) vertebrae. The most inferior functional disc is between the L5 and S1 vertebrae. The discs vary in thickness in different regions. They are thicker in the cervical and lumbar regions and thinnest in the superior thoracic region. Their relative thickness is related to the range of movement, and their varying shapes produce the secondary curvatures of the vertebral column. The discs are thicker anteriorly in the cervical and lumbar regions, and their thickness is most uniform in the thoracic region.

Uncovertebral "joints" (of Luschka) are located between the uncus of the bodies (uncinate processes) of the C3–C6 vertebrae and the beveled inferolateral surfaces of the vertebral bodies superior to them (Fig. 4.9). The joints are at the lateral and posterolateral margins of the IV discs. The articulating surfaces of these joint-like structures are covered with cartilage and contain a capsule filled with fluid. They are considered to be synovial joints by some; others consider them to be degenerative spaces (fissures) in the discs occupied by extracellular fluid. The uncovertebral "joints" are frequent sites of spur formation (projecting processes of bone) that may cause neck pain.

The **anterior longitudinal ligament** is a strong, broad fibrous band that covers and connects the anterolateral aspects of the vertebral bodies and IV discs (Figs. 4.8A and 4.10A). The ligament extends from the pelvic surface of the sacrum to the anterior tubercle of the C1 vertebra (atlas) and the occipital bone anterior to the foramen magnum. The anterior longitudinal ligament maintains the stability of the intervertebral joints and limits extension of the vertebral column.

The **posterior longitudinal ligament** is a much narrower, somewhat weaker band compared to the anterior longitudinal ligament. The ligament runs within the vertebral canal along the posterior aspect of the vertebral bodies (Fig. 4.8A,C). It is attached mainly to the IV discs and less so to the posterior edges of the vertebral bodies from C2 (axis)

Nucleus pulposus
Anulus fibrosus
Articular cavity of uncovertebral joint
Uncus of vertebral (uncinate process)
Body

FIGURE 4.9. **Uncovertebral joints.** These joints are at the posterolateral margin of the cervical IV discs.

to the sacrum. The posterior longitudinal ligament helps prevent hyperflexion of the vertebral column and posterior herniation of the IV discs. It is well innervated with nociceptive (pain) nerve endings.

JOINTS OF VERTEBRAL ARCHES

The joints of the vertebral arches are the **zygapophysial joints** (facet joints). These articulations are synovial, plane joints between the superior and the inferior articular processes

(G. *zygapophyses*) of adjacent vertebrae. Each joint is surrounded by a thin, loose **joint (articular) capsule,** which is attached to the margins of the articular surfaces of the articular processes of adjacent vertebrae (Fig. 4.10B,C). Accessory ligaments unite the laminae, transverse processes, and spinous processes and help stabilize the joints. The zygapophysial joints permit gliding movements between the articular processes; the shape and disposition of the articular surfaces determine the type of movement possible. The zygapophysial

A Anterolateral view

B Superior view

C Posterolateral view

D Lateral view

FIGURE 4.10.   **Joints and ligaments of vertebral column. A.** The pedicles of the superior vertebrae have been sawn through, and their bodies have been removed. A rib and its costovertebral joint and associated ligaments are also shown. **B.** In this transverse section of an IV disc, the nucleus pulposus has been removed to show the hyaline cartilage plate covering the superior surface of the vertebral body. **C.** The vertebral arch of the superior vertebra has been removed to show the posterior longitudinal ligament. **D.** Ligaments of the cervical region.

joints are innervated by articular branches that arise from the medial branches of the posterior rami of spinal nerves (Fig. 4.11). Each posterior ramus supplies two adjacent joints; therefore, each joint is supplied by two spinal nerves.

ACCESSORY LIGAMENTS OF INTERVERTEBRAL JOINTS

The laminae of adjacent vertebral arches are joined by broad, pale, yellow elastic fibrous tissue called the **ligamenta flava** (L. *flavus*, yellow), which extend almost vertically from the lamina above to the lamina below (Fig. 4.10A). The ligaments bind the laminae of the adjoining vertebrae together, forming alternating sections of the posterior wall of the vertebral canal. The ligamenta flava resist separation of the vertebral laminae by arresting abrupt flexion of the vertebral column and thereby preventing injury to the IV discs.

The strong elastic ligamenta flava help preserve the normal curvatures of the vertebral column and assist with straightening the column after flexing. Adjacent spinous processes are united by weak, almost membranous **interspinous ligaments** and strong fibrous **supraspinous ligaments** (Fig. 4.10B,C). The supraspinous ligament merges superiorly with the **nuchal ligament** (L. *ligamentum nuchae*), the strong median ligament of the neck. The nuchal ligament is composed of thickened fibroelastic tissue extending from the external occipital protuberance and posterior border of the foramen magnum to the spinous

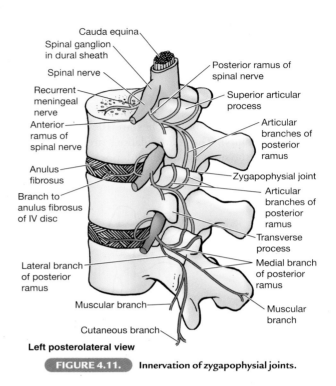

Left posterolateral view

FIGURE 4.11.   Innervation of zygapophysial joints.

processes of the cervical vertebrae. Because of the shortness of the C3–C5 spinous processes, the nuchal ligament substitutes for bone in providing muscular attachments. The **intertransverse ligaments** (Fig. 4.10C), connecting adjacent

---

Aging of Vertebrae and Intervertebral Discs

 During middle and older age, there is an overall decrease in bone density and strength, particularly centrally within the vertebral body, that results in the superior and inferior surfaces of the vertebrae becoming increasingly concave. The nuclei pulposi dehydrate and lose elastin and proteoglycans while gaining collagen. As a result, the IV discs lose their turgor, becoming stiffer and more resistant to deformation. The lamellae of the anulus thicken and often develop fissures and cavities. Although the margins of adjacent vertebral bodies approach more closely as the superior and inferior surfaces of the body become concave, it has been shown that the IV discs increase in size with age. Not only do the IV discs become increasingly convex but also, between the ages of 20 and 70, their diameter increases (Bogduk, 1997). Aging of the IV discs combined with the changing shape of the vertebrae results in an increase in compressive forces at the periphery of the vertebral bodies, where the discs attach. In response, osteophytes (bony

spurs) commonly develop around the margins of the vertebral bodies.

Injury and Disease of Zygapophysial Joints

 When the zygapophysial joints are injured or develop osteophytes during aging (osteoarthritis), the related spinal nerves are often affected. This causes pain along the distribution pattern of the dermatomes and spasm in the muscles derived from the associated myotomes (a myotome consists of all the muscles or parts of muscles receiving innervation from one spinal nerve). *Denervation of lumbar zygapophysial joints* is a procedure that may be used for treatment of back pain caused by disease of these joints. The nerves are sectioned near the joints or are destroyed by radiofrequency *percutaneous rhizolysis* (root dissolution). The denervation process is directed at the articular branches of two adjacent posterior rami of the spinal nerves because each joint receives innervation from both the nerve exiting that level and the superjacent nerve.

A Superior view
- Anterior tubercle of atlas
- Dens of axis
- **Anterior cavity of median atlanto-axial joint**
- Superior articular facet of atlas
- **Transverse ligament of atlas**
- **Posterior cavity of median atlanto-axial joint**
- Posterior arch of atlas (C1)
- Vertebral canal
- Spinous process of axis (C2)

B Median section
- Dura mater (cut edge)
- Apical ligament of dens
- **Anterior atlanto-occipital membrane**
- Anterior cavity of median atlanto-axial joint
- Dens of axis
- Body of axis (C2)
- Anterior longitudinal ligament
- Tectorial membrane
- Superior longitudinal band of cruciate ligament
- Transverse ligament of atlas
- Vertebral artery
- Posterior atlanto-occipital membrane
- Inferior longitudinal band of cruciate ligament
- Posterior atlanto-axial memebrane
- Ligamentum flavum
- Interspinous ligament
- Posterior longitudinal ligament (cut edge and posterior surface)

C Posterior view
- Bands of cruciate ligament
  - Superior longitudinal band
  - Transverse ligament of atlas
  - Inferior longitudinal band
- **Tectorial membrane**
- **Alar ligament**
- Joint capsule of atlanto-occipital joint
- Atlas
- Atlanto-axial joint (lateral)
- Foramen transversarium
- Axis
- Tectorial membrane

FIGURE 4.12. **Craniovertebral joints. A.** Ligaments of the atlanto-occipital and atlanto-axial joints. The large vertebral foramen of the atlas (C1 vertebra) is divided into two foramina by the transverse ligament of atlas. The larger posterior foramen is for the spinal cord, and the smaller anterior foramen is for the dens of the axis (C2 vertebra). **B.** The hemisected craniovertebral region shows the median joints and membranous continuities of the ligamenta flava and longitudinal ligaments in the craniovertebral region. **C.** Bands of cruciate ligament.

transverse processes, consist of scattered fibers in the cervical region and fibrous cords in the thoracic region. In the lumbar region, they are thin and membranous.

CRANIOVERTEBRAL JOINTS

The craniovertebral joints include the atlanto-occipital joints, between the atlas (C1 vertebra) and the occipital bone of the cranium, and the atlanto-axial joints, between the C1 and the C2 vertebrae. *Atlanto*, a Greek prefix, refers to the atlas. These craniovertebral articulations are synovial joints that have no IV discs. Their design allows a wider range of movement than in the rest of the vertebral column.

Atlanto-occipital Joints. The atlanto-occipital joints, between the lateral masses of C1 (atlas) and the occipital condyles (Fig. 4.12C), permit nodding of the head, such as the neck flexion and extension that occurs when indicating approval (the "yes" movement). The main movement is flexion, with a little lateral flexion (bending) and rotation. These joints also permit sideways tilting of the head. The atlanto-occipital joints are synovial joints of the condyloid type and have thin, loose joint capsules. The cranium and C1 are also connected by **anterior** and **posterior atlanto-occipital membranes,** which extend from the anterior and posterior arches of C1 to the anterior and posterior margins of the foramen magnum (Fig. 4.12B). The anterior and posterior atlanto-occipital membranes help prevent excessive movement of these joints.

Atlanto-axial Joints. There are three atlanto-axial articulations: two (right and left) **lateral atlanto-axial joints** between the lateral masses of C1 and the superior facets of C2 (Fig. 4.12C), and one **median atlanto-axial joint** between the dens of C2 and the anterior arch and transverse ligament of the atlas (Fig. 4.12A, B). The median atlanto-axial joint is a pivot joint, whereas the lateral atlanto-axial joints are plane-type synovial joints. Movement at all three atlanto-axial joints permits the head to be turned from side to side, as occurs when rotating the head to indicate disapproval (the "no" movement). During this movement, the cranium and C1 vertebra rotate on the C2 vertebra as a unit. During rotation of the head, the dens of C2 is the pivot, which is held in a socket formed anteriorly by the anterior arch of the atlas and posteriorly by the transverse ligament of the atlas.

The **transverse ligament of the atlas** is a strong band extending between the tubercles on the medial aspects of the lateral masses of the C1 vertebrae (Fig. 4.12A). Vertically oriented but much weaker superior and inferior **longitudinal bands** pass from the transverse ligament to the occipital bone superiorly and to the body of C2 inferiorly. Together, the transverse ligament and the longitudinal bands form the **cruciate ligament** (formerly the cruciform ligament), so named because of its resemblance to a cross (Fig. 4.12C).

The **alar ligaments** extend from the sides of the dens to the lateral margins of the foramen magnum. These short, rounded cords attach the cranium to the C2 vertebra and

serve as check ligaments, preventing excessive rotation at the joints.

The **tectorial membrane** is the strong superior continuation of the posterior longitudinal ligament across the median atlanto-axial joint through the foramen magnum to the central floor of the cranial cavity. It runs from the body of C2 to the internal surface of the occipital bone and covers the alar ligaments and transverse ligaments of the atlas (Fig. 4.12B,C).

Movements of Vertebral Column

The following movements of the vertebral column are possible (Fig. 4.13): flexion, extension, lateral flexion and rotation. The range of movement of the vertebral column varies according to the region and the individual. The normal range of movement possible in healthy young adults is typically reduced by 50% or more as they age. The mobility of the column results primarily from the compressibility and elasticity of the IV discs. The range of movement of the vertebral column is limited by the:

- Thickness, elasticity, and compressibility of the IV discs.
- Shape and orientation of the zygapophysial joints.
- Tension of the joint capsules of the above joints.
- Resistance of the back muscles and ligaments (such as the ligamenta flava and the posterior longitudinal ligament).
- Attachment to the thoracic (rib) cage.
- Bulk of the surrounding tissues.

FIGURE 4.13.   Movements of vertebral column.

Herniation of Nucleus Pulposus

Herniation or protrusion of the gelatinous nucleus pulposus into or through the anulus fibrosus is a well-recognized cause of low back and lower limb pain. If degeneration of the posterior longitudinal ligament and wearing of the anulus fibrosus has occurred, the nucleus pulposus may herniate into the vertebral canal and compress the spinal cord or nerve roots of spinal nerves in the cauda equina (Fig. B4.7). Herniations usually occur posterolaterally, where the anulus is relatively thin and does not receive support from the posterior or anterior longitudinal ligaments. A posterolateral herniation is more likely to be symptomatic because of the proximity of the spinal nerve roots.

The *localized back pain* of a herniated disc results from pressure on the longitudinal ligaments and periphery of the anulus fibrosus and from local inflammation, resulting from chemical irritation by substances from the ruptured nucleus pulposus. *Chronic pain* resulting from the spinal nerve roots being compressed by the herniated disc is referred to the area (dermatome) supplied by that nerve. Posterolateral herniation is most common in the lumbar region; approximately 95% of protrusions occur at the L4–L5 or L5–S1 levels. In patients of advanced years, the nerve roots are more likely being compressed by increased ossification (osteophytes) of the IV foramen as they exit. *Sciatica*, pain in the lower back and hip and radiating down the back of the thigh into the leg, is often caused by a herniated lumbar IV disc or osteophytes that compress the L5 or S1 component of the sciatic nerve. The spinal nerve roots descend to the IV foramen from which the spinal nerve formed by their merging will exit. The nerve that exits a given IV foramen passes through the superior bony half of the foramen and thus lies above and is not affected by a herniating disc at that level. However, the nerve roots passing to the IV foramen immediately and farther below pass directly across the area of herniation (i.e., herniation of the L4–L5 disc affects the L5 nerve root) (Fig. B4.6*B*).

Symptom-producing IV disc protrusions occur in the cervical region almost as often as in the lumbar region. In the cervical region, the IV discs are centrally placed in the anterior border of the IV foramen, and a herniating disc compresses the nerve actually exiting at that level. Recall, however, that cervical spinal nerves exit superior to the vertebra of the same number. Cervical disc protrusions result in pain in the neck, shoulder, arm, and hand.

Cauda equina
Compressed spinal nerve root
Herniation of nucleus pulposus
Defect in anulus fibrosus
Nucleus pulposus
Anulus fibrosus

A Transverse section

B Transverse MRI

C Median MRI

Vertebral canal
Posterior longitudinal ligament
Nucleus pulposus
Anulus fibrosus
Herniation of nucleus pulposus

D Median section

FIGURE B4.7.

Rupture of Transverse Ligament of Atlas

When the transverse ligament of the atlas ruptures, the dens is set free, resulting in *atlanto-axial subluxation* or incomplete dislocation of the median atlanto-axial joint. When complete dislocation occurs, the dens may be driven into the upper cervical region of the spinal cord, causing *quadriplegia* (paralysis of all four limbs), or into the medulla of the brainstem, causing death.

Rupture of Alar Ligaments

The alar ligaments are weaker than the transverse ligament of the atlas. Consequently, combined flexion and rotation of the head may tear one or both alar ligaments. Rupture of an alar ligament results in an increase of approximately 30% in the range of movement to the opposite side.

The back muscles producing movements of the vertebral column are discussed subsequently; however, the movements are not produced exclusively by the back muscles. They are assisted by gravity and the action of the anterolateral abdominal muscles (see Chapter 2). Movements between adjacent vertebrae occur at the resilient nuclei pulposi of the IV discs and at the zygapophysial joints.

The orientation of the latter joints permits some movements and restricts others. Although movements between adjacent vertebrae are relatively small, especially in the thoracic region, the summation of all the small movements produces a considerable range of movement of the vertebral column as a whole (e.g., when flexing to touch the toes). Movements of the vertebral column are freer in the cervical and lumbar regions than in the thoracic region. Flexion, extension, lateral flexion, and rotation of the neck are especially free because the:

- IV discs, although thin relative to most other discs, are thick relative to the small size of the vertebral bodies at this level.
- Articular surfaces of the zygapophysial joints are relatively large and the joint planes are almost horizontal.
- Joint capsules of the zygapophysial joints are loose.
- Neck is relatively slender (with less surrounding soft tissue bulk).

Flexion of the vertebral column is greatest in the cervical region. The sagittally oriented joint planes of the lumbar region are conducive to flexion and extension. Extension of the vertebral column is most marked in the lumbar region and usually is more extensive than flexion; however, the interlocking articular processes here prevent rotation. The lumbar region, like the cervical region, has large IV discs (the largest ones occur here) relative to the size of the vertebral bodies. Lateral flexion of the vertebral column is greatest in the cervical and lumbar regions.

The thoracic region, in contrast, has IV discs that are thin relative to the size of the vertebral bodies. Relative stability is also conferred on this part of the vertebral column through its connection to the sternum by the ribs and costal cartilages. The joint planes here lie on an arc that is centered on the vertebral body, permitting rotation in the thoracic region. This rotation of the upper trunk, in combination with the rotation permitted in the cervical region and that at the atlanto-axial joints, enables the torsion of the axial skeleton that occurs as one looks back over the shoulder. However, flexion is limited in the thoracic region, including lateral flexion.

Vasculature of Vertebral Column

Vertebrae are supplied by *periosteal* and *equatorial branches* of the major cervical and segmental arteries and their spinal branches. *Spinal branches* supplying the vertebrae are branches of the (Fig. 4.14):

- Vertebral and ascending cervical arteries in the neck.
- Posterior intercostal arteries in the thoracic region.

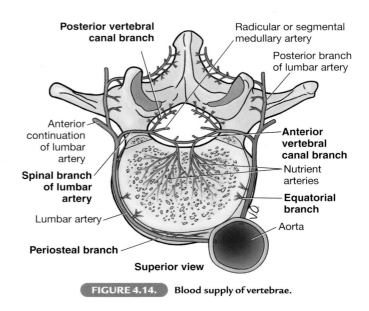

FIGURE 4.14.   Blood supply of vertebrae.

- Subcostal and lumbar arteries in the abdomen.
- Iliolumbar and lateral and medial sacral arteries in the pelvis.

Periosteal and **equatorial branches** arise from these arteries as they cross the external (anterolateral) surfaces of the vertebrae. **Spinal branches** enter the IV foramina and divide into **anterior** and **posterior vertebral canal branches** that pass to the vertebral body and vertebral arch, respectively, and give rise to ascending and descending branches that anastomose with spinal canal branches of adjacent levels. Anterior vertebral canal branches send nutrient arteries into the vertebral bodies. The spinal branches continue as terminal *radicular arteries* distributed to the posterior and anterior roots of the spinal nerves and their coverings or as *segmental medullary arteries* that continue to the spinal cord.

Spinal veins form venous plexuses along the vertebral column both inside (**internal vertebral epidural venous plexus**) and outside (**external vertebral venous plexus**) the vertebral canal (Fig. 4.15). The large, tortuous **basivertebral veins** form within the vertebral bodies and emerge from foramina on the surfaces of the vertebral bodies (mostly the posterior aspect) and drain into the external and especially the internal vertebral venous plexuses. The **intervertebral veins** receive veins from the spinal cord and vertebral venous plexuses as they accompany the spinal nerves through the IV foramina to drain into the *vertebral veins* of the neck and *segmental veins* of the trunk.

Innervation of Vertebral Column

Other than the zygapophysial joints (innervated by articular branches of the medial branches of the posterior rami), the vertebral column is innervated by (**recurrent**) **meningeal**

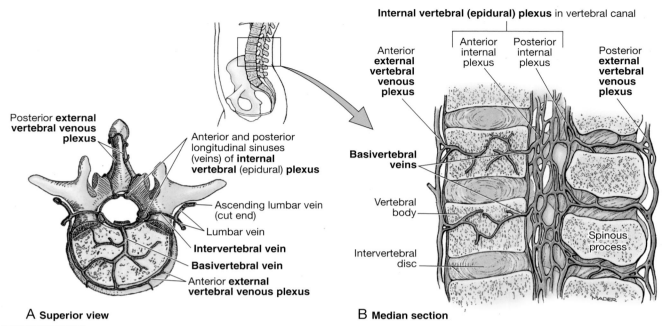

Internal vertebral (epidural) plexus in vertebral canal

Posterior **external vertebral venous plexus**

Anterior and posterior longitudinal sinuses (veins) of **internal vertebral** (epidural) **plexus**

Ascending lumbar vein (cut end)

Lumbar vein

Intervertebral vein

Basivertebral vein

Anterior **external vertebral venous plexus**

A Superior view

Anterior **external vertebral venous plexus**

Anterior internal plexus

Posterior internal plexus

Posterior **external vertebral venous plexus**

Basivertebral veins

Vertebral body

Intervertebral disc

Spinous process

B Median section

FIGURE 4.15. **Venous drainage of vertebral column. A.** The venous drainage parallels the arterial supply and enters the external and internal vertebral venous plexuses. There is also anterolateral drainage from the external aspects of the vertebrae into segmental veins. **B.** The dense plexus of thin-walled vessels within the vertebral canal, the internal vertebral venous plexuses, consists of valveless anastomoses between anterior and posterior longitudinal venous sinuses.

branches of the spinal nerves (Fig. 4.16). Most of the meningeal branches run back through the IV foramen, but some branches remain outside the canal. The branches outside the canal supply the anuli fibrosi and anterior longitudinal ligament; those inside the canal supply the periosteum, ligamenta flava, anuli fibrosi posteriorly, posterior longitudinal ligament, spinal dura mater, and blood vessels within the vertebral canal.

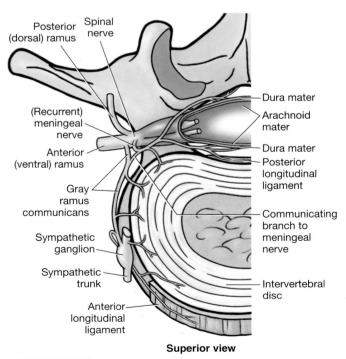

Posterior (dorsal) ramus

Spinal nerve

(Recurrent) meningeal nerve

Anterior (ventral) ramus

Gray ramus communicans

Sympathetic ganglion

Sympathetic trunk

Anterior longitudinal ligament

Dura mater

Arachnoid mater

Dura mater

Posterior longitudinal ligament

Communicating branch to meningeal nerve

Intervertebral disc

Superior view

FIGURE 4.16. **Innervation of periosteum and ligaments of vertebral column and meninges.**

Back Pain

Back pain in general, and lower back pain in particular, is an immense health problem. Five categories of structures receive innervation in the back and can be sources of pain:
- Fibroskeletal structures: periosteum, ligaments, and anuli fibrosi of IV discs.
- Meninges: coverings of the spinal cord.
- Synovial joints: capsules of the zygapophysial joints.
- Muscles: intrinsic muscles of the back.
- Nervous tissue: spinal nerves or nerve roots exiting the IV foramina.

Of these, the first two structures are innervated by (recurrent) meningeal branches of the spinal nerves and the next two are innervated by the posterior rami. Pain from nervous tissue—that is, caused by compression or irritation of spinal nerves or nerve roots—is typically *referred pain.*

SPINAL CORD AND MENINGES

The spinal cord, spinal meninges, spinal nerve roots, and neurovascular structures that supply them are in the **vertebral canal** (Fig. 4.17). The **spinal cord,** the major reflex center and conduction pathway between the body and the brain, is a cylindrical structure that is slightly flattened anteriorly and posteriorly. It is protected by the vertebrae and their associated ligaments and muscles, the spinal meninges, and the cerebrospinal fluid (CSF). The spinal cord begins as a continuation of the **medulla oblongata** (commonly called the medulla), the caudal part of the brainstem. In the newborn, the inferior end of the spinal cord usually is opposite the IV disc between the L2 and the L3 vertebrae. In adults, the spinal cord usually ends opposite the IV disc between the L1 and the L2 vertebrae; however, its tapering end, the **conus medullaris,** may terminate as high as T12 or as low as L3. Thus the spinal cord occupies only the superior two thirds of the vertebral canal. The spinal cord is enlarged in two regions for innervation of the limbs:

- The **cervical enlargement** extends from the C4 through the T1 segments of the spinal cord, and most of the

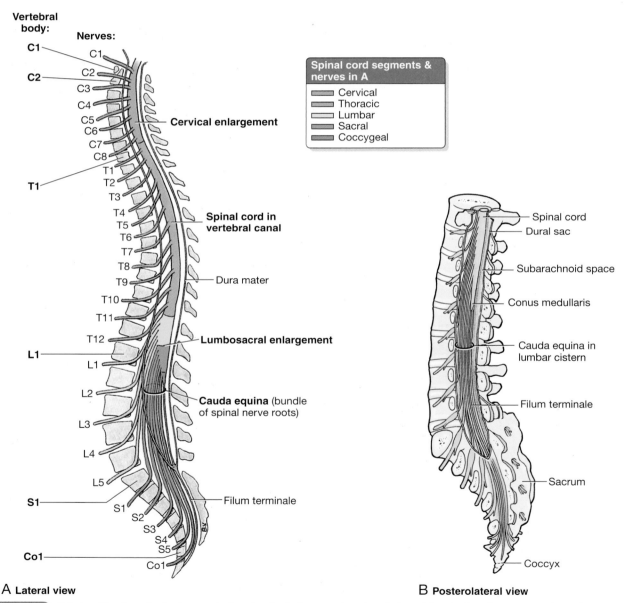

Spinal cord segments & nerves in A	
▭	Cervical
▭	Thoracic
▭	Lumbar
▭	Sacral
▭	Coccygeal

A Lateral view

B Posterolateral view

FIGURE 4.17. **Relationship of vertebral column, spinal cord and spinal nerves.** Note the relation of the spinal cord segments and spinal nerves to the vertebral column.

anterior rami of the spinal nerves arising from it form the *brachial plexus of nerves,* which innervates the upper limbs (Chapter 6).

- The **lumbosacral (lumbar) enlargement** extends from the L1 through the S3 segments of the spinal cord, and the anterior rami of the spinal nerves arising from it contribute to the *lumbar* and *sacral plexuses of nerves,* which innervate the lower limbs (Chapter 5). The spinal nerve roots arising from the lumbosacral enlargement and conus medullaris form the **cauda equina,** the bundle of spinal nerve roots running through the *lumbar cistern* (subarachnoid space).

Structure of Spinal Nerves

A total of 31 pairs of spinal nerves are attached to the spinal cord: 8 cervical, 12 thoracic, 5 lumbar, 5 sacral, and 1 coccygeal (Fig. 4.17A). Multiple rootlets attach to the posterior and anterior surfaces of the spinal cord and converge to form **posterior** and **anterior roots of the spinal nerves** (Fig. 4.18A,B). The part of the spinal cord to which the rootlets of one pair of roots attach is a **segment of the spinal cord.** The posterior roots of the spinal nerves contain afferent (or sensory) fibers from skin; subcutaneous and deep tissues; and, often, viscera. The anterior roots of spinal nerves contain efferent (motor) fibers to skeletal muscle and many contain presynaptic autonomic fibers. The cell bodies of somatic axons contributing to the anterior roots are in the **anterior horns of gray matter** of the spinal cord (Fig. 4.18C), whereas the cell bodies of axons making up the posterior roots are outside the spinal cord in the **spinal ganglia** (posterior root ganglia) at the distal ends of the posterior roots. The posterior and anterior nerve roots unite at their points of exit from the vertebral canal to form a **spinal nerve.** The C1 nerves lack posterior roots in 50% of people, and the coccygeal nerve (Co1) may be absent. Each spinal nerve divides almost immediately into a **posterior (dorsal) ramus** and **anterior (ventral) ramus** (Fig. 4.18A). The posterior rami supply the skin and deep muscles of the back; the anterior rami supply the limbs and the rest of the trunk.

In adults, the spinal cord is shorter than the vertebral column; hence there is a progressive obliquity of the spinal nerve roots as the cord descends (Fig. 4.17). Because of the increasing distance between the spinal cord segments and the corresponding vertebrae, the length of the nerve roots increases progressively as the inferior end of the vertebral column is approached. The lumbar and sacral nerve rootlets are the longest. They descend until they reach the IV foramina of exit in the lumbar and sacral regions of the vertebral column, respectively. The bundle of spinal nerve roots in the **lumbar cistern** (subarachnoid space) within the vertebral canal caudal to the termination of the spinal cord resembles a horse's tail, hence its name, *cauda equina* (L. horse tail) (Figs. 4.17B and 4.18D).

The inferior end of the spinal cord has a conical shape and tapers into the *conus medullaris.* From its inferior end, the **filum terminale** descends among the spinal nerve roots in the cauda equina. It consists primarily of pia mater but its proximal end also includes vestiges of neural tissue, connective tissue, and neuroglial tissue. The filum terminale takes on layers of arachnoid and dura mater as it penetrates the inferior end of the dural sac and passes through the **sacral hiatus** to attach ultimately to the coccyx posteriorly. The filum terminale serves as an anchor for the end of the **dural sac,** the continuation of the dura inferior to the conus medullaris.

Spinal Meninges and Cerebrospinal Fluid

Collectively, the dura mater, arachnoid mater, and pia mater surrounding the spinal cord form the **spinal meninges.** These membranes and CSF surround, support, and protect the spinal cord and the spinal nerve roots, including those in the cauda equina.

The **spinal dura mater,** composed of tough, fibrous, and some elastic tissue, is the outermost covering membrane of the spinal cord (Fig. 4.18). The spinal dura mater is separated from the vertebrae by the **extradural (epidural) space** (Fig. 4.19 and Table 4.5). The dura forms the **spinal dural sac,** a long tubular sheath within the vertebral canal (Fig. 4.17). The spinal dural sac adheres to the margin of the foramen magnum of the cranium, where it is continuous with the cranial dura mater. The spinal dural sac is pierced by the spinal nerves and is anchored inferiorly to the coccyx by the *filum terminale.* The spinal dura extends into the IV foramina and along the posterior and anterior nerve roots distal to the spinal ganglia to form **dural root sheaths,** or sleeves (Fig. 4.18A). These sheaths blend with the epineurium (outer connective tissue covering of spinal nerves) that adheres to the periosteum lining the IV foramina.

The **spinal arachnoid mater** is a delicate, avascular membrane composed of fibrous and elastic tissue that lines the dural sac and the dural root sheaths. It encloses the CSF-filled subarachnoid space containing the spinal cord, spinal nerve roots, and spinal ganglia (Fig. 4.18B,C). The arachnoid mater is not attached to the dura but is held against the inner surface of the dura by the pressure of the CSF. In a *lumbar spinal puncture,* the needle traverses the dura and arachnoid mater simultaneously. Their apposition is the **dura–arachnoid interface,** often erroneously referred to as the "subdural space" (Fig. 4.19). No actual space occurs naturally at this site; it is rather a weak cell layer (Haines, 2006). Bleeding into this layer creates a pathological space at the dura–arachnoid junction in which a *subdural hematoma* is formed. In the cadaver, because of the absence of CSF, the arachnoid falls away from the internal surface of the dura and lies loosely on the spinal cord. The arachnoid mater is separated from the pia mater on the surface of the spinal cord by the *subarachnoid space* containing CSF (Figs. 4.18 and 4.19; Table 4.5). Delicate

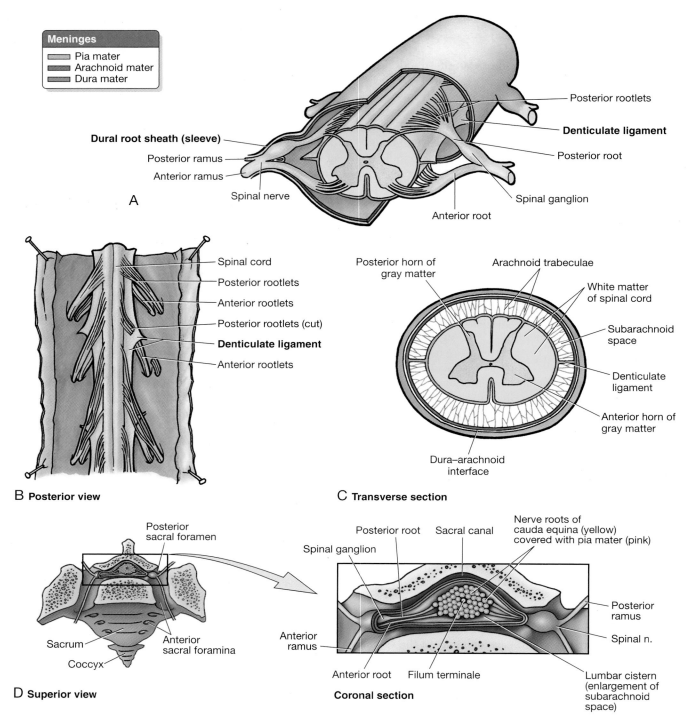

Meninges
- Pia mater
- Arachnoid mater
- Dura mater

Posterior rootlets

Denticulate ligament

Dural root sheath (sleeve)

Posterior ramus

Anterior ramus

Spinal nerve

Posterior root

Spinal ganglion

Anterior root

A

Spinal cord

Posterior rootlets

Anterior rootlets

Posterior rootlets (cut)

Denticulate ligament

Anterior rootlets

B **Posterior view**

Posterior horn of gray matter

Arachnoid trabeculae

White matter of spinal cord

Subarachnoid space

Denticulate ligament

Anterior horn of gray matter

Dura–arachnoid interface

C **Transverse section**

Posterior sacral foramen

Sacrum

Coccyx

Anterior sacral foramina

D **Superior view**

Posterior root

Spinal ganglion

Sacral canal

Nerve roots of cauda equina (yellow) covered with pia mater (pink)

Posterior ramus

Spinal n.

Anterior ramus

Anterior root

Filum terminale

Lumbar cistern (enlargement of subarachnoid space)

Coronal section

FIGURE 4.18. **Spinal cord and spinal meninges. A.** Spinal cord within its meninges. **B.** The meninges have been cut and spread out. The pia mater covers the spinal cord and projects laterally as the denticulate ligament. **C.** Transverse section of spinal cord demonstrating spinal meninges and associated spaces. **D.** Coronal section through first sacral foramina. In common use, the term "mater" is often omitted, referring simply to "dura," "arachnoid," and "pia."

Posterior spinal artery

Posterior spinal veins

Anterior spinal artery

Anterior and posterior segmental medullary arteries

Anterior spinal veins

Subarachnoid space

Spinal branch (arises from the vertebral, intercostal, lumbar, or sacral artery, depending on level of spinal cord)

Dura-arachnoid interface

Anterior and posterior radicular arteries

Vertebral canal

Internal vertebral venous plexus and fat in extradural space

Intervertebral foramen

Meninges
- Pia mater
- Arachnoid mater
- Dura mater

Anterolateral view

FIGURE 4.19.   Spinal cord in situ: vasculature and meninges with associated spaces.

TABLE 4.5 SPACES ASSOCIATED WITH SPINAL MENINGES

Space	Location	Contents
Extradural (epidural)	Between wall of vertebral canal and dura mater	Fat (loose connective tissue); internal vertebral venous plexuses; inferior to L2 vertebra, the roots of spinal nerves
Subarachnoid	Between arachnoid and pia mater	CSF; arachnoid trabeculae; radicular, segmental, medullary, and spinal arteries; veins

strands of connective tissue, the **arachnoid trabeculae,** span the subarachnoid space connecting the arachnoid and pia (Fig. 4.18C).

The **spinal pia mater,** the innermost covering membrane of the spinal cord, consists of flattened cells with long, equally flattened processes that closely follow all the surface features of the spinal cord (Fig. 4.11B,C). The pia mater also directly covers the roots of the spinal nerves and spinal blood vessels. Inferior to the conus medullaris, the pia continues as the filum terminale.

The spinal cord is suspended in the dural sac by the filum terminale and especially by the right and left sawtooth

denticulate ligaments (L. *denticulus,* a small tooth), which run longitudinally along each side of the spinal cord. These ligaments consist of a fibrous sheet of pia mater extending midway between the posterior and the anterior nerve roots. Between 20 and 22 of these processes, shaped much like sharks' teeth, attach to the internal surface of the arachnoid-lined dural sac. The superior processes (uppermost part) of the right and left denticulate ligament attach to the cranial dura mater immediately superior to the foramen magnum. The inferior process extends from the conus medullaris passing between the T12 and the L1 nerve roots.

SUBARACHNOID SPACE

The subarachnoid space lies between the arachnoid mater and the pia mater and is filled with CSF (Figs. 4.17*B*, 4.18*C*, and 4.19; and Table 4.5). The enlargement of the subarachnoid space in the dural sac, caudal to the conus medullaris, and containing CSF and the cauda equina is the **lumbar cistern** (Fig. 4.18*D*).

Lumbar Spinal Puncture

To obtain a sample of CSF from the lumbar cistern, a *lumbar puncture needle,* fitted with a stylet, is inserted into the subarachnoid space. Lumbar spinal puncture (spinal tap) is performed with the patient leaning forward or lying on the side with the back flexed. Flexion of the vertebral column facilitates insertion of the needle by stretching the ligamenta flava and spreading the laminae and spinous processes apart (Fig. B4.8). Under aseptic conditions, the needle is inserted in the midline between the spinous processes of the L3 and L4 (or the L4 and L5) vertebrae. At these levels in adults, there is reduced danger of damaging the spinal cord.

Epidural Anesthesia (Blocks)

An anesthetic agent can be injected into the extradural (epidural) space using the position described for lumbar spinal puncture. The anesthetic has a direct effect on the spinal nerve roots of the cauda equina after they exit from the dural sac (Fig. B4.8). The patient loses sensation inferior to the level of the block.

An anesthetic agent can also be injected into the extradural space in the sacral canal through the sacral hiatus (caudal epidural anesthesia) or through the posterior sacral foramina (trans-sacral epidural anesthesia) (Fig. B4.9). The distance the agent ascends (and hence the number of nerves affected) depends on the amount injected and on the position assumed by the patient.

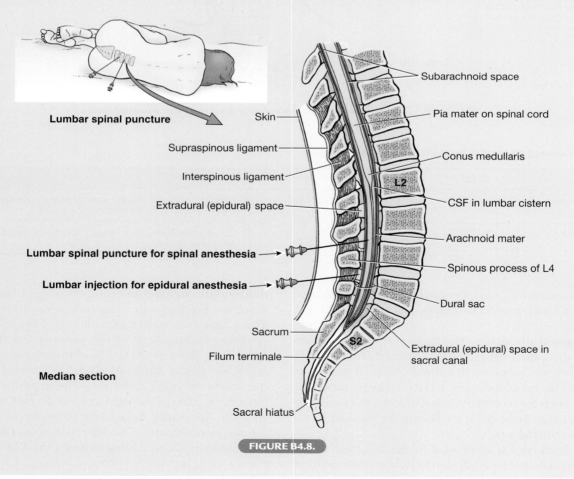

Lumbar spinal puncture

Median section

Skin
Supraspinous ligament
Interspinous ligament
Extradural (epidural) space
Lumbar spinal puncture for spinal anesthesia
Lumbar injection for epidural anesthesia
Sacrum
Filum terminale
Sacral hiatus

Subarachnoid space
Pia mater on spinal cord
Conus medullaris
L2
CSF in lumbar cistern
Arachnoid mater
Spinous process of L4
Dural sac
S2
Extradural (epidural) space in sacral canal

FIGURE B4.8.

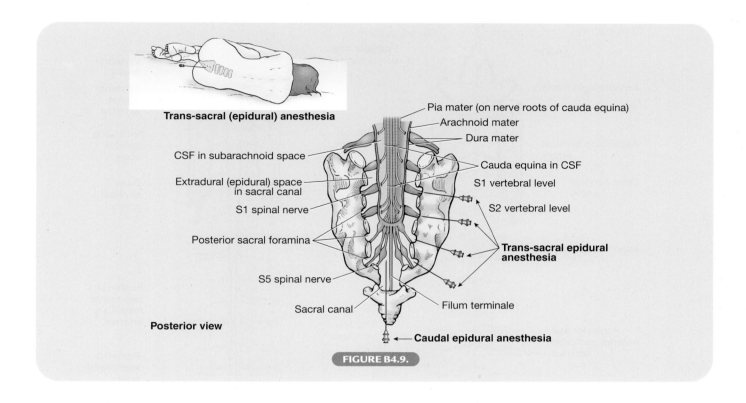

Trans-sacral (epidural) anesthesia

Pia mater (on nerve roots of cauda equina)
Arachnoid mater
Dura mater
CSF in subarachnoid space
Cauda equina in CSF
Extradural (epidural) space in sacral canal
S1 vertebral level
S1 spinal nerve
S2 vertebral level
Posterior sacral foramina
Trans-sacral epidural anesthesia
S5 spinal nerve
Sacral canal
Filum terminale
Posterior view
Caudal epidural anesthesia

FIGURE B4.9.

Vasculature of Spinal Cord and Spinal Nerve Roots

The arteries supplying the spinal cord are branches of the vertebral, ascending cervical, deep cervical, intercostal, lumbar, and lateral sacral arteries (Figs. 4.19 and 4.20). Three longitudinal arteries supply the spinal cord: an **anterior spinal artery,** formed by the union of branches of vertebral arteries, and paired **posterior spinal arteries,** each of which is a branch of either the vertebral artery or the posterior inferior cerebellar artery.

The spinal arteries run longitudinally from the medulla of the brainstem to the conus medullaris of the spinal cord. By themselves, the anterior and posterior spinal arteries supply only the short superior part of the spinal cord. The circulation to much of the spinal cord depends on segmental medullary and radicular arteries running along the spinal nerve roots. The **anterior** and **posterior segmental medullary arteries** are derived from spinal branches of ascending cervical, deep cervical, vertebral, posterior intercostal, and lumbar arteries that supply the spinal cord. The medullary segmental arteries enter the vertebral canal through the IV foramina and are located chiefly where the need for a good blood supply to the spinal cord is greatest: the cervical and lumbosacral enlargements. The **great anterior segmental medullary artery** (of Adamkiewicz) reinforces the circulation to two thirds of the spinal cord, including the lumbosacral enlargement. It is much larger than the other segmental

medullary arteries and usually arises on the left side at low thoracic or upper lumbar levels.

Posterior and anterior roots of the spinal nerves and their coverings are supplied by **posterior** and **anterior radicular arteries,** which run along the nerve roots. These vessels do not reach the posterior or anterior spinal arteries. Segmental medullary arteries occur irregularly in the place of radicular arteries; they are larger vessels that make it to the spinal arteries.

The 3 **anterior** and 3 **posterior spinal veins** are arranged longitudinally; they communicate freely with each other and are drained by up to 12 **anterior** and **posterior medullary** and **radicular veins.** The veins draining the spinal cord join the **internal vertebral venous plexus** in the epidural space (Fig. 4.15). This venous plexus passes superiorly through the foramen magnum to communicate with the dural venous sinuses and veins in the cranium (see Chapter 7). The internal vertebral plexus also communicates with the **external vertebral venous plexus** on the external surface of the vertebrae.

MUSCLES OF BACK

Most body weight is anterior to the vertebral column, especially in obese people. For this reason, the many strong muscles attached to the spinous and transverse processes of vertebrae are necessary to support and move the vertebral column. There are two major groups of muscles in the back.

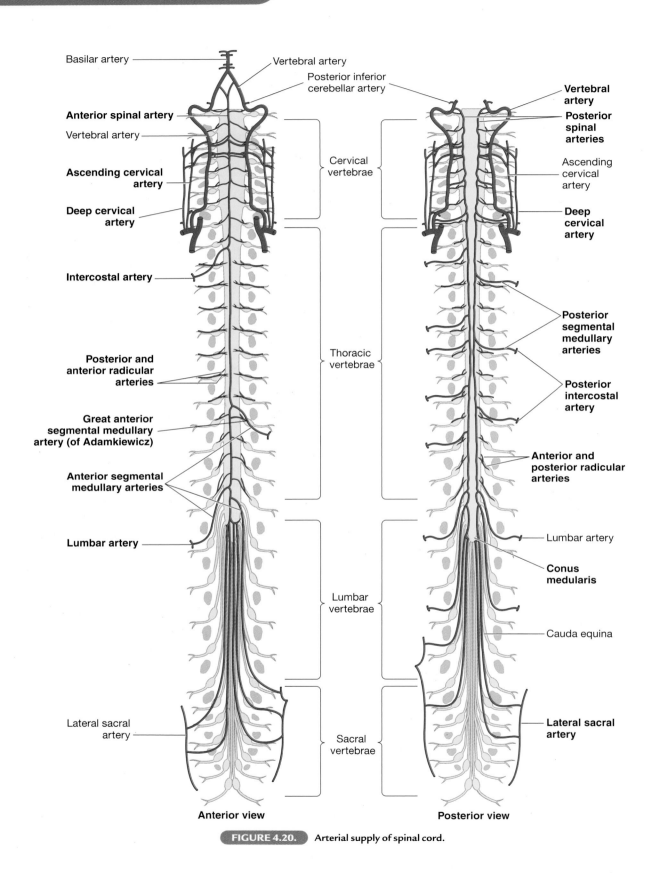

FIGURE 4.20.   Arterial supply of spinal cord.

Ischemia of Spinal Cord

The segmental reinforcements of blood supply from the segmental medullary arteries are important in supplying blood to the anterior and posterior spinal arteries. Fractures, dislocations, and fracture–dislocations may interfere with the blood supply to the spinal cord from the spinal and medullary arteries. Deficiency of blood supply (ischemia) of the spinal cord affects its function and can lead to muscle weakness and paralysis.

The spinal cord may also suffer circulatory impairment if the segmental medullary arteries, particularly the great anterior segmental medullary artery (of Adamkiewicz), are narrowed by *obstructive arterial disease*. Sometimes the aorta is purposely occluded ("cross-clamped") during surgery. Patients undergoing such surgeries, and those with ruptured aneurysms of the aorta or occlusion of the great anterior segmental medullary artery, may lose all sensation and voluntary movement inferior to the level of impaired blood supply to the spinal cord (*paraplegia*). This is secondary to death of neurons in the part of the spinal cord supplied by the anterior spinal artery.

When systemic blood pressure drops severely for 3 to 6 minutes, blood flow from the segmental medullary arteries to the anterior spinal artery supplying the midthoracic region of the spinal cord may be reduced or stopped. These patients may also lose sensation and voluntary movement in the areas supplied by the affected level of the spinal cord.

Alternative Circulation Pathways

The *vertebral venous plexuses* are important because blood may return from the pelvis or abdomen through these plexuses and reach the heart via the superior vena cava when the inferior vena cava is obstructed. These veins also can provide a route for metastasis of cancer cells to the vertebrae or the brain from an abdominal or pelvic tumor (e.g., prostate cancer).

The **extrinsic back muscles** include *superficial* and *intermediate muscles* that produce and control limb and respiratory movements, respectively. The **intrinsic back muscles** include muscles that specifically act on the vertebral column, producing its movements and maintaining posture.

Extrinsic Back Muscles

The **superficial extrinsic back muscles** (trapezius, latissimus dorsi, levator scapulae, and rhomboids) connect the upper limbs to the trunk (see Chapter 6). These muscles, although located in the back region, for the most part, receive their nerve supply from the anterior rami of cervical nerves and act on the upper limb. The trapezius receives its motor fibers from a cranial nerve, the spinal accessory nerve (CN XI). The **intermediate extrinsic back muscles** (serratus posterior superior and inferior) are thin muscles and are commonly designated superficial respiratory muscles but are more likely proprioceptive rather than motor in function. They are described with muscles of the thoracic wall (see Chapter 1).

Intrinsic Back Muscles

The intrinsic back muscles (*muscles of back proper,* deep back muscles) are innervated by the posterior rami of spinal nerves and act to maintain posture and control movements of the vertebral column. These muscles, extending from the pelvis to the cranium, are enclosed by deep fascia that attaches medially to the nuchal ligament, the tips of the spinous processes of the vertebrae, the supraspinous ligament, and the median crest of the sacrum. The fascia attaches laterally to the cervical and lumbar transverse processes and to the angles of the ribs. The thoracic and lumbar parts of the deep fascia constitute the **thoracolumbar fascia** (Fig. 4.21). The deep back muscles are grouped according to superficial, intermediate, and deep layers according to their relationship to the surface (Table 4.6).

SUPERFICIAL LAYER OF INTRINSIC BACK MUSCLES

The **splenius muscles** (L. *musculi splenii*) are thick and flat and lie on the lateral and posterior aspects of the neck, covering the vertical muscles somewhat like a bandage, which explains their name (L. *splenion,* bandage). The splenii arise from the midline and extend superolaterally to the cervical vertebrae (**splenius cervicis**) and cranium (**splenius capitis**). These muscles cover the deep neck muscles (Fig. 4.22B; Table 4.6).

INTERMEDIATE LAYER OF INTRINSIC BACK MUSCLES

The **erector spinae muscles** (sacrospinalis) lie in a "groove" on each side of the vertebral column between the

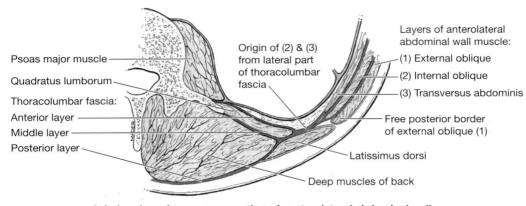

Inferior view of transverse section of posterolateral abdominal wall

FIGURE 4.21. Transverse section of the intrinsic back muscles and layers of thoracolumbar fascia.

spinous processes and the angles of the ribs (Fig. 4.22). The massive **erector spinae,** the chief extensor of the vertebral column, divides into three muscle columns:

- Iliocostalis: lateral column.
- Longissimus: intermediate column.
- Spinalis: medial column.

Each column is divided regionally into three parts according to its superior attachments (e.g., iliocostalis lumborum, iliocostalis thoracis, and iliocostalis cervicis). The common

origin of the three erector spinae columns is through a broad tendon that attaches inferiorly to the posterior part of the iliac crest, the posterior aspect of the sacrum, the sacroiliac ligaments, and the sacral and inferior lumbar spinous processes. Although the muscle columns are generally identified as isolated muscles, each column is actually composed of many overlapping shorter fibers—a design that provides stability, localized action, and segmental vascular and neural supply. The attachments, nerve supply, and actions of the erector spinae are described in Table 4.6.

Surface Anatomy of Back Muscles

In the midline of the back there is a posterior median furrow that overlies the tips of the spinous processes of the vertebrae (Fig. SA4.3). The furrow is continuous superiorly with the nuchal groove in the neck. The erector spinae muscles produce prominent vertical bulges on each side of the furrow. The superficially located trapezius (D, descending [superior] part; T, transverse [middle] part; A, ascending [inferior] part) and latissimus dorsi muscles connecting the upper limbs to the vertebral column are also clearly visible.

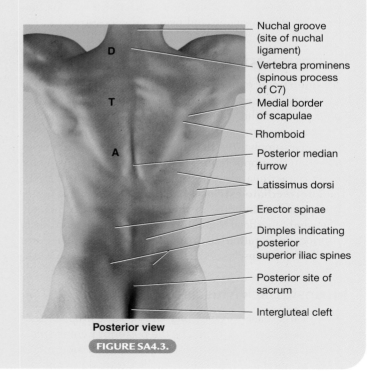

Posterior view

FIGURE SA4.3.

DEEP LAYER OF INTRINSIC BACK MUSCLES

Deep to the erector spinae muscles is an obliquely disposed group of muscles—the **transversospinales muscle group,** which is composed of the semispinalis, multifidus, and rotatores. These muscles originate from transverse processes of vertebrae and pass to spinous processes of more superior vertebrae. They occupy the "gutter" between the transverse and spinous processes (Fig. 4.23; Table 4.7).

- The semispinalis is superficial, spanning four to six segments.
- The multifidus is deeper, spanning two to four segments.
- The rotatores are deepest, spanning one to two segments.

The **semispinalis,** as its name indicates, arises from approximately half of the vertebral column. It is divided into three parts according to the vertebral level of their superior attachments: semispinalis capitis, semispinalis cervicis, and semispinalis thoracis.

The **semispinalis capitis** is responsible for the longitudinal bulge on each side in the back of the neck near the median plane. It ascends from the cervical and thoracic transverse processes to the occipital bone.

The **semispinalis thoracis and cervicis** pass superomedially from the transverse processes to the thoracic and cervical spinous processes of more superior vertebrae.

The **multifidus** consists of short, triangular muscular bundles that are thickest in the lumbar region. Each bundle passes obliquely superiorly and medially and attaches along the whole length of the spinous process of the adjacent superior vertebra.

The **rotatores**—best developed in the thoracic region—are the deepest of the three layers of transversospinales muscles. They arise from the transverse process of one vertebra and insert into the root of the spinous processes of the next one or two vertebrae superiorly.

The **interspinales**, **intertransversarii**, and **levatores costarum** are the smallest of the deep back muscles. The interspinales and intertransversarii muscles connect spinous and transverse processes, respectively. These muscles are small and placed in positions of poor mechanical advantage. Hence it has been proposed that the smaller muscles of small–large muscle pairs function more as organs of proprioception and that larger muscles are the producers of motion.

MUSCLES PRODUCING MOVEMENTS OF INTERVERTEBRAL JOINTS

The principal muscles producing movements of the cervical, thoracic, and lumbar IV joints and structures limiting these movements are summarized in Tables 4.8 and 4.9. The back muscles are relatively inactive in the stand-easy position. It is

TABLE 4.6 SUPERFICIAL AND INTERMEDIATE LAYERS OF INTRINSIC BACK MUSCLES

Muscle	Origin	Insertion	Nerve Supply	Main Action(s)
Superficial layer of intrinsic back muscles				
Splenius	Arises from nuchal ligament and spinous processes of C7–T6 vertebrae	*Splenius capitis:* fibers run superolaterally to mastoid process of temporal bone and lateral third of superior nuchal line of occipital bone *Splenius cervicis:* tubercles of transverse processes of C1–C3 or C4 vertebrae	Posterior rami of spinal nerves	*Acting alone:* laterally flex neck and rotate head to side of active muscles *Acting together:* extend head and neck
Intermediate layer of intrinsic back muscles (erector spinae)				
Iliocostalis Longissimus Spinalis	Arises by broad tendon from posterior part of iliac crest, posterior surface of sacrum, sacro-iliac ligaments, sacral and inferior lumbar spinous processes, and supraspinous ligament	*Iliocostalis* (lumborum, thoracis, and cervicis): fibers run superiorly to angles of lower ribs and cervical transverse processes *Longissimus* (thoracis, cervicis, and capitis): fibers run superiorly to ribs between tubercles and angles to transverse processes in thoracic and cervical regions and to mastoid process of temporal bone *Spinalis* (thoracis, cervicis, and capitis): fibers run superiorly to spinous processes in upper thoracic region and to cranium	Posterior rami of spinal nerves	*Acting bilaterally:* extend vertebral column and head; as back is flexed, control movement by gradually lengthening their fibers *Acting unilaterally:* laterally flex vertebral column

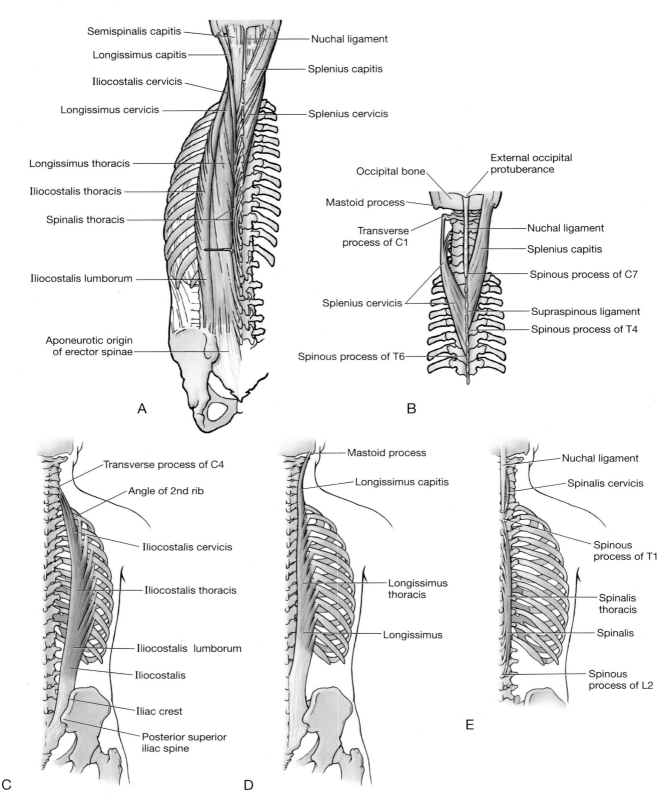

Posterior views

FIGURE 4.22. **Superficial and intermediate layers of intrinsic back muscles. A.** Overview. **B.** Splenius capitis and splenius cervicis. **C.** Iliocostalis. **D.** Longissimus. **E.** Spinalis.

TABLE 4.7 DEEP LAYERS OF INTRINSIC BACK MUSCLES

Muscle	Origin	Insertion	Nerve Supply	Main Action(s)
Deep layer of intrinsic back muscles (transversospinales)				
Semispinalis (thoracis, cervicis, and capitis)	Arises from transverse processes of C4–T10 vertebrae	Fibers run superomedially to occipital bone and spinous processes in upper thoracic and cervical regions, spanning 4–6 segments	Posterior rami of spinal nerves	Extends head and thoracic and cervical regions of vertebral column and rotates them contralaterally
Multifidus	Arises from posterior sacrum, posterior superior iliac spine of ilium, aponeurosis of erector spinae, sacro-iliac ligaments, mammillary processes of lumbar vertebrae, transverse processes of T1–T3, and articular processes of C4–C7	Thickest in lumbar region, fibers pass obliquely superomedially to entire length of spinous processes of vertebrae located 2–4 segments superior to origin		Unilateral contraction rotates to contralateral side; stabilizes vertebrae during local movements of vertebral column
Rotatores (brevis and longus)	Arise from transverse processes of vertebrae; are best developed in thoracic region	Fibers pass superomedially to attach to junction of lamina and transverse process or spinous process of vertebra immediately (brevis) or 2 segments (longus) superior to vertebra of origin		May function as organs of proprioception; possibly stabilize vertebrae and assist with local extension and rotatory movements of vertebral column
Minor deep layer of intrinsic back muscles				
Interspinales	Superior surfaces of spinous processes of cervical and lumbar vertebrae	Inferior surfaces of spinous processes of vertebrae superior to vertebra of origin	Posterior rami of spinal nerves	Aid in extension and rotation of vertebral column
Intertransversarii	Transverse processes of cervical and lumbar vertebrae	Transverse processes of adjacent vertebrae	Posterior and anterior rami of spinal nerves[a]	Aid in lateral flexion of vertebral column; acting bilaterally, stabilize vertebral column
Levatores costarum	Tips of transverse processes of C7 and T1–T11 vertebrae	Pass inferolaterally and insert on rib between its tubercle and angle	Posterior rami of C8–T11 spinal nerves	Elevate ribs, assisting respiration; assist with lateral flexion of vertebral column

[a]Most back muscles are innervated by posterior rami of the spinal nerves, but a few are innervated by anterior rami.

actually the interaction of anterior (abdominal) and posterior (back) muscles that provides the stability and produces motion of the axial skeleton.

Smaller muscles generally have higher densities of *muscle spindles* (sensors of proprioception—the sense of one's position—that are interdigitated among the muscle's fibers) than do large muscles. It has been presumed that this is because small muscles are used for the most precise movements, such as fine postural movements or manipulation, and therefore require more proprioceptive feedback. The movements described for small muscles are assumed from the location of their attachments, from the direction of the muscle fibers, and from activity measured by *electromyography*. Muscles such as the rotatores, however, are so small and are placed in positions of such relatively poor mechanical advantage that their ability to produce the movements described is somewhat questionable. Furthermore, such small muscles often are redundant to other larger muscles having superior mechanical advantage. Hence it has been proposed that the smaller muscles of small–large muscle pairs function more as "kinesiological monitors" (organs of proprioception) and that the larger muscles are the producers of motion.

Back muscles
- Superficial extrinsic
- Intermediate extrinsic
- Erector spinae (intermediate intrinsic)
- Transversospinales (deep intrinsic)

A Posterior view

- Superior nuchal line
- External occipital protuberance
- Obliquus capitis superior
- Mastoid process
- Rectus capitis posterior major
- Semispinalis capitis
- Obliquus captitis inferior
- Semispinalis thoracis
- Rotatores
- Levatores costarum
- Lumbar intertransversarii
- Multifidus

B Transverse section

- Spinalis
- Longissimus
- Iliocostalis
- Rotatores
- Multifidus
- Semispinalis
- Serratus posterior
- Latissimus dorsi
- Trapezius

C Posterior views

- Semispinalis capitis (cut)
- Semispinalis cervicis
- Semispinalis thoracis

D

- Multifidus
- Rotatores
- Multifidus

E

- Cervical interspinales
- Cervical intertransversarii
- Levatores costarum
- Lumbar interspinales
- Lumbar intertransversarii

FIGURE 4.23. **Deep layer of intrinsic back muscles. A.** Overview. **B.** Transverse section. The erector spinae consists of three columns and the transversospinales consists of three layers: semispinalis (**C**), multifidus (**D**), and rotatores (**A**). **E.** Interspinales, intertransversarii, and levatores costarum.

TABLE 4.8 PRINCIPAL MUSCLES PRODUCING MOVEMENT OF CERVICAL INTERVERTEBRAL JOINTS

A Muscles producing flexion

B Muscles producing lateral flexion

Key
- Sternocleidomastoid (SCM)
- Longus colli
- Scalenes
- Intertransversarii
- Splenius capitis
- Splenius cervicis and levator scapulae
- Semispinalis cervicis and iliocostalis cervicis
- Longissimus capitis
- Multifidus
- Semispinalis capitis
- Trapezius

C   D   E

C–E, Muscles producing extension

	Flexion	Extension	Lateral Bending	Rotation
Acting muscles	Bilateral action of: • Longus colli • Scalene • Sternocleidomastoid	Bilateral action of deep neck muscles: • Semispinalis cervicis and iliocostalis cervicis • Splenius cervicis and levator scapulae • Splenius capitis • Multifidus • Longissimus capitis • Semispinalis capitis • Trapezius	Unilateral action of: • Iliocostalis cervicis • Longissimus capitis and cervicis • Splenius capitis • Splenius cervicis • Intertransversarii and scalenes	Ipsilateral action of: • Rotatores • Semispinalis capitis and cervicis • Multifidus • Splenius cervicis Contralateral action of: • Sternocleidomastoid
Limiting structures	Limiting structures • Ligaments: posterior atlanto-axial, posterior longitudinal, flavum, tectorial membrane • Posterior neck muscles • Anulus fibrosus (tension posteriorly)	• Ligaments: anterior longitudinal, anterior atlanto-axial • Anterior neck muscles • Anulus fibrosus (tension anteriorly) • Spinous processes (contact between adjacent processes)	• Ligaments: alar ligament tension limits movement to contralateral side • Anulus fibrosus (tension anteriorly) • Zygapophysial (facet) joints	• Ligaments: alar ligament tension limits movement to ipsilateral side • Anulus fibrosus

TABLE 4.9 PRINCIPAL MUSCLES PRODUCING MOVEMENTS OF THORACIC AND LUMBAR INTERVERTEBRAL JOINTS

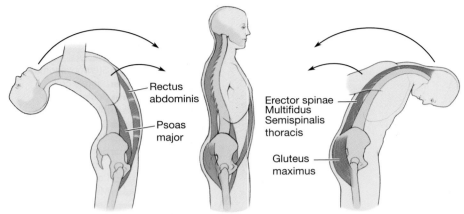

A **Flexion (starting from extended position)** B **Neutral** C **Extension (starting from flexed position)**

Rectus abdominis

Psoas major

Erector spinae
Multifidus
Semispinalis thoracis

Gluteus maximus

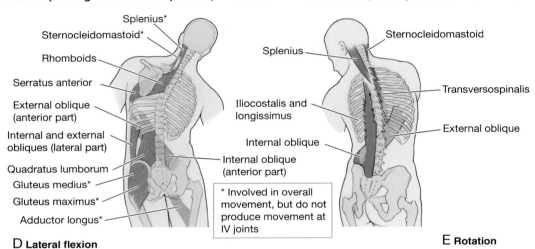

Splenius*
Sternocleidomastoid*
Rhomboids
Serratus anterior
External oblique (anterior part)
Internal and external obliques (lateral part)
Quadratus lumborum
Gluteus medius*
Gluteus maximus*
Adductor longus*

D **Lateral flexion**

Splenius
Iliocostalis and longissimus
Internal oblique
Internal oblique (anterior part)

Sternocleidomastoid
Transversospinalis
External oblique

E **Rotation**

* Involved in overall movement, but do not produce movement at IV joints

(Muscles shown contract to bend/rotate to opposite [left] side)

	Flexion	Extension	Lateral Bending	Rotation
Acting muscles	Bilateral action of: • Rectus abdominis • Psoas major • Gravity	Bilateral action of: • Erector spinae • Multifidus • Semispinalis thoracis	Unilateral action of: • Iliocostalis thoracis and lumborum • Longissimus thoracis • Multifidus • External and internal oblique • Quadratus lumborum • Rhomboids • Serratus anterior	Unilateral action of: • Rotatores • Multifidus • Iliocostalis • Longissimus • External oblique acting synchronously with opposite internal oblique • Splenius thoracis
Limiting structures	• Ligaments: supraspinous, interspinous, flavum • Capsules of zygapophysial (facet) joints • Extensor muscles • Vertebral bodies (apposition anteriorly) • IV disc (compression anteriorly) • Anulus fibrosus (tension posteriorly)	• Ligaments: anterior longitudinal • Capsules of zygapophysial joints • Abdominal muscles • Spinous processes (contact between adjacent processes) • Anulus fibrosus (tension anteriorly) • IV discs (compression posteriorly)	• Ligaments: contralateral side • Contralateral muscles that laterally bend trunk • Contact between iliac crest and thorax • Anulus fibrosus (tension of contralateral fibers) • IV disc (compression ipsilaterally)	• Ligaments: costovertebral • Ipsilateral external oblique, contralateral internal oblique • Articular facets (apposition) • Anulus fibrosus

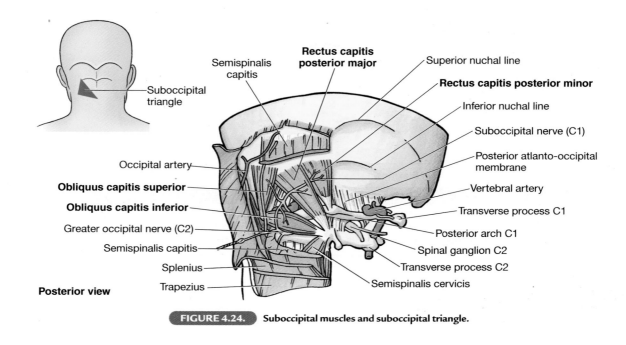

FIGURE 4.24. Suboccipital muscles and suboccipital triangle.

Suboccipital and Deep Neck Muscles

The **suboccipital region**—superior part of the back of the neck—is the triangular area (*suboccipital triangle*) inferior to the occipital region of the head, including the posterior aspects of the C1 and C2 vertebrae.

The **suboccipital triangle** lies deep to the trapezius and semispinalis capitis muscles (Fig. 4.24). The four small muscles in the suboccipital region—rectus capitis posterior major and minor and obliquus capitis superior and inferior—are innervated by the posterior ramus of C1, the **suboccipital nerve.** These muscles are mainly postural muscles, but they act on the head—directly or indirectly—as indicated by *capitis* in their name.

- **Rectus capitis posterior major** arises from the spinous process of the C2 vertebra and inserts into the lateral part of the inferior nuchal line of the occipital bone.
- **Rectus capitis posterior minor** arises from the posterior tubercle on the posterior arch of the C1 vertebra and inserts into the medial third of the inferior nuchal line.
- **Obliquus capitis inferior** arises from the spinous process of the C2 vertebra and inserts into the transverse process of the C1 vertebra. The name of this muscle is somewhat misleading because it is the only "capitis" muscle that has no attachment to the cranium.
- **Obliquus capitis superior** arises from the transverse process of C1 and inserts into the occipital bone between the superior and the inferior nuchal lines.

The boundaries and contents of the suboccipital triangle are:

- Superomedially, rectus capitis posterior major.
- Superolaterally, obliquus capitis superior.
- Inferolaterally, obliquus capitis inferior.
- Floor, posterior atlanto-occipital membrane and posterior arch of C1.
- Roof, semispinalis capitis.
- Contents, *vertebral artery* and *suboccipital nerve* (C1).

TABLE 4.10 PRINCIPAL MUSCLES PRODUCING MOVEMENT OF ATLANTO-OCCIPITAL JOINTS

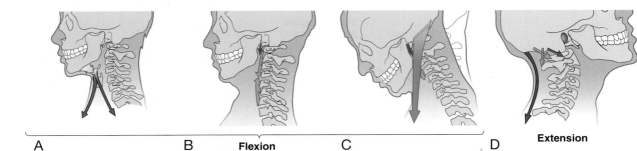

A   B   **Flexion**   C   D   **Extension**

Key

Suprahyoid muscles	Longus capitis	Rectus capitis posterior major
Infrahyoid muscles	Sternocleidomastoid	Rectus capitis posterior minor
Rectus capitis anterior	Trapezius	Obliquus capitis superior

Flexion	Extension	Lateral Bending (not shown)
Longus capitis	Rectus capitis posterior major and minor	Sternocleidomastoid
Rectus capitis anterior	Oblıquus capitis superior	
Anterior fibers of sternocleidomastoid	Splenius capitis	Rectus capitis lateralis
Suprahyoid and infrahyoid muscles	Longissimus capitis	Longissimus capitis
	Trapezius	Splenius capitis

The actions of the suboccipital group of muscles are to extend the head on C1 and rotate the head and the C1 on C2 vertebrae. The principal muscles producing movements of the craniovertebral joints are summarized in Tables 4.10 and 4.11. The motor innervation of the muscles and the cutaneous innervation of the posterior aspect of the head and neck are summarized in Figure 4.25 and Table 4.12.

Reduced Blood Supply to Brainstem

The winding course of the vertebral arteries through the foramina transversaria of the cervical vertebrae and through the suboccipital triangle becomes clinically significant when blood flow through them is reduced, as occurs with *arteriosclerosis*. Under these conditions, prolonged turning of the head may cause light-headedness, dizziness, and other symptoms resulting from interference with the blood supply to the brainstem.

TABLE 4.11 PRINCIPAL MUSCLES PRODUCING MOVEMENT OF ATLANTO-AXIAL JOINTS[a]

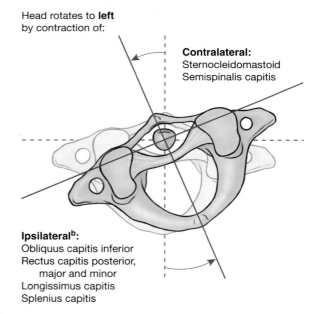

Head rotates to **left** by contraction of:

Contralateral:
Sternocleidomastoid
Semispinalis capitis

Ipsilateral[b]:
Obliquus capitis inferior
Rectus capitis posterior, major and minor
Longissimus capitis
Splenius capitis

[a]Rotation is the specialized movement at these joints. Movement of one joint involves the other.

[b]Same side to which head is rotated.

FIGURE 4.25.   Sensory innervation of suboccipital region and head. **A.** Dermatomes. **B.** Cutaneous innervation.

TABLE 4.12 NERVE SUPPLY OF POSTERIOR ASPECT OF HEAD AND NECK

Nerve	Origin	Course	Distribution
Suboccipital	Posterior ramus of C1 spinal nerve	Runs between cranium and C1 vertebra to reach suboccipital triangle	Muscles of suboccipital triangle
Greater occipital	Posterior ramus of C2 spinal nerve	Emerges inferior to obliquus capitis inferior and ascends to posterior scalp	Skin over neck and occipital bone
Lesser occipital	Anterior rami of spinal nerves C2–C3	Pass directly to skin	Skin of superior posterolateral neck and scalp posterior to ear
Posterior rami, nerves C3–C7	Posterior rami of spinal nerves C3–C7	Pass segmentally to muscles and skin	Intrinsic muscles of back and overlying skin adjacent to vertebral column

Back Sprains and Strains

Back sprain is an injury in which only ligamentous tissue, or the attachment of ligament to bone, is involved, without dislocation or fracture. It results from excessively strong contractions related to movements of the vertebral column, such as excessive extension or rotation.

Back strain involves some degree of stretching or microscopic tearing of muscle fibers. The muscles usually involved are those producing movements of the lumbar IV joints, especially the erector spinae. If the weight is not properly balanced on the vertebral column, strain is exerted on the muscles. This is the most common cause of low back pain.

As a protective mechanism, the back muscles go into spasm after an injury or in response to inflammation (e.g., of ligaments). A spasm is a sudden involuntary contraction of one or more muscle groups. Spasms result in cramps, pain, and interference with function, producing involuntary movement and distortion of the vertebral column.

Using the back as a lever when lifting puts an enormous strain on the vertebral column and its ligaments and muscles. These strains can be minimized if the lifter crouches, holds the back as straight as possible, and uses the muscles of the buttocks and lower limbs to assist with the lifting.

Medical Imaging of Back

Conventional radiographs are very good for high-contrast structures such as bone (Fig. 4.26A). The advent of digital radiography allows improved contrast resolution.

Myelography is a radiopaque contrast study that allows visualization of the spinal cord and spinal nerve roots (Fig. 4.26B). In this procedure, largely replaced by MRI, contrast material is injected into the spinal subarachnoid space. This technique shows the extent of the subarachnoid space and its extensions around the spinal nerve roots within the dural sheaths.

Computerized tomography (CT) differentiates between the white and the gray matter of the brain and spinal cord. It has also improved the radiological assessment of fractures of the vertebral column, particularly in determining the degree of compression of the spinal cord. The dense vertebrae attenuate much of the X-ray beam and, therefore, appear white on the scans (Figs. 4.26D and 4.27).

Uncovertebral joint
Superior lip vertebral body C5
Pedicle
1st rib
Transverse process of T2
Clavicle
Spinous process of T2

C3
C7

A Anteroposterior view

Pedicle
L3 vertebral body
Dye in dural root sheaths (extensions of subarachnoid space around spinal nerve roots)
Cauda equina
Lumbar cistern within dural sac

B Anteroposterior view

MP C1 D C1 MP
C2
St IV St
VA C3
C4
C5
C6
Sc C7
Lu T1 Lu

C Coronal MRI

Left common iliac artery
Intervertebral disc
Psoas major
Superior articular process of L5
Zygapophysial joint
Cauda equina in lumbar cistern
Inferior articular process of L4
Lamina
Spinous process

D Transverse CT

FIGURE 4.26. **Imaging of the vertebral column. A.** Anteroposterior radiograph of cervical region. *Arrowheads*, margins of the column of air (*black*) in the trachea; *boxed area*, column of articular processes and the overlapping transverse processes. **B.** Myelogram of lumbar region. **C.** Coronal MRI scan of cervical region. *D*, dens of axis; *IV*, intervertebral; *Lu*, lung; *MP*, mastoid process; *Sc*, scalenes; *St*, sternocleidomastoid; *VA*, vertebral artery. **D.** Transverse (axial) CT scan of L4–L5 IV disc.

The IV discs have a higher density than the surrounding adipose tissue in the extradural space and the CSF in the subarachnoid space. Three-dimensional reconstruction of CT images is shown in Figure 4.27C.

Magnetic resonance imaging (MRI), like CT, is a computer-assisted imaging procedure, but X-rays are not used as with CT. MRI produces extremely good images of the vertebral column, spinal cord, and CSF (Fig. 4.26C). MRI clearly demonstrates the components of IV discs and shows their relationship to the vertebral bodies and longitudinal ligaments. Herniations of the nucleus pulposus and its relationship to the spinal nerve roots also are well defined. MRI is the imaging procedure of choice for evaluating IV disc disorders.

A Inferior view

B Inferior view

Key for A and B							
1	Linea alba	6	Latissimus dorsi	11	Multifidus	16	Spinous process
2	Rectus abdominis	7	Descending aorta	12	Rotatores	17	Cauda equina
3	External oblique	8	Inferior vena cava	13	Iliocostalis	18	Psoas major
4	Internal oblique	9	Spinalis	14	4th lumbar vertebra	19	Quadratus lumborum
5	Transversus abdominis	10	Longissimus	15	Transverse process		

Key for C	
AA	Anterior arch of C1
AT	Anterior tubercle of C1
C1–C4	Vertebrae
D	Dens (odontoid process) of C2
FJ	Zygapophysial (facet) joint
La	Lamina
PA	Posterior arch of C1
PT	Posterior tubercle of C1
SF	Superior articular facet of C1
SP	Spinous process
T	Foramen transversarium
VC	Vertebral canal

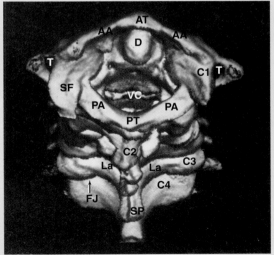

C Posterior view

FIGURE 4.27.   **Computed tomographic (CT) imaging. A.** Transverse section of cadaveric specimen at L4 vertebra. **B.** Transverse (axial) CT scan at L4 vertebra. **C.** 3D reconstructed CT image of cervical spine.

 Go to http://thePoint.lww.com/ECA4e for helpful study tools, including USMLE-style questions, case studies, images, and more!

BONES OF LOWER LIMB / 318

Hip Bone / 318

Femur / 318

Patella / 322

Tibia / 322

Fibula / 322

Tarsus, Metatarsus, and Phalanges / 323

■ Surface Anatomy of Lower Limb Bones / 327

FASCIA, VESSELS, AND NERVES OF LOWER LIMB / 329

Subcutaneous Tissue and Fascia / 329

Venous Drainage of Lower Limb / 331

Lymphatic Drainage of Lower Limb / 332

Cutaneous Innervation of Lower Limb / 333

THIGH AND GLUTEAL REGIONS / 336

Anterior Thigh Muscles / 336

Medial Thigh Muscles / 337

NEUROVASCULAR STRUCTURES AND RELATIONSHIPS IN ANTEROMEDIAL THIGH / 341

Femoral Triangle and Adductor Canal / 341

Femoral Nerve / 342

Femoral Sheath / 342

Femoral Artery / 343

Femoral Vein / 346

Obturator Artery and Nerve / 346

GLUTEAL REGION AND POSTERIOR THIGH / 346

Gluteal Muscles / 347

Gluteal Bursae / 348

Posterior Thigh Muscles / 349

Nerves of Gluteal Region and Posterior Thigh / 349

Vasculature of Gluteal and Posterior Thigh Regions / 352

POPLITEAL FOSSA / 356

Fascia of Popliteal Fossa / 356

Vessels in Popliteal Fossa / 356

Nerves in Popliteal Fossa / 357

LEG / 357

Anterior Compartment of Leg / 357

Lateral Compartment of Leg / 360

Posterior Compartment of Leg / 363

FOOT / 371

Deep Fascia of Foot / 371

Muscles of Foot / 372

Nerves of Foot / 376

Arteries of Foot / 376

Venous Drainage of Foot / 377

Lymphatic Drainage of Foot / 377

WALKING: THE GAIT CYCLE / 377

JOINTS OF LOWER LIMB / 379

Hip Joint / 379

Knee Joint / 385

Tibiofibular Joints / 389

Ankle Joint / 395

Joints of Foot / 398

Arches of Foot / 400

MEDICAL IMAGING OF LOWER LIMB / 403

The lower limbs (extremities) are specialized for locomotion, supporting body weight, and maintaining balance. The lower limbs are connected to the trunk by the **pelvic girdle,** a bony ring composed of the sacrum and right and left hip bones joined anteriorly at the **pubic symphysis** (L. *symphysis pubis*). The lower limb has six major regions (Fig. 5.1):

1. **Gluteal region** (L. *regio glutealis*) is the transitional zone between the trunk and free lower limbs. It includes the **buttocks** (L. *nates, clunes*) and **hip region** (L. *regio coxae*), which overlies the hip joint and greater trochanter of the femur.
2. **Femoral region** (L. *regio femoris*), also referred to as the thigh, contains most of the **femur,** which connects the hip and knee joints.
3. **Knee region** (L. *regio genus*) contains the distal femur, the proximal tibia and fibula, and the *patella* (knee cap) as

well as the joints between these bony structures; the fat-filled hollow posterior to the knee (L. *poples*) is called the *popliteal fossa.*

4. **Leg region** (L. *regio cruris*) connects the knee and ankle joints and contains the **tibia** and **fibula;** the **calf** (L. *sura*) of the leg is the posterior prominence. Often laypersons refer incorrectly to the entire lower limb as "the leg."
5. **Ankle** or **talocrural region** (L. *regio talocruralis*) includes the narrow distal part of the leg and ankle (talocrural) joint.
6. **Foot region** (L. *regio pedis*), the distal part of the lower limb, contains the *tarsus, metatarsus,* and *phalanges* (toe bones). The superior surface is the **dorsum of the foot,** and the inferior, ground-contacting surface is the **sole** or **plantar region.** The **toes** are the **digits of the foot;** the **great toe** (L. *hallux*) has only two phalanges, and the other digits have three.

A Anterior view

B Lateral view

FIGURE 5.1.   **Lower limb. A.** Regions and bones of lower limb. **B.** Center of gravity in a relaxed standing position.

BONES OF LOWER LIMB

Body weight is transferred from the vertebral column through the *sacro-iliac joints* to the pelvic girdle and from the pelvic girdle through the hip joints to the femurs (L. *femora*) and then through the femurs to the knee joints. Weight is then transferred from the knee joint to the ankle joint by the tibia. The fibula does not articulate with the femur and does not bear weight. At the ankle, the weight is transferred to the talus. The talus is the keystone of a longitudinal arch formed by the tarsal and metatarsal bones of each foot, which distribute the weight evenly between the heel and the forefoot when standing. To support the erect bipedal posture better, the femurs are oblique (directed inferomedially) within the thighs so that when standing the knees are adjacent and are placed directly inferior to the trunk, returning the center of gravity to the vertical lines of the supporting legs and feet (Figs. 5.1 and 5.2). The femurs of females are slightly more oblique than those of males, reflecting the greater width of their pelves.

Hip Bone

Each mature **hip bone** is formed by the fusion of three primary bones: *ilium, ischium,* and *pubis* (Figs. 5.3A). At puberty, these bones are still separated by a **triradiate cartilage.** The cartilage disappears and the bones begin to fuse at 15 to 17 years of age; fusion is complete between 20 and 25 years of age.

The **ilium,** the superior and largest part of the hip bone, contributes to the superior part of the **acetabulum** (Fig. 5.3), the cup-like cavity (socket) on the lateral aspect of the hip bone for articulation with the head of the femur. The ilium consists of a **body,** which joins the pubis and ischium to the acetabulum, and an **ala** (wing), which is bordered superiorly by the **iliac crest.**

The **ischium** forms the posteroinferior part of the acetabulum and hip bone. The ischium consists of a **body,** where it joins the ilium and superior ramus of the pubis to form the acetabulum. The **ramus of the ischium** joins the inferior ramus of the pubis to form the **ischiopubic ramus** (Fig. 5.3B).

The **pubis** forms the anterior part of the acetabulum and the anteromedial part of the hip bone. The right pubis has a **body** that articulates with the left pubis at the pubic symphysis. It also has two **rami,** superior and inferior.

To place the hip bone or bony pelvis in the anatomical position (Fig. 5.3B,C), situate it so that the:

- Anterior superior iliac spine (ASIS) and anterosuperior aspect of the pubis lie in the same coronal (frontal) plane.
- Symphysial surface of the pubis is vertical, parallel to the median plane.

Fractures of Hip Bone

Fractures of the hip bone are "pelvic fractures," although the term *hip fracture* is most commonly applied, unfortunately, to fractures of the femoral heads, neck, or trochanters.

Avulsion fractures of the hip bone may occur during sports that require sudden acceleration or deceleration of forces. A small part of the bone with a piece of tendon or ligament attached is "avulsed" (torn away)—for example, the anterior superior and inferior iliac spines, and the ischial tuberosities.

- Internal aspect of the body of the pubis faces almost directly superiorly.
- Acetabulum faces inferolaterally, with the acetabular notch directed inferiorly.
- Obturator foramen lies inferomedial to the acetabulum.

Femur

The **femur** is the longest and heaviest bone in the body. The femur consists of a **shaft** (body) and superior or proximal and inferior or distal ends (Fig. 5.2). Most of the shaft is smoothly rounded, except for a prominent double-edged ridge on its posterior aspect, the **linea aspera,** which diverges inferiorly. The proximal end of the femur consists of a head, neck, and greater and lesser trochanters. The **head of the femur** is covered with articular cartilage, except for a medially placed depression or pit, the **fovea for the ligament of the head.** The **neck of the femur** is trapezoidal; the narrow end supports the head and its broader base is continuous with the shaft.

Where the neck joins the shaft are two large, blunt elevations—the trochanters. The conical **lesser trochanter,** with its rounded tip, extends medially from the posteromedial part of the junction of the femoral neck and shaft (Fig. 5.2A). The **greater trochanter** is a large, laterally placed mass that projects superomedially where the neck joins the shaft. The **intertrochanteric line** is a roughened ridge running from the greater to the lesser trochanter. A similar but smoother ridge, the **intertrochanteric crest,** joins the trochanters posteriorly (Fig. 5.2B).

The distal end of the femur ends in two spirally curved **femoral condyles (medial and lateral).** The femoral condyles articulate with the tibial condyles to form the knee joint.

A Anterior view

Iliac crest
Tubercle of iliac crest
Anterior superior iliac spine (ASIS)
Anterior inferior iliac spine
Greater trochanter
Neck of femur
Intertrochanteric line
Lesser trochanter
Femur
Patella
Lateral epicondyle
Lateral condyle of femur
Apex of head
Head
Neck
Fibula
Tibia
Lateral malleolus
Calcaneus
Cuboid

Hip bone
Iliac fossa
Iliopubic eminence
Superior ramus of pubis
Pubic tubercle
Pubic crest
Body of pubis
Pubic symphysis
Obturator foramen
Head of femur
Shaft of femur
Base of patella
Adductor tubercle
Medial epicondyle
Apex of patella
Medial condyle of femur
Medial condyle of tibia
Intercondylar eminence
Tibial tuberosity
Anterior border
Lateral surface
Medial surface
Medial malleolus
Talus
Navicular
3 2 1 Cuneiforms
1st metatarsal
Proximal phalanx
Distal phalanx

B Anterior view of proximal femur

Greater trochanter
Intertrochanteric line
Shaft of femur
Fovea for ligament of head
Head of femur
Neck of femur
Lesser trochanter

C Anterior view of patella

Base
Lateral border
Medial border
Apex

D Posterior view of patella

Base
Medial articular surface
Lateral articular surface
Apex

FIGURE 5.2.   Bones of lower limb.

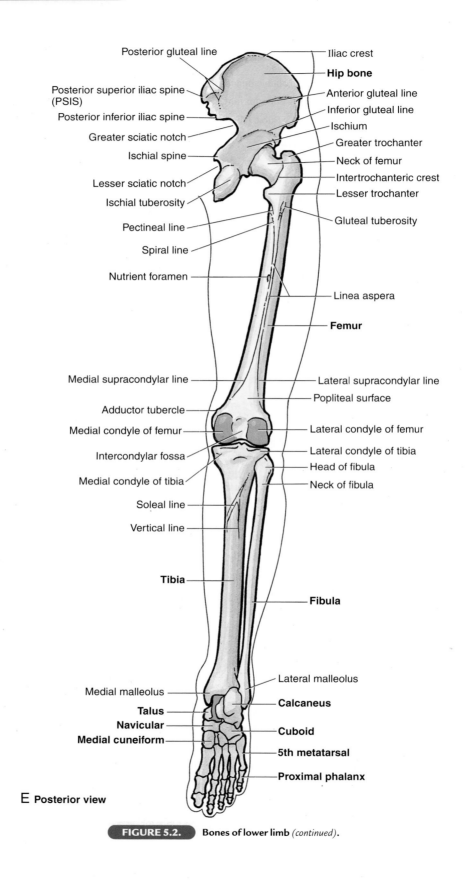

Posterior gluteal line

Iliac crest

Hip bone

Posterior superior iliac spine (PSIS)

Anterior gluteal line

Posterior inferior iliac spine

Inferior gluteal line

Greater sciatic notch

Ischium

Ischial spine

Greater trochanter

Lesser sciatic notch

Neck of femur

Intertrochanteric crest

Ischial tuberosity

Lesser trochanter

Pectineal line

Gluteal tuberosity

Spiral line

Nutrient foramen

Linea aspera

Femur

Medial supracondylar line

Lateral supracondylar line

Popliteal surface

Adductor tubercle

Medial condyle of femur

Lateral condyle of femur

Intercondylar fossa

Lateral condyle of tibia

Head of fibula

Medial condyle of tibia

Neck of fibula

Soleal line

Vertical line

Tibia

Fibula

Lateral malleolus

Medial malleolus

Calcaneus

Talus

Navicular

Cuboid

Medial cuneiform

5th metatarsal

Proximal phalanx

E **Posterior view**

FIGURE 5.2. Bones of lower limb *(continued)*.

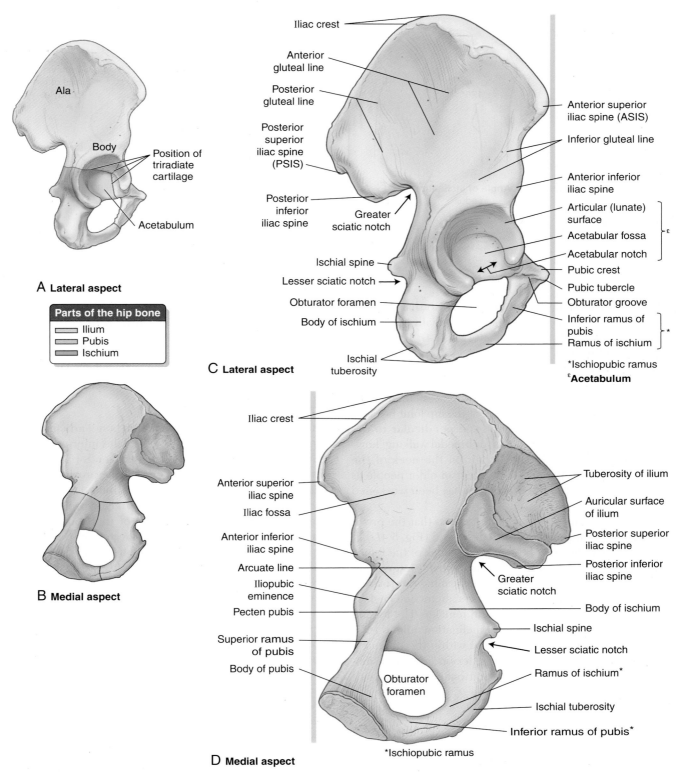

A **Lateral aspect**

Parts of the hip bone
- Ilium
- Pubis
- Ischium

B **Medial aspect**

C **Lateral aspect**

*Ischiopubic ramus
ᵋ**Acetabulum**

D **Medial aspect**

*Ischiopubic ramus

FIGURE 5.3.   **Hip bone. A. and B.** Parts of hip bone of a 13-year-old. **C. and D.** Right hip bone of an adult in anatomical position. In this position, the anterior superior iliac spine (ASIS) and the anterior aspect of the pubis lie in the same vertical plane (indicated in *blue*).

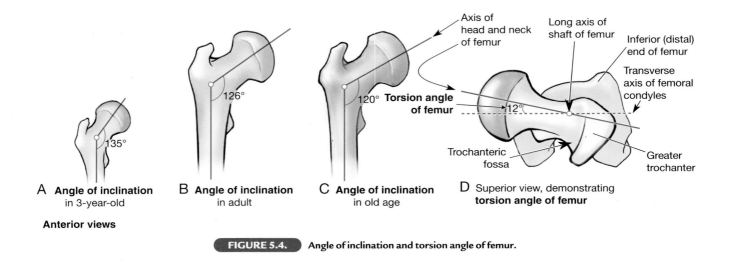

A **Angle of inclination** in 3-year-old

B **Angle of inclination** in adult

C **Angle of inclination** in old age

D Superior view, demonstrating **torsion angle of femur**

Anterior views

FIGURE 5.4. Angle of inclination and torsion angle of femur.

The proximal femur is bent (L-shaped) so that the long axis of the head and neck project superomedially at an angle to that of the obliquely oriented shaft (Fig. 5.4). This obtuse **angle of inclination** in the adult is 115 to 140 degrees, averaging 126 degrees. The angle is less in females because of the increased width between the acetabula and the greater obliquity of the shaft. The angle of inclination allows greater mobility of the femur at the hip joint because it places the head and neck more perpendicular to the acetabulum. This is advantageous for bipedal walking; however, it imposes considerable strain on the neck of the femur. Fractures of the neck may occur in older people as a result of a slight stumble if the neck has been weakened by osteoporosis.

When the femur is viewed superiorly, so that the proximal end is superimposed over the distal end (Fig. 5.4D), it can be seen that the axis of the head and neck of the femur and the transverse axis of the femoral condyles intersect at the long axis of the shaft of the femur forming the **torsion angle,** or **angle of declination**. The mean torsion angle is 7 degrees in males and 12 degrees in females. The torsion angle, combined with the angle of inclination, allows rotatory movements of the femoral head within the obliquely placed acetabulum to convert into flexion and extension, abduction and adduction, and rotational movements of the thigh.

Patella

The patella (knee cap) is a large sesamoid bone that is formed intratendinously after birth. This triangular bone, located anterior to the knee joint, articulates with the patellar surface of the femur (Fig. 5.2A). The subcutaneous **anterior surface** of the patella is convex; the thick **base** (superior border) slopes inferoanteriorly; the two lateral and medial **borders** converge inferiorly to form the pointed **apex**; and the **articular surface** (posterior surface) has a smooth articular area that is divided into medial and lateral articular surfaces by a vertical ridge (Fig. 5.2C,D).

Tibia

The large, weight-bearing **tibia** (shin bone) articulates with the femoral condyles superiorly, the talus inferiorly, and the fibula laterally at its proximal and distal ends (Fig. 5.2). The distal end of the tibia is smaller than the proximal end and has facets for articulation with the fibula and talus. The **medial malleolus** is an inferiorly directed projection from the medial side of the distal end of the tibia. The large **nutrient foramen** of the tibia is located on the posterior aspect of the proximal third of the bone (Fig. 5.5B). From it, the **nutrient canal** runs inferiorly in the tibia before it opens into the medullary (marrow) cavity. For other bony features see Figure 5.5.

Fibula

The slender **fibula** lies posterolateral to the tibia and serves mainly for muscle attachment (Figs. 5.2 and 5.5). At its proximal end the fibula consists of an enlarged **head** superior to a narrow neck. At its distal end, the fibula enlarges to form the **lateral malleolus,** which is more prominent and more posteriorly placed than the medial malleolus and extends approximately 1 cm farther distally. The fibula is not directly involved in weight bearing; however, its lateral malleolus helps hold the talus in its socket. The shafts of the tibia and fibula are connected by an **interosseous membrane** throughout most of their lengths.

A Anterior view

B Posterior view

FIGURE 5.5. **Right tibia and fibula.** The shafts are connected by the interosseous membrane composed of strong obliquely oriented fibers.

Tarsus, Metatarsus, and Phalanges

The **bones of the foot** include the tarsus, metatarsus, and phalanges (Figs. 5.2 and 5.6).

TARSUS

The tarsus consists of seven bones: calcaneus, talus, cuboid, navicular, and three cuneiforms. Only the talus articulates with the leg bones. The **calcaneus** (heel bone) is the largest and strongest bone in the foot. It articulates with the talus superiorly and the cuboid anteriorly (Fig. 5.6A). The calcaneus transmits most of the body weight from the talus to the ground. The **sustentaculum tali**, projecting from the superior border of the medial surface of the calcaneus, supports the head of the talus (Fig. 5.6B). The lateral surface of the calcaneus has an oblique ridge (Fig. 5.6C), the **fibular trochlea.** The posterior part of the calcaneus has a prominence, the **calcaneal tuberosity** (L. *tuber calcanei*), which has medial, lateral, and anterior tubercles (Fig. 5.6B).

The **talus** (ankle bone) has a **head, neck,** and **body** (Fig. 5.6C). The talus rests on the anterior two thirds of the calcaneus. The superior surface, the **trochlea of the talus,** bears the weight of the body transmitted from the tibia and articulates with the two malleoli. The head of the talus articulates anteriorly with the navicular. The rounded **head of talus** rests partially on the **sustentaculum tali** (talar shelf) of the calcaneus (Fig. 5.6B,E).

The **navicular** (L. little ship), a flattened, boat-shaped bone, is located between the talar head and the cuneiforms. The medial surface of the navicular projects inferiorly as the **tuberosity of navicular.** If the tuberosity is too prominent, it may press against the medial part of the shoe and cause foot pain.

The **cuboid** is the most lateral bone in the distal row of the tarsus. Anterior to the **tuberosity of cuboid** (Fig. 5.6B), on the lateral and plantar surfaces of the bone, is a groove for the tendon of the fibularis longus muscle (Fig. 5.6B,C).

There are three cuneiforms: **medial** (first), **intermediate** (second), and **lateral** (third). Each cuneiform (L. *cuneus,*

A Dorsal view

B Plantar view

C Lateral view

D Lateral view

E Medial view

F Medial view

FIGURE 5.6. **Bones of foot.** *Blue,* articular cartilages.

Femoral Fractures

The neck of the femur is most frequently fractured, especially in females secondary to osteoporosis. Fractures of the proximal femur can occur at several locations—for example, transcervical and intertrochanteric (Fig. B5.1A,B). The femoral shaft is large and strong; however, a violent direct injury, such as may be sustained in an automobile accident, may fracture it, causing, for example, a spiral fracture (Fig. B5.1C). Fractures of the distal femur may be complicated by separation of the condyles, resulting in misalignment of the knee joint.

Coxa Vara and Coxa Valga

The angle of inclination varies with age, sex, and development of the femur (e.g., consequent to a congenital defect in ossification of the femoral neck). It also may change with any pathological process that weakens the neck of the femur (e.g., rickets). When the angle of inclination is decreased, the condition is **coxa vara** (Fig. B5.2A); when it is increased, the condition is **coxa valga** (Fig. B5.2B). Coxa vara causes a mild passive abduction of the hip.

A Transcervical fracture of femoral neck

B Intertrochanteric fracture

C Spiral fracture

Anterior views

FIGURE B5.1.

Posterior views

A Coxa vara (decreased angle of inclination)

B Coxa valga (increased angle of inclination)

FIGURE B5.2.

wedge-shaped) articulates with the navicular posteriorly and the base of the appropriate metatarsal anteriorly. In addition, the lateral cuneiform articulates with the cuboid.

METATARSUS

The **metatarsus** consists of five metatarsals, which connect the tarsus and phalanges. They are numbered from the medial side of the foot (Fig. 5.6B,C). The **first metatarsal** is shorter and stouter than the others. The **second metatarsal** is the longest. Each metatarsal has a **base** (proximally), a **shaft,** and a **head** (distally). The bases of the

metatarsals articulate with the cuneiform and cuboid bones, and the heads articulate with the proximal phalanges. The bases of the first and fifth metatarsals have large tuberosities; the **tuberosity of the fifth metatarsal** projects over the lateral margin of the cuboid (Fig. 5.6C).

PHALANGES

There are 14 **phalanges.** The first digit (great toe) has two phalanges (proximal and distal); the other four digits have three each: proximal, middle, and distal (Fig. 5.6A,B). Each **phalanx** has a **base** (proximally), a **shaft,** and a **head** (distally).

Tibial and Fibular Fractures

The tibial shaft is narrowest at the junction of its inferior and middle thirds, which is the most common site of fracture. Because its anterior surface is subcutaneous, the tibial shaft is the most frequent site of a *compound fracture*, one in which the skin is perforated and blood vessels are torn (Fig. B5.3A), or a diagonal fracture (Fig. B5.3B). Fracture of the tibia through the nutrient canal predisposes to nonunion of the bone fragments, resulting from damage to the nutrient artery. *Fibular fractures* commonly occur just proximal to the lateral malleolus and often are associated with fracture–dislocations of the ankle joint (Fig. B5.3C). When a person slips, forcing the foot into an excessively inverted position, the ankle ligaments tear, forcibly tilting the talus against the lateral malleolus and shearing it off.

Bone Grafts

The fibula is a common source of bone for grafting. Even after a segment of the fibular shaft has been removed, walking, running, and jumping can be normal. Free vascularized fibulas have been used to restore skeletal integrity to limbs in which congenital bone defects exist and to replace segments of bone after trauma or excision of a malignant tumor. The periosteum and nutrient artery are generally removed with the piece of bone so that the graft will remain alive and grow when transplanted to another site. The transplanted piece of fibula, secured in its new site, eventually restores the blood supply of the bone to which it has been attached.

Fractures Involving Epiphysial Plates

The primary ossification center for the superior end of the tibia appears shortly after birth and joins the shaft of the tibia during adolescence (usually 16 to 18 years of age). Tibial fractures in children are more serious if they involve the epiphysial plates because continued normal growth of the bone may be jeopardized. The tibial tuberosity usually forms by inferior bone growth from the superior epiphysial center at approximately 10 years of age, but a separate center for the tibial tuberosity may appear at approximately 12 years of age. Disruption of the epiphysial plate at the tibial tuberosity may cause inflammation of the tuberosity and chronic recurring pain during adolescence (*Osgood-Schlatter disease*), especially in young athletes (Fig. B5.4).

Anterior views

A **Compound (open) fracture with external bleeding**

B **Diagonal fracture with shortening**

Fibula (F)

Tibia (T)

Talus (A)

Inversion

Posterior view

C **Fibular fracture with excessive inversion of foot**

FIGURE B5.3.

Osgood-Schlatter Disease (lateral radiograph)
Tibial tuberosity elongated and fragmented with overlying soft tissue swelling

FIGURE B5.4.

Fractures of Foot Bones

Calcaneal fractures occur in people who fall on their heels (e.g., from a ladder). Usually the bone breaks into several fragments (*comminuted fracture*) that disrupt the subtalar joint, where the talus articulates with the calcaneus (Fig. B5.5A). *Fractures of the talar neck* may occur during severe dorsiflexion of the ankle (e.g., when a person is pressing extremely hard on the brake pedal of a car during a head-on collision). Metatarsal and phalangeal fractures are a common injury in endurance athletes and may also occur when a heavy object falls on the foot. Metatarsal fractures are also common in dancers, especially female ballet dancers using the *demipointe* technique. The "dancer's fracture" usually occurs when the dancer loses balance, putting the full body weight on the metatarsal and fracturing the bone (Fig. B5.5B).

Calcaneus

A Lateral view, comminuted fracture of calcaneus

4th metatarsal

5th metatarsal

Tuberosity of 5th metatarsal

Cuboid

B Dorsum of foot, fractures of metatarsals

FIGURE B5.5.

Surface Anatomy of Lower Limb Bones

Pelvic Girdle and Femur

When your hands are on your hips, they rest on the **iliac crests,** the curved superior borders of the alae (wings) of the ilium. The anterior third of the crest is easily palpated because it is subcutaneous. The highest point of the crest is at the level of the intervertebral (IV) disc between the L4 and the L5 vertebrae. The iliac crest ends anteriorly at the rounded **anterior superior iliac spine** (ASIS), which is easy to palpate, especially in thin persons, because it is subcutaneous and often visible (Fig. SA5.1A,B). The ASIS is used as the proximal point for measurement of leg length to the medial malleolus of the tibia. The iliac crest ends posteriorly at the **posterior superior iliac spine** (PSIS), which may be difficult to palpate (Fig. SA5.1C). Its position is easy to locate because it lies at the bottom of a skin dimple, approximately 4 cm lateral to the midline demarcating the sacro-iliac joints. The dimple exists because the skin and fascia attach to the PSIS.

The ischial tuberosity is easily palpated in the inferior part of the buttock when the thigh is flexed. It bears body weight when sitting. The thick gluteus maximus and fat obscure the tuberosity when the thigh is extended. The **gluteal fold,** a prominent skin fold containing fat, coincides with the inferior border of the gluteus maximus muscle.

The **greater trochanter of the femur** is easily palpable on the lateral side of the hip approximately 10 cm inferior to the iliac crest (Fig. SA5.1B,C).

Highest level of iliac crest
Supracristal plane
Anterior superior iliac spine
Buttock
Site of tip of greater trochanter of femur
Gluteal fold
Thigh

A Lateral view

FIGURE SA5.1.

Because it lies close to the skin, the greater trochanter causes discomfort when you lie on your side on a hard surface. In the anatomical position, a line joining the tips of the greater trochanters normally passes through the centers of the femoral heads and pubic tubercles. The **shaft of the femur** usually is not palpable because it is covered with large muscles. The **medial and lateral condyles** of the femur are subcutaneous and easily palpated when the knee is flexed or extended. The patellar surface of the femur is where the **patella** slides during flexion and extension of the leg. The lateral and medial margins of the patellar surface can be palpated when the knee is flexed. The **adductor tubercle,** a small prominence of bone, may be felt at the superior part of the medial femoral condyle.

Tibia and Fibula

The **tibial tuberosity,** an oval elevation on the anterior surface of the tibia, is palpable approximately 5 cm distal (inferior) to the apex of the patella (Fig. SA5.1*B*). The subcutaneous **anterior border and medial surface of the tibia** is also easy to palpate. The skin covering it is freely movable. The prominence at the ankle, the **medial malleolus,** is also subcutaneous, and its inferior end is blunt. The **medial** and **lateral tibial condyles** can be palpated anteriorly at the sides of the patellar ligament, especially when the knee is flexed. The **head of the fibula** can be palpated easily at the level of the superior part of the tibial tuberosity because its knob-like head is subcutaneous at the posterolateral aspect

B **Anterior view**

Green = palpable features of lower limb bones

C **Posterior view**

FIGURE SA5.1. *(continued)*

of the knee. The **neck of fibula** can be palpated just distal to the fibular head. Only the distal quarter of the shaft of the fibula is palpable. Feel your **lateral malleolus,** noting that it is subcutaneous and that its inferior end is sharp. Note that the tip of the lateral malleolus extends farther distally and more posteriorly than does the tip of the **medial malleolus.**

Bones of Foot

The **head of talus** is palpable anteromedial to the proximal part of the lateral malleolus when the foot is inverted and anterior to the medial malleolus when the foot is everted. Eversion of the foot makes the head of talus more prominent as it moves away from the navicular. The head of talus occupies the space between the sustentaculum tali and the tuberosity of navicular. When the foot is plantarflexed, the superior surface of the **body of the talus** can be palpated on the anterior aspect of the ankle, anterior to the inferior end of the tibia (Fig. SA5.1*D*).

The weight-bearing **medial tubercle of the calcaneus** on the plantar surface of the foot is broad and large but may not be palpable because of the thick overlying skin and subcutaneous tissue (Fig. SA5.1*E*). The **fibular trochlea,** a lateral extension of the calcaneus, may be detectable as a small tubercle on the lateral subcutaneous aspect of the calcaneus, anteroinferior to the tip of the lateral malleolus. The **sustentaculum tali** is the only part of the medial aspect of the calcaneus that may be palpated as a small prominence just distal to the tip of the medial malleolus.

The **tuberosity of the navicular** is easily seen and palpated on the medial aspect of the foot, inferoanterior to the tip of the medial malleolus. Usually, palpation of bony prominences on the plantar surface of the foot is difficult because of the thick skin, fascia, and pads of fat. The cuboid and cuneiforms are difficult to identify individually by palpation. The **cuboid** can be felt on the lateral aspect of the foot, posterior to the base of the fifth metatarsal. The **medial cuneiform** can be indistinctly palpated between the tuberosity of the navicular and the base of the first metatarsal.

The **head of the first metatarsal** forms a prominence on the medial aspect of the foot. The medial and lateral **sesamoids** inferior to the head of this metatarsal can be felt to slide when the first digit is moved passively over them. The **tuberosity of the fifth metatarsal** forms a prominent

landmark on the lateral aspect of the foot and can be palpated easily at the midpoint of the lateral border of the foot. The shafts of the **metatarsals** and **phalanges** can be felt on the dorsum of the foot between the extensor tendons.

D Dorsum of foot

E Plantar aspect of foot

FIGURE SA5.1. *(continued)*

FASCIA, VESSELS, AND CUTANEOUS NERVES OF LOWER LIMB

Subcutaneous Tissue and Fascia

The **subcutaneous tissue (superficial fascia)** lies deep to the skin and consists of loose connective tissue that contains a variable amount of fat, cutaneous nerves, super-ficial veins, lymphatic vessels, and lymph nodes (Fig. 5.7). The subcutaneous tissue of the hip and thigh is continuous with that of the inferior part of the anterolateral abdominal wall and buttock. At the knee, the subcutaneous tissue loses its fat and blends with the deep fascia, but fat is present in the subcutaneous tissue of the leg.

The **deep fascia** is especially strong, investing the limb like an elastic stocking (Fig. 5.7*A*). The deep fascia limits outward extension of contracting muscles, making muscular

Anterior superior iliac spine

Inguinal ligament

Falciform margin of saphenous opening

Great saphenous vein

Subcutaneous tissue

Iliotibial tract

Level of section in Figure 5.8A

Fascia lata

Saphenous opening

Pubic tubercle

Cribriform fascia in saphenous opening

Bursae

Deep fascia of leg (crural fascia)

Level of section in Figure 5.8B

Extensor retinacula

A **Anterior view**

Iliac crest

Iliac tubercle

Tensor fasciae latae

Gluteus maximus

Site of ischial tuberosity (deep to muscle when thigh is extended)

Fascia lata

Iliotibial tract

Patella

Anterolateral tibial tubercle (Gerdy tubercle)

Tibia

B **Lateral view**

FIGURE 5.7. Fascia of lower limb. **A.** Deep fascia. **B.** Iliotibial tract.

contraction more efficient in compressing veins to push blood toward the heart. The *deep fascia of the thigh* is called **fascia lata** (L. *lata,* broad). The fascia lata attaches to and is continuous with:

- The inguinal ligament, pubic arch, body of pubis, and pubic tubercle superiorly. The membranous layer of subcutaneous tissue (Scarpa fascia) of the inferior abdominal wall also attaches to the fascia lata just inferior to the inguinal ligament.
- The iliac crest laterally and posteriorly.
- The sacrum, coccyx, sacrotuberous ligament, and ischial tuberosity posteriorly.
- The exposed parts of the bones around the knee and the deep fascia of the leg distally.

The fascia lata is substantial because it encloses the large thigh muscles, especially laterally where it is thickened to form the **iliotibial tract** (Fig. 5.7B). This broad band of fibers is also the aponeurosis of the *tensor fasciae latae* and *gluteus maximus* muscles. The iliotibial tract extends from

the iliac tubercle to the anterolateral tibial tubercle (Gerdy tubercle) on the lateral condyle of the tibia.

The thigh muscles are separated into three **fascial compartments:** anterior, medial, and posterior. The walls of these compartments are formed by the fascia lata and three fascial intermuscular septa that arise from the deep aspect of the fascia lata and attach to the linea aspera of the femur (Fig. 5.8A). The **lateral intermuscular septum** is strong; the other two septa are relatively weak. The lateral intermuscular septum extends from the iliotibial tract to the lateral lip of the linea aspera and lateral supracondylar line of the femur.

The **saphenous opening** in the fascia lata is a gap or hiatus in the fascia lata inferior to the medial part of the inguinal ligament, about 4 cm inferolateral to the pubic tubercle (Fig. 5.7A). Its medial margin is smooth, but its superior, lateral, and inferior margins form a sharp edge, the **falciform margin.** The sieve-like **cribriform fascia** (L. *cribrum,* a sieve) is a localized membranous layer of subcutaneous tissue that spreads over the saphenous opening,

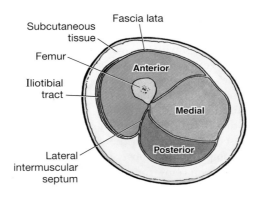

A Inferior view of transverse section of thigh

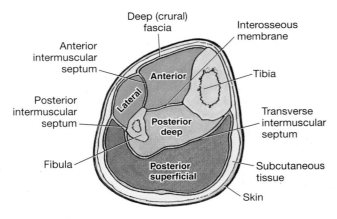

B Inferior view of transverse section of leg

FIGURE 5.8. Fascial compartments. **A.** Thigh. **B.** Leg. See Figure 5.7 for level of sections.

enclosing it. The **great** saphenous vein and some efferent lymphatics pass through the saphenous opening and cribriform fascia to enter the femoral vein and the deep inguinal lymph nodes, respectively.

The **deep fascia of the leg or crural fascia** (L. *crus,* leg) is continuous with the fascia lata and attaches to the anterior and medial borders of the tibia, where it is continuous with its periosteum (Fig. 5.7A). The crural fascia is thick in the proximal part of the anterior aspect of the leg, where it forms part of the proximal attachments of the underlying muscles. Although thin in the distal part of the leg, the crural fascia is thickened where it forms the **extensor retinacula. Anterior** and **posterior intermuscular septa** pass from the deep surface of the crural fascia and attach to the corresponding margins of the fibula. The *interosseous membrane* and the *intermuscular septa* divide the leg into three compartments (Fig. 5.8B): anterior (dorsiflexor), lateral (fibular), and posterior (plantarflexor). The **transverse intermuscular septum** divides the plantarflexor muscles in the posterior compartment into superficial and deep parts.

Venous Drainage of Lower Limb

The lower limb has superficial and deep veins; the superficial veins are in the subcutaneous tissue, and the deep veins are deep to the deep fascia and accompany all major arteries. Superficial and deep veins have valves, but they are more numerous in deep veins.

The two major **superficial veins** are the great and small saphenous veins (Fig. 5.9). The **great saphenous vein** is formed by the union of the **dorsal digital vein of the great toe** and the **dorsal venous arch** of the foot. The great saphenous vein (Fig. 5.9A,B):

- Ascends anterior to the medial malleolus.
- Passes posterior to the medial condyle of the femur (about a hand's breadth posterior to the medial border of the patella).
- Anastomoses freely with the small saphenous vein.
- Traverses the saphenous opening in the fascia lata.
- Empties into the **femoral vein**.

A Anteromedial view

FIGURE 5.9. Superficial venous and lymphatic drainage of lower limb. **A.** Normal superficial veins distended after exercise.

The **small saphenous vein** arises on the lateral side of the foot from the union of the dorsal digital vein of the fifth digit with the **dorsal venous arch** (Fig. 5.9*A,B*). The small saphenous vein (Fig. 5.9*D*):

- Ascends posterior to the lateral malleolus as a continuation of the lateral marginal vein.
- Passes along the lateral border of the calcaneal tendon.
- Inclines to the midline of the fibula and penetrates the deep fascia.
- Ascends between the heads of the gastrocnemius muscle.
- Empties into the popliteal vein in the popliteal fossa.

Perforating veins penetrate the deep fascia close to their origin from the superficial veins (Fig. 5.9*C*). They contain *valves* that allow blood to flow only from the superficial veins to the deep veins. The perforating veins pass through the deep fascia at an oblique angle so that when muscles contract and pressure increases inside the deep fascia, the perforating veins are compressed. Compression of the perforating veins also prevents blood from flowing from the deep to the superficial veins. This pattern of venous blood flow, from superficial to deep, is important for proper venous return from the limb because it enables muscular contractions to propel blood toward the heart against the pull of gravity (*musculovenous pump*).

The **deep veins** in the lower limb accompany all the major arteries (L. *venae comitantes*) and their branches. Instead of occurring as a single vein in the limbs, the deep veins are usually paired, frequently interconnecting veins that flank the artery they accompany. They are contained within a vascular sheath with the artery, whose pulsations also help compress and move blood in the veins (Fig. 5.10*A,B*). The deep veins from the leg flow into the popliteal vein posterior to the knee, which becomes the femoral vein in the thigh. The profunda femoris vein joins the terminal portion of the femoral vein. The femoral vein passes deep to the inguinal ligament to become the external iliac vein in the pelvis.

Lymphatic Drainage of Lower Limb

The lower limb has superficial and deep lymphatic vessels. The **superficial lymphatic vessels** converge on and accompany the saphenous veins and their tributaries. The

B Anteromedial view   **C Medial view**   **D Posterolateral view**

FIGURE 5.9.   *(continued)* **Superficial venous and lymphatic drainage of lower limb. B.** Great saphenous vein and superficial lymphatic drainage. *Arrows,* superficial lymphatic drainage to the inguinal nodes. **C.** Perforating veins. **D.** Small saphenous vein and superficial lymphatic drainage (*arrows*) to the popliteal lymph nodes.

Figure 5.10. Deep venous drainage.

lymphatic vessels accompanying the great saphenous vein end in the **superficial inguinal lymph nodes** (Fig. 5.9B). Most lymph from these nodes passes to the **external iliac lymph nodes,** located along the external iliac vein, but some lymph may also pass to the **deep inguinal lymph nodes,** located on the medial aspect of the femoral vein. The lymphatic vessels accompanying the small saphenous vein enter the **popliteal lymph nodes,** which surround the popliteal vein in the fat of the popliteal fossa (Fig. 5.9D). The **deep lymphatic vessels** of the leg accompany deep veins and enter the popliteal lymph nodes. Most lymph from these nodes ascends through deep lymphatic vessels to the deep inguinal lymph nodes. Lymph from the deep nodes passes to the external iliac lymph nodes.

Cutaneous Innervation of Lower Limb

Cutaneous nerves in the subcutaneous tissue supply the skin of the lower limb (Fig. 5.11A,B). These nerves, except for some in the proximal part of the limb, are branches of the lumbar and sacral plexuses (see Chapters 3 and 4). The area of skin supplied by cutaneous branches from a single spinal nerve is a **dermatome** (Fig. 5.11C–F). Dermatomes L1–L5 extend as a series of bands from the posterior midline of the trunk into the limbs, passing laterally and inferiorly around the limb to its anterior and medial aspects, reflecting the medial rotation that occurs developmentally. Dermatomes S1 and S2 pass inferiorly down the posterior aspect of the limb, separating near the ankle to pass to the lateral and medial margins of the foot (Fig. 5.11F).

Although simplified into distinct zones in dermatome maps, adjacent dermatomes overlap, except at the **axial line,** the line of junction of dermatomes supplied from discontinuous spinal levels.

Two different dermatome maps are commonly used. The pattern according to Foerster (1933) is preferred by many because of its correlation with clinical findings (Fig. 5.11C,D) and that of Keegan and Garrett (1948) by others for its correlation with limb development (Fig. 5.11E,F).

FIGURE 5.11. **Cutaneous innervation of lower limb. A. and B.** Peripheral cutaneous nerve distribution. **C–F.** Dermatomes. Two different dermatome maps are frequently used: **C** and **D**, Foerster, 1933; **E** and **F**, Keegan and Garrett, 1948.

Abnormalities of Sensory Function

 In most instances, a peripheral nerve sensitizing an area of skin represents more than one segment of the spinal cord. Therefore, to interpret abnormalities of peripheral sensory function, peripheral nerve distribution of the major cutaneous nerves must be interpreted as anatomically different from dermatome distribution of the spinal cord segments (Fig. 5.11). Neighboring dermatomes may overlap.

Pain sensation is tested by using a sharp object and asking the patient if pain is felt. If there is no sensation, the spinal cord segment(s) involved can be determined.

Compartment Syndromes in Leg and Fasciotomy

  The fascial compartments of the lower limbs are generally closed spaces, ending proximally and distally at the joints. Trauma to muscles and/or vessels in the compartments from burns, sustained intense use of muscles, or blunt trauma may produce hemorrhage, edema, and inflammation of the muscles. Because the septa and deep fascia of the leg forming the boundaries of the leg compartments are strong, the increased volume consequent to any of these processes increases intracompartmental pressure.

The pressure may reach levels high enough to compress structures significantly in the compartment(s) concerned. The small vessels of muscles and nerves (vasa nervorum) are particularly vulnerable to compression. Structures distal to the compressed area may become ischemic and permanently injured (e.g., loss of motor function in muscles whose blood supply and/or innervation is affected). Increased pressure in a confined anatomical space adversely affects the circulation and threatens the function and viability of tissue within or distally (**compartment syndromes**).

Loss of distal leg pulses is an obvious sign of arterial compression, as is lowering of the temperature of tissues distal to the compression. A **fasciotomy** (incision of overlying fascia or a septum) may be performed to relieve the pressure in the compartment(s) concerned.

Saphenous Cutdown and Saphenous Nerve Injury

  Even when it is not visible in infants, in obese people, or in patients in shock whose veins are collapsed, the great saphenous vein can always be located by making a skin incision anterior to the medial malleolus. This procedure, called a **saphenous cutdown,** is used to insert a cannula for prolonged administration of blood, plasma expanders, electrolytes, or drugs.

The saphenous nerve accompanies the great saphenous vein anterior to the medial malleolus. Should this nerve be cut during a saphenous cutdown or caught by a ligature during closure of a surgical wound, the patient may complain of pain or numbness along the medial border of the foot.

Varicose Veins, Thrombosis, and Thrombophlebitis

 Frequently, the great saphenous vein and its tributaries become **varicose** (dilated so that the cusps of their valves do not close). *Varicose veins* are common in the posteromedial parts of the lower limb and may cause discomfort (Fig. B5.6). In a healthy vein the valves allow blood to flow toward the heart while keeping blood from flowing away from the heart. Valves in varicose veins are incompetent due to dilation or rotation and no longer function properly. As a result, blood flows inferiorly in the veins, producing varicose veins.

Deep venous thrombosis (DVT) of one or more of the deep veins of the lower limb is characterized by swelling, warmth, and *erythema* (inflammation) and infection. **Venous stasis** (stagnation) is an important cause of thrombus formation. Venous stasis can be caused by:

- Incompetent, loose fascia that fails to resist muscle expansion, diminishing the effectiveness of the musculovenous pump.

Varicose veins (medial view)

FIGURE B5.6.   Varicose veins.

- External pressure on the veins from bedding during a prolonged hospital stay or from a tight cast or bandage.
- Muscular inactivity (e.g., during an overseas flight).

DVT with inflammation around the involved veins (**thrombophlebitis**) may develop. A large thrombus that breaks free from a lower limb vein may travel to a lung, forming a **pulmonary thromboembolism** (obstruction of a pulmonary artery). A large embolus may obstruct a main pulmonary artery and may cause death.

Enlarged Inguinal Lymph Nodes

 Lymph nodes enlarge when diseased. **Abrasions** and minor sepsis, caused by pathogenic microorganisms or their toxins in the blood or other tissues, may produce moderate enlargement of the superficial inguinal lymph nodes (**lymphadenopathy**) in otherwise healthy people. Because these enlarged nodes are located in subcutaneous tissue, they are usually easy to palpate.

When inguinal lymph nodes are enlarged, their entire field of drainage—the trunk inferior to the umbilicus, including the perineum, as well as the entire lower limb—should be examined to determine the cause of their enlargement. In female patients, the relatively remote possibility of metastasis of cancer from the uterus should also be considered because some lymphatic drainage from the uterine fundus may flow along lymphatics accompanying the round ligament of the uterus through the inguinal canal to reach the superficial inguinal lymph nodes.

Regional Nerve Blocks of Lower Limbs

  Interruption of the conduction of impulses in peripheral nerves (nerve block) may be achieved by making perineural injections of anesthetics close to the nerves whose conductivity is to be blocked.

The femoral nerve (L2–L4) can be blocked 2 cm inferior to the inguinal ligament, approximately a finger's breadth lateral to the femoral artery. **Paresthesia** (tingling, burning, tickling) radiates to the knee and over the medial side of the leg if the saphenous nerve (terminal branch of femoral) is affected.

THIG AND GLUTEAL REGIONS

In evolution, the development of a prominent gluteal region is closely associated with the assumption of bipedalism and an erect posture. Modification of the shape of the femur necessary for bipedal walking allows the superior placement of the abductors of the thigh into the gluteal region. The remaining thigh muscles are organized into three compartments—*anterior* or *extensor, medial* or *adductor,* and *posterior* or *flexor*—by intermuscular septa (Fig. 5.8*A*). Generally, the anterior group is innervated by the femoral nerve, the medial group by the obturator nerve, and the posterior group by the tibial portion of the sciatic nerve.

Anterior Thigh Muscles

The large **anterior compartment of the thigh** contains the **anterior thigh muscles,** *flexors of the hip,* and *extensors of the knee.* The attachments, nerve supply, and main actions of these muscles are summarized in Figure 5.12 and Table 5.1. The anterior thigh muscles are:

- **Pectineus**: a flat quadrangular muscle, located in the anterior part of the superomedial aspect of the thigh, that adducts and flexes the thigh and assists with medial rotation of the thigh.

- **Iliopsoas** (the chief flexor of the thigh): formed by the merger of two muscles, the psoas major and iliacus. The fleshy parts of the two muscles lie in the posterior wall of the abdomen and greater pelvis, merging as they enter the thigh by passing deep to the inguinal ligament and attaching to the lesser trochanter of the femur. It is in a unique position not only to produce movement but also to stabilize (fixate). This muscle is also a postural muscle, active during standing in maintaining normal lumbar lordosis and, indirectly, the compensatory thoracic kyphosis (curvature of vertebral columns).

- **Sartorius,** the tailor's muscle (L. *sartus,* patched or repaired): a long, ribbon-like muscle that is the most superficial muscle in the anterior thigh; it passes obliquely (lateral to medial) across the superoanterior part of the thigh. It acts across both the hip and the knee joints, and when acting bilaterally, the muscles bring the lower limbs into the cross-legged sitting position. None of the actions is strong; therefore, it is mainly a synergist, acting with other thigh muscles that produce these movements.

- **Quadriceps femoris** (L. four-headed femoral muscle): the great extensor of the leg that forms the main bulk of the anterior thigh muscles. It covers almost all the anterior aspect and sides of the femur. This muscle has four parts:
  - **Rectus femoris,** the "kicking muscle" (L. *rectus,* straight): it crosses the hip joint and helps the iliopsoas

flex this joint. Its ability to extend the knee is compromised during hip flexion.

- **Vastus lateralis:** the largest component of the quadriceps, located on the lateral aspect of the thigh.
- **Vastus intermedius:** lies deep to the rectus femoris between the vastus medialis and the vastus lateralis.
- **Vastus medialis:** covers the medial aspect of the thigh.

A small, flat muscle, the **articularis genu** (articular muscle of knee), a derivative of the vastus intermedius (Fig. 5.12*E*), attaches superiorly to the inferior part of the anterior aspect of the femur and inferiorly to the synovial membrane of the knee joint and the wall of the *suprapatellar bursa*. The muscle pulls the synovial membrane superiorly during extension of the leg, thereby preventing folds of the membrane from being compressed between the femur and the patella within the knee joint.

The tendons of the four parts of the quadriceps unite in the distal part of the thigh to form the **quadriceps tendon** (Fig. 5.12*B*). The **patellar ligament** (L. *ligamentum patellae*), attached to the **tibial tuberosity,** is the continuation of the quadriceps tendon in which the patella is embedded. The

vastus medialis and lateralis also attach independently to the patella and form aponeuroses, the **medial** and **lateral patellar retinacula,** which reinforce the joint capsule of the knee on each side of the patella en route to attachment to the anterior border of the *tibial plateau*. The patella provides additional leverage for the quadriceps in placing the tendon more anteriorly, farther from the joint's axis, causing it to approach the tibia from a position of greater mechanical advantage.

Medial Thigh Muscles

The medial thigh muscles—collectively called the **adductor group**—are in the medial compartment of the thigh and are innervated primarily by the obturator nerve (Fig. 5.12; Table 5.2). The adductor group consists of:

- **Adductor longus:** the most anterior muscle in the group.
- **Adductor brevis:** deep to the pectineus and adductor longus muscles.
- **Adductor magnus:** the largest adductor muscle, composed of adductor and hamstring parts; the parts differ in their attachments, nerve supply, and main actions.

TABLE 5.1 ANTERIOR THIGH MUSCLES

Muscle	Proximal Attachment	Distal Attachment	Innervation[a]	Main Action(s)
Pectineus	Superior ramus of pubis	Pectineal line of femur, just inferior to lesser trochanter	Femoral nerve (**L2**, L3); may receive branch from obturator nerve	Adducts and flexes thigh; assists with medial rotation of thigh
Sartorius	Anterior superior iliac spine and superior part of notch inferior to it	Superior part of medial surface of tibia	Femoral nerve (L2, L3)	Flexes, abducts, and laterally rotates thigh at hip joint; flexes leg at knee joint
Iliopsoas				
Psoas major[b]	Sides of T12–L5 vertebrae and discs between them; transverse processes of all lumbar vertebrae	Lesser trochanter of femur	Anterior rami of lumbar nerves (**L1, L2,** L3)	Acting conjointly in flexing thigh at hip joint and in stabilizing this joint; psoas major is also a postural muscle that helps control deviation of the trunk and is active during standing
Iliacus	Iliac crest, iliac fossa, ala of sacrum, and anterior sacro-iliac ligaments	Tendon of psoas major, lesser trochanter, and femur distal to it	Femoral nerve (**L2**, L3)	
Quadriceps femoris				
Rectus femoris	Anterior inferior iliac spine and ilium superior to acetabulum	Via common tendinous (quadriceps tendon) and independent attachments to base of patella; indirectly via patellar ligament to tibial tuberosity; medial and lateral vasti also attach to tibia and patella via aponeuroses (medial and lateral patellar retinacula)	Femoral nerve (L2, **L3, L4**)	Extends leg at knee joint; rectus femoris also steadies hip joint and helps iliopsoas flex thigh
Vastus lateralis	Greater trochanter and lateral lip of linea aspera			
Vastus medialis	Intertrochanteric line and medial lip of linea aspera of femur			
Vastus intermedius	Anterior and lateral surfaces of shaft of femur			

[a]The spinal cord segmental innervation is indicated (e.g., "**L1, L2,** L3" means that the nerves supplying the psoas major are derived from the first three lumbar segments of the spinal cord). Numbers in boldface (**L1, L2**) indicate the main segmental innervation. Damage to one or more of the listed spinal cord segments or to the motor nerve roots arising from them results in paralysis of the muscles concerned.

[b]The psoas minor is a small muscle that attaches proximally to the T12–L1 vertebrae and IV discs and distally to the pectineal line and iliopectineal eminence.

Anterior views

A

B

C

D **Anterior view**

E **Sagittal section**

F **Anterior view**

G **Posterior view**

FIGURE 5.12.   **Anterior and medial thigh muscles. A.** Surface anatomy of the thigh. **B.** Muscles. **C.** Iliopsoas (psoas major and iliacus) and pectineus.
D. Quadriceps femoris. Most of the rectus femoris has been removed to show the vastus intermedius. **E.** Articularis genu (articular muscle of knee).
F. and G. Muscle attachment sites.

FIGURE 5.13. Medial thigh muscles. **A.** Superficial. **B.** Deep. **C.** Muscle attachments.

TABLE 5.2 MEDIAL THIGH MUSCLES

Muscle[a]	Proximal Attachment[b]	Distal Attachment[b]	Innervation[c]	Main Action(s)
Adductor longus	Body of pubis inferior to pubic crest	Middle third of linea aspera of femur	Obturator nerve (L2, **L3**, L4)	Adducts thigh
Adductor brevis	Body and inferior ramus of pubis	Pectineal line and proximal part of linea aspera of femur		Adducts thigh and to some extent flexes it
Adductor magnus	*Adductor part:* inferior ramus of pubis, ramus of ischium *Hamstring part:* ischial tuberosity	*Adductor part:* gluteal tuberosity, linea aspera, medial supracondylar line *Hamstring part:* adductor tubercle of femur	*Adductor part:* obturator nerve (L2, **L3**, L4) *Hamstring part:* tibial part of sciatic nerve (**L4**)	Adducts thigh; its adductor part also flexes thigh, and its hamstring part extends it
Gracilis	Body and inferior ramus of pubis	Superior part of medial surface of tibia	Obturator nerve (**L2**, L3)	Adducts thigh; flexes leg, and helps rotate it medially
Obturator externus	Margins of obturator foramen and obturator membrane	Trochanteric fossa of femur	Obturator nerve (L3, **L4**)	Laterally rotates thigh; steadies head of femur in acetabulum

[a]Collectively, the first four muscles listed are the adductors of the thigh, but their actions are more complex (e.g., they act as flexors of the hip joint during flexion of the knee joint and are active during walking).

[b]See Figure 5.13C for muscle attachments.

[c]The spinal cord segmental innervation is indicated (e.g., "L2, **L3, L4**" means that the nerves supplying the adductor magnus are derived from the second to fourth lumbar segments of the spinal cord). Numbers in boldface (**L3, L4**) indicate the main segmental innervation.

- **Gracilis:** a long, strap-like muscle lying along the medial side of the thigh and knee; it is the only adductor muscle to cross and act at the knee joint as well as the hip joint.
- **Obturator externus:** a deeply placed fan-shaped muscle in the superomedial part of the thigh.

The **adductor hiatus** is an opening between the distal aponeurotic attachment of the adductor part of the adductor magnus and the tendon of the hamstring part (Fig. 5.13*B*).

The adductor hiatus transmits the femoral artery and vein from the anterior compartment of the thigh to the popliteal fossa posterior to the knee. The main action of the adductor group of muscles is to adduct the thigh. They are used to stabilize the stance when standing on both feet, to correct lateral sway of the trunk, and when there is a side-to-side shift. The adductors contribute to flexion of the extended thigh and to extension of the flexed thigh when running or against resistance.

Hip and Thigh Contusions

Sports broadcasters and trainers refer to a "hip pointer," which is a *contusion of the iliac crest* that usually occurs at its anterior part. This is one of the most common injuries to the hip region, usually occurring in association with sports, such as the various forms of football, ice hockey, and volleyball.

Contusions cause bleeding from ruptured capillaries and infiltration of blood into the muscles, tendons, and other soft tissues. The term *hip pointer* may also refer to avulsion of bony muscle attachments, for example, of the sartorius or rectus femoris to the anterior superior and inferior iliac spines respectively. However, these injuries should be called *avulsion fractures*.

Another term commonly used is "charley horse," which may refer either to the cramping of an individual thigh muscle because of ischemia, or to contusion and rupture of blood vessels sufficient to form a *hematoma*. The injury is usually the consequence of tearing of fibers of the rectus femoris; sometimes the quadriceps tendon is also partially torn. A charley horse is associated with localized pain and/or muscle stiffness and commonly follows direct trauma.

Patellar Tendon Reflex

Tapping the patellar ligament with a reflex hammer normally elicits the **patellar reflex** ("knee jerk"). This myotatic (deep tendon) reflex is routinely tested during a physical examination by having the person sit with the legs dangling. A firm strike on the ligament with a reflex hammer usually causes the leg to extend. If the reflex is normal, a hand on the person's quadriceps should feel the muscle contract. This tendon reflex tests the integrity of the femoral nerve and the L2–L4 spinal cord segments. *Diminution or absence of the patellar tendon reflex* may result from any lesion that interrupts the innervation of the quadriceps (e.g., peripheral nerve disease).

Paralysis of Quadriceps

A person with **paralyzed quadriceps muscles** cannot extend the leg against resistance and usually presses on the distal end of the thigh during walking to prevent inadvertent flexion of the knee joint. Weakness of the vastus medialis or vastus lateralis, resulting from arthritis or trauma to the knee joint, can result in abnormal patellar movement and loss of joint stability.

Chondromalacia Patellae

Chondromalacia patellae (runner's knee) is a common knee problem for marathon runners, but can also occur in running sports such as basketball. The soreness and aching around or deep to the patella results from *quadriceps imbalance*. Chondromalacia patellae may also result from a blow to the patella or extreme flexion of the knee.

Transplantation of Gracilis

Because the gracilis is a relatively weak member of the adductor group of muscles, it can be removed without noticeable loss of its actions on the leg. Surgeons often transplant the gracilis, or part of it, with its nerve and blood vessels to replace a damaged muscle in the forearm or to create a replacement for a nonfunctional external anal sphincter, for example.

Groin Pull

Sports broadcasters refer to a "pulled groin" or "groin injury." These terms refer to a strain, stretching, and probably some tearing of the proximal attachments of the flexor and adductor thigh muscles. The proximal attachments of these muscles are in the inguinal region (groin). Groin pulls usually occur in sports that require quick starts (e.g., sprinting or soccer) or extreme stretching (e.g., gymnastics).

NEUROVASCULAR STRUCTURES AND RELATIONSHIPS IN ANTEROMEDIAL THIGH

Femoral Triangle and Adductor Canal

The femoral triangle is a subfascial space in the anterosuperior third of the thigh (Fig. 5.14). It appears as a triangular depression inferior to the inguinal ligament when the thigh is flexed, abducted, and laterally rotated. The femoral triangle is bounded:

- Superiorly by the inguinal ligament, which forms the *base of the femoral triangle.*
- Medially by the adductor longus.
- Laterally by the sartorius; the *apex* is where the medial border of the sartorius crosses the lateral border of the adductor longus.

The muscular *floor of the femoral triangle* is formed by the iliopsoas laterally and pectineus medially (Fig. 5.14*C*). The *roof of the femoral triangle* is formed by fascia lata, cribriform fascia, subcutaneous tissue, and skin. Deep to the inguinal ligament, the **retroinguinal space** is an important passageway connecting the trunk/abdominopelvic cavity to the lower limb. It is created as the inguinal ligament spans the gap between the ASIS and the pubic tubercle (Fig. 5.15). The space is divided into two compartments by the iliopsoas fascia. The lateral compartment is the muscular compartment, through which the iliopsoas muscle and femoral nerve pass; the medial compartment allows the passage of the veins, arteries, and lymphatics between the greater pelvis and the femoral triangle.

The contents of the femoral triangle, from lateral to medial, are the (Fig. 5.14):

- Femoral nerve and its (terminal) branches.
- Femoral artery and several of its branches.

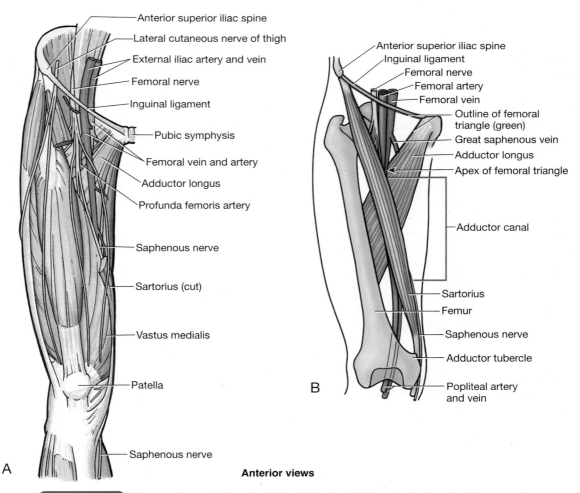

A.

- Anterior superior iliac spine
- Lateral cutaneous nerve of thigh
- External iliac artery and vein
- Femoral nerve
- Inguinal ligament
- Pubic symphysis
- Femoral vein and artery
- Adductor longus
- Profunda femoris artery
- Saphenous nerve
- Sartorius (cut)
- Vastus medialis
- Patella
- Saphenous nerve

B.

- Anterior superior iliac spine
- Inguinal ligament
- Femoral nerve
- Femoral artery
- Femoral vein
- Outline of femoral triangle (green)
- Great saphenous vein
- Adductor longus
- Apex of femoral triangle
- Adductor canal
- Sartorius
- Femur
- Saphenous nerve
- Adductor tubercle
- Popliteal artery and vein

Anterior views

FIGURE 5.14. Nerves and vessels of anterior thigh. A. Overview. B. Femoral triangle and adductor canal.

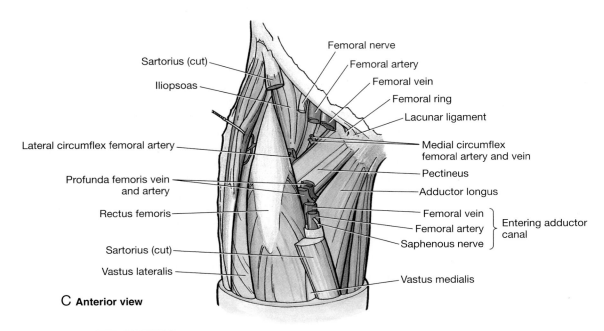

Sartorius (cut)

Iliopsoas

Lateral circumflex femoral artery

Profunda femoris vein
and artery

Rectus femoris

Sartorius (cut)

Vastus lateralis

C Anterior view

Femoral nerve

Femoral artery

Femoral vein

Femoral ring

Lacunar ligament

Medial circumflex
femoral artery and vein

Pectineus

Adductor longus

Femoral vein ⎱
Femoral artery ⎰ Entering adductor canal
Saphenous nerve

Vastus medialis

FIGURE 5.14.   **Nerves and vessels of anterior thigh** (*continued*). **C.** Floor of femoral triangle.

- Femoral vein and its proximal tributaries (e.g., the great saphenous vein and deep femoral veins).
- Femoral canal.
- Deep inguinal lymph nodes and associated lymphatic vessels.

The femoral triangle is bisected by the femoral artery and vein, which pass to and from the adductor canal at its apex (Fig. 5.14*B*). The **adductor canal** (subsartorial canal, Hunter canal) extends from the apex of the femoral triangle, where the sartorius crosses over the adductor longus, to the adductor hiatus in the tendon of adductor magnus. It provides an intermuscular passage for the femoral artery and vein, the saphenous nerve, and the nerve to vastus medialis, delivering the femoral vessels to the popliteal fossa where they become popliteal vessels. The adductor canal is bounded anteriorly and laterally by the vastus medialis; posteriorly by the adductor longus and adductor magnus; and medially by the sartorius, which overlies the groove between the above muscles, forming the roof of the canal.

Femoral Nerve

The **femoral nerve** (L2–L4) is the largest branch of the lumbar plexus. The nerve originates in the abdomen within the psoas major and descends posterolaterally through the pelvis to the midpoint of the inguinal ligament. It then passes deep to this ligament and enters the femoral triangle, lateral to the femoral vessels (Figs. 5.14 and 5.15). After entering the triangle, the femoral nerve divides into several terminal branches to the anterior thigh muscles. It also sends articular branches to the hip and knee joints and provides cutaneous branches to the anteromedial thigh. The terminal

cutaneous branch of the femoral nerve, the **saphenous nerve,** descends through the femoral triangle, lateral to the femoral sheath containing the femoral vessels. The saphenous nerve accompanies the femoral artery and vein through the adductor canal and becomes superficial by passing between the sartorius and the gracilis when the femoral vessels transverse the adductor hiatus (Fig. 5.13*A,B*). The saphenous nerve runs anteroinferiorly to supply the skin and fascia on the anteromedial aspects of the knee, leg, and foot.

Femoral Sheath

The **femoral sheath** is a funnel-shaped, fascial tube of varying length (usually 3 to 4 cm) that passes deep to the inguinal ligament and encloses proximal parts of the femoral vessels and creates the femoral canal medial to them (Fig. 5.15). The sheath is formed by an inferior prolongation of the transversalis and iliopsoas fascia from the abdomen/greater pelvis. The femoral sheath does not enclose the femoral nerve. The sheath terminates inferiorly by becoming continuous with the tunica adventitia, the loose connective tissue covering of the femoral vessels. When a long femoral sheath occurs, its medial wall is pierced by the great saphenous vein and lymphatic vessels. The femoral sheath allows the femoral artery and vein to glide deep to the inguinal ligament during movements of the hip joint. The femoral sheath is subdivided into three compartments by vertical septa of extraperitoneal connective tissue that extend from the abdomen along the femoral vessels. The compartments of the femoral sheath are the *lateral compartment* for the femoral artery; *intermediate compartment* for the femoral vein; and *medial compartment,* which constitutes the femoral canal.

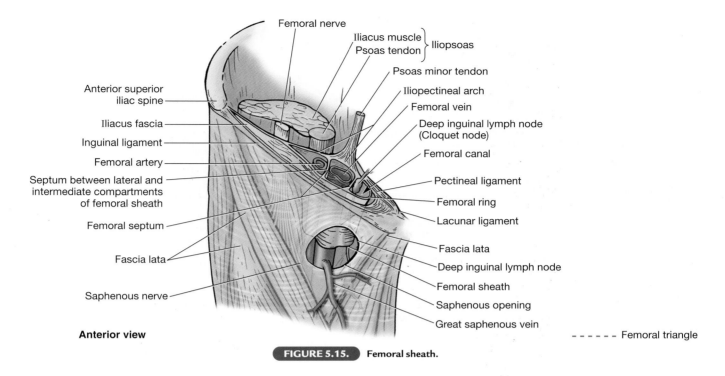

Femoral nerve

Iliacus muscle
Psoas tendon } Iliopsoas

Psoas minor tendon

Iliopectineal arch

Femoral vein

Deep inguinal lymph node
(Cloquet node)

Femoral canal

Pectineal ligament

Femoral ring

Lacunar ligament

Fascia lata

Deep inguinal lymph node

Femoral sheath

Saphenous opening

Great saphenous vein

Anterior superior
iliac spine

Iliacus fascia

Inguinal ligament

Femoral artery

Septum between lateral and
intermediate compartments
of femoral sheath

Femoral septum

Fascia lata

Saphenous nerve

Anterior view

– – – – – – Femoral triangle

FIGURE 5.15.   **Femoral sheath.**

The **femoral canal** is the smallest of the three compartments. It is short and conical and lies between the medial edge of the femoral sheath and the femoral vein. The femoral canal:

- Extends distally to the level of the proximal edge of the saphenous opening.
- Allows the femoral vein to expand when venous return from the lower limb is increased or when increased intra-abdominal pressure causes a temporary stasis in the vein.
- Contains loose connective tissue, fat, a few lymphatic vessels, and sometimes a deep inguinal lymph node (Cloquet node).

The base of the femoral canal, formed by the small (approximately 1 cm wide) proximal opening at its abdominal end, is the oval **femoral ring** (Fig. 5.15). This opening is closed by extraperitoneal fatty tissue that forms the femoral septum. The boundaries of the femoral ring are as follows: *laterally*, a **femoral septum** between the femoral canal and the femoral vein; *posteriorly*, the superior ramus of the pubis covered by the pectineus and its fascia; *medially*, the lacunar ligament; and *anteriorly*, the medial part of the inguinal ligament.

Femoral Artery

The **femoral artery,** the chief artery to the lower limb, is the continuation of the external iliac artery distal to the inguinal ligament (Figs. 5.14 and 5.16; Table 5.3). The femoral artery:

- Enters the femoral triangle deep to the midpoint of the inguinal ligament (midway between the ASIS and the pubic tubercle), lateral to the femoral vein.
- Lies deep to the fascia lata and descends on the adjacent borders of the iliopsoas and pectineus.
- Bisects the femoral triangle and exits at its apex to enter the adductor canal, deep to the sartorius.
- Exits the adductor canal by passing through the adductor hiatus and becoming the *popliteal artery.*

The **profunda femoris artery** (deep artery of the thigh) is the largest branch of the femoral artery and the chief artery to the thigh. It arises from the femoral artery in the femoral triangle (Figs. 5.14C and 5.16; Table 5.3). In the middle third of the thigh, it is separated from the femoral artery and vein by the adductor longus. It gives off three or four **perforating arteries** that wrap around the posterior aspect of the femur and supply the adductor magnus, hamstring, and vastus lateralis muscles.

The *circumflex femoral arteries* are usually branches of the profundus femoris artery thigh, but they may arise from the femoral artery. They encircle the thigh, anastomose with each other and other arteries, and supply the thigh muscles and the proximal end of the femur. The **medial circumflex femoral artery** supplies most of the blood to the head and neck of the femur via its branches, the **posterior retinacular arteries.** It passes deeply between the iliopsoas and pectineus to reach the posterior part of the thigh. The **lateral circumflex femoral artery** passes laterally across the joint capsule, mainly supplying muscles on the lateral side of the thigh (Fig. 5.16; Table 5.3).

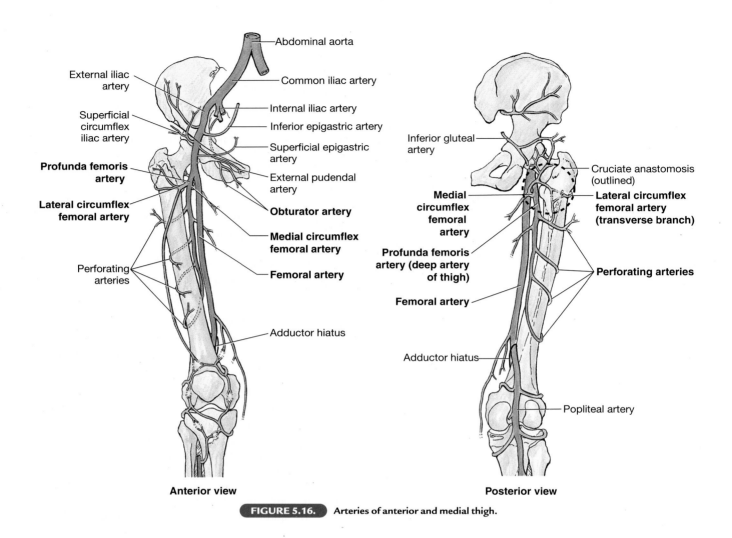

FIGURE 5.16. Arteries of anterior and medial thigh.

TABLE 5.3 ARTERIES OF ANTERIOR AND MEDIAL THIGH

Artery	Origin	Course	Distribution
Femoral	Continuation of external iliac artery distal to inguinal ligament	Descends through femoral triangle; enters adductor canal; terminates as it traverses adductor hiatus; becomes popliteal artery	Anterior and anteromedial aspects of thigh
Profunda femoris (deep artery of thigh)	Femoral artery 1–5 cm inferior to inguinal ligament	Passes inferiorly in medial compartment of thigh, deep to adductor longus	Perforating branches pass through adductor magnus to supply muscles in medial, posterior, and lateral part of anterior compartments
Lateral circumflex femoral	Profunda femoris artery; may arise from femoral artery	Passes laterally deep to sartorius and rectus femoris and dividing into ascending, transverse, and descending arteries	Ascending branch supplies anterior part of gluteal region; transverse branch winds around femur; descending branch joins genicular periarticular anastomosis
Medial circumflex femoral	Profunda femoris artery; may arise from femoral artery	Passes medially and posteriorly between pectineus and iliopsoas; enters gluteal region; and divides into two branches	Supplies most blood to head and neck of femur; transverse branch takes part in cruciate anastomosis of thigh; ascending branch joins inferior gluteal artery
Obturator	Internal iliac artery or (in ~20%) as an accessory or replaced obturator artery from the inferior epigastric artery	Passes through obturator foramen; enters medial compartment of thigh; and divides into anterior and posterior branches	Anterior branch supplies obturator externus, pectineus, adductors of thigh, and gracilis; posterior branch supplies muscles attached to ischial tuberosity

Femoral Hernia

The femoral ring is a weak area in the lower anterior abdominal wall that is the site of a *femoral hernia,* a protrusion of abdominal viscera (often a loop of small intestine) through the femoral ring into the femoral canal (Fig. B5.7). A femoral hernia is more common in women than in men. The hernial sac compresses the contents of the femoral canal and distends its wall. Initially, the hernia is relatively small because it is contained within the femoral canal, but it can enlarge by passing through the saphenous opening into the subcutaneous tissue of the thigh. *Strangulation of a femoral hernia* may occur and interfere with the blood supply to the herniated intestine, and vascular impairment may result in death of the tissues.

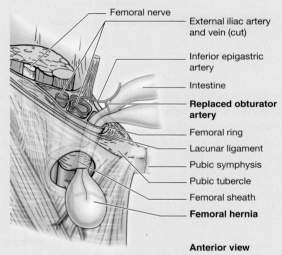

Femoral nerve
External iliac artery and vein (cut)
Inferior epigastric artery
Intestine
Replaced obturator artery
Femoral ring
Lacunar ligament
Pubic symphysis
Pubic tubercle
Femoral sheath
Femoral hernia

Anterior view

Late stage femoral hernia

FIGURE B5.7.

Replaced or Accessory Obturator Artery

An enlarged pubic branch of the inferior epigastric artery either takes the place of the obturator artery (**replaced obturator artery**) or joins it as an **accessory obturator artery** in approximately 20% of people (Fig B5.7). This artery runs close to or across the femoral ring to reach the obturator foramen and could be closely related to the neck of a femoral hernia. Consequently, this artery could be involved in a *strangulated femoral hernia.* Surgeons placing staples during endoscopic repair of both inguinal and femoral hernias must also be vigilant concerning the possible presence of this common arterial variant.

Femoral Pulse and Cannulation of Femoral Artery

The pulse of the femoral artery is usually palpable just inferior to the midpoint of the inguinal ligament. Normally, the pulse is strong; however, if the common or external iliac arteries are partially occluded, the pulse may be diminished. The femoral artery may be compressed at the midpoint of the inguinal ligament to control arterial bleeding after lower limb trauma (Fig. B5.8).

The femoral artery may be cannulated just inferior to the midpoint of the inguinal ligament (e.g., for cardioangiography—radiography of the heart and great vessels after the introduction of contrast material). For *left cardiac angiography,* a long slender catheter is inserted percutaneously into the femoral artery and passed superiorly in the aorta to the openings of the coronary arteries (see Chapter 1). Blood may also be taken from the femoral artery for blood gas analysis.

Femoral artery
Superior ramus of pubis

Compression of femoral artery Medial view (right side)

FIGURE B5.8.

Cannulation of Femoral Vein

The femoral vein usually is not palpable, but its position can be located by feeling the pulsations of the femoral artery, which lies just lateral to it. In thin people, the femoral vein may be close to the surface and may be mistaken for the great saphenous vein. It is thus important to know that the femoral vein has no tributaries at this level, except for the great saphenous vein that joins it approximately 3 cm inferior to the inguinal ligament. To secure blood samples and take pressure recordings from the chambers of the right side of the heart and/or from the pulmonary artery and to perform *right cardiac angiography,* a long slender catheter is inserted into the femoral vein as it passes through the femoral triangle. Under fluoroscopic control, the catheter is passed superiorly through the external and common iliac veins into the inferior vena cava and right atrium of the heart.

Femoral Vein

The **femoral vein** is the continuation of the popliteal vein proximal to the adductor hiatus (Fig. 5.14*A*). As it ascends through the adductor canal, the femoral vein lies posterolateral and then posterior to the femoral artery (Fig. 5.14*B*). The femoral vein enters the femoral sheath lateral to the femoral canal and ends posterior to the inguinal ligament, where it becomes the external iliac vein. In the inferior part of the femoral triangle, the femoral vein receives the profunda femoris vein, the great saphenous vein, and other tributaries. The *profunda femoris vein* (*deep vein of thigh*), formed by the union of three or four perforating veins, enters the femoral vein inferior to the inguinal ligament and inferior to the termination of the great saphenous vein.

Obturator Artery and Nerve

The **obturator artery** usually arises from the internal iliac artery (Fig. 5.16; Table 5.3). In approximately 20% of people, an enlarged pubic branch of the inferior epigastric artery either takes the place of the obturator artery (*replaced obturator artery*) or joins it as an *accessory obturator artery*. The obturator artery passes through the obturator foramen, enters the medial compartment of the thigh, and divides into anterior and posterior branches, which straddle the adductor brevis muscle. The obturator artery supplies the obturator externus, pectineus, adductors of thigh, and gracilis. Its posterior branch gives off an acetabular branch that supplies the head of the femur.

The **obturator nerve** (L2–L4) descends along the medial border of the psoas muscle and enters the thigh through the obturator foramen. It divides into anterior and posterior branches, which, like the arteries, straddle the adductor brevis. The anterior branch supplies the adductor longus, adductor brevis, gracilis, and pectineus; the posterior branch supplies the obturator externus and adductor magnus.

GLUTEAL REGION AND POSTERIOR THIGH

The gluteal region (hip and buttocks) is the prominent area posterior to the pelvis. It is bounded superiorly by the iliac crest, greater trochanter, and ASIS and inferiorly by the *gluteal fold.* The gluteal fold also demarcates the superior boundary of the thigh (Fig. 5.17). The *intergluteal cleft* separates the buttocks from each other.

The parts of the bony pelvis—hip bones, sacrum, and coccyx—are bound together by *gluteal ligaments.* The **sacrotuberous** and **sacrospinous ligaments** convert the sciatic notches in the hip bones into the greater and lesser sciatic foramina (Fig. 5.18). The **greater sciatic foramen** is

Posterior view

FIGURE 5.17. Surface landmarks of gluteal region.

the passageway for structures entering or leaving the pelvis, whereas the **lesser sciatic foramen** is a passageway for structures entering or leaving the perineum.

It is helpful to think of the greater sciatic foramen as the "door" through which arteries and nerves leave the pelvis and enter the gluteal region.

Posterior view

FIGURE 5.18. Sacrotuberous and sacrospinous ligaments.

A **Lateral view**

B **Posterior view**

E **Posterior view**

C **Posterior view**

D **Posterior view**

F **Anterior view**

FIGURE 5.19. **Gluteal muscles. A.** Attachments of tensor fasciae latae (tensor of fascia lata) and gluteus maximus into the iliotibial tract. **B.** Gluteus maximus. **C.** Deep dissection of gluteus medius and lateral rotators of the hip joint. **D.** Deeper dissection of gluteus minimus and obturator internus. **E. and F.** Attachments of the muscles.

Gluteal Muscles

The gluteal muscles are organized into two layers: superficial and deep (Fig. 5.19; Table 5.4). The superficial layer consists of three large glutei (maximus, medius, and minimus) and the tensor fasciae latae. The main actions of the **gluteus maximus** are extension and lateral rotation of the thigh. It functions primarily between the flexed and the standing positions, as when rising from the sitting position, straightening from the bending position, walking uphill and up stairs, and running. The **gluteus medius** and **minimus** are fan-shaped muscles that lie deep to the gluteus maximus. They are abductors and medial rotators of the thigh. The **tensor fasciae latae** lies on the lateral side of the hip, enclosed between two layers of fascia lata. The tensor fasciae latae is primarily a flexor of the thigh; however, it generally does not act independently. To produce flexion, it acts in concert with the iliopsoas and rectus femoris. The tensor fasciae latae also tenses the fascia lata and iliotibial tract, thereby helping support the femur on the tibia when standing. The deep layer consists of smaller muscles, the **piriformis, obturator internus, superior** and **inferior gemelli,** and **quadratus femoris** (Fig. 5.20). These

muscles, covered by the inferior half of the gluteus maximus, are lateral rotators of the thigh, but they also stabilize the hip joint, working with the strong ligaments of the hip joint to steady the femoral head in the acetabulum.

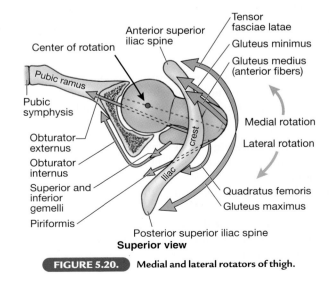

Superior view

FIGURE 5.20.   **Medial and lateral rotators of thigh.**

TABLE 5.4 MUSCLES OF GLUTEAL REGION

Muscle	Proximal Attachment	Distal Attachment	Innervation[a]	Main Action(s)
Gluteus maximus	Ilium posterior to posterior gluteal line; dorsal surface of sacrum and coccyx; and sacrotuberous ligament	Most fibers end in iliotibial tract, which inserts into lateral condyle of tibia; some fibers insert on gluteal tuberosity of femur	Inferior gluteal nerve (L5, **S1, S2**)	Extends thigh and assists in its lateral rotation; steadies thigh and assists in rising from sitting position
Gluteus medius	External surface of ilium between anterior and posterior gluteal lines	Lateral surface of greater trochanter of femur	Superior gluteal nerve (L4, L5, S1)	Abduct and medially rotate thigh; keep pelvis level when opposite leg is raised
Gluteus minimus	External surface of ilium between anterior and inferior gluteal lines	Anterior surface of greater trochanter of femur		
Tensor fasciae latae (tensor of fascia lata)	Anterior superior iliac spine; anterior part of iliac crest	Iliotibial tract, which attaches to lateral condyle of tibia (Gerdy tubercle)		Flexes thigh
Piriformis (passes through greater sciatic foramen)	Anterior surface of 2nd–4th sacral segments; superior margin of greater sciatic notch and sacrotuberous ligament	Superior border of greater trochanter of femur	Branches of anterior rami of **S1**, S2	Laterally rotate extended thigh; abduct flexed thigh; steady femoral head in acetabulum (stabilizes hip joint)
Obturator internus (passes through lesser sciatic foramen)	Pelvic surface of ilium and ischium; and obturator membrane	Medial surface of greater trochanter (trochanteric fossa) of femur[b]	Nerve to obturator internus (L5, **S1**)	
Gemelli, superior and inferior	*Superior:* ischial spine *Inferior:* ischial tuberosity		*Superior:* same as obturator internus *Inferior:* same as quadratus femoris	
Quadratus femoris	Lateral border of ischial tuberosity	Quadrate tubercle on intertrochanteric crest of femur and area inferior to it	Nerve to quadratus femoris (L5, S1)	Laterally rotates thigh; steadies femoral head in acetabulum

[a]The spinal cord segmental innervation is indicated (e.g., "**S1**, S2" means that the nerves supplying the piriformis are derived from the first two sacral segments of the spinal cord). Numbers in boldface (**S1**) indicate the main segmental innervation.

[b]Gemelli muscles blend with the tendon of the obturator internus muscle as it attaches to the greater trochanter of the femur.

Gluteal Bursae

Gluteal bursae, membranous sacs containing a capillary layer of synovial fluid, separate the gluteus maximus from adjacent structures (Fig. 5.21). The bursae are located in areas subject to friction—for example, between a muscle and a bony prominence—to reduce friction and permit free movement. The bursae associated with the gluteus maximus are as follows:

- The **trochanteric bursa** separates the superior part of the gluteus maximus from the greater trochanter of the femur.
- The **ischial bursa** separates the inferior part of the gluteus maximus from the ischial tuberosity.
- The **gluteofemoral bursa** separates the iliotibial tract from the superior part of the proximal attachment of the vastus lateralis.

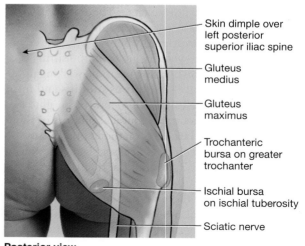

Skin dimple over left posterior superior iliac spine

Gluteus medius

Gluteus maximus

Trochanteric bursa on greater trochanter

Ischial bursa on ischial tuberosity

Sciatic nerve

Posterior view

FIGURE 5.21. Gluteal bursae.

TABLE 5.5 POSTERIOR THIGH MUSCLES

Muscle[a]	Proximal Attachment[b]	Distal Attachment[b]	Innervation[c]	Main Action(s)
Semitendinosus	Ischial tuberosity	Medial surface of superior part of tibia	Tibial division of sciatic nerve (**L5**, **S1**, S2)	Extend thigh; flex leg and rotate it medially when knee is flexed; when thigh and leg are flexed, can extend trunk
Semimembranosus		Posterior part of medial condyle of tibia; reflected attachment forms oblique popliteal ligament (to lateral femoral condyle)		
Biceps femoris, long and short heads	*Long head:* ischial tuberosity *Short head:* linea aspera and lateral supracondylar line of femur	Lateral side of head of fibula; tendon is split at this site by fibular collateral ligament of knee	*Long head:* tibial division of sciatic nerve (L5, **S1**, S2) *Short head:* common fibular division of sciatic nerve (L5, **S1**, S2)	Flexes leg and rotates it laterally when knee is flexed; extends thigh (e.g., when starting to walk)

[a]Collectively these three muscles are known as hamstrings.

[b]See Figure 5.22B for muscle attachments.

[c]The spinal cord segmental innervation is indicated (e.g., "L5, **S1,** S2" means that the nerves supplying the biceps femoris are derived from the fifth lumbar segment and first two sacral segments of the spinal cord). Numbers in boldface (**S1**) indicate the main segmental innervation.

Posterior Thigh Muscles

Three of the four muscles in the posterior aspect of the thigh are **hamstrings** (Fig. 5.22; Table 5.5): **semitendinosus, semimembranosus,** and **biceps femoris (long head).** The hamstrings span and act on two joints (extension at the hip joint and flexion at the knee joint), arise from the ischial tuberosity deep to the gluteus maximus, and are innervated by the tibial division of the sciatic nerve. Both actions cannot be performed maximally at the same time. A fully flexed knee shortens the hamstrings so they cannot further contract to extend the thigh. Similarly, a fully extended hip shortens the hamstrings so they cannot act on the knee. When the thighs and legs are fixed, the hamstrings can help extend the trunk at the hip joint. They are active in thigh extension under all situations except full flexion of the knee, including maintenance of the relaxed standing posture.

The **short head of biceps femoris,** the fourth muscle in the posterior compartment, is not a hamstring as it crosses only the knee joint and is innervated by the fibular division of the sciatic nerve.

Nerves of Gluteal Region and Posterior Thigh

Several nerves arise from the sacral plexus and either supply the gluteal region (e.g., superior and inferior gluteal nerves) or pass through it to supply the perineum (e.g., pudendal nerve) and thigh (e.g., sciatic nerve). The skin of the gluteal region is richly innervated by the superficial gluteal nerves, the **superior, middle,** and **inferior clunial nerves** (Fig. 5.11B). The deep gluteal nerves are the **sciatic, posterior cutaneous nerve of the thigh, superior gluteal** and **inferior gluteal nerves, nerve to the quadratus femoris, pudendal nerve,** and **nerve to the obturator internus** (Fig. 5.23; Table 5.6). All of these nerves are branches of the sacral plexus and leave the pelvis through the greater sciatic foramen (Fig. 5.23C). Except for the superior gluteal nerve, they all emerge inferior to the piriformis muscle. The pudendal nerve supplies no structures in the gluteal region; it supplies structures in the perineum (see Chapter 3).

The **sciatic nerve** is the largest nerve in the body and is the continuation of the main part of the sacral plexus (Fig. 5.23D). The sciatic nerve runs inferolaterally under cover of the gluteus maximus, midway between the greater trochanter and the ischial tuberosity (Fig. 5.21). It descends from the gluteal region into the posterior thigh, where it lies on the adductor magnus and is crossed posteriorly by the long head of the biceps femoris (Fig. 5.23D). The sciatic nerve is so large that it receives a named branch of the inferior gluteal artery, **the artery to the sciatic nerve.** The sciatic nerve is really two nerves loosely bound together in the same connective tissue sheath: the *tibial nerve,* derived from anterior (preaxial) divisions of anterior rami, and the *common fibular (peroneal) nerve,* derived from posterior (postaxial) divisions of the anterior rami (Fig. 5.23D). The two nerves separate in the inferior third of the thigh; however, in 12% of people, the nerves separate as they leave the pelvis. In these cases, the tibial nerve passes inferior to the piriformis, and the common fibular nerve pierces this muscle or passes superior to it (Fig. 5.23E). The sciatic nerve supplies no structures in the gluteal region; it innervates the posterior thigh muscles, all leg and foot muscles, and the skin of most of the leg and foot. It also supplies articular branches to all lower limb joints.

Posterior views

FIGURE 5.22. **Muscles of posterior aspect of thigh. A.** Surface anatomy. **B.** Muscle attachments. **C.** A superficial dissection. **D.** Deep dissection showing the semimembranosus and the short head of the biceps femoris. **E.** Deeper dissection showing adductor magnus.

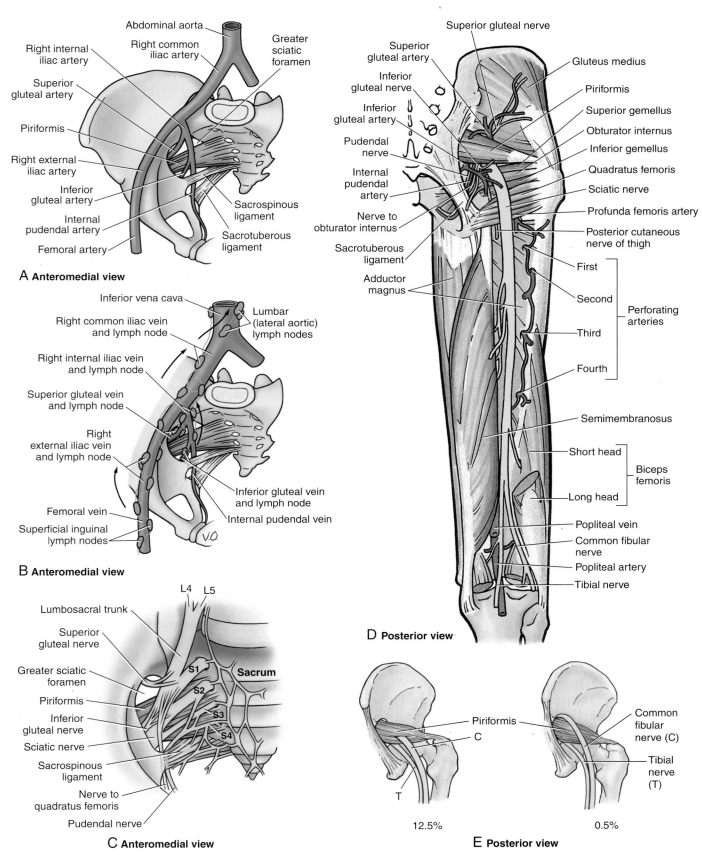

A Anteromedial view

Abdominal aorta
Right common iliac artery
Greater sciatic foramen
Right internal iliac artery
Superior gluteal artery
Piriformis
Right external iliac artery
Inferior gluteal artery
Internal pudendal artery
Femoral artery
Sacrospinous ligament
Sacrotuberous ligament

B Anteromedial view

Inferior vena cava
Right common iliac vein and lymph node
Lumbar (lateral aortic) lymph nodes
Right internal iliac vein and lymph node
Superior gluteal vein and lymph node
Right external iliac vein and lymph node
Femoral vein
Superficial inguinal lymph nodes
Inferior gluteal vein and lymph node
Internal pudendal vein
V.O.

C Anteromedial view

L4 L5
Lumbosacral trunk
Superior gluteal nerve
Greater sciatic foramen
Piriformis
Inferior gluteal nerve
Sciatic nerve
Sacrospinous ligament
Nerve to quadratus femoris
Pudendal nerve
S1 S2 S3 S4
Sacrum

D Posterior view

Superior gluteal nerve
Superior gluteal artery
Inferior gluteal nerve
Inferior gluteal artery
Pudendal nerve
Internal pudendal artery
Nerve to obturator internus
Sacrotuberous ligament
Adductor magnus
Gluteus medius
Piriformis
Superior gemellus
Obturator internus
Inferior gemellus
Quadratus femoris
Sciatic nerve
Profunda femoris artery
Posterior cutaneous nerve of thigh
First
Second
Third
Fourth
Perforating arteries
Semimembranosus
Short head
Long head
Biceps femoris
Popliteal vein
Common fibular nerve
Popliteal artery
Tibial nerve

E Posterior view

Piriformis
C
T
12.5%
Common fibular nerve (C)
Tibial nerve (T)
0.5%

FIGURE 5.23.   **Nerves and vasculature of gluteal region and posterior thigh. A.** Arteries. **B.** Veins and lymphatics. **C.** Formation of sciatic nerve in pelvis. **D.** Course of arteries and nerves in posterior thigh. **E.** Anomalous relationships of sciatic nerve to piriformis.

TABLE 5.6 NERVES OF THE GLUTEAL AND POSTERIOR THIGH REGIONS

Nerve	Origin	Course	Distribution[a]
Clunial: superior, middle, and inferior	*Superior:* posterior rami of L1–L3 nerves *Middle:* posterior rami of S1–S3 nerves *Inferior:* posterior cutaneous nerve of thigh	*Superior:* cross iliac crest *Middle:* exit through posterior sacral foramina and enter gluteal region *Inferior:* curve around inferior border of gluteus maximus	Supplies skin of gluteal region (buttocks) as far as greater trochanter
Sciatic	Sacral plexus (L4–S3)	Leaves pelvis through greater sciatic foramen inferior to piriformis; enters gluteal region; descends deep to biceps femoris; bifurcates into tibial and common fibular nerves at apex of popliteal fossa	Supplies no muscles in gluteal region; supplies all muscles in posterior compartment of thigh
Posterior cutaneous nerve of thigh	Sacral plexus (S1–S3)	Leaves pelvis through greater sciatic foramen inferior to piriformis; runs deep to gluteus maximus; emerges from its inferior border; descends in posterior thigh deep to fascia lata	Supplies skin of buttock through inferior clunial branches and skin over posterior aspect of thigh and calf; lateral perineum, upper medial thigh via perineal branch
Superior gluteal	Sacral plexus (L4–S1)	Leaves pelvis through greater sciatic foramen superior to piriformis; runs between gluteus medius and minimus	Innervates gluteus medius, gluteus minimus, and tensor fasciae latae
Inferior gluteal	Sacral plexus (L5–S2)	Leaves pelvis through greater sciatic foramen inferior to piriformis; divides into several branches	Innervates gluteus maximus
Nerve to quadratus femoris	Sacral plexus (L4, L5–S1)	Leaves pelvis through greater sciatic foramen deep to sciatic nerve	Innervates hip joint, inferior gemellus, and quadratus femoris
Pudendal	Sacral plexus (S2–S4)	Enters gluteal region through greater sciatic foramen inferior to piriformis; descends posterior to sacrospinous ligament; enters perineum through lesser sciatic foramen	Supplies most innervation to the perineum; supplies no structures in gluteal region
Nerve to obturator internus	Sacral plexus (L5–S2)	Enters gluteal region through greater sciatic foramen inferior to piriformis; descends posterior to ischial spine; enters lesser sciatic foramen; passes to obturator internus	Supplies superior gemellus and obturator internus

[a]See Figure 5.11 for cutaneous innervation of the lower limb.

Vasculature of Gluteal and Posterior Thigh Regions

The **arteries of the gluteal region** arise, directly or indirectly, from the *internal iliac arteries,* but the patterns of origin are variable (Fig. 5.23 *A,D* and 5.24; Table 5.7). The major gluteal branches of the internal iliac artery are the superior and inferior gluteal arteries and the internal pudendal artery. The **superior** and **inferior gluteal arteries** leave the pelvis through the greater sciatic foramen and pass superior and inferior to the piriformis, respectively (Fig. 5.23*A,D*). The **internal pudendal artery** enters the gluteal region through the greater sciatic foramen inferior to the piriformis and enters the perineum through the lesser sciatic foramen (Fig. 5.23*A*). It does not supply the buttock. After birth, the posterior compartment of the thigh has no major artery exclusive to the compartment; it receives blood from the inferior gluteal, medial circumflex femoral, and

perforating and popliteal arteries. The *profunda femoris artery* (deep artery of thigh) is the chief artery of the thigh, giving off *perforating arteries* (Fig. 5.24; Table 5.7), which pierce the adductor magnus to enter the posterior compartment and supply the hamstrings. A continuous anastomotic chain thus extends from the gluteal to the popliteal region, which gives rise to branches to the muscles and to the sciatic nerve.

The *veins of the gluteal region* are tributaries of the **internal iliac veins** that drain blood from the gluteal region (Fig. 5.23*B*). The **superior** and **inferior gluteal veins** accompany the corresponding arteries through the greater sciatic foramen, superior and inferior to the piriformis, respectively. They communicate with tributaries of the femoral vein, thereby providing an alternate route for the return of blood from the lower limb if the femoral vein is occluded or has to be ligated. The **internal pudendal veins** accompany the internal pudendal arteries and join to

TABLE 5.7 ARTERIES OF THE GLUTEAL AND POSTERIOR THIGH REGIONS

Artery	Course	Distribution
Superior gluteal[a]	*Superficial branch:* enters gluteal region through greater sciatic foramen, superior to piriformis; divides into superficial and deep branches; anastomoses with inferior gluteal and medial circumflex femoral arteries *Deep branch:* runs between gluteus medius and minimus	*Superficial branch:* gluteus maximus *Deep branch:* gluteus medius and minimus and tensor fasciae latae
Inferior gluteal[a]	Enters gluteal region through greater sciatic foramen, inferior to piriformis; descends on medial side of sciatic nerve; anastomoses with superior gluteal artery and participates in cruciate anastomosis of thigh, involving first perforating artery of profunda femoris and medial and lateral circumflex femoral arteries	Gluteus maximus, obturator internus, quadratus femoris, and superior parts of hamstrings
Internal pudendal[a]	Enters gluteal region through greater sciatic foramen; descends posterior to ischial spine; enters perineum through lesser sciatic foramen	External genitalia and muscles in the perineal region; does not supply gluteal region
Perforating[b]	Enters posterior compartment by perforating aponeurotic portion of adductor magnus attachment and medial intermuscular septum; after providing muscular branches to hamstrings, continues on to anterior compartment by piercing lateral intermuscular septum	Supplies majority (central portions) of hamstring muscles, then continues to supply vastus lateralis in anterior compartment

[a]Arise from the internal iliac artery.

[b]Arise from profunda femoris artery.

enter the internal iliac vein. The pudendal veins drain blood from the perineum (see Chapter 3). *Perforating veins* accompany the arteries of the same name to drain blood from the posterior compartment of the thigh into the *profunda femoris vein.* They also communicate inferiorly with the popliteal vein and superiorly with the inferior gluteal vein.

Lymph from the deep tissues of the gluteal region follows the gluteal vessels to the **gluteal lymph nodes** and from them to the internal, external, and common **iliac lymph nodes** and then to the **lumbar (caval) lymph nodes** (Fig. 5.23B). *Lymph from superficial tissues* of the gluteal region enters the *superficial inguinal lymph nodes.* The superficial inguinal nodes send efferent lymphatic vessels to the **external iliac nodes**.

Posterior view

FIGURE 5.24.   Arteries of gluteal and posterior thigh regions.

Trochanteric and Ischial Bursitis

Diffuse deep pain in the lateral thigh region, especially during stair climbing or rising from a seated position, may be caused by **trochanteric bursitis.** It is characterized by point tenderness over the greater trochanter; however, the pain often radiates along the iliotibial tract. **Ischial bursitis** results from excessive friction between the ischial bursae and the ischial tuberosities (e.g., as from cycling). Because the tuberosities bear the body weight during sitting, these pressure points may lead to *pressure sores* in debilitated people, particularly paraplegic persons.

Injury to Superior Gluteal Nerve

Injury to the superior gluteal nerve results in a disabling *gluteus medius limp* to compensate for weakened abduction of the thigh by the gluteus medius and minimus. Also a *gluteal gait,* a compensatory list of the body to the weakened side, may be present. Medial rotation of the thigh is also severely impaired.

When a person is asked to stand on one leg, the gluteus medius and minimus normally contract as soon as the contralateral foot leaves the floor, preventing tipping of the pelvis to the unsupported side (Fig. B5.9*A*). When a person with paralysis of the superior gluteal nerve is asked to stand on one leg, the pelvis descends on the unsupported side (Fig. B5.9*B*), indicating that the gluteus medius on the contralateral side is weak or nonfunctional. This is referred to clinically as a **positive Trendelenburg test.**

When the pelvis descends on the unsupported side, the lower limb becomes, in effect, too long and does not clear the ground when the foot is brought forward in the swing phase of walking. To compensate, the individual leans away from the unsupported side, raising the pelvis to allow adequate room for the foot to clear the ground as it swings forward. This results in a characteristic "waddling" or gluteal gait. Other ways to compensate are to lift the foot higher as it is brought forward or to swing the foot outward.

Hamstring Injuries

Hamstrings strains (pulled and/or torn hamstrings) are common in people who run and/or kick hard. The muscular exertion required to excel in these sports may tear part of the proximal attachment of the hamstrings to the ischial tuberosity.

Injury to Sciatic Nerve

A pain in the buttock may result from compression of the sciatic nerve by the piriformis muscle (**piriformis syndrome**). *Incomplete section of the sciatic nerve* (e.g., from a stab wound) may also involve the inferior gluteal and/or the posterior femoral cutaneous nerves. Recovery from a sciatic lesion is slow and usually incomplete. With respect to the sciatic nerve, the buttock has a side of safety (its lateral side) and a side of danger (its medial side). Wounds or surgery on the medial side may injure the sciatic nerve and its branches to the hamstrings. Paralysis of these muscles results in impairment of thigh extension and leg flexion.

Intragluteal Injections

The gluteal region is a common site for intramuscular injection of drugs because the gluteal muscles are thick and large, providing a large area for venous absorption of drugs. Injections into the buttock are safe only in the superolateral quadrant of the buttock (Fig. B5.10). Complications of improper technique include nerve injury, hematoma, and abscess formation.

Abductors of thigh
Active   Paralyzed

Iliotibial tract

A   B

Posterior views

FIGURE B5.9.   Trendelenburg test.

Greater trochanter of femur   Piriformis

Posterior superior iliac spine

Iliac crest

Gluteus medius

Safe area (green)

Gluteus maximus

Superior border of greater trochanter

Right sciatic n.

V. Oxorn

Posterior view
Safe area (green) for intragluteal injections

FIGURE B5.10.

A Posterior view

Sciatic nerve

Semimembranosus (1)

Biceps femoris (5)

Popliteal fossa (P)

Common fibular nerve

Semitendinosus (2)

Tibial nerve

Head of fibula

Gastrocnemius, medial head (3)

Gastrocnemius, lateral head (4)

Medial sural cutaneous nerve

Lateral sural cutaneous nerve

Communicating sural nerve

Fibularis longus

Sural nerve

Lateral sural cutaneous nerve

Fibularis brevis

Calcaneal tendon

Fibularis longus tendon

Lateral malleolus

B Posterolateral view

Semitendinosus

Sciatic nerve

Tibial nerve

Common fibular (peroneal) nerve

Popliteal vein and artery

Biceps femoris

Semi- membranosus

Superior lateral genicular vein and artery

Superior medial genicular artery and vein

Gastrocnemius, lateral head

Gastrocnemius, medial head

Lateral sural cutaneous nerve

Medial sural cutaneous nerve

Sural communicating nerve

Small saphenous vein

Sural nerve

C Posterior view

Descending branch of lateral femoral circumflex artery

Femoral artery

Descending genicular artery

Adductor hiatus

Popliteal artery

Saphenous branch

Superior lateral genicular artery

Superior medial genicular artery

Inferior lateral genicular artery

Middle genicular artery

Anterior tibial recurrent artery

Inferior medial genicular artery

Anterior tibial artery

Posterior tibial artery

D Anterior view

FIGURE 5.25.   **Popliteal fossa. A. and B.** Surface anatomy. *Line,* outline of fossa; *numbers,* defined in part **B. C.** Boundaries and contents. **D.** Genicular anastomosis.

POPLITEAL FOSSA

The **popliteal fossa** is a mostly fat-filled diamond-shaped space posterior to the knee (Fig. 5.25). All important vessels and nerves from the thigh to the leg pass through this fossa.

The popliteal fossa is bounded by:

- Biceps femoris superolaterally.
- Semimembranosus superomedially, medial to which is the semitendinosus tendon.
- Lateral and medial heads of the gastrocnemius, inferolaterally and inferomedially respectively.
- Skin and popliteal fascia posteriorly (roof).
- Popliteal surface of the femur, posterior capsule of the knee joint, and the popliteus fascia covering the popliteus muscle (floor).

The contents of the popliteal fossa include the (Fig. 5.25C):

- Termination of the small saphenous vein.
- Popliteal artery and vein and their branches and tributaries.
- Tibial and common fibular nerves.
- Posterior cutaneous nerve of the thigh.
- Popliteal lymph nodes and lymphatic vessels.
- Fat.

Fascia of Popliteal Fossa

The *subcutaneous tissue* overlying the fossa contains fat, the small saphenous vein (unless it has penetrated the deep fascia at a more inferior level), and three cutaneous nerves: the terminal branch(es) of the *posterior cutaneous nerve of the thigh* and the *medial and lateral sural cutaneous nerves.* The **popliteal fascia** is a strong sheet of deep fascia that forms a protective covering for neurovascular structures passing from the thigh through the popliteal fossa to the leg. The popliteal fascia is continuous with the *fascia lata* superiorly and the *deep fascia of the leg* inferiorly. When the leg is extended, the popliteal fascia stretches and the semimembranosus moves laterally, providing further protection to the contents of the fossa.

Vessels in Popliteal Fossa

The **popliteal artery,** the continuation of the femoral artery, begins where the femoral artery passes through the adductor hiatus (Fig. 5.25D). The popliteal artery passes through the popliteal fossa and ends at the inferior border of the popliteus by dividing into the **anterior** and **posterior tibial arteries**. The deepest structure in the popliteal fossa, the popliteal artery, runs close to the joint capsule of the knee joint. Five genicular branches of the popliteal artery supply the joint capsule and ligaments of the knee joint. The genicular arteries are the **superior lateral, superior**

medial, middle, inferior lateral, and inferior medial genicular arteries (Fig. 5.25D). They participate in the formation of the **genicular anastomosis** (L. *genu,* knee), a network of vessels around the knee that provide collateral circulation capable of maintaining blood supply to the leg during full knee flexion. Other contributors to the anastomosis are shown in Figure 5.25D. The muscular branches of the popliteal artery supply the hamstring, gastrocnemius, soleus, and plantaris muscles. The superior muscular branches of the popliteal artery have clinically important anastomoses with the terminal part of the deep artery of thigh and gluteal arteries.

The **popliteal vein** is formed at the distal border of the popliteus as a continuation of the *posterior tibial veins* (Fig. 5.26A). Throughout its course, the vein lies superficial to and in the same fibrous sheath as the popliteal artery (Fig. 5.26B). Superiorly, the popliteal vein becomes the *femoral vein* as it traverses the adductor hiatus (Fig. 5.26A). The small saphenous vein passes from the posterior aspect of the lateral malleolus to the popliteal fossa, where it pierces the deep popliteal fascia and enters the popliteal vein.

The **superficial popliteal lymph nodes** are usually small and lie in the subcutaneous tissue. The **deep popliteal lymph nodes** surround the vessels and receive lymph from the joint capsule of the knee and the lymphatic vessels that accompany the deep veins of the leg (Fig. 5.26). Lymphatic vessels from the popliteal lymph nodes follow the femoral vessels to the *deep inguinal lymph nodes.*

A **Posterior view**   B **Posterolateral view**

FIGURE 5.26.   **Venous and lymphatic drainage of leg. A.** Deep veins. **B.** Superficial veins and lymphatic drainage of subcutaneous tissues.

Nerves in Popliteal Fossa

The *sciatic nerve* usually ends at the superior angle of the popliteal fossa by dividing into the tibial and common fibular nerves (Fig. 5.25C). The **tibial nerve**—the medial, larger terminal branch of the sciatic nerve—is the most superficial of the three main central components of the popliteal fossa (nerve, vein, and artery). The tibial nerve bisects the fossa as it passes from its superior to its inferior angle. While in the fossa, the tibial nerve gives branches to the soleus, gastrocnemius, plantaris, and popliteus muscles. A **medial sural cutaneous nerve** is also derived from the tibial nerve in the popliteal fossa (Fig. 5.25C). It is joined by the **sural communicating branch of the common fibular nerve** at a highly variable level to form the **sural nerve.** This nerve supplies skin on the posterior and lateral aspects of the leg and lateral side of the foot. The **lateral sural cutaneous nerve** is a branch of the common fibular nerve that supplies the skin of the lateral aspect of the leg.

The **common fibular nerve** (Fig. 5.25C)—the lateral, smaller terminal branch of the sciatic nerve—begins at the superior angle of the popliteal fossa and follows closely the medial border of the biceps femoris and its tendon along the superolateral boundary of the popliteal fossa. The common fibular nerve leaves the fossa by passing superficial to the lateral head of the gastrocnemius and winding around the fibular neck, where it is vulnerable to injury. Here it divides into its terminal branches, the superficial and deep fibular nerves. The most inferior branches of the *posterior cutaneous nerve of the thigh* supply the skin that overlies the popliteal fossa.

Popliteal Pulse

Because the popliteal artery is deep in the popliteal fossa, it may be difficult to feel the *popliteal pulse*. To palpate this pulse the person is placed in the prone position with the knee flexed to relax the popliteal fascia and hamstrings. The pulsations are best felt in the inferior part of the fossa. Weakening or loss of the popliteal pulse is a sign of femoral artery obstruction.

Popliteal Aneurysm

A *popliteal aneurysm* (abnormal dilation of all or part of the popliteal artery) usually causes edema (swelling) and pain in the popliteal fossa. If the femoral artery has to be ligated, blood can bypass the occlusion through the genicular anastomosis and reach the popliteal artery distal to the ligation.

LEG

The leg contains the *tibia* and *fibula,* bones that connect the knee and ankle. The tibia, the weight-bearing bone, is larger and stronger than the fibula. The leg bones are connected by the *interosseous membrane.* The leg is divided into three compartments, anterior, lateral, and posterior, which are formed by the anterior and posterior *intermuscular septa,* the *interosseous membrane,* and the two leg bones (Fig. 5.28).

Anterior Compartment of Leg

The **anterior compartment**, or dorsiflexor (*extensor*) compartment, is located anterior to the *interosseous membrane,* between the lateral surface of the tibial shaft and the medial surface of the fibular shaft (Figs. 5.27 and 5.28; Table 5.8). The anterior compartment is bounded anteriorly by the deep fascia of the leg and skin. Inferiorly, two band-like thickenings of the deep fascia form retinacula that bind the tendons of the anterior compartment muscles, preventing them from bow-stringing anteriorly during dorsiflexion of the ankle joint. The **superior extensor retinaculum** is a strong, broad band of deep fascia (Fig. 5.27A) passing from the fibula to the tibia, proximal to the malleoli. The **inferior extensor retinaculum,** a Y-shaped band of deep fascia, attaches laterally to the anterosuperior surface of the calcaneus and medially to the medial malleolus and medial cuneiform. It forms a strong loop around the tendons of the fibularis tertius and extensor digitorum longus muscles. The four muscles in the anterior compartment are (Figs. 5.27):

- Tibialis anterior.
- Extensor digitorum longus.
- Extensor hallucis longus.
- Fibularis tertius.

These muscles are mainly dorsiflexors of the ankle joint and extensors of the toes (Table 5.8).

The **deep fibular peroneal nerve**, one of the two terminal branches of the common fibular nerve, is the nerve of the anterior compartment (Fig. 5.27B,D). The deep fibular nerve arises between the fibularis longus muscle and the neck of the fibula. After entering the compartment, the nerve accompanies the anterior tibial artery.

The **anterior tibial artery** supplies structures in the anterior compartment (Fig. 5.27D). The smaller terminal branch of the popliteal artery, the anterior tibial artery, begins at the inferior border of the popliteus muscle. It passes anteriorly through a gap in the superior part of the interosseous membrane and descends on the anterior surface of this membrane between the tibialis anterior and the extensor digitorum longus. It ends at the ankle joint, midway between the malleoli (Fig. 5.27D), where it becomes the **dorsalis pedis artery** (dorsal artery of foot).

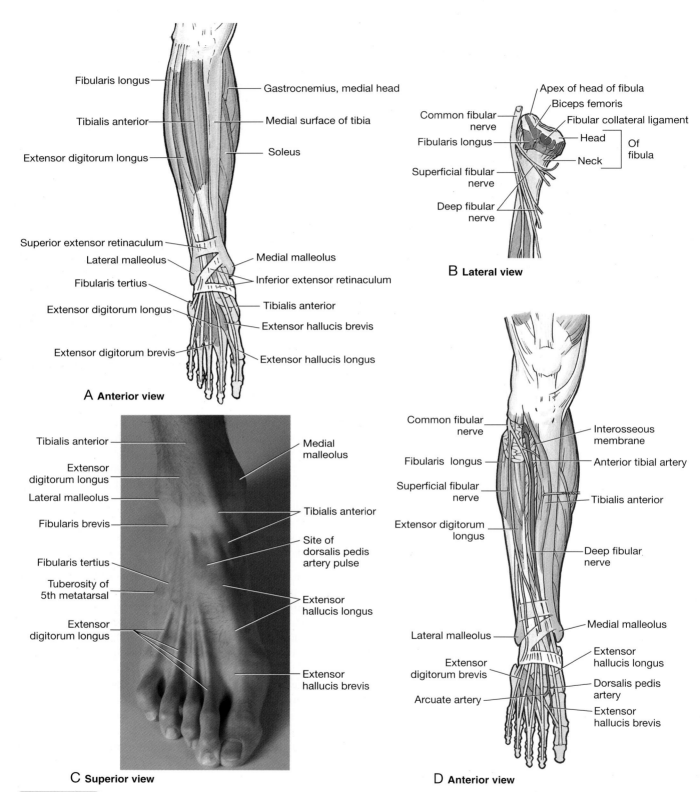

Fibularis longus

Tibialis anterior

Extensor digitorum longus

Superior extensor retinaculum

Lateral malleolus

Fibularis tertius

Extensor digitorum longus

Extensor digitorum brevis

Gastrocnemius, medial head

Medial surface of tibia

Soleus

Medial malleolus

Inferior extensor retinaculum

Tibialis anterior

Extensor hallucis brevis

Extensor hallucis longus

A Anterior view

Apex of head of fibula

Biceps femoris

Common fibular nerve

Fibular collateral ligament

Fibularis longus

Head

Neck

Of fibula

Superficial fibular nerve

Deep fibular nerve

B Lateral view

Tibialis anterior

Extensor digitorum longus

Lateral malleolus

Fibularis brevis

Fibularis tertius

Tuberosity of 5th metatarsal

Extensor digitorum longus

Medial malleolus

Tibialis anterior

Site of dorsalis pedis artery pulse

Extensor hallucis longus

Extensor hallucis brevis

C Superior view

Common fibular nerve

Fibularis longus

Superficial fibular nerve

Extensor digitorum longus

Lateral malleolus

Extensor digitorum brevis

Arcuate artery

Interosseous membrane

Anterior tibial artery

Tibialis anterior

Deep fibular nerve

Medial malleolus

Extensor hallucis longus

Dorsalis pedis artery

Extensor hallucis brevis

D Anterior view

FIGURE 5.27. **Anterior compartment of leg and dorsum of foot. A.** Muscles. **B.** Nerves. **C.** Surface anatomy. **D.** Nerves and vessels. The muscles have been separated to display these structures.

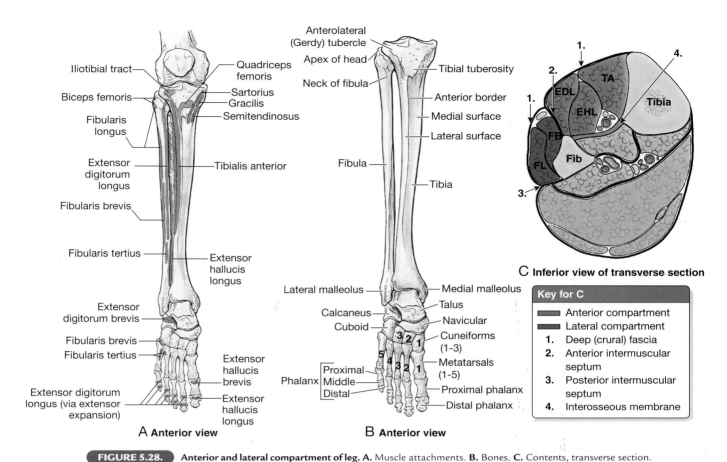

FIGURE 5.28. Anterior and lateral compartment of leg. **A.** Muscle attachments. **B.** Bones. **C.** Contents, transverse section.

TABLE 5.8 MUSCLES OF THE ANTERIOR AND LATERAL COMPARTMENTS OF THE LEG

Muscle	Proximal Attachment	Distal Attachment	Innervation[a]	Main Action(s)
Anterior compartment				
Tibialis anterior (TA)	Lateral condyle and superior half of lateral surface of tibia and interosseous membrane	Medial and inferior surfaces of medial cuneiform and base of 1st metatarsal	Deep fibular nerve (**L4**, L5)	Dorsiflexes ankle; inverts foot; supports medial longitudinal arch of foot
Extensor hallucis longus (EHL)	Middle part of anterior surface of fibula and interosseous membrane	Dorsal aspect of base of distal phalanx of great toe (hallux)		Extends great toe; dorsiflexes ankle
Extensor digitorum longus (EDL)	Lateral condyle of tibia and superior three fourths of anterior surface of interosseous membrane	Middle and distal phalanges of lateral four digits	Deep fibular nerve (L5, S1)	Extends lateral four digits; dorsiflexes ankle
Fibularis tertius	Inferior third of anterior surface of fibula and interosseous membrane	Dorsum of base of 5th metatarsal		Dorsiflexes ankle; aids in eversion of foot
Lateral compartment				
Fibularis longus (FL)	Head and superior two thirds of lateral surface of fibula	Base of 1st metatarsal and medial cuneiform	Superficial fibular nerve (**L5**, **S1**, S2)	Evert foot; weakly plantarflex ankle. FL supports transverse arch of foot.
Fibularis brevis (FB)	Inferior two thirds of lateral surface of fibula	Dorsal surface of tuberosity of base of 5th metatarsal		

[a]The spinal cord segmental innervation is indicated (e.g., "**L4**, L5" means that the nerves supplying the tibialis anterior are derived from the fourth and fifth lumbar segments of the spinal cord). Numbers in boldface (**L4**) indicate the main segmental innervation. Damage to one or more of the listed spinal cord segments or to the motor nerve roots arising from them results in paralysis of the muscles concerned.

A **Lateral view**

B **Lateral view**

FIGURE 5.29.   Lateral compartment of leg and lateral aspect of foot. **A.** Muscles. **B.** Surface anatomy. **C.** Retinacula and synovial sheaths of the tendons (*blue*).

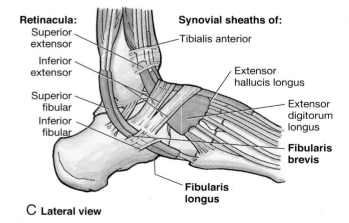

C **Lateral view**

Lateral Compartment of Leg

The **lateral compartment,** or *evertor compartment,* is bounded by the lateral surface of the fibula, the anterior and posterior intermuscular septa, and the deep fascia of the leg (Table 5.8). The lateral compartment contains two muscles—the **fibularis longus** and **brevis**—that pass posterior to the lateral malleolus (Fig. 5.29).

The **superficial fibular nerve,** the nerve in the lateral compartment, is a terminal branch of the common fibular nerve (Fig. 5.25*B,C*). After supplying the two muscles, it continues as a cutaneous nerve, supplying the skin on the distal part of the anterior surface of the leg and nearly all the dorsum of the foot.

The lateral compartment of the leg does not have an artery coursing through it (Fig. 5.27D and 5.28C). The muscles are supplied proximally by perforating branches of the **anterior tibial artery** and distally by perforating branches of the **fibular artery**. These perforating arteries have accompanying veins (L. *venae comitantes*).

Tibialis Anterior Strain (Shin Splints)

 Shin splints—edema and pain in the area of the distal two thirds of the tibia—result from repetitive microtrauma of the tibialis anterior (TA), which causes small tears in the periosteum covering the shaft of the tibia and/or of fleshy attachments to the overlying deep fascia of the leg. Shin splints are a mild form of the anterior compartment syndrome.

Shin splints commonly occur during traumatic injury or athletic overexertion of muscles in the anterior compartment, especially TA. Often persons who lead sedentary lives develop shin splints when they participate in walk-a-thons (long-distance walks).

Shin splints also occur in trained runners who do not warm up and cool down sufficiently. Muscles in the anterior compartment swell from sudden overuse, and the edema and muscle–tendon inflammation reduce the blood flow to the muscles. The swollen muscles are painful and tender to pressure.

Containment and Spread of Compartmental Infections in Leg

 The fascial compartments of the lower limbs are generally closed spaces, ending proximally and distally at the joints. Because the septa and deep fascia of the leg forming the boundaries of the leg compartments are strong, the increased volume consequent to infection with *suppuration* (formation of pus) increases intracompartmental pressure. Inflammations within the anterior and posterior compartments of the leg spread chiefly in a distal direction; however, a purulent (pus-forming) infection in the lateral compartment of the leg can ascend proximally into the popliteal fossa, presumably along the course of the fibular nerve. Fasciotomy may be necessary to relieve compartmental pressure and débride (remove by scraping) pockets of infection.

Injury to Common Fibular Nerve and Footdrop

 Because of its superficial position, *the common fibular is the nerve most often injured in the lower limb*, mainly because it winds subcutaneously around the fibular neck, leaving it vulnerable to direct trauma. This nerve may also be severed during fracture of the fibular neck or severely stretched when the knee joint is injured or dislocated.

Severance of the common fibular nerve results in flaccid paralysis of all muscles in the anterior and lateral compartments of the leg (dorsiflexors of ankle and evertors of foot). The loss of dorsiflexion of the ankle causes **footdrop**, which is exacerbated by unopposed inversion of the foot. This has the effect of making the limb "too long": The toes do not clear the ground during the swing phase of walking (Fig. B5.11A).

There are several other conditions that may result in a lower limb that is "too long" functionally—for example, pelvic tilt and spastic paralysis or contraction of the soleus. There are at least three means of compensating for this problem:

1. A *waddling gait,* in which the individual leans to the side opposite the long limb, "hiking" the hip (Fig. B5.11B).
2. A *swing-out gait,* in which the long limb is swung out laterally (abducted) to allow the toes to clear the ground (Fig. B5.11C).
3. A high-stepping *steppage gait,* in which extra flexion is employed at the hip and knee to raise the foot as high as necessary to keep the toes from hitting the ground (Fig. B5.11D).

Because the dropped foot makes it difficult to make the heel strike the ground first as in a normal gait, a steppage gait is commonly employed in the case of flaccid paralysis. Sometimes an extra "kick" is added as the free limb swings forward in an attempt to flip the forefoot upward just before setting the foot down.

The braking action normally produced by eccentric contraction of the dorsiflexors is also lost in flaccid paralysis footdrop. Therefore, the foot is not lowered to the ground in a controlled manner after heel strike; instead, the foot slaps the ground suddenly, producing a distinctive *clop* and greatly increasing the shock both received by the forefoot and transmitted up the tibia to the knee. Individuals with a common fibular nerve injury may also experience a variable loss of sensation on the anterolateral aspect of the leg and the dorsum of the foot.

Foot drop

Compensating for foot drop

A Toes do not clear ground during swing phase

B Waddling gait

C Swing-out gait

D Steppage gait

FIGURE B5.11.

Deep Fibular Nerve Entrapment

 Excessive use of muscles supplied by the deep fibular nerve (e.g., during skiing, running, and dancing) may result in muscle injury and edema in the anterior compartment. This entrapment may cause compression of the deep fibular nerve and pain in the anterior compartment.

Compression of the nerve by tight-fitting ski boots, for example, may occur where the nerve passes deep to the inferior extensor retinaculum and the extensor hallucis brevis. Pain occurs in the dorsum of the foot and usually radiates to the web space between the first and second toes. Because ski boots are a common cause of this type of nerve entrapment, this condition has been called the "ski boot syndrome"; however, the syndrome also occurs in soccer players and runners and can also result from tight shoes.

Superficial Fibular Nerve Entrapment

Chronic ankle sprains may produce recurrent stretching of the superficial fibular nerve, which may cause pain along the lateral side of the leg and the dorsum of the ankle and foot. Numbness and *paresthesia* (tickling or tingling) may be present and increase with activity.

Palpation of Dorsalis Pedis Pulse

The *dorsalis pedis artery pulse* is evaluated during a physical examination of the peripheral vascular system. Dorsalis pedis pulses may be palpated with the feet slightly dorsiflexed. The pulses are usually easy to palpate because these dorsal arteries are subcutaneous and pass along a line from the extensor retinaculum to a point just lateral to the extensor hallucis longus tendons (Fig. B5.12). A diminished or absent dorsalis pedis pulse usually suggests vascular insufficiency resulting from arterial disease. The five P signs of acute arterial occlusion are *pain, pallor, paresthesia, paralysis,* and *pulselessness.* Some healthy adults (and even children) have *congenitally nonpalpable dorsalis pedis pulses;* the variation is usually bilateral. In these cases, the dorsalis pedis artery is replaced by an extended perforating fibular artery of smaller caliber than the typical dorsalis pedis artery, but running in the same location.

Extensor hallucis longus

Dorsalis pedis artery

Tibialis anterior tendon

Dorsalis pedis pulse

FIGURE B5.12.

Posterior Compartment of Leg

The **posterior compartment,** or plantarflexor compartment, is the largest of the three leg compartments. The posterior compartment and the *calf muscles* within it are divided into superficial and deep subcompartments/muscle groups by the **transverse intermuscular septum** (Figs.5.8*B*, 5.30 and 5.31*C*). The tibial nerve and posterior tibial and fibular vessels supply both parts of the posterior compartment but run in the deep part, just deep (anterior) to the transverse intermuscular septum.

SUPERFICIAL MUSCLE GROUP

The superficial muscle group, including the **gastrocnemius, soleus,** and **plantaris,** forms a powerful muscular mass in the calf (Figs. 5.30 and 5.31; Table 5.9). The two-headed **gastrocnemius** and the **soleus** share a common tendon, the **calcaneal tendon** (L. *tendo calcaneus,* Achilles tendon), which attaches to the calcaneus. Collectively, these two muscles form the three-headed **triceps surae** (L. *sura,* calf). The triceps surae elevates the heel and thus depresses the forefoot, generating as much as 93% of the plantarflexion force.

The calcaneal tendon typically spirals a quarter turn (90 degrees) during its descent, so that the gastrocnemius fibers attach laterally and the soleal fibers attach medially. This arrangement is thought to be significant to the tendon's elastic ability to absorb energy (shock) and recoil, releasing the energy as part of the propulsive force it exerts. Although they share a common tendon, the two muscles of the triceps surae are capable of acting alone, and often do so: "You stroll with the soleus but win the long jump with the gastrocnemius."

To test the triceps surae, the foot is plantarflexed against resistance (e.g., by "standing on the toes," in which case body weight [gravity] provides resistance). If normal, the calcaneal tendon and triceps surae can be seen and palpated.

A *subcutaneous calcaneal bursa,* located between the skin and the calcaneal tendon, allows the skin to move over the taut tendon. A deep *bursa of the calcaneal tendon* (retrocalcaneal bursa), located between the tendon and the calcaneus, allows the tendon to glide over the bone.

The **gastrocnemius** is the most superficial muscle in the posterior compartment and forms the proximal, most prominent part of the *calf* (Fig. 5.30*B*; Table 5.9). It is a fusiform, two-headed, two-joint muscle with the medial head slightly larger and extending more distally than its lateral partner. The heads come together at the inferior margin of the popliteal fossa, where they form the inferolateral and inferomedial boundaries of this fossa.

The gastrocnemius crosses and is capable of acting on both the knee and the ankle joints; however, it cannot exert its full power on both joints at the same time. It functions most effectively when the knee is extended and is maximally activated when knee extension is combined with dorsiflexion. It is incapable of producing plantarflexion when the knee is fully flexed.

The **soleus** is located deep to the gastrocnemius and is the "workhorse" of plantarflexion (Figs. 5.30*C*; Table 5.9). It is a large muscle, flatter than the gastrocnemius, that is named for its resemblance to a sole—the flat fish that reclines on its side on the sea floor. The soleus has a continuous proximal attachment in the shape of an inverted U to the posterior aspects of the fibula and tibia and a tendinous arch between them, the **tendinous arch of soleus** (L. *arcus tendineus soleus*) (Fig. 5.30*C*). The popliteal artery and tibial nerve exit the popliteal fossa by passing through this arch, the popliteal artery simultaneously bifurcating into its terminal branches, the anterior and posterior tibial arteries.

The soleus can be palpated on each side of the gastrocnemius when the individual is standing on tiptoes (Fig. 5.30*A*). The soleus may act with the gastrocnemius in plantarflexing the ankle joint; it cannot act on the knee joint and acts alone when the knee is flexed. The soleus has many parts, each with fiber bundles in different directions.

When the foot is planted, the soleus pulls posteriorly on the bones of the leg. This is important to standing because the line of gravity passes anterior to the leg's bony axis. The soleus is thus an antigravity muscle (the predominant plantarflexor for standing and strolling), which contracts antagonistically but cooperatively (alternately) with the dorsiflexor muscles of the leg to maintain balance.

The **plantaris** is a small muscle with a short belly and a long tendon (Fig. 5.30*C*; Table 5.9). This vestigial muscle is absent in 5% to 10% of people. Because of its minor role, the plantaris tendon can be removed for grafting (e.g., during reconstructive surgery of the tendons of the hand) without causing disability.

DEEP MUSCLE GROUP

Four muscles make up the deep group in the posterior compartment (Fig. 5.30*D* and 5.31; Table 5.9):

- Popliteus
- Flexor digitorum longus
- Flexor hallucis longus
- Tibialis posterior

The **popliteus** is a thin, triangular muscle in the floor of the popliteal fossa (Fig. 5.30*C,D*). The popliteus acts on the knee joint, whereas the other muscles act on the ankle and foot joints. The **flexor hallucis longus** is the powerful flexor of all the joints of the great toe. Immediately after the triceps surae has delivered the thrust of plantarflexion to the ball of the foot (the prominence of the sole underlying the heads of the first and second metatarsals), the flexor hallucis longus delivers a final thrust via flexion of the great toe for the preswing (toe-off) of the gait cycle.

Posterior views

FIGURE 5.30. **Muscles of posterior compartment of leg. A.** Surface anatomy. *Numbers* are identified in part **B. B.** Gastrocnemius. **C.** Soleus, popliteus, and plantaris. **D.** Muscles of deep compartment.

TABLE 5.9 MUSCLES OF POSTERIOR COMPARTMENT OF LEG

Muscle	Proximal Attachment	Distal Attachment	Innervation[a]	Main Action(s)
Superficial muscle group				
Gastrocnemius: Lateral head (LG) Medial head (MG)	*Lateral head:* lateral aspect of lateral condyle of femur *Medial head:* popliteal surface of femur, superior to medial condyle	Posterior surface of calcaneus via calcaneal tendon	Tibial nerve (S1, S2)	Plantarflexes ankle when knee is extended; raises heel during walking, and flexes leg at knee joint
Soleus (SOL)	Posterior aspect of head of fibula, superior quarter of posterior surface of fibula, soleal line, and medial border of tibia			Plantarflexes ankle; steadies leg on foot
Plantaris (P)	Inferior end of lateral supra-condylar line of femur and oblique popliteal ligament			Weakly assists gastrocnemius in plantarflexing ankle
Deep muscle group				
Popliteus	Lateral surface of lateral condyle of femur and lateral meniscus	Posterior surface of tibia, superior to soleal line	Tibial nerve (L4, L5, S1)	Weakly flexes knee and unlocks it by laterally rotating femur on fixed tibia, or medially rotating tibia of unplanted limb

TABLE 5.9 MUSCLES OF POSTERIOR COMPARTMENT OF LEG (*continued*)

Muscle	Proximal Attachment	Distal Attachment	Innervation[a]	Main Action(s)
Flexor hallucis longus (FHL)	Inferior two thirds of posterior surface of fibula and inferior part of interosseous membrane	Base of distal phalanx of great toe (hallux)	Tibial nerve (**S2**, S3)	Flexes great toe at all joints; weakly plantarflexes ankle; supports medial longitudinal arch of foot
Flexor digitorum longus (FDL)	Medial part of posterior surface of tibia inferior to soleal line and by a broad tendon to fibula	Bases of distal phalanges of lateral four digits		Flexes lateral four digits; plantarflexes ankle; supports longitudinal arches of foot
Tibialis posterior (TP)	Interosseous membrane, posterior surface of tibia inferior to soleal line, and posterior surface of fibula	Primarily to tuberosity of navicular; also to cuneiforms, cuboid and bases of 2nd–4th metatarsals	Tibial nerve (L4, L5)	Plantarflexes ankle; inverts foot; supports medial longitudinal arch of foot

[a]The spinal cord segmental innervation is indicated (e.g., "**S2**, S3" means that the nerves supplying the flexor hallucis longus are derived from the second and third sacral segments of the spinal cord). Numbers in boldface (**S2**) indicate the main segmental innervation.

The **flexor digitorum longus** is smaller than the flexor hallucis longus, even though it moves four digits. It passes diagonally into the sole of the foot, superficial to the tendon of the flexor hallucis longus, and divides into four tendons, which pass to the distal phalanges of the lateral four toes (Fig. 5.32). The **tibialis posterior,** the deepest muscle in the group, lies between the flexor digitorum longus and the flexor hallucis longus in the same plane as the tibia and fibula within the deep subcompartment (Fig. 5.30*D*). When the foot is off the ground, it can act synergistically with the tibialis anterior to invert the foot, their otherwise antagonistic functions cancelling each other. However, the primary role of the tibialis posterior is to support or maintain (fix) the medial longitudinal arch during weight bearing; consequently the muscle contracts statically throughout the stance phase of gait.

The **tibial nerve** (L4, L5, and S1–S3) is the larger of the two terminal branches of the *sciatic nerve* (Fig. 5.31*B* and 5.33). It runs through the popliteal fossa with the popliteal artery and vein passing between the heads of the gastrocnemius. These structures pass deep to the tendinous arch of the soleus. The tibial nerve supplies all muscles in the posterior compartment of the leg (Tables 5.9 and 5.10). At the ankle, the nerve lies between the flexor hallucis longus and the flexor digitorum longus. Posteroinferior to the medial malleolus, the tibial nerve divides into the medial and lateral plantar nerves. A branch of the tibial nerve, the *medial sural cutaneous nerve,* usually unites with the *sural communicating branch of the common fibular nerve* to form the **sural nerve** (Fig. 5.33*B*; Table 5.10). This nerve supplies the skin of the lateral and posterior part of the inferior third of the leg and the lateral side of the foot. Articular branches of the tibial nerve supply the knee joint and medial calcaneal branches supply the skin of the heel (Fig. 5.34).

The **posterior tibial artery** (Fig. 5.33*A*; Table 5.11), the larger terminal branch of the popliteal artery, provides the

blood supply to the posterior compartment of the leg and to the foot. It begins at the distal border of the popliteus and passes deep to the tendinous arch of the soleus. After giving off the **fibular artery,** its largest branch, the posterior tibial artery passes inferomedially on the posterior surface of the tibialis posterior. During its descent, it is accompanied by the tibial nerve and veins. The posterior tibial artery runs posterior to the medial malleolus (Fig. 5.33*B*). Deep to the

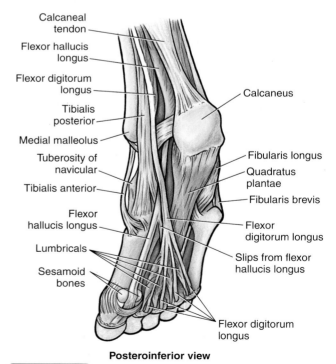

Calcaneal tendon
Flexor hallucis longus
Flexor digitorum longus
Tibialis posterior
Medial malleolus
Tuberosity of navicular
Tibialis anterior
Flexor hallucis longus
Lumbricals
Sesamoid bones

Calcaneus
Fibularis longus
Quadratus plantae
Fibularis brevis
Flexor digitorum longus
Slips from flexor hallucis longus
Flexor digitorum longus

Posteroinferior view

FIGURE 5.32. Relationships of muscles of deep posterior compartment posterior to medial malleolus and in sole of foot.

Synovial sheaths in B

1 Extensor hallucis longus
2 Tibialis anterior
3 Tibialis posterior
4 Flexor digitorum longus
5 Flexor hallucis longus

FIGURE 5.33. **Nerves and vessels of the posterior leg. A.** Vessels and nerves are exposed by removal of most of soleus muscle. **B.** Structures passing posterior to medial malleolus. Synovial sheaths of the tendons are *blue*; each is named in key.

flexor retinaculum and the origin of the abductor hallucis, the posterior tibial artery divides into *medial* and *lateral plantar arteries*, the arteries of the sole of the foot.

The fibular artery arises inferior to the distal border of the popliteus and the tendinous arch of soleus (Fig. 5.33A). It descends obliquely toward the fibula and then passes along its medial side, usually within the flexor hallucis longus. The fibular artery gives muscular branches to the muscles in the posterior and lateral compartments of the leg. It also gives rise to the *nutrient artery of the fibula*. The perforating branch pierces the *interosseous membrane* and passes to the dorsum of the foot. The large **nutrient artery of tibia** arises from the origin of the anterior or posterior tibial artery. It pierces the tibialis posterior and enters the nutrient foramen in the proximal third of the posterior surface of the tibia (Fig. 5.35).

Gastrocnemius Strain

 Gastrocnemius strain (tennis leg) is a painful calf injury resulting from partial tearing of the medial belly of the gastrocnemius at or near its musculotendinous junction. It is caused by over-stretching the muscle by concomitant full extension of the knee and dorsiflexion of the ankle joint.

Posterior Tibial Pulse

The posterior tibial pulse can usually be palpated between the posterior surface of the medial malleolus and the medial border of the calcaneal tendon (Fig. B5.13). Because the posterior tibial artery passes deep to the flexor reti-naculum, it is important when palpating this pulse to have the person relax the retinaculum by inverting the foot. Failure to do this may lead to the erroneous conclusion that the pulse is absent.

Medial malleolus
Posterior tibial artery
Calcaneal tendon

FIGURE B5.13.

Both arteries are examined simultaneously for equality of force. Palpation of the posterior tibial pulses is essential for examining patients with occlusive *peripheral arterial disease.* Although posterior tibial pulses are absent in approximately 15% of normal young people, absence of posterior tibial pulses is a sign of occlusive peripheral arterial disease in people older than 60 years. For example, *intermittent claudication,* characterized by leg pain and cramps, develops during walking and disappears after rest. These conditions result from ischemia of the leg muscles caused by narrowing or occlusion of the leg arteries.

Injury to Tibial Nerve

Injury to the tibial nerve is uncommon because of its deep and protected position in the popliteal fossa; however, the nerve may be injured by deep lacerations in the fossa. *Posterior dislocation of the knee joint* may also damage the tibial nerve. *Severance of the tibial nerve* produces paralysis of the flexor muscles in the leg and the intrinsic muscles in the sole of the foot. People with a tibial nerve injury are unable to plantarflex their ankle or flex their toes. Loss of sensation also occurs on the sole of the foot.

Absence of Plantarflexion

If the muscles of the calf are paralyzed, the calcaneal tendon is ruptured, or normal push-off is painful, a much less effective and efficient push-off (from the midfoot) can still be accomplished by the actions of the gluteus maximus and hamstrings in extending the thigh at the hip joint and the quadriceps in extending the knee. Because push-off from the forefoot is not possible (in fact, the ankle will be passively dorsiflexed as the body's weight moves anterior to the foot), those attempting to walk in the absence of plantarflexion often rotate the foot as far laterally (externally) as possible during the stance phase to disable passive dorsiflexion and allow a more effective push-off through hip and knee extension exerted at the midfoot.

Calcaneal Tendon Reflex

The *ankle (jerk) reflex* is elicited by striking the calcaneal tendon briskly with a reflex hammer while the person's legs are dangling over the side of the examining table. This tendon reflex tests the S1 and S2 nerve roots. If the S1 nerve root is cut or compressed, the ankle reflex is virtually absent.

Inflammation and Rupture of Calcaneal Tendon

Inflammation of the calcaneal tendon constitutes 9% to 18% of running injuries. Microscopic tears of collagen fibers in the tendon, particularly just superior to its attachment to the calcaneus, result in *tendinitis,* which causes pain during walking.

Calcaneal tendon rupture is often sustained by people with a history of calcaneal tendinitis. After complete rupture of the tendon, passive dorsiflexion is excessive, and the person cannot plantarflex against resistance.

Calcaneal Bursitis

Calcaneal bursitis results from inflammation of the bursa of calcaneal tendon located between the calcaneal tendon and the superior part of the posterior surface of the calcaneus. Calcaneal bursitis causes pain posterior to the heel and occurs commonly during long-distance running, basketball, and tennis. It is caused by excessive friction on the bursa as the calcaneal tendon continuously slides over it.

FIGURE 5.34. Nerves of leg.

TABLE 5.10 NERVES OF LEG

Nerve	Origin	Course	Distribution
Saphenous	Femoral nerve	Descends with femoral vessels through femoral triangle and adductor canal; then descends with great saphenous vein	Supplies skin on medial side of leg and foot
Sural	Formed by the union of cutaneous branches from the tibial and common fibular nerves	Descends between heads of gastrocnemius; becomes superficial at middle of leg; descends with small saphenous vein; passes inferior to lateral malleolus to lateral side of foot	Supplies skin on posterior and lateral aspects of leg and lateral side of foot
Tibial	Sciatic nerve	Forms as sciatic bifurcates at apex of popliteal fossa; descends through popliteal fossa and lies on popliteus; runs inferiorly on tibialis posterior with posterior tibial vessels; terminates beneath flexor retinaculum by dividing into medial and lateral plantar nerves	Supplies posterior muscles of leg and knee joint
Common fibular	Sciatic nerve	Forms as sciatic bifurcates at apex of popliteal fossa and follows medial border of biceps femoris and its tendon; passes over posterior aspect of head of fibula; then winds around neck of fibula deep to fibularis longus, where it divides into deep and superficial fibular nerves	Supplies skin on lateral part of posterior aspect of leg via its branch, the lateral sural cutaneous nerve; also supplies knee joint via its articular branch
Superficial fibular	Common fibular nerve	Arises between fibularis longus and neck of fibula; descends in lateral compartment of leg; pierces deep fascia at distal third of leg to become subcutaneous	Supplies lateral muscles of leg and skin on distal third of anterior surface of leg and dorsum of foot, except skin of first interdigital cleft
Deep fibular	Common fibular nerve	Arises between fibularis longus and neck of fibula; passes through extensor digitorum longus and descends on interosseous membrane; crosses distal end of tibia and enters dorsum of foot	Supplies anterior muscles of leg, and skin of first interdigital cleft; sends articular branches to joints it crosses

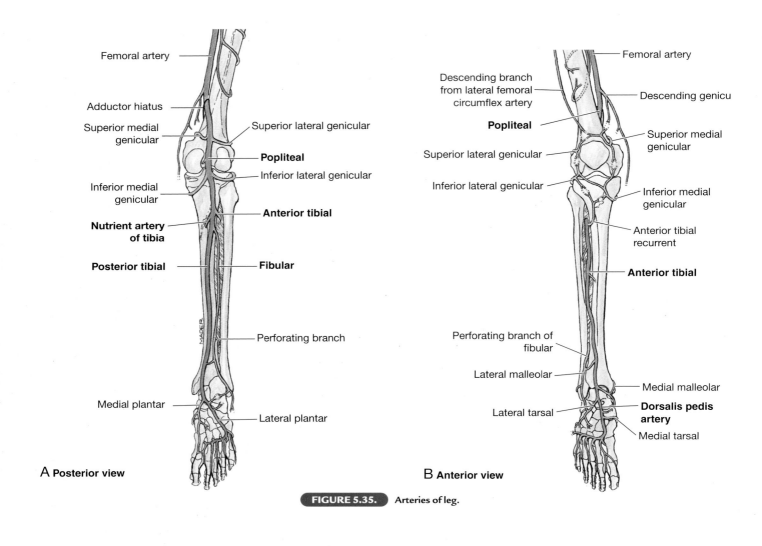

A Posterior view

B Anterior view

FIGURE 5.35. Arteries of leg.

TABLE 5.11 ARTERIES OF LEG

Artery	Origin	Course	Distribution
Popliteal	Continuation of femoral artery at adductor hiatus in adductor magnus	Passes through popliteal fossa to leg; ends at inferior border of popliteus muscle by dividing into anterior and posterior tibial arteries	Superior, middle, and inferior genicular arteries to knee; muscular branches to hamstrings and muscles of superficial posterior compartment of leg
Anterior tibial	Popliteal artery	Passes into anterior compartment through gap in superior part of interosseous membrane; descends on this membrane between tibialis anterior and extensor digitorum longus	Anterior compartment of leg
Dorsalis pedis (dorsal artery of foot)	Continuation of anterior tibial artery distal to inferior extensor retinaculum	Descends anteromedially to first interosseous space; divides into deep plantar and 1st dorsal metatarsal arteries	Muscles on dorsum of foot; pierces first dorsal interosseous muscle as deep plantar artery to contribute to formation of plantar arch
Posterior tibial	Popliteal	Passes through posterior compartment of leg; terminates distal to flexor retinaculum by dividing into medial and lateral plantar arteries	Posterior and lateral compartments of leg; circumflex fibular branch joins anastomoses around knee; nutrient artery passes to tibia
Fibular	Posterior tibial	Descends in posterior compartment adjacent to posterior intermuscular septum	Posterior compartment of leg: perforating branches supply lateral compartment of leg

FOOT

The **foot,** distal to the ankle, provides a platform for supporting the weight of the body when standing and has an important role in locomotion. The skeleton of the foot consists of 7 tarsals, 5 metatarsals, and 14 phalanges (Fig. 5.36). The foot and its bones may be considered in terms of three anatomical and functional parts:

- The **hindfoot:** talus and calcaneus.
- The **midfoot:** navicular, cuboid, and cuneiforms.
- The **forefoot:** metatarsals and phalanges.

The regions of the foot include:

- The **plantar region** (sole): the part contacting the ground.
- The **dorsal region of foot** (dorsum of the foot): the part directed superiorly.
- The **heel region** (heel): the sole underlying the calcaneus.

- The **ball of the foot:** the sole underlying the heads of the medial two metatarsals.

The **great toe** (L. *hallux*) is also called the **first toe** (L. *digitus primus*); the **little toe** (L. *digitus minimus*) is also called the **fifth toe** (L. *digitus quintus*).

Deep Fascia of Foot

The **deep fascia** is thin on the dorsum of the foot, where it is continuous with the *inferior extensor retinaculum*. Over the lateral and posterior aspects, the deep fascia of the foot is continuous with the **plantar fascia,** the deep fascia of the sole, which has a thick central part (the **plantar aponeurosis**) and weaker medial and lateral parts (Fig. 5.37). The plantar fascia holds parts of the foot together, helps protect the sole from injury, and helps support the longitudinal arches of the foot. The plantar aponeurosis arises posteriorly from the calcaneus and distally divides into five bands that become continuous with the fibrous digital sheaths that enclose the flexor tendons that pass to the toes. Inferior to the heads of the metatarsals, the aponeurosis is reinforced by transverse fibers forming the *superficial transverse metatarsal ligament.* In the forefoot and midfoot, vertical intermuscular septa extend superiorly from the margins of the plantar aponeurosis toward the first and fifth metatarsals, forming three *compartments of the sole* (Fig. 5.38):

- **Medial compartment of the sole**, covered superficially by *medial plantar fascia,* contains the abductor hallucis, flexor hallucis brevis, tendon of the flexor hallucis longus, and medial plantar nerve and vessels.
- **Central compartment of the sole,** covered by the *plantar aponeurosis,* contains the flexor digitorum brevis, flexor digitorum longus, quadratus plantae, lumbricals,

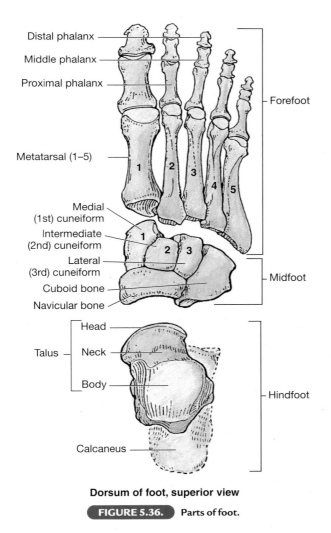

Dorsum of foot, superior view

Distal phalanx
Middle phalanx
Proximal phalanx
Metatarsal (1–5)
Medial (1st) cuneiform
Intermediate (2nd) cuneiform
Lateral (3rd) cuneiform
Cuboid bone
Navicular bone
Talus
Head
Neck
Body
Calcaneus
Forefoot
Midfoot
Hindfoot

FIGURE 5.36. Parts of foot.

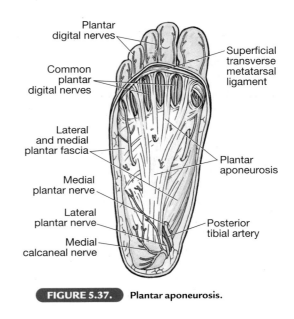

Plantar digital nerves
Common plantar digital nerves
Lateral and medial plantar fascia
Medial plantar nerve
Lateral plantar nerve
Medial calcaneal nerve
Superficial transverse metatarsal ligament
Plantar aponeurosis
Posterior tibial artery

FIGURE 5.37. Plantar aponeurosis.

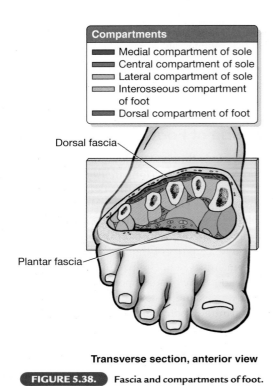

Compartments

■ Medial compartment of sole
■ Central compartment of sole
▢ Lateral compartment of sole
▢ Interosseous compartment
    of foot
■ Dorsal compartment of foot

Dorsal fascia

Plantar fascia

Transverse section, anterior view

FIGURE 5.38.   **Fascia and compartments of foot.**

adductor hallucis, distal part of tendon flexor hallucis longus, and lateral plantar nerve and vessels.

• **Lateral compartment of the sole,** covered by the thinner *lateral plantar fascia*, contains the abductor and flexor digiti minimi brevis.

In the forefoot only, a fourth compartment, the **interosseous compartment of the foot,** contains the metatarsals, the dorsal and plantar interosseous muscles, and the deep plantar and metatarsal vessels.

Muscles of Foot

Of the 20 individual muscles of the foot, 14 are located on the plantar aspect, 2 are on the dorsal aspect, and 4 are intermediate in position. From the plantar aspect, muscles of the sole are arranged in four layers within four compartments. The muscles of the foot are illustrated in Figure 5.40, and their attachments, innervation, and actions are described in Table 5.12.

Despite their compartmental and layered arrangement, the **plantar muscles** function primarily as a group during the support phase of stance, maintaining the arches of the foot (see Fig 5.43, Table 5.15). They basically resist forces that tend to reduce the longitudinal arch as weight is received at the heel (posterior end of the arch) and is then transferred to the ball of the foot and great toe (anterior end of the arch).

The muscles become most active in the later portion of the movement to stabilize the foot for propulsion (push-off), a time when forces also tend to flatten the foot's transverse arch. Concurrently, they are also able to refine further the efforts of the long muscles, producing supination and pronation in enabling the platform of the foot to adjust to uneven ground.

The muscles of the foot are of little importance individually because fine control of the individual toes is not important to most people. Rather than producing actual movement, they are most active in fixing the foot or in increasing the pressure applied against the ground by various aspects of the sole or toes to maintain balance.

Despite its name, the adductor hallucis is probably most active during the push-off phase of stance in pulling the lateral four metatarsals toward the great toe, fixing the transverse arch of the foot, and resisting forces that would spread the metatarsal heads as weight and force are applied to the forefoot (Table 5.15).

In Table 5.12, note that the:

• **P**lantar interossei **AD**duct (**PAD**) and arise from a single metatarsal as unipennate muscles.
• **D**orsal interossei **AB**duct (**DAB**) and arise from two metatarsals as bipennate muscles.

The *tibial nerve* divides posterior to the medial malleolus into the *medial* and *lateral plantar nerves* (Fig. 5.41; Table 5.13). These nerves supply the intrinsic muscles of the plantar aspect of the foot.

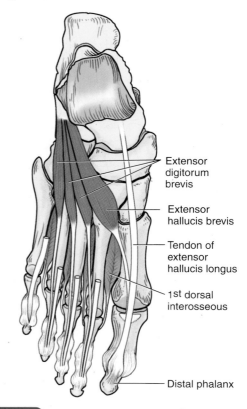

Extensor digitorum brevis

Extensor hallucis brevis

Tendon of extensor hallucis longus

1st dorsal interosseous

Distal phalanx

FIGURE 5.39.   **Extensor digitorum brevis and extensor hallucis brevis.**

TABLE 5.12 MUSCLES OF SOLE OF FOOT

Muscle	Proximal Attachment	Distal Attachment	Innervation[a]	Main Action(s)
First layer				
Abductor hallucis	Medial tubercle of tuberosity of calcaneus, flexor retinaculum, and plantar aponeurosis	Medial side of base of proximal phalanx of 1st digit	Medial plantar nerve (S2, **S3**)	Abducts and flexes 1st digit (great toe, hallux)
Flexor digitorum brevis	Medial tubercle of tuberosity of calcaneus, plantar aponeurosis, and intermuscular septa	Both sides of middle phalanges of lateral four digits		Flexes lateral four digits
Abductor digiti minimi	Medial and lateral tubercles of tuberosity of calcaneus, plantar aponeurosis, and intermuscular septa	Lateral side of base of proximal phalanx of 5th digit	Lateral plantar nerve (S2, **S3**)	Abducts and flexes 5th digit
Second layer				
Quadratus plantae	Medial surface and lateral margin of plantar surface of calcaneus	Posterolateral margin of tendon of flexor digitorum longus	Lateral plantar nerve (S2, **S3**)	Assists flexor digitorum longus in flexing lateral four digits
Lumbricals	Tendons of flexor digitorum longus	Medial aspect of expansion over lateral four digits	*Medial one:* medial plantar nerve (S2, **S3**) *Lateral three:* lateral plantar nerve (S2, **S3**)	Flex proximal phalanges; extend middle and distal phalanges of lateral four digits
Third layer				
Flexor hallucis brevis	Plantar surfaces of cuboid and lateral cuneiform	Both sides of base of proximal phalanx of 1st digit	Medial plantar nerve (S2, **S3**)	Flexes proximal phalanx of 1st digit
Adductor hallucis	*Oblique head:* bases of metatarsals 2–4 *Transverse head:* plantar ligaments of 3rd–5th metatarsophalangeal joints	Tendons of both heads attach to lateral side of base of proximal phalanx of 1st digit	Deep branch of lateral plantar nerve (S2, **S3**)	Adducts 1st digit; assists in maintaining transverse arch of foot
Flexor digiti minimi brevis	Base of 5th metatarsal	Base of proximal phalanx of 5th digit	Superficial branch of lateral plantar nerve (S2, **S3**)	Flexes proximal phalanx of 5th digit, thereby assisting with its flexion
Fourth layer				
Plantar interossei (three muscles)	Bases and medial sides of metatarsals 3–5	Medial sides of bases of proximal phalanges of 3rd–5th digits	Lateral plantar nerve (S2, **S3**)	Adduct digits (3–5) and flex metatarsophalangeal joints
Dorsal interossei (four muscles)	Adjacent sides of metatarsals 1–5	*First:* medial side of proximal phalanx of 2nd digit *Second to fourth:* lateral sides of 2nd–4th digits		Abduct digits (2–4) and flex metatarsophalangeal joints

[a]The spinal cord segmental innervation is indicated (e.g., "S2, **S3**" means that the nerves supplying the abductor hallucis are derived from the second and third sacral segments of the spinal cord). Numbers in boldface (**S3**) indicate the main segmental innervation.

The *medial plantar nerve* Courses within the medial compartment of the sole between the first and the second muscle layers. Initially, the lateral plantar artery and nerve run laterally between the muscles of the first and second layers of plantar muscles. Their deep branches then pass medially between the muscles of the third and fourth layers.

Two closely connected muscles on the dorsum of the foot are the **extensor digitorum brevis (EDB)** and **extensor hallucis brevis (EHB)** (Fig. 5.39). The EHB is actually part of the EDB. These muscles form a fleshy mass on the lateral part of the dorsum of the foot, anterior to the lateral malleolus, and aid the extensor digitorum and extensor hallucis longus to extend digits one through four.

Flexor hallucis longus
Flexor digitorum longus
Flexor digitorum brevis
Abductor digiti minimi
Flexor digiti minimi brevis
Adductor hallucis, flexor hallucis brevis
Abductor hallucis, flexor hallucis brevis
Adductor hallucis
Fibularis longus
Tibialis anterior
Quadratus plantae
Abductor digiti minimi
Tibialis posterior
Flexor digitorum brevis, plantar aponeurosis

A

Lateral plantar artery
Lateral plantar nerve
Abductor digiti minimi
Medial plantar artery
Medial plantar nerve
Flexor digitorum brevis
Abductor hallucis

B

Flexor digiti minimi brevis
Lumbricals
Quadratus plantae
Lateral plantar nerve
Lateral plantar artery
Tendon of flexor hallucis longus
Tendon of flexor digitorum longus
Medial plantar artery
Medial plantar nerve

C

*Adductor hallucis, transverse head
Adductor hallucis, oblique head
Fibularis longus
*Ligamentous origin
Sesamoid bones
Flexor hallucis brevis
Abductor hallucis (cut)
Long plantar ligament
Tibialis anterior

D

1st
2nd
3rd
4th
3rd
2nd
1st

E

Interosseous muscles in E

■	Dorsal interossei (4), bipennate
■	Plantar interossei (3), unipennate

Plantar views

FIGURE 5.40.   **Muscles of sole of foot. A.** Muscle attachments. **B.** First layer. **C.** Second layer. **D.** Third layer. **E.** Fourth layer.

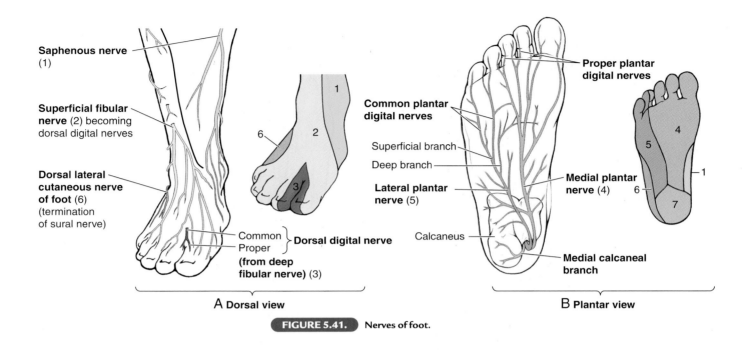

FIGURE 5.41. Nerves of foot.

TABLE 5.13 NERVES OF FOOT

Nerve[a]	Origin	Course	Distribution[a]
Saphenous (1)	Femoral nerve	Arises in femoral triangle and descends through thigh and leg; accompanies great saphenous vein anterior to medial malleolus; ends on medial side of foot	Supplies skin on medial side of foot as far anteriorly as head of 1st metatarsal
Superficial fibular (2)	Common fibular nerve	Pierces deep fascia in distal third of leg to become cutaneous; then sends branches to foot and digits	Supplies skin on dorsum of foot and all digits, except lateral side of fifth digit and first interdigital cleft
Deep fibular (3)		Passes deep to extensor retinaculum to enter dorsum of foot	Supplies extensor digitorum/extensor hallucis brevis and skin of first interdigital cleft
Medial plantar (4)	Larger terminal branch of tibial nerve	Passes distally in foot between abductor hallucis and flexor digitorum brevis; divides into muscular and cutaneous branches	Supplies skin of medial side of sole of foot and sides of first three digits; also supplies abductor hallucis, flexor digitorum brevis, flexor hallucis brevis, and first lumbrical
Lateral plantar (5)	Smaller terminal branch of tibial nerve	Passes laterally in foot between quadratus plantae and flexor digitorum brevis muscles; divides into superficial and deep branches	Supplies quadratus plantae, abductor digiti minimi, and flexor digiti minimi brevis; deep branch supplies plantar and dorsal interossei, lateral three lumbricals, and adductor hallucis; supplies skin on sole lateral to a line splitting 4th digit
Sural (6)	Formed by the union of cutaneous branches from the tibial and common fibular nerves	Passes inferior to lateral malleolus to lateral side of foot	Lateral aspect of hindfoot and midfoot
Calcaneal branches (7)	Tibial and sural nerves	Pass from distal part of posterior aspect of leg to skin on heel	Skin of heel

[a]Numbers refer to the above figure.

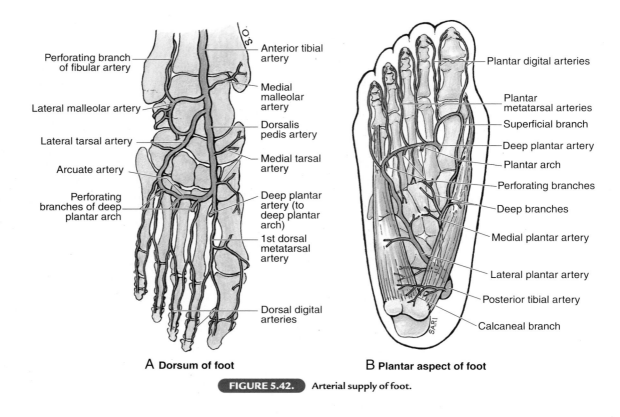

A Dorsum of foot   **B** Plantar aspect of foot

FIGURE 5.42.   Arterial supply of foot.

Nerves of Foot

The *tibial nerve* divides posterior to the medial malleolus into the **medial** and **lateral plantar nerves** (Fig. 5.41; Table 5.13). These nerves supply the intrinsic muscles of the foot, except for the extensor digitorum brevis and extensor hallucis brevis, which are supplied by the **deep fibular nerve**. The cutaneous innervation of the foot is supplied:

- Medially by the **saphenous nerve,** which extends distally to the head of the first metatarsal.
- Superiorly (dorsum of foot) by the **deep fibular nerve** (the web of skin between the contiguous sides of the first and second toes) and the **superficial fibular nerve** (remainder of dorsum of foot).
- Inferiorly (sole of foot) by the **medial** and **lateral plantar nerves;** the common border of their distribution extends along the fourth metatarsal and digit.
- Laterally by the **sural nerve,** including part of the heel.
- Posteriorly (heel) by the **calcaneal branches of the tibial and sural nerves**.

Arteries of Foot

The arteries of the foot are terminal branches of the anterior and posterior *tibial arteries* (Fig. 5.42), the dorsal and plantar arteries, respectively. The **dorsalis pedis artery** (dorsal artery of foot), often a major source of blood supply to the forefoot, is the direct continuation of the **anterior tibial artery**. The dorsalis pedis artery begins midway between the malleoli (at the ankle joint) and runs anteromedially, deep to the inferior extensor retinaculum between the extensor hallucis longus and the extensor digitorum longus tendons on the dorsum of the foot. The dorsalis pedis artery gives off the **lateral tarsal artery** and then passes distally to the first interosseous space, where it gives off the **arcuate artery** and then divides into the **first dorsal metatarsal artery** and a **deep plantar artery** (Fig. 5.42A). The deep plantar artery passes deeply between the heads of the first dorsal interosseous muscle to enter the sole of the foot, where it joins the lateral plantar artery to form the **deep plantar arch** (Fig. 5.42B). The **arcuate artery** gives off the **second, third,** and **fourth dorsal metatarsal arteries,** which run to the clefts of the toes, where each of them divides into two **dorsal digital arteries** (Fig. 5.42A).

The sole of the foot has prolific blood supply from the **posterior tibial artery,** which divides deep to the flexor retinaculum. The terminal branches pass deep to the abductor hallucis as the *medial* and *lateral plantar arteries,* which accompany similarly named nerves. The **medial plantar artery** supplies the muscles of the great toe and the skin on the medial side of the sole and has digital branches that accompany digital branches of the medial plantar nerve.

Initially, the **lateral plantar artery** and nerve course laterally between the muscles of the first and second layers of plantar muscles (Fig. 5.42*B*). The **deep plantar arch** begins opposite the base of the fifth metatarsal as the continuation of the *lateral plantar artery,* coursing between the third and the fourth muscle layers. The arch is completed medially by union with the *deep plantar artery,* a branch of the dorsal artery of the foot. As it crosses the foot, the deep plantar arch gives rise to four **plantar metatarsal arteries;** three **perforating branches;** and many branches to the skin, fascia, and muscles in the sole. The plantar digital arteries arise from the plantar metatarsal arteries near the base of the proximal phalanx, supplying adjacent digits. The more medial metatarsal arteries are joined by superficial digital branches of the medial plantar artery.

Venous Drainage of Foot

There are both superficial and deep veins in the foot. The **deep veins** consist of interanastomosing paired veins accompanying all the arteries internal to the deep fascia. The **superficial veins** are subcutaneous, are unaccompanied by arteries, and drain most of the blood from the foot. Dorsal digital veins continue proximally as **dorsal metatarsal veins,** which join to form the subcutaneous **dorsal venous arch**, proximal to which a **dorsal venous network** covers the remainder of the dorsum of the foot (Fig. 5.10). Superficial veins from a **plantar venous network** drain around either the medial or the lateral border of the foot to converge with the dorsal venous arch and network to form medial and lateral marginal veins, which become the *great* and *small saphenous veins,* respectively.

Lymphatic Drainage of Foot

The lymphatics of the foot begin in the subcutaneous plexuses. The collecting vessels consist of superficial and deep lymphatic vessels, which follow the superficial veins and major vascular bundles, respectively. Superficial lymphatic vessels are most numerous in the sole. The *medial superficial lymphatic vessels* leave the foot medially along the *great saphenous vein* and accompany it to the *superficial inguinal lymph nodes* (Fig. 5.9*A*), located along the vein's termination, and then to the *deep inguinal lymph nodes.* The *lateral superficial lymphatic vessels* drain the lateral side of the foot and accompany the *small saphenous vein* to the popliteal fossa, where they enter the *popliteal lymph nodes* (Fig. 5.26*B*). The *deep lymphatic vessels* from the foot also drain into the popliteal lymph nodes. Lymphatic vessels from them follow the femoral vessels to the deep inguinal lymph nodes. All lymph from the lower limb then passes to the iliac lymph nodes.

WALKING: THE GAIT CYCLE

Locomotion is a complex function. The movements of the lower limb during walking on a level surface may be divided into alternating swing and stance phases. The **gait cycle** consists of one cycle of swing and stance by one limb. The **stance phase** begins with **heel strike,** when the heel strikes the ground and begins to assume the body's full weight, and ends with **push-off** from the forefoot. The **swing phase** begins after push-off, when the toes leave the ground, and ends when the heel strikes the ground. The swing phase occupies approximately 40% of the walking cycle and the stance phase, 60%. In running, the time and percentage of the gait cycle represented by the stance phase are reduced. Walking is a remarkably efficient activity, taking advantage of gravity and momentum so that a minimum of physical exertion is required. The muscle actions during the gait cycle are summarized in Figure 5.43 and Table 5.14.

Plantar Fasciitis

Straining and inflammation of the plantar aponeurosis, a condition called *plantar fasciitis,* may result from running and high-impact aerobics, especially when inappropriate footwear is worn. It causes pain on the plantar surface of the heel and on the medial aspect of the foot. Point tenderness is located at the proximal attachment of the plantar aponeurosis to the medial tubercle of the calcaneus and on the medial surface of this bone. The pain increases with passive extension of the great toe and may be further exacerbated by dorsiflexion of the ankle and/or weight bearing. If a *calcaneal spur* (abnormal bony process) protrudes from the medial tubercle, plantar fasciitis is likely to cause pain on the medial side of the foot when walking. Usually, a bursa develops at the end of the spur, which may become inflamed and tender.

Hemorrhaging Wounds of Sole of Foot

Puncture wounds of the sole of the foot involving the deep plantar arch and its branches usually result in severe bleeding. Ligature of the arch is difficult because of its depth and the structures surrounding it.

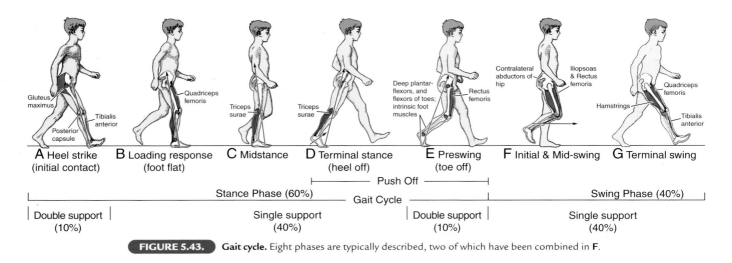

A Heel strike
(initial contact)   **B** Loading response
(foot flat)   **C** Midstance   **D** Terminal stance
(heel off)   **E** Preswing
(toe off)   **F** Initial & Mid-swing   **G** Terminal swing

Push Off

Stance Phase (60%) ——— Gait Cycle ——— Swing Phase (40%)

Double support
(10%) | Single support
(40%) | Double support
(10%) | Single support
(40%)

FIGURE 5.43.   **Gait cycle.** Eight phases are typically described, two of which have been combined in **F**.

TABLE 5.14 MUSCLE ACTION DURING GAIT CYCLE

	Phase of Gait	Mechanical Goals	Active Muscle Groups
S T A N C E P H A S E	Heel strike (initial contact)	Lower forefoot to ground	Ankle dorsiflexors (eccentric contraction)
		Continue deceleration (reverse forward swing)	Hip extensors
		Preserve longitudinal arch of foot	Intrinsic muscles of foot
			Long tendons of foot
	Loading response (flat foot)	Accept weight	Knee extensors
		Decelerate mass	Ankle plantarflexors
		Stabilize pelvis	Hip abductors
		Preserve longitudinal arch of foot	Intrinsic muscles of foot
			Long tendons of foot
	Midstance	Stabilize knee	Knee extensors
		Control dorsiflexion (preserve momentum)	Ankle plantarflexors (eccentric contraction)
		Stabilize pelvis	Hip abductors
		Preserve longitudinal arch of foot	Intrinsic muscles of foot
	Terminal stance (heel off)	Accelerate mass	Ankle plantarflexors (concentric contraction)
		Stabilize pelvis	Hip abductors
		Preserve arches of foot; fix forefoot	Intrinsic muscles of foot
			Long tendons of foot
	Preswing (toe off)	Accelerate mass	Long flexors of digits
		Preserve arches of foot; fix forefoot	Intrinsic muscles of foot
			Long tendons of foot
		Decelerate thigh; prepare for swing	Flexor of hip (eccentric contraction)
S W I N G P H A S E	Initial swing	Accelerate thigh, vary cadence	Flexor of hip (concentric contraction)
		Clear foot	Ankle dorsiflexors
	Midswing	Clear foot	Ankle dorsiflexors
	Terminal swing	Decelerate thigh	Hip extensors (eccentric contraction)
		Decelerate leg	Knee flexors (eccentric contraction)
		Position foot	Ankle dorsiflexors
		Extend knee to place foot (control stride); prepare for contact	Knee extensors

Modified from Rose J, Gamble JG. *Human Walking,* 2nd ed. Baltimore, Lippincott Williams & Wilkins, 1994.

Sural Nerve Grafts

Pieces of the sural nerve are often used for nerve grafts in procedures such as repairing nerve defects resulting from wounds. The surgeon is usually able to locate this nerve in relation to the small saphenous vein. Because of variations in the level of formation of the sural nerve, the surgeon may have to make incisions in both legs and then select the better specimen.

Plantar Reflex

The **plantar reflex** (L4, L5, S1, and S2 nerve roots) is a myotatic (deep tendon) reflex. The lateral aspect of the sole is stroked with a blunt object, such as a tongue depressor, beginning at the heel and crossing to the base of the great toe. Flexion of the toes is a normal response. Slight fanning of the lateral four toes and dorsiflexion of the great toe is an abnormal response (*Babinski sign*), indicating brain injury or cerebral disease, except in infants. Because the corticospinal tracts (motor function) are not fully developed in newborns, a Babinski sign is usually elicited and may be present until children are 4 years of age.

Contusion of Extensor Digitorum Brevis

Clinically, knowing the location of the belly of the extensor digitorum brevis is important for distinguishing this muscle from abnormal edema. Contusion and tearing of the muscle fibers and associated blood vessels result in a *hematoma*, producing edema anteromedial to the lateral malleolus. Most people who have not seen this inflamed muscle assume they have a severely sprained ankle.

Medial Plantar Nerve Entrapment

Compressive irritation of the medial plantar nerve as it passes deep to the flexor retinaculum or curves deep to the abductor hallucis may cause aching, burning, numbness, and tingling (paresthesia) on the medial side of the sole and in the region of the navicular tuberosity. Medial plantar nerve compression may occur during repetitive eversion of the foot (e.g., during gymnastics and running). Because of its frequency in runners, these symptoms have been called "jogger's foot."

JOINTS OF LOWER LIMB

The joints of the lower limb include the articulations of the pelvic girdle (lumbosacral joints, sacro-iliac joints, and pubic symphysis), which are discussed in Chapter 3. The remaining joints of the lower limb are the hip joint, knee joint, tibiofibular joints, ankle joint, and foot joints.

Hip Joint

The **hip joint** forms the connection between the lower limb and the pelvic girdle. It is a strong and stable multiaxial ball-and-socket type of synovial joint. The femoral head is the ball, and the acetabulum is the socket (Fig. 5.44). The hip joint is designed for stability over a wide range of movement. During standing, the entire weight of the upper body is transmitted through the hip bones to the heads and necks of the femurs.

ARTICULAR SURFACES

The round **head of the femur** articulates with the cup-like acetabulum of the hip bone. The head is covered with **articular cartilage,** except for the pit or *fovea for the ligament of the head of femur.* The rim of the acetabulum consists of a semilunar articular part covered with articular cartilage, the **lunate surface of the acetabulum.** Because the depth of the acetabulum is increased by the fibrocartilaginous **acetabular labrum** (L. *labrum,* lip) and the **transverse acetabular ligament** (bridging the *acetabular notch*), more than half of the head fits within the acetabulum (Fig. 5.44A,C). Centrally, a deep nonarticular part, the **acetabular fossa,** is thin and formed mainly by the ischium.

JOINT CAPSULE

The external **fibrous layer of the joint capsule** attaches proximally on the hip bone to the bony rim of the acetabulum and the **transverse acetabular ligament**. Distally, it attaches to the femoral neck only anteriorly at the intertrochanteric line and at the root of the greater trochanter (Fig. 5.44). Posteriorly, the fibrous layer has an arched border that crosses the neck proximal to the intertrochanteric crest but is not attached to it (Fig. 5.44B). The joint capsule covers approximately the proximal two thirds of the neck of the femur posteriorly. A protrusion of the **synovial membrane** beyond the free posterior margin of the joint capsule onto the femoral neck forms a bursa for the obturator externus tendon.

Most fibers of the fibrous layer take a spiral course from the hip bone to the intertrochanteric line; some deep fibers,

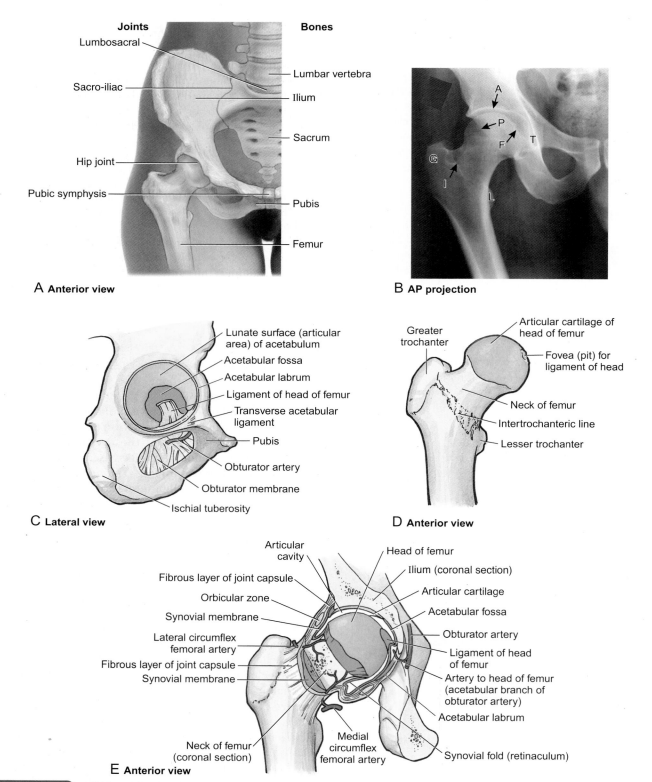

Joints

Lumbosacral

Sacro-iliac

Hip joint

Pubic symphysis

Bones

Lumbar vertebra

Ilium

Sacrum

Pubis

Femur

A **Anterior view**

B **AP projection**

Lunate surface (articular area) of acetabulum

Acetabular fossa

Acetabular labrum

Ligament of head of femur

Transverse acetabular ligament

Pubis

Obturator artery

Obturator membrane

Ischial tuberosity

C **Lateral view**

Greater trochanter

Articular cartilage of head of femur

Fovea (pit) for ligament of head

Neck of femur

Intertrochanteric line

Lesser trochanter

D **Anterior view**

Articular cavity

Fibrous layer of joint capsule

Orbicular zone

Synovial membrane

Lateral circumflex femoral artery

Fibrous layer of joint capsule

Synovial membrane

Neck of femur (coronal section)

Medial circumflex femoral artery

Head of femur

Ilium (coronal section)

Articular cartilage

Acetabular fossa

Obturator artery

Ligament of head of femur

Artery to head of femur (acetabular branch of obturator artery)

Acetabular labrum

Synovial fold (retinaculum)

E **Anterior view**

FIGURE 5.44. **Articular surfaces and blood supply of hip joint. A.** Joints and bones of pelvic girdle and hip. **B.** Radiograph of hip joint. *A,* roof of acetabulum; *F,* fovea (pit) for the ligament of the head of femur; *G,* greater trochanter; *I,* intertrochanteric crest; *L,* lesser trochanter; *P,* posterior rim of acetabulum; *T,* "teardrop" appearance caused by superimposition of structures at the inferior margin of the acetabulum. **C.** Acetabular region of hip bone. **D.** Bony features of proximal femur. **E.** Blood supply of head and neck of femur. A section of bone has been removed from the femoral neck.

Anterior inferior iliac spine

Iliofemoral ligament

Acetabular rim

Sacrospinous ligament

Sacrotuberous ligament

Obturator membrane

Intertrochanteric line

Pubofemoral ligament

A Anterior view

Greater sciatic foramen

Sacrospinous ligament

Acetabular rim

Ischiofemoral ligament

Greater trochanter

Orbicular zone

Synovial protrusion

Intertrochanteric crest

Lesser sciatic foramen

Lesser trochanter

Sacrotuberous ligament

Ischial tuberosity

B Posterior view

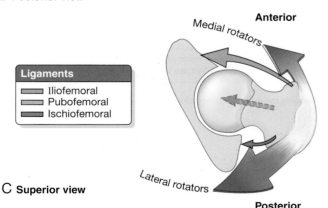

Anterior

Medial rotators

Ligaments

☐ Iliofemoral
☐ Pubofemoral
☐ Ischiofemoral

Lateral rotators

C Superior view

Posterior

FIGURE 5.45. **Ligaments of hip joint. A.** Iliofemoral and pubofemoral ligaments. **B.** Ischiofemoral ligament. **C.** Transverse section through right hip joint demonstrates the reciprocal pull of the medial and lateral rotators (*reddish brown arrows*) and the intrinsic ligaments of the hip joint (see key). Relative strengths are indicated by arrow width.

most marked in the posterior part of capsule, wind circularly around the neck, forming an **orbicular zone** (Fig. 5.45*B*). Thick parts of the fibrous layer form the ligaments of the hip joint, which pass in a spiral fashion from the pelvis to the femur. Extension winds the spiraling ligaments and fibers more tightly, constricting the capsule and drawing the femoral head tightly into the acetabulum.

The hip joint is reinforced (Fig. 5.45):

- *Anteriorly and superiorly* by the strong Y-shaped **iliofemoral ligament** (Bigelow ligament), which attaches to the anterior inferior iliac spine and acetabular rim proximally and the intertrochanteric line distally. The iliofemoral ligament prevents hyperextension of the hip joint during standing by screwing the femoral head into the acetabulum.
- *Inferiorly and anteriorly* by the **pubofemoral ligament,** which arises from the obturator crest of the pubic bone and passes laterally and inferiorly to merge with the fibrous layer of the joint capsule. This ligament blends with the medial part of the iliofemoral ligament and tightens during extension and abduction of the hip joint. The pubofemoral ligament prevents overabduction of the hip joint.
- *Posteriorly* by the weak **ischiofemoral ligament,** which arises from the ischial part of the acetabular rim and spirals superolaterally to the neck of the femur, medial to the base of the greater trochanter.

Both muscles (medial and lateral rotators of the thigh) and ligaments pull the femoral head medially into the acetabulum. They are reciprocally balanced when doing so (Fig. 5.45*C*).

The **synovial membrane of the hip joint** lines the fibrous layer as well as any intracapsular bony surfaces not lined with articular cartilage (Fig. 5.44*D*). Thus, where the fibrous layer attaches to the femur, the synovial membrane reflects proximally along the femoral neck to the edge of the femoral head. The **synovial folds** (retinacula), which reflect superiorly along the femoral neck as longitudinal bands, contain subsynovial **retinacular arteries** (branches of the medial and a few from the lateral femoral circumflex artery), which supply the head and neck of the femur. The **ligament of head of femur,** primarily a synovial fold conducting a blood vessel, is weak and of little importance in strengthening the hip joint (Fig. 5.44*E*). Its wide end attaches to the margins of the acetabular notch and the *transverse acetabular ligament;* its narrow end attaches to the femur at the *fovea for the ligament of the head of femur.* Usually, the ligament contains a small artery to the head of the femur. A fat pad in the acetabular fossa fills the part of the fossa that is not occupied by the ligament of the head of femur. Both the ligament and the fat pad are covered with synovial membrane.

Functional groups of muscles
acting at hip joint

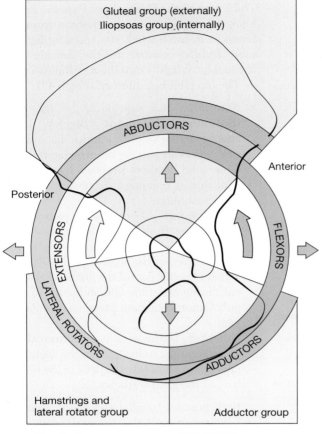

Flexors
Iliopsoas Sartorius Tensor fasciae latae Rectus femoris Pectineus Adductor longus Adductor brevis Adductor magnus, anterior part Gracilis
Adductors
Adductor longus Adductor brevis Adductor magnus Gracilis Pectineus Obturator externus
Lateral rotators
Obturator externus Obturator internus Gemelli Piriformis Quadratus femoris Gluteus maximus
Extensors

Hamstrings:
   Semitendinosus
   Semimembranosus
   Long head of biceps femoris
Adductor magnus, posterior part
Gluteus maximus

Abductors
Gluteus medius Gluteus minimus Tensor fasciae latae
Medial rotators
Gluteus medius } Gluteus minimus } Anterior parts Tensor fasciae latae

Circular Zones

Lateral view

The zones represent the position of origin of the functional groups relative to the center of the femoral head in the acetabulum (point of rotation). Pull is applied on the femur (femoral trochanters or shaft) from these positions.

Colored Arrows

The arrows show the direction of rotation of the femoral head caused by activity of the functional groups.

FIGURE 5.46. Relative positions of muscles producing movements of hip joint.

HIP MOVEMENTS

Hip movements are flexion–extension, abduction–adduction, medial–lateral rotation, and circumduction (Fig. 5.46; Table 5.15). Movements of the trunk at the hip joints are also important, such as those occurring when a person lifts the trunk from the supine position during sit-ups or keeps the pelvis level when one foot is off the ground. The degree of flexion and extension possible at the hip joint depends on the position of the knee. If the knee is flexed, relaxing the hamstrings, the thigh can be actively flexed until it almost reaches the anterior abdominal wall. Not all this movement occurs at the hip joint; some results from flexion of the vertebral column. During extension of the hip joint, the fibrous layer of the joint capsule, especially the iliofemoral ligament, is taut; therefore, the hip can usually be extended only slightly beyond the vertical except by movement of the bony

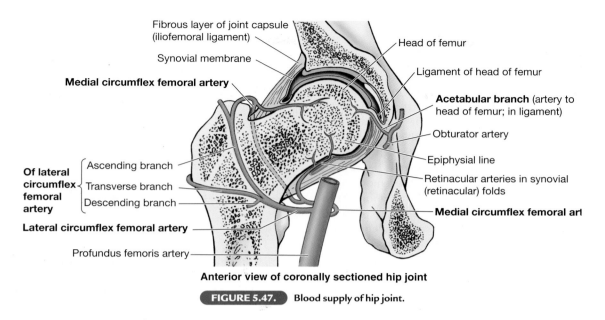

Anterior view of coronally sectioned hip joint

FIGURE 5.47. Blood supply of hip joint.

pelvis (flexion of the lumbar vertebrae). Abduction of the hip joint is usually somewhat freer than adduction. Lateral rotation is much more powerful than medial rotation.

BLOOD SUPPLY

The arteries supplying the hip joint are the (Fig. 5.47):

- **Medial** and **lateral circumflex femoral arteries,** which are usually branches of the *profunda femoris artery* but are occasionally branches of the femoral artery. The main blood supply is from the retinacular arteries arising as branches from the circumflex femoral arteries (especially the *medial circumflex femoral artery*).

- **Artery to the head of femur,** a branch of the obturator artery that traverses the ligament of the head.

NERVE SUPPLY

Hilton's law states that the nerve supplying the muscles extending directly across and acting at a given joint also innervate the joint. Therefore, the nerve supply of the hip joint is from the:

- *Femoral nerve* or its muscular branches, anteriorly.
- *Obturator nerve,* inferiorly.
- *Superior gluteal nerve,* superiorly.
- *Nerve to quadratus femoris,* posteriorly.

TABLE 5.15 STRUCTURES LIMITING MOVEMENTS OF HIP JOINT

Movement	Limiting Structures
Flexion	Soft tissue apposition Tension of joint capsule posteriorly Tension of gluteus maximus
Extension	*Ligaments:* iliofemoral, ischiofemoral, and pubofemoral Tension of iliopsoas
Abduction	*Ligaments:* pubofemoral, ischiofemoral, and inferior band of iliofemoral Tension of hip adductors
Adduction	Soft tissue apposition (thighs) Tension of iliotibial band, superior joint capsule, superior band of iliofemoral ligament, and hip abductors (especially when contralateral hip joint is abducted or flexed)
Internal rotation	*Ligaments:* ischiofemoral and posterior joint capsule Tension of external rotators of hip joint
External rotation	*Ligaments:* iliofemoral, pubofemoral, and anterior joint capsule

Modified from Clarkson HM. *Musculoskeletal Assessment. Joint Range of Motion and Manual of Muscle Strength,* 2nd ed. Baltimore: Lippincott Williams & Wilkins, 2000.

Fractures of Femoral Neck ("Hip Fractures")

Fracture of the neck of the femur often disrupts the blood supply to the head of the femur. The medial circumflex femoral artery supplies most of the blood to the head and neck of the femur. Its retinacular arteries often are torn when the femoral neck is fractured or the hip joint is dislocated. In some cases, the blood supplied to the femoral head through the artery to the ligament of the femoral head may be the only remaining source of blood to the proximal fragment. This artery is frequently inadequate for maintaining the femoral head; consequently, the fragment may undergo *aseptic vascular necrosis*, the result of deficient blood supply. These fractures are especially common in individuals older than 60 years, especially in women because their femoral necks are often weak and brittle as a result of *osteoporosis*.

Normal hip

Hip bone
Cartilage
Femur

Osteophytes and eroded articular cartilage

Hip with moderate arthritis

Hip prosthesis

FIGURE B5.14.

Surgical Hip Replacement

The hip joint is subject to severe traumatic injury and degenerative disease. *Osteoarthritis of the hip joint,* characterized by pain, edema, limitation of motion, and erosion of articular cartilage, is a common cause of disability. During hip replacement, a metal prosthesis anchored to the person's femur by bone cement replaces the femoral head and neck (Fig. B5.14). A plastic socket is cemented to the hip bone to replace the acetabulum.

Dislocation of Hip Joint

Congenital dislocation of the hip joint is common, occurring in approximately 1.5 per 1,000 live births; it affects more girls and is bilateral in approximately half the cases. Dislocation occurs when the femoral head is not properly located in the acetabulum. The affected limb appears (and functions as if) shorter because the dislocated femoral head is more superior than on the normal side, resulting in a positive *Trendelenburg sign* (hip appears to drop to one side during walking). Inability to abduct the thigh is characteristic of congenital dislocation.

Acquired dislocation of the hip joint is uncommon because this joint is so strong and stable. Nevertheless, dislocation may occur during an automobile accident when the hip is flexed, adducted, and medially rotated, the usual position of the lower limb when a person is riding in a car. Posterior dislocations are most common. The fibrous layer of the joint capsule ruptures inferiorly and posteriorly, allowing the femoral head to pass through the tear in the capsule and over the posterior margin of the acetabulum onto the lateral surface of the ilium, shortening and medially rotating the affected limb. Because of the close relationship of the *sciatic nerve* to the hip joint, it may be injured (stretched and/or compressed) during posterior dislocation or fracture–dislocation of the hip joint.

FIGURE 5.48. Bones of right knee joint. **A. and C.** Bony features. **B. and D.** Radiographs. *Letters* are defined in *A*.

Knee Joint

The knee is primarily a hinge type of synovial joint, allowing flexion and extension; however, the hinge movements are combined with gliding and rolling and with rotation about a vertical axis. Although the knee joint is well constructed, its function is commonly impaired when it is hyperextended (e.g., in body-contact sports such as hockey).

ARTICULAR SURFACES

The **articular surfaces of the knee joint** are characterized by their large size and incongruent shapes (Fig. 5.48). The knee joint consists of three articulations:

- Two **femorotibial articulations** (**lateral** and **medial**) between the lateral and the medial femoral and tibial condyles.
- One intermediate **femoropatellar articulation** between the patella and the femur.

The fibula is not involved in the knee joint. The stability of the knee joint depends on the:

- Strength and actions of surrounding muscles and their tendons.
- Ligaments connecting the femur and tibia.

Of these supports, the muscles are most important; therefore, many sport injuries are preventable through appropriate conditioning and training. The most important muscle in stabilizing the knee joint is the large *quadriceps femoris,* particularly the inferior fibers of the vastus medialis and lateralis.

JOINT CAPSULE

The **joint capsule** consists of an external *fibrous layer* (fibrous capsule) and an internal *synovial membrane* that lines all internal surfaces of the articular cavity not covered with articular cartilage.

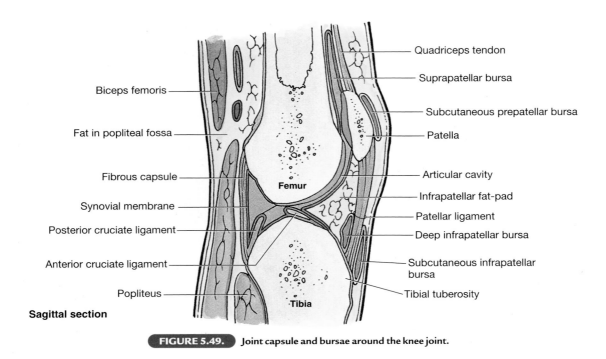

Biceps femoris

Fat in popliteal fossa

Fibrous capsule

Femur

Synovial membrane

Posterior cruciate ligament

Anterior cruciate ligament

Popliteus

Tibia

Sagittal section

Quadriceps tendon

Suprapatellar bursa

Subcutaneous prepatellar bursa

Patella

Articular cavity

Infrapatellar fat-pad

Patellar ligament

Deep infrapatellar bursa

Subcutaneous infrapatellar bursa

Tibial tuberosity

FIGURE 5.49. Joint capsule and bursae around the knee joint.

The fibrous layer has a few thickened parts that make up intrinsic ligaments but, for the most part, it is thin. The fibrous layer attaches to the femur superiorly (Fig. 5.49), just proximal to the articular margins of the condyles. Posteriorly, it encloses the condyles and the *intercondylar fossa* (Fig. 5.48C). The fibrous layer has an opening posterior to the lateral tibial condyle to allow the popliteus tendon to pass out of the joint capsule to attach to the tibia (Fig. 5.50B). Inferiorly, the fibrous layer attaches to the margin of the articular surface of the tibia (tibial plateau), except where the popliteus tendon crosses the bone. The quadriceps tendon, patella, and patellar ligament serve as a capsule anteriorly—that is, the fibrous layer is continuous with the lateral and medial margins of these structures (Fig. 5.49).

The extensive *synovial membrane* lines the internal aspect of the fibrous capsule and attaches to the periphery of the patella and the edges of the *menisci* (Fig. 5.49). It lines the fibrous layer laterally and medially, but centrally it becomes separated from the fibrous layer. The synovial membrane reflects from the posterior aspect of the joint anteriorly into the intercondylar region, covering the cruciate ligaments and the **infrapatellar fat pad,** so they are excluded from the articular cavity (Fig. 5.49). This creates a median infrapatellar synovial fold, a vertical fold of synovial membrane that approaches the posterior aspect of the patella. Thus, it almost subdivides the articular cavity into right and left femorotibial articular cavities. Fat-filled lateral and medial alar folds of synovial membrane extend into the joint from the infrapatellar fold. More reflections or plicae have been identified with arthroscopy. If these plicae

become inflamed they can cause pain on movement and may be arthroscopically removed.

Superior to the patella, the knee joint cavity extends deep to the vastus intermedius as the **suprapatellar bursa.** The synovial membrane of the joint capsule is continuous with the synovial lining of this bursa (Fig. 5.49). Muscle slips deep to the vastus intermedius form the *articularis genu muscle* (articular muscle of the knee), which attaches to the synovial membrane and retracts the suprapatellar bursa during extension of the knee.

LIGAMENTS

The joint capsule is strengthened by five extracapsular or capsular (intrinsic) ligaments (Fig. 5.50): patellar ligament, fibular collateral ligament, tibial collateral ligament, oblique popliteal ligament, and arcuate popliteal ligament.

The **patellar ligament,** the distal part of the quadriceps tendon, is a strong, thick fibrous band passing from the apex and adjoining margins of the patella to the tibial tuberosity. Laterally, it receives the *medial* and *lateral patellar retinacula,* aponeurotic expansions of the vastus medialis and lateralis and overlying deep fascia. The retinacula play an important role in maintaining alignment of the patella relative to the patellar articular surface of the femur. The *collateral ligaments of the knee* are taut when the knee is fully extended; however, as flexion proceeds, they become increasingly slack, permitting rotation at the knee.

The **fibular collateral ligament** (FCL), rounded and cord-like, is strong. It extends inferiorly from the lateral

A **Anterior view**

B **Posterior view**

FIGURE 5.50. **Relations and ligaments of knee joint. A.** Anterior view of flexed knee with patellar ligament cut and reflected superiorly. **B.** Posterior view.

epicondyle of femur to the lateral surface of the head of the fibula (Fig. 5.50*A*,*B*). The tendon of the popliteus passes deep to the FCL, separating it from the lateral meniscus. The tendon of the biceps femoris is split into two parts by this ligament.

The **tibial collateral ligament** (TCL) is a strong flat band that extends from the medial epicondyle of the femur to the medial condyle and superior part of the medial surface of the tibia. At its midpoint, the deep fibers of the TCL are firmly attached to the medial meniscus.

The **oblique popliteal ligament** is a reflected expansion of the tendon of the semimembranosus that strengthens the joint capsule posteriorly. It arises posterior to the medial tibial condyle and passes superolaterally to attach to the central part of the posterior aspect of the joint capsule.

The **arcuate popliteal ligament** arises from the posterior aspect of the fibular head, passes superomedially over the tendon of the popliteus, and spreads over the posterior surface of the knee joint.

The *intra-articular structures* within the knee joint consist of the cruciate ligaments and menisci. The popliteus tendon is also intra-articular during part of its course.

The **cruciate ligaments** (L. *crux*, a cross) join the femur and tibia, criss-crossing within the joint capsule but outside the articular cavity (Figs. 5.50 and 5.51). The cruciate ligaments cross each other obliquely like the letter *X*. During medial rotation of the tibia on the femur, the cruciate ligaments wind around each other; thus, the amount of medial rotation possible is limited to about 10 degrees. Because

they become unwound during lateral rotation, nearly 60 degrees of lateral rotation is possible when the knee is flexed more than 90 degrees. The crossing-over point of the cruciate ligaments serves as the pivot for rotatory movements at the knee. Because of their oblique orientation, in every position one cruciate ligament, or parts of one or both ligaments, is tense.

The **anterior cruciate ligament** (ACL), the weaker of the two cruciate ligaments, arises from the anterior intercondylar area of the tibia, just posterior to the attachment of the medial meniscus (Fig. 5.51). It extends superiorly, posteriorly, and laterally to attach to the posterior part of the medial side of the lateral condyle of the femur. The ACL has a relatively poor blood supply and limits posterior rolling of the femoral condyles on the tibial plateau during flexion, converting it to spin. It also prevents posterior displacement of the femur on the tibia and hyperextension of the knee joint. When the joint is flexed at a right angle, the tibia cannot be pulled anteriorly because it is held by the ACL.

The **posterior cruciate ligament** (PCL), the stronger of the two cruciate ligaments, arises from the posterior intercondylar area of the tibia (Fig. 5.51). The PCL passes superiorly and anteriorly on the medial side of the ACL to attach to the anterior part of the lateral surface of the medial condyle of the femur. The PCL limits anterior rolling of the femur on the tibial plateau during extension, converting it to spin. It also prevents anterior displacement of the femur on the tibia or posterior displacement of the tibia on the femur and helps prevent hyperflexion of the

FIGURE 5.51. Cruciate ligaments and menisci of knee joint. **A.** Anterior cruciate ligament. **B.** Posterior cruciate ligament. In **A.** and **B.** the femur has been sectioned longitudinally and the near half has been removed with the proximal part of the corresponding cruciate ligament. **C.** Attachments to tibial plateau. The patella and quadriceps tendon are transected, and the patellar fragment and patellar ligament are reflected anteriorly. **D.** The numbers on this MRI image of the right knee are defined in part **C.**

knee joint. In the weight-bearing flexed knee, the PCL is the main stabilizing factor for the femur (e.g., when walking downhill).

The **menisci of the knee joint** are crescentic plates of fibrocartilage on the articular surface of the tibia that deepen the surface and play a role in shock absorption (Fig. 5.51*C*). The menisci are thicker at their external margins and taper to thin, unattached edges in the interior of the joint. Wedge-shaped in transverse section, the menisci are firmly attached at their ends to the *intercondylar area of the tibia.* Their external margins attach to the fibrous layer of the capsule of the knee joint. The **coronary ligaments** are capsular fibers that attach the margins of the menisci to the tibial condyles. A slender fibrous band, the **transverse ligament of knee,** joins the anterior edges of the menisci (Fig. 5.51*C*), allowing them to move together during knee movements. The **medial meniscus** is C-shaped and broader posteriorly than anteriorly. Its anterior end (horn) attaches to the anterior intercondylar area of the tibia, anterior to the attachment of the ACL. Its posterior end attaches to the posterior intercondylar area, anterior

to the attachment of the PCL. The medial meniscus firmly adheres to the deep surface of the tibial collateral ligament. The **lateral meniscus** is nearly circular and is smaller and more freely movable than the medial meniscus. The tendon of the popliteus separates the lateral meniscus from the fibular collateral ligament. A strong tendinous slip, the **posterior meniscofemoral ligament,** joins the lateral meniscus to the PCL and the medial femoral condyle (Fig. 5.50*B*).

MOVEMENTS OF KNEE JOINT

Flexion and extension are the main knee movements; some rotation occurs when the knee is flexed (Table 5.16). When the leg is fully extended with the foot on the ground, the knee passively "locks" because of medial rotation of the femur on the tibia. This position makes the lower limb a solid column and more adapted for weight bearing. When the knee is "locked", the thigh and leg muscles can relax briefly without making the knee joint too unstable. To "unlock" the knee, the popliteus contracts, rotating the femur laterally

TABLE 5.16 STRUCTURES LIMITING MOVEMENTS OF KNEE JOINT

Movement	Limiting Structures
Flexion (femoropatellar and femorotibial)	Soft tissue apposition posteriorly Tension of vastus lateralis, medialis, and intermedius Tension of rectus femoris (especially with hip joint extended)
Extension (femoropatellar and femorotibial)	*Ligaments:* anterior cruciate and posterior cruciate, fibular and tibial collateral, posterior joint capsule, and oblique popliteal ligament
Internal rotation (femorotibial with knee flexed)	*Ligaments:* anterior cruciate and posterior cruciate
External rotation (femorotibial with knee flexed)	*Ligaments:* fibular and tibial collateral

Modified from Clarkson HM: *Musculoskeletal Assessment. Joint Range of Motion and Manual of Muscle Strength,* 2nd ed. Baltimore: Lippincott Williams & Wilkins, 2000.

about 5 degrees on the tibial plateau so that flexion of the knee can occur. The menisci must be able to move on the tibial plateau as the points of contact between the femur and the tibia change.

Three paired facets (superior, middle, and inferior) on the posterior surface of the patella articulate with the patellar surface of the femur successively during flexion and extension of the knee (Fig. 5.52).

BURSAE AROUND KNEE

There are at least 12 bursae around the knee joint because most tendons run parallel to the bones and pull lengthwise across the joint during knee movements (Fig. 5.53; Table 5.17). The **subcutaneous prepatellar** and **infrapatellar bursae** are located at the convex surface of the joint, allowing the skin to be able to move freely during knee movements. Four bursae communicate with the articular cavity of the knee joint: **suprapatellar bursa** (deep to the distal quadriceps), *popliteus bursa, anserine bursa,* and *gastrocnemius bursa.*

ARTERIES AND NERVES OF KNEE JOINT

The genicular branches that form the periarticular **genicular anastomosis** around the knee are from the femoral, popliteal, anterior and posterior recurrent branches of the anterior tibial, and circumflex fibular arteries (Fig. 5.25C,D). The middle genicular branches of the popliteal artery penetrate the fibrous layer of the joint capsule and supply the cruciate ligaments, synovial membrane, and peripheral margins of the menisci.

The *nerves of the knee joint* are articular branches from the femoral, tibial, and common fibular nerves and the obturator and saphenous nerves.

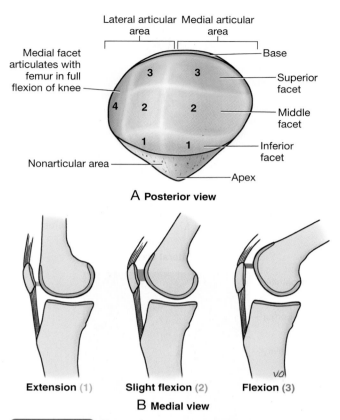

FIGURE 5.52. **Femoropatellar articulation. A.** Articular surfaces of patella. **B.** Articulation of patella with femur during flexion and extension of knee.

Tibiofibular Joints

The tibia and fibula are connected by two joints: the *superior tibiofibular joint* and the *tibiofibular syndesmosis* (inferior tibiofibular joint). In addition, an *interosseous membrane* joins the shafts of the two bones (Fig. 5.54). Movement at the proximal joint is impossible without movement at the distal one. The fibers of the interosseous membrane and all ligaments of tibiofibular articulations run inferiorly from the tibia to the fibula, resisting the downward pull placed on the fibula by most muscles attached to it. However, they allow slight upward movement of the fibula during dorsiflexion of the ankle.

The **superior tibiofibular joint** is a plane type of synovial joint between the flat facet on the fibular head and a similar facet located posterolaterally on the lateral tibial condyle. The tense joint capsule surrounds the joint and attaches to the margins of the articular surfaces of the fibula and tibia. The joint capsule is strengthened by **anterior** and **posterior ligaments of head of fibula** (Fig. 5.54B). The synovial membrane lines the fibrous capsule. Slight gliding movements occur during dorsiflexion of the foot.

The **tibiofibular syndesmosis** is a compound fibrous joint (Fig. 5.54C). The integrity of this articulation is

FIGURE 5.53. Bursae around knee joint and proximal leg.

TABLE 5.17 BURSAE AROUND KNEE JOINT

Bursae	Locations	Comments
Suprapatellar	Between femur and tendon of quadriceps femoris	Held in position by articular muscle of knee; communicates freely with synovial cavity of knee joint
Popliteus	Between tendon of popliteus and lateral condyle of tibia	Opens into synovial cavity of knee joint inferior to lateral meniscus
Anserine	Separates tendons of sartorius, gracilis, and semitendinosus from tibia and tibial collateral ligament	Area where tendons of these muscles attach to tibia; resembles a goose's foot (L. *pes*, foot; L. *anserinus*, goose)
Gastrocnemius	Lies deep to proximal attachment of tendon of medial head of gastrocnemius	An extension of synovial cavity of knee joint
Semimembranosus	Between medial head of gastrocnemius and semimembranosus tendon	Related to distal attachment of semimembranosus
Subcutaneous prepatellar	Between skin and anterior surface of patella	Allows free movement of skin over patella during movements of leg
Subcutaneous infrapatellar	Between skin and tibial tuberosity	Helps knee withstand pressure when kneeling
Deep infrapatellar	Between patellar ligament and anterior surface of tibia	Separated from knee joint by infrapatellar fat pad

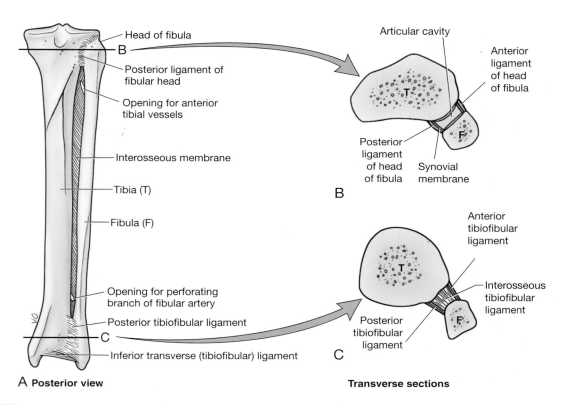

A Posterior view

Transverse sections

Head of fibula

B

Posterior ligament of fibular head

Opening for anterior tibial vessels

Interosseous membrane

Tibia (T)

Fibula (F)

Opening for perforating branch of fibular artery

Posterior tibiofibular ligament

C

Inferior transverse (tibiofibular) ligament

Articular cavity

Anterior ligament of head of fibula

Posterior ligament of head of fibula

Synovial membrane

B

Anterior tibiofibular ligament

Interosseous tibiofibular ligament

Posterior tibiofibular ligament

C

FIGURE 5.54. Tibiofibular joints. **A.** Superior tibiofibular joint and tibiofibular syndesmosis, posterior view. The level of the transverse sections shown in parts **B** and **C** are identified. **B.** Transverse section through the superior tibiofibular joint. **C.** Transverse section through the tibiofibular syndesmosis. *F*, fibula; *T*, tibia.

essential for stability of the ankle joint because it keeps the lateral malleolus firmly against the lateral surface of the talus. The strong **interosseous tibiofibular ligament** is continuous superiorly with the interosseous membrane and forms the principal connection between the distal ends of the tibia and fibula. The joint is also strengthened anteriorly and posteriorly by the **anterior** and **posterior tibiofibular ligaments.** The

distal, deep continuation of the posterior inferior tibiofibular ligament, the **inferior transverse (tibiofibular) ligament,** forms a strong connection between the medial and lateral malleoli and the posterior "wall" of the malleolar mortise, for the trochlea (superior articular surface) of the talus (see Fig. 5.55B). Slight movement of the joint occurs to accommodate the talus during dorsiflexion of the foot.

Genu Varum and Genu Valgum

The femur is placed diagonally within the thigh, whereas the tibia is almost vertical within the leg, creating an angle, the **Q-angle,** at the knee between the long axes of the bones. The Q-angle is assessed by drawing a line from the ASIS to the middle of the patella and extrapolating a second (vertical) line through the middle of the patella and tibial tuberosity (Fig. B5.15A). The Q-angle is typically greater in adult females, owing to their wider pelves. A medial angulation of the leg in relation to the thigh, in which the femur is abnormally vertical and the Q-angle

is small, is a deformity called *genu varum* (bowleg) that causes unequal weight distribution (Fig. B5.15B). Excess pressure is placed on the medial aspect of the knee joint, which results in *arthrosis* (destruction of knee cartilage). A lateral angulation of the leg (Fig. B5.15C) in relation to the thigh (exaggeration of knee angle) is *genu valgum* (knock-knee). Consequently, in genu valgum, excess stress is placed on the lateral structures of the knee. The patella, normally pulled laterally by the tendon of the vastus lateralis, is pulled even farther laterally when the leg is extended in the presence of genu varum so that its articulation with the femur is abnormal.

FIGURE B5.15. Alignment of lower limb bones. Normal alignment (**A**), genu varum (**B**), and genu valgum (**C**) are shown. *ASIS,* anterior superior iliac spine.

Patellofemoral Syndrome

Pain deep to the patella often results from excessive running, especially downhill; hence, this type of pain is often called "runner's knee." The pain results from repetitive microtrauma caused by abnormal tracking of the patella relative to the patellar surface of the femur, a condition known as the **patellofemoral syndrome.** This syndrome may also result from a direct blow to the patella and from **osteoarthritis of the patellofemoral compartment** (degenerative wear and tear of articular cartilages). In some cases, strengthening of the vastus medialis corrects *patellofemoral dysfunction.* This muscle tends to prevent lateral dislocation of the patella resulting from the Q-angle because the vastus medialis attaches to and pulls on the medial border of the patella. Hence, weakness of the vastus medialis predisposes the individual to patellofemoral dysfunction and patellar dislocation.

Patellar Dislocation

When the patella is dislocated, it nearly always dislocates laterally. Patellar dislocation is more common in women, presumably because of their greater Q-angle, which, in addition to representing the oblique placement of the femur relative to the tibia, represents the angle of pull of the quadriceps relative to the axis of the patella and tibia (the term *Q-angle* was actually coined in reference to

the angle of pull of the quadriceps). The tendency toward lateral dislocation is normally counterbalanced by the medial, more horizontal pull of the powerful vastus medialis. In addition, the more anterior projection of the lateral femoral condyle and deeper slope for the larger lateral patellar facet provide a mechanical deterrent to lateral dislocation. An imbalance of the lateral pull and the mechanisms resisting it results in abnormal tracking of the patella within the patellar groove and chronic patellar pain, even if actual dislocation does not occur.

Popliteal Cysts

Popliteal cysts (Baker cysts) are abnormal fluid-filled sacs of synovial membrane in the region of the popliteal fossa. A popliteal cyst is almost always a complication of chronic knee joint effusion. The cyst may be a herniation of the gastrocnemius or semimembranosus bursa through the fibrous layer of the joint capsule into the popliteal fossa, communicating with the synovial cavity of the knee joint by a narrow stalk. Synovial fluid may also escape from the knee joint (*synovial effusion*) or a bursa around the knee and collect in the popliteal fossa. Here it forms a new synovial-lined sac, or popliteal cyst. Popliteal cysts are common in children but seldom cause symptoms. In adults, popliteal cysts can be large, extending as far as the midcalf, and may interfere with knee movements.

Knee Joint Injuries

Knee joint injuries are common because the knee is a low-placed, mobile, weight-bearing joint and its stability depends almost entirely on its associated ligaments and muscles. The most common knee injuries in contact sports are ligament sprains, which occur when the foot is fixed on the ground. If a force is applied against the knee when the foot cannot move, ligament injuries are likely to occur. The tibial (TCL) and fibular (FCL) collateral ligaments are tightly stretched when the leg is extended, preventing disruption of the sides of the joint. The firm attach-

ment of the TCL to the medial meniscus is of clinical significance because tearing of this ligament frequently results in concomitant tearing of the medial meniscus. The injury is frequently caused by a blow to the lateral side of the extended knee or excessive lateral twisting of the flexed knee, which disrupts the TCL and concomitantly tears and/or detaches the medial meniscus from the joint capsule. This injury is common in athletes who twist their flexed knees while running (e.g., in football and soccer). The anterior cruciate ligament (ACL), which serves as a pivot for rotatory movements of the knee, is taut during flexion and may also tear subsequent to the rupture of the TCL, creating an

Anterior cruciate ligament (torn)
Tibial collateral ligament (torn)
Medial meniscus (torn)

A **"Unhappy triad" of knee injuries**

B **Anterior drawer sign (ACL)**

Half of bone is removed to show ligaments

Anterior cruciate ligament (torn)

The anterior cruciate ligament (*ACL*) prevents the femur from sliding posteriorly on the tibia and hyperextension of the knee and limits medial rotation of the femur when the foot is on the ground and the leg is flexed.

C **Posterior drawer sign (PCL)**

Posterior cruciate ligament (torn)

The posterior cruciate ligament (*PCL*) prevents the femur from sliding anteriorly on the tibia, particularly when the knee is flexed.

FIGURE B5.16.

Normal lateral meniscus of the knee

ACL graft (*black arrow*) with femoral anchoring screw visible (*white arrow*)

Trimming of a torn lateral meniscus (*LM*)

D

Metal femoral component

Plastic tibial component

Metal tibial component

E

F Prepatellar bursitis

FIGURE B5.16. (*continued*)

"unhappy triad" of injuries (Fig. B5.16A). *ACL rupture,* one of the most common knee injuries in skiing accidents, for example, causes the free tibia to slide anteriorly under the femur, a sign known as the *anterior drawer sign* (Fig. 5.16B). Although strong, posterior cruciate ligament (*PCL*) *rupture* may occur when a person lands on the tibial tuberosity when the knee is

flexed. PCL ruptures usually occur in conjunction with tibial or fibular ligament tears. The *posterior drawer sign,* in which the free tibia slides posteriorly under the fixed femur, occurs as a result of PCL rupture (Fig. B5.16C).

Arthroscopy of Knee Joint

Arthroscopy is an endoscopic examination that allows visualization of the interior of the knee joint cavity with minimal disruption of tissue (Fig. B5.16D). The arthroscope and one (or more) additional cannula(e) are inserted through tiny incisions known as portals. The second cannula is for passage of specialized tools (e.g., manipulative probes or forceps) or equipment for trimming, shaping, or removing damaged tissue. This technique allows removal of torn menisci and loose bodies in the joint such as bone chips, and débridement (the excision of devitalized articular cartilaginous material in advanced cases of arthritis). Ligament repair or replacement may also be performed using an arthroscope.

Knee Replacement

If a person's knee is diseased (from osteoarthritis, for example), an artificial knee joint may be inserted (*total knee replacement arthroplasty*) (Fig. B5.16E). The artificial knee joint consists of plastic and metal components that are cemented to the femoral and tibial bone ends after removal of the defective areas.

Bursitis in Knee Region

Prepatellar bursitis ("housemaid's knee") is usually a friction bursitis caused by friction between the skin and the patella. If the inflammation is chronic, the bursa becomes distended with fluid and forms a swelling anterior to the knee (Fig. B5.16F). *Subcutaneous infrapatellar bursitis* results from excessive friction between the skin and the tibial tuberosity; the edema occurs over the proximal end of the tibia. *Deep infrapatellar bursitis* results in edema between the patellar ligament and the tibia, superior to the tibial tuberosity.

The suprapatellar bursa communicates with the articular cavity of the knee joint; consequently, abrasions or penetrating wounds (e.g., a stab wound) superior to the patella may result in *suprapatellar bursitis* caused by bacteria entering the bursa from the torn skin. The infection may spread to the knee joint.

A **Anterior view**   **Posterior view**

FIGURE 5.55. Bones of leg and ankle joint. **A.** Bones in situ. **B.** Posteroanterior radiograph. **C.** Lateral radiograph.

B **Posteroanterior view (slightly oblique)**

C **Lateral view**

Ankle Joint

The **ankle joint (talocrural articulation)** is a hinge-type synovial joint. It is located between the distal ends of the tibia and fibula and the superior part of the talus (Fig. 5.55).

ARTICULAR SURFACES

The distal ends of the tibia and fibula (along with the inferior transverse part of the posterior tibiofibular ligament) form a *malleolar mortise* (deep socket) into which the pulley-shaped *trochlea of the talus* fits (Fig. 5.55*B*). The **trochlea** (L. pulley) is the rounded superior articular surface of the talus. The medial surface of the lateral malleolus articulates with the lateral surface of the talus. The tibia articulates with the talus in two places:

- Its inferior surface forms the roof of the malleolar mortise, transferring the body's weight to the talus.
- Its medial malleolus articulates with the medial surface of the talus.

The malleoli grip the talus tightly as it rocks in the mortise during movements of the ankle joint. The grip of the malleoli on the trochlea is strongest during dorsiflexion of the foot because this movement forces the wider, anterior part of the trochlea posteriorly, spreading the tibia and fibula slightly apart. This spreading is limited by the strong interosseous tibiofibular ligament and the anterior and posterior tibiofibu-lar ligaments that unite the tibia and fibula. The ankle joint is relatively unstable during plantarflexion because the trochlea is narrower posteriorly and therefore lies loosely within the mortise during plantarflexion.

JOINT CAPSULE

The joint capsule is thin anteriorly and posteriorly but is supported on each side by strong collateral ligaments (Fig. 5.56). The fibrous layer of the capsule is attached superiorly to the borders of the articular surfaces of the tibia and malleoli and inferiorly to the talus. The synovial membrane lining the fibrous layer of the joint capsule extends superiorly between the tibia and the fibula as far as the interosseous tibiofibular ligament.

Fibula

Anteror tibiofiular ligament

Anterior talofibular ligament

Interosseous talocalcaneal ligament

Posterior tibiofibular ligament

Lateral malleolus

Posterior talofibular ligament

Calcaneofibular ligament

Bifurcate ligament

Lateral talocalcaneal ligament

Cuboid

Calcaneus

A **Lateral view**

Medial malleolus

Tibia

Anterior tibiotalar part of medial ligament of ankle

Talus

Posterior tibiotalar
Tibionavicular
Tibiocalcaneal — Parts of medial ligament of ankle

Navicular

Spring ligament

Medial talocalcaneal ligament

Sustenaculum tali

Calcaneus

B **Medial view**

Long plantar ligament

Tibia

Fibula

Interosseous membrane

Groove for tibialis posterior and flexor digitorum longus

Posterior tibiofibular ligament

Inferior transverse ligament

Medial malleolus

Talus

Tibial fibers of posterior talofibular ligament

Parts of medial ligament of ankle [Posterior tibiotalar — Tibiocalcaneal —

Lateral malleolus

Groove for tendon of flexor hallucis longus

Posterior talofibular ligament

Sustenaculum tali

Calcaneofibular ligament

Medial and posterior talocalcaneal ligaments

Calcaneal tendon

Calcaneus

C **Posterior view**

FIGURE 5.56. Ligaments of ankle and talocalcaneal joints.

LIGAMENTS

The ankle joint is reinforced laterally by the **lateral ligament of the ankle,** which consists of three separate ligaments (Fig. 5.56*A,C*):

- **Anterior talofibular ligament,** a flat, weak band that extends anteromedially from the lateral malleolus to the neck of the talus.
- **Posterior talofibular ligament,** a thick, fairly strong band that runs horizontally medially, and slightly posteriorly from the malleolar fossa of the fibula to the lateral tubercle of the talus.

- **Calcaneofibular ligament,** a round cord that passes posteroinferiorly from the tip of the lateral malleolus to the lateral surface of the calcaneus.

The joint capsule of the ankle joint is reinforced medially by the large, strong **medial ligament of the ankle** (deltoid ligament) that attaches proximally to the medial malleolus and fans out from it to attach distally to the talus, calcaneus, and navicular via four adjacent and continuous parts (Fig. 5.56): the **tibionavicular part,** the **tibiocalcaneal part,** and the **anterior** and **posterior tibiotalar parts.** The medial ligament stabilizes the ankle joint during eversion of

Medial malleolus
Medial ligament of ankle
Sustentaculum tali
Tibialis posterior
Flexor digitorum longus
Flexor hallucis longus
Medial plantar nerve and artery
Abductor hallucis
Quadratus plantae
Lateral plantar nerve and artery
Flexor digitorum brevis

Tibia
Fibula
Talus
Calcaneus

Interosseous membrane
Ankle joint
Trochlea of talus
Posterior talofibular ligament
Lateral malleolus
Subtalar joint
Fibularis brevis
Fibularis longus
Abductor digiti minimi
Fat

Coronal section

FIGURE 5.57.   Ankle and subtalar joints, coronal section.

the foot and prevents subluxation (partial dislocation) of the ankle joint.

MOVEMENTS

The main movements of the ankle joint are dorsiflexion and plantarflexion of the foot. When the foot is plantarflexed, some "wobble" (small amounts of abduction, adduction, inversion, and eversion) is possible in this unstable position. Structures limiting movements of the ankle joint are outlined in Table 5.18.

- *Dorsiflexion of the ankle* is produced by muscles in the anterior compartment of the leg (Table 5.8). Dorsiflexion is usually limited by passive resistance of the triceps surae to stretching and by tension in the medial and lateral ligaments.
- *Plantarflexion of ankle* is produced by muscles in the posterior and lateral compartments of the leg (Table 5.9).

ARTERIES AND NERVES

The arteries are derived from malleolar branches of the fibular and anterior and posterior tibial arteries. The nerves are derived from the tibial nerve and deep fibular nerve.

Tibial Nerve Entrapment

Entrapment and compression of the tibial nerve (*tarsal tunnel syndrome*) occurs when there is edema and tightness in the ankle involving the synovial sheaths of the tendons of muscles in the posterior compartment of the leg. The area involved is from the medial malleolus to the calcaneus. The heel pain results from compression of the tibial nerve by the flexor retinaculum.

Ankle Sprains

The ankle is the most frequently injured major joint in the body. *Ankle sprains* (torn fibers of ligaments) are most common. A sprained ankle is nearly always an *inversion injury,* involving twisting of the weight-bearing plantarflexed foot. The *anterior talofibular ligament* (part of the lateral ligament) is most commonly torn during ankle sprains, either partially or completely, resulting in instability of the ankle joint. The *calcaneofibular ligament* may also be torn.

TABLE 5.18   STRUCTURES LIMITING MOVEMENTS OF ANKLE JOINT

Movement	Limiting Structures
Plantarflexion	*Ligaments:* anterior talofibular, anterior part of medial, anterior joint capsule Contact of talus with tibia Tension of dorsiflexors of ankle
Dorsiflexion	*Ligaments:* medial, calcaneofibular, posterior talofibular, posterior joint capsule Contact of talus with tibia Tension of plantarflexors of ankle

Modified from Clarkson HM. *Musculoskeletal Assessment. Joint Range of Motion and Manual of Muscle Strength,* 2nd ed. Baltimore: Lippincott Williams & Wilkins, 2000.

Pott Fracture–Dislocation of Ankle

A **Pott fracture–dislocation of the ankle** occurs when the foot is forcibly everted. This action pulls on the extremely strong medial ligament, often tearing off the medial malleolus (Fig. B5.17). The talus then moves laterally, shearing off the lateral malleolus or, more commonly, breaking the fibula superior to the tibiofibular syndesmosis. If the tibia is carried anteriorly, the posterior margin of the distal end of the tibia is also sheared off by the talus.

Tibial (*T*) and fibular (*F*) fractures

Fibular fracture with excessive inversion of foot

Posterior views

FIGURE B5.17.

- First metatarsal
- Fibularis longus (tendon)
- Medial cuneiform
- **Plantar calcaneonavicular (spring) ligament**
- Medial ligament of ankle
- Sustentaculum tali
- **Plantar calcaneocuboid ligament (short plantar ligament)**
- **Long plantar ligament**
- Calcaneous

Plantar surface

FIGURE 5.58. **Plantar ligaments.** Deep dissection of right foot.

Joints of Foot

The joints of the foot involve the tarsals, metatarsals, and phalanges (Figs. 5.57 and 5.59; Table 5.19). The important intertarsal joints are the *subtalar (talocalcaneal) joint* and the *transverse tarsal joint (calcaneocuboid and talonavicular joints)*. Inversion and eversion of the foot are the main movements involving these joints. The other intertarsal joints and the *tarsometatarsal* and *intermetatarsal joints* are relatively small and are so tightly joined by ligaments that only slight movement occurs between them. In the foot, flexion and extension occurs in the forefoot at the metatarsophalangeal and interphalangeal joints. All of the foot bones proximal to the metatarsophalangeal joints are united by dorsal and plantar ligaments.

The **subtalar joint** occurs where the talus rests on and articulates with the calcaneus (Fig. 5.57). The subtalar joint is a synovial joint that is surrounded by a weak joint capsule, which is supported by medial, lateral, posterior, and interosseous *talocalcaneal ligaments*. The **interosseous talocalcaneal ligament** lies within the *tarsal sinus*, which separates the subtalar and calcaneonavicular joints and is especially strong. The **transverse tarsal joint** is a compound joint formed by the **talonavicular part of the talocalcaneonavicular** and the **calcaneocuboid joints**—two separate joints aligned transversely. Transection across the transverse tarsal joint is a standard method for *surgical amputation of the foot*.

The major ligaments of the plantar aspect of the foot are (Fig. 5.58) the:

- **Plantar calcaneonavicular (spring) ligament,** which extends across and fills a wedge-shaped gap between the sustentaculum tali and the inferior margin of the posterior articular surface of the navicular. This ligament supports the head of the talus and plays important roles in the transfer of weight from the talus and in maintaining the longitudinal arch of the foot.
- **Long plantar ligament,** which passes from the plantar surface of the calcaneus to the groove on the cuboid. Some of its fibers extend to the bases of the metatarsals, thereby forming a tunnel for the tendon of the fibularis longus. The long plantar ligament is important in maintaining the longitudinal arch of the foot.
- **Plantar calcaneocuboid (short plantar) ligament,** which is located deep to the long plantar ligament. It extends from the anterior aspect of the inferior surface of the calcaneus to the inferior surface of the cuboid. It is also involved in maintaining the longitudinal arch of the foot.

The structures limiting movements of the feet and toes are summarized in Table 5.20.

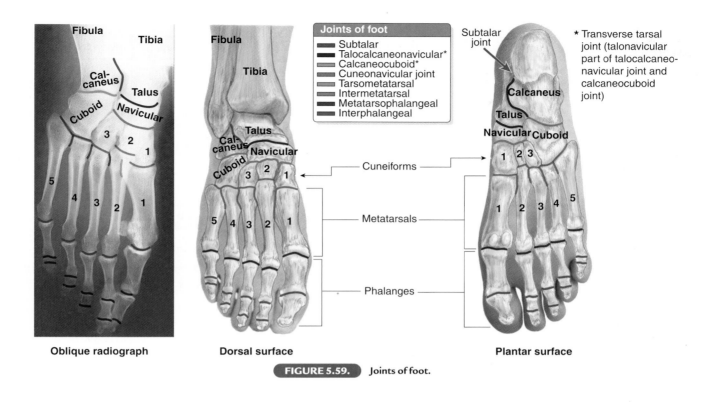

FIGURE 5.59. Joints of foot.

TABLE 5.19 JOINTS OF FOOT

Joint	Articulating Surfaces	Joint Capsule	Ligaments	Blood Supply	Nerve Supply
Subtalar (talocalcaneal, anatomical subtalar joint) *Type:* Plane synovial joint *Movements:* Inversion and eversion of foot	Inferior surface of body of talus (posterior calcaneal articular facet) articulates with superior surface (posterior talar articular surface) of calcaneus	Attached to margins of articular surfaces	Medial, lateral, and posterior talocalcaneal ligaments support capsule; interosseous talocalcaneal ligament binds bones together	Posterior tibial and fibular arteries	
Talocalcaneonavicular *Type:* Synovial joint; talonavicular part is ball-and-socket type *Movements:* Gliding and rotatory	Head of talus articulates with calcaneus and navicular bones	Incompletely encloses joint	Plantar calcaneonavicular (spring) ligament supports head of talus		*Plantar aspect:* medial or lateral plantar nerve *Dorsal aspect:* deep fibular nerve
Calcaneocuboid *Type:* Plane synovial joint *Movements:* Inversion and eversion of foot; circumduction	Anterior end of calcaneus articulates with posterior surface of cuboid	Encloses joint	Dorsal and plantar calcaneocuboid, and long plantar ligaments support joint capsule	Anterior tibial artery via lateral tarsal artery, a branch of dorsal artery of the foot	
Cuneonavicular joint *Type:* Plane synovial joint *Movements:* Little	Anterior navicular articulates with bases of cuneiform bones	Common capsule encloses joint	Dorsal and plantar cuneonavicular ligaments		
Tarsometatarsal *Type:* Plane synovial joint(s) *Movements:* Gliding or sliding	Anterior tarsal bones articulate with bases of metatarsal bones	Separate joint capsules enclose each joint	Dorsal, plantar, and interosseous tarsometatarsal ligaments bind bones together		Deep fibular; medial and lateral plantar nerves; sural nerve

TABLE 5.19 JOINTS OF FOOT (*continued*)

Joint	Articulating Surfaces	Joint Capsule	Ligaments	Blood Supply	Nerve Supply
Intermetatarsal *Type:* Plane synovial joint *Movements:* Little	Bases of metatarsal bones articulate with each other	Separate joint capsules enclose each joint	Dorsal, plantar, and interosseous tarsometatarsal ligaments bind bones together	Lateral metatarsal artery, (a branch of dorsalis pedis artery of foot)	Digital nerves
Metatarsophalangeal *Type:* Condyloid synovial joint *Movements:* Flexion, extension, and some abduction, adduction, and circumduction	Heads of metatarsal bones articulate with bases of proximal phalanges		Collateral ligaments support capsule on each side; plantar ligaments support plantar part of capsule		
Interphalangeal *Type:* Hinge synovial joint *Movements:* Flexion and extension	Head of one phalanx articulates with base of one distal to it		Collateral and plantar ligaments support joints	Digital branches of plantar arch	

TABLE 5.20 STRUCTURES LIMITING MOVEMENTS OF FOOT AND TOES

Movement	Joint	Limiting Structures
Inversion	Subtalar, transverse tarsal	*Ligaments:* lateral ligament of ankle, talocalcaneal ligament, lateral joint capsule Tension of evertor muscles of ankle
Eversion	Subtalar, transverse tarsal	*Ligaments:* medial ligament of ankle, medial talocalcaneal ligament, medial joint capsule Tension of tibialis posterior, flexor hallucis longus, flexor digitorum longus Contact of talus with calcaneus
Flexion	MTP, PIP, DIP	*MTP:* tension of posterior joint capsule, extensor muscles, collateral ligaments *PIP:* soft tissue apposition, tension of collateral ligaments and posterior joint capsule *DIP:* tension in collateral and oblique retinacular ligaments, and posterior joint capsule
Extension	MTP, PIP, DIP	*MTP:* tension of plantar joint capsule, plantar ligaments, and flexor muscles *PIP:* tension in plantar joint capsule *DIP:* ligaments and plantar joint capsule
Abduction	MTP	*Ligaments:* collateral ligaments, medial joint capsule Tension of adductor muscles Skin between web spaces
Adduction	MTP	Apposition of toes

DIP, distal interphalangeal joints (toes 2–5); *MTP,* metatarsophalangeal joints; *PIP,* proximal interphalangeal joints.

Modified from Clarkson HM. *Musculoskeletal Assessment. Joint Range of Motion and Manual of Muscle Strength,* 2nd ed. Baltimore: Lippincott Williams & Wilkins, 2000.

Arches of Foot

The foot is composed of numerous bones connected by ligaments that provide considerable flexibility which allow it to deform with each ground contact, thereby absorbing much of the shock. Furthermore, the tarsal and metatarsal bones are arranged in longitudinal and transverse arches passively supported and actively restrained by flexible tendons that add to the weight-bearing capabilities and resiliency of the foot (Fig. 5.60). The arches distribute weight over the foot (*pedal platform*), acting not only as shock absorbers but also as springboards for propelling it during walking, running, and jumping. The resilient arches add to the foot's ability to adapt to changes in surface contour. The weight of the body is transmitted to the talus from the tibia. Then it is transmitted posteriorly to the calcaneus and anteriorly to the "ball of the foot" (the sesamoid bones of the first metatarsal and the head of the second metatarsal), and that weight/pressure is shared laterally with the heads of the third through fifth metatarsals as necessary for balance and

A Plantar view

Sesamoid bones of 1st metatarsal and head of 2nd metatarsal

Heads of 3rd–5th metatarsals

Tuberosity of calcaneus

Medial cuneiform

1st metatarsal

Navicular

Talus

Calcaneus

Medial view

Talus

Calcaneus

Cuboid

5th metatarsal

Lateral view

B

Dynamic support

Tibialis anterior

Tibialis posterior

Flexor hallucis longus

Fibularis longus

Intrinsic plantar muscles

Passive support (Four (1-4) layers)

Plantar aponeurosis (1)

Plantar calcaneonavicular ligament (4)

Long plantar ligament (2)

Short plantar ligament (3)

C Medial view

FIGURE 5.60.   **Arches of foot. A.** Weight-bearing areas of foot. **B.** Medial and lateral longitudinal arches. **C.** Passive (*purple*) and dynamic (*gray*) supports of the foot.

comfort (Fig. 5.60A). Between these weight-bearing points are the relatively elastic arches of the foot, which become slightly flattened by the body weight during standing, but they normally resume their curvature (recoil) when body weight is removed.

The **longitudinal arch of the foot** is composed of medial and lateral parts (Fig. 5.60B). Functionally, both parts act as a unit, with the transverse arch spreading the weight in all directions. The **medial longitudinal arch** is higher and more important than the lateral longitudinal arch. The medial longitudinal arch is composed of the calcaneus, talus, navicular, three cuneiforms, and three metatarsals. *The talar head is the keystone of the medial lon-*

gitudinal arch. The tibialis anterior, attaching to the first metatarsal and medial cuneiform (Fig. 5.60C), helps strengthen the medial longitudinal arch. The fibularis longus tendon, passing from lateral to medial, also helps support this arch. The **lateral longitudinal arch** is much flatter than the medial part of the arch and rests on the ground during standing. It is composed of the calcaneus, cuboid, and lateral two metatarsals.

The **transverse arch of the foot** runs from side to side. It is formed by the cuboid, cuneiforms, and bases of the metatarsals. The medial and lateral parts of the longitudinal arch serve as pillars for the transverse arch. The tendon of the fibularis longus and tibialis posterior, crossing the sole of the foot obliquely, help maintain the curvature of the transverse arch.

The integrity of the bony arches of the foot is maintained by both passive factors and dynamic supports (Fig. 5.60C). The passive factors include the shape of the united bones and the four successive layers of fibrous tissue: plantar aponeurosis, long plantar ligament, plantar calcaneocuboid (short plantar) ligament, and calcaneonavicular (spring) ligament. The dynamic supports include the active (reflexive) bracing action of the intrinsic muscles of the foot and the active and tonic contraction of the muscles with long tendons extending into the foot (flexor hallucis and flexor digitorum longus for the longitudinal arch and fibularis longus and tibialis anterior for the transverse arch). Of these factors, the plantar ligaments and plantar aponeurosis bear the greatest stress and are most important in maintaining the arches.

Hallux Valgus

Hallux valgus is a foot deformity caused by degenerative joint disease; it is characterized by lateral deviation of the great toe (L. *hallux*). In some people, the deviation is so great that the first toe overlaps the second toe. These individuals are unable to move their first digit away from their second digit because the sesamoid bones under the head of the first metatarsal are displaced and lie in the space between the heads of the first and second metatarsals. In addition, a subcutaneous bursa may form owing to pressure and friction against the shoe. When tender and inflamed, the bursa is called a bunion (Fig. B5.18).

Bunion

Corns

Hallux valgus

Hallux valgus bunion and corns

FIGURE B5.18.

Pes Planus (Flatfeet)

Acquired flatfeet ("fallen arches") are likely to be secondary to dysfunction of the tibialis posterior owing to trauma, degeneration with age, or denervation. In the absence of normal passive or dynamic support, the plantar calcaneonavicular ligament fails to support the head of the talus. Consequently, the talar head displaces inferomedially and becomes prominent. As a result, some flattening of the medial part of the longitudinal arch occurs, along with lateral deviation of the forefoot (Fig. B5.19). Flatfeet are common in older people, particularly if they undertake much unaccustomed standing or gain weight rapidly, adding stress on the muscles and increasing the strain on the ligaments supporting the arches.

Flatfoot footprint

Talus

View of fallen arch

FIGURE B5.19.

Medical Imaging of Lower Limb

Transverse sections (A and B) and MRI scans (C and D) of thigh, inferior views

Key					
AB	Adductor brevis	FA	Femoral artery	PS	Posteromedial intermuscular septum
AL	Adductor longus	FL	Fascia lata	RF	Rectus femoris
AM	Adductor magnus	FV	Femoral vein	S	Sartorius
AS	Anteromedial intermuscular septum	G	Gracilis	SM	Semimembranosus
		GSV	Great saphenous vein	SN	Sciatic nerve
BFL	Long head of biceps femoris	IT	Iliotibial tract	ST	Semitendinosus
BFS	Short head of biceps femoris	LS	Lateral intermuscular septum	TN	Tibial nerve
BPA	Branch of profunda femoris artery	ONA	Anterior branch of obturator nerve	VI	Vastus intermedius
CFN	Common fibular nerve	ONP	Posterior branch of obturator nerve	VL	Vastus lateralis
F	Femur	PFA	Profunda femoris artery	VM	Vastus medialis

FIGURE 5.61.   Transverse sections (A and B) and MRI scans (C and D) of thigh.

Transverse sections (A-C) and MRI scans (D-F) of leg, inferior views

FIGURE 5.62. Transverse sections (A–C) and MRI scans (D–F) of leg.

Key	
AC	Anterior inter-muscular septum
AV	Anterior tibial vessels and deep fibular nerve
CT	Calcaneal tendon
EDL	Extensor digitorum longus
EHL	Extensor hallucis longus
F	Fibula
FA	Fibular artery
FB	Fibularis brevis
FDL	Flexor digitorum longus
FHL	Flexor hallucis longus
FL	Fibularlis longus
GA	Gastrocnemius aponeurosis
G	Gracilis
GM	Gluteus maximus
GSV	Great saphenous vein
HF	Head of fibula
IN	Interosseous membrane
ITF	Inferior tibiofibular joint
LG	Lateral head of gastrocnemius
MG	Medial head of gastrocnemius
MM	Medial malleolus
P	Popliteus
PC	Posterior inter-muscular septum
PL	Plantaris
SOL	Soleus
SSV	Small saphenous vein
T	Tibia
TA	Tibialis anterior
Ta	Talus
TP	Tibialis posterior
TV	Tibial nerve and posterior tibial vessels

 Go to *http://thePoint.lww.com/ECA4e for helpful study tools, including USMLE-style questions, case studies, images, and more!*

Upper Limb

BONES OF UPPER LIMB / 406

Clavicle / 407

Scapula / 407

Humerus / 410

Ulna and Radius / 410

Bones of Hand / 411

■ Surface Anatomy of Upper Limb Bones / 415

SUPERFICIAL STRUCTURES OF UPPER LIMB / 417

Fascia of Upper Limb / 417

Cutaneous Nerves of Upper Limb / 419

Venous Drainage of Upper Limb / 421

Lymphatic Drainage of Upper Limb / 422

ANTERIOR AXIOAPPENDICULAR MUSCLES / 422

POSTERIOR AXIOAPPENDICULAR AND SCAPULOHUMERAL MUSCLES / 423

Superficial Posterior Axioappendicular Muclses /424

Deep Posterior Axioappendicular Muscles /424

Scapulohumeral Muscles /427

■ Surface Anatomy of Pectoral and Scapular Regions (Anterior and Posterior Axioappendicular and Scapulohumeral Muscles) / 428

AXILLA / 427

Axillary Artery and Vein / 429

Axillary Lymph Nodes / 432

Brachial Plexus / 433

ARM / 440

Muscles of Arm / 440

Arteries and Veins of Arm /443

Nerves of Arm / 443

Cubital Fossa / 446

■ Surface Anatomy of Arm and Cubital Fossa / 447

FOREARM / 446

Muscles of Forearm / 446

Nerves of Forearm / 456

Arteries and Veins of Forearm / 456

HAND / 461

Fascia of Palm / 461

Muscles of Hand / 462

Flexor Tendons of Extrinsic Muscles / 466

Arteries and Veins of Hand / 466

Nerves of Hand / 468

■ Surface Anatomy of Forearm and Hand / 473

JOINTS OF UPPER LIMB / 475

Sternoclavicular Joint / 475

Acromioclavicular Joint / 476

Glenohumeral Joint / 476

Elbow Joint / 482

Proximal Radio-Ulnar Joint / 483

Distal Radio-Ulnar Joint / 485

Joints of Hand / 488

MEDICAL IMAGING OF UPPER LIMB / 492

The upper limb is characterized by its mobility and ability to grasp, strike, and conduct fine motor skills (*manipulation*). These characteristics are especially marked in the hand. Efficiency of hand function results in a large part from the ability to place it in the proper position by movements at the scapulothoracic, glenohumeral, elbow, radio-ulnar, and wrist joints. The upper limb consists of four segments, which are further subdivided into regions (Figs. 6.1 and 6.2):

- **Shoulder,** which includes the pectoral, scapular, and lateral supraclavicular regions. The **pectoral (shoulder) girdle** is a bony ring, incomplete posteriorly, formed by the scapulae and clavicles and completed anteriorly by the manubrium of the sternum.
- **Arm** (L. *brachium*) is between the shoulder and the elbow and is centered around the humerus. It consists of the anterior and posterior regions of the arm.

- **Forearm** (L. *antebrachium*) is between the elbow and the wrist and contains the ulna and radius. It consists of the anterior and posterior regions of the forearm.
- **Hand** (L. *manus*) is distal to the forearm and contains the carpus, metacarpus, and phalanges. It is composed of the wrist, palm, dorsum of hand, and digits (fingers, including the opposable thumb), and is richly supplied with sensory endings for touch, pain, and temperature.

BONES OF UPPER LIMB

The pectoral girdle and bones of the free part of the upper limb form the **superior appendicular skeleton,** which articulates with the axial skeleton only at the sternoclavicular

FIGURE 6.1. Segments and bones of upper limb.

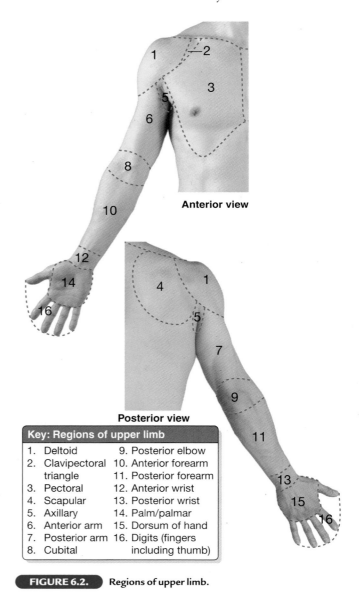

Anterior view

Posterior view

Key: Regions of upper limb	
1. Deltoid	9. Posterior elbow
2. Clavipectoral triangle	10. Anterior forearm
3. Pectoral	11. Posterior forearm
4. Scapular	12. Anterior wrist
5. Axillary	13. Posterior wrist
6. Anterior arm	14. Palm/palmar
7. Posterior arm	15. Dorsum of hand
8. Cubital	16. Digits (fingers including thumb)

FIGURE 6.2. Regions of upper limb.

joint, allowing great mobility (Fig. 6.3). The pectoral girdle is supported, stabilized, and propelled by **axioappendicular muscles,** which attach to the ribs, sternum, and vertebrae of the *axial skeleton*.

Clavicle

The **clavicle** (collar bone) connects the upper limb to the trunk. Its **sternal end** articulates with the **manubrium of the sternum** at the *sternoclavicular* (SC) *joint*. Its **acromial end** articulates with the *acromion of the scapula* at the *acromioclavicular* (AC) *joint* (Figs. 6.3 and 6.4). The medial two thirds of the shaft of the clavicle are convex anteriorly, whereas the lateral third is flattened and concave anteriorly. These curvatures increase the resilience of the clavicle and give it the appearance of an elongated capital S. The clavicle:

- Serves as a strut (rigid support) from which the scapula and free limb are suspended, keeping the limb away from the thorax so that the arm has maximum freedom of motion. Fixing the strut in position, especially after its elevation, enables elevation of the ribs for deep inspiration.
- Forms one of the boundaries of the *cervicoaxillary canal* (passageway between neck and arm), affording protection to the neurovascular bundle supplying the upper limb.
- Transmits shocks (traumatic impacts) from the upper limb to the axial skeleton.

Although designated as a long bone, the clavicle has no medullary (marrow) cavity. It consists of spongy (trabecular) bone with a shell of compact bone.

Scapula

The **scapula** (shoulder blade) is a triangular flat bone that lies on the posterolateral aspect of the thorax, overlying the second through seventh ribs (Figs. 6.3 and 6.4). The convex **posterior surface** of the scapula is unevenly divided by the **spine of the scapula** into a small **supraspinous fossa** and a much larger **infraspinous fossa**. The concave **costal surface** of the scapula has a large **subscapular fossa.** The triangular **body of the scapula** is thin and translucent superior and inferior to the scapular spine.

The scapula has **medial** (axillary), **lateral** (vertebral), and **superior borders** and **superior** and **inferior angles.** The lateral border of scapula is the thickest part of the bone, which includes the **head of the scapula** where the glenoid cavity is located. The **neck of the scapula** is just inferior to the head (Fig. 6.4*B*). The superior border of the scapula is marked near the junction of its medial two thirds and lateral third by the **suprascapular notch.**

The spine of the scapula continues laterally as the flat expanded **acromion,** which forms the subcutaneous point of the shoulder and articulates with the acromial end of the clavicle (Fig. 6.3*C*).

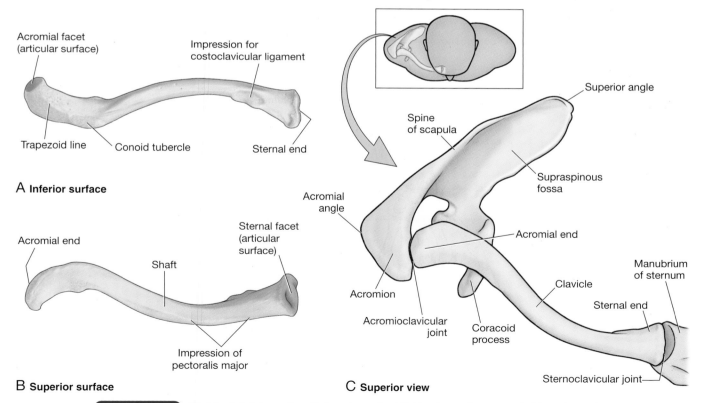

A Inferior surface

Acromial facet (articular surface) · Impression for costoclavicular ligament · Trapezoid line · Conoid tubercle · Sternal end

B Superior surface

Acromial end · Shaft · Sternal facet (articular surface) · Impression of pectoralis major

C Superior view

Spine of scapula · Superior angle · Supraspinous fossa · Acromial angle · Acromial end · Acromion · Acromioclavicular joint · Coracoid process · Clavicle · Manubrium of sternum · Sternal end · Sternoclavicular joint

FIGURE 6.3. Clavicle. **A.** Inferior surface. **B.** Superior surface. **C.** Muscle attachments to clavicle and scapula.

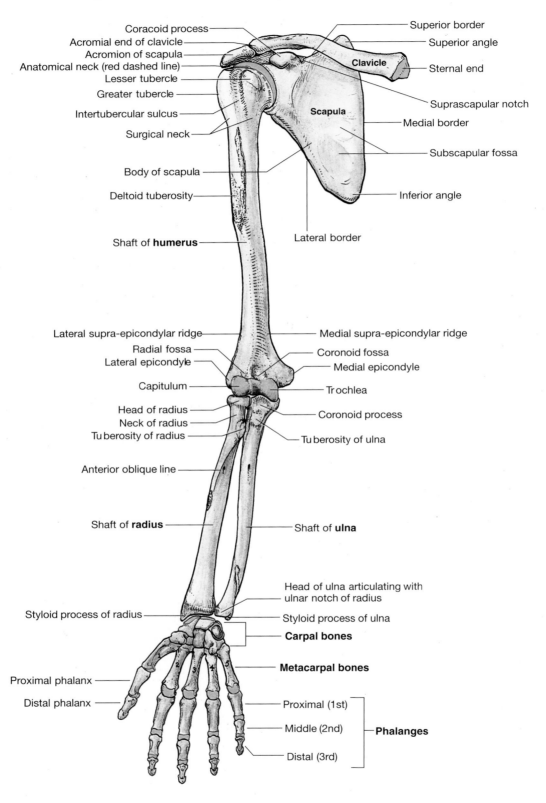

Coracoid process

Acromial end of clavicle

Acromion of scapula

Anatomical neck (red dashed line)

Lesser tubercle

Greater tubercle

Intertubercular sulcus

Surgical neck

Body of scapula

Deltoid tuberosity

Shaft of **humerus**

Superior border

Superior angle

Clavicle

Sternal end

Suprascapular notch

Scapula

Medial border

Subscapular fossa

Inferior angle

Lateral border

Lateral supra-epicondylar ridge

Radial fossa

Lateral epicondyle

Capitulum

Head of radius

Neck of radius

Tuberosity of radius

Anterior oblique line

Shaft of **radius**

Styloid process of radius

Proximal phalanx

Distal phalanx

Medial supra-epicondylar ridge

Coronoid fossa

Medial epicondyle

Trochlea

Coronoid process

Tuberosity of ulna

Shaft of **ulna**

Head of ulna articulating with ulnar notch of radius

Styloid process of ulna

Carpal bones

Metacarpal bones

Proximal (1st)

Middle (2nd)

Distal (3rd)

Phalanges

A **Anterior view**

FIGURE 6.4A.   Bones of upper limb.

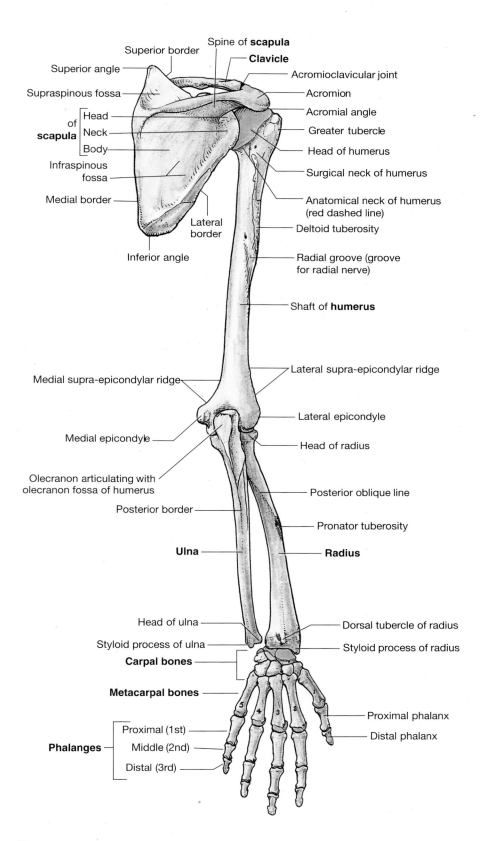

Spine of **scapula**

Superior border

Superior angle

Clavicle

Acromioclavicular joint

Supraspinous fossa

Acromion

Acromial angle

of   Head
scapula Neck

Greater tubercle

Head of humerus

Body

Surgical neck of humerus

Infraspinous
fossa

Anatomical neck of humerus
(red dashed line)

Medial border

Deltoid tuberosity

Lateral
border

Radial groove (groove
for radial nerve)

Inferior angle

Shaft of **humerus**

Medial supra-epicondylar ridge

Lateral supra-epicondylar ridge

Lateral epicondyle

Medial epicondyle

Head of radius

Olecranon articulating with
olecranon fossa of humerus

Posterior oblique line

Posterior border

Pronator tuberosity

Ulna

Radius

Head of ulna

Dorsal tubercle of radius

Styloid process of ulna

Styloid process of radius

Carpal bones

Metacarpal bones

Proximal phalanx

Distal phalanx

Proximal (1st)

Middle (2nd)
Phalanges

Distal (3rd)

B **Posterior view**

FIGURE 6.4B.   *(continued)*

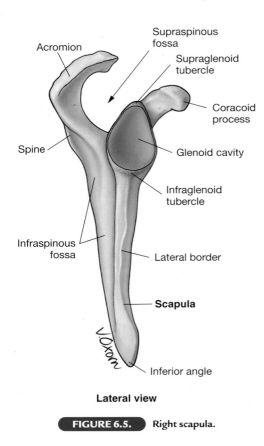

Lateral view

FIGURE 6.5.   Right scapula.

Extension

FIGURE 6.6.   Bones of right elbow during extension and flexion of elbow joint.

Superolaterally, the lateral surface of the scapula has a **glenoid cavity,** which articulates with the head of the humerus at the glenohumeral (shoulder) joint (Fig. 6.5). The glenoid (G. socket) cavity is a shallow, concave, oval fossa, which is directed anterolaterally and slightly superiorly and is considerably smaller than the head of the humerus for which it serves as a socket. The beak-like **coracoid process** is superior to the glenoid cavity and projects anterolaterally.

Humerus

The **humerus** (arm bone), the largest bone in the upper limb, articulates with the scapula at the glenohumeral joint and the radius and ulna at the elbow joint (Fig. 6.4). Proximally, the ball-shaped **head of the humerus** articulates with the glenoid cavity of the scapula. The **intertubercular sulcus** (bicipital groove) of the proximal end of the humerus separates the **lesser tubercle** from the **greater tubercle.** Just distal to the humeral head, the **anatomical neck of the humerus** separates the head from the tubercles. Distal to the tubercles is the narrow **surgical neck of the humerus.**

The **shaft of the humerus** has two prominent features: the **deltoid tuberosity** laterally and the **radial groove** (groove for radial nerve, spiral groove) posteriorly for the radial nerve and deep artery of the arm. The inferior end of the humeral shaft widens as the sharp medial and lateral **supra-epicondylar** (supracondylar) **ridges** form and then

end distally in the prominent **medial epicondyle** and **lateral epicondyle.**

The distal end of the humerus, including the trochlea, capitulum, olecranon, coronoid, and radial fossae, makes up the **condyle of the humerus.** It has two articular surfaces: a lateral **capitulum** (L. little head) for articulation with the head of the radius and a medial **trochlea** (L. pulley) for articulation with the trochlear notch of the ulna. Superior to the trochlea anteriorly is the **coronoid fossa,** which receives the coronoid process of the ulna during full flexion of the elbow (Figs. 6.4*A* and 6.6). Posteriorly, the **olecranon fossa** accommodates the olecranon of the ulna during extension of the elbow. Superior to the capitulum anteriorly, the shallow **radial fossa** accommodates the edge of the head of the radius when the elbow is fully flexed.

Ulna and Radius

The **ulna,** the stabilizing bone of the forearm, is the medial and longer of the two forearm bones (Fig. 6.4). Its proximal end has two prominent projections—the **olecranon** posteriorly and the **coronoid process** anteriorly; they form the walls of the **trochlear notch.** The trochlear notch of the ulna articulates with the trochlea of the humerus. Inferior to the coronoid process is the **tuberosity of the ulna.** On the lateral side of the coronoid process is a smooth, rounded concavity, the **radial notch,** which articulates with the head of radius (Fig. 6.7*A*). Distal to the radial notch is a prominent ridge, the **supinator crest,** and between it and the distal part of the coronoid process is a concavity, the **supinator fossa.** Proximally, the **shaft of the ulna** is thick, but it tapers, diminishing in diameter distally. At its narrow distal end is the rounded **head of ulna** with the small, conical **ulnar styloid process** (Fig. 6.4). The ulna does not articulate directly with the carpal bones. It is separated from the carpals by a fibrocartilaginous articular disc.

A **Lateral view**

B **Posterior view**

FIGURE 6.7.   **Ulna and radius. A.** Proximal part of ulna.
B. Distal end of radius.

The **radius** is the lateral and shorter of the two forearm bones. Its proximal end consists of a cylindrical head, a short neck, and a projection from the medial surface, the radial tuberosity (Fig. 6.4A). Proximally, the smooth superior

aspect of the **head of the radius** is concave for articulation with the capitulum of humerus. The head also articulates medially with the radial notch of ulna (Fig. 6.7A). The **neck of the radius** is the narrow part between the head and the radial tuberosity. The radial tuberosity demarcates the proximal end (head and neck) from the shaft. The **shaft of the radius** has a lateral convexity and gradually enlarges as it passes distally. The medial aspect of the distal end of the radius forms a concavity, the **ulnar notch,** which accommodates the head of the ulna (Fig. 6.7B). Its lateral aspect terminates distally as the **radial styloid process.** The radial styloid process is larger than the ulnar styloid process and extends farther distally. The **dorsal tubercle of the radius** lies between two of the shallow grooves for passage of the tendons of forearm muscles.

Bones of Hand

The **wrist,** or **carpus,** is composed of eight **carpal bones** (carpals) arranged in proximal and distal rows of four (Figs. 6.8 and 6.9). These small bones give flexibility to the wrist. The carpus is markedly convex from side to side posteriorly and concave anteriorly. Augmenting movement at the wrist, the two rows of carpals glide on each other; each carpal also glides on those adjacent to it. The proximal surfaces of the proximal row of carpals articulate with the inferior end of the radius and the articular disc of the wrist joint. The distal surfaces of these bones articulate with the distal row of carpals.

From lateral to medial, the four bones in the proximal row of carpals are the:

- **Scaphoid** (G. *skaphé,* skiff, boat): a boat-shaped bone that has a prominent **scaphoid tubercle.**

A **Anterior view**

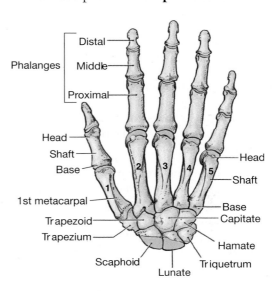

B **Posterior view**

FIGURE 6.8.   **Bones of hand.**

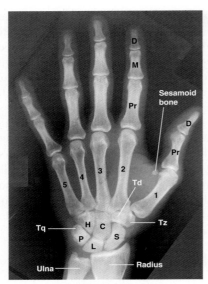

Anteroposterior view

FIGURE 6.9.   Radiograph of right hand.

Key
Scaphoid (S)
Lunate (L)
Triquetrum (Tq)
Pisiform (P)
Trapezium (Tz)
Trapezoid (Td)
Capitate (C)
Hamate (H)
Metacarpals
    (1–5)
Phalanges:
Proximal (Pr)
Middle (M)
Distal (D)

- **Lunate** (L. *luna*, moon): a moon-shaped bone that is broader anteriorly than posteriorly.
- **Triquetrum** (L. *triquetrus*, three-cornered): a pyramidal bone on the medial aspect of the carpus.
- **Pisiform** (L. *pisum*, pea): a small, pea-shaped bone that lies on the palmar surface of the triquetrum.

The proximal surfaces of the distal row of carpals articulate with the proximal row of carpals, and their distal surfaces articulate with the metacarpals. From lateral to medial, the four bones in the distal row of carpals are the:

- **Trapezium** (G. *trapeze*, table): a four-sided bone on the lateral side of the carpus.
- **Trapezoid:** a wedge-shaped bone that resembles a trapezium.
- **Capitate** (L. *caput*, head): the head-shaped bone that is the largest bone in the carpus.
- **Hamate** (L. *hamulus*, a little hook): a wedge-shaped bone, which has a hooked process, the **hook of hamate,** that extends anteriorly.

The **metacarpus** forms the skeleton of the palm of the hand between the carpus and the phalanges (Fig. 6.9). It is composed of five **metacarpal bones.** Each metacarpal consists of a base, shaft, and head. The proximal **bases of the metacarpals** articulate with the carpal bones, and the distal **heads of the metacarpals** articulate with the proximal phalanges and form the knuckles. The first metacarpal (of the thumb) is the thickest and shortest of these bones.

Each digit has three **phalanges** (**proximal, middle,** and **distal**) except for the first (thumb), which has only two

(**proximal** and **distal**). Each phalanx has a **base** proximally, a **shaft (body),** and a **head** distally. The distal phalanges are flattened and expanded at their distal ends, which underlie the nail beds.

Fracture of Clavicle

The clavicle is commonly fractured, often by an indirect force transmitted from an outstretched hand through the bones of the forearm and arm to the shoulder during a fall. A fracture may also result from a fall directly on the shoulder. The weakest part of the clavicle is at the junction of its middle and lateral thirds. After fracture of the clavicle, the sternocleidomastoid (SCM) muscle elevates the medial fragment of bone (Fig. B6.1).

The trapezius muscle is unable to hold up the lateral fragment owing to the weight of the upper limb, and thus the shoulder drops. In addition to being depressed, the lateral fragment of the clavicle may be pulled medially by the adductor muscles of the arm, such as the pectoralis major. Overriding of the bone fragments shortens the clavicle.

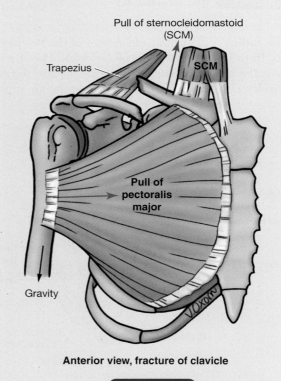

Anterior view, fracture of clavicle

FIGURE B6.1.

Ossification of Clavicle

The clavicle is the first long bone to ossify (via *intramembranous ossification*), beginning during the fifth and sixth embryonic weeks from medial and lateral primary ossification centers that are close together in the shaft of the clavicle. The ends of the clavicle later pass through a cartilaginous phase (*endochondral ossification*); the cartilages form growth zones similar to those of other long bones.

A secondary ossification center appears at the sternal end and forms a scale-like epiphysis that begins to fuse with the shaft (diaphysis) between 18 and 25 years of age and is completely fused to it between 25 and 31 years of age. This is the last of the epiphyses of long bones to fuse. An even smaller scale-like epiphysis may be present at the acromial end of the clavicle; it must not be mistaken for a fracture.

Sometimes fusion of the two ossification centers of the clavicle fails to occur; as a result, a bony defect forms between the lateral and the medial thirds of the clavicle. Awareness of this possible congenital defect should prevent diagnosis of a fracture in an otherwise normal clavicle. When doubt exists, both clavicles are radiographed because this defect is usually bilateral.

Fracture of Scapula

Fracture of the scapula is usually the result of severe trauma, as occurs in pedestrian–vehicle accidents. Usually there are also fractured ribs. Most fractures require little treatment because the scapula is covered on both sides by muscles. Most fractures involve the protruding subcutaneous acromion.

Fractures of Humerus

Fractures of the surgical neck of the humerus are especially common in elderly people with *osteoporosis* (Fig. B6.2). Even a low-energy fall on the hand, with the force being transmitted up the forearm bones of the extended limb, may result in a fracture. *Transverse fractures of the shaft of humerus* frequently result from a direct blow to the arm. Fracture of the distal part of the humerus, near the supracondylar ridges, is a *supracondylar fracture*. Because nerves are in contact with the humerus, they may be injured when the associated part of the humerus is fractured: surgical neck, axillary nerve; radial groove, radial nerve; distal humerus, median nerve; and medial epicondyle, ulnar nerve.

Anterior views

Fractures of the humerus			
1	Surgical neck	5	Spiral
2	Transverse	6	Supracondylar
3	Medial epicondyle	7	Greater tubercle
4	Anatomical neck	8	Comminuted

FIGURE B6.2.

Fractures of Ulna and Radius

Fractures of both the ulna and the radius are the result of severe injury. A direct injury usually produces transverse fractures at the same level, often in the middle third of the bones. Because the shafts of these bones are firmly bound together by the interosseous membrane, a fracture of one bone is likely to be associated with dislocation of the nearest joint. *Fracture of the distal end or the radius is the most common fracture in people older than 50 years.* A complete fracture of the distal 2 cm of the radius, called a **Colles fracture,** is the most common fracture of the forearm (Fig. B6.3). The distal fragment of the radius is displaced dorsally and often **comminuted** (broken into pieces). The fracture results from forced dorsiflexion of the hand, usually as the result of trying to ease a fall by outstretching the upper limb. Often, the ulnar styloid process is **avulsed** (broken off). Normally, the radial styloid process projects farther distally than the ulnar styloid process; consequently, when a Colles fracture occurs, this relationship is reversed because of shortening of the radius. This clinical condition is often referred to as a *dinner fork (silver fork) deformity* because a posterior angulation occurs in the forearm just proximal to the wrist and the normal anterior curvature of the relaxed hand. The posterior bending is produced by the posterior displacement and tilt of the distal fragment of the radius.

Fractures of Hand

Fracture of the scaphoid often results from a fall on the palm with the hand abducted (Fig. B6.4). The fracture occurs across the narrow part ("waist") of the scaphoid. Pain occurs primarily on the lateral side of the wrist, especially during dorsiflexion and abduction of the hand. Initial radiographs of the wrist may not reveal a fracture, but radiographs taken 10 to 14 days later reveal a fracture because bone resorption has occurred. Owing to the poor blood supply to the proximal part of the scaphoid, union of the fractured parts may take several months. *Avascular necrosis of the proximal fragment of the scaphoid* (pathological death of bone resulting from poor blood supply) may occur and produce *degenerative joint disease of the wrist.*

Radial artery
Palmar carpal branch
Scaphoid (fractured and necrotic)
Trapezoid
Radius
Ulna
Triquetrum
Lunate
Pisiform
Hook of hamate
Capitate
Trapezium

Fracture of scaphoid

FIGURE B6.4.

Fracture of the hamate may result in nonunion of the fractured bony parts because of the traction produced by the attached muscles. Because the ulnar nerve is close to the hook of the hamate, the nerve may be injured by this fracture, causing decreased grip strength of the hand. The ulnar artery may also be damaged when the hamate is fractured.

Severe crushing injuries of the hand may produce multiple metacarpal fractures, resulting in instability of the hand. Similar injuries of the distal phalanges are common (e.g., when a finger is caught in a car door). A *fracture of a distal phalanx* is usually comminuted, and a painful hematoma (collection of blood) develops. *Fractures of the proximal and middle phalanges* are usually the result of crushing or hyperextension injuries.

Avulsed ulnar styloid process

Distal fragment of radius overrides the rest of the bone

Palmar view

Lateral view

Colles fracture of distal radius ("dinner fork deformity")

FIGURE B6.3.

Surface Anatomy of Upper Limb Bones

Most bones of the upper limb offer a palpable segment or surface, enabling the skilled examiner to discern abnormalities owing to trauma or malformation (Fig. SA6.1A). The **clavicle** is subcutaneous and can be palpated throughout its length. Its sternal end projects superior to the manubrium. Between the elevated sternal ends of the clavicle is the **jugular notch** (suprasternal notch). The acromial end of the clavicle often rises higher than the acromion, forming a palpable elevation at the **acromioclavicular joint**. The acromial end can be palpated 2 to 3 cm medial to the lateral border of the acromion, particularly when the arm is alternately flexed and extended (Fig. SA6.1A).

The **coracoid process of scapula** can be felt deeply at the lateral end of the clavicle in the clavipectoral (deltopectoral) triangle (Fig. SA6.1B). The **acromion of the scapula** is felt easily and is often visible. The lateral and posterior borders of the acromion meet to form the **acromial angle**

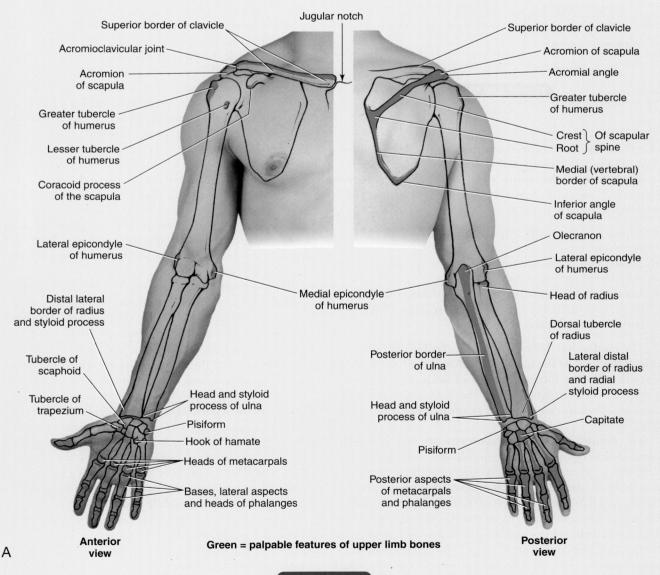

Jugular notch

Superior border of clavicle
Acromioclavicular joint
Acromion of scapula
Greater tubercle of humerus
Lesser tubercle of humerus
Coracoid process of the scapula
Lateral epicondyle of humerus
Distal lateral border of radius and styloid process
Tubercle of scaphoid
Tubercle of trapezium
Head and styloid process of ulna
Pisiform
Hook of hamate
Heads of metacarpals
Bases, lateral aspects and heads of phalanges
Medial epicondyle of humerus

Superior border of clavicle
Acromion of scapula
Acromial angle
Greater tubercle of humerus
Crest ⎱ Of scapular
Root ⎰ spine
Medial (vertebral) border of scapula
Inferior angle of scapula
Olecranon
Lateral epicondyle of humerus
Head of radius
Dorsal tubercle of radius
Lateral distal border of radius and radial styloid process
Posterior border of ulna
Head and styloid process of ulna
Pisiform
Capitate
Posterior aspects of metacarpals and phalanges

A   **Anterior view**

Green = palpable features of upper limb bones

Posterior view

FIGURE SA6.1A.

Coracoid process

Greater tubercle

Lesser tubercle

Intertubercular groove

Shaft of humerus

FIGURE SA6.1B.

(Fig. SA6.1A). Inferior to the acromion, the *deltoid muscle* forms the rounded curve of the shoulder.

The **crest of the spine of scapula** is subcutaneous throughout and can be easily palpated. When the upper limb is in the anatomical position, the:

- Superior angle of the scapula lies at the level of the T2 vertebra.
- Medial end of the root of the scapular spine is opposite the spinous process of the T3 vertebra.
- Inferior angle of the scapula lies at the level of the T7 vertebra, near the inferior border of the seventh rib and seventh intercostal space.

The **medial border of scapula** is palpable inferior to the root of the spine of the scapula as it crosses the third through seventh ribs. The **lateral border of scapula** is not easily palpated because it is covered by the teres major and minor muscles. The **inferior angle of scapula** is easily felt and is often visible.

The **greater tubercle of humerus** may be felt with the person's arm by the side on deep palpation through the deltoid muscle, inferior to the lateral border of the acromion. In this position, the tubercle is the most lateral bony point of the shoulder. When the arm is abducted, the greater tubercle is pulled beneath the acromion and is no longer palpable. The **lesser tubercle of the humerus** may be felt with difficulty by deep palpation through the anterior deltoid, approximately 1 cm laterally and slightly inferior to the tip of the coracoid process. Rotation of the arm facilitates palpa-

tion of this tubercle. The location of the **intertubercular sulcus or groove,** between the greater and the lesser tubercles, is identifiable during flexion and extension of the elbow joint by palpating in an upward direction along the tendon of the long head of the biceps brachii as it moves through the intertubercular sulcus. The **shaft of humerus** may be felt with varying distinctness through the muscles surrounding it. The **medial** and **lateral epicondyles** of the humerus are palpated on the medial and lateral aspects of the elbow region.

The **olecranon** and **posterior border of the ulna** can be palpated easily. When the elbow joint is extended, observe that the tip of the olecranon and the humeral epicondyles lie in a straight line. When the elbow is flexed, the olecranon forms the apex of an approximately equilateral triangle, of which the epicondyles form the angles at its base. The **head of radius** can be palpated and felt to rotate in the depression on the posterolateral aspect of the extended elbow, just distal to the lateral epicondyle of the humerus. The **radial styloid process** can be palpated on the lateral side of the wrist in the **anatomical snuff box** (see Fig. SA6.4C); it is larger and approximately 1 cm more distal than the ulnar styloid process. The **dorsal tubercle of radius** is easily felt around the middle of the dorsal aspect of the distal end of the radius (Fig. SA6.1C). The **head of ulna** forms a rounded subcutaneous prominence that can be easily seen and palpated on the medial side of the dorsal aspect of the wrist. The pointed subcutaneous **ulnar styloid process** may be felt slightly distal to the ulnar head when the hand is supinated.

The **pisiform** can be felt on the anterior aspect of the medial border of the wrist and can be moved from side to side when the hand is relaxed (Fig. SA6.1D). The **hook of hamate** can be palpated on deep pressure over the medial side of the palm, about 2 cm distal and lateral to the pisiform. The **tubercles of the scaphoid** and **trapezium** can be palpated at the base and medial aspect of the **thenar eminence** (ball of thumb) when the hand is extended.

The **metacarpals,** although overlain by the long extensor tendons of the digits, can be palpated on the dorsum of the hand (Fig. SA6.1C). The **heads of the metacarpals** form the knuckles; the third metacarpal head is the most prominent. The dorsal aspects of the phalanges can be palpated easily. The knuckles of the fingers are formed by the **heads of the proximal and middle phalanges.**

When measuring upper limb length, or segments of it, the acromial angle, lateral epicondyle of the humerus, styloid process of the radius, and tip of the third finger are most commonly used as measuring points, with the limb relaxed (dangling) but with the palm directed anteriorly.

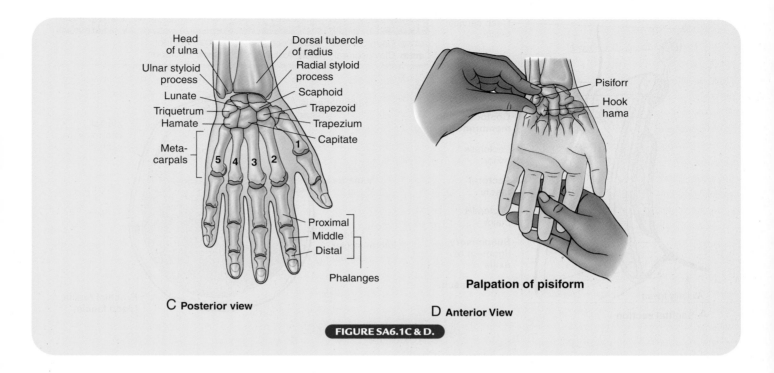

Head of ulna
Ulnar styloid process
Lunate
Triquetrum
Hamate
Meta-carpals

Dorsal tubercle of radius
Radial styloid process
Scaphoid
Trapezoid
Trapezium
Capitate

5 4 3 2 1

Proximal
Middle
Distal

Phalanges

C Posterior view

Pisiforr
Hook hama

Palpation of pisiform

D Anterior View

FIGURE SA6.1C & D.

SUPERFICIAL STRUCTURES OF UPPER LIMB

Deep to the skin is subcutaneous tissue (superficial fascia) containing fat and deep fascia surrounding the muscles. If no structure (muscle or tendon, for example) intervenes between the skin and the bone, the deep fascia usually attaches to bone.

Fascia of Upper Limb

The **pectoral fascia** invests the pectoralis major and is continuous inferiorly with the fascia of the anterior abdominal wall. The pectoral fascia leaves the lateral border of the pectoralis major and becomes the **axillary fascia** (Fig. 6.10*A,B*), which forms the floor of the axilla. Deep to the pectoral fascia and the pectoralis major, another fascial layer, the **clavipectoral fascia,** descends from the clavicle, enclosing the subclavius and then the pectoralis minor, becoming continuous inferiorly with the axillary fascia. The part of the clavipectoral fascia between the pectoralis minor and the subclavius, the **costocoracoid membrane,** is pierced by the lateral pectoral nerve, which primarily supplies the pectoralis major. The part of the clavipectoral fascia inferior to the pectoralis minor, the **suspensory ligament of axilla** (Fig. 6.10*A*), supports the axillary fascia and pulls it and the skin inferior to it upward during abduction of the arm, forming the **axillary fossa.**

The scapulohumeral muscles that cover the scapula and form the bulk of the shoulder are also ensheathed by deep fascia. The **deltoid fascia** invests the deltoid and is continuous with the pectoral fascia anteriorly and the dense infraspinous fascia posteriorly (Fig. 6.10*B*). The muscles that cover the anterior and posterior surfaces of the scapula are covered superficially by deep fascia, which is attached to the margins of the scapula. This arrangement creates osseofibrous *subscapular, supraspinous,* and *infraspinous compartments.*

The **brachial fascia,** a sheath of deep fascia, encloses the arm like a snug sleeve (Fig. 6.10*B*); it is continuous superiorly with the deltoid, pectoral, axillary, and infraspinous fasciae. The brachial fascia is attached inferiorly to the epicondyles of the humerus and the olecranon of the ulna and is continuous with the antebrachial fascia, the deep fascia of the forearm. Two septa, the **medial** and **lateral intermuscular septa,** extend from the deep surface of the brachial fascia and attach to the central shaft and medial and lateral supra-epicondylar ridges of the humerus. These septa divide the arm into **anterior (flexor)** and **posterior (extensor) fascial** compartments, each of which contains muscles serving similar functions and sharing common innervation (Fig. 6.10*C*).

In the forearm, similar fascial compartments are surrounded by the **antebrachial fascia** and separated by the *interosseous membrane* connecting the radius and ulna (Fig. 6.10*D*). The antebrachial fascia thickens posteriorly over the distal ends of the radius and ulna to form a transverse band, the **extensor retinaculum,** which holds the extensor

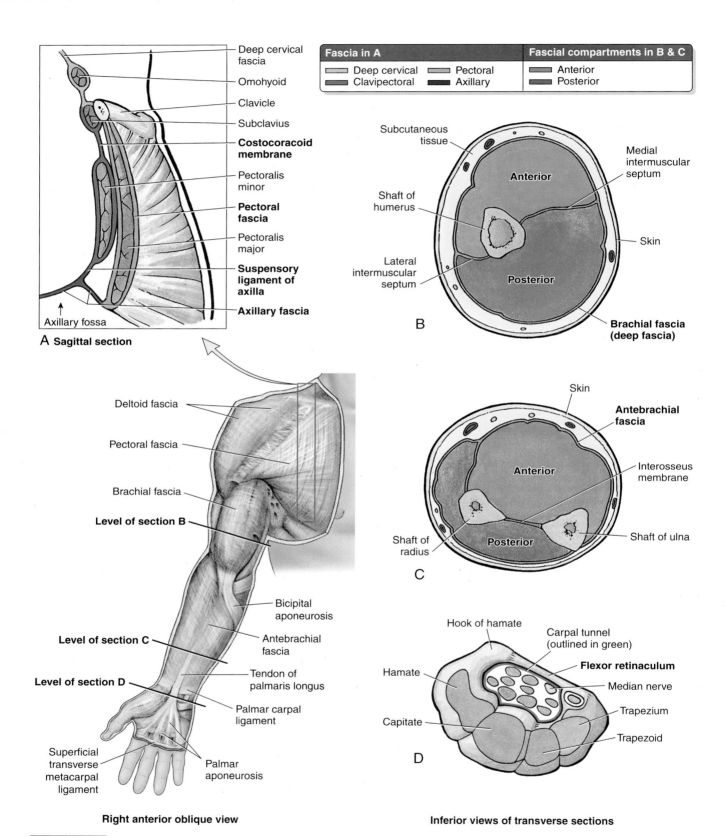

FIGURE 6.10. **Fascia of upper limb. A.** Axillary and pectoral fascia. **B.** Fascial compartments of arm. **C.** Fascial compartments of forearm. **D.** Flexor retinaculum and carpal tunnel.

tendons in position. The antebrachial fascia also forms an anterior thickening, which is continuous with the extensor retinaculum but is officially unnamed; some authors identify it as the *palmar carpal ligament*. Immediately distal, but at a deeper level to the latter, the antebrachial fascia is also continued as the **flexor retinaculum** (transverse carpal ligament). This fibrous band extends between the anterior prominences of the outer carpal bones and converts the anterior concavity of the carpus into the **carpal tunnel** through which the flexor tendons and median nerve pass (Fig. 6.10E).

The deep fascia of the upper limb continues beyond the extensor and flexor retinacula as the **palmar fascia**. The central part of the palmar fascia, the *palmar aponeurosis,* is thick, tendinous, and triangular. The aponeurosis forms four distinct thickenings that radiate to the bases of the fingers and become continuous with the fibrous tendon sheaths of the digits (Fig. 6.10E). The bands are traversed distally by the **superficial transverse metacarpal ligament,** which forms the base of the palmar aponeurosis. Strong *skin ligaments* extend from the palmar aponeurosis to the skin, holding the palmar skin close to the aponeurosis.

Cutaneous Nerves of Upper Limb

Cutaneous nerves in the subcutaneous tissue supply the skin of the upper limb. The **dermatomes** of the limb follow a general pattern that is easy to understand if one notes that developmentally the limbs grow as lateral protrusions of the

FIGURE 6.11. Segmental (dermatomal) innervation. **A.** and **B.** Foerster (1933) map. **C.** and **D.** Keegan and Garrett (1948) map.

Peripheral (cutaneous nerve) innervation

A Anterior view   **B Posterior view**

FIGURE 6.12.   Peripheral (cutaneous) innervation of upper limb.

trunk, with the first digit (thumb or great toe) located on the cranial side. Thus, the lateral surface of the upper limb is more cranial than the medial surface. There are two dermatome maps in common use. One corresponds to the concepts of limb development (Keegan & Garrett, 1948), and the other is based on clinical findings and is generally preferred by neurologists (Foerster, 1933). Both maps are approximations, delineating dermatomes as distinct zones when actually there is much overlap between adjacent dermatomes and much variation. In both maps, observe the progression of the segmental innervation (dermatomes) of the various cutaneous areas around the limb (Fig. 6.11):

- C3 and C4 nerves supply the region at the base of the neck, extending laterally over the shoulder.
- C5 nerve supplies the arm laterally (i.e., superior aspect of the abducted limb).
- C6 nerve supplies the forearm laterally and the thumb.
- C7 nerve supplies the middle and ring fingers (or middle three fingers) and the middle of the posterior surface of the limb.

- C8 nerve supplies the little finger, the medial side of the hand, and the forearm (i.e., the inferior aspect of the abducted limb).
- T1 nerve supplies the middle of the forearm to the axilla.
- T2 nerve supplies a small part of the arm and the skin of the axilla.

Most cutaneous nerves of the upper limb are derived from the **brachial plexus,** a major nerve network formed by the anterior rami of the C5–T1 spinal nerves. The cutaneous nerves to the shoulder are derived from the **cervical plexus,** a nerve network consisting of a series of nerve loops formed between adjacent anterior rami of the first four cervical nerves. The cervical plexus lies deep to the sternocleidomastoid (SCM) on the lateral aspect of the neck. The cutaneous nerves of the arm and forearm are as follows (Fig. 6.12):

- **Supraclavicular nerves** (C3, C4) pass anterior to the clavicle, immediately deep to the platysma, and supply the skin over the clavicle and the superolateral aspect of the pectoralis major.

- **Posterior cutaneous nerve of the arm** (C5–C8), a branch of the *radial nerve*, supplies the skin on the posterior surface of the arm.
- **Posterior cutaneous nerve of the forearm** (C5–C8), also a branch of the *radial nerve*, supplies the skin on the posterior surface of the forearm.
- **Superior lateral cutaneous nerve of the arm** (C5, C6), the terminal branch of the *axillary nerve*, emerges from beneath the posterior margin of the deltoid to supply the skin over the lower part of this muscle and on the lateral side of the midarm.
- **Inferior lateral cutaneous nerve of the arm** (C5, C6), a branch of the *radial nerve*, supplies the skin over the inferolateral aspect of the arm; it is frequently a branch of the posterior cutaneous nerve of the forearm.
- **Lateral cutaneous nerve of the forearm** (C6, C7), the terminal branch of the *musculocutaneous nerve*, supplies the skin on the lateral side of the forearm.
- **Medial cutaneous nerve of the arm** (C8–T2) arises from the *medial cord of the brachial plexus*, often uniting in the axilla with the lateral cutaneous branch of the second intercostal nerve. It supplies the skin on the medial side of the arm.
- **Intercostobrachial nerve** (T2), a lateral cutaneous branch of the *second intercostal nerve*, also contributes to the innervation of the skin on the medial surface of the arm.
- **Medial cutaneous nerve of the forearm** (C8, T1) arises from the *medial cord of the brachial plexus* and supplies the skin on the anterior and medial surfaces of the forearm.

Venous Drainage of Upper Limb

The main superficial veins of the upper limb, the cephalic and basilic veins, originate in the subcutaneous tissue on the dorsum of the hand from the **dorsal venous network** (Fig. 6.13). **Perforating veins** form communications between the superficial and the deep veins.

The **cephalic vein** (G. *kephalé*, head) ascends in the subcutaneous tissue from the lateral aspect of the dorsal venous network, proceeding along the lateral border of the wrist and the anterolateral surface of the forearm and arm. Anterior to the elbow, the cephalic vein communicates with the **median cubital vein**, which passes obliquely across the anterior aspect of the elbow and joins the basilic vein. Superiorly, the cephalic vein passes between the deltoid and the pectoralis major muscles and enters the *clavipectoral triangle*, where it pierces the costocoracoid membrane, part of the clavipectoral fascia, and joins the terminal part of the axillary vein.

The **basilic vein** ascends in the subcutaneous tissue from the medial end of the dorsal venous network along the medial side of the forearm and inferior part of the arm. It then passes deeply near the junction of the middle and inferior thirds of the arm, piercing the brachial fascia and running superiorly parallel to the brachial artery, where it

FIGURE 6.13. Superficial venous and lymphatic drainage of upper limb. *Green arrows,* superficial lymphatic drainage to lymph nodes.

merges with the accompanying veins (L. *venae comitantes*) of the brachial artery to form the axillary vein (Fig. 6.13A). The **median antebrachial vein** (median vein of forearm) ascends in the middle of the anterior aspect of the forearm.

Deep veins lie internal to the deep fascia and usually occur as paired, continually interanastomosing, accompanying veins that travel with and bear the same name as the major arteries of the upper limb.

Lymphatic Drainage of Upper Limb

Superficial lymphatic vessels arise from **lymphatic plexuses** in the skin of the fingers, palm, and dorsum of the hand and ascend mostly with superficial veins, such as the cephalic and basilic veins (Fig. 6.13). Some lymphatic vessels accompanying the basilic vein enter the **cubital lymph nodes,** located proximal to the medial epicondyle. Efferent vessels from these nodes ascend in the arm and terminate in the **humeral (lateral) axillary lymph nodes.** Most lymphatic vessels accompanying the cephalic vein cross the proximal part of the arm and anterior aspect of the shoulder to enter the **apical axillary lymph nodes.** Some vessels enter the more superficial **deltopectoral lymph nodes.**

Deep lymphatic vessels, less numerous than superficial vessels, accompany the major deep veins and terminate in the **humeral (lateral) axillary lymph nodes.**

ANTERIOR AXIOAPPENDICULAR MUSCLES

Four **anterior axioappendicular (thoracoappendicular or pectoral) muscles** move the pectoral girdle: pectoralis major, pectoralis minor, subclavius, and serratus anterior (Fig. 6.14). The attachments, nerve supply, and main actions of these muscles are summarized in Figure 6.15 and Table 6.1.

The fan-shaped **pectoralis major** covers the superior part of the thorax. It has **clavicular** and **sternocostal heads.** The sternocostal head is much larger and its lateral border forms most of the anterior wall of the axilla, with its inferior border forming the *anterior axillary fold* (see "Axilla," later in this chapter). The pectoralis major and adjacent deltoid form the narrow **deltopectoral groove,** in which the cephalic vein runs. However, the muscles diverge slightly from each other superiorly and, along with the clavicle, form the **clavipectoral (deltopectoral) triangle** (Fig. 6.14A).

The triangular **pectoralis minor** lies in the anterior wall of the axilla (Fig. 6.14B), where it is almost completely covered by the pectoralis major. The pectoralis minor stabilizes the scapula and is used when stretching the upper limb forward to touch an object that is just out of reach. With the coracoid process, the pectoralis minor forms a "bridge" under which vessels and nerves pass to the arm. Thus, the pectoralis minor is a useful anatomical and surgical landmark for structures in the axilla.

The **subclavius** lies almost horizontally when the arm is in the anatomical position (Fig. 6.14B). This small, round muscle is located inferior to the clavicle and affords some

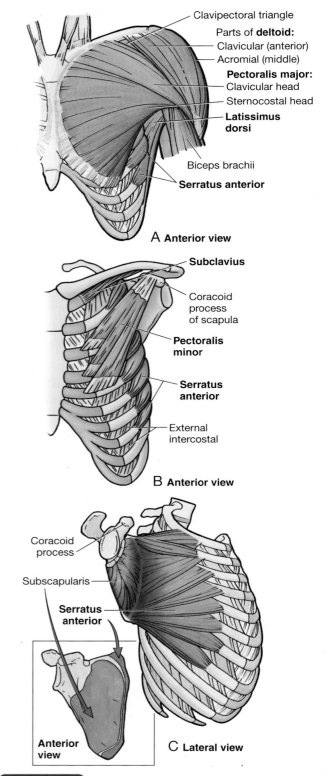

FIGURE 6.14. Anterior axioappendicular muscles. **A.** Pectoralis major and deltoid. **B.** Pectoralis minor and subclavius. **C.** Serratus anterior. *Inset,* Scapular attachments of subscapularis (*red*); serratus anterior (*blue*).

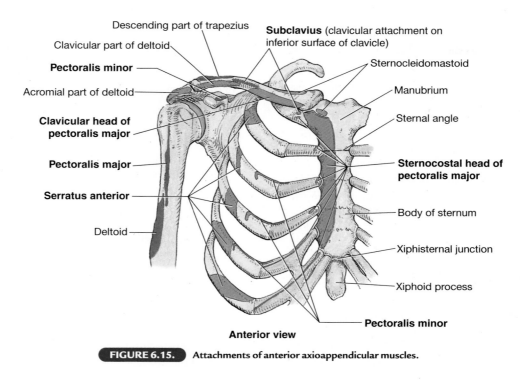

Descending part of trapezius
Clavicular part of deltoid
Pectoralis minor
Acromial part of deltoid
**Clavicular head of
pectoralis major**
Pectoralis major
Serratus anterior
Deltoid

Subclavius (clavicular attachment on
inferior surface of clavicle)
Sternocleidomastoid
Manubrium
Sternal angle
**Sternocostal head of
pectoralis major**
Body of sternum
Xiphisternal junction
Xiphoid process
Pectoralis minor

Anterior view

FIGURE 6.15.   Attachments of anterior axioappendicular muscles.

TABLE 6.1 ANTERIOR AXIOAPPENDICULAR MUSCLES

Muscle	Medial Attachment	Lateral Attachment	Innervation[a]	Main Action(s)
Pectoralis major	*Clavicular head:* anterior surface of medial half of clavicle *Sternocostal head:* anterior surface of sternum, superior six costal cartilages, aponeurosis of external oblique muscle	Lateral lip of intertubercular sulcus (groove) of humerus	Lateral and medial pectoral nerves; clavicular head (C5, **C6**), sternocostal head (**C7, C8,** T1)	Adducts and medially rotates humerus; draws scapula anteriorly and inferiorly Acting alone, clavicular head flexes humerus and sternocostal head extends it from the flexed position
Pectoralis minor	3rd–5th ribs near their costal cartilages	Medial border and superior surface of coracoid process of scapula	Medial pectoral nerve (C8, T1)	Stabilizes scapula by drawing inferiorly and anteriorly against thoracic wall
Subclavius	Junction of 1st rib and its costal cartilage	Inferior surface of middle third of clavicle	Subclavian nerve (**C5,** C6)	Anchors and depresses clavicle
Serratus anterior	External surfaces of lateral parts of 1st–8th ribs	Anterior surface of medial border of scapula	Long thoracic nerve (C5, **C6, C7**)	Protracts scapula and holds against thoracic wall; rotates scapula

[a]The spinal cord segmental innervation is indicated (e.g., "**C5,** C6" means that the nerves supplying the subclavius are derived from the fifth and sixth cervical segments of the spinal cord). Numbers in boldface (**C5**) indicate the main segmental innervation. Damage to one or more of the listed spinal cord segments or to the motor nerve roots arising from them results in paralysis of the muscles concerned.

protection to the subclavian vessels and the superior trunk of the brachial plexus if the clavicle fractures.

The **serratus anterior** overlies the lateral part of the thorax and forms the medial wall of the axilla (Fig. 6.14*C*). This broad sheet of thick muscle was given its name because of the sawtooth appearance of its fleshy slips or digitations (L. *serratus,* a saw). By keeping the scapula closely applied to the thoracic wall, the serratus anterior anchors this bone, enabling other muscles to use it as a fixed bone for movements of the humerus.

POSTERIOR AXIOAPPENDICULAR AND SCAPULOHUMERAL MUSCLES

The **posterior axioappendicular muscles** (superficial and intermediate groups of extrinsic back muscles) attach the superior appendicular skeleton of the upper limb to the axial skeleton. The *intrinsic back muscles,* which maintain posture and control movements of the vertebral column,

Paralysis of Serratus Anterior

When the serratus anterior is paralyzed because of *injury to the long thoracic nerve*, the medial border of the scapula moves laterally and posteriorly away from the thoracic wall. This gives the scapula the appearance of a wing. When the arm is raised, the medial border and inferior angle of the scapula pull markedly away from the posterior thoracic wall, a deformation known as a *winged scapula* (Fig. B6.5). The arm cannot be abducted above the horizontal position because the serratus anterior is unable to rotate the glenoid cavity superiorly to allow complete abduction of the limb.

Venipuncture

Because of the prominence and accessibility of the superficial veins, they are commonly used for *venipuncture* (to draw blood or inject a solution). By applying a tourniquet to the arm, the venous return is occluded and the veins distend and

Winged scapula

Right winged scapula

FIGURE B6.5.

usually are visible and/or palpable. Once a vein is punctured, the tourniquet is removed so that when the needle is removed the vein will not bleed extensively. The **median cubital vein** is commonly used for venipuncture. The veins forming the *dorsal venous network* and the cephalic and basilic veins are commonly used for long-term introduction of fluids (*intravenous feeding*). The cubital veins are also a site for the introduction of cardiac catheters.

are described in Chapter 4. The posterior shoulder muscles are divided into three groups:

- *Superficial posterior axioappendicular (extrinsic shoulder) muscles:* trapezius and latissimus dorsi (Fig. 6.16 and Table 6.2).
- *Deep posterior axioappendicular (extrinsic shoulder) muscles:* levator scapulae and rhomboids (Fig. 6.16 and Table 6.2).
- *Scapulohumeral (intrinsic shoulder) muscles:* deltoid, teres major, and the four rotator cuff muscles, supraspinatus, infraspinatus, teres minor, and subscapularis (Fig. 6.17 and Table 6.3).

Superficial Posterior Axioappendicular Muscles

The **trapezius** provides a direct attachment of the pectoral girdle to the trunk. This large triangular muscle covers the posterior aspect of the neck and the superior half of the trunk (Fig. 6.16*A* and Table 6.2). The trapezius attaches the pectoral girdle to the cranium and vertebral column and assists in suspending the upper limb. The fibers of the trapezius are divided into three parts that have different actions at the scapulothoracic joint between the scapula and the thoracic wall:

- **Descending (superior) part** elevates the scapula.
- **Middle part** retracts the scapula (i.e., pulls it posteriorly).

- **Ascending (inferior) part** depresses the scapula and lower the shoulder.

The descending (superior) and ascending (inferior) parts of trapezius act together in rotating the scapula on the thoracic wall. The trapezius also braces the shoulders by pulling the scapulae posteriorly and superiorly, fixing them in position with tonic contraction; consequently, weakness of this muscle causes drooping of the shoulders.

The **latissimus dorsi** is a large, fan-shaped muscle that covers a wide area of the back (Fig. 6.16 and Table 6.2). It passes from the trunk to the humerus and acts directly on the glenohumeral (shoulder) joint and indirectly on the pectoral girdle (scapulothoracic joint). In conjunction with the pectoralis major, the latissimus dorsi raises the trunk to the arm, which occurs when the limb is fixed and the body moves, as when performing chin-ups (hoisting oneself so the chin touches an overhead bar) or climbing a tree. These movements are also used when the trunk is fixed and the limb moves, as when chopping wood, paddling a canoe, and swimming.

Deep Posterior Axioappendicular Muscles

The superior third of the **levator scapulae** lies deep to the SCM; the inferior third is deep to the trapezius (Fig. 6.16 and Table 6.2). True to its name, the levator scapulae acts with the superior part of trapezius to elevate the scapula. With the rhomboids and pectoralis minor, the levator scapulae

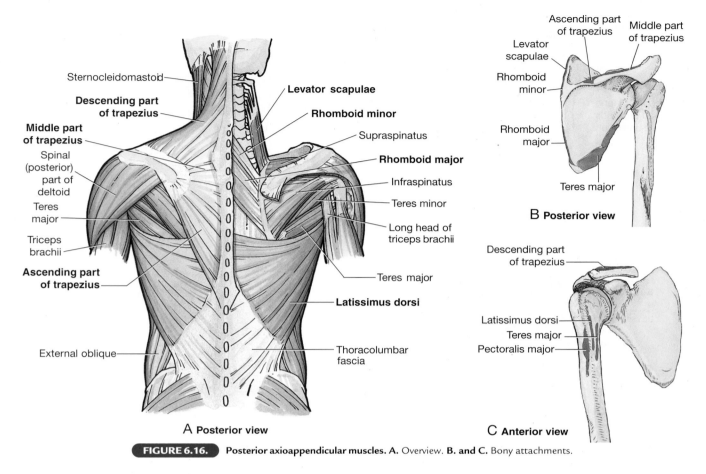

FIGURE 6.16. Posterior axioappendicular muscles. **A.** Overview. **B.** and **C.** Bony attachments.

TABLE 6.2 POSTERIOR AXIOAPPENDICULAR MUSCLES

Muscle	Medial Attachment	Lateral Attachment	Innervation[a]	Main Action(s)
Superficial posterior thoracoappendicular (extrinsic shoulder) muscles				
Trapezius	Medial third of superior nuchal line; external occipital protuberance; nuchal ligament; spinous processes of C7–T12 vertebrae	Lateral third of clavicle; acromion and spine of scapula	Spinal accessory nerve (CN XI) (motor fibers) and C3, C4 (pain and proprioceptive fibers)	*Descending (superior) part* elevates; *ascending (inferior) part* depresses; and *middle part* (or all parts together) retracts scapula; descending and ascending parts act together to rotate glenoid cavity superiorly
Latissimus dorsi	Spinous processes of inferior 6 thoracic vertebrae, thoracolumbar fascia, iliac crest, and inferior 3 or 4 ribs	Floor of intertubercular sulcus (groove) of humerus	Thoracodorsal nerve (**C6, C7,** C8)	Extends, adducts, and medially rotates humerus; raises body toward arms during climbing
Deep posterior thoracoappendicular (extrinsic shoulder) muscles				
Levator scapulae	Posterior tubercles of transverse processes of C1–C4 vertebrae	Medial border of scapula superior to root of spine	Dorsal scapular (C5) and cervical (C3, C4) nerves	Elevates scapula and tilts its glenoid cavity inferiorly by rotating scapula
Rhomboid minor and major	*Minor:* nuchal ligament; spinous processes of C7 and T1 vertebrae *Major:* spinous processes of T2–T5 vertebrae	*Minor:* triangular area at medial end of scapular spine *Major:* medial border of scapula from level of spine to inferior angle	Dorsal scapular nerve (C4, **C5**)	Retract scapula and rotate it to depress glenoid cavity; fix scapula to thoracic wall

[a]The spinal cord segmental innervation is indicated (e.g., "**C6, C7,** C8" means that the nerves supplying the latissimus dorsi are derived from the sixth through eighth cervical segments of the spinal cord). Numbers in boldface (**C6, C7**) indicate the main segmental innervation. Damage to one or more of the listed spinal cord segments or to the motor nerve roots arising from them results in paralysis of the muscles concerned.

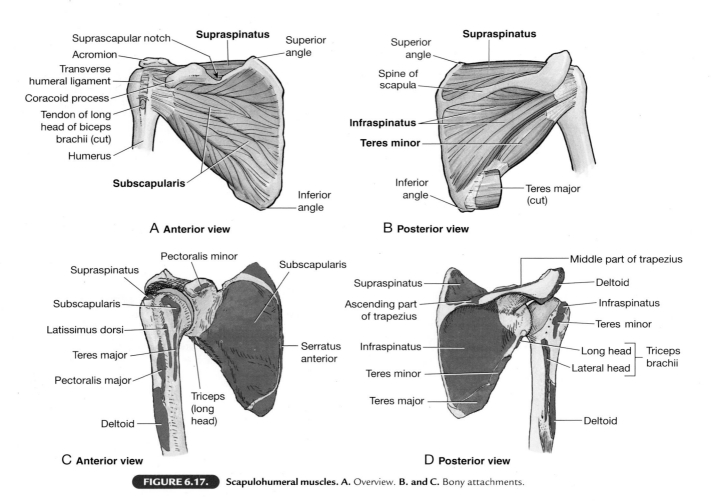

FIGURE 6.17. Scapulohumeral muscles. **A.** Overview. **B.** and **C.** Bony attachments.

TABLE 6.3 SCAPULOHUMERAL (INTRINSIC SHOULDER) MUSCLES

Muscle	Proximal Attachment	Distal Attachment	Innervation[a]	Main Action(s)
Deltoid	Lateral third of clavicle; acromion and spine of scapula	Deltoid tuberosity of humerus	Axillary nerve (**C5,** C6)	Clavicular (anterior) part flexes and medially rotates arm; acromial (middle) part abducts arm; spinal (posterior) part extends and laterally rotates arm
Supraspinatus[b]	Supraspinous fossa of scapula	Superior facet ⎫ of greater tubercle of humerus	Suprascapular nerve (C4, **C5,** C6)	Initiates and assists deltoid in abduction of arm and acts with other rotator cuff muscles[b]
Infraspinatus[b]	Infraspinous fossa of scapula	Middle facet ⎬	Suprascapular nerve (**C5,** C6)	Laterally rotate arm; help hold humeral head in glenoid cavity of scapula
Teres minor[b]	Middle part of lateral border of scapula	Inferior facet ⎭	Axillary nerve (**C5,** C6)	
Teres major	Posterior surface of inferior angle of scapula	Medial lip of intertubercular groove of humerus	Lower subscapular nerve (C5, **C6**)	Adducts and medially rotates arm
Subscapularis[b]	Subscapular fossa (most of anterior surface of scapula)	Lesser tubercle of humerus	Upper and lower subscapular nerves (C5, **C6,** C7)	Medially rotates and adducts arm; helps hold humeral head in glenoid cavity

[a]The spinal cord segmental innervation is indicated (e.g., "**C5,** C6" means that the nerves supplying the deltoid are derived from the fifth and sixth cervical segments of the spinal cord). Numbers in boldface (**C5**) indicate the main segmental innervation. Damage to one or more of the listed spinal cord segments or to the motor nerve roots arising from them results in paralysis of the muscles concerned.

[b]Collectively, the supraspinatus, infraspinatus, teres minor, and subscapularis muscles are referred to as the rotator cuff, or SITS, muscles. Their primary function during all movements of the glenohumeral (shoulder) joint is to hold the humeral head in the glenoid cavity of the scapula.

rotates the scapula, depressing the glenoid cavity. Acting bilaterally, they extend the neck; acting unilaterally, the muscle may contribute to lateral flexion of the neck.

The two **rhomboids** (major and minor) lie deep to the trapezius and form parallel bands that pass inferolaterally from the vertebrae to the medial border of the scapula (Table 6.2). The thin flat **rhomboid major** is approximately two times wider than the thicker **rhomboid minor** lying superior to it. The rhomboids retract and rotate the scapula, depressing the glenoid cavity. They also assist the serratus anterior in holding the scapula against the thoracic wall and fixing the scapula during movements of the upper limb.

Scapulohumeral Muscles

The six **scapulohumeral muscles** (the deltoid, teres major, supraspinatus, infraspinatus, subscapularis, and teres minor) are relatively short muscles that pass from the scapula to the humerus and act on the glenohumeral joint (Fig. 6.17 and Table 6.3).

The **deltoid** is a thick powerful muscle forming the rounded contour of the shoulder. The muscle is divided into *clavicular (anterior), acromial (middle),* and *spinal (posterior) parts* that can act separately or as a whole (Fig. SA6.2 and Table 6.3). When all three parts contract simultaneously, the arm is abducted. The clavicular and spinal parts act like guy ropes to steady the arm as it is abducted. When the arm is fully adducted, the line of pull of the deltoid coincides with the axis of the humerus; thus, it pulls directly upward on the bone and cannot initiate or produce abduction. The deltoid is, however, able to act as a shunt muscle, resisting inferior displacement of the head of the humerus from the glenoid cavity. From the fully adducted position, abduction must be initiated by the supraspinatus or by leaning to the side, allowing gravity to initiate the movement. The deltoid becomes fully effective as an abductor after the initial 15 degrees of abduction.

The **teres major** is a thick rounded muscle that lies on the inferolateral third of the scapula (Table 6.3). It adducts and medially rotates the arm, but along with the deltoid and rotator cuff muscles it is an important stabilizer of the humeral head in the glenoid cavity during movement.

Four of the scapulohumeral muscles (intrinsic shoulder muscles)—*S*upraspinatus, *I*nfraspinatus, *T*eres minor, and *S*ubscapularis (referred to as **SITS** muscles)—are called **rotator cuff muscles** because they form a musculotendinous rotator cuff around the glenohumeral joint (Fig. 6.17 and Table 6.3). All except the supraspinatus are rotators of the humerus. The supraspinatus, besides being part of the rotator cuff, initiates and assists the deltoid in the first 15 degrees of abduction of the arm. The tendons of the SITS or rotator cuff muscles blend with the joint capsule of the glenohumeral joint, reinforcing it as the musculotendinous rotator cuff, which protects the joint and gives it stability.

Injury to Axillary Nerve

Atrophy of the deltoid occurs when the axillary nerve (C5 and C6) is severely damaged (e.g., as might occur when the surgical neck of the humerus is fractured). As the deltoid atrophies unilaterally, the rounded contour of the shoulder disappears, resulting in visible asymmetry of the shoulder outlines. This gives the shoulder a flattened appearance and produces a slight hollow inferior to the acromion. A loss of sensation may occur over the lateral side of the proximal part of the arm, the area supplied by the superior lateral cutaneous nerve of the arm. To test the deltoid (or the function of the axillary nerve) the arm is abducted, against resistance, starting from approximately 15 degrees.

Rotator Cuff Injuries and Supraspinatus

Injury or disease may damage the rotator cuff, producing instability of the glenohumeral joint. Rupture or tear of the supraspinatus tendon is the most common injury of the rotator cuff. *Degenerative tendinitis of the rotator cuff* is common, especially in older people. These syndromes are discussed in detail later in this chapter, in relationship to the glenohumeral (shoulder) joint.

Tonic contraction of these muscles holds the relatively large head of the humerus firmly against the small and shallow glenoid cavity during arm movements. Bursae around the glenohumeral (shoulder) joint, between the tendons of the rotator cuff muscles and the fibrous layer of the joint capsule, reduce friction on the tendons passing over the bones or other areas of resistance.

AXILLA

The **axilla** is the pyramidal space inferior to the glenohumeral joint and superior to the skin and axillary fascia at the junction of the arm and thorax (Fig. 6.18).

The shape and size of the axilla vary, depending on the position of the arm; it almost disappears when the arm is fully abducted. The axilla provides a passageway for vessels and nerves going to and from the upper limb. The axilla has an apex, base, and four walls, three of which are muscular:

- The *apex of the axilla* is the **cervico-axillary canal,** the passageway between the neck and the axilla. It is bounded by the first rib, clavicle, and superior edge of the scapula.

Surface Anatomy of Pectoral and Scapular Regions (Anterior and Posterior Axioappendicular and Scapulohumeral Muscles)

The large vessels and nerves to the upper limb pass posterior to the convexity in the clavicle. The **clavipectoral (deltopectoral) triangle** is the slightly depressed area just inferior to the lateral part of the clavicle (Fig. SA6.2A). The clavipectoral triangle is bounded by the clavicle superiorly, the deltoid laterally, and the **clavicular head of pectoralis major** medially. When the arm is abducted and then adducted against resistance, the two heads of the **pectoralis major** are visible and palpable. As this muscle extends from the thoracic wall to the arm, it forms the **anterior axillary fold.** Digitations of the serratus anterior appear inferolateral to the pectoralis major. The **coracoid process** of the scapula is covered by the **anterior part of deltoid;** however, the tip of the process can be felt on deep palpation in the clavipectoral triangle.

The **deltoid** forms the contour of the shoulder (Fig. SA6.2B); as its name indicates, it is shaped like the inverted Greek letter delta.

A **Anterior view**

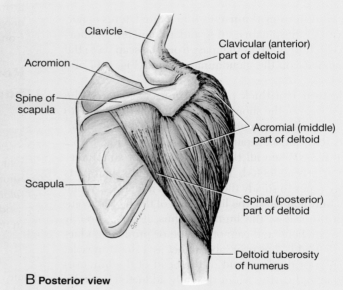

B **Posterior view**

Key	
AF	Axillary fossa
AX	Anterior axillary fold
C	Clavicle
CL	Clavicular head of pectoralis major
CP	Clavipectoral triangle
DA	Acromial (middle) part of deltoid
DC	Clavicular (anterior) part of deltoid
DS	Spinal (posterior) part of deltoid
LD	Latissimus dorsi
M	Manubrium
PX	Posterior axillary fold
SA	Serratus anterior
ST	Sternocostal head of pectoralis major
T	Triangle of auscultation
TA	Ascending part of trapezius
TD	Descending part of trapezius
TJ	Teres major
TM	Middle part of trapezius

C **Posterior view**

FIGURE SA6.2.

The superior border of the **latissimus dorsi** and a part of the **rhomboid major** are overlapped by the **trapezius** (Fig. SA6.2C). The area formed by the superior border of latissimus dorsi, the medial border of the scapula, and the inferolateral border of the trapezius is called the *triangle of auscultation*. This gap in the thick back musculature is a good place to examine posterior segments of the lungs with a stethoscope. When the scapulae are drawn anteriorly by folding the arms across the thorax and the trunk is flexed, the triangle of auscultation enlarges. The **teres major** forms a raised oval area on the inferolateral third of the posterior aspect of the scapula when the arm is adducted against resistance. The **posterior axillary fold** is formed by the teres major and the tendon of the latissimus dorsi. Between the anterior and posterior axillary folds lies the axillary fossa (Fig. SA6.2A).

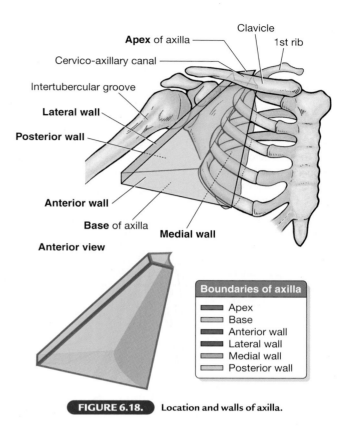

FIGURE 6.18.   Location and walls of axilla.

The arteries, veins, lymphatics, and nerves traverse this superior opening to pass to or from the arm.

- The *base of the axilla* is formed by the concave skin, subcutaneous tissue, and axillary (deep) fascia extending from the arm to the thoracic wall forming the **axillary fossa** (armpit).
- The *anterior wall of the axilla* is formed by the pectoralis major and minor and the pectoral and clavipectoral fascia associated with them. The **anterior axillary fold** is the inferiormost part of the anterior wall.
- The *posterior wall of the axilla* is formed chiefly by the scapula and subscapularis on its anterior surface and inferiorly by the teres major and latissimus dorsi. The **posterior axillary fold** is the inferiormost part of the posterior wall that may be grasped.
- The *medial wall of the axilla* is formed by the thoracic wall and the overlying serratus anterior.
- The *lateral wall of the axilla* is the narrow bony wall formed by the *intertubercular sulcus* of the humerus.

The axilla contains the axillary artery and its branches, axillary vein and its tributaries, nerves of the cords and branches of the brachial plexus, lymphatic vessels, and several groups of *axillary lymph nodes*, all embedded in *axillary fat*. Proximally, the neurovascular structures are ensheathed in a sleeve-like extension of the cervical prevertebral fascia, the axillary sheath.

Axillary Artery and Vein

The **axillary artery** begins at the lateral border of the first rib as the continuation of the subclavian artery and ends at the inferior border of the teres major (Fig. 6.19 and Table 6.4). It passes posterior to the pectoralis minor into the arm and becomes the brachial artery when it passes distal to the inferior border of the teres major. For descriptive purposes, the axillary artery is divided into three parts relative to the pectoralis minor (the part number also indicates the number of its branches):

- The **first part of the axillary artery** is located between the lateral border of the first rib and the medial border of the pectoralis minor; it is enclosed in the *axillary sheath* and has one branch: the *superior thoracic artery.*
- The **second part of the axillary artery** lies posterior to the pectoralis minor and has two branches: the *thoracoacromial artery* and *lateral thoracic artery*, which pass medial and lateral to the muscle, respectively.
- The **third part of the axillary artery** extends from the lateral border of the pectoralis minor to the inferior border of the teres major and has three branches. The *subscapular artery* is the largest branch of the axillary artery. Opposite the origin of this artery, the *anterior circumflex humeral artery* and *posterior circumflex humeral artery* arise.

The **axillary vein** lies initially (distally) on the anteromedial side of the axillary artery, with its terminal part anteroinferior to the artery (Fig. 6.20). This large vein is formed by the union of the *accompanying brachial veins* and the basilic vein at the inferior border of the teres major. The axillary vein ends at the lateral border of the first rib, where it becomes the **subclavian vein.** The veins of the axilla are more abundant than the arteries, are highly variable, and frequently anastomose.

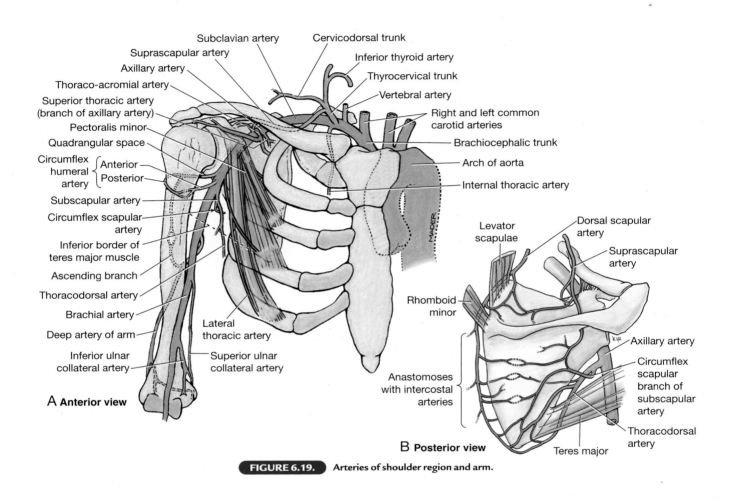

FIGURE 6.19.   Arteries of shoulder region and arm.

TABLE 6.4   ARTERIES OF PROXIMAL UPPER LIMB (SHOULDER REGION AND ARM)

Artery	Origin		Course
Internal thoracic	Inferior surface of first part		Descends, inclining anteromedially, posterior to sternal end of clavicle and 1st costal cartilage; enters thorax to descend in parasternal plane; gives rise to perforating branches, anterior intercostal, musculophrenic, and superior epigastric arteries
Thyrocervical trunk	Anterior surface of first part	Subclavian artery	Ascends as a short trunk often giving rise to two branches: inferior thyroid artery and cervicodorsal trunk. Arising from the cervicodorsal trunk are the suprascapular and dorsal scapular arteries (may also arise directly from thyrocervical trunk).
Suprascapular	Thyrocervical (or as direct branch of subclavian artery)		Passes inferolaterally crossing anterior scalene muscle, phrenic nerve, subclavian artery, and brachial plexus, running laterally posterior and parallel to clavicle; next passes over transverse scapular ligament to supraspinous fossa; then lateral to scapular spine (deep to acromion) to infraspinous fossa on posterior surface of scapula

TABLE 6.4 ARTERIES OF PROXIMAL UPPER LIMB (SHOULDER REGION AND ARM) (*cont'd.*)

Artery	Origin		Course
Superior thoracic	First part		Runs anteromedially along superior border of pectoralis minor; then passes between it and pectoralis major to thoracic wall; helps supply 1st and 2nd intercostal spaces and superior part of serratus anterior
Thoraco-acromial	Second part	Axillary artery	Curls around superomedial border of pectoralis minor; pierces costocoracoid membrane (clavipectoral fascia); divides into four branches: pectoral, deltoid, acromial, and clavicular
Lateral thoracic			Descends along axillary border of pectoralis minor; follows it onto thoracic wall, supplying lateral aspect of breast
Circumflex humeral (**anterior** and **posterior**)	Third part		Encircle surgical neck of humerus, anastomosing with each other laterally; larger posterior branch traverses quadrangular space
Subscapular			Descends from level of inferior border of subscapularis along lateral border of scapula, dividing within 2–3 cm into terminal branches, the circumflex scapular and thoracodorsal arteries
Circumflex scapular	Subscapular artery		Curves around lateral border of scapula to enter infraspinous fossa, anastomosing with suprascapular artery
Thoracodorsal			Continues course of subscapular artery, descending with thoracodorsal nerve to enter apex of latissimus dorsi
Deep brachial artery of arm	Just inferior to teres major	Brachial artery	Accompanies radial nerve along radial groove of humerus, supplying posterior compartment of arm and participating in periarticular arterial anastomoses around elbow joint
Superior ulnar collateral	Near middle of arm		Accompanies ulnar nerve to posterior aspect of elbow; anastomoses with posterior ulnar recurrent artery
Inferior ulnar collateral	Superior to medial epicondyle of humerus		Passes anterior to medial epicondyle of humerus to anastomose with anterior ulnar recurrent artery

Compression of Axillary Artery

Compression of the third part of the axillary artery against the humerus may be necessary when profuse bleeding occurs. If compression is required at a more proximal site, the axillary artery can be compressed at its origin at the lateral border of the first rib by exerting downward pressure in the angle between the clavicle and the attachment of the SCM. See also the section on thoracic outlet syndrome (p. xxx).

Arterial Anastomoses Around Scapula

Many arterial anastomoses (communications between arteries) occur around the scapula (Table 6.4). Several arteries join to form networks on the anterior and posterior surfaces of the scapula: the dorsal scapular, suprascapular, and subscapular (via the circumflex scapular branch). The importance of the *collateral circulation* made possible by these anastomoses becomes apparent when ligation of a lacerated subclavian or axillary artery is necessary. For example, the axillary artery may have to be ligated between the first rib and subscapular artery; in other cases, vascular stenosis (narrowing) of the axillary artery may result from an atherosclerotic lesion that causes reduced blood flow. In either case, the direction of blood flow in the subscapular artery is reversed, enabling blood to reach the third part of the axillary artery. Note that the subscapular artery receives blood through several anastomoses with the suprascapular artery, transverse cervical artery, and intercostal arteries. *Slow occlusion of an artery* (e.g., resulting from disease) often enables sufficient collateral circulation to develop, preventing *ischemia* (deficiency of blood). Sudden occlusion usually does not allow sufficient time for adequate collateral circulation to develop; as a result, ischemia of the upper limb occurs. *Abrupt surgical ligation of the axillary artery* between the origins of the subscapular artery and the deep artery of the arm will cut off the blood supply to the arm because the collateral circulation is inadequate.

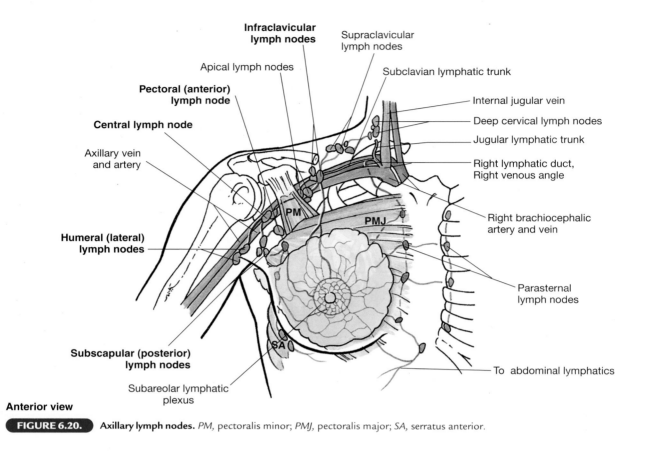

FIGURE 6.20. **Axillary lymph nodes.** *PM,* pectoralis minor; *PMJ,* pectoralis major; *SA,* serratus anterior.

Injury to Axillary Vein

Wounds in the axilla often involve the axillary vein because of its large size and exposed position. When the arm is fully abducted, the axillary vein overlaps the axillary artery anteriorly. A wound in the proximal part of the vein is particularly dangerous, not only because of profuse bleeding but also because of the risk of air entering the vein and producing *air emboli* (air bubbles) in the blood.

Axillary Lymph Nodes

Many lymph nodes are found in the axillary fat. There are five principal groups of axillary lymph nodes: pectoral, subscapular, humeral, central, and apical (Figs. 6.20 and 6.21).

The **pectoral (anterior) nodes** consist of three to five nodes that lie along the medial wall of the axilla, around the lateral thoracic vein and inferior border of the pectoralis minor. The pectoral nodes receive lymph mainly from the anterior thoracic wall, including most of the breast (see Chapter 1).

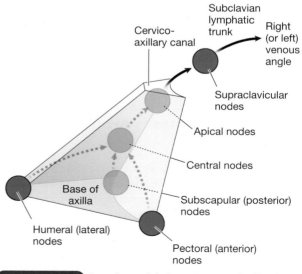

FIGURE 6.21. Location and drainage pattern of axillary lymph nodes, schematic illustration.

The **subscapular (posterior) nodes** consist of six or seven nodes that lie along the posterior axillary fold and subscapular blood vessels. These nodes receive lymph from the posterior aspect of the thoracic wall and scapular region.

The **humeral (lateral) nodes** consist of four to six nodes that lie along the lateral wall of the axilla, medial and posterior to the axillary vein. These humeral nodes receive nearly all the lymph from the upper limb, except that carried by lymphatic vessels accompanying the cephalic vein, which primarily drain to the apical axillary and infraclavicular nodes (Figs. 6.20 and 6.21).

Efferent lymphatic vessels from the pectoral, subscapular, and humeral nodes pass to the **central nodes.** The central nodes consist of three or four large nodes situated deep to the pectoralis minor near the base of the axilla, in association with the second part of the axillary artery. Efferent vessels from the central nodes pass to the apical nodes.

The **apical nodes** are located at the apex of the axilla along the medial side of the axillary vein and the first part of the axillary artery. The apical nodes receive lymph from all other groups of axillary nodes as well as from lymphatics accompanying the proximal cephalic vein. Efferent vessels from the apical nodes traverse the *cervicoaxillary canal* and unite to form the **subclavian lymphatic trunk,** although some vessels may drain en route through the **clavicular (infraclavicular and supraclavicular) nodes.** The subclavian lymphatic trunk may be joined by the jugular and bronchomediastinal trunks on the right side to form the **right lymphatic duct,** or it may enter the **right venous angle** independently (Fig. 6.20). On the left side, the subclavian trunk most commonly joins the **thoracic duct.**

Brachial Plexus

The **brachial plexus** is a major network of nerves supplying the upper limb. It begins in the lateral cervical region (posterior triangle) and extends into the axilla. The brachial plexus is formed by the union of the anterior rami of the C5–T1 nerves, which constitute the **roots of brachial plexus** (Fig. 6.22 and Table 6.5). The roots usually pass through the gap between the anterior and middle scalene muscles with the subclavian artery. The sympathetic fibers carried by each root of the plexus are received from gray rami of the middle and inferior cervical ganglia as the roots pass between the scalene muscles (see Chapter 8).

Enlargement of Axillary Lymph Nodes

An infection in the upper limb can cause the axillary nodes to enlarge and become tender and inflamed, a condition called *lymphangitis* (inflammation of lymphatic vessels). The humeral group of nodes is usually the first ones to be involved. Lymphangitis is characterized by warm, red streaks in the skin of the limb. Infections in the pectoral region and breast, including the superior part of the abdomen, can also produce enlargement of the axillary nodes. These nodes are also the most common site of metastases (spread) of cancer of the breast.

Spinal accessory nerve (CN XI)
Levator scapulae
Middle scalene
Trapezius
Superior trunk of brachial plexus
Superficial cervical artery
Dorsal scapular artery
Posterior scalene
Middle trunk of brachial plexus
Inferior trunk of brachial plexus
Suprascapular { Nerve / Artery / Vein }

C5 and C6 roots of brachial plexus (anterior rami)
Phrenic nerve
Sternocleidomastoid
Internal jugular vein (IJV)
Thyrocervical trunk
Anterior scalene
Subclavian artery
External jugular vein (EJV)
Clavicle
1st rib
Subclavian vein

Anterior view of right side

FIGURE 6.22.   Brachial plexus and subclavian vessels in lateral cervical region (posterior triangle) of neck.

FIGURE 6.23. Schematic illustrations of brachial plexus.

Roots (formed by anterior rami)

Trunks

Divisions

Cords

Terminal branches

1. Dorsal scapular nerve
2. Suprascapular nerve
3. Subclavian nerve
4. Long thoracic nerve
5. Lateral pectoral nerve
6. Medial pectoral nerve
7. Medial cutaneous nerve of arm
8. Medial cutaneous nerve of forearm
9. Upper subscapular nerve
10. Thoracodorsal nerve
11. Lower subscapular nerve

AD: Anterior division
PD: Posterior division

1–4: Supraclavicular branches
5–11: Infraclavicular branches

TABLE 6.5 BRACHIAL PLEXUS AND NERVES OF UPPER LIMB

Nerve	Origin[a]	Course	Structures Innervated
Supraclavicular branches			
Dorsal scapular	Posterior aspect of anterior ramus of **C5** with a frequent contribution from C4	Pierces middle scalene; descends deep to levator scapulae and rhomboids	Rhomboids; occasionally supplies levator scapulae
Long thoracic	Posterior aspect of anterior rami of **C5, C6,** C7	Superior two rami pierce middle scalene; passes through cervicoaxillary canal, descending posterior to C8 and T1 anterior rami; runs inferiorly on superficial surface of serratus anterior	Serratus anterior
Suprascapular	Superior trunk, receiving fibers from **C5,** C6, and often C4	Passes laterally across lateral cervical region (posterior triangle of neck), superior to brachial plexus; then through scapular notch deep to transverse scapular ligament	Supraspinatus and infraspinatus muscles; glenohumeral (shoulder) joint
Subclavian nerve (nerve to subclavius)	Superior trunk, receiving fibers from C5, **C6,** and often C4	Descends posterior to clavicle and anterior to brachial plexus and subclavian artery; often giving an *accessory root to phrenic nerve*	Subclavius and sternoclavicular joint (accessory phrenic root innervates diaphragm)

TABLE 6.5 BRACHIAL PLEXUS AND NERVES OF UPPER LIMB (*continued*)

Nerve	Origin[a]	Course	Structures Innervated
Infraclavicular branches			
Lateral pectoral	Side branch of lateral cord, receiving fibers from C5, **C6,** C7	Pierces costocoracoid membrane to reach deep surface of pectoral muscles; a *communicating branch to the medial pectoral nerve* passes anterior to axillary artery and vein	Primarily pectoralis major, but some lateral pectoral nerve fibers pass to pectoralis minor via branch to medial pectoral nerve
Musculocutaneous	Terminal branch of lateral cord, receiving fibers from C5–C7	Exits axilla by piercing coracobrachialis; descends between biceps brachii and brachialis, supplying both; continues as *lateral cutaneous nerve of forearm*	Muscles of anterior compartment of arm (coracobrachialis, biceps brachii, and brachialis); skin of lateral aspect of forearm
Median	*Lateral root of median nerve* is a terminal branch of lateral cord (C6, C7 fibers); *medial root of median nerve* is a terminal branch of medial cord (C8, T1 fibers)	Lateral and medial roots merge to form median nerve lateral to axillary artery; descends through arm adjacent to brachial artery, with nerve gradually crossing anterior to artery to lie medial to artery in cubital fossa	Muscles of anterior forearm compartment (except for flexor carpi ulnaris and ulnar half of flexor digitorum profundus), five intrinsic muscles in thenar half of palm and palmar skin
Medial pectoral		Passes between axillary artery and vein; then pierces pectoralis minor and enters deep surface of pectoralis major; although it is called *medial* for its origin from medial cord, it lies lateral to lateral pectoral nerve	Pectoralis minor and sternocostal part of pectoralis major
Medial cutaneous nerve of arm	Side branches of medial cord, receiving fibers from C8, T1	Smallest nerve of plexus; runs along medial side of axillary and brachial veins; communicates with *intercostobrachial nerve*	Skin of medial side of arm, as far distal as medial epicondyle of humerus and olecranon of ulna
Median cutaneous nerve of forearm		Initially runs with ulnar nerve (with which it may be confused) but pierces deep fascia with basilic vein and enters subcutaneous tissue, dividing into anterior and posterior branches	Skin of medial side of forearm, as far distal as wrist
Ulnar	Larger terminal branch of medial cord, receiving fibers from C8, T1, and often C7	Descends medial arm; passes posterior to medial epicondyle of humerus; then descends ulnar aspect of forearm to hand	Flexor carpi ulnaris and ulnar half of flexor digitorum profundus (forearm); most intrinsic muscles of hand; skin of hand medial to axial line of digit 4
Upper subscapular	Side branch of posterior cord, receiving fibers from **C5**	Passes posteriorly, entering subscapularis directly	Superior portion of subscapularis
Lower subscapular	Side branch of posterior cord, receiving fibers from **C6**	Passes inferolaterally, deep to subscapular artery and vein	Inferior portion of subscapularis and teres major
Thoracodorsal	Side branch of posterior cord, receiving fibers from C6, **C7,** C8	Arises between upper and lower subscapular nerves and runs inferolaterally along posterior axillary wall to apical part of latissimus dorsi	Latissimus dorsi
Axillary	Terminal branch of posterior cord, receiving fibers from **C5,** C6	Exits axillary fossa posteriorly, passing through quadrangular space[b] with posterior circumflex humeral artery; gives rise to *superior lateral brachial cutaneous nerve;* then winds around surgical neck of humerus deep to deltoid	Glenohumeral (shoulder) joint; teres minor and deltoid muscles; skin of superolateral arm (over inferior part of deltoid)
Radial	Larger terminal branch of posterior cord (largest branch of plexus), receiving fibers from C5–T1	Exits axillary fossa posterior to axillary artery; passes posterior to humerus in radial groove with profunda brachii artery between lateral and medial heads of triceps; perforates lateral intermuscular septum; enters cubital fossa, dividing into *superficial* (cutaneous) and *deep* (motor) *radial nerves*	All muscles of posterior compartments of arm and forearm; skin of posterior and inferolateral arm, posterior forearm, and dorsum of hand lateral to axial line of digit 4

[a]Boldface **C5** indicates primary component of the nerve.

[b]Bounded superiorly by the subscapularis, head of humerus, and teres minor; inferiorly by the teres major; medially by the long head of the triceps; and laterally by the coracobrachialis and surgical neck of the humerus.

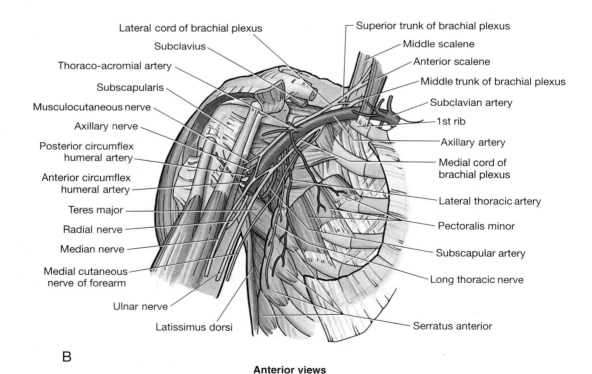

A

Coracoid process
Clavicle
Subscapularis
Axillary artery
Axillary vein
Biceps brachii { Short head / Long head
2nd rib
Musculocutaneous nerve
Lateral pectoral nerve
Coracobrachialis
Medial pectoral nerve
Teres major
Pectoralis minor
Median nerve
Latissimus dorsi
Ulnar nerve
Brachial artery
Sternocostal head of pectoralis major (cut)
Serratus anterior

B

Lateral cord of brachial plexus
Superior trunk of brachial plexus
Subclavius
Middle scalene
Thoraco-acromial artery
Anterior scalene
Subscapularis
Middle trunk of brachial plexus
Musculocutaneous nerve
Subclavian artery
Axillary nerve
1st rib
Posterior circumflex humeral artery
Axillary artery
Anterior circumflex humeral artery
Medial cord of brachial plexus
Teres major
Lateral thoracic artery
Radial nerve
Pectoralis minor
Median nerve
Subscapular artery
Medial cutaneous nerve of forearm
Long thoracic nerve
Ulnar nerve
Serratus anterior
Latissimus dorsi

Anterior views

FIGURE 6.24. **Boundaries and contents of axilla. A.** Relationship of nerves and vessels to pectoralis minor. **B.** Boundaries and contents, superficial dissection.

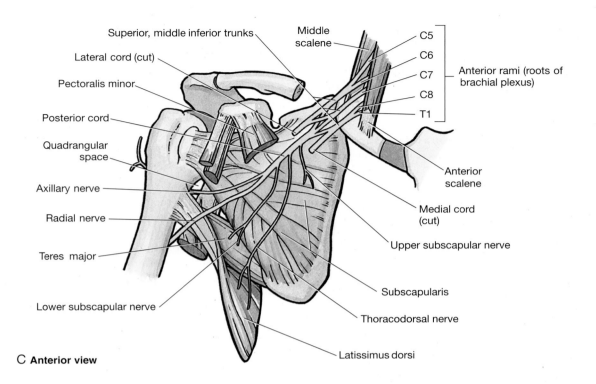

C **Anterior view**

D **Transverse section**

FIGURE 6.24. **Boundaries and contents of axilla.** (*Continued*) **C.** Posterior wall of axilla with posterior cord of brachial plexus and its branches. **D.** Transverse section of shoulder and axilla.

In the inferior part of the neck, the roots of the brachial plexus unite to form three trunks (Fig. 6.23):

- A **superior trunk**, from the union of the C5 and C6 roots.
- A **middle trunk**, which is a continuation of the C7 root.
- An **inferior trunk**, from the union of the C8 and T1 roots.

Each trunk of the brachial plexus divides into anterior and posterior divisions as the plexus passes through the *cervicoaxillary canal* posterior to the clavicle. **Anterior divisions of the trunks** supply the *anterior (flexor) compartments* of the upper limb, and **posterior divisions of the trunks** supply the *posterior (extensor) compartments* of the upper limb.

The divisions of the trunks form three cords of the brachial plexus within the axilla (Fig. 6.24):

- Anterior divisions of the superior and middle trunks unite to form the **lateral cord.**
- The anterior division of the inferior trunk continues as the **medial cord.**

- Posterior divisions of all three trunks unite to form the **posterior cord.**

The cords of the brachial plexus are named for their position in relation to the second part of the axillary artery (e.g., the lateral cord is lateral to the axillary artery, most easily seen when the limb is abducted).

The brachial plexus is divided into **supraclavicular** and **infraclavicular parts** by the clavicle (Figs. 6.23 and 6.24 and Table 6.5):

- Four *branches of the supraclavicular part of the plexus* arise from the roots (anterior rami) and trunks of the plexus (dorsal scapular nerve, long thoracic nerve, nerve to the subclavius, and suprascapular nerve) and are approachable through the neck. *Muscular branches* arise from the anterior rami of C5–T1 to supply the scalene and longus colli muscles.
- *Branches of the infraclavicular part of the plexus* arise from the cords of the brachial plexus and are approachable through the axilla.

Variations of Brachial Plexus

Variations in the brachial plexus formation are common. In addition to the five anterior rami (C5–T1) that form the roots of the plexus, small contributions may be made by the anterior rami of C4 or T2. When the superiormost root (anterior ramus) of the plexus is C4 and the inferiormost root is C8, it is called a *prefixed brachial plexus*. Alternatively, when the superior root is C6 and the inferior root is T2, it is a *postfixed brachial plexus*. In the latter type, the inferior trunk of the plexus may be compressed by the first rib, producing neurovascular symptoms in the upper limb. Variations also may occur in the formation of trunks, divisions, and cords; in the origin and/or combination of branches; and in the relationship to the axillary artery and scalene muscles.

Brachial Plexus Injuries

Injuries to the brachial plexus affect movements and cutaneous sensations in the upper limb. Disease, stretching, and wounds in the lateral cervical region (posterior triangle of the neck) or in the axilla may produce brachial plexus injuries (see Chapter 8). Signs and symptoms depend on which part of the plexus is involved. Injuries to the brachial plexus result in loss of muscular movement (*paralysis*) and loss of cutaneous sensation (*anesthesia*).

In *complete paralysis*, no movement is detectable. In *incomplete paralysis*, not all muscles are paralyzed; therefore, the person can move, but the movements are weak compared to those on the uninjured side.

Injuries to superior parts of the brachial plexus (C5 and C6) usually result from an excessive increase in the angle between the neck and the shoulder. These injuries can occur in a person who is thrown from a motorcycle or a horse and lands on the shoulder in a way that widely separates the neck and shoulder (Fig. B6.6A). When thrown, the person's shoulder often hits something (e.g., a tree or the ground) and stops but the head and trunk continue to move. This stretches or ruptures superior parts of the brachial plexus or **avulses** (tears) the roots of the plexus from the spinal cord. Injury to the superior trunk is apparent by the characteristic position of the limb ("waiter's tip position") in which the limb hangs by the side in medial rotation (Fig. B6.6B). *Upper brachial plexus injuries* can also occur in a newborn when excessive stretching of the neck occurs during delivery (Fig. B6.6C). As a result of *injuries to the superior parts of the brachial plexus (Erb-Duchenne palsy)*, paralysis of the muscles of the shoulder and arm supplied by C5–C6 occurs. The usual clinical appearance is an upper limb with an adducted shoulder, medially rotated arm, and extended elbow. The lateral aspect of the upper limb also experiences loss of sensation. Chronic microtrauma to the superior trunk of the brachial plexus

A   B   C

D   E   F

FIGURE B6.6.

from carrying a heavy backpack can produce motor and sensory deficits in the distribution of the musculocutaneous and radial nerves.

Injuries to inferior parts of the brachial plexus (Klumpke paralysis) are much less common. These injuries may occur when the upper limb is suddenly pulled superiorly—for example, when a person grasps something to break a fall or when a baby's limb is pulled excessively during delivery (Fig. B6.6D,E). These events injure the inferior trunk of the plexus (C8 and T1) and may avulse the roots of the spinal nerves from the spinal cord. The short muscles of the hand are affected and a *claw hand* results (Fig. B6.6F).

Brachial Plexus Block

Injection of an anesthetic solution into or immediately surrounding the axillary sheath interrupts nerve impulses and produces anesthesia of the structures supplied by the branches of the cords of the plexus. Combined with an occlusive tourniquet technique to retain the anesthetic agent, this procedure enables surgeons to operate on the upper limb without using a general anesthetic. The brachial plexus can be anesthetized using a number of approaches, such as interscalene, supraclavicular, and axillary.

ARM

The arm extends from the shoulder to the elbow. Two types of movement occur between the arm and the forearm at the elbow joint: flexion–extension and pronation–supination. The muscles performing these movements are clearly divided into anterior (*flexor*) and posterior (*extensor*) groups. The chief action of both groups is at the elbow joint, but some muscles also act at the glenohumeral joint.

Muscles of Arm

Of the four arm muscles, three flexors (biceps brachii, brachialis, and coracobrachialis) are in the anterior (flexor) compartment and are supplied by the musculocutaneous nerve (Figs. 6.24A, and 6.25), and one extensor (triceps brachii) is in the posterior compartment, supplied by the radial nerve. A small triangular muscle on the posterior aspect of the elbow, the anconeus, covers the posterior aspect of the ulna proximally. Figure 6.26 and Table 6.6 list the attachments, nerve supply, and main actions of the arm muscles.

The **biceps brachii** has two heads (*bi,* two + L. *caput,* head): a **long head** and a **short head.** A broad band, the transverse humeral ligament, passes from the lesser to the greater tubercle of the humerus and converts the intertubercular groove into a canal for the tendon of the long head of the biceps. When the elbow is extended, the biceps is a simple flexor of the forearm; however, as the elbow flexion approaches 90 degrees and more power is needed, the biceps with the forearm in supination produces flexion, but with the forearm in pronation the biceps is the primary (most powerful) supinator of the forearm. A triangular membranous band, the **bicipital aponeurosis** (Fig. 6.25), runs from the biceps tendon across the cubital fossa and merges with the antebrachial (deep) fascia covering the flexor muscles in the medial side of the forearm.

The **brachialis,** a flattened fusiform muscle, lies posterior (deep) to the biceps (Fig. 6.25B). It is the only pure flexor, producing the greatest amount of flexion force. It flexes the forearm in all positions and during slow and quick movements. When the forearm is extended slowly, the brachialis steadies the movement by slowly relaxing.

The **coracobrachialis,** an elongated muscle in the superomedial part of the arm, is a useful landmark for locating other structures in the arm (Fig. 6.25B). The musculocutaneous nerve pierces it, and the distal part of its attachment indicates the location of the nutrient foramen of the humerus. The coracobrachialis helps flex and adduct the arm and stabilize the glenohumeral (shoulder) joint.

FIGURE 6.25. Muscles, arteries, and nerves of anterior arm. **A.** Superficial dissection. **B.** Deep dissection.

The **triceps brachii** is a large fusiform muscle in the posterior compartment of the arm that arises by **long, lateral,** and **medial heads** (Figs. 6.27 and 6.28; Table 6.6). The triceps is the main extensor of the elbow. Because its long head crosses the glenohumeral joint, the triceps helps stabilize the adducted glenohumeral joint by serving as a shunt muscle, resisting inferior displacement of the head of the humerus along with the deltoid and coracobrachialis. Just proximal to the distal attachment of the triceps is a friction-reducing *subtendinous olecranon bursa,* between the triceps tendon and

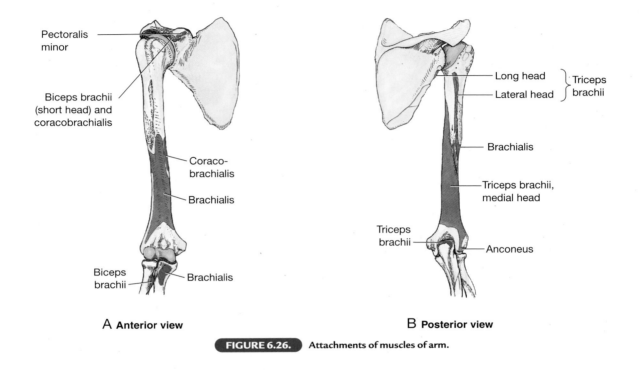

A Anterior view   **B** Posterior view

FIGURE 6.26.   Attachments of muscles of arm.

TABLE 6.6 MUSCLES OF ARM

Muscle	Proximal Attachment	Distal Attachment	Innervation[a]	Main Action(s)
Biceps brachii	*Short head:* tip of coracoid process of scapula *Long head:* supraglenoid tubercle of scapula	Tuberosity of radius and fascia of forearm via bicipital aponeurosis	Musculocutaneous nerve[b] (C5, **C6**)	Supinates forearm and, when it is supinated, flexes forearm; flexes arm; short head resists dislocation of shoulder
Brachialis	Distal half of anterior surface of humerus	Coronoid process and tuberosity of ulna		Flexes forearm in all positions
Coracobrachialis	Tip of coracoid process of scapula	Middle third of medial surface of humerus	Musculocutaneous nerve (C5, **C6**, C7)	Helps flex and adduct arm; resists dislocation of shoulder
Triceps brachii	*Long head:* infraglenoid tubercle of scapula *Lateral head:* posterior surface of humerus, superior to radial groove *Medial head:* posterior surface of humerus, inferior to radial groove	Proximal end of olecranon of ulna and fascia of forearm	Radial nerve (C6, **C7, C8**)	Chief extensor of forearm; long head extends arm and resists dislocation of humerus (especially important during abduction)
Anconeus	Lateral epicondyle of humerus	Lateral surface of olecranon and superior part of posterior surface of ulna	Radial nerve (C7, C8, T1)	Assists triceps in extending forearm; stabilizes elbow joint; abducts ulna during pronation

[a]The spinal cord segmental innervation is indicated (e.g., "C5, **C6**" means that the nerves supplying the biceps brachii are derived from the fifth and sixth cervical segments of the spinal cord). Numbers in boldface (**C6**) indicate the main segmental innervation. Damage to one or more of the listed spinal cord segments or to the motor nerve roots arising from them results in paralysis of the muscles concerned.

[b]Some of the lateral part of the brachialis is innervated by a branch of the radial nerve.

A

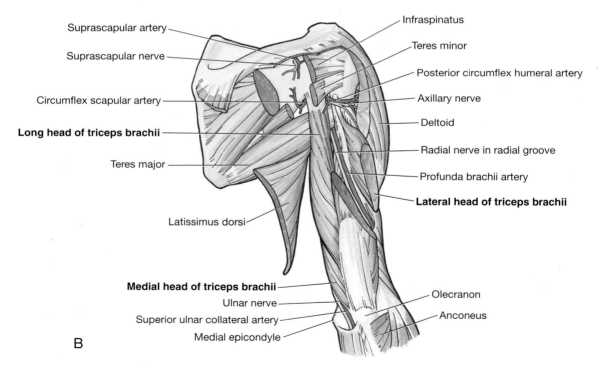

B

Posterior views

FIGURE 6.27. Muscles, arteries, and nerves of posterior arm. **A.** Superficial dissection. **B.** Deep dissection.

FIGURE 6.28. Transverse section to illustrate relationships of muscles and neurovascular structures of arm.

the olecranon. The **anconeus** muscle helps the triceps extend the forearm and also abducts the ulna during pronation of the forearm (Fig. 6.26*B* and Table 6.6).

Arteries and Veins of Arm

The **brachial artery** provides the main arterial supply to the arm and is the continuation of the axillary artery (Figs. 6.25*A* and 6.28; Table 6.4). It begins at the inferior border of the teres major and ends in the cubital fossa opposite the neck of the radius under cover of the bicipital aponeurosis, where it divides into the radial and ulnar arteries. The brachial artery, relatively superficial and palpable throughout its course, lies anterior to the triceps and brachialis. At first, it lies medial to the humerus, where its pulsations are palpable in the **medial bicipital groove.** It then passes anterior to the medial supraepicondylar ridge and trochlea of the humerus. As it passes inferolaterally, the brachial artery accompanies the median nerve, which crosses anterior to the artery. During its course through the arm, the brachial artery gives rise to unnamed *muscular branches* and the *humeral nutrient artery,* which arise from its lateral aspect. The main named branches of the brachial artery that arise from its medial aspect are the **profunda brachii artery (deep artery of arm)** (Fig. 6.27*B*) and the **superior** and **inferior ulnar collateral arteries.** The latter vessels help form the periarticular **arterial anastomoses of the elbow region** (Table 6.4).

Two sets of *veins of the arm,* superficial and deep, anastomose freely with each other. The two main **superficial veins of the arm,** the *cephalic* and *basilic veins,* are described earlier (Figs. 6.13 and 6.28). Paired deep veins, collectively constituting the **brachial vein,** accompany the brachial artery. The brachial vein begins at the elbow by union of the *accompanying veins of the ulnar and radial arteries* and ends by merging with the basilic vein to form the axillary vein. Both superficial and deep veins have valves, but the deep veins have more.

Nerves of Arm

Four main nerves pass through the arm: median, ulnar, musculocutaneous, and radial (Figs. 6.24–6.28; Table 6.5). The **median nerve** in the arm is formed in the axilla by the union of medial and lateral roots from the medial and lateral cords of the brachial plexus, respectively (Fig. 6.24*A,B*). The nerve runs distally in the arm, initially on the lateral side of the brachial artery until it reaches the middle of the arm, where it crosses to the medial side and contacts the brachialis. The median nerve then descends into the cubital fossa, where it lies deep to the bicipital aponeurosis and median cubital vein. The median and ulnar nerves supply no branches to the arm; however, they supply articular branches to the elbow joint.

The **ulnar nerve** in the arm arises from the medial cord of the brachial plexus, conveying fibers mainly from the C8 and T1 nerves (Fig. 6.24). It passes distally, anterior to the insertion of teres major and to the long head of triceps, on the medial side of the brachial artery. Around the middle of the arm, it pierces the medial intermuscular septum with the superior ulnar collateral artery and descends between the septum and the medial head of triceps. The ulnar nerve passes posterior to the medial epicondyle of the humerus to enter the forearm (Figs. 6.26A and 6.27B).

The **musculocutaneous nerve** arises from the lateral cord of the brachial plexus, pierces the coracobrachialis, and then continues distally between the brachialis and the biceps (Fig. 6.24A,B). After supplying all three muscles of the anterior compartment of the arm, the nerve emerges lateral to the biceps brachii as the *lateral cutaneous nerve of the forearm* (Fig. 6.25A).

The **radial nerve** enters the arm posterior to the brachial artery, medial to the humerus, and anterior to the long head of triceps (Figs. 6.24B,C and 6.27B). The radial nerve descends inferolaterally with the profunda brachii artery and curves around the humeral shaft in the radial groove. The radial nerve pierces the lateral intermuscular septum and continues inferiorly in the anterior compartment between the brachialis and the brachioradialis. In the cubital fossa, it divides into *deep* and *superficial branches* (Fig. 6.29). The radial nerve supplies the muscles in the posterior compartments of the arm and forearm and the overlying skin.

Biceps Tendinitis

The tendon of the long head of the biceps, enclosed by a synovial sheath, moves back and forth in the intertubercular sulcus (groove) of the humerus. Wear and tear of this mechanism can cause shoulder pain. Inflammation of the tendon (**biceps tendinitis**) usually is the result of repetitive microtrauma in sports involving throwing (e.g., baseball).

Rupture of Tendon of Long Head of Biceps

Rupture of the tendon of the long head of the biceps usually results from wear and tear of an inflamed tendon (*biceps tendinitis*). Normally, the tendon is torn from its attachment to the supraglenoid tubercle of the scapula. The rupture is commonly dramatic and is associated with a snap or pop. The detached muscle belly forms a ball near the center of the distal part of the anterior aspect of the arm (Popeye deformity) (Fig. B6.7).

Bicipital Myotatic Reflex

The biceps reflex is one of several deep-tendon reflexes that are routinely tested during physical examination. The relaxed limb is passively pronated and partially extended at the elbow. The examiner's thumb is firmly placed on the biceps tendon, and the reflex hammer is briskly tapped at the base of the nail bed of the examiner's thumb (Fig. B6.8). A normal (positive) response is an involuntary contraction of the biceps, felt as a momentarily tensed tendon, usually with a brief jerk-like flexion of the elbow. A positive response confirms the integrity of the musculocutaneous nerve and the C5 and C6 spinal cord segments. Excessive, diminished, or prolonged (hung) responses may indicate central or peripheral nervous system disease.

Rupture of biceps tendon (*arrows*)

FIGURE B6.7.

Biceps brachii

Biceps tendon

FIGURE B6.8.   Method of eliciting biceps reflex.

Injury to Radial Nerve

 Injury to the radial nerve superior to the origin of its branches to the triceps brachii results in *paralysis of the triceps, brachioradialis, supinator, and extensor muscles of the wrist and fingers.* Loss of sensation occurs in areas of skin supplied by this nerve. When the radial nerve is injured in the radial groove, the triceps is usually not completely paralyzed but only weakened because only the medial head is affected; however, the muscles in the posterior compartment of the forearm that are supplied by more distal branches of the radial nerve are paralyzed. The characteristic clinical sign of radial nerve injury is **wrist-drop** (inability to extend the wrist and fingers at the metacarpophalangeal joints) (Fig. B6.9). Instead, the wrist is flexed because of unopposed tonus of the flexor muscles and gravity.

Wrist-drop

FIGURE B6.9.

Injury to Musculocutaneous Nerve

 Injury to the musculocutaneous nerve in the axilla is usually inflicted by a weapon such as a knife. A musculocutaneous nerve injury results in *paralysis of the coracobrachialis, biceps, and brachialis;* consequently, flexion of the elbow and supination of the forearm are greatly weakened. Loss of sensation may occur on the lateral surface of the forearm supplied by the lateral cutaneous nerve of the forearm.

Occlusion or Laceration of Brachial Artery

Although collateral pathways confer some protection against gradual, temporary, and partial occlusion, sudden complete occlusion or laceration of the brachial artery creates a surgical emergency because paralysis of muscles results from ischemia within a few hours. After this, fibrous scar tissue develops and causes the involved muscles to shorten permanently, producing a flexion deformity—*ischemic compartment syndrome* (Volkmann ischemic

contracture). Flexion of the fingers and sometimes the wrist results in loss of hand power.

Measuring Blood Pressure

A *sphygmomanometer* is used to measure arterial blood pressure. A cuff is placed around the arm and inflated with air until it compresses the *brachial artery* against the humerus and occludes it. A stethoscope is placed over the artery in the *cubital fossa*, the pressure in the cuff is gradually released, and the examiner detects the sound of blood beginning to spurt through the artery. The first audible spurt indicates *systolic blood pressure.* As the pressure is completely released, the point at which the pulse can no longer be heard indicates *diastolic blood pressure.*

Compression of Brachial Artery

The best place to compress the brachial artery to control hemorrhage is near the middle of the arm. The biceps must be pushed laterally to detect pulsations of the artery (Fig. B6.10). Because the arterial anastomoses around the elbow provide a functionally and surgically important collateral circulation, the brachial artery may be clamped distal to the inferior ulnar collateral artery without producing tissue damage. The anatomical basis for this is that the ulnar and radial arteries still receive sufficient blood through the anastomoses. Ischemia of the elbow and forearm results from clamping the brachial artery proximal to the deep artery of the arm for an extended period.

Brachial artery

Compression of brachial artery
FIGURE B6.10.

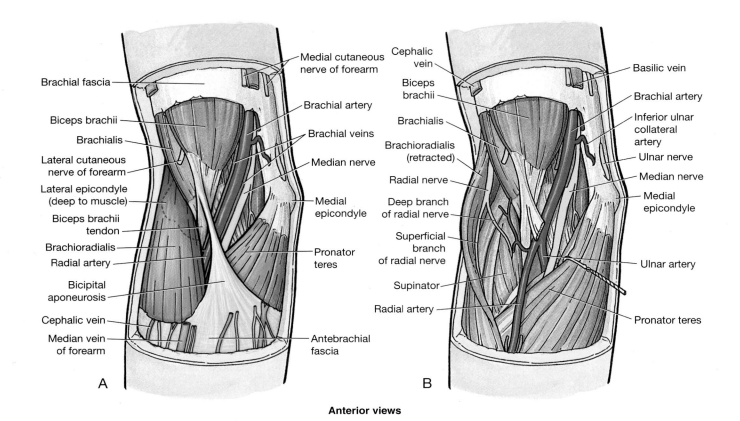

Anterior views

FIGURE 6.29.   **Cubital fossa. A.** Superficial dissection. **B.** Deep dissection.

Cubital Fossa

The **cubital fossa** is the shallow triangular depression on the anterior surface of the elbow (Fig. 6.29A). The boundaries of the cubital fossa are:

- Superiorly, an imaginary line connecting the medial and lateral epicondyles.
- Medially, the pronator teres.
- Laterally, the brachioradialis.

The *floor of the cubital fossa* is formed by the brachialis and supinator muscles. The *roof of the cubital fossa* is formed by the continuity of brachial and antebrachial (deep) fascia, reinforced by the bicipital aponeurosis, subcutaneous tissue, and skin.

The *contents of the cubital fossa* are the (Fig. 6.29B):

- Terminal part of the brachial artery and the commencement of its terminal branches, the radial and ulnar arteries; the brachial artery lies between the biceps tendon and the median nerve.
- (Deep) accompanying veins of the arteries.
- Biceps brachii tendon.
- Median nerve.
- Radial nerve, dividing into superficial and deep branches.

In the subcutaneous tissue overlying the cubital fossa are the *median cubital vein* (Fig. 6.13A), lying anterior to the brachial artery, and the *medial and lateral cutaneous nerves of the forearm,* related to the basilic and cephalic veins (Fig. 6.29).

FOREARM

The **forearm** lies between the elbow and the wrist and contains two bones, the *radius* and *ulna,* which are joined by an interosseous membrane (Fig. 6.30A). The role of forearm movement, occurring at the elbow and radio-ulnar joints, is to assist the shoulder in the application of force and in controlling the placement of the hand in space.

Muscles of Forearm

The tendons of the forearm muscles pass through the distal part of the forearm and continue into the wrist, hand, and fingers. The flexors and pronators of the forearm are in the anterior compartment and are served mainly by the *median nerve;* the one and a half exceptions are innervated by the *ulnar nerve.* The extensors and supinators of the forearm are in the posterior compartment and are all innervated by the *radial nerve* (Fig. 6.30).

Surface Anatomy of Arm and Cubital Fossa

The borders of the *deltoid* are visible when the arm is abducted against resistance. The **distal attachment of the deltoid** can be palpated on the lateral surface of the humerus. The **three heads of the triceps** form a bulge on the posterior aspect of the arm and are identifiable when the forearm is extended from the flexed position against resistance (Fig. SA6.3*A*). The **triceps tendon** may be felt as it descends along the posterior aspect of the arm to the **olecranon**. The **biceps brachii** forms a bulge on the anterior aspect of the arm; its belly becomes more prominent when the elbow is flexed and supinated against resistance (Fig. SA6.3*B*). Medial and lateral **bicipital grooves** separate the bulges formed by the biceps and triceps. The cephalic vein runs superiorly in the lateral bicipital groove and the basilic vein ascends in the medial bicipital groove. The **biceps tendon** can be palpated in the cubital fossa, immediately lateral to the midline. The proximal part of the **bicipital aponeurosis** can be palpated where it passes obliquely over the brachial artery and median nerve. The **brachial artery** may be felt pulsating deep to the medial border of the biceps.

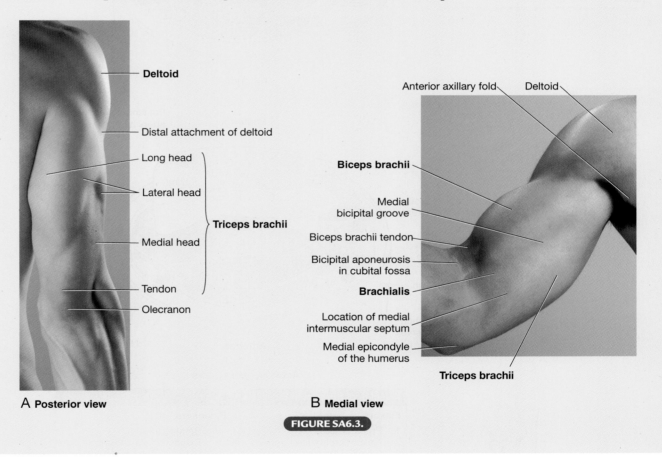

A Posterior view

B Medial view

FIGURE SA6.3.

FLEXOR–PRONATOR MUSCLES OF FOREARM

The **flexor–pronator muscles** are in the anterior compartment of the forearm (Figs. 6.30 and 6.31). The tendons of most flexor muscles pass across the anterior surface of the wrist and are held in place by the **palmar carpal ligament** and the *flexor retinaculum (transverse carpal ligament)*, thickenings of the antebrachial fascia. The flexor muscles are arranged in three layers or groups (Figs. 6.31 and 6.32; Table 6.7):

• A **superficial layer or group** of four muscles: **pronator teres, flexor carpi radialis, palmaris longus,** and **flexor carpi ulnaris** (FCU). These muscles are all attached proximally by a *common flexor tendon* to the medial epicondyle of the humerus, the *common flexor origin*.

Posterior

Radius

Ulna

Interosseous membrane

Muscle compartments of forearm
- Flexor–pronator
- Extensor–supinator

A

Anterior

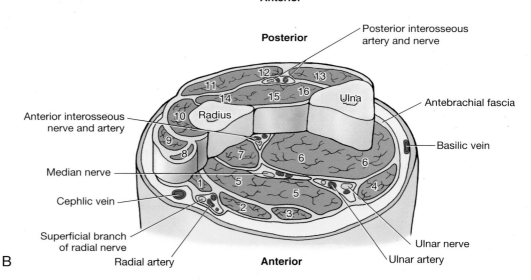

Posterior

Posterior interosseous artery and nerve

Ulna

Antebrachial fascia

Basilic vein

Anterior interosseous nerve and artery

Radius

Median nerve

Cephlic vein

Superficial branch of radial nerve

Radial artery

Ulnar nerve

Ulnar artery

B

Anterior

Anterosuperior views

Plane of section A and B

Muscles of forearm in B

Flexors		Extensors	
1	Pronator teres	8	Brachioradialis
2	Flexor carpi radialis	9	Extensor carpi radialis longus
3	Palmaris longus	10	Extensor carpi radialis brevis
4	Flexor carpi ulnaris	11	Extensor digitorum
5	Flexor digitorum superficialis	12	Extensor digiti minimi
6	Flexor digitorum profundus	13	Extensor carpi ulnaris
7	Flexor pollicis longus	14	Abductor pollicis longus
		15	Extensor pollicis brevis
		16	Extensor pollicis longus and extensor indicis

FIGURE 6.30.   Transverse section of the anterior and posterior compartments of forearm. **A.** Compartments. **B.** Contents of compartments.

Anterior views

FIGURE 6.31.   Muscles of anterior compartment of forearm. **A.** First layer. **B.** Second layer. **C.** Third layer.

- An **intermediate layer or group,** consisting of one muscle: **flexor digitorum superficialis** (FDS).
- A **deep layer or group** of three muscles: **flexor digitorum profundus** (FDP), **flexor pollicis longus** (FPL), and **pronator quadratus**.

The five superficial and intermediate muscles cross the elbow joint; the three deep muscles do not.

Functionally, the *brachioradialis* is a flexor of the forearm, but it is located in the extensor (posterior) compartment and is thus supplied by the radial nerve (Table 6.7). Therefore, the brachioradialis is a major exception to the generalization that the radial nerve supplies only extensor muscles and that all flexors lie in the anterior compartment.

The **long flexors of the digits** (FDS and FDP) also flex the metacarpophalangeal and wrist joints.

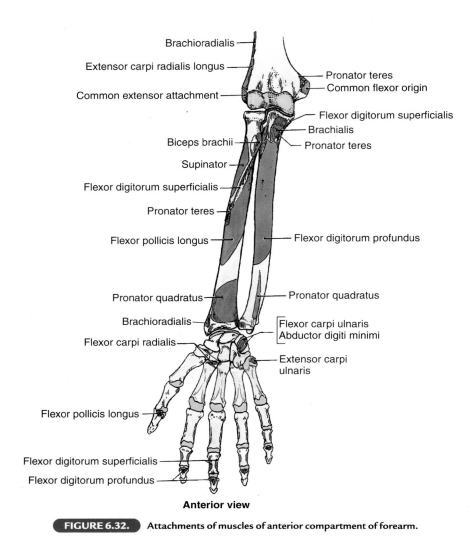

Brachioradialis

Extensor carpi radialis longus

Pronator teres

Common flexor origin

Common extensor attachment

Flexor digitorum superficialis

Brachialis

Biceps brachii

Pronator teres

Supinator

Flexor digitorum superficialis

Pronator teres

Flexor pollicis longus

Flexor digitorum profundus

Pronator quadratus

Pronator quadratus

Brachioradialis

Flexor carpi ulnaris
Abductor digiti minimi

Flexor carpi radialis

Extensor carpi ulnaris

Flexor pollicis longus

Flexor digitorum superficialis

Flexor digitorum profundus

Anterior view

FIGURE 6.32. Attachments of muscles of anterior compartment of forearm.

TABLE 6.7 MUSCLES OF ANTERIOR COMPARTMENT OF FOREARM

Muscle	Proximal Attachment	Distal Attachment	Innervation[a]	Main Action	
Superficial (first) layer					
Pronator teres (PT)	*Ulnar head:* coronoid process of ulna *Humeral head:* Medial epicondyle of humerus	Middle of convexity of lateral surface of radius	Median nerve (C6, **C7**)	Pronates and flexes forearm (at elbow)	
Flexor carpi radialis (FCR)	Medial epicondyle of humerus	Base of 2nd (3rd) metacarpal		Flexes and abducts hand (at wrist)	
Palmaris longus		Distal half of flexor retinaculum, palmar aponeurosis	Median nerve (C7, C8)	Flexes hand (at wrist) and tenses palmar aponeurosis	
Flexor carpi ulnaris (FCU): **Humeral head** **Ulnar head**	Olecranon and posterior border (via aponeurosis)	Pisiform, hook of hamate, 5th metacarpal	Ulnar nerve (C7, **C8**)	Flexes and adducts hand (at wrist)	

TABLE 6.7 MUSCLES OF ANTERIOR COMPARTMENT OF FOREARM (*continued*)

Muscle	Proximal Attachment	Distal Attachment	Innervation[a]	Main Action
Intermediate (second) layer				
Flexor digitorum superficialis (FDS)	*Humero-ulnar head*: medial epicondyle of humerus and coronoid process of ulna *Radial head*: oblique line of radius	Shafts (bodies) of middle phalanges of medial four digits	Median nerve (C7, C8, T1)	Flexes proximal interphalangeal joints of middle four digits; acting more strongly, it also flexes proximal phalanges at metacarpophalangeal joints
Deep (third) layer				
Flexor digitorum profundus (FDP)	Proximal three quarters of medial and anterior surfaces of ulna and interosseous membrane	Bases of distal phalanges of 2nd, 3rd, 4th, and 5th digits	*Lateral part (to digits 2 and 3)*: Median nerve (**C8**, T1) (anterior interosseous branch) *Medial part (to digits 4 and 5)*: Ulnar nerve (C8, **T1**)	Flexes distal interphalangeal joints of digits 2, 3, 4, and 5; assists with wrist flexion
Flexor pollicis longus (FPL)	Anterior surface of radius and adjacent interosseous membrane	Base of distal phalanx of thumb	Anterior interosseous nerve, from median nerve (**C8**, T1)	Flexes phalanges of 1st digit (thumb)
Pronator quadratus	Distal quarter of anterior surface of ulna	Distal quarter of anterior surface of radius		Pronates forearm; deep fibers bind radius and ulna together

[a]The spinal cord segmental innervation is indicated (e.g., "C6, **C7**" means that the nerves supplying the pronator teres are derived from the sixth and seventh cervical segments of the spinal cord). Numbers in boldface (**C7**) indicate the main segmental innervation. Damage to one or more of the listed spinal cord segments or to the motor nerve roots arising from them results in paralysis of the muscles concerned.

The FDP flexes the fingers in slow action; this action is reinforced by the FDS when speed and flexion against resistance are required. When the wrist is flexed at the same time that the metacarpophalangeal and interphalangeal joints are flexed, the long flexor muscles of the fingers are operating over a shortened distance between attachments, and the action resulting from their contraction is consequently weaker. Extending the wrist increases their operating distance, and thus their contraction is more efficient in producing a strong grip. Tendons of the long flexors of the digits pass through the distal part of the forearm, wrist, and palm and continue to the medial four fingers. The FDS flexes the middle phalanges; the FDP flexes the distal phalanges.

The **pronator quadratus** is the prime mover for pronation. The pronator quadratus initiates pronation and is assisted by the *pronator teres* when more speed and power are needed. The pronator quadratus also helps the interosseous membrane hold the radius and ulna together, particularly when upward thrusts are transmitted through the wrist (e.g., during a fall on the hand).

EXTENSOR MUSCLES OF FOREARM

The extensor muscles are in the posterior (extensor–supinator) compartment of the forearm, and all are innervated by branches of the radial nerve (Figs. 6.30 and 6.33; Table 6.8).

These muscles may be organized into three functional groups:

- Muscles that extend and abduct or adduct the hand at the wrist joint: extensor carpi radialis longus, extensor carpi radialis brevis, and extensor carpi ulnaris.
- Muscles that extend the medial four digits: extensor digitorum, extensor indicis, and extensor digiti minimi.
- Muscles that extend or abduct the thumb: abductor pollicis longus (APL), extensor pollicis brevis (EPB), and extensor pollicis longus (EPL).

The extensor tendons are held in place in the wrist region by the **extensor retinaculum,** which prevents bowstringing of the tendons when the hand is extended at the wrist joint. As the tendons pass over the dorsum of the wrist, they are covered with **synovial tendon sheaths,** which reduce friction for the extensor tendons as they traverse the osseofibrous tunnels formed by the attachment of the extensor retinaculum to the distal radius and ulna (Fig. 6.34).

The extensor muscles are organized anatomically into superficial and deep layers. Four *superficial extensors* (extensor carpi radialis brevis, extensor digitorum, extensor digiti minimi, and extensor carpi ulnaris) are attached proximally by a *common extensor tendon* to the lateral epicondyle (Fig. 6.33A; Table 6.8).

A Posterior view

- Olecranon
- Anconeus
- Flexor carpi ulnaris
- **Extensor carpi ulnaris**
- Extensor digiti minimi
- **Brachioradialis**
- Lateral epicondyle
- **Extensor carpi radialis longus**
- **Extensor carpi radialis brevis**
- **Extensor digitorum**
- Abductor pollicis longus
- Extensor pollicis brevis
- Anatomical snuff box
- Extensor pollicis longus

B Lateral view

- **Extensor indicis**
- Extensor retinaculum
- **Extensor carpi radialis brevis**
- **Extensor carpi radialis longus**
- Dorsal carpal branch
- Dorsalis indicis artery
- 1st dorsal interosseous (retracted)
- **Abductor pollicis longus**
- **Extensor pollicis brevis**
- **Extensor pollicis longus**
- Radial artery in anatomical snuff box
- Dorsalis pollicis arteries
- Adductor pollicis
- Radialis indicis artery

C Posterior view

- Lateral epicondyle
- Anconeus
- **Supinator**
- Posterior interosseous nerve
- Posterior interosseous artery
- **Abductor pollicis longus**
- **Extensor pollicis longus**
- **Extensor indicis**
- **Extensor pollicis brevis**
- Dorsal tubercle of radius
- Styloid process of radius
- Radial artery
- Base of 1st metacarpal
- Dorsal carpal arch
- Dorsalis pollicis artery
- Dorsal metacarpal arteries

FIGURE 6.33. **Muscles and neurovascular structures of posterior compartment of forearm. A.** Superficial dissection. **B.** Anatomical snuff box. **C.** Deep dissection.

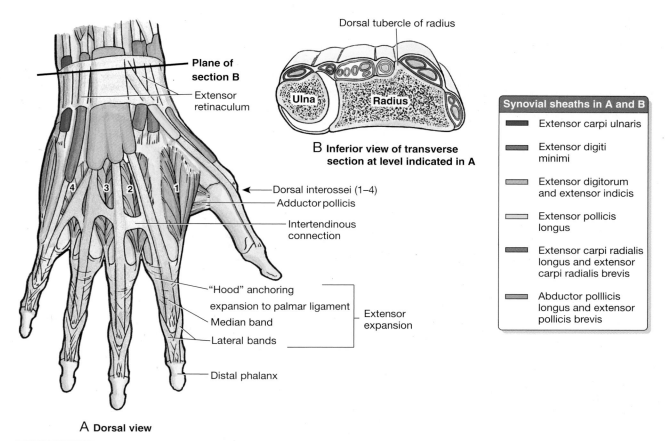

Dorsal tubercle of radius

Plane of
section B

Extensor
retinaculum

Ulna   Radius

B **Inferior view of transverse
section at level indicated in A**

Dorsal interossei (1–4)
Adductor pollicis
Intertendinous
connection

"Hood" anchoring
expansion to palmar ligament
Median band   Extensor
Lateral bands   expansion

Distal phalanx

A **Dorsal view**

Synovial sheaths in A and B
Extensor carpi ulnaris
Extensor digiti minimi
Extensor digitorum and extensor indicis
Extensor pollicis longus
Extensor carpi radialis longus and extensor carpi radialis brevis
Abductor polllicis longus and extensor pollicis brevis

FIGURE 6.34.   Synovial sheaths of extensor tendons on distal forearm and dorsum of hand. **A.** Illustration with color-coded synovial sheaths. **B.** Transverse section through distal end of radius and ulna to show extensor tendons in their synovial sheaths.

The proximal attachment of the other two superficial extensors (brachioradialis and extensor carpi radialis longus) is to the lateral supra-epicondylar ridge of the humerus and the adjacent lateral intermuscular septum (Fig. 6.35). The four flat tendons of the extensor digitorum pass deep to the extensor retinaculum to the medial four fingers (Fig. 6.34A). The common tendons of the index and little fingers are joined on their medial sides near the knuckles by the respective tendons of the extensor indicis and extensor digiti minimi (extensors of index and little fingers, respectively). The extensor indicis tendon joins the tendons of extensor digitorum to pass deep to the extensor retinaculum through the **tendinous sheath of extensor digitorum and extensor indicis** (common extensor synovial sheath). On the dorsum of the hand, the tendons of extensor digitorum spread out as they run toward the fingers. Adjacent tendons are linked proximal to the metacarpophalangeal joints by three oblique **intertendinous connections** that restrict independent extension of the fingers (Fig. 6.34A). Consequently, normally no finger can remain fully flexed as the other ones are fully extended.

On the distal ends of the metacarpals and along the phalanges, the four tendons of extensor digitorum flatten to form **extensor expansions** (Figs. 6.34 and 6.36). Each extensor expansion (dorsal expansion or hood) is a triangular tendinous aponeurosis that wraps around the dorsum and sides of a head of the metacarpal and base of the proximal phalanx. The visor-like "hood" of the extensor expansion over the head of the metacarpal is anchored on each side to the **palmar ligament** (a thickened portion of the fibrous layer of the joint capsule of the metacarpophalangeal joints). In forming the extensor expansion, each extensor digitorum tendon divides into a **median band,** which passes to the base of the middle phalanx, and two **lateral bands,** which pass to the base of the distal phalanx. The tendons of the interosseous and lumbrical muscles of the hand join the lateral bands of the extensor expansion (Fig. 6.36).

The **retinacular ligament** is a delicate fibrous band that runs from the proximal phalanx and fibrous digital sheath obliquely across the middle phalanx and two interphalangeal joints (Fig. 6.36B). During flexion of the distal interphalangeal joint, the retinacular ligament becomes taut.

Brachioradialis

Ext. carpi rad. longus

Triceps brachii

Common extensor origin (on anterior aspect)

Anconeus

Flexor carpi ulnaris

Supinator

Flexor digitorum profundus

Extensor pollicis longus

Pronator teres

Abductor pollicis longus

Extensor indicis

Extensor pollicis brevis

Brachioradialis

Extensor carpi radialis brevis

Extensor carpi ulnaris

Extensor carpi radialis longus

Extensor pollicis brevis

Extensor pollicis longus

Dorsal expansion (extensor expansion)

Posterior view

FIGURE 6.35.   Attachments of muscles of posterior compartment of forearm.

TABLE 6.8 MUSCLES OF POSTERIOR COMPARTMENT OF FOREARM

Muscle	Proximal Attachment	Distal Attachment	Innervation[a]	Main Action
Superficial layer				
Brachioradialis	Proximal two thirds of lateral supra-epicondylar ridge of humerus	Lateral surface of distal end of radius proximal to styloid process	Radial nerve (C5, **C6**, C7)	Relatively weak flexion of forearm, maximal when forearm is in midpronated position
Extensor carpi radialis longus	Lateral supra-epicondylar ridge of humerus	Dorsal aspect of base of 2nd metacarpal	Radial nerve (C6, C7)	Extend and abduct hand at the wrist joint; extensor carpi radialis brevis active during fist clenching
Extensor carpi radialis brevis	Lateral epicondyle of humerus (common extensor origin)	Dorsal aspect of base of 3rd metacarpal	Deep branch of radial nerve (**C7**, C8)	
Extensor digitorum		Extensor expansions of medial four fingers	Posterior interosseous nerve (**C7**, C8), continuation of deep branch of radial nerve	Extends medial four fingers primarily at metacarpophalangeal joints, secondarily at interphalangeal joints
Extensor digiti minimi		Extensor expansion of 5th finger		Extends 5th finger primarily at metacarpophalangeal joint, secondarily at interphalangeal joint
Extensor carpi ulnaris	Lateral epicondyle of humerus; posterior border of ulna via a shared aponeurosis	Dorsal aspect of base of 5th metacarpal		Extends and adducts hand at wrist joint (also active during fist clenching)

TABLE 6.8　MUSCLES OF POSTERIOR COMPARTMENT OF FOREARM (*continued*)

Muscle	Proximal Attachment	Distal Attachment	Innervation[a]	Main Action
Deep layer				
Supinator	Lateral epicondyle of humerus; radial collateral and anular ligaments; supinator fossa; crest of ulna	Lateral, posterior, and anterior surfaces of proximal third of radius	Deep branch of radial nerve (C7, **C8**)	Supinates forearm; rotates radius to turn palm anteriorly or superiorly (if elbow is flexed)
"Outcropping" muscles of deep layer				
Abductor pollicis longus	Posterior surface of proximal halves of ulna, radius, and interosseous membrane	Base of 1st metacarpal	Posterior interosseous nerve (C7, **C8**), continuation of deep branch of radial nerve	Abducts thumb and extends it at carpometacarpal joint
Extensor pollicis longus	Posterior surface of middle third of ulna and interosseous membrane	Dorsal aspect of base of distal phalanx of thumb		Extends distal phalanx of thumb at interphalangeal joint; extends metacarpophalangeal and carpometacarpal joints
Extensor pollicis brevis	Posterior surface of distal third of radius and interosseous membrane	Dorsal aspect of base of proximal phalanx of thumb		Extends proximal phalanx of thumb at metacarpophalangeal joint; extends carpometacarpal joint
Extensor indicis	Posterior surface of distal third of ulna and interosseous membrane	Extensor expansion of 2nd finger		Extends 2nd finger (enabling its independent extension); helps extend hand at wrist

[a]The spinal cord segmental innervation is indicated (e.g., "**C7**, C8" means that the nerves supplying the extensor carpi radialis brevis are derived from the seventh and eighth cervical segments of the spinal cord). Numbers in boldface (**C7**) indicate the main segmental innervation. Damage to one or more of the listed spinal cord segments or to the motor nerve roots arising from them results in paralysis of the muscles concerned.

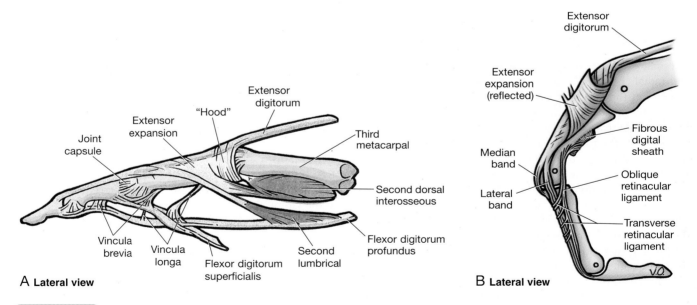

FIGURE 6.36. **Extensor expansion and vincula. A.** Parts of extensor expansion. The vincula are fibrous bands that convey small vessels to the tendons. **B.** Retinacular ligaments.

The taut retinacular ligament pulls the proximal interphalangeal joint into flexion. Similarly, on extending the proximal joint, the distal joint is pulled by the retinacular ligament into nearly complete extension.

The deep extensor muscles of forearm (APL, EPB, and **extensor pollicis longus**) act on the thumb. The **extensor indicis** confers independence to the index finger in that it may act alone or together with the extensor digitorum to extend the index finger (Figs. 6.33 and 6.35; Table 6.8). The three muscles acting on the thumb (APL, EPB, and EPL) are deep to the superficial extensors and emerge ("crop out") from a furrow in the lateral part of the forearm that divides the extensors. Because of this characteristic, they are referred to as *outcropping muscles*. The tendons of the APL and EPB bound the triangular **anatomical snuff box** laterally, and the tendon of the EPL bounds it medially (Fig. 6.33*A,B*). The snuff box is visible as a hollow on the lateral aspect of the wrist when the thumb is extended fully; this draws the APL, EPB, and EPL tendons up and produces a concavity between them. Observe that the:

- *Radial artery* lies on the floor of the snuff box.
- *Radial styloid process* can be palpated proximally and the base of the first metacarpal can be palpated distally in the snuff box.
- *Scaphoid and trapezium* can be felt in the floor of the snuff box between the radial styloid process and the first metacarpal.

Nerves of Forearm

The major **nerves of the forearm** are the median, ulnar, and radial (Figs. 6.37 and 6.38). Although the radial nerve appears in the cubital region, it soon enters the posterior compartment of the forearm. Besides the cutaneous branches, there are only two nerves of the anterior aspect of the forearm: the median and ulnar nerves. Their origins are described in Table 6.5 and their courses and distributions in Figure 6.38 and Table 6.9.

The **median nerve** is the principal nerve of the anterior compartment of the forearm. It enters the forearm with the brachial artery and lies medial to it. The median nerve leaves the cubital fossa by passing between the heads of the pronator teres, giving branches to them, and then passes deep to the FDS, continuing distally through the middle of the forearm, between the FDS and the FDP (Fig. 6.37). Near the wrist, the median nerve becomes superficial by passing between the tendons of the FDS and flexor carpi radialis (FCR) deep to the palmaris longus tendon. The **anterior interosseous nerve is its major branch** (Fig. 6.37). Articular and muscular branches and a palmar cutaneous branch are also derived from the median nerve.

The **ulnar nerve** passes posterior to the medial epicondyle of the humerus and enters the forearm by passing between the heads of the FCU (Fig. 6.37), giving branches to them. It then passes inferiorly between the FCU and the FDP, supplying the ulnar (medial) part of the muscle that sends tendons to digits 4 and 5. The ulnar nerve becomes superficial at the wrist, running on the medial side of the ulnar artery and the lateral side of the FCU tendon. The ulnar nerve emerges from beneath the FCU tendon just proximal to the wrist and passes superficial to the flexor retinaculum to enter the hand, where it supplies the skin on the medial side of the hand. The branches of the ulnar nerve in the forearm (articular, muscular, and palmar and dorsal cutaneous branches) are described in Table 6.9.

The **radial nerve** leaves the posterior compartment of the arm to cross the anterior aspect of the lateral epicondyle of the humerus. In the cubital region, the radial nerve divides into deep and superficial branches (Fig. 6.37). The *deep branch of radial nerve* arises anterior to the lateral epicondyle and pierces the supinator. The deep branch winds around the lateral aspect of the neck of the radius and enters the posterior (extensor–pronator) compartment of the forearm, where it continues as the *posterior interosseous nerve* (Fig. 6.38*C;* Table 6.9). The superficial branch of the radial nerve is a cutaneous and articular nerve that descends in the forearm under cover of the brachioradialis (Fig. 6.37). The *superficial branch of the radial nerve* (sensory or cutaneous) emerges in the distal part of the forearm and crosses the roof of the anatomical snuff box. It is distributed to skin on the dorsum of the hand and to a number of joints in the hand.

Arteries and Veins of Forearm

The brachial artery ends in the distal part of the cubital fossa opposite the neck of the radius by dividing into the ulnar and radial arteries, the main arteries of the forearm (Fig. 6.37). The branches of the ulnar and radial arteries are illustrated in Figure 6.39 and described in Table 6.10.

The **ulnar artery** descends through the anterior (flexor–pronator) compartment of the forearm, deep to the pronator teres. Pulsations of the ulnar artery can be palpated on the lateral side of the FCU tendon, where it lies anterior to the ulnar head (Fig. 6.37). The ulnar nerve is on the medial side of the ulnar artery.

When the brachioradialis is pulled laterally, the entire length of the artery is visible until the distal part of the forearm. The radial artery leaves the forearm by winding around the lateral aspect of the wrist and crossing the floor of the anatomical snuff box to reach the hand. The pulsation of the **radial artery** is usually measured on the distal radius between the tendons of flexor carpi radialis and abductor pollicis longus (Fig. 6.37).

There are superficial and deep veins in the forearm: *superficial veins* ascend in the subcutaneous tissue; *deep veins* accompany the deep arteries (e.g., radial and ulnar).

Biceps brachii

Brachialis

Lateral cutaneous
nerve of forearm

Brachioradialis

Radial nerve

Branches
of radial
nerve
Deep
Superficial

Supinator

Anterior interosseous
artery and nerve

Radial artery

Flexor pollicis longus

Site for taking radial pulse

Superficial palmar
branch of radial artery

Recurrent branch of
median nerve

Palmar
digital
nerves

Median nerve

Ulnar nerve

Brachial artery

Bicipital aponeurosis

Medial epicondyle

Tendon of biceps brachii

Ulnar artery

Common interosseous artery

Flexor carpi ulnaris

Ulnar nerve

Flexor digitorum profundus

Median nerve

Tendon of flexor carpi ulnaris

Site for taking ulnar pulse

Deep branch of ulnar artery

Deep branch of ulnar nerve

Superficial branch of ulnar nerve

Deep branch of ulnar nerve

Deep palmar arch

Anterior view

FIGURE 6.37.   Muscles, vessels, and nerves of anterior aspect of forearm and hand.

FIGURE 6.38. Nerves of forearm. **A–C.** Motor innervation. **D.** and **E.** Cutaneous innervation.

TABLE 6.9 NERVES OF FOREARM

Nerve	Origin	Course in Forearm
Median	By union of lateral root of median nerve (C6, C7, from lateral cord of brachial plexus) with medial root (C8, T1) from medial cord	Enters cubital fossa medial to brachial artery; exits by passing between heads of pronator teres; descends in fascial plane between flexors digitorum superficialis and profundus; runs deep to palmaris longus tendon as it approaches flexor retinaculum to traverse carpal tunnel
Anterior interosseous	Median nerve in distal part of cubital fossa	Descends on anterior aspect of interosseous membrane with artery of same name, between FDP and FPL, to pass deep to pronator quadratus
Palmar cutaneous branch of median nerve	Median nerve of middle to distal forearm, proximal to flexor retinaculum	Passes superficial to flexor retinaculum to reach skin of central palm
Ulnar	Larger terminal branch of medial cord of brachial plexus (C8, T1, often receives fibers from C7)	Enters forearm by passing between heads of flexor carpi ulnaris, after passing posterior to medial epicondyle of humerus; descends forearm between FCU and FDP; becomes superficial in distal forearm
Palmar cutaneous branch of ulnar nerve	Ulnar nerve near middle of forearm	Descends anterior to ulnar artery; perforates deep fascia in distal forearm; runs in subcutaneous tissue to palmar skin medial to axis of 4th digit
Dorsal cutaneous branch of ulnar nerve	Ulnar nerve in distal half of forearm	Passes posteroinferiorly between ulna and flexor carpi ulnaris; enters subcutaneous tissue to supply skin of dorsum medial to axis of 4th digit
Radial	Larger terminal branch of posterior cord of brachial plexus (C5–T1)	Enters cubital fossa between brachioradialis and brachialis; anterior to lateral epicondyle divides into terminal superficial and deep branches
Posterior cutaneous nerve of forearm	Radial nerve, as it traverses radial groove of posterior humerus	Perforates lateral head of triceps; descends along lateral side of arm and posterior aspect of forearm to wrist
Superficial branch of radial nerve	Sensory terminal branch of radial nerve, in cubital fossa	Descends between pronator teres and brachioradialis, emerging from latter to arborize over anatomical snuff box and supply skin of dorsum lateral to axis of 4th finger
Deep branch of radial/ posterior interosseous nerve	Motor terminal branch of radial nerve, in cubital fossa	Deep branch exits cubital fossa winding around neck of radius, penetrating and supplying supinator; emerges in posterior compartment of forearm as posterior interosseous nerve; descends on membrane with artery of same name
Lateral cutaneous nerve of forearm	Continuation of musculocutaneous nerve distal to muscular branches	Emerges lateral to biceps brachii on brachialis, running initially with cephalic vein; descends along lateral border of forearm to wrist
Medial cutaneous nerve of forearm	Medial cord of brachial plexus, receiving C8 and T1 fibers	Perforates deep fascia of arm with basilic vein proximal to cubital fossa; descends medial aspect of forearm in subcutaneous tissue to wrist

FCU, flexor carpi ulnaris; *FDP*, flexor digitorum profundus; *FPL*, flexor pollicis longus.

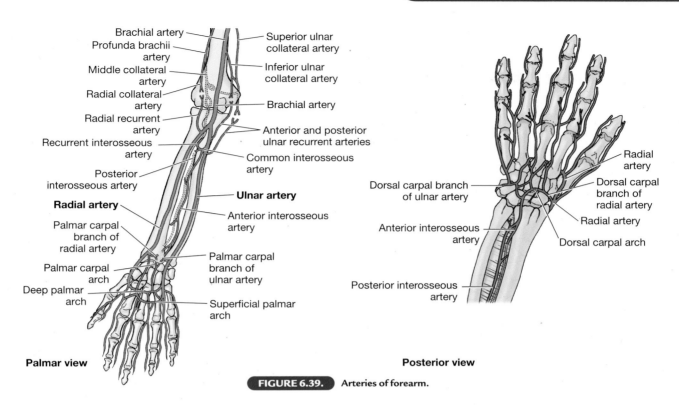

FIGURE 6.39.   Arteries of forearm.

TABLE 6.10   ARTERIES OF FOREARM AND WRIST

Artery	Origin	Course in Forearm
Ulnar	As larger terminal branch of brachial artery in cubital fossa	Descends inferomedially and then directly inferiorly deep to superficial pronator teres, palmaris longus, and flexor digitorum superficialis to reach medial side of forearm; passes superficial to flexor retinaculum at wrist in ulnar (Guyon) canal to enter hand
Anterior ulnar recurrent artery	Ulnar artery just distal to elbow joint	Passes superiorly between brachialis and pronator teres, supplying both; then anastomoses with inferior ulnar collateral artery anterior to medial epicondyle
Posterior ulnar recurrent artery	Ulnar artery distal to anterior ulnar recurrent artery	Passes superiorly, posterior to medial epicondyle and deep to tendon of flexor carpi ulnaris; then anastomoses with superior ulnar collateral artery
Common interosseous	Ulnar artery in cubital fossa, distal to bifurcation of brachial artery	Passes laterally and deeply, terminating by dividing into anterior and posterior interosseous arteries
Anterior interosseous	As terminal branches of common interosseous artery, between radius and ulna	Passes distally on anterior aspect of interosseous membrane to proximal border of pronator quadratus; pierces membrane and continues distally to join dorsal carpal arch on posterior aspect of interosseous membrane
Posterior interosseous		Passes to posterior aspect of interosseous membrane, giving rise to recurrent interosseous artery; runs distally between superficial and deep extensor muscles, supplying both
Recurrent interosseous	Posterior interosseous artery, between radius and ulna	Passes superiorly, posterior to proximal radio-ulnar joint, to anastomose with middle collateral artery (from deep artery of arm)
Palmar carpal branch	Ulnar artery in distal forearm	Runs across anterior aspect of wrist, deep to tendons of flexor digitorum profundus, to anastomose with the palmar carpal branch of the radial artery, forming **palmar carpal arch**
Dorsal carpal branch	Ulnar artery, proximal to pisiform	Passes across dorsal surface of wrist, deep to extensor tendons, to anastomose with dorsal carpal branch of radial artery, forming **dorsal carpal arch**
Radial	As smaller terminal branch of brachial artery in cubital fossa	Runs inferolaterally under cover of brachioradialis; lies lateral to flexor carpi radialis tendon in distal forearm; winds around lateral aspect of radius and crosses floor of anatomical snuff box to pierce 1st dorsal interosseous muscle
Radial recurrent	Lateral side of radial artery, just distal to brachial artery bifurcation	Ascends between brachioradialis and brachialis, supplying both (and elbow joint); then anastomoses with radial collateral artery (from profunda brachii artery)
Palmar carpal branch	Distal radial artery near distal border of pronator quadratus	Runs across anterior wrist deep to flexor tendons to anastomose with the palmar carpal branch of ulnar artery to form palmar carpal arch
Dorsal carpal branch	Distal radial artery in proximal part of snuff box	Runs medially across wrist deep to pollicis and extensor radialis tendons, anastomoses with ulnar dorsal carpal branch forming dorsal carpal arch

Muscle Testing of FDS and FDP

 To test the FDS, one finger is flexed at the proximal interphalangeal joint against resistance and the other three fingers are held in an extended position to inactivate the FDP (Fig. B6.11A). *To test the FDP,* the proximal interphalangeal joint is held in the extended position while the person attempts to flex the distal interphalangeal joint (Fig. B6.11B).

A Flexor digitorum superficialis (FDS)
muscle test

B Flexor digitorum profundus (FDP)
muscle test

FIGURE B6.11.

Elbow Tendinitis or Lateral Epicondylitis

Elbow tendinitis (tennis elbow) is a painful musculoskeletal condition that may follow repetitive use of the superficial extensor muscles of the forearm. Pain is felt over the lateral epicondyle and radiates down the posterior surface of the forearm. People with elbow tendinitis often feel pain when they open a door or lift a glass. Repeated forceful flexion and extension of the wrist strain the attachment of the common extensor tendon, producing inflammation of the periosteum of the lateral epicondyle (*lateral epicondylitis*).

Synovial Cyst of Wrist

 Sometimes a nontender cystic swelling appears on the hand, most commonly on the dorsum of the wrist (Fig. B6.12). The thin-walled cyst contains clear mucinous fluid. Clinically, this type of swelling is called a "ganglion" (G. swelling or knot). These synovial cysts are close to and often communicate with the synovial sheaths. The distal attachment of the extensor carpi radialis brevis (ECRB) tendon is a common site for such a cyst. A cystic swelling of the common flexor synovial sheath on the anterior aspect of the wrist can enlarge enough to produce compression of the median nerve by narrowing the carpal tunnel (*carpal tunnel syndrome*).

Synovial
cyst

Tendons

Synovial cyst

Synovial cyst

FIGURE B6.12.

Mallet or Baseball Finger

Sudden severe tension on a long extensor tendon may avulse part of its attachment to the phalanx. The most common result of this injury is *mallet* or *baseball finger.* This deformity results from the distal interphalangeal joint suddenly being forced into extreme flexion (hyperflexion) when the tendon is attempting to extend the distal phalanx—for example, when a baseball is miscaught (hyperflexing it) or the finger is jammed into a base pad. These actions avulse the attachment of the tendon from the base of the distal phalanx. As a result, the person is unable to extend the distal interphalangeal joint (Fig. B6.13).

Mallet finger

FIGURE B6.13. Mallet finger.

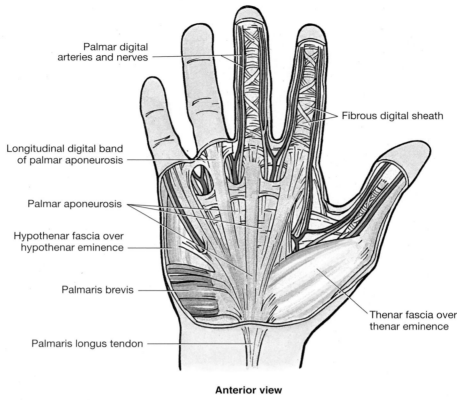

Palmar digital arteries and nerves

Fibrous digital sheath

Longitudinal digital band of palmar aponeurosis

Palmar aponeurosis

Hypothenar fascia over hypothenar eminence

Palmaris brevis

Thenar fascia over thenar eminence

Palmaris longus tendon

Anterior view

FIGURE 6.40. Palmar aponeurosis, fibrous digital sheaths, nerves, and vessels.

HAND

The wrist, the proximal part of the hand, is at the junction of the forearm and hand. The *skeleton of the hand* consists of *carpals* in the wrist, *metacarpals* in the hand proper, and *phalanges* in the fingers, which are numbered from 1 to 5, beginning with the thumb and ending with the little finger. The palmar aspect of the hand features a central concavity that separates two eminences: a lateral more prominent **thenar eminence** at the base of the thumb, and a medial, smaller **hypothenar eminence** proximal to the base of the fifth finger (Fig. 6.40).

Fascia of Palm

The **fascia of the palm** is continuous with the antebrachial fascia and the fascia of the dorsum of the hand. The **palmar fascia** is thin over the thenar and hypothenar eminences, but it is thick centrally where it forms the fibrous palmar aponeurosis, and in the fingers where it forms the digital sheaths (Fig. 6.40). The **palmar aponeurosis,** a strong, well-defined part of the deep fascia of the palm, covers the soft tissues and overlies the long flexor tendons. The proximal end or apex of the triangular palmar aponeurosis is continuous with the flexor retinaculum and the palmaris

longus tendon. Distal to the apex, the palmar aponeurosis forms four longitudinal digital bands that radiate from the apex and attach distally to the bases of the proximal phalanges, where they become continuous with the fibrous digital sheaths (Fig. 6.40). The **fibrous digital sheaths** are ligamentous tubes that enclose the flexor tendon(s) and the synovial sheaths that surround them as they pass along the palmar aspect of their respective digit.

A **medial fibrous septum** extends deeply from the medial border of the palmar aponeurosis to the fifth metacarpal. Medial to this septum is the medial or **hypothenar compartment** containing the hypothenar muscles (Figs. 6.40 and 6.41). Similarly, a **lateral fibrous septum** extends deeply from the lateral border of the palmar aponeurosis to the third metacarpal. Lateral to the septum is the lateral or **thenar compartment** containing the thenar muscles. Between the hypothenar and the thenar compartments is the **central compartment** containing the flexor tendons and their sheaths, the lumbrical muscles, the superficial palmar arterial arch, and the digital vessels and nerves (Fig. 6.41). The deepest muscular plane of the palm is the **adductor compartment** containing the adductor pollicis. Between the flexor tendons and the fascia covering the deep palmar muscles are two potential spaces: the **thenar space** and the **midpalmar space** (Fig. 6.41). These spaces

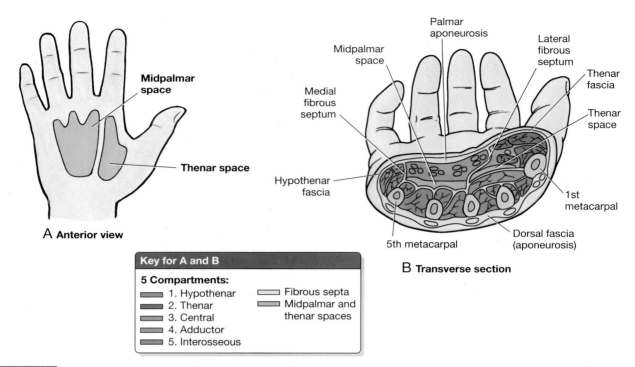

Midpalmar space

Thenar space

A **Anterior view**

Palmar aponeurosis

Midpalmar space

Lateral fibrous septum

Thenar fascia

Medial fibrous septum

Thenar space

Hypothenar fascia

1st metacarpal

5th metacarpal

Dorsal fascia (aponeurosis)

B **Transverse section**

Key for A and B

5 Compartments:
1. Hypothenar
2. Thenar
3. Central
4. Adductor
5. Interosseous

Fibrous septa
Midpalmar and thenar spaces

FIGURE 6.41. **Compartments and spaces of palm. A.** Schematic illustration showing location of thenar and midpalmar spaces. **B.** Transverse section showing compartments and spaces.

are bounded by fibrous septa passing from the edges of the palmar aponeurosis to the metacarpals. Between the two spaces is the especially strong lateral fibrous septum, which is attached to the third metacarpal. The midpalmar space is continuous with the anterior compartment of the forearm via the carpal tunnel.

Muscles of Hand

The intrinsic muscles of the hand are located in five compartments (Fig. 6.41; Table 6.11):

- Thenar muscles in the *thenar compartment:* abductor pollicis brevis, flexor pollicis brevis, and opponens pollicis.
- Hypothenar muscles in the *hypothenar compartment:* abductor digiti minimi, flexor digiti minimi brevis, and opponens digiti minimi.
- Adductor pollicis in the *adductor compartment.*
- The short muscles of the hand, the lumbricals, in the *central compartment* with the long flexor tendons.
- The interossei in separate *interosseous compartments* between the metacarpals.

THENAR MUSCLES

The **thenar muscles** form the *thenar eminence* on the lateral surface of the palm and are chiefly responsible for opposition of the thumb (Fig. 6.42A). Normal movement of

the thumb is important for the precise activities of the hand. The high degree of freedom of movements of the thumb results from the first metacarpal being independent, with mobile joints at both ends. Several muscles are required to control its freedom of movement (Fig. 6.45):

- *Abduction:* **APL** and **abductor pollicis brevis** (APB).
- *Adduction:* **adductor pollicis** (AD) and first dorsal interosseous.
- *Extension:* EPL, EPB, and APL.
- *Flexion:* **flexor pollicis longus** (FPL) and **flexor pollicis brevis** (FPB).
- *Opposition:* **opponens pollicis.**

Opposition occurs at the carpometacarpal joint of the thumb. The complex movement of opposition begins with the thumb in the extended position and initially involves abduction and medial rotation of the first metacarpal ("cupping" of the palm) produced by the action of the opponens pollicis and then flexion at the metacarpophalangeal joint. The reinforcing action of the adductor pollicis and flexor pollicis longus increases the pressure that the opposed thumb can exert on the fingertips.

HYPOTHENAR MUSCLES

The **hypothenar muscles** (abductor digiti minimi, flexor digiti minimi brevis, and opponens digiti minimi) are in the

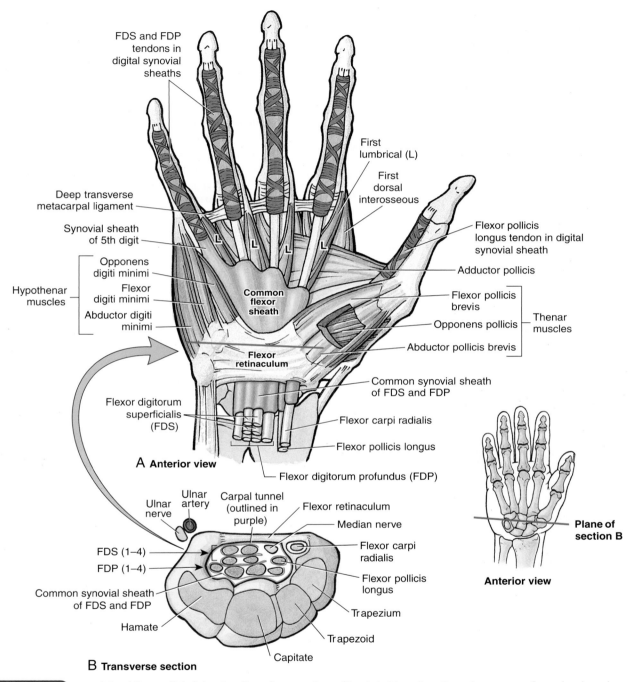

FDS and FDP tendons in digital synovial sheaths

First lumbrical (L)

First dorsal interosseous

Deep transverse metacarpal ligament

Synovial sheath of 5th digit

Flexor pollicis longus tendon in digital synovial sheath

Adductor pollicis

Opponens digiti minimi

Hypothenar muscles

Flexor digiti minimi

Common flexor sheath

Flexor pollicis brevis

Abductor digiti minimi

Opponens pollicis

Thenar muscles

Abductor pollicis brevis

Flexor retinaculum

Common synovial sheath of FDS and FDP

Flexor digitorum superficialis (FDS)

Flexor carpi radialis

Flexor pollicis longus

A Anterior view

Flexor digitorum profundus (FDP)

Ulnar nerve

Ulnar artery

Carpal tunnel (outlined in purple)

Flexor retinaculum

Median nerve

Flexor carpi radialis

FDS (1–4)

FDP (1–4)

Flexor pollicis longus

Common synovial sheath of FDS and FDP

Trapezium

Hamate

Trapezoid

Capitate

Plane of section B

Anterior view

B Transverse section

FIGURE 6.42. **Synovial and fibrous digital sheaths of long flexor tendons of hand. A.** Dissection of muscles, common flexor sheath, and synovial sheaths of digits 1–5 (*blue*). **B.** Transverse section of wrist shows carpal tunnel and its contents.

hypothenar compartment and produce the *hypothenar eminence* on the medial side of the palm (Fig. 6.42). The **palmaris brevis** is a small muscle in the subcutaneous tissue of the hypothenar eminence (Fig. 6.40); it is not in the hypothenar compartment. It wrinkles the skin of the hypothenar eminence, deepening the hollow of the palm, thereby aiding the palmar grip. The palmaris brevis covers

and protects the ulnar nerve and artery. It is attached proximally to the medial border of the palmar aponeurosis and to the skin on the medial border of the hand.

SHORT MUSCLES OF HAND

The **short hand muscles** are the lumbricals and interossei (Figs. 6.42–6.44; Table 6.11). The four slender **lumbrical**

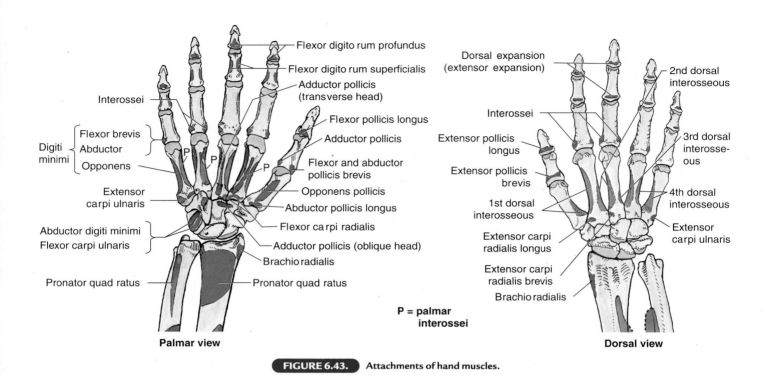

Palmar view

- Flexor digito rum profundus
- Flexor digito rum superficialis
- Adductor pollicis (transverse head)
- Interossei
- Digiti minimi
  - Flexor brevis
  - Abductor
  - Opponens
- Flexor pollicis longus
- Adductor pollicis
- Flexor and abductor pollicis brevis
- Extensor carpi ulnaris
- Opponens pollicis
- Abductor pollicis longus
- Abductor digiti minimi
- Flexor carpi ulnaris
- Flexor carpi radialis
- Adductor pollicis (oblique head)
- Brachio radialis
- Pronator quad ratus
- Pronator quad ratus

Dorsal view

- Dorsal expansion (extensor expansion)
- 2nd dorsal interosseous
- Interossei
- Extensor pollicis longus
- Extensor pollicis brevis
- 3rd dorsal interosseous
- 1st dorsal interosseous
- 4th dorsal interosseous
- Extensor carpi radialis longus
- Extensor carpi ulnaris
- Extensor carpi radialis brevis
- Brachio radialis

P = palmar interossei

FIGURE 6.43.   Attachments of hand muscles.

TABLE 6.11 INTRINSIC MUSCLES OF HAND

Muscle	Proximal Attachment	Distal Attachment	Innervation[a]	Main Action
Thenar muscles				
Opponens pollicis	Flexor retinaculum and tubercles of scaphoid and trapezium	Lateral side of 1st metacarpal	Recurrent branch of median nerve (**C8**, T1)	To oppose thumb, it draws 1st metacarpal medially to center of palm and rotates it medially
Abductor pollicis brevis		Lateral side of base of proximal phalanx of thumb		Abducts thumb; helps oppose it
Flexor pollicis brevis: Superficial head Deep head				Flexes thumb
Adductor pollicis: Oblique head	Bases of 2nd and 3rd metacarpals, capitate, adjacent carpals	Medial side of base of proximal phalanx of thumb	Deep branch of ulnar nerve (C8, **T1**)	Adducts thumb toward lateral border of palm
Transverse head	Anterior surface of shaft of 3rd metacarpal			
Hypothenar muscles				
Abductor digiti minimi	Pisiform	Medial side of base of proximal phalanx of 5th finger	Deep branch of ulnar nerve (C8, **T1**)	Abducts 5th finger; assists in flexion of its proximal phalanx
Flexor digiti minimi brevis	Hook of hamate and flexor retinaculum			Flexes proximal phalanx of 5th finger
Opponens digiti minimi		Medial border of 5th metacarpal		Draws 5th metacarpal anterior and rotates it, bringing 5th finger into opposition with thumb

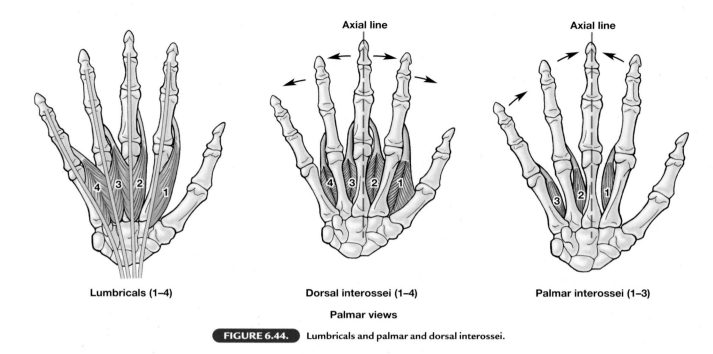

Palmar views

FIGURE 6.44. Lumbricals and palmar and dorsal interossei.

TABLE 6.11 INTRINSIC MUSCLES OF HAND (*continued*)

Muscle	Proximal Attachment	Distal Attachment	Innervation[a]	Main Action
Short muscles				
Lumbricals				
1 and 2	Lateral two tendons of flexor digitorum profundus (as unipennate muscles)	Lateral sides of extensor expansions of 2nd–5th fingers	Median nerve (C8, **T1**)	Flex metacarpophalangeal joints; extend interphalangeal joints of 2nd–5th fingers
3 and 4	Medial three tendons of flexor digitorum profundus (as bipennate muscles)		Deep branch of ulnar nerve (C8, **T1**)	
Dorsal interossei, 1–4	Adjacent sides of two metacarpals (as bipennate muscles)	Bases of proximal phalanges; extensor expansions of 2nd–4th fingers		Abduct 2nd–4th fingers from axial line; act with lumbricals in flexing metacarpophalangeal joints and extending interphalangeal joints
Palmar interossei, 1–3	Palmar surfaces of 2nd, 4th, and 5th metacarpals (as unipennate muscles)	Bases of proximal phalanges; extensor expansions of 2nd, 4th, and 5th fingers		Adduct 2nd, 4th, and 5th fingers toward axial line; assist lumbricals in flexing metacarpophalangeal joints and extending interphalangeal joints

[a]The spinal cord segmental innervation is indicated (e.g., "**C8**, T1" means that the nerves supplying the opponens pollicis are derived from the eighth cervical segment and first thoracic segment of the spinal cord). Numbers in boldface (**C8**) indicate the main segmental innervation. Damage to one or more of the listed spinal cord segments or to the motor nerve roots arising from them results in paralysis of the muscles concerned.

muscles were named because of their worm-like appearance (L. *lumbricus,* earthworm). The lumbricals flex the fingers at the metacarpophalangeal joints and extend the interphalangeal joints. The four **dorsal interosseous muscles** (dorsal interossei) are located between the metacarpals; the three **palmar interosseous muscles** (palmar interossei) are on the palmar surfaces of the second, fourth, and fifth metacarpals (Fig. 6.44). The first dorsal interosseous muscle is easy to palpate; oppose the thumb firmly against the index finger and it can be felt easily in the web between them. The four dorsal interossei abduct the fingers and the three palmar interossei adduct them. As a mnemonic device use the following acronyms: **d**orsal **ab**duct (**DAB**) and **p**almar **ad**duct (**PAD**). Acting together, the dorsal and palmar

| Abduction | Adduction | Extension | Flexion | Opposition | Reposition |

FIGURE 6.45. Movements of thumb.

interossei and lumbricals produce flexion at the metacarpophalangeal joints and extension of the interphalangeal joints (Z-movement). This occurs because of their attachment to the lateral bands of the extensor expansions.

Flexor Tendons of Extrinsic Muscles

The tendons of the flexor digitorum superficialis (FDS) and flexor digitorum profundus (FDP) enter the **common flexor sheath** deep to the flexor retinaculum (Fig. 6.42). The tendons enter the central compartment of the hand and fan out to enter the respective **digital synovial sheaths.** The common flexor and digital sheaths enable the tendons to slide freely past each other during movements of the fingers. Near the base of the proximal phalanx, the tendon of the FDS splits and surrounds the tendon of the FDP (Fig. 6.48A). The halves of the FDS tendon are attached to the margins of the anterior aspect of the shaft of the middle phalanx. The tendon of the FDP, after passing through the split in the FDS tendon, the *tendinous chiasm,* passes distally to attach to the anterior aspect of the base of the distal phalanx (Fig. 6.36).

The **fibrous digital sheaths** are strong ligamentous tunnels containing the flexor tendons and their synovial sheaths (Figs. 6.46). The sheaths extend from the heads of the metacarpals to the bases of the distal phalanges. These sheaths prevent the tendons from pulling away from the digits (bow-stringing). The fibrous digital sheaths attach to the bones to form **osseofibrous tunnels** through which the tendons pass to reach the digits. The **anular** and **cruciform parts (ligaments) of the fibrous sheath** (often referred to clinically as "pulleys") are thickened reinforcements of these sheaths. The long flexor tendons are supplied by small blood vessels that pass to them within synovial folds (*vincula*) from the periosteum of the phalanges (Figs. 6.36A and 6.46).

The tendon of FPL passes deep to the flexor retinaculum to the thumb within its own synovial sheath. At the head of the metacarpal, the tendon runs between two *sesamoid*

Fibrous digital sheath
- Cruciate part (ligament)
- Anular part (ligament)

FIGURE 6.46. Fibrous digital sheaths of digits. **A.** Anular and cruciate parts. **B.** Close-up of the anular part showing relationships of synovial sheath and mesotendon (vincula).

bones, one in the combined tendon of the FPB and APB and the other in the tendon of the AD.

Arteries and Veins of Hand

The ulnar and radial arteries and their branches provide all the blood to the hand (Figs. 6.47 and 6.48; Table 6.12). The *ulnar artery* enters the hand anterior to the flexor retinaculum between the pisiform and the hook of hamate via the *ulnar canal* (Guyon canal). The **ulnar artery** lies lateral to the ulnar nerve. It gives rise to the deep (palmar) branch

Radialis indicis

Proper palmar digital artery gives rise to a dorsal branch

Dorsal branches of proper palmar digital arteries

Dorsalis indicis

Common palmar digital arteries

Dorsal digital arteries

Superficial palmar arch

Dorsal metacarpal arteries

Princeps pollicis

Palmar metacarpal arteries

Perforating branches

Dorsalis pollicis

Deep palmar arch

Dorsal carpal arch

Dorsal branch

Palmar carpal arch

Dorsal carpal branch of ulnar artery

Secondary site for taking radial pulse

Superficial branch

Site for taking ulnar artery pulse

Anterior interosseous artery

Radial artery

Site for taking radial artery pulse

Ulnar artery

Anterior interosseous artery

Posterior interosseous artery

Radial artery

Radius

Radialis indicis

Anterior view

Lateral view (isolated 3rd digit)

Posterior view

FIGURE 6.47.   Arteries of hand.

TABLE 6.12 ARTERIES OF HAND

Artery	Origin	Course
Superficial palmar arch	Direct continuation of ulnar artery; arch is completed on lateral side by superficial branch of radial artery or another of its branches	Curves laterally deep to palmar aponeurosis and superficial to long flexor tendons; curve of arch lies across palm at level of distal border of extended thumb
Deep palmar arch	Direct continuation of radial artery; arch is completed on medial side by deep branch of ulnar artery	Curves medially, deep to long flexor tendons; is in contact with bases of metacarpals
Common palmar digitals	Superficial palmar arch	Pass distally on lumbricals to webbing of fingers
Proper palmar digitals	Common palmar digital arteries	Run along sides of 2nd–5th digits
Princeps pollicis	Radial artery as it turns into palm	Descends on palmar aspect of 1st metacarpal; divides at base of proximal phalanx into two branches that run along sides of thumb
Radialis indicis	Radial artery; but may arise from princeps pollicis artery	Passes along lateral side of index finger to its distal end
Dorsal carpal arch	Radial and ulnar arteries	Arches within fascia on dorsum of hand
Palmar carpal arch	Radial and ulnar arteries	Arches on anterior aspect of wrist

and then continues superficial to the long flexor tendons, where it is the main contributor to the **superficial palmar arch**. The *superficial palmar arch* gives rise to three **common palmar digital arteries** that anastomose with **palmar metacarpal arteries** from the deep palmar arch. Each common palmar digital artery divides into a pair of **proper palmar digital arteries** that run along the adjacent sides of the second to fourth fingers. The **radial artery** curves dorsally around the scaphoid and trapezium in the

floor of the *anatomical snuff box* (Fig. 6.33 A,B) and enters the palm by passing between the heads of the first dorsal interosseous muscle. It then turns medially and passes between the heads of the adductor pollicis (Fig. 6.49). The radial artery ends by anastomosing with the deep branch of the ulnar artery to form the **deep palmar arch** (Figs. 6.47 and 6.49). This arch, formed mainly by the radial artery, lies across the metacarpals just distal to their bases. The deep palmar arch gives rise to three *palmar metacarpal arteries*

A **Anterior view**

B **Anteroposterior view**

FIGURE 6.48.   **Nerves and arteries of hand. A.** Superficial dissection showing the superficial palmar arch and the distribution of median and ulnar nerves. **B.** Anteroposterior angiogram of hand. 1, Proper palmar digital artery. 2, Common palmar digital artery. 3, Superficial palmar arch. 4, Deep palmar arch. 5, Ulnar artery. 6, Radial artery.

and the *princeps pollicis artery*. The *radialis indicis artery* passes along the lateral side of the index finger (Fig. 6.47).

The *superficial* and *deep palmar venous arches,* associated with the superficial and deep palmar (arterial) arches, drain into the deep veins of the forearm. The dorsal digital veins drain into three dorsal metacarpal veins, which unite to form the *dorsal venous network.* Superficial to the metacarpus, this network is prolonged proximally on the lateral side as the *cephalic vein.* The *basilic vein* arises from the medial side of the dorsal venous network.

Nerves of Hand

The median, ulnar, and radial nerves supply the hand. The **median nerve** enters the hand through the carpal tunnel, deep to the flexor retinaculum (Figs. 6.48 and 6.49), along with the tendons of the FDS, FDP, and FPL. The **carpal tunnel** is the passageway deep to the flexor retinaculum between the tubercles of the scaphoid and the trapezoid bones on the lateral side and the pisiform and the hook of hamate on the medial side. Distal to the carpal tunnel, the median nerve supplies two and a half thenar muscles and the first and second lumbricals (Table 6.11). It also sends sensory fibers to the skin on the lateral palmar surface, the sides

of the first three digits, the lateral half of the fourth digit, and the dorsum of the distal halves of these digits. Note, however, that the *palmar cutaneous branch of the median nerve,* which supplies the central palm, arises proximal to the flexor retinaculum and passes superficial to it (i.e., it does not pass through the carpal tunnel).

The **ulnar nerve** leaves the forearm by emerging from deep to the tendon of the FCU (Figs. 6.48 and 6.49). It continues distally to the wrist via the *ulnar (Guyon) canal.* Here the ulnar nerve is bound by fascia to the anterior surface of the flexor retinaculum. It then passes alongside the lateral border of the pisiform; the ulnar artery is on its lateral side. Just proximal to the wrist, the ulnar nerve gives off a *palmar cutaneous branch* that passes superficial to the flexor retinaculum and palmar aponeurosis; it supplies skin on the medial side of the palm. The ulnar nerve also gives off a *dorsal cutaneous branch,* which supplies the medial half of the dorsum of the hand, the fifth finger, and the medial half of the fourth finger (Fig. 6.50). The ulnar nerve ends at the distal border of the flexor retinaculum by dividing into superficial and deep branches (Fig. 6.49). The *superficial branch of the ulnar nerve* supplies cutaneous branches to the anterior surfaces of the medial one and a half fingers. The *deep branch of the ulnar nerve* supplies the hypothenar

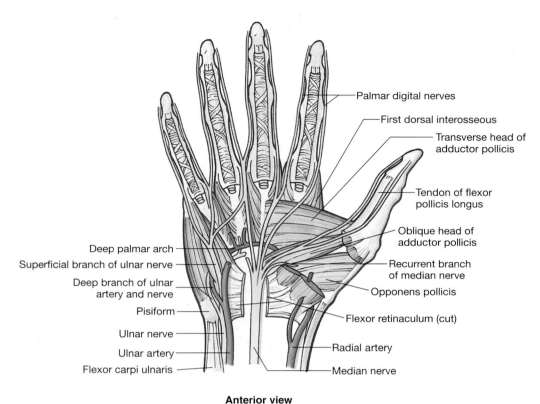

Anterior view

FIGURE 6.49. Deep dissection showing muscles, nerves, and deep palmar arch.

muscles, the medial two lumbricals, the adductor pollicis, the deep head of FPB, and all the interossei (Table 6.11). The deep branch also supplies several joints (wrist, intercarpal, carpometacarpal, and intermetacarpal). The ulnar nerve is referred to as the *nerve of fine movements* because it innervates muscles that are concerned with intricate hand movements.

The **radial nerve** supplies no hand muscles. Its terminal branches, superficial and deep, arise in the cubital fossa. The *superficial branch of the radial nerve* is entirely sensory (Fig. 6.50). It pierces the deep fascia near the dorsum of the wrist to supply the skin and fascia over the lateral two thirds of the dorsum of the hand, the dorsum of the thumb, and the proximal parts of the lateral one and a half digits.

FIGURE 6.50. Cutaneous innervation of hand.

Dupuytren Contracture of Palmar Fascia

Dupuytren contracture is a disease of the palmar fascia resulting in progressive shortening, thickening, and fibrosis of the palmar fascia and palmar aponeurosis. The fibrous degeneration of the longitudinal digital bands of the aponeurosis on the medial side of the hand pulls the fourth and fifth fingers into partial flexion at the metacarpophalangeal and proximal interphalangeal joints (Fig. B6.14).

Dupuytren contracture

FIGURE B6.14.

The contracture is frequently bilateral. Treatment of Dupuytren contracture usually involves surgical excision of all fibrotic parts of the palmar fascia to free the fingers.

Hand Infections

Because the palmar fascia is thick and strong, swellings resulting from hand infections usually appear on the dorsum of the hand, where the fascia is thinner. The potential fascial spaces of the palm are important because they may become infected. The fascial spaces determine the extent and direction of the spread of pus formed in the infected areas. Depending on the site of infection, pus will accumulate in the thenar, hypothenar, or adductor compartments. Antibiotic therapy has made infections that spread beyond one of these fascial compartments rare, but an untreated infection can spread proximally through the carpal tunnel into the forearm anterior to the pronator quadratus and its fascia.

Laceration of Palmar Arches

Bleeding is usually profuse when the palmar (arterial) arches are lacerated. It may not be sufficient to ligate (tie off) only one forearm artery when the arches are lacerated because these vessels usually have numerous communications in the forearm and hand and thus bleed from both ends. To obtain a bloodless surgical operating field for treating complicated hand injuries, it may be necessary to compress the brachial artery and its branches proximal to the elbow (e.g., using a pneumatic tourniquet). This procedure prevents blood from reaching the ulnar and radial arteries through the anastomoses around the elbow.

The superficial and deep palmar (arterial) arches are not palpable, but their surface markings are visible. The superficial palmar arch occurs at the level of the distal border of the fully extended thumb. The deep palmar arch lies approximately 1 cm proximal to the superficial palmar arch. The location of these arches should be borne in mind in wounds of the palm and when palmar incisions are made (Fig. 6.48*B*).

Palmar Wounds and Surgical Incisions

The location of superficial and deep palmar arches should be kept in mind when examining wounds of the palm and when making palmar incisions. Furthermore, it is important to know that the superficial palmar arch is at the same level as the distal extremity of the common flexor sheath. Incisions or wounds along the medial surface of the thenar eminence may injure the recurrent branch of the median nerve to the thenar muscles.

Ischemia of Digits

Intermittent bilateral attacks of *ischemia of the digits*, marked by cyanosis and often accompanied by paresthesia and pain, are characteristically brought on by cold and emotional stimuli. The condition may result from an anatomical abnormality or an underlying disease. When the cause of the condition is idiopathic (unknown) or primary, it is called *Raynaud syndrome* (disease).

The arteries of the upper limb are innervated by sympathetic nerves. Postsynaptic fibers from the sympathetic ganglia enter nerves that form the brachial plexus and are distributed to the digital arteries through branches arising from the plexus. When treating ischemia resulting from Raynaud syndrome, it may be necessary to perform a cervicodorsal *presynaptic sympathectomy* (excision of a segment of a sympathetic nerve) to dilate the digital arteries.

Tenosynovitis

Injuries such as puncture of a finger by a rusty nail can cause infection of the digital synovial sheaths. When inflammation of the tendon and synovial sheath (**tenosynovitis**) occurs, the digit swells and movement becomes painful. Because the tendons of the second through fourth digits nearly always have separate synovial sheaths, the infection usually is confined to the infected digit. If the infection is untreated, however, the proximal ends of these sheaths may rupture, allowing the infection to spread to the midpalmar space (Fig. 6.41). Because the synovial sheath of the little finger is usually continuous with the common flexor sheath, tenosynovitis in this finger may spread to the common sheath and thus through the palm and carpal tunnel to the anterior forearm. Likewise, tenosynovitis in the thumb may spread through the continuous synovial sheath of the FPL (radial bursa). How far an infection spreads from the digits depends on variations in their connections with the common flexor sheath.

The tendons of the APL and EPB are in the same tendinous sheath on the dorsum of the wrist. Excessive friction of these tendons results in fibrous thickening of the sheath and stenosis of the osseofibrous tunnel, **Quervain tenovaginitis stenosans.** This condition causes pain in the wrist that radiates proximally to the forearm and distally to the thumb.

If the tendons of the FDS and FDP enlarge (forming a nodule) proximal to the tunnel, the person is unable to extend the finger. When the finger is extended passively, a snap is audible. Flexion produces another snap as the thickened tendon moves. This condition is called **digital tenovaginitis stenosans** (trigger finger or snapping finger) (Fig. B6.15).

Thickened anular ligament of fibrous digital sheath

Nodule

Long flexor tendon

Digital tenovaginitis stenosans (trigger finger)

FIGURE B6.15.

Carpal Tunnel Syndrome

Carpal tunnel syndrome results from any lesion that significantly reduces the size of the carpal tunnel or, more commonly, increases the size of some of the structures (or their coverings) that pass through it (e.g., inflammation of the synovial sheaths). The median nerve is the most sensitive structure in the carpal tunnel and, therefore, is the most affected (Fig. 6.42B). The median nerve has two terminal sensory branches that supply the skin of the hand; hence **paresthesia** (tingling), **hypothesia** (diminished sensation), or **anesthesia** (absence of tactile sensation) may occur in the lateral three and a half digits. Recall, however, that the *palmar cutaneous branch of the median nerve* arises proximal to and does not pass through the carpal tunnel; thus sensation in the central palm remains unaffected. This nerve also has one terminal motor branch, the recurrent branch, which innervates the three thenar muscles.

Wasting of the thenar eminence and progressive loss of coordination and strength in the thumb (owing to weakness of the APB and opponens pollicis) may occur if the cause of the compression is not alleviated. Individuals with carpal tunnel syndrome are unable to oppose the thumb (Fig. B6.16). To relieve the compression and resulting symptoms, partial or complete surgical division of the flexor retinaculum, a procedure called **carpal tunnel release,** may be necessary. The incision for carpal tunnel release is made toward the medial side of the wrist and flexor retinaculum to avoid possible injury to the recurrent branch of the median nerve.

Trauma to Median Nerve

Lesions of the median nerve usually occur in two places: the forearm and wrist. The most common site is where the nerve passes through the carpal tunnel. Laceration of the wrist often causes median nerve injury because this nerve is relatively close to the surface. This results in paralysis and wasting of the thenar muscles and the first two lumbricals. Hence opposition of the thumb is not possible and fine control movements of the second and third digits are impaired. Sensation is also lost over the thumb and adjacent two and a half fingers.

Median nerve injury resulting from a perforating wound in the elbow region results in loss of flexion of the proximal and distal interphalangeal joints of the second and third digits. The ability to flex the metacarpophalangeal joints of these digits is also affected because digital branches of the median nerve supply the first and second lumbricals. This results in a deformity in which thumb movements are limited to flexion and extension of the thumb in the plane of the palm. This condition is caused by the inability to oppose and by limited abduction of the thumb (Fig. B6.16).

when trying to make a fist. Furthermore, the person cannot extend the interphalangeal joints when trying to straighten the fingers. This characteristic appearance of the hand is known as a *claw hand* (Fig. B6.17A). This deformity results from atrophy of the interosseous muscles of the hand. The claw is produced by the unopposed action of the extensors and FDP.

Compression of the ulnar nerve also may occur at the wrist where it passes between the pisiform and the hook of hamate. The depression between these bones is converted by the pisohamate ligament into an osseofibrous ulnar tunnel (Guyon tunnel). **Ulnar canal syndrome** is manifest by hypoesthesia in the medial one and one half fingers (Fig. B6.17B) and weakness of the intrinsic hand muscles. Clawing of the fourth and fifth fingers may occur, but in contrast to proximal ulnar nerve injury, their ability to flex is unaffected and there is no radial deviation of the hand.

A Inability to oppose thumb (movement occurs at carpometacarpal joint)

Emaciation of thenar eminence, thumb adducted and extended

B Wasting of thenar eminence

FIGURE B6.16.

A Claw hand

Palmar digital branches
Palmar branch

B Sensory distribution of ulnary nerve

FIGURE B6.17. Ulnar nerve injury.

Ulnar Nerve Injury

Ulnar nerve injury usually occurs in one of four places: (1) posterior to the medial epicondyle of the humerus (most common), (2) in the cubital tunnel formed by the tendinous arch connecting the humeral and ulnar heads of the FCU, (3) at the wrist, and (4) in the hand. Ulnar nerve injury occurring at the elbow or wrist or in the hand may result in extensive motor and sensory loss to the hand. An injury to the nerve in the distal part of the forearm denervates most intrinsic hand muscles. The power of wrist adduction is impaired, and when an attempt is made to flex the wrist joint, the hand is drawn to the lateral side by the FCR in the absence of the "balance" provided by the FCU. After ulnar nerve injury, the person has difficulty making a fist because, in the absence of opposition, the metacarpophalangeal joints become hyperextended, and he or she cannot flex the fourth and fifth fingers at the distal interphalangeal joints

Radial Nerve Injury

Although the radial nerve supplies no muscles in the hand, radial nerve injury in the arm by a fracture of the humeral shaft can produce serious disability of the hand. This injury is proximal to the branches to the extensors of the wrist, so wrist drop is the primary clinical manifestation. The hand is flexed at the wrist and lies flaccid, and the digits also remain in the flexed position at the metacarpophalangeal joints. The extent of anesthesia is minimal, even in serious radial nerve injuries, and usually is confined to a small area on the lateral part of the dorsum of the hand. Severance of the deep branch results in an inability to extend the thumb and the metacarpophalangeal joints of the other digits. Loss of sensation does not occur because the deep branch is entirely muscular and articular in distribution.

Surface Anatomy of Forearm and Hand

The cubital fossa, the triangular hollow area on the anterior surface of the elbow, is bounded medially by the prominence formed by the flexor–pronator group of muscles that are attached to the medial epicondyle. To estimate the position of these muscles, put your thumb posterior to your medial epicondyle and place your fingers on your forearm as shown in Figure SA6.4*A*.

A common place for measuring the radial pulse rate is where the radial artery lies on the anterior surface of the distal end of the radius, lateral to the FCR tendon (Fig. SA6.4*B*). Here the artery can be felt pulsating between the tendons of the FCR and the APL and where it can be compressed against the radius. The **tendons of the FCR and palmaris longus** can be palpated anterior to the wrist.

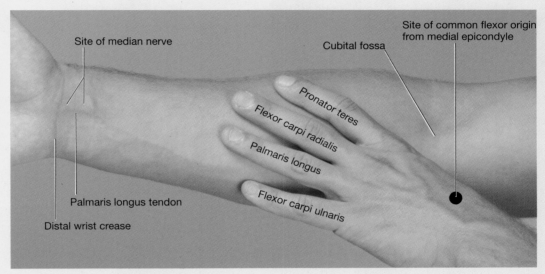

Site of median nerve
Site of common flexor origin from medial epicondyle
Cubital fossa
Pronator teres
Flexor carpi radialis
Palmaris longus
Flexor carpi ulnaris
Palmaris longus tendon
Distal wrist crease

A Anterior view of supinated forearm

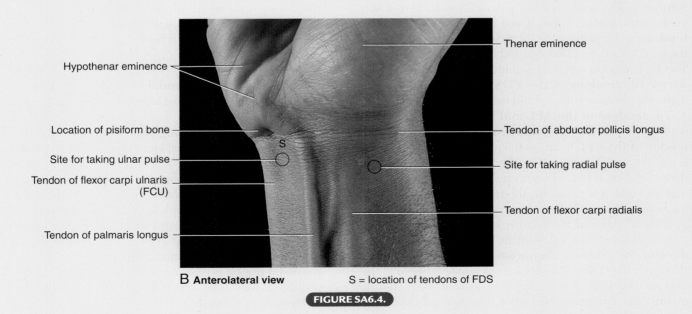

Hypothenar eminence
Location of pisiform bone
Site for taking ulnar pulse
Tendon of flexor carpi ulnaris (FCU)
Tendon of palmaris longus
S
Thenar eminence
Tendon of abductor pollicis longus
Site for taking radial pulse
Tendon of flexor carpi radialis

B Anterolateral view   S = location of tendons of FDS

FIGURE SA6.4.

C Posterior view

D Anterior view

FIGURE SA6.4. *(continued)*

These tendons are a little lateral to the middle of the wrist and are usually observed by flexing the closed fist against resistance. The tendon of the palmaris longus serves as a guide to the median nerve, which lies deep to it. The **FCU tendon** can be palpated as it crosses the anterior aspect of the wrist near the medial side and inserts into the pisiform. The FCU tendon serves as a guide to the ulnar nerve and artery. The **tendons of the FDS** can be palpated as the digits are alternately flexed and extended (Fig SA6.4*B*).

The **tendons of the APL and EPB** indicate the lateral (anterior) boundary of the **anatomical snuff box,** and the **tendon of the EPL** indicates the medial (posterior) boundary of the box (Fig. SA6.4*C*). The radial artery crosses the floor of the snuff box, where its pulsations may be felt. The scaphoid and, less distinctly, the trapezium are palpable in the floor of the snuff box.

If the dorsum of the hand is examined with the wrist extended against resistance and the digits abducted, the **tendons of the extensor digitorum** to the fingers stand out (Fig. SA6.4*C*). These tendons are not visible far beyond the knuckles because they flatten here to form the extensor expansions of the fingers. Under the loose subcutaneous

tissue and extensor tendons, the metacarpals can be palpated. The knuckles that become visible when a fist is made are produced by the **heads of the metacarpals.**

The palmar skin presents several more or less constant *flexion creases* where the skin is firmly bound to the deep fascia (Fig. SA6.4*D*):

- *Wrist creases:* **proximal, middle, distal.** The *distal wrist crease* indicates the proximal border of the flexor retinaculum.
- *Palmar creases:* **radial longitudinal crease** (the "life line" of palmistry), proximal and distal transverse palmar creases.
- *Transverse digital flexion creases:* The **proximal digital crease** is located at the root of the digit, approximately 2 cm distal to the metacarpophalangeal joint. The proximal digital crease of the thumb crosses obliquely, proximal to the first metacarpophalangeal joint. The **middle digital crease** lies over the proximal interphalangeal joint, and the **distal digital crease** lies proximal to the distal interphalangeal joint. The thumb, having two phalanges, has only two flexion creases.

JOINTS OF UPPER LIMB

Movement of the pectoral girdle involves the sternoclavicular, acromioclavicular, and glenohumeral joints, usually all moving simultaneously (Fig. 6.51). Functional defects in any of these joints impair movements of the pectoral girdle. Mobility of the scapula is essential for the freedom of movement of the upper limb. When testing *the range of motion of the pectoral girdle*, both scapulothoracic (movement of the scapula on the thoracic wall) and glenohumeral movements must be considered. Although the initial 30 degrees may occur without scapular motion, in the overall movement of fully elevating the arm, the movement occurs in a 2:1 ratio. For every 3 degrees of elevation, approximately 2 degrees occurs at the glenohumeral joint and 1 degree at the scapulothoracic joint. This is known as *scapulohumeral rhythm.* The important movements of the pectoral girdle are scapular movements: elevation and depression, protraction (lateral or forward movement of the scapula), and retraction (medial or backward movement of the scapula) and rotation of the scapula.

Sternoclavicular Joint

The **sternoclavicular (SC) joint** is a synovial articulation between the sternal end of the clavicle and the manubrium of the sternum and the first costal cartilage. The SC joint is a saddle type of joint but functions as a ball-and-socket joint (Fig. 6.51). The SC joint is divided into two compartments by an **articular disc.** The disc is firmly attached to the *anterior* and *posterior SC ligaments,* thickenings of the fibrous layer of the joint capsule, as well as to the *interclavicular ligament* (Fig. 6.51*B*). The great strength of the SC joint is a consequence of these attachments. Thus, although the articular disc serves as a shock absorber of forces transmitted along the clavicle from the upper limb, dislocation of the clavicle is unusual whereas fracture of the clavicle is common. The SC joint, the only articulation between the upper limb and the axial skeleton, can be readily palpated because the sternal end of the clavicle lies superior to the manubrium of the sternum.

The **joint capsule** surrounds the SC joint, including the epiphysis at the sternal end of the clavicle. The *fibrous layer of the capsule* is attached to the margins of the articular surfaces, including the periphery of the articular disc. A *synovial*

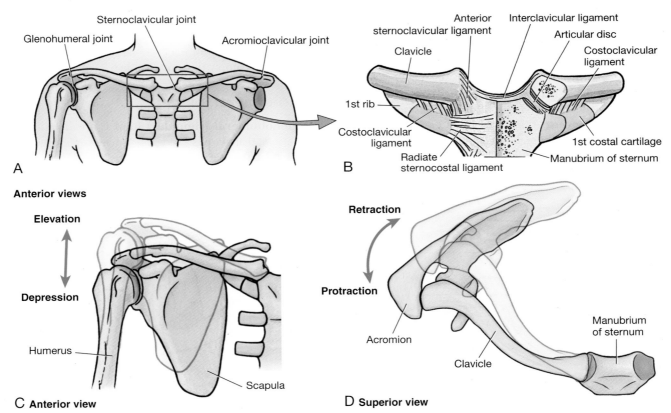

A   **Anterior views**

C   **Anterior view**

D   **Superior view**

FIGURE 6.51.   **Sternoclavicular and acromioclavicular joints. A.** Joints of pectoral girdle. Red box shows area illustrated in **B. B.** Structure of sternoclavicular joint. **C. and D.** Range of motion of clavicle permitted by movements at sternoclavicular and acromioclavicular joints. Elevation and depression (**C**), protraction and retraction (**D**).

membrane lines the internal surfaces of the fibrous layer of the capsule. **Anterior** and **posterior SC ligaments** reinforce the joint capsule anteriorly and posteriorly. The **interclavicular ligament** strengthens the capsule superiorly. It extends from the sternal end of one clavicle to the sternal end of the other clavicle; it is also attached to the superior border of the manubrium. The **costoclavicular ligament** anchors the inferior surface of the sternal end of the clavicle to the first rib and its costal cartilage, limiting elevation of the pectoral girdle.

Although the SC joint is extremely strong, it is significantly mobile to allow movements of the pectoral girdle and upper limb. During full elevation of the limb, the clavicle is raised to approximately a 60-degree angle. The SC joint can also be moved anteriorly or posteriorly over a range up to 25 to 30 degrees.

The SC joint is supplied by internal thoracic and suprascapular arteries (Table 6.4). Branches of the medial supraclavicular nerve and the subclavian nerve supply the SC joint (Table 6.5).

Acromioclavicular Joint

The **acromioclavicular (AC) joint** is a plane synovial articulation (Fig. 6.52). It is located 2 to 3 cm from the "point" of the shoulder formed by the lateral part of the acromion of the scapula. The acromial end of the clavicle articulates with the acromion. The articular surfaces, covered with fibrocartilage, are separated by an incomplete wedge-shaped *articular disc.*

The sleeve-like, relatively loose *fibrous layer of the joint capsule* is attached to the margins of the articular surfaces. A *synovial membrane* lines the internal surface of the fibrous layer of the capsule. Although relatively weak, the joint capsule is strengthened superiorly by fibers of the trapezius.

The **AC ligament,** a fibrous band extending from the acromion to the clavicle, strengthens the AC joint superiorly (Fig. 6.52A). Most of its strength comes from the coracoclavicular ligament. It maintains its integrity and prevents the acromion from being driven under the clavicle even when the AC joint is separated. The strong, extra-articular **coracoclavicular ligament** (subdivided into conoid and trapezoid ligaments) is located several centimeters from the AC joint, which anchors the clavicle to the coracoid process of the scapula (Fig. 6.54D). The apex of the vertical **conoid ligament** is attached to the root of the *coracoid process.* Its wide attachment (base) is to the *conoid tubercle* on the inferior surface of the clavicle. The nearly horizontal **trapezoid ligament** is attached to the superior surface of the coracoid process and extends laterally and posteriorly to the trapezoid line on the inferior surface of the clavicle. In addition to augmenting the AC joint, the coracoclavicular ligament provides the means by which the scapula and free limb are (passively) suspended from the clavicle.

The acromion of the scapula rotates on the acromial end of the clavicle. These movements are associated with motion at the physiological scapulothoracic joint. The axioappendicular muscles that attach to and move the scapula cause the acromion to move on the clavicle (Fig. 6.53). Factors limiting scapular movements are listed in Table 6.13. The AC joint is supplied by the suprascapular and thoraco-acromial arteries (Table 6.4). Supraclavicular, lateral pectoral, and axillary nerves supply the joint (Table 6.5).

Glenohumeral Joint

The **glenohumeral (shoulder) joint** is a ball-and-socket, synovial joint that permits a wide range of movement; however, its mobility makes the joint relatively unstable (Fig. 6.54).

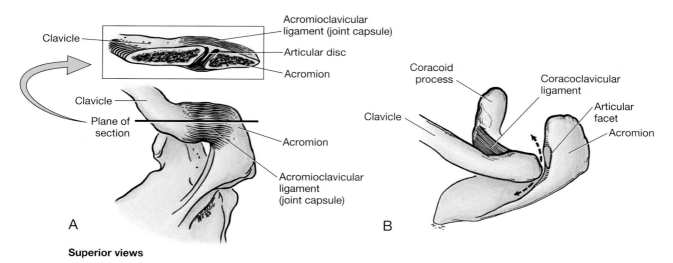

Superior views

FIGURE 6.52.   **Acromioclavicular joint. A.** Joint capsule and articular disc. **B.** Coracoclavicular ligament and articular facet of acromion.

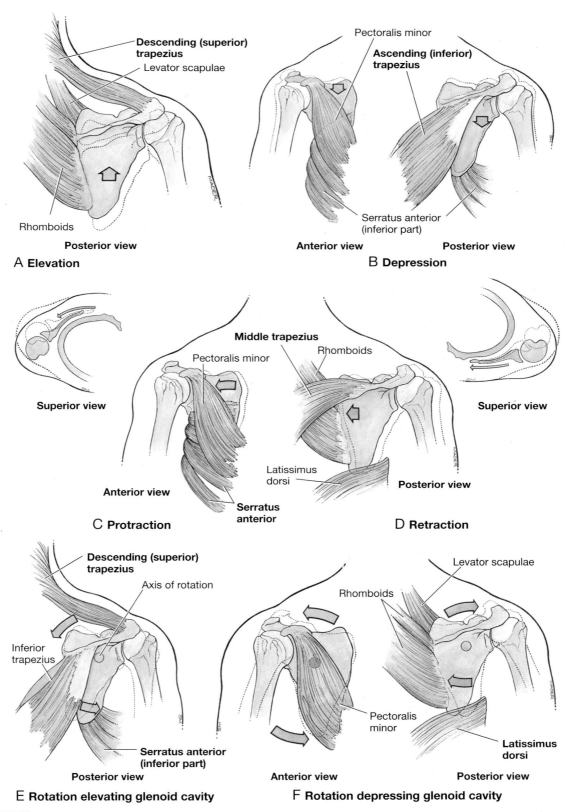

Descending (superior) trapezius
Levator scapulae
Rhomboids
Posterior view
A **Elevation**

Pectoralis minor
Ascending (inferior) trapezius
Serratus anterior (inferior part)
Anterior view   Posterior view
B **Depression**

Superior view
Middle trapezius
Pectoralis minor
Rhomboids
Serratus anterior
Anterior view
C **Protraction**

Latissimus dorsi
Posterior view
Superior view
D **Retraction**

Descending (superior) trapezius
Axis of rotation
Inferior trapezius
Serratus anterior (inferior part)
Posterior view
E **Rotation elevating glenoid cavity**

Levator scapulae
Rhomboids
Pectoralis minor
Latissimus dorsi
Anterior view   Posterior view
F **Rotation depressing glenoid cavity**

FIGURE 6.53. **Scapular movements.** Scapula moves on the thoracic wall at the conceptual "scapulothoracic joint." *Dotted lines,* the starting position of each movement.

A AP View

B Coronal section

C Lateral view

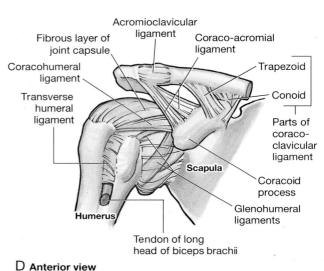

D Anterior view

FIGURE 6.54. **Glenohumeral and acromioclavicular joints. A.** Radiograph. **B.** Coronal section of glenohumeral joint. **C.** Lateral view of glenoid cavity and related structures following disarticulation of humerus. **D.** Ligaments.

ARTICULATION AND JOINT CAPSULE OF GLENOHUMERAL JOINT

The large spherical *humeral head* articulates with the relatively small and shallow *glenoid cavity* of the scapula, which is deepened slightly by the ring-like, fibrocartilaginous **glenoid labrum** (L. lip). Both articular surfaces are covered with hyaline cartilage (Fig. 6.54*B,C*). The glenoid cavity accepts little more than a third of the humeral head, which is held in the cavity by the tonus of the musculotendinous **rotator cuff** (supraspinatus, infraspinatus, teres minor, and subscapularis).

The loose *fibrous layer of the joint capsule* surrounds the glenohumeral joint and is attached medially to the margin of the glenoid cavity and laterally to the anatomical neck of the humerus. Superiorly, the fibrous layer encloses the proximal attachment of the long head of biceps brachii to the supraglenoid tubercle of the scapula within the joint. The inferior part of the joint capsule, the only part not reinforced by the rotator cuff muscles, is its weakest area. Here the capsule is particularly lax and lies in folds when the arm is adducted; however, it becomes taut when the arm is abducted (Figs. 6.54*B,D*).

The *synovial membrane* lines the internal surface of the fibrous capsule and reflects from it onto the glenoid labrum and the humerus as far as the articular margin of its head. The synovial membrane also forms a tubular sheath for the tendon of the long head of the biceps brachii. Anteriorly, there is a communication between the *subscapular bursa* and the synovial cavity of the joint.

TABLE 6.13 STRUCTURES LIMITING MOVEMENTS OF PECTORAL GIRDLE

Movement	Joint(s)	Limiting Structures (Tension)
Flexion (0–180°)	Sternoclavicular Acromioclavicular Glenohumeral Scapulothoracic	*Ligaments:* posterior part of coracohumeral, trapezoid, and posterior part of joint capsule of glenohumeral joint *Muscles:* rhomboids, levator scapulae, extensor and external rotator muscles, rotator muscles of glenohumeral joint
Abduction (0–180°)	Sternoclavicular Acromioclavicular Glenohumeral Scapulothoracic	*Ligaments:* middle and inferior glenohumeral, trapezoid, and inferior part of joint capsule of glenohumeral joint *Muscles:* rhomboids, levator scapulae, adductor muscles of glenohumeral joint *Bony apposition* between greater tubercle of humerus and superior part of glenoid cavity/labrum or lateral aspect of acromion
Extension	Glenohumeral	*Ligaments:* anterior part of coracohumeral and anterior part of joint capsule of glenohumeral joint *Muscles:* clavicular head of pectoralis major
Medial (internal) rotation	Glenohumeral	*Ligaments:* posterior glenohumeral joint capsule *Muscles:* infraspinatus and teres minor
Lateral (external) rotation	Glenohumeral	*Ligaments:* glenohumeral, coracohumeral, anterior glenohumeral joint capsule *Muscles:* latissimus dorsi, teres major, pectoralis major, subscapularis

Modified from Clarkson HM. *Musculoskeletal Assessment. Joint Range of Motion and Manual of Muscle Strength,* 2nd ed. Baltimore: Lippincott Williams & Wilkins, 2000.

LIGAMENTS OF GLENOHUMERAL JOINT

The **glenohumeral ligaments,** evident only on the internal aspect of the capsule, strengthen the anterior aspect of the capsule (Fig. 6.54*C*). The **coracohumeral ligament,** a strong band that passes from the base of the coracoid process to the anterior aspect of the greater tubercle, strengthens the capsule superiorly (Fig. 6.54*D*). The glenohumeral ligaments are intrinsic ligaments that are part of the fibrous layer of the capsule. The **transverse humeral ligament** is a broad fibrous band that runs from the greater to the lesser tubercle, bridging over the intertubercular sulcus (groove) and converting the groove into a canal for the tendon of the long head of biceps brachii and its synovial sheath.

The **coraco-acromial arch** is an extrinsic, protective structure formed by the smooth inferior aspect of the *acromion* and *coracoid process* of the scapula, with the **coraco-acromial ligament** spanning between them (Fig. 6.54*C*). The coraco-acromial arch overlies the head of the humerus, preventing its superior displacement from the glenoid cavity. The arch is so strong that a forceful superior thrust of the humerus will not fracture it; the shaft of the humerus or clavicle fractures first.

MOVEMENTS OF GLENOHUMERAL JOINT

The glenohumeral joint has more freedom of movement than any other joint in the body. This freedom results from the laxity of its joint capsule and the configuration of the spherical humeral head and shallow glenoid cavity. The glenohumeral joint allows movements around the three axes and permits flexion–extension, abduction–adduction, rotation (medial and lateral) of the humerus, and circumduction. Table 6.13 lists structures that limit movements of the glenohumeral joint. Lateral rotation of the humerus increases the range of abduction. When the arm is abducted without rotation, the greater tubercle contacts the *coraco-acromial arch,* preventing further abduction. If the arm is then laterally rotated 180 degrees, the tubercles are rotated posteriorly and more articular surface becomes available to continue elevation. Stiffening or fixation of the joints of the pectoral girdle (*ankylosis*) results in a much more restricted range of movement, even if the glenohumeral joint is normal.

The muscles moving the joint are the *axioappendicular muscles,* which may act indirectly on the joint (i.e., act on the pectoral girdle), and the *scapulohumeral muscles,* which act directly on the joint (Tables 6.1–6.3). Other muscles serve the glenohumeral joint as *shunt muscles,* acting to resist dislocation without producing movement at the joint, or maintain the head of the humerus in the glenoid cavity. For example, when the arms are at one's side the deltoid functions as a shunt muscle.

BLOOD SUPPLY AND INNERVATION OF GLENOHUMERAL JOINT

The glenohumeral joint is supplied by the *anterior* and *posterior circumflex humeral arteries* and branches of the *suprascapular artery* (Table 6.4). The *suprascapular, axillary,* and *lateral pectoral nerves* supply the glenohumeral joint (Table 6.5).

BURSAE AROUND GLENOHUMERAL JOINT

Several **bursae** containing capillary films of *synovial fluid* are located near the joint where tendons rub against bone, ligaments, or other tendons and where skin moves over a bony prominence. Some bursae communicate with the joint cavity; hence, opening a bursa may mean entering the cavity of the joint.

The **subacromial bursa,** sometimes referred to as the *subdeltoid bursa* (Fig. 6.54C), is located between the acromion, coraco-acromial ligament, and deltoid superiorly and the supraspinatus tendon and joint capsule of the glenohumeral joint inferiorly. Thus it facilitates movement of the supraspinatus tendon under the coraco-acromial arch and of the deltoid over the joint capsule and the greater tubercle of the humerus.

The **subscapular bursa** is located between the tendon of the subscapularis and the neck of the scapula. This bursa protects the tendon where it passes inferior to the root of the coracoid process and over the neck of the scapula. It usually communicates with the cavity of the glenohumeral joint through an opening in the fibrous layer of the joint capsule.

Rotator Cuff Injuries

The musculotendinous rotator cuff is commonly injured during repetitive use of the upper limb above the horizontal (e.g., during throwing and racquet sports, swimming, and weight lifting). Recurrent inflammation of the rotator cuff, especially the relatively avascular area of the supraspinatus tendon, is a common cause of shoulder pain and results in tears of the rotator cuff (Fig. B6.18). Repetitive use of the rotator cuff muscles (e.g., by baseball pitchers) may allow the humeral head and rotator cuff to impinge on the coracoacromial arch, producing irritation of the arch and inflammation of the rotator cuff. As a result, *degenerative tendinitis of the rotator* cuff develops. Attrition of the supraspinatus tendon also occurs. Because the supraspinatus muscle is no longer functional with a complete tear of the rotator cuff, the person cannot initiate abduction of the upper limb. If the arm is passively abducted 15 degrees or more, the person can usually maintain or continue the abduction using the deltoid.

Dislocation of Acromioclavicular Joint

Although its extrinsic (coracoclavicular) ligament is strong, the AC joint itself is weak and easily injured by a direct blow. In contact sports such as football, soccer, and hockey, it is not uncommon for *dislocation of the AC joint* to result from a hard fall on the shoulder or on the outstretched upper limb (Fig. B6.19). Dislocation of the AC joint also can occur when a hockey player is, for example, driven violently into the boards. An AC dislocation, often called a "shoulder separation," is severe when both the AC and the coracoclavicular ligaments are torn. When the coracoclavicular ligament tears, the shoulder separates from the clavicle and falls because of the weight of the upper limb. Dislocation of the AC joint makes the acromion more prominent, and the clavicle may move superior to this process.

Rupture of supraspinatus tendon

Supraspinatus

Acromion

Subacromial bursa (distended with inflammatory fluid)

Coracoid

Clavicle

Rotator cuff injury

FIGURE B6.18.   Rotator cuff injury.

Dislocation of acromioclavicular joint without ligament rupture

Dislocation of acromioclavicular joint with rupture of coracoclavicular ligament

FIGURE B6.19.

A **Anterior dislocation of right glenohumeral joint**   **B** **Subacromial bursa**

Dislocation of Glenohumeral Joint

Because of its freedom of movement and instability, the glenohumeral joint is commonly dislocated by direct or indirect injury. Most dislocations of the humeral head occur in the downward (inferior) direction but are described clinically as anterior or (more rarely) posterior dislocations, indicating whether the humeral head has descended anterior or posterior to the infraglenoid tubercle and the long head of triceps. **Anterior dislocation of the glenohumeral joint** occurs most often in young adults (Fig. B6.20A), particularly athletes. It is usually caused by excessive extension and lateral rotation of the humerus. The head of the humerus is driven inferoanteriorly, and the fibrous layer of the joint capsule and glenoid labrum may be stripped from the anterior aspect of the glenoid cavity. A hard blow to the humerus when the glenohumeral joint is fully abducted tilts the head of the humerus inferiorly onto the inferior weak part of the joint capsule. This may tear the capsule and dislocate the joint so that the humeral head comes to lie inferior to the glenoid cavity and anterior to the infraglenoid tubercle. Subsequently, the strong flexor and adductor muscles of the glenohumeral joint usually pull the humeral head anterosuperiorly into a subcoracoid position. Unable to use the arm, the person commonly supports it with the other hand. The **axillary nerve** may be injured when the glenohumeral joint dislocates because of its close relation to the inferior part of the capsule of this joint (Fig. B6.20B).

Calcific Supraspinatus Tendinitis

Inflammation and calcification of the *subacromial bursa* result in pain, tenderness, and limitation of movement of the glenohumeral joint. This condition is also known as *calcific scapulohumeral bursitis*. Deposition of calcium in the supraspinatus tendon may irritate the overlying subacromial bursa, producing an inflammatory reaction, *subacromial bursitis*. As long as the glenohumeral joint is adducted, no pain usually results because in this position the painful lesion is away from the inferior surface of the acromion. In most people, the pain occurs during 50 to 130 degrees of abduction (*painful arc syndrome*) because during this arc the supraspinatus tendon is in intimate contact with the inferior surface of the acromion. The pain usually develops in males 50 years of age and older after unusual or excessive use of the glenohumeral joint.

Adhesive Capsulitis of Glenohumeral Joint

Adhesive fibrosis and scarring between the inflamed capsule of the glenohumeral joint, rotator cuff, subacromial bursa, and deltoid usually cause **adhesive capsulitis** ("frozen shoulder"). A person with this condition has difficulty abducting the arm but can obtain an apparent abduction of up to 45 degrees by elevating and rotating the scapula. Injuries that may initiate this condition include glenohumeral dislocations, calcific supraspinatus tendinitis, partial tearing of the rotator cuff, and bicipital tendinitis.

FIGURE 6.55. Elbow and proximal radio-ulnar joints. **A.** Anteroposterior radiograph. **B.** Lateral radiograph. **C.** Medial ligaments. **D.** Lateral ligaments. **E.** Anular ligament. **F.** Articular surfaces of proximal end of ulna.

Elbow Joint

The **elbow joint,** a hinge type of synovial joint, is located 2 to 3 cm inferior to the humeral epicondyles.

ARTICULATION AND JOINT CAPSULE OF ELBOW JOINT

The spool-shaped *trochlea* and spheroidal *capitulum* of the humerus articulate with the *trochlear notch* of the ulna and

the slightly concave superior aspect of the *head of radius,* respectively; therefore, there are *humero-ulnar* and *humeroradial articulations* (Fig. 6.55A,C).

The *fibrous layer of the joint capsule* surrounding the joint is attached to the humerus at the margins of the lateral and medial ends of the articular surfaces of the capitulum and trochlea. Anteriorly and posteriorly, it is carried superiorly, proximal to the coronoid and olecranon fossae (Fig. 6.57). The *synovial membrane* lines the internal surface of the fibrous layer of the joint capsule and the intracapsular non-articular parts of the humerus. It is continuous inferiorly with the synovial membrane of the proximal radio-ulnar joint. The joint capsule is weak anteriorly and posteriorly but is strengthened on each side by ligaments.

LIGAMENTS OF ELBOW JOINT

The **collateral ligaments of the elbow joint** are strong triangular bands that are medial and lateral thickenings of the fibrous layer of the joint capsule (Fig. 6.55B,D,E). The lateral, fan-like **radial collateral ligament** extends from the lateral epicondyle of the humerus and blends distally with the **anular ligament of the radius.** This ligament encircles and holds the head of the radius in the radial notch of the ulna, forming the proximal radio-ulnar joint and permitting pronation and supination of the forearm. The medial, triangular **ulnar collateral ligament** extends from the medial epicondyle of the humerus to the coronoid process and olecranon of the ulna. It consists of three bands: (1) the *anterior cord-like band* is the strongest, (2) the *posterior fan-like band* is the weakest, and (3) the slender *oblique band* deepens the socket for the trochlea of the humerus (Fig. 6.55C).

MOVEMENTS OF ELBOW JOINT

Flexion and extension occur at the elbow joint. The long axis of the fully extended ulna makes an angle of approximately 170 degrees with the long axis of the humerus. This angle is called the **carrying angle** and is named for the way the forearm angles away from the body when something is carried, such as a pail of water (Fig. 6.56). The obliquity of the angle is more pronounced in women than in men. Table 6.14 lists structures limiting movements of the elbow joint.

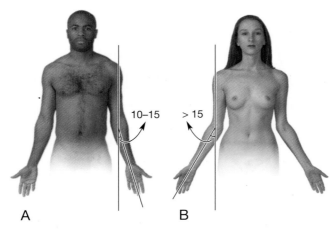

FIGURE 6.56. **Carrying angle of elbow joint.** Note the angle is greater in the woman.

FIGURE 6.57. Coronal section through humero-ulnar articulation of elbow joint showing relationships of bursae.

BLOOD SUPPLY AND INNERVATION OF ELBOW JOINT

The arteries supplying the elbow are derived from the anastomosis of arteries around the elbow joint (Fig. 6.39; Table 6.10). The elbow joint is supplied by the musculocutaneous, radial, and ulnar nerves.

BURSAE AROUND ELBOW JOINT

The clinically important bursae are the (Figs. 6.57 and 6.58B):

- **Intratendinous olecranon bursa,** which is sometimes present in the tendon of triceps brachii.
- **Subtendinous olecranon bursa,** which is located between the olecranon and the triceps tendon, just proximal to its attachment to the olecranon.
- **Subcutaneous olecranon bursa,** which is located in the subcutaneous connective tissue over the olecranon.

The *bicipitoradial bursa* (biceps bursa) separates the biceps tendon from the anterior part of the radial tuberosity.

Proximal Radio-Ulnar Joint

The **proximal (superior) radio-ulnar joint** is a pivot type of synovial joint that allows movement of the head of the radius on the ulna (Figs. 6.55B,E and 6.58).

A Superior view of transverse section of proximal radio-ulnar joint

Olecranon (cut)
Radial notch of ulna
Anular ligament
Head of radius
Trochlear articulating surface

B Inferior view of transverse section, pronated position

Bicipitoradial bursa
Radius
Biceps brachii tendon
Ulna
Supinator
Supinator crest

C Anteroposterior radiograph

Olecranon
Capitulum
Head of radius
Proximal radio-ulnar joint
Coronoid process
Tuberosity of radius
Radius
Ulna
Distal radio-ulnar joint
Radial styloid process
Site of articular disc of distal radio-ulnar joint
1 2 3 4 5

D Supination

Axis of rotary movement
Proximal radio-ulnar joint
Anular ligament of radius
Ulna
Radius
Distal radio-ulnar joint

E Pronation

Proximal radio-ulnar joint
Ulna
Radius
Distal radio-ulnar joint

FIGURE 6.58. **Proximal and distal radio-ulnar joints. A.** Anular ligament. The head of the radius rotates in the "socket" formed by the anular ligament. **B.** Actions of supinator and biceps brachii in producing supination are shown. **C.** Radiograph. **D.** Position of radius and ulna in supination. **E.** Position of radius and ulna in pronation.

ARTICULATION AND JOINT CAPSULE OF PROXIMAL RADIO-ULNAR JOINT

The head of the radius articulates with the radial notch of the ulna. The radial head is held in place by the *anular ligament of the radius.* The *fibrous layer of the joint capsule* encloses the joint and is continuous with that of the elbow joint. The *synovial membrane* lines the internal surface of the fibrous layer and non-articulating aspects of the bones. The synovial membrane is an inferior prolongation of the synovial membrane of the elbow joint (Fig. 6.55C).

TABLE 6.14 STRUCTURES LIMITING MOVEMENTS OF ELBOW AND RADIO-ULNAR JOINTS

Joint(s)	Movement	Limiting Structures (Tension)
Humeroulnar Humeroradial	**Extension**	*Muscles:* flexor muscles of elbow *Joint capsule:* anteriorly *Bony apposition* between olecranon of ulna and olecranon fossa of humerus
Humeroulnar Humeroradial	**Flexion**	*Muscle:* triceps brachii *Joint capsule:* posteriorly *Soft tissue apposition* between anterior forearm and arm *Bony apposition* between head of radius and radial fossa of humerus
Humeroradial Proximal radio-ulnar Distal radio-ulnar Interosseous membrane	**Pronation**	*Muscles:* supinator, biceps brachii *Ligaments:* quadrate, dorsal inferior radio-ulnar, interosseous membrane *Bony apposition* of the radius on ulna
Humeroradial Proximal radio-ulnar Distal radio-ulnar	**Supination**	*Muscles:* pronator teres, pronator quadratus *Ligaments:* quadrate, anterior inferior radio-ulnar, interosseous membrane

Modified from Clarkson HM. *Musculoskeletal Assessment. Joint Range of Motion and Manual of Muscle Strength,* 2nd ed. Baltimore: Lippincott Williams & Wilkins, 2000.

LIGAMENTS OF PROXIMAL RADIO-ULNAR JOINT

The **anular ligament** attaches to the ulna, anterior and posterior to the radial notch, which forms a collar that, with the radial notch, forms a ring that completely encircles the head of the radius (Fig. 6.58A). The deep surface of the anular ligament is lined with synovial membrane, which continues distally as a **sacciform recess of the proximal radio-ulnar joint** on the neck of the radius. This arrangement allows the radius to rotate within the anular ligament without binding, stretching, or tearing of the synovial membrane.

Distal Radio-Ulnar Joint

The **distal (inferior) radio-ulnar joint** is a pivot type of synovial joint. The radius moves around the relatively fixed distal end of the ulna (Fig. 6.58; Table 6.15).

ARTICULATION AND JOINT CAPSULE OF DISTAL RADIO-ULNAR JOINT

The rounded head of the ulna articulates with the ulnar notch on the medial side of the distal end of the radius. A fibrocartilaginous **articular disc of the distal radio-ulnar joint** binds the ends of the ulna and radius together and is the main uniting structure of the joint (Figs. 6.58 and 6.59B). The base of the disc attaches to the medial edge of the ulnar notch of the radius, and its apex is attached to the lateral side of the base of the styloid process of ulna. The proximal surface of this triangular disc articulates with the distal aspect of the head of the ulna. Hence the joint cavity is L-shaped in a coronal section, with the vertical bar of the *L* between the radius and the ulna and the horizontal bar between the ulna and the articular disc. The articular disc separates the cavity of the distal radio-ulnar joint from the cavity of the wrist joint.

The *fibrous layer of the joint capsule* encloses the joint but is deficient superiorly. The *synovial membrane* extends superiorly between the radius and the ulna to form the **sacciform recess of the distal radio-ulnar joint** (Fig. 6.59B). This redundancy of the synovial membrane accommodates the twisting of the capsule that occurs when the distal end of the radius travels around the relatively fixed distal end of the ulna during pronation and supination of the forearm.

LIGAMENTS OF DISTAL RADIO-ULNAR JOINT

Anterior and posterior ligaments strengthen the fibrous layer of the joint capsule. These relatively weak transverse bands extend from the radius to the ulna across the anterior and posterior surfaces of the joint.

MOVEMENTS OF PROXIMAL AND DISTAL RADIO-ULNAR JOINTS

During pronation and supination of the forearm, the head of the radius rotates within the cup-shaped anular ligament and the distal end of the radius rotates around the head of the ulna (Fig. 6.58). **Supination** turns the palm anteriorly, or superiorly when the forearm is flexed. **Pronation** turns the palm posteriorly, or inferiorly when the forearm is flexed. During pronation and supination, it is the radius that rotates (Fig. 6.58D,E). Table 6.14 lists the structures that limit movements of the proximal and distal radio-ulnar joint.

Supination is produced by the supinator (when resistance is absent) and by the biceps brachii (when resistance is present), with some assistance from the EPL and extensor carpi radialis longus (ECRL). *Pronation* is produced by the pronator quadratus (primarily) and pronator teres (secondarily), with some assistance from the FCR, palmaris longus, and brachioradialis (when the forearm is in the mid-pronated position).

Bursitis of Elbow

The *subcutaneous olecranon bursa* is exposed to injury during falls on the elbow and to infection from abrasions of the skin covering the olecranon. Repeated excessive pressure and friction produces a friction *subcutaneous olecranon bursitis* (e.g., "student's elbow") (Fig. B6.21). *Subtendinous olecranon bursitis* results from excessive friction between the triceps tendon and the olecranon—for example, resulting from repeated flexion–extension of the forearm as occurs during certain assembly-line jobs. The pain is severe during flexion of the forearm because of pressure exerted on the inflamed subtendinous olecranon bursa by the triceps tendon.

Avulsion of Medial Epicondyle

Avulsion of the medial epicondyle in children can result from a fall that causes severe abduction of the extended elbow. The resulting traction on the ulnar collateral ligament pulls the medial epicondyle distally. The anatomical basis of avulsion of the medial epicondyle is that the epiphysis for the medial epicondyle may not fuse with the distal end of the humerus until up to age 20. *Traction injury of the ulnar nerve* is a complication of the abduction type of avulsion of the medial epicondyle.

Dislocation of Elbow Joint

Posterior dislocation of the elbow joint may occur when children fall on their hands with their elbows flexed. Dislocations of the elbow may result from hyperextension or a blow that drives the ulna posteriorly or posterolaterally. The distal end of the humerus is driven through the weak anterior part of the fibrous layer of the joint capsule as the radius and ulna dislocate posteriorly. Injury to the ulnar nerve may also occur.

Subcutaneous olecranon bursitis

FIGURE B6.21.

ARTERIES AND NERVES OF PROXIMAL AND DISTAL RADIO-ULNAR JOINTS

The proximal radio-ulnar joint is supplied by the radial portion of the **periarticular arterial anastomosis of the elbow joint** (Fig. 6.39; Table 6.10). It is innervated by the musculocutaneous, median, and radial nerves (Table 6.9). Pronation is essentially a function of the median nerve, whereas supination is a function of the musculocutaneous and radial nerves. The anterior and posterior *interosseous arteries* and *nerves* supply the distal radio-ulnar joint (Fig. 6.47).

TABLE 6.15 STRUCTURES LIMITING MOVEMENTS OF WRIST AND CARPAL JOINTS

Movement	Limiting Structures (Tension)
Flexion	*Ligaments:* posterior radiocarpal and posterior part of joint capsule
Extension	*Ligaments:* anterior radiocarpal and anterior part of joint capsule *Bony apposition* between radius and carpal bones
Abduction	*Ligaments:* ulnar collateral ligament and medial part of joint capsule *Bony apposition* between styloid process of radius and scaphoid
Adduction	*Ligaments:* radial collateral and lateral part of joint capsule

Modified from Clarkson HM. *Musculoskeletal Assessment. Joint Range of Motion and Manual of Muscle Strength,* 2nd ed. Baltimore: Lippincott Williams & Wilkins, 2000.

Ulnar Collateral Ligament Reconstruction

 Rupture, tearing, and stretching of the ulnar collateral ligament (UCL) are increasingly common injuries related to athletic throwing (primarily baseball pitching, but also football passing, javelin throwing, and playing water polo). Reconstruction of the UCL, commonly known as a "Tommy John procedure" (for the first pitcher to undergo the surgery), involves an autologous transplant of a long tendon from the contralateral forearm or leg (e.g., the palmaris longus or plantaris tendon). A 10- to 15-cm length of tendon is passed through holes drilled through the medial epicondyle of the humerus and the lateral aspect of the coronoid process of the ulna (Fig. B6.22).

A Medial view

B Medial view

C Medial view

FIGURE B6.22.

Subluxation and Dislocation of the Radial Head

 Preschool children, particularly girls, are vulnerable to transient subluxation (incomplete temporary dislocation) of the head of the radius ("pulled elbow"). The history of these cases is typical. The child is suddenly lifted (jerked) by the upper limb when the forearm is pronated (Fig. B6.23). The child may cry out and refuse to use the limb, which is protected by holding it with the elbow flexed and the forearm pronated. The sudden pulling of the upper limb tears the distal attachment of the anular ligament, where it is loosely attached to the neck of the radius. The radial head then moves distally, partially out of the anular ligament. The proximal part of the torn ligament may become trapped between the head of the radius and the capitulum of the humerus. The source of pain is the pinched anular ligament. The treatment of subluxation consists of supination of the child's forearm while the elbow is flexed. The tear in the anular ligament soon heals when the limb is placed in a sling for about 2 weeks.

Humerus

Anular ligament

Force causes radial head to subluxate from anular ligament

Lump caused by displaced head of radius

Muscle pulls radial head superiorly

Subluxation and dislocation
Anterior view

FIGURE B6.23.

TABLE 6.16 WRIST AND CARPAL JOINTS

Joint	Type	Articulation	Joint Capsule	Ligaments	Movements	Blood Supply	Nerve Supply
Wrist (radiocarpal)	Condyloid synovial joint	Distal end of radius and articular disc with proximal row of carpal bones (except pisiform)	Fibrous layer of joint capsule surrounds joint and attaches to distal ends of radius and ulna and proximal row of carpal bones; lined by synovial membrane	Anterior and posterior ligaments strengthen fibrous capsule; ulnar collateral ligament attaches to styloid process of ulna and triquetrum; radial collateral ligament attaches to styloid process of radius and scaphoid	Flexion–extension, abduction–adduction, circumduction	Dorsal and palmar carpal arches	
Carpal (inter-carpal)	Plane synovial joint	Between carpal bones of proximal row; joints between carpal bones of distal row *Midcarpal joint:* synovial joint between proximal and distal rows of carpal bones *Pisiform joint:* synovial joint between pisiform and triquetrum	Fibrous layer of joint capsule surrounds joints; lined by synovial membrane; pisiform joint is separate from other carpal joints	Carpal bones united by anterior, posterior, and interosseous ligaments	Small amount of gliding movement possible; flexion and abduction of hand occur at midcarpal joint	Dorsal and palmar carpal arches	Anterior interosseous branch of median nerve, posterior interosseous branch of radial nerve, and dorsal and deep branches of ulnar nerve
Car-pometacarpal (CMC) and intermetacarpal (IM)	Plane synovial joints, except for CMC joint of thumb (saddle-shaped synovial joint)	Carpals and metacarpals with each other; CMC joint of thumb between trapezium and base of 1st metacarpal	Fibrous layer of joint capsule sur-rounds joints; lined on internal surface by syn-ovial membrane	Bones united by anterior, poste-rior, and interosseous lig-aments	Flexion–extension and abduction–adduction of CMC joint of 1st digit; almost no movement at 2nd and 3rd digits; 4th digit slightly mobile; 5th digit very mobile	Dorsal and palmar metacarpal arteries and deep carpal and deep palmar arches	

Joints of Hand

The carpal and digital joints are described in Table 6.16, and structures limiting movement are summarized in Table 6.15.

The **wrist** (carpus), the proximal segment of the hand, is a complex of eight carpal bones. The carpus articulates proximally with the forearm at the wrist joint and distally with the five metacarpals (Fig. 6.59). The joints formed by the carpus include the *wrist (radiocarpal joint), inter-carpal, carpometacarpal,* and *intermetacarpal joints.* Aug-menting movement at the wrist joint, the two rows of carpals glide on each other; in addition, each bone glides on those adjacent to it.

Each digit has three phalanges except the thumb, which has two. The proximal phalanges articulate with the metacarpal bones at the metacarpophalangeal joints. The joint between the proximal and the middle phalanx is the proximal interphalangeal joint and that between the middle and the distal phalanx is the distal interphalangeal joint (Figs. 6.59 and 6.60). The thumb has one interpha-langeal joint.

A Anterior view, right hand

Deep transverse metacarpal ligament

Palmar ligament (plate)

Collateral ligament

Palmar ligament (plate)

Collateral ligament

Radiate carpal ligaments

1st metacarpal

Capsule of carpometacarpal joint of thumb

Radial collateral ligament

Styloid process

Hook of hamate

Pisohamate ligament

Pisiform

Ulnar collateral ligament

Styloid process

Ulna   Radius

B Coronal section

Intercarpal joints

Interosseous metacarpal ligament

1st metacarpal

Carpometacarpal joint of 5th digit

Carpometacarpal joint of thumb

Pisotriquetral joint

Midcarpal joint (dotted line)

Radial collateral ligament

Ulnar collateral ligament

Fibrous layer of joint capsule

Articular disc of distal radio-ulnar joint

Synovial membrane

Radiocarpal joint

Sacciform recess

Distal radio-ulnar joint

Ulna

Radius

Carpal bones

C	Capitate
H	Hamate
L	Lunate
M	Trapezium
P	Pisiform
S	Scaphoid
T	Triquetrum
Z	Trapezoid

C Anteroposterior (AP) radiograph

Distal interphalangeal joint

Proximal interphalangeal joint

Metacarpophalangeal joint

Distal phalanx

Proximal phalanx

Sesamoid bone

Muscle and soft tissue

1st metacarpal

Trapezium (T)

Styloid process of radius

Distal radio-ulnar joint

Phalanges — Distal / Middle / Proximal

Metacarpal — Head / Shaft / Base

Hook of hamate

Pisiform

Styloid process of ulna

Head of ulna

FIGURE 6.59.   **Wrist and hand joints. A.** Ligaments. **B.** Coronal section of distal radio-ulnar, wrist, and carpal joints. **C.** Radiograph.

Lateral views

FIGURE 6.60. Ligaments of metacarpophalangeal and interphalangeal joints. **A.** Collateral ligaments and palmar ligaments (plates) of second digit. **B.** Collateral ligament with metacarpophalangeal joint in extension is lax. **C.** Collateral ligament is taut with metacapophalangeal joint in flexion. **D.** Joints of digit.

TABLE 6.17 METACARPOPHALANGEAL AND INTERPHALANGEAL JOINTS

Joint	Type	Articulation	Joint Capsule	Ligaments	Movements	Blood Supply	Nerve Supply
Metacarpopha-langeal	Condyloid synovial joints	Heads of metacarpals with base of proximal phalanges	Fibrous layer of joint capsule encloses each joint; lined on internal surface by synovial membrane	Strong palmar ligaments attached to phalanges and metacarpals; deep transverse metacarpal ligaments unite 2nd–5th joints holding heads of metacarpals together; collateral ligaments pass from heads of metacarpals to bases of phalanges	Flexion–extension, abduction–adduction, and circumduction of 2nd–5th digits; flexion–extension of thumb occurs but abduction–adduction is limited	Deep digital arteries arising from superficial palmar arches	Digital nerves arising from ulnar and median nerves
Interphalangeal	Hinge synovial joints	Heads of phalanges with bases of more distally located phalanges	Fibrous capsule encloses each joint; lined on internal surface by synovial membrane	Similar to metacarpopha-langeal joints, except they unite phalanges	Flexion–extension	Digital arteries	Digital nerves arising from ulnar and median nerves

TABLE 6.18 STRUCTURES LIMITING MOVEMENTS OF HAND JOINTS

Movement	Joint(s)	Limiting Structures (Tension)
Flexion	CMC (thumb)	*Ligaments:* posterior part of joint capsule *Muscles:* extensor and abductor pollicis brevis *Apposition* between thenar eminence and palm
	MCP (digits 1–5)	*Ligaments:* collateral, posterior part of joint capsule *Apposition* between proximal phalanx and metacarpal
	PIP (digits 2–5)	*Ligaments:* collateral, posterior part of joint capsule *Apposition* between middle and proximal phalanges
	DIP (digits 2–5)	*Ligaments:* collateral, oblique retinacular, and posterior part of joint capsule
	IP (thumb)	*Ligaments:* collateral and posterior part of joint capsule *Apposition* between distal and proximal phalanges
Extension	CMC (thumb)	*Ligaments:* anterior part of joint capsule *Muscles:* 1st dorsal interosseous, flexor pollicis brevis
	MCP (digits 1–5)	*Ligaments:* anterior part of joint capsule, palmar ligament
	PIP and DIP (digits 2–5)	
	IP (thumb)	
Abduction	CMC and MCP	*Muscles:* 1st dorsal interosseous, adductor pollicis *Fascia and skin* of 1st web space
	MCP (digits 2–5)	*Ligaments:* collateral *Fascia and skin* of web spaces
Adduction	CMC and MCP (thumb)	*Apposition* between thumb and index finger
	MCP (digits 2–5)	*Apposition* between adjacent digits

Modified from Clarkson HM. *Musculoskeletal Assessment. Joint Range of Motion and Manual of Muscle Strength,* 2nd ed. Baltimore: Lippincott Williams & Wilkins, 2000.

CMC, carpometacarpal joint; *DIP,* distal interphalangeal joint; *IP,* interphalangeal joint; *MCP,* metacarpophalangeal joint; *PIP,* proximal interphalangeal joint.

Wrist Fractures and Dislocations

Fracture of the distal end of the radius (*Colles fracture*), the most common fracture in people over 50 years of age, is discussed in the blue box "Fracture of Ulna and Radius" (p. xxx). *Fracture of the scaphoid,* relatively common in young adults, is discussed in the blue box "Fractures of Hand" (p. xxx).

Anterior dislocation of the lunate is an uncommon but serious injury that usually results from a fall on the dorsiflexed wrist. The lunate is pushed out of its place in the floor of the carpal tunnel toward the palmar surface of the wrist. The displaced lunate may compress the median nerve and lead to *carpal tunnel syndrome* (discussed earlier in this chapter). Because of its poor blood supply, *avascular necrosis of the lunate* may occur. In some cases, excision of the lunate may be required. In *degenerative joint disease of the wrist,* surgical fusion of carpals (**arthrodesis**) may be necessary to relieve the severe pain.

Lateral view
Dorsal displacement
of radial epiphysis

FIGURE B6.24.

Fracture–separation of the distal radial epiphysis is common in children because of frequent falls in which forces are transmitted from the hand to the radius. In a lateral radiograph of a child's wrist, dorsal displacement of the distal radial epiphysis is obvious (Fig. B6.24). When the epiphysis is placed in its normal position during reduction, the prognosis for normal bone growth is good.

Without knowledge of bone growth and the appearance of bones in radiographic and other diagnostic images at various ages, a displaced epiphyseal plate could be mistaken for a fracture, and separation of an epiphysis could be interpreted as a displaced piece of fractured bone. Knowledge of the patient's age and location of epiphyses can prevent these errors.

Medical Imaging of Upper Limb

Anterior

Posterior

A   **Transverse section**

Transverse CT

Key					
1	Biceps brachii	6	Radial artery	11	Median nerve
2	Cephalic vein	7	Humerus	12	Ulnar nerve
3	Brachialis	8	Musculocutaneous nerve	13	Basilic vein
4	Lateral intermuscular septum	9	Brachial artery	14	Medial intermuscular septum
5	Profunda brachii artery	10	Brachial veins	15	Lateral head of triceps brachii

16	Medial head of triceps brachii
17	Long head of triceps brachii
a	Cortex of humerus
b	Medullary (marrow) cavity of humerus

FIGURE 6.61. Transverse sections of specimens with correlated transverse MRI or CT scans of left upper limb. A. Arm.

B   **Transverse section**   Anterior → Posterior   **Transverse MRI**

Key

1	Basilic vein	8	Median nerve	15	Flexor digitorum profundus	22	Extensor pollicis longus
2	Flexor carpi ulnaris	9	Flexor carpi radialis	16	Ulna	23	Posterior interosseous
3	Ulnar nerve	10	Flexor pollicis longus	17	Radius		vessels and nerve
4	Flexor digitorum superficialis	11	Brachioradialis	18	Extensor carpi radialis longus	24	Extensor digiti minimi
5	Palmaris longus	12	Radial artery	19	Extensor carpi radialis brevis	25	Extensor digitorum
6	Ulnar vein	13	Radial nerve	20	Interosseous membrane	26	Abductor pollicis longus
7	Ulnar artery	14	Cephalic vein	21	Extensor carpi ulnaris		

C   **Transverse section**   Anterior → Posterior   **Transverse CT**

Key

1	Muscles of hypothenar eminence	7	Flexor pollicis longus tendon	14	Capitate
2	Ulnar artery	8	Flexor carpi radialis tendon	15	Trapezoid
3	Ulnar nerve	9	Muscles of the thenar eminence	16	Trapezium
4	Palmaris longus tendon	10	Abductor pollicis longus tendon	17	First metacarpal
5	Flexor digitorum superfcialis and	11	Extensor pollicis brevis tendon	18	Extensor carpi ulnaris tendon
	profundus tendon	12	Triquetrum	19	Extensor carpi radialis tendon
6	Median nerve	13	Hamate	h	Hook of hamate

FIGURE 6.61.   Transverse sections of specimens with correlated transverse MRI or CT scans of left upper limb *(continued)*. **B.** Forearm. **C.** Carpal tunnel.

Acromioclavicular joint — Subclavius

Deltoid

Subcutaneous tissue

Quadrangular space

Long head of triceps brachii

A **Coronal MRI**

Subclavius

Coracoclavicular ligament

Articulating surfaces of glenohumeral joint

Subscapularis

1st rib

Axillary vein

Intercostal muscle

Axillary fat

B **Transverse CT**

C **Transverse CT**

Key							
A	Acromion	D	Deltoid muscle	H	Head of humerus		
AC	Acromioclavicular joint	G	Glenoid cavity (fossa)	N	Surgical neck of humerus		
Cl	Clavicle	GH	Glenohumeral joint	SP	Spine of scapula		
Co	Coracoid process	Gr	Greater tubercle of humerus	SsN	Suprascapular notch		

FIGURE 6.62. **Imaging of glenohumeral and acromioclavicular joints. A.** Coronal MRI. The white (signal-intense) parts of the identified bones are the fatty matrix of cancellous bone; the thin black outlines (absence of signal) of the bones are the compact bone that forms their outer surface. **B.** Transverse CT scan through acromioclavicular joint. **C.** Transverse CT scan through glenohumeral joint.

 Go to *http://thePoint.lww.com/ECA4e for helpful study tools, including USMLE-style questions, case studies, images, and more!*

Head

CRANIUM / 496

Facial Aspect of Cranium / 496

Lateral Aspect of Cranium / 496

Occipital Aspect of Cranium / 498

Superior Aspect of Cranium / 498

External Surface of Cranial Base / 499

Internal Surface of Cranial Base / 502

SCALP / 502

CRANIAL MENINGES / 503

Dura Mater / 504

Arachnoid Mater and Pia Mater / 509

Meningeal Spaces / 511

BRAIN / 512

Parts of Brain / 512

Ventricular System of Brain / 512

Vasculature of Brain / 517

FACE / 519

Muscles of Face / 519

Nerves of Face / 519

Superficial Vasculature of Face and Scalp / 522

Parotid Gland / 526

ORBITS / 529

Eyelids and Lacrimal Apparatus / 530

Eyeball / 533

Extra-ocular Muscles of Orbit / 540

Nerves of Orbit / 544

Vasculature of Orbit / 545

TEMPORAL REGION / 549

Temporal Fossa / 549

Infratemporal Fossa / 550

TEMPOROMANDIBULAR JOINT / 555

ORAL REGION / 557

Oral Cavity / 557

Oral Vestibule / 557

Teeth and Gingivae / 558

Palate / 560

Tongue / 563

Salivary Glands / 567

PTERYGOPALATINE FOSSA / 570

NOSE / 573

External Nose / 573

Nasal Cavities / 573

Paranasal Sinuses / 574

EAR / 578

External Ear / 578

Middle Ear / 580

Internal Ear / 583

MEDICAL IMAGING OF HEAD / 589

The **head** consists of the *brain*, its protective coverings, and the *ears* and *face*. The **cranium** (skull) is the skeleton of the head (Fig. 7.1). Learning the features of the cranium serves as an important framework to facilitate the understanding of the head region.

In the *anatomical position*, the cranium is oriented so that the inferior margin of the orbit (eye sockets or orbital cavity) and the superior margin of the external acoustic meatus of both sides lie in the same horizontal plane (Fig. 7.1*B*). This standard craniometric reference is the **orbitomeatal plane** (Frankfort plane).

CRANIUM

The *cranium* consists of two parts: the neurocranium and viscerocranium (Fig. 7.1). The **neurocranium** (cranial vault) is the bony covering (case) of the brain and its membranous coverings, the cranial meninges. It also contains the proximal parts of the cranial nerves and the vasculature of the brain. The neurocranium has a dome-like roof, the **calvaria** (skullcap), and a floor or **cranial base** (basicranium). The neurocranium is formed by eight bones: four singular bones centered on the midline (*frontal, ethmoid, sphenoid,* and *occipital*) and two sets of bones occurring as bilateral pairs (*temporal* and *parietal*). Most calvarial bones are united by fibrous interlocking *sutures;* however, during childhood, some bones (sphenoid and occipital) are united by hyaline cartilage (*synchondroses*).

The **viscerocranium** (facial skeleton) is made up of the facial bones that mainly develop in the mesenchyme of the embryonic pharyngeal arches (Moore & Persaud, 2008). The viscerocranium forms the anterior part of the cranium and consists of bones surrounding the mouth, nose, and most of the orbits (Fig. 7.1*A*). It consists of 15 irregular bones: three singular bones lying in the midline (*mandible, ethmoid,* and *vomer*) and six paired bones occurring bilaterally (*maxilla; inferior nasal concha* (turbinate)*;* and *zygomatic, palatine, nasal,* and *lacrimal bones*).

Facial Aspect of Cranium

Features of the anterior or **fascial (frontal) aspect of the cranium** are the frontal and zygomatic bones, orbits, nasal region, maxillae, and mandible (Fig. 7.1*A*).

The **frontal bone** forms the skeleton of the forehead, articulating inferiorly with the nasal and zygomatic bones. It also articulates with the lacrimal, ethmoid, and sphenoid bones and forms the roof of the orbit and part of the floor of the anterior part of the cranial cavity. The intersection of the frontal and nasal bones is the **nasion** (L. *nasus,* nose). The **supra-orbital margin** of the frontal bone, the angular boundary between the squamous (flat) and the

orbital parts, has either a **supra-orbital foramen** or **notch.** Just superior to the supra-orbital margin is a ridge, the **superciliary arch.** In some adult crania, a remnant of the developmental frontal suture, the **metopic suture,** is visible in the midline of the **glabella,** the smooth area between the superciliary arches.

The **zygomatic bones**, forming the prominences of the cheeks, lie on the inferolateral sides of the orbits and rest on the maxillae. A small **zygomaticofacial foramen** pierces the lateral aspect of each bone. Inferior to the nasal bones is the pear-shaped **piriform aperture,** the anterior nasal opening of the cranium. The bony **nasal septum** can be observed, dividing the nasal cavity into right and left parts. On the lateral wall of each nasal cavity are curved bony plates, the **nasal conchae** (the middle and inferior nasal conchae are shown in Fig. 7.1*A*).

The **maxillae** form the upper jaw and are united at the **intermaxillary suture** in the median plane. Their **alveolar processes** include the tooth sockets (alveoli) and constitute the supporting bone for the **maxillary teeth.** The maxillae surround most of the piriform aperture and form the infra-orbital margins medially. They have a broad connection with the zygomatic bones laterally and have an **infra-orbital foramen** inferior to each orbit.

The **mandible** is the U-shaped bone forming the lower jaw; it has alveolar processes for the **mandibular teeth.** It consists of a horizontal part, the **body,** and a vertical part, the **ramus.** Inferior to the second premolar teeth are **mental foramina.** Forming the prominence of the chin is the **mental protuberance,** a triangular elevation of bone inferior to the **mandibular symphysis,** the region where the halves of the infantile mandible fuse.

The bones of the orbit are illustrated and described later in this chapter (Fig. 7.22). Within the orbits are the **superior** and **inferior orbital fissures** and **optic canals.**

Lateral Aspect of Cranium

The **lateral aspect of the cranium** is formed by both the neurocranium and the viscerocranium (Fig. 7.1*B*). The main features of the neurocranial part are the **temporal fossa,** which is bounded superiorly and posteriorly by **superior** and **inferior temporal lines,** anteriorly by the frontal and zygomatic bones, and inferiorly by the zygomatic arch. The **zygomatic arch** is formed by the union of the **temporal process of the zygomatic bone** and the **zygomatic process of the temporal bone.** The *infratemporal fossa* is an irregular space inferior and deep to the zygomatic arch and the mandible and posterior to the maxilla.

In the anterior part of the temporal fossa, superior to the midpoint of the zygomatic arch, is the **pterion** (G. *pteron,* wing). It is usually indicated by an H-shaped formation of sutures that unite the frontal, parietal, sphenoid (greater wing), and temporal bones.

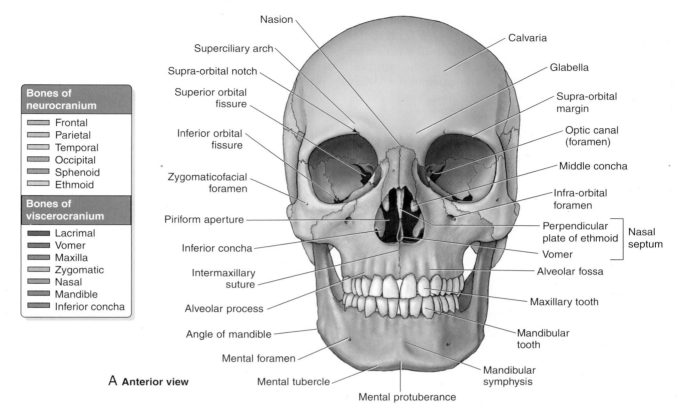

Bones of neurocranium
- Frontal
- Parietal
- Temporal
- Occipital
- Sphenoid
- Ethmoid

Bones of viscerocranium
- Lacrimal
- Vomer
- Maxilla
- Zygomatic
- Nasal
- Mandible
- Inferior concha

Nasion
Superciliary arch
Supra-orbital notch
Superior orbital fissure
Inferior orbital fissure
Zygomaticofacial foramen
Piriform aperture
Inferior concha
Intermaxillary suture
Alveolar process
Angle of mandible
Mental foramen

Calvaria
Glabella
Supra-orbital margin
Optic canal (foramen)
Middle concha
Infra-orbital foramen
Perpendicular plate of ethmoid } Nasal septum
Vomer
Alveolar fossa
Maxillary tooth
Mandibular tooth
Mandibular symphysis

A **Anterior view**
Mental tubercle
Mental protuberance

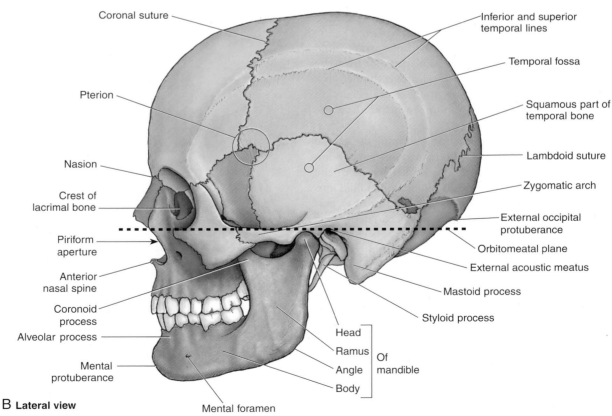

Coronal suture
Pterion
Nasion
Crest of lacrimal bone
Piriform aperture
Anterior nasal spine
Coronoid process
Alveolar process
Mental protuberance

Inferior and superior temporal lines
Temporal fossa
Squamous part of temporal bone
Lambdoid suture
Zygomatic arch
External occipital protuberance
Orbitomeatal plane
External acoustic meatus
Mastoid process
Styloid process

Head
Ramus } Of
Angle } mandible
Body

B **Lateral view**
Mental foramen

FIGURE 7.1.   **Adult cranium (skull).** In **B** the pterion is the area of junction of four bones within the temporal fossa.

The **external acoustic opening** is the entrance to the **external acoustic meatus** (ear canal), which leads to the tympanic membrane (eardrum). The **mastoid process** of the temporal bone lies posteroinferior to the external acoustic meatus. Anteromedial to the mastoid process is the slender **styloid process** of the temporal bone.

Occipital Aspect of Cranium

The posterior or **occipital aspect of the cranium** is formed by the rounded posterior aspect of the head or **occiput** (L. back of head). The occipital bone, parts of the parietal bones, and mastoid parts of the temporal bones form this part of the

cranium (Fig. 7.2A). The **external occipital protuberance** is usually an easily palpable elevation in the median plane. The **superior nuchal line,** marking the superior limit of the neck, extends laterally from each side of this protuberance; the **inferior nuchal line** is less distinct. In the center of the occiput, the **lambda** indicates the junction of the sagittal and lambdoid sutures. The lambda can sometimes be felt as a depression.

Superior Aspect of Cranium

The **superior aspect of the cranium,** usually somewhat oval in form, broadens posterolaterally at the **parietal eminences** (Fig. 7.2B). The four bones forming the *calvaria,*

Fractures of Cranium

The convexity of the calvaria (skullcap) distributes and thereby minimizes the effects of a blow to it. However, hard blows to the head in thin areas are likely to produce *depressed fractures,* in which a fragment of bone is depressed inward, compressing and/or injuring the brain (Fig. B7.1). In *comminuted fractures,* the bone is broken into several pieces. *Linear calvarial fractures,* the most frequent type, usually occur at the point of impact, but fracture lines often radiate away from it in two or more directions. If the area of the calvaria is thick at the site of impact, the bone usually bends inward without fracturing; however, a fracture may occur some distance from the site of direct trauma where the calvaria is thinner. In a *contrecoup (counterblow) fracture,* the fracture occurs on the opposite side of the cranium rather than at the point of impact.

Basilar fractures involve the bones forming the cranial base (e.g., occipital bone around the foramen magnum, temporal and sphenoid bones, and the roof of the orbit). As a result of leakage of cerebrospinal fluid into the nose (CSF rhinorrhea) and ear (CSF otorrhea), cranial nerve and blood vessel injury may occur, depending on the site of the fracture.

Fracture of the pterion can be life-threatening because it overlies the frontal (anterior) branches of the middle meningeal vessels, which lie in the grooves on the internal aspect of the lateral wall of the calvaria. A hard blow to the side of the head may fracture the thin bones forming the pterion, rupturing the frontal branch of the middle meningeal artery crossing the pterion. The resulting *hematoma* exerts pressure on the underlying cerebral cortex. Untreated *middle meningeal artery hemorrhage* may cause death in a few hours.

Lateral view

Median section

1. Linear fracture
2. Depressed fracture
3. Comminuted fracture
4. Basilar fracture

FIGURE B7.1.   **Fractures of cranium.**

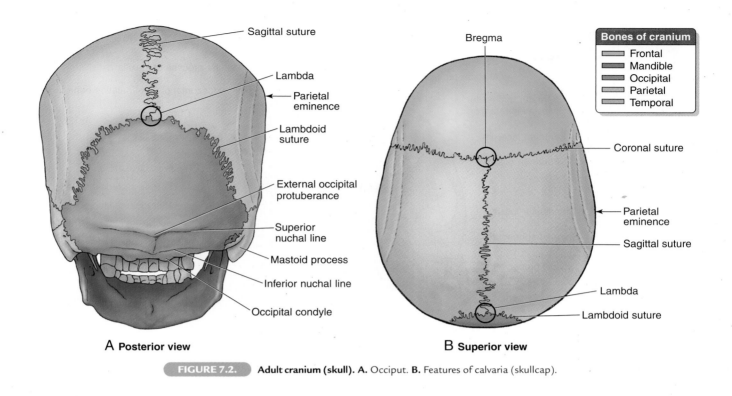

A Posterior view

B Superior view

FIGURE 7.2.   **Adult cranium (skull). A.** Occiput. **B.** Features of calvaria (skullcap).

the dome-like roof of the neurocranium, are visible from this aspect: the frontal bone anteriorly, the right and left parietal bones laterally, and the occipital bone posteriorly. The **coronal suture** unites the frontal and parietal bones, the **sagittal suture** unites the right and left parietal bones, and the **lambdoid suture** unites the occipital bone with the right and left parietal and temporal bones. The **bregma** is the landmark formed by the intersection of the sagittal and coronal sutures. The **vertex**, the superior point of the cranium, is near the midpoint of the sagittal suture (Fig 7.2A).

External Surface of Cranial Base

The **external aspect of the cranial base** or basicranium features the **alveolar arch of the maxillae** (the free border of the **alveolar processes** surrounding and supporting the maxillary teeth); the **palatine processes** of the maxillae; and the palatine, sphenoid, vomer, temporal, and occipital bones (Fig. 7.3A). The *hard palate* (bony palate) is formed by the **palatine processes of the maxillae** anteriorly and the **horizontal plates of the palatine bones** posteriorly. Posterior to the central incisor teeth is the **incisive fossa.** Posterolaterally are the **greater** and **lesser palatine foramina.** The posterior edge of the palate forms the inferior boundary of the **choanae** (posterior nasal apertures), which are separated from each other by the **vomer.** The vomer is a thin flat bone that forms a part of the bony **nasal septum** (Fig. 7.1A). Wedged between the frontal,

temporal, and occipital bones is the **sphenoid bone,** which consists of a body and three pairs of processes: the **greater** and **lesser wings** and the **pterygoid processes** (Figs. 7.3A and D). The pterygoid processes, consisting of **medial** and **lateral pterygoid plates,** extend inferiorly on each side of the sphenoid from the junction of the body and greater wings (Fig. 7.3A). The opening of the bony part of the pharyngotympanic (auditory) tube and the *sulcus (groove) for the cartilaginous part of the tube* lies medial to the **spine of the sphenoid,** inferior to the junction of the greater wing of the sphenoid and the **petrous** (L. rock-like) part of the temporal bone. Depressions in the **squamous** (L. flat) **part of the temporal bone,** called the **mandibular fossae,** accommodate the heads of the mandible when the mouth is closed.

The cranial base is formed posteriorly by the **occipital bone,** which articulates with the sphenoid anteriorly. The parts of the occipital bone encircle the large **foramen magnum.** On the lateral parts of the occipital bone are two large protuberances, the **occipital condyles,** by which the cranium articulates with the vertebral column (Fig. 7.3D). The large opening between the occipital bone and the petrous part of the temporal bone is the **jugular foramen.** The internal carotid artery enters the carotid canal at the **external opening of the carotid canal** just anterior to the jugular foramen. The **mastoid processes** provide for muscle attachments. The **stylomastoid foramen** lies posterior to the base of the styloid process.

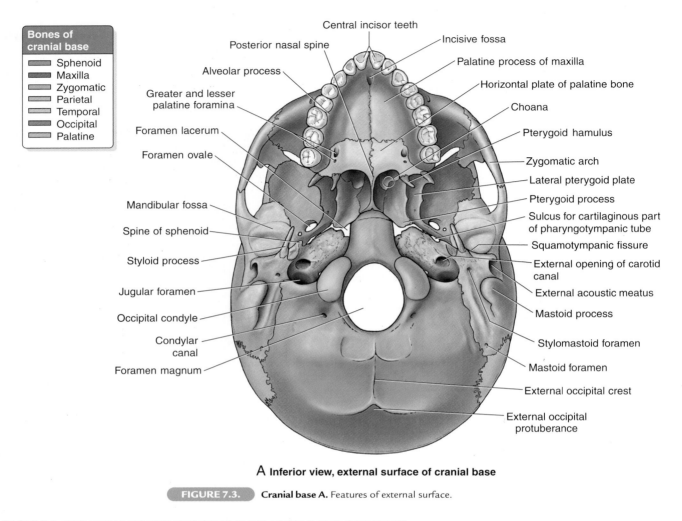

Bones of cranial base

- Sphenoid
- Maxilla
- Zygomatic
- Parietal
- Temporal
- Occipital
- Palatine

Central incisor teeth
Posterior nasal spine
Incisive fossa
Alveolar process
Palatine process of maxilla
Greater and lesser palatine foramina
Horizontal plate of palatine bone
Choana
Foramen lacerum
Pterygoid hamulus
Foramen ovale
Zygomatic arch
Lateral pterygoid plate
Mandibular fossa
Pterygoid process
Spine of sphenoid
Sulcus for cartilaginous part of pharyngotympanic tube
Squamotympanic fissure
Styloid process
External opening of carotid canal
Jugular foramen
External acoustic meatus
Occipital condyle
Mastoid process
Condylar canal
Stylomastoid foramen
Foramen magnum
Mastoid foramen
External occipital crest
External occipital protuberance

A Inferior view, external surface of cranial base

FIGURE 7.3. **Cranial base A.** Features of external surface.

TABLE 7.1 FORAMINA/APERTURES OF CRANIAL FOSSAE AND CONTENTS

Foramina/Apertures	Contents
Anterior cranial fossa	
Foramen cecum	Nasal emissary vein (1% of population; in danger of injury during surgery)
Cribriform foramina in cribriform plate	Axons of olfactory cells in olfactory epithelium that form olfactory nerves (CNI)
Anterior and posterior ethmoidal foramina	Vessels and nerves with same names as foramina
Middle cranial fossa	
Optic canals	Optic nerves (CN II) and ophthalmic arteries
Superior orbital fissure	Ophthalmic veins; ophthalmic nerve (CN V_1); CN III, IV, and VI; and sympathetic fibers
Foramen rotundum	Maxillary nerve (CN V_2)
Foramen ovale	Mandibular nerve (CN V_3) and accessory meningeal artery
Foramen spinosum	Middle meningeal artery and vein and meningeal branch of CN V_3
Foramen lacerum[a]	Internal carotid artery and its accompanying sympathetic and venous plexuses
Groove or hiatus of greater petrosal nerve	Greater petrosal nerve and petrosal branch of middle meningeal artery
Posterior cranial fossa	
Foramen magnum	Medulla and meninges, vertebral arteries, CN XI, dural veins, anterior and posterior spinal arteries
Jugular foramen	CN IX, X, and XI; superior bulb of internal jugular vein; inferior petrosal and sigmoid sinuses; and meningeal branches of ascending pharyngeal and occipital arteries
Hypoglossal canal	Hypoglossal nerve (CN XII)
Condylar canal	Emissary vein that passes from sigmoid sinus to vertebral veins in neck
Mastoid foramen	Mastoid emissary vein from sigmoid sinus and meningeal branch of occipital artery

[a]Structures actually pass horizontally across (rather than vertically through) the area of the foramen lacerum, an artifact of dry skulls, which is closed by cartilage in life.

B **Superior view, cranial fossae**

Contents of
anterior fossa

Anterior fossa

Contents of
middle fossa

Middle fossa

Contents of
posterior fossa

Posterior fossa

C **Inferior view of brain**

Frontal crest

Anterior ethmoidal
foramen (obscured)

Orbital part of
frontal bone (orbital plate)

Lesser wing of sphenoid

Sphenoidal crest

Superior orbital fissure

Greater wing of sphenoid

Foramen rotundum

Foramen ovale

Groove for middle
meningeal artery

Dorsum sellae*

Petrous ridge

Jugular foramen

Hypoglossal canal

Foramen magnum

Cerebellar fossa

*Components of sella turcica

Foramen cecum

Crista galli

Cribriform plate

Posterior ethmoidal
foramen (obscured)

Tuberculum sellae*

Prechiasmatic sulcus

Optic canal

Anterior clinoid process

Hypophysial fossa*

Posterior clinoid
process

Foramen spinosum

Foramen lacerum

Internal acoustic meatus

Clivus

Groove for
sigmoid sinus

Internal occipital
crest

Groove for
transverse sinus

Internal occipital
protuberance

**Bones of Internal
Cranial Base in D**

Frontal
Sphenoid
Ethmoid
Parietal
Temporal
Occipital

D **Superior view, internal surface of cranial base**

FIGURE 7.3. (*continued*) **Cranial base. B.** Cranial fossae of internal surface of cranial base. **C.** Lobes and cerebellum of brain related
to cranial fossae. **D.** Features of internal surface.

Internal Surface of Cranial Base

The **internal surface of the cranial base** has three large depressions that lie at different levels: the *anterior, middle,* and *posterior cranial fossae,* which form the bowl-shaped floor of the cranial cavity (Fig. 7.3*B*). The anterior cranial fossa is at the highest level, and the posterior cranial fossa is at the lowest level.

The **anterior cranial fossa** is formed by the frontal bone anteriorly, the ethmoid bone centrally, and the body and lesser wings of the sphenoid posteriorly (Fig. 7.3*D*). The greater part of the anterior cranial fossa is formed by ridged **orbital plates of the frontal bone,** which support the frontal lobes of the brain and form the roofs of the orbits (Figs. 7.3*B,C*). The **frontal crest** is a median bony extension of the frontal bone (Fig. 7.3*D*). At its base is the **foramen cecum of the frontal bone,** which gives passage to vessels during fetal development. The **crista galli** (L. cock's comb) is a median ridge of bone that projects superiorly from the ethmoid. On each side of the crista galli is the sieve-like **cribriform plate of the ethmoid.**

The butterfly-shaped **middle cranial fossa** has a *central part* composed of the *sella turcica* (Turkish saddle) on the body of the sphenoid and large depressed *lateral parts* on each side. The **sella turcica** is surrounded by the **anterior** and **posterior clinoid processes** (*clinoid* means "bedpost"). The sella turcica is composed of three parts:

* The **tuberculum sellae** (horn of saddle), the slight elevation anteriorly on the body of the sphenoid.
* The **hypophysial fossa** (pituitary fossa), a saddle-like depression for the pituitary gland (L. *hypophysis*) in the middle.
* The **dorsum sellae** (back of saddle) posteriorly, formed by a square plate of bone on the body of the sphenoid. Its prominent superolateral angles are the *posterior clinoid processes.*

The bones forming the larger, lateral parts of the middle cranial fossa are the greater wings of the sphenoid, squamous parts of the temporal bones laterally, and petrous parts of the temporal bones posteriorly. The lateral parts of the middle cranial fossa support the temporal lobes of the brain (Figs. 7.3*B,C*). The boundary between the middle and the posterior cranial fossae is formed by the *superior border of the petrous part of the temporal bones* (*petrous ridge*) laterally and the dorsum sellae of the sphenoid medially (Fig. 7.3*D*). The **sphenoidal crests** are the sharp posterior margins of the *lesser wings of the sphenoid bones,* which overhang the lateral parts of the fossae anteriorly. The *sphenoidal crests* end medially in two sharp bony projections: the *anterior clinoid processes.* The **prechiasmatic sulcus** extends between the right and the left **optic canals.** The **foramen lacerum** lies posterolateral to the hypophysial fossa. In life, it is closed by a cartilage plate. On each side of the body of the sphenoid, four foramina perforate the roots of the greater wings of the sphenoid (Fig. 7.3*D*):

* **Superior orbital fissure:** an opening between the greater and the lesser wings that communicates with the orbit.
* **Foramen rotundum**: a circular foramen located posterior to the medial end of the superior orbital fissure.
* **Foramen ovale**: an oval foramen located posterolateral to the foramen rotundum.
* **Foramen spinosum**: located posterolateral to the foramen ovale.

The **posterior cranial fossa,** the largest and deepest of the cranial fossae, contains the cerebellum, pons, and medulla oblongata (Figs. 7.3*B,C*). This fossa is formed mostly by the occipital bone, but parts of the sphenoid and temporal bones make smaller contributions to it (Fig. 7.3*D*). From the dorsum sellae there is a marked incline, the **clivus,** which leads to the **foramen magnum.** Posterior to this large foramen, the **internal occipital crest** is a landmark that divides the posterior part of the fossae into two **cerebellar fossae;** the crest ends superiorly in the **internal occipital protuberance.** Broad grooves in this fossa are formed by the *transverse* and *sigmoid sinuses.* At the base of the petrous ridges of the temporal bones are the **jugular foramina.** Anterosuperior to the jugular foramen is the **internal acoustic meatus.** The **hypoglossal canals** lie superior to the anterolateral margin of the foramen magnum.

SCALP

The **scalp** consists of skin and subcutaneous tissue that covers the neurocranium from the superior nuchal lines on the occipital bone to the supra-orbital margins of the frontal bone (Fig. 7.1*A*). Laterally, the scalp extends over the temporal fascia to the zygomatic arches. The neurovascular structures of the scalp are discussed with those of the face.

The scalp is composed of five layers, the first three of which are connected intimately, thus moving as a unit (e.g., when wrinkling the forehead). Each letter in the word *scalp* serves as a memory key for one of its five layers that cover the neurocranium (Fig. 7.4*A*):

* **S**kin, thin except in the occipital region, contains many sweat and sebaceous glands and hair follicles; it has an abundant arterial supply and good venous and lymphatic drainage.
* **C**onnective tissue, forming the thick, dense, richly vascularized, subcutaneous layer, is well supplied with cutaneous nerves.

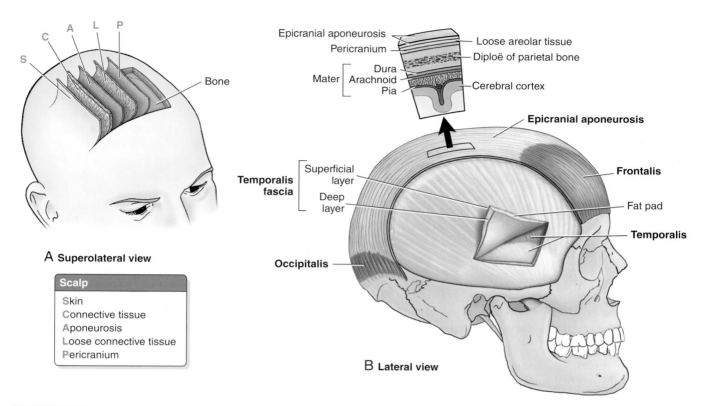

Scalp. A. Layers of the scalp. **B.** Epicranial aponeurosis. The epicranial aponeurosis, frontalis, occipitalis, and superior auricular muscle constitue the *epicranius.*

- **A**poneurosis (**epicranial aponeurosis**), a strong tendinous sheet that covers the calvaria, serves as the attachment for the frontal and occipital bellies of the occipitofrontalis muscle and the superior auricular muscle (Fig. 7.4*B*); collectively these structures form the musculoaponeurotic *epicranius.*
- **L**oose connective tissue, a sponge-like layer, has potential spaces that may distend with fluid as a result of injury or infection (Fig. 7.4*A*); this layer allows free movement of the **scalp proper** (the first three layers) over the underlying calvaria.
- **P**ericranium, a dense layer of connective tissue, forms the external periosteum of the neurocranium; it is firmly attached but can be stripped fairly easily from the calvaria of living people, except where the pericranium is continuous with the fibrous tissue in the cranial sutures.

CRANIAL MENINGES

The **cranial meninges** are coverings of the brain that lie immediately internal to the cranium. The meninges protect the brain; form the supporting framework for arteries, veins, and venous sinuses; and enclose a fluid-filled cavity, the

Scalp Injuries and Infections

The loose connective tissue layer is the *danger area of the scalp* because pus or blood spreads easily in it. Infection in this layer can also pass into the cranial cavity through *emissary veins,* which pass through the calvaria and reach intracranial structures such as the meninges. An infection cannot pass into the neck because the occipital belly of the occipitofrontalis muscle attaches to the occipital bone and mastoid parts of the temporal bones. Neither can the infection spread laterally beyond the zygomatic arches because the epicranial aponeurosis is continuous with the temporal fascia that attaches to these arches. An infection or fluid (e.g., pus or blood) can enter the eyelids and the root of the nose because the frontal belly of the occipitofrontalis muscle inserts into the skin and subcutaneous tissue and does not attach to the bone. Consequently, "black eyes" can result from an injury to the scalp or forehead. *Ecchymosis,* or purple patches, develop as a result of extravasation of blood into the subcutaneous tissue and skin of the eyelids and surrounding regions.

subarachnoid space. The meninges are composed of three membranous connective tissue layers (Fig. 7.5):

- **Dura mater** (dura): tough, thick external fibrous layer.
- **Arachnoid mater** (arachnoid): thin intermediate layer.
- **Pia mater** (pia): delicate internal vascular layer.

The arachnoid and pia are continuous membranes that make up the **leptomeninx.** The arachnoid is separated from the pia by the subarachnoid space, which contains **cerebrospinal fluid** (CSF). This is a clear liquid similar in constitution to blood; it provides nutrients but has less protein and a different ion concentration. CSF is formed predominantly by the *choroid plexuses* within the four ventricles of the brain. CSF leaves the ventricular system of the brain and enters the subarachnoid space, where it cushions and nourishes the brain. (See Fig. 7.12.)

Dura Mater

The **dura mater** (dura), a two-layered membrane that is adherent to the internal surface of the cranium, consists of (Figs. 7.5 and 7.10):

- An external *periosteal layer,* formed by the periosteum covering the internal surface of the calvaria.

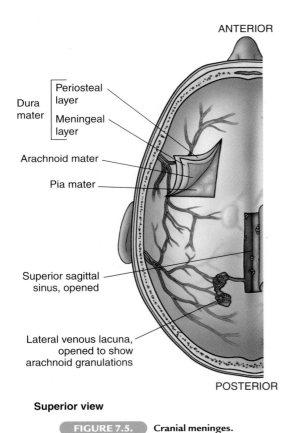

ANTERIOR

Dura mater
Periosteal layer
Meningeal layer

Arachnoid mater

Pia mater

Superior sagittal sinus, opened

Lateral venous lacuna, opened to show arachnoid granulations

POSTERIOR

Superior view

FIGURE 7.5. Cranial meninges.

- An internal *meningeal layer,* a strong fibrous membrane that is continuous at the foramen magnum with the dura covering the spinal cord.

DURAL INFOLDINGS OR REFLECTIONS

The internal **meningeal layer of the dura** reflects away from the external **periosteal layer of the dura** to form **dural infoldings** (reflections), which divide the cranial cavity into compartments and support parts of the brain (Fig. 7.6). The dural infoldings are the *falx cerebri, tentorium cerebelli, falx cerebelli,* and *diaphragma sellae.*

The **falx cerebri** (cerebral falx), the largest dural infolding, is a sickle-shaped partition that lies in the **longitudinal cerebral fissure** that separates the right and left cerebral hemispheres (Figs. 7.6A and 7.10C). The falx cerebri attaches in the median plane to the internal surface of the calvaria, from the *frontal crest* of the frontal bone and the crista galli of the ethmoid bone anteriorly to the internal occipital protuberance posteriorly. The falx cerebri ends posteriorly by becoming continuous with the tentorium cerebelli.

The **tentorium cerebelli** (cerebellar tentorium) is a wide crescentic septum that separates the occipital lobes of the cerebral hemispheres from the cerebellum (Figs. 7.6A,B). The tentorium cerebelli attaches anteriorly to the clinoid processes of the sphenoid bone, anterolaterally to the petrous part of the temporal bone, and posterolaterally to the internal surface of the occipital bone and part of the parietal bone. The falx cerebri attaches to the tentorium cerebelli in the midline and holds it up, giving it a tent-like appearance (L. *tentorium,* tent). The concave anteromedial border of the tentorium cerebelli is free, leaving a gap called the **tentorial notch** through which the brainstem extends from the posterior into the middle cranial fossa (Fig. 7.6A). The tentorium cerebelli divides the cranial cavity into *supratentorial* and *infratentorial compartments* (Fig. 7.6B).

The **falx cerebelli** (cerebellar falx) is a vertical dural infolding that lies inferior to the tentorium cerebelli in the posterior part of the posterior cranial fossa (Fig. 7.6B). It partially separates the cerebellar hemispheres.

The **diaphragma sellae** (sellar diaphragm), the smallest dural infolding, is a circular sheet of dura that is suspended between the clinoid processes, forming a partial roof over the hypophysial fossa. The diaphragma sellae covers the pituitary gland in this fossa and has an aperture for passage of the infundibulum (pituitary stalk) and hypophysial veins (Figs. 7.8A,B.)

DURAL VENOUS SINUSES

The **dural venous sinuses** are endothelial-lined spaces between the periosteal and meningeal layers of the dura

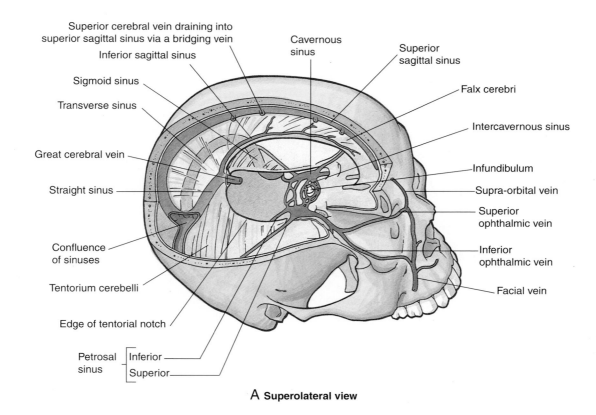

Superior cerebral vein draining into
superior sagittal sinus via a bridging vein

Inferior sagittal sinus

Sigmoid sinus

Transverse sinus

Great cerebral vein

Straight sinus

Confluence
of sinuses

Tentorium cerebelli

Edge of tentorial notch

Petrosal sinus — Inferior
Superior

Cavernous sinus

Superior sagittal sinus

Falx cerebri

Intercavernous sinus

Infundibulum

Supra-orbital vein

Superior ophthalmic vein

Inferior ophthalmic vein

Facial vein

A Superolateral view

(Figs. 7.6*A,B*). They form where dural infoldings attach (Fig. 7.10). Large veins from the surface of the brain and from the diploë empty into these sinuses, and all blood from the brain and fom the diplöe ultimately drains through them into the internal jugular veins (IJVs).

The **superior sagittal sinus** lies in the convex attached (superior) border of the falx cerebri (Figs. 7.6 and 7.10). It begins at the crista galli and ends near the internal occipital protuberance at the **confluence of sinuses**. The superior sagittal sinus receives the superior cerebral veins and communicates on each side through slit-like openings with the **lateral venous lacunae,** lateral expansions of the superior sagittal sinus (Fig. 7.5).

Arachnoid granulations (collections of arachnoid villi) are tufted prolongations of the arachnoid that protrude through the meningeal layer of the dura mater into the dural venous sinuses, and lateral venous lacunae. The arachnoid granulations transfer CSF to the venous system (Fig. 7.12*A*).

The **inferior sagittal sinus,** much smaller than the superior sagittal sinus, runs in the inferior, free concave border of the falx cerebri and ends in the straight sinus (Figs. 7.6*A,B* and 7.7*A*).

The **straight sinus** is formed by the union of the inferior sagittal sinus with the great cerebral vein. It runs inferoposteriorly along the line of attachment of the falx cerebri to the tentorium cerebelli to join the *confluence of sinuses* (Figs. 7.6*A,B*).

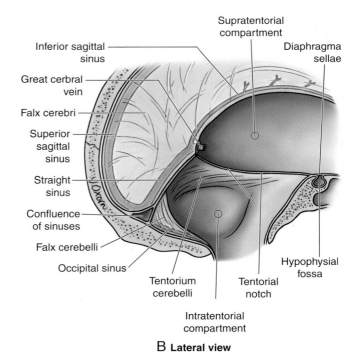

Inferior sagittal sinus

Great cerbral vein

Falx cerebri

Superior sagittal sinus

Straight sinus

Confluence of sinuses

Falx cerebelli

Occipital sinus

Tentorium cerebelli

Supratentorial compartment

Diaphragma sellae

Hypophysial fossa

Tentorial notch

Intratentorial compartment

B Lateral view

FIGURE 7.6. **Dural infoldings (reflections) and dural venous sinuses. A.** The brain and part of the calvaria are removed to demonstrate the sinuses related to the falx cerebri and tentorium cerebelli. **B.** Straight sinus and falx cerebri.

Superior ophthalmic vein

Intercavernous sinuses

Sphenoparietal sinus

Cavernous sinus

Basilar plexus

Superior petrosal sinus

Inferior petrosal sinus

Beginning of internal jugular vein

Sigmoid sinus

Great cerebral vein

Left transverse sinus

Inferior sagittal sinus (cut end)

Straight sinus

Superior sagittal sinus

Tentorium cerebelli

A Superior view

Superior sagittal sinus

Falx cerebri

Inferior sagittal sinus

Supra-orbital vein

Superior ophthalmic vein

Cavernous sinus

Emissary veins

Inferior ophthalmic vein

Pterygoid venous plexus

Maxillary vein

Facial vein

Drainage
← To superior petrosal sinus
← To inferior petrosal sinus

B Medial view

FIGURE 7.7. **Dural venous sinuses. A.** Dural venous sinuses of internal surface of cranial base. **B.** Schematic illustration of anterior part of the left half of the cranial cavity and facial skeleton.

The **transverse sinuses** pass laterally from the *confluence of sinuses* in the posterior attached margin of the tentorium cerebelli, grooving the occipital bones and the posteroinferior angles of the parietal bones (Fig. 7.7*A*). The transverse sinuses leave the tentorium cerebelli at the posterior aspect of the petrous temporal bone and become the sigmoid sinuses.

The **sigmoid sinuses** follow S-shaped courses in the posterior cranial fossa, forming deep grooves in the temporal and occipital bones. Each sigmoid sinus turns anteriorly and then continues inferiorly as the IJV after traversing the jugular foramen.

The **occipital sinus** lies in the attached border of the falx cerebelli and ends superiorly in the confluence of sinuses (Fig. 7.6*B*). The occipital sinus communicates inferiorly with the internal vertebral venous plexus.

The **cavernous sinus** is located bilaterally on each side of the sella turcica on the body of the sphenoid bone (Figs. 7.6*A* and 7.7*A,B*). The cavernous sinus consists of a venous plexus of thin-walled veins that extend from the superior orbital fissure anteriorly to the apex of the petrous part of the temporal bone posteriorly. The cavernous sinus receives blood from the superior and inferior ophthalmic veins, super-

ficial middle cerebral vein, and sphenoparietal sinus. The venous channels in the cavernous sinuses communicate with each other through **intercavernous sinuses** anterior and posterior to the infundibulum of the pituitary gland. The cavernous sinuses drain posteroinferiorly through the *superior* and *inferior petrosal sinuses* and via emissary veins to the *pterygoid venous plexuses* (Figs. 7.7*A,B*).

The **internal carotid artery** (Figs. 7.8*A–C*), surrounded by the *carotid plexus of sympathetic nerves*, courses through the cavernous sinus and is crossed by the *abducent nerve (CN VI)*. From superior to inferior, the lateral wall of each cavernous sinus contains the *oculomotor nerve (CN III)*, *trochlear nerve (CN IV)*, and *CN V₁ and CN V₂ divisions of the trigeminal nerve*.

The **superior petrosal sinuses** run from the posterior ends of the cavernous sinuses to join the transverse sinuses, where these sinuses curve inferiorly to form the sigmoid sinuses (Fig. 7.7*A*). Each superior petrosal sinus lies in the anterolateral attached margin of the tentorium cerebelli, which attaches to the superior border of the petrous part of the temporal bone.

The **inferior petrosal sinuses** commence at the posterior end of the cavernous sinus and drain the cavernous

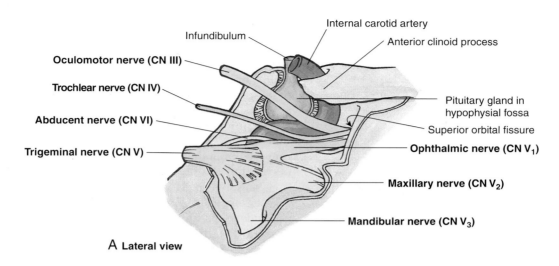

Internal carotid artery

Infundibulum

Oculomotor nerve (CN III)

Trochlear nerve (CN IV)

Abducent nerve (CN VI)

Trigeminal nerve (CN V)

Anterior clinoid process

Pituitary gland in hypophysial fossa

Superior orbital fissure

Ophthalmic nerve (CN V₁)

Maxillary nerve (CN V₂)

Mandibular nerve (CN V₃)

A **Lateral view**

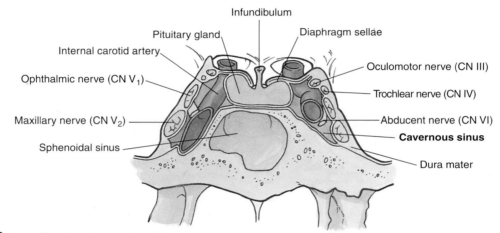

Infundibulum

Pituitary gland

Diaphragm sellae

Internal carotid artery

Oculomotor nerve (CN III)

Ophthalmic nerve (CN V₁)

Trochlear nerve (CN IV)

Abducent nerve (CN VI)

Maxillary nerve (CN V₂)

Cavernous sinus

Sphenoidal sinus

Dura mater

B **Posterior view of coronal section**

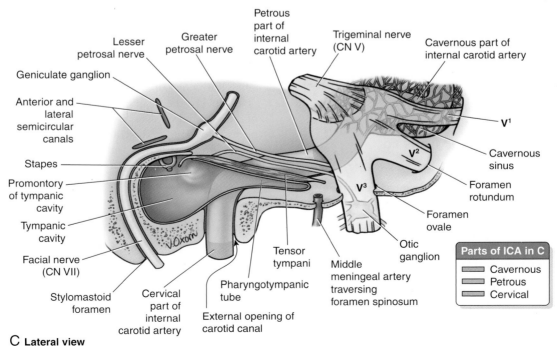

Petrous part of internal carotid artery

Greater petrosal nerve

Lesser petrosal nerve

Trigeminal nerve (CN V)

Cavernous part of internal carotid artery

Geniculate ganglion

Anterior and lateral semicircular canals

Stapes

Promontory of tympanic cavity

Tympanic cavity

Facial nerve (CN VII)

Stylomastoid foramen

Cervical part of internal carotid artery

External opening of carotid canal

Tensor tympani

Pharyngotympanic tube

Middle meningeal artery traversing foramen spinosum

Otic ganglion

V¹

Cavernous sinus

Foramen rotundum

V²

V³

Foramen ovale

Parts of ICA in C

Cavernous

Petrous

Cervical

C **Lateral view**

FIGURE 7.8. **Internal carotid artery and associated structures. A.** Observe the relationships of the oculomotor, trochlear, trigeminal, and abducent nerves. **B.** Cavernous sinuses. **C.** Petrous and cavernous parts of the internal carotid artery (ICA).

sinuses directly into the origin of the IJVs. The *basilar plexus* connects the inferior petrosal sinuses and communicates inferiorly with the internal vertebral venous plexus (Fig. 7.7*B*). **Emissary veins** connect the dural venous sinuses with veins outside the cranium (Figs. 7.7*B* and 7.10*C*). The size and number of emissary veins vary.

VASCULATURE AND NERVE SUPPLY OF DURA MATER

The **arteries of the dura** supply more blood to the calvaria than to the dura. The largest of these vessels, the **middle meningeal artery** (Figs. 7.9*A* and 7.10*A*), is a branch of the maxillary artery. The middle meningeal artery enters the middle cranial fossa through the *foramen spinosum,* runs laterally in the fossa, and turns supero-anteriorly on the greater wing of the sphenoid, where it divides into frontal and parietal branches. The **frontal (anterior) branch** runs

superiorly to the pterion and then curves posteriorly to ascend toward the vertex of the cranium. The **parietal (posterior) branch** runs posterosuperiorly and ramifies over the posterior aspect of the cranium. The **veins of the dura** accompany the meningeal arteries (Fig. 7.10*A*).

The **innervation of the dura** is largely by the three divisions of CN V (Fig. 7.9*B*). Sensory branches are also conveyed from the vagus (CN X) and hypoglossal (CN XII) nerves, but the fibers probably are peripheral branches from sensory ganglia of the superior three cervical nerves. The sensory endings are more numerous in the dura along each side of the superior sagittal sinus and in the tentorium cerebelli than they are in the floor of the cranium. Pain fibers are most numerous where arteries and veins course in the dura. Pain arising from the dura is generally referred, perceived as a headache arising in cutaneous or mucosal regions supplied by the involved cervical nerve or division of the trigeminal nerve.

Occlusion of Cerebral Veins and Dural Venous Sinuses

Occlusion of cerebral veins and dural venous sinuses may result from thrombi (clots), thrombophlebitis (venous inflammation), or tumors. The facial veins make clinically important connections with the cavernous sinus through the superior ophthalmic veins (Fig. 7.6*A*). Blood from the medial angle of the eye, nose, and lips usually drains inferiorly into the facial vein. However, because the facial vein has no valves, blood may pass superiorly to the superior ophthalmic vein and enter the cavernous sinus. In people with *thrombophlebitis of the facial vein,* pieces of an infected thrombus may extend into the cavernous sinus, producing *thrombophlebitis of the cavernous sinus.*

Metastasis of Tumor Cells to Dural Sinuses

The basilar and occipital sinuses communicate through the foramen magnum with the internal vertebral venous plexuses (Fig. 7.7*D*). Because these venous channels are valveless, compression of the thorax, abdomen, or pelvis, as occurs during heavy coughing and straining, may force venous blood from these regions into the internal vertebral venous system and subsequently into the dural venous sinuses. As a result, pus in abscesses and tumor cells in these regions may spread to the vertebrae and brain.

Fractures of Cranial Base

In fractures of the cranial base, the internal carotid artery may be torn, producing an *arteriovenous fistula* within the cavernous sinus. Arterial blood rushes into the cavernous sinus, enlarging it and forcing retrograde blood into its venous tributaries, especially the ophthalmic veins. As a result, the eyeball protrudes (*exophthalmos*) and the conjunctiva becomes engorged (chemosis). The protruding eyeball pulsates in synchrony with the radial pulse, a phenomenon known as *pulsating exophthalmos.* Because CNs III, IV, V$_1$, V$_2$, and VI lie in or close to the lateral wall of the cavernous sinus, they may also be affected when the sinus is injured (Fig. 7.6*B*).

A blow to the head can detach the periosteal layer of dura from the calvaria without fracturing the cranial bones. However, in the cranial base, the two dural layers are firmly attached and difficult to separate from the bones. Consequently, a fracture of the cranial base usually tears the dura and results in leakage of CSF.

Dural Origin of Headaches

The dura is sensitive to pain, especially where it is related to the dural venous sinuses and meningeal arteries. Although the causes of headache are numerous, distention of the scalp or meningeal vessels (or both) is believed to be one cause of headache. Many headaches appear to be dural in

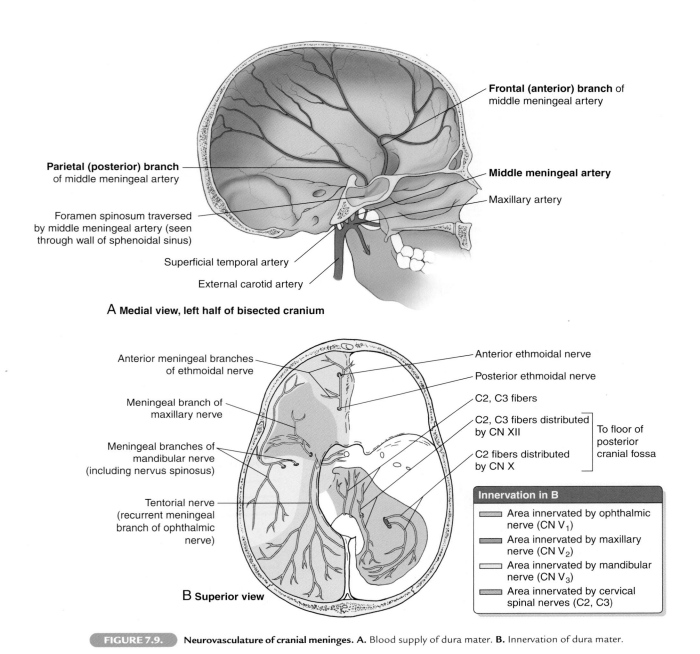

Frontal (anterior) branch of middle meningeal artery

Parietal (posterior) branch of middle meningeal artery

Middle meningeal artery

Foramen spinosum traversed by middle meningeal artery (seen through wall of sphenoidal sinus)

Maxillary artery

Superficial temporal artery

External carotid artery

A **Medial view, left half of bisected cranium**

Anterior meningeal branches of ethmoidal nerve

Anterior ethmoidal nerve

Meningeal branch of maxillary nerve

Posterior ethmoidal nerve

C2, C3 fibers

C2, C3 fibers distributed by CN XII

Meningeal branches of mandibular nerve (including nervus spinosus)

C2 fibers distributed by CN X

To floor of posterior cranial fossa

Tentorial nerve (recurrent meningeal branch of ophthalmic nerve)

Innervation in B

☐ Area innervated by ophthalmic nerve (CN V$_1$)

☐ Area innervated by maxillary nerve (CN V$_2$)

☐ Area innervated by mandibular nerve (CN V$_3$)

☐ Area innervated by cervical spinal nerves (C2, C3)

B **Superior view**

FIGURE 7.9. **Neurovasculature of cranial meninges. A.** Blood supply of dura mater. **B.** Innervation of dura mater.

origin, such as the headache occurring after a lumbar spinal puncture for removal of CSF. These headaches are thought to result from stimulation of sensory nerve endings in the dura. When CSF is removed, the brain sags slightly, pulling on the dura; this may cause pain and headache. For this reason, patients are asked to keep their heads down after lumbar puncture to minimize the pull on the dura, reducing the chances of headache.

Arachnoid Mater and Pia Mater

The **arachnoid mater** and **pia mater (leptomeninx)** develop from a single layer of mesenchyme surrounding the embryonic brain. CSF-filled spaces form within this layer and coalesce to form the *subarachnoid space* (Fig. 7.10A–C). Web-like **arachnoid trabeculae** pass between the arachnoid and the pia. The avascular arachnoid mater, although closely applied to the meningeal layer of the dura, is held against the inner surface of the dura by the pressure of the CSF. The **pia mater** is a thin membrane that is highly vascularized by a network of fine blood vessels and adheres to the surface of the brain and follows its contours (Fig. 7.10C).

A Superior view

B Coronal section, open superior sagittal sinus

C Coronal section

D Coronal section

FIGURE 7.10. **Layers, formations, and relations of cranial meninges. A.** Meningeal layers in situ and branches of middle meningeal vessels. **B.** Meningeal layers and dural sinus formation. **C.** Relationship of meninges to cranium and to right *(R)* and left *(L)* cerebral hemispheres. **D.** Enlarged detail of C.

When the cerebral arteries penetrate the cerebral cortex, the pia follows them for a short distance, forming a pial coat and a periarterial space.

Meningeal Spaces

Of the three meningeal "spaces" commonly mentioned in relation to the cranial meninges, only one exists as a space in the absence of pathology:

- The **dura–cranium interface** (extradural or epidural space) is not a natural space between the cranium and the external periosteal layer of the dura because the dura is attached to the bones. It becomes a space only pathologically—for example, when blood from torn meningeal vessels pushes the periosteum away from the cranium and accumulates.
- The **dura–arachnoid junction** or interface (subdural space) is likewise not a natural space between the dura and the arachnoid. A space may develop in the dural border cell layer as the result of trauma, such as after a blow to the head (Haines, 2006).
- The **subarachnoid space,** between the arachnoid and pia, is a real space that contains CSF, trabecular cells, cerebral arteries, and bridging superior cerebral veins that drain into the superior sagittal sinus (Fig. 7.10*B*).

Head Injuries and Intracranial Hemorrhage

Extradural or epidural hemorrhage is arterial in origin. Blood from torn branches of a middle meningeal artery collects between the external periosteal layer of the dura and the calvaria, usually after a hard blow to the head. This results in the formation of an *extradural* or *epidural hematoma* (Fig. B7.2). Typically, a brief *concussion* (loss of consciousness) occurs, followed by a lucid interval of some hours. Later, drowsiness and coma occur. The brain is compressed as the blood mass increases, necessitating evacuation of the blood and occlusion of the bleeding vessels.

A dural border hematoma classically is called a subdural hematoma; however, this term is a misnomer because there is no naturally occurring space at the dura–arachnoid junction. Hematomas at this junction are usually caused by extravasated blood that splits open the dural border cell layer (Fig. B7.2). The blood does not collect within a preexisting space but rather creates a space at the dura-arachnoid junction (Haines, 2006). Dural border hemorrhage usually follows a blow to the head that jerks the brain inside the cranium and injures it. The precipitating trauma may be trivial or forgotten but a hematoma may develop over many weeks from venous bleeding. Dural border hemorrhage is typically venous in origin and commonly results from tearing of a superior cerebral vein bridging in as it enters the superior sagittal sinus.

Subarachnoid hemorrhage is an extravasation (escape) of blood, usually arterial, into the subarachnoid space (Fig. B7.2). Most subarachnoid hemorrhages result from *rupture of a saccular aneurysm* (sac-like dilation on an artery). Some subarachnoid hemorrhages are associated with head trauma involving cranial fractures and cerebral lacerations. Bleeding into the subarachnoid space results in meningeal irritation, a severe headache, stiff neck, and often loss of consciousness.

Extradural or epidural hematoma   **Dural border (subdural) hematoma**   **Subarachnoid hemorrhage**

FIGURE B7.2.

BRAIN

The following is a brief discussion of the parts of the brain, vasculature, and ventricular system. The brain is composed of the *cerebrum, cerebellum,* and *brainstem* (midbrain, pons, and medulla oblongata) (Figs. 7.11*A,B*). Of the 12 cranial nerves, *11 cranial nerves arise from the brain* (Fig. 7.11*D*). They have motor, parasympathetic, and/or sensory functions. Generally, these nerves are surrounded by a dural sheath as they leave the cranium; the dural sheath becomes continuous with the connective tissue of the epineurium. For a summary of the cranial nerves, see Chapter 9.

Cerebral Injuries

Cerebral contusion (bruising) results from brain trauma in which the pia is stripped from the injured surface of the brain and may be torn, allowing blood to enter the subarachnoid space. The bruising results from the sudden impact of the moving brain against the stationary cranium or from the suddenly moving cranium against the stationary brain. Cerebral contusion may result in an extended loss of consciousness.

Cerebral lacerations are often associated with depressed cranial fractures or gunshot wounds. Lacerations result in rupture of blood vessels and bleeding into the brain and subarachnoid space, causing increased intracranial pressure and cerebral compression. Cerebral compression may be produced by:
- Intracranial collections of blood.
- Obstruction of CSF circulation or absorption.
- Intracranial tumors or abscesses.
- Brain swelling caused by *brain edema,* an increase in brain volume resulting from an increase in water and sodium content.

Parts of Brain

When the calvaria and dura mater are removed, **gyri** (folds), **sulci** (grooves), and **fissures** (clefts) of the cerebral cortex are visible through the delicate arachnoid–pia layer. The parts of brain include (Figs. 7.11*A–C*):

- The **cerebrum** includes the cerebral hemispheres. The **cerebral hemispheres** form the largest part of the brain and are separated by the falx cerebri (Fig. 7.10*C*). Each cerebral hemisphere is divided into four lobes: frontal, parietal, temporal, and occipital. The frontal lobes occupy the anterior cranial fossa, the temporal lobes occupy the lateral parts of the middle cranial fossae, and the occipital lobes extend posteriorly over the tentorium cerebelli (Figs. 7.3*B* and 7.12*B*).
- The **diencephalon** is composed of the epithalamus, thalamus, and hypothalamus and forms the central core of the brain (Fig. 7.11*B*).
- The **midbrain,** the rostral part of the brainstem, lies at the junction of the middle and posterior cranial fossae. CN III and IV are associated with the midbrain.
- The **pons,** the part of the brainstem between the midbrain rostrally and the medulla oblongata caudally, lies in the anterior part of the posterior cranial fossa. CN V is associated with the pons.
- The **medulla oblongata** (**medulla**), the most caudal part of the brainstem, is continuous with the spinal cord and lies in the posterior cranial fossa. CN IX, X, and XII are associated with the medulla, whereas CN VI–VIII are located at the junction of the pons and medulla.
- The **cerebellum** is the large brain mass lying posterior to the pons and medulla and inferior to the posterior part of the cerebrum. It lies beneath the tentorium cerebelli in the posterior cranial fossa and consists of two hemispheres united by a narrow middle part, the **vermis.**

Ventricular System of Brain

The ventricular system of the brain consists of two lateral ventricles and the midline third and fourth ventricles (Fig. 7.12*A*). The **lateral ventricles** (first and second ventricles) open into the third ventricle through the **interventricular foramina** (of Monro). The **third ventricle,** a slit-like cavity between the right and the left halves of the diencephalon, is continuous with the **cerebral aqueduct,** a narrow channel in the midbrain connecting the third and fourth ventricles. The **fourth ventricle,** lying in the posterior parts of the pons and medulla, extends inferoposteriorly. Inferiorly, it tapers to a narrow channel that continues into the spinal cord as the central canal. CSF drains from the fourth ventricle through a single **median aperture** (of Magendie) and paired **lateral apertures** (of Luschka) into the subarachnoid space. These apertures are the only means by which CSF enters the subarachnoid space. If they are blocked, the ventricles distend, producing compression of the cerebral hemispheres. At certain areas, mainly at the base of the brain, the arachnoid and pia mater are widely separated by large pools (cisterns) of CSF (Fig. 7.12*B*). Major **subarachnoid cisterns** include the:

- **Cerebellomedullary cistern,** the largest of the cisterns, located between the cerebellum and the medulla; receives CSF from the apertures of the fourth ventricle; divided

A Lateral view

Central sulcus
Postcentral gyrus
Precentral gyrus
Occipital pole
Lateral sulcus (fissure)
Frontal pole
Temporal pole
Transverse fissure
Pons
Cerebellum
Medulla (oblongata)

B Medial view

Corpus callosum
Interthalamic adhesion
Fornix
Choroid plexus
Septum pellucidum
Thalamus
Pineal body (epithalamus)
Parieto-occipital sulcus (fissure)
Calcarine sulcus
Cerebral aqueduct
Cerebellum
4th ventricle
Median aperture
Central canal
Anterior commissure
Hypothalamus
Midbrain
Pons
Medulla (oblongata)

Lobes and structures
- Frontal lobe
- Parietal lobe
- Temporal lobe
- Occipital lobe
- Cerebellum
- Diencephalon
- Brainstem:
  - Midbrain
  - Pons
  - Medulla (oblongata)
- Cranial nerves:
  - CN I – CN XII

C Superior view

Cerebral hemispheres
Left   Right
Longitudinal fissure
Precentral gyrus
Central sulcus
Postcentral gyrus

D Inferior (ventral) view

Olfactory nerves (fila) collectively comprising olfactory nerve (CN I)
Optic nerve (CN II)
Oculomotor nerve (CN III)
Trochlear nerve (CN IV)
Trigeminal nerve (CN V)
Abducent nerve (CN VI)
Facial nerve (CN VII)
Hypoglossal nerve (CN XII)
Spinal cord
Glossopharyngeal nerve (CN IX)
Vagus nerve (CN X)
Spinal accessory nerve (CN XI)

FIGURE 7.11. **Structure of brain. A.** Right cerebral hemisphere, cerebellum, and brainstem. **B.** Parts of brain identified on median section. *Arrow,* site of interventricular foramen. **C.** Right and left cerebral hemispheres. **D.** Brainstem and cranial nerves. Because the brain is usually studied in detail in a separate neuroanatomy course, the brain is covered by only a superficial survey of its gross structure in the typical anatomy course, with attention primarily focused on the relationship between the brain and its environment.

into the **posterior cerebellomedullary cistern** (L. *cisterna magna*) and the **lateral cerebellomedullary cistern.**

- **Pontocerebellar cistern** (pontine cistern), an extensive space ventral to the pons and continuous inferiorly with the spinal subarachnoid space.
- **Interpeduncular cistern** (basal cistern), located in the interpeduncular fossa between the cerebral peduncles of the midbrain.
- **Chiasmatic cistern,** inferior and anterior to the optic chiasm.
- **Quadrigeminal cistern** (cistern of the great cerebral vein), located between the posterior part of the corpus callosum and the superior surface of the cerebellum.

CSF is secreted (at the rate of 400–500 mL/day) by choroidal epithelial cells of the **choroid plexuses** in the lateral, third, and fourth ventricles (Fig. 7.12*B*). The choroid plexuses consist of vascular fringes of pia mater (tela choroidea) covered by cuboidal epithelial cells. Some CSF leaves the fourth ventricle to pass inferiorly into the subarachnoid space around the spinal cord and posterosuperiorly over the cerebellum. However, most CSF flows into the interpeduncular and quadrigeminal cisterns. CSF from the various cisterns flows superiorly through the sulci and fissures on the medial and superolateral surfaces of the cerebral hemispheres. CSF also passes into the extensions of the subarachnoid space around the cranial nerves.

The main site of CSF absorption into the venous system is through the **arachnoid granulations,** protrusions of arachnoid villi into the walls of dural venous sinuses, especially the superior sagittal sinus and its lateral venous lacunae (Figs. 7.10*A–C* and 7.12*A*). Along with the meninges and calvaria, CSF protects the brain by providing a cushion against blows to the head. The CSF in the subarachnoid space provides the buoyancy that prevents the weight of the brain from compressing the cranial nerve roots and blood vessels against the internal surface of the cranium.

Cisternal Puncture

 CSF may be obtained, for diagnostic purposes, from the posterior cerebellomedullary cistern, using a procedure known as *cisternal puncture*. The subarachnoid space or the ventricular system may also be entered for measuring or monitoring CSF pressure, injecting antibiotics, or administering contrast media for radiography.

Hydrocephalus

 Overproduction of CSF, obstruction of its flow, or interference with its absorption results in an excess of CSF in the ventricles and enlargement of the head, a condition known as *hydrocephalus* (Fig. B7.3). Excess CSF dilates the ventricles; thins the brain; and, in infants, separates the bones of the calvaria because the sutures and fontanelles are still open.

Leakage of Cerebrospinal Fluid

Fractures in the floor of the middle cranial fossa may result in leakage of CSF from the external acoustic meatus (*CSF otorrhea*) if the meninges superior to the middle ear are torn and the tympanic membrane (eardrum) is ruptured.

Fractures in the floor of the anterior cranial fossa may involve the cribriform plate of the ethmoid, resulting in leakage of CSF through the nose (*CSF rhinorrhea*).

CSF otorrhea and CSF rhinorrhea may be primary indications of a cranial base fracture and increase the risk of *meningitis* because an infection could spread to the meninges from the ear or nose.

Hydrocephalus

FIGURE B7.3.

Arachnoid granulations

Subarachnoid space
containing CSF

Superior
sagittal
sinus

Choroid plexus

**Lateral
ventricles**

3rd ventricle

Cerebral
aqueduct

Lateral
apertures

4th ventricle

Median aperture

Central canal
(of spinal cord)

A **Medial view, ventricles viewed from left**

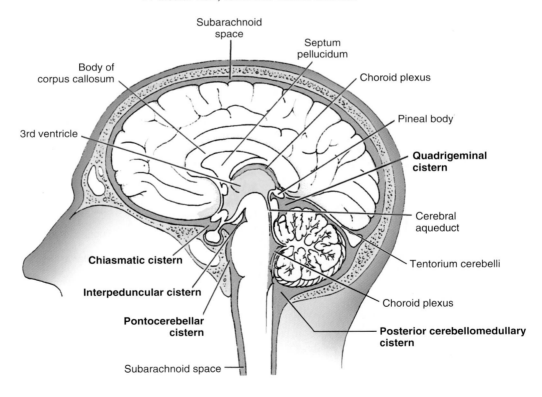

Subarachnoid
space

Septum
pellucidum

Body of
corpus callosum

Choroid plexus

Pineal body

3rd ventricle

**Quadrigeminal
cistern**

Cerebral
aqueduct

Tentorium cerebelli

Chiasmatic cistern

Interpeduncular cistern

Choroid plexus

**Pontocerebellar
cistern**

**Posterior cerebellomedullary
cistern**

Subarachnoid space

B **Medial view**

FIGURE 7.12.   **Ventricular system of brain. A.** Ventricles. *Arrows,* direction of cerebrospinal fluid (*CSF*) flow. **B.** Subarachnoid cisterns.

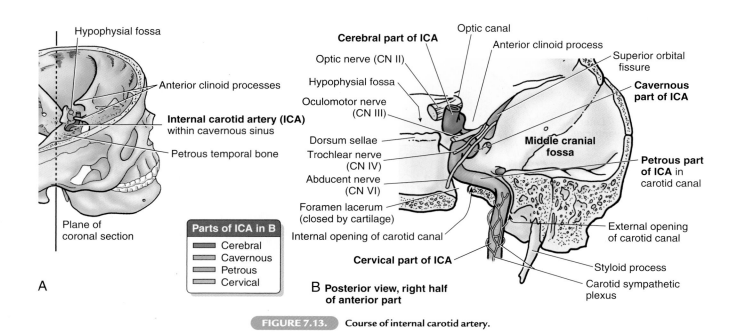

FIGURE 7.13. Course of internal carotid artery.

*Components of cerebral arterial circle (of Willis)

Inferior view

FIGURE 7.14. **Blood supply of brain.** Cerebral arterial circle and cranial nerves.

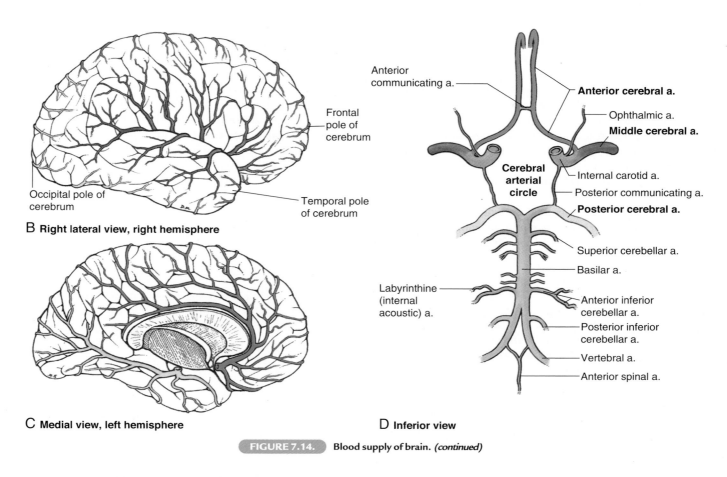

B **Right lateral view, right hemisphere**

C **Medial view, left hemisphere**

D **Inferior view**

FIGURE 7.14. Blood supply of brain. *(continued)*

TABLE 7.2 ARTERIAL SUPPLY OF CEREBRAL HEMISPHERES

Artery	Origin	Distribution
Internal carotid	Common carotid artery at superior border of thyroid cartilage	Gives branches to walls of cavernous sinus, pituitary gland, and trigeminal ganglion; provides primary supply to brain
Anterior cerebral	Internal carotid artery	Cerebral hemispheres, except for occipital lobes
Anterior communicating	Anterior cerebral artery	Cerebral arterial circle (of Willis)
Middle cerebral	Continuation of internal carotid artery distal to anterior cerebral artery	Most of lateral surface of cerebral hemispheres
Vertebral	Subclavian artery	Cranial meninges and cerebellum
Basilar	Formed by union of vertebral arteries	Brainstem, cerebellum, and cerebrum
Posterior cerebral	Terminal branch of basilar artery	Interior aspect of cerebral hemisphere and occipital lobe
Posterior communicating	Posterior cerebral artery	Optic tract, cerebral peduncle, internal capsule, and thalamus

Vasculature of Brain

Although it accounts for only about 2.5% of body weight, the brain receives about one sixth of the cardiac output and one fifth of the oxygen consumed by the body at rest. The blood supply to the brain is from the internal carotid and vertebral arteries (Figs. 7.13 and 7.14; Table 7.2).

The **internal carotid arteries** arise in the neck from the common carotid arteries and enter the cranial cavity with the carotid plexus of sympathetic nerves through the carotid canals. The intracranial course of the internal carotid artery can be seen in Figures 7.8 and 7.13B. The cervical part of the artery ascends to the entrance to the carotid canal in the petrous temporal bone. The petrous part of the artery turns horizontally and medially in the carotid canal to emerge superior to the foramen lacerum, entering the cranial cavity. The cavernous part of the artery runs on the lateral side of the sphenoid in the carotid groove as it traverses the cavernous sinuses. Inferior to the anterior clinoid process, the artery makes a 180-degree turn to join the cerebral arterial circle. The internal carotid arteries course anteriorly through the cavernous sinuses, with the abducent nerves (CN VI) and in close proximity to the oculomotor (CN III) and trochlear (CN IV) nerves. The terminal branches of the internal carotids are the **anterior** and **middle cerebral arteries** (Fig. 7.14).

The **vertebral arteries** begin in the root of the neck as branches of the first part of the subclavian arteries, pass through the transverse foramina of the first six cervical vertebrae, and perforate the dura and arachnoid to pass through the foramen magnum. The intracranial parts of the vertebral arteries unite at the caudal border of the pons to form the **basilar artery** (Figs. 7.14*A,B*; Table 7.2). The basilar artery runs through the pontocerebellar cistern to the superior border of the pons, where it ends by dividing into the two **posterior cerebral arteries.**

In addition to supplying branches to deeper parts of the brain, the cortical branches of each cerebral artery supply a surface and a pole of the cerebrum. The cortical branches of the:

- *Anterior cerebral arteries* supply most of the medial and superior surfaces and the frontal pole.

Strokes

An *ischemic stroke* denotes the sudden development of neurological deficits that are related to impaired cerebral blood flow. The most common causes of strokes are spontaneous cerebrovascular accidents such as cerebral embolism, cerebral thrombosis, cerebral hemorrhage, and subarachnoid hemorrhage (Rowland, 2000). The cerebral arterial circle is an important means of collateral circulation in the event of gradual obstruction of one of the major arteries forming the circle. Sudden occlusion, even if only partial, results in neurological deficits. In elderly persons, the anastomoses are often inadequate when a large artery (e.g., internal carotid) is occluded, even if the occlusion is gradual (in which case function is impaired at least to some degree).

Hemorrhagic stroke follows the rupture of an artery or a *saccular aneurysm,* a sac-like dilation on a weak part of the arterial wall. The most common type of saccular aneurysm is a *berry aneurysm,* occurring in the vessels of or near the cerebral arterial circle and the medium arteries at the base of the brain (Fig. B7.4). In time, especially in people with hypertension (high blood pressure), the weak part of the arterial wall expands and may rupture, allowing blood to enter the subarachnoid space.

Transient Ischemic Attacks

Transient ischemic attacks (TIAs) refer to neurological symptoms resulting from ischemia (deficient blood supply) of the brain. The symptoms of a TIA may be ambiguous: staggering, dizziness, light-headedness, fainting, and paresthesias (e.g., tingling in a limb). Most TIAs last a few minutes, but some persist for up to an hour. Individuals with TIAs are at increased risk for myocardial infarction and ischemic stroke (Brust, 2005).

Anterior communicating artery

Middle cerebral artery

Internal carotid artery

Posterior communicating artery

Posterior cerebral artery

Basilar artery

Aneurysms (green)

Posterior inferior cerebellar artery

Berry aneurysm

FIGURE B7.4.

- *Middle cerebral arteries* supply the lateral surface and temporal pole.
- *Posterior cerebral arteries* supply the inferior surface and occipital pole.

The **cerebral arterial circle** (of Willis) at the base of the brain is an important anastomosis between the four arteries (two vertebral and two internal carotid arteries) that supply the brain. The arterial circle is formed by the *posterior cerebral, posterior communicating, internal carotid, anterior cerebral,* and *anterior communicating arteries.* The various components of the cerebral arterial circle give numerous small branches to the brain. Variations in the origin and size of the vessels forming the cerebral arterial circle are common (e.g., the posterior communicating arteries may be absent, or there may be two anterior communicating arteries). In approximately one in three people, one posterior cerebral artery is a major branch of the internal carotid artery.

The thin-walled, valveless **cerebral veins** draining the brain pierce the arachnoid and meningeal layer of dura to end in the nearest dural venous sinuses. The sinuses drain for the most part into the IJVs. The superior cerebral veins on the superolateral surface of the brain drain into the superior sagittal sinus (Fig. 7.6A); cerebral veins on the posteroinferior aspect drain into the straight, transverse, and superior petrosal sinuses. The **great cerebral vein** (of Galen), a single midline vein, is formed inside the brain by the union of two internal cerebral veins and ends by merging with the inferior sagittal sinus to form the straight sinus (Figs. 7.6A,B).

FACE

The face is the anterior aspect of the head from the forehead to the chin and from one ear to the other. The basic shape of the face is determined by the underlying bones, the facial muscles, and the subcutaneous tissue. The skin of the face is thin, pliable, and firmly attached to the underlying cartilages of the external ear and nose.

Facial Injuries

Because the face does not have a distinct layer of deep fascia and the subcutaneous tissue is loose between the attachments of facial muscles, *facial lacerations* tend to gape (part widely). Consequently, the skin must be sutured carefully to prevent scarring. The looseness of the subcutaneous tissue also enables fluid and blood to accumulate in the loose connective tissue after bruising of the face. Facial inflammation causes considerable swelling.

Muscles of Face

The facial muscles (muscles of facial expression) are in the subcutaneous tissue of the anterior and posterior scalp, face, and neck (Fig. 7.15, Table 7.3). Most of these muscles attach to bone or fascia and produce their effects by pulling the skin. They move the skin and change facial expressions to convey mood. The *muscles of facial expression* also surround the orifices of the mouth, eyes, and nose and act as sphincters and dilators that close and open the orifices.

The **orbicularis oris** is the sphincter of the mouth and is the first of a series of sphincters associated with the alimentary (digestive) tract. The **buccinator** (L. trumpeter), active in smiling, also keeps the cheek taut, thereby preventing it from folding and being injured during chewing. The orbicularis oris and buccinator work with the tongue to keep food between the teeth during mastication (chewing). The buccinator is also active during sucking, whistling, and blowing (e.g., when playing a wind instrument).

The **orbicularis oculi** closes the eyelids and assists the flow of lacrimal fluid (tears). It has three parts: the *palpebral part,* which gently closes the eyelids; the *lacrimal part,* which passes posterior to the lacrimal sac, aiding drainage of tears; and the *orbital part,* which tightly closes the eyelids to protect the eyeballs against glare and dust.

Nerves of Face

Cutaneous (sensory) innervation of the face is provided primarily by the *trigeminal nerve* (CN V—Fig. 7.16), whereas the motor innervation to the muscles of facial expression is provided by the *facial nerve* (CN VII—Fig. 7.15B) and the motor innervation to the muscles of mastication by the *mandibular nerve,* the motor root of the trigeminal nerve.

The cutaneous nerves of the neck overlap those of the face (Fig. 7.16B). Cutaneous branches of the cervical nerves from the *cervical plexus* extend over the ear, the posterior aspect of the neck and scalp. The *great auricular nerve* innervates the inferior aspect of the auricle and much of the area overlying the angle of the mandible.

The **trigeminal nerve** (CN V) is the sensory nerve for the face and the motor nerve for the muscles of mastication and several small muscles (Fig. 7.16; Table 7.4). Three large groups of peripheral processes from nerve cell bodies of the **trigeminal ganglion**—the large sensory ganglion of CN V—form the **ophthalmic nerve** (CN V$_1$), the **maxillary nerve** (CN V$_2$), and the sensory component of the **mandibular nerve** (CN V$_3$). These nerves are named according to their main regions of termination: the eye, maxilla, and mandible, respectively. The first two divisions (CN V$_1$ and CN V$_2$) are wholly sensory. CN V$_3$ is largely sensory but also receives motor fibers (axons) from the motor

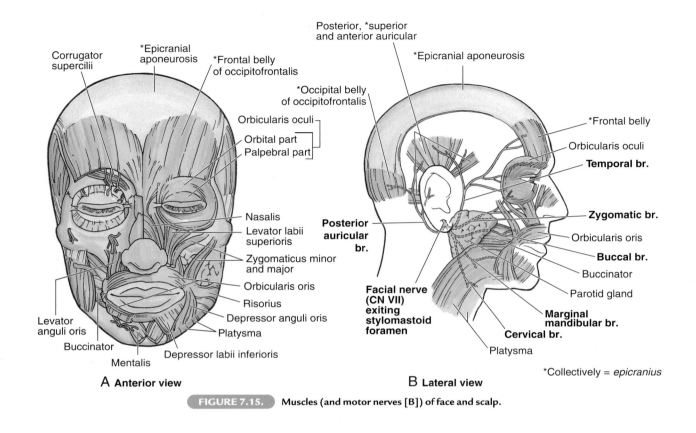

FIGURE 7.15.   Muscles (and motor nerves [B]) of face and scalp.

TABLE 7.3 MAJOR FUNCTIONAL MUSCLES OF FACE AND SCALP

Muscle[a]	Origin	Insertion	Main Action(s)
Occipitofrontalis			
Frontal belly	Epicranial aponeurosis	Skin and subcutaneous tissue of eyebrows and forehead	Elevates eyebrows and wrinkles skin of forehead; protracts scalp (indicating surprise or curiosity)
Occipital belly	Lateral two thirds of superior nuchal line	Epicranial aponeurosis	Retracts scalp; increasing effectiveness of frontal belly
Orbicularis oculi (orbital sphincter)	Medial orbital margin; medial palpebral ligament; lacrimal bone	Skin around margin of orbit; superior and inferior tarsi (tarsal plates)	Closes eyelids: palpebral part does so gently; orbital part tightly (winking)
Orbicularis oris (oral sphincter)	Medial maxilla and mandible; deep surface of peri-oral skin; angle of mouth	Mucous membrane of lips	Tonus closes mouth; phasic contraction compresses and protrudes lips (kissing) or resists distension (when blowing)
Buccinator (cheek muscle)	Mandible, alveolar processes of maxilla and mandible, pterygomandibular raphe	Angle of mouth (modiolus); orbicularis oris	Presses cheek against molar teeth; works with tongue to keep food between occlusal surfaces and out of oral vestibule; resists distension (when blowing)
Platysma	Subcutaneous tissue of infraclavicular and supraclavicular regions	Base of mandible; skin of cheek and lower lip; angle of mouth; orbicularis oris	Depresses mandible (against resistance); tenses skin of inferior face and neck (conveying tension and stress)

[a]All facial muscles are innervated by the facial nerve (CN VII) via its posterior auricular branch or via the temporal, zygomatic, buccal, marginal mandibular, or cervical branches of the parotid plexus.

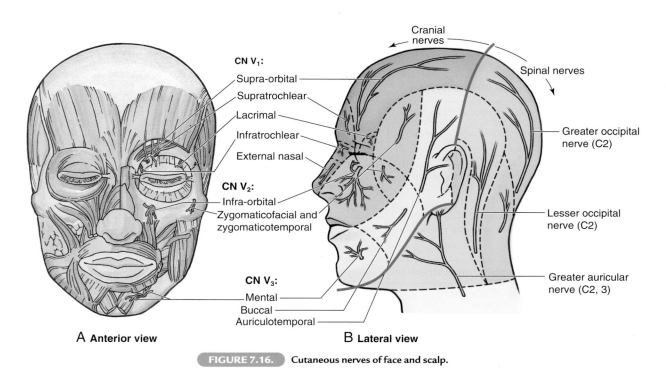

FIGURE 7.16. Cutaneous nerves of face and scalp.

TABLE 7.4 CUTANEOUS NERVES OF FACE AND SCALP

Nerve	Origin	Course	Distribution
Cutaneous nerves derived from ophthalmic nerve (CN V₁)			
Supra-orbital	Branch from bifurcation of *frontal nerve,* approximately in middle of orbital roof	Continues anteriorly along roof of orbit, emerging via supra-orbital notch or foramen; ascends forehead, breaking into branches	Mucosa of *frontal sinus;* skin and conjunctiva of middle of *superior eyelid;* skin and pericranium of *anterolateral forehead and scalp* to vertex
Supratrochlear	Branch from bifurcation of *frontal nerve,* approximately in middle of orbital roof	Continues anteromedially along roof of orbit, passing lateral to trochlea and ascending forehead	Skin and conjunctiva of medial aspect of *superior eyelid;* skin and pericranium of *anteromedial forehead*
Lacrimal	Branch of *CN V₁* proximal to superior	Runs superolaterally through orbit, receiving secretomotor fibers via a communicating branch from the zygomaticotemporal nerve	*Lacrimal gland* (secretomotor fibers); small area of skin and conjunctiva of *lateral part of superior eyelid*
Infratrochlear	Terminal branch (with anterior ethmoidal nerve) of *nasociliary nerve*	Follows medial wall of orbit, passing inferior to trochlea	Skin lateral to *root of nose;* skin and conjunctiva of *eyelids adjacent to medial canthus, lacrimal sac,* and lacrimal caruncle
External nasal	Terminal branch of *anterior ethmoidal nerve*	Emerges from nasal cavity by passing between nasal bone and lateral nasal cartilage	Skin of nasal *ala, vestibule, and dorsum of nose,* including *apex*
Cutaneous nerves derived from maxillary nerve (CN V₂)			
Infra-orbital	Continuation of *CN V₂* distal to its entrance into the orbit via the inferior orbital fissure	Traverses infra-orbital groove and canal in orbital floor, giving rise to superior alveolar branches; then emerges via infra-orbital foramen, immediately dividing into inferior palpebral, internal and external nasal, and superior labial branches	Mucosa of *maxillary sinus;* premolar, canine, and incisor *maxillary teeth;* skin and conjunctiva of *inferior eyelid;* skin of *cheek, lateral nose,* and antero-inferior *nasal septum;* skin and oral mucosa of *upper lip*
Zygomaticofacial	Smaller terminal branch (with zygomaticotemporal nerve) of *zygomatic nerve*	Traverses zygomaticofacial canal in zygomatic bone at inferolateral angle of orbit	Skin on prominence of *cheek*
Zygomaticotemporal	Larger terminal branch (with zygomaticofacial nerve) of *zygomatic nerve*	Sends communicating branch to lacrimal nerve in orbit; then passes to temporal fossa via zygomaticotemporal canal in zygomatic bone	Skin overlying *anterior part of temporal fossa*

TABLE 7.4 CUTANEOUS NERVES OF FACE AND SCALP *(continued)*

Nerve	Origin	Course	Distribution
Cutaneous nerves derived from mandibular nerve (CN V₃)			
Auriculotemporal	In infratemporal fossa via two roots from *posterior trunk of CN V₃* that encircle middle meningeal artery	Passes posteriorly deep to ramus of mandible and superior deep part of parotid gland, emerging posterior to temporo-mandibular joint	Skin anterior to auricle and posterior two thirds of *temporal region;* skin of tragus and adjacent helix of *auricle;* skin of roof of *external acoustic meatus;* and skin of superior *tympanic membrane*
Buccal	In infratemporal fossa as sensory branch of *anterior trunk of CN V₃*	Passes between two parts of lateral ptery-goid muscle, emerging anteriorly from cover of ramus of mandible and masseter, uniting with buccal branches of facial nerve	Skin and oral mucosa of *cheek* (overlying and deep to anterior part of buccinator); *buccal gingiva* (gums) adjacent to second and third molars
Mental	Terminal branch of *inferior alveolar nerve* (branch of V₃)	Emerges from mandibular canal via mental foramen in anterolateral aspect of body of mandible	Skin of *chin;* oral mucosa of *lower lip*
Cutaneous nerves derived from anterior rami of cervical spinal nerves			
Great auricular	Spinal nerves C2 and C3 via cervical plexus	Ascends vertically across sternocleidomas-toid, posterior to external jugular vein	Skin overlying angle of mandible and inferior lobe of auricle; parotid sheath
Lesser occipital		Follows posterior border of sternocleido-mastoid; then ascends posterior to auricle	Scalp posterior to auricle
Cutaneous nerves derived from posterior rami of cervical spinal nerves			
Greater occipital nerve	As medial branch of posterior ramus of spinal nerve C2	Emerges between axis and obliquus capitis inferior; then pierces trapezius	Scalp of occipital region
Third occipital nerve	As lateral branch of posterior ramus of spinal nerve C3	Pierces trapezius	Scalp of lower occipital and suboccipital regions

root of CN V (Table 7.4). The major cutaneous branches of the trigeminal nerve (Table 7.4) are:

- Ophthalmic nerve (CN V₁): lacrimal, supra-orbital, supratrochlear, infratrochlear, and external nasal nerves.
- Maxillary nerve (CN V₂): infra-orbital, zygomaticotempo-ral, and zygomaticofacial nerves.
- Mandibular (CN V₃): auriculotemporal, buccal, and men-tal nerves.

The **motor nerves of the face** are the *facial nerve* (CN VII) to the muscles of facial expression and the **mandibular nerve** (CN V₃) to the muscles of mastication (masseter, tem-poral, medial, and lateral pterygoids) These nerves also supply some more deeply placed muscles (described later in this chapter in relation to the mouth, middle ear, and neck). The **facial nerve** (CN VII) emerges from the cranium via the *stylomastoid foramen* (Fig. 7.15*B*; Tables 7.1 and 7.3). Its extracranial branches (temporal, zygomatic, buccal, marginal mandibular, cervical, and posterior auricular nerves) supply the superficial muscle of the neck and chin (platysma), mus-cles of facial expression, muscle of the cheek (buccinator), muscles of the ear (auricular), and muscles of the scalp (occipital and frontal bellies of occipitofrontal muscle).

Innervation of the scalp anterior to the auricles is by branches of all three divisions of the **trigeminal nerve** (CN

V₁, CN V₂, CN V₃) (Fig. 7.16*B*; Table 7.4). Posterior to the auricles, innervation of the scalp is by spinal cutaneous nerves (C2 and C3).

Superficial Vasculature of Face and Scalp

The face is richly supplied by superficial arteries and exter-nal veins, as is evident in blushing and blanching (becoming pale). The terminal branches of both arteries and veins anas-tomose freely, including anastomoses across the midline with contralateral partners. Most arteries supplying the face are branches of the *external carotid arteries* (Fig. 7.17; Table 7.5). Most external facial veins are drained by veins that accompany the arteries of the face. As with most superficial veins, they are subject to many variations and have abundant anastomoses that allow drainage to occur by alternate routes during periods of temporary compression. The alternate routes include both superficial pathways and deep drainage.

The **facial artery** provides the major arterial supply to the face (Figs. 7.17*B* and 7.18; Table 7.5). It arises from the external carotid artery and winds its way to the inferior bor-der of the mandible, just anterior to the masseter. It then courses over the face to the medial angle (canthus) of the eye. The facial artery sends branches to the upper and lower lips (**superior** and **inferior labial arteries**). The

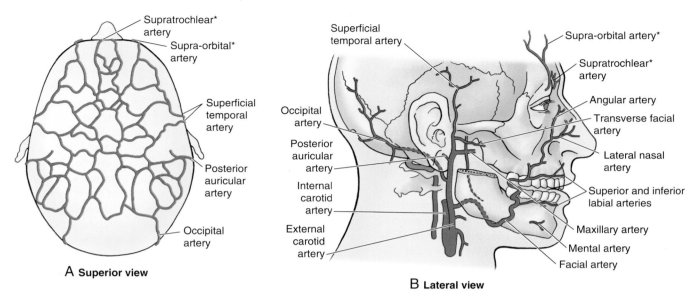

A **Superior view**

B **Lateral view**

*Source = internal carotid artery (all other labeled arteries are from external carotid artery)

FIGURE 7.17. Arteries of face and scalp.

TABLE 7.5 SUPERFICIAL ARTERIES OF FACE AND SCALP

Nerve	Origin	Course	Distribution
Facial	External carotid artery	Ascends deep to submandibular gland; winds around inferior border of mandible and enters face	Muscles of facial expression and face
Inferior labial	Facial artery near angle of mouth	Runs medially in lower lip	Lower lip
Superior labial		Runs medially in upper lip	Upper lip and ala (side) and septum of nose
Lateral nasal	Facial artery as it ascends alongside nose	Passes to ala of nose	Skin on ala and dorsum of nose
Angular	Terminal branch of facial artery	Passes to medial angle (canthus) of eye	Superior part of cheek and inferior eyelid
Occipital	External carotid artery	Passes medial to posterior belly of digastric and mastoid process; accompanies occipital nerve in occipital region	Scalp of back of head, as far as vertex
Posterior auricular		Passes posteriorly, deep to parotid gland, along styloid process between mastoid process and ear	Auricle and scalp posterior to auricle
Superficial temporal	Smaller terminal branch of external carotid artery	Ascends anterior to ear to temporal region and ends in scalp	Facial muscles and skin of frontal and temporal regions
Transverse facial	Superficial temporal artery within parotid gland	Crosses face superficial to masseter and inferior to zygomatic arch	Parotid gland and duct, muscles and skin of face
Mental	Terminal branch of inferior alveolar artery	Emerges from mental foramen and passes to chin	Facial muscles and skin of chin
Supra-orbital	Terminal branch of ophthalmic artery, a branch of internal carotid artery	Passes superiorly from supra-orbital foramen	Muscle and skin of forehead and scalp
Supratrochlear		Passes superiorly from supratrochlear notch	Muscles and skin of scalp

Trigeminal Neuralgia

Trigeminal neuralgia (tic douloureux) is a sensory disorder of the sensory root of *CN V* characterized by sudden attacks of excruciating, lightning-like jabs of facial pain. A *paroxysm* (sudden sharp pain) can last for 15 minutes or more. The maxillary nerve (CN V$_2$) is most frequently involved; then the mandibular nerve (CN V$_3$); and, least frequently, the ophthalmic nerve (CN V$_1$). The pain often is initiated by touching a sensitive *trigger zone* of the skin.

The cause of trigeminal neuralgia is unknown; however, some investigators believe that most affected people have an anomalous blood vessel that compresses the sensory root of CN V. When the aberrant artery is moved away from the root, the symptoms usually disappear. Other researchers believe the condition is caused by pathological processes affecting neurons of the trigeminal ganglion. In some cases, it is necessary to section the sensory root for relief of trigeminal neuralgia.

Lesions of Trigeminal Nerve

Lesions of the entire trigeminal nerve cause widespread anesthesia involving the:

- Corresponding anterior half of the scalp.
- Face, except for an area overlying the angle of the mandible.
- Cornea and conjunctiva.
- Mucous membranes of the nose and paranasal sinuses, mouth, and anterior part of the tongue. Paralysis of the muscles of mastication also occurs.

Bell Palsy

Injury to the facial nerve (CN VII) or its branches produces paralysis of some or all the facial muscles on the affected side (Bell palsy).

The affected areas sag and facial expression is distorted (Fig. B7.5). The loss of tonus of the orbicularis oculi causes the inferior eyelid to evert (fall away from the surface of the eyeball). As a result, the lacrimal fluid is not spread over the cornea, preventing adequate lubrication, hydration, and flushing of the cornea. This makes the cornea vulnerable to ulceration. If the injury weakens or paralyzes the buccinator and orbicularis oris, food will accumulate in the oral vestibule during chewing, usually requiring continual removal with a finger. When the sphincters or dilators of the mouth are affected, displacement of the mouth (drooping of the corner) is produced by gravity and contraction of unopposed contralateral facial muscles, resulting in food and saliva dribbling out of the side of the mouth. Weakened lip muscles affect speech. Affected people cannot whistle or blow a wind instrument effectively. They frequently dab their eyes and mouth with a handkerchief to wipe the fluid (tears and saliva), which runs from the drooping eyelid and mouth.

Bell palsy

FIGURE B7.5.

facial artery also sends branches to the side of the nose (**lateral nasal artery**) and then terminates as the **angular artery,** which supplies the medial angle of the eye.

The **superficial temporal artery** is the smaller terminal branch of the external carotid artery; the other branch is the *maxillary artery*. The superficial temporal artery emerges on the face between the temporomandibular joint (TMJ) and the auricle and ends in the scalp by dividing into **frontal** and **parietal branches** (Fig. 7.18). The **transverse facial artery** arises from the superficial temporal artery within the parotid gland and crosses the face superficial to the masseter. It divides into numerous branches that supply the parotid gland and duct, the masseter, and the skin of the face. It anastomoses with branches of the facial artery.

The **arteries of the scalp** course within the subcutaneous connective tissue layer between the skin and the epicranial aponeurosis. They anastomose freely with one another. The arterial walls are firmly attached to the dense

Parietal branch of superficial temporal artery

Epicranial aponeurosis

Temporalis

Superficial temporal vein and artery

Auriculotemporal nerve (CN V₃)

Occipital belly

External acoustic meatus

Mastoid process

Posterior auricular branch (CN VII)

Buccal branch (CN VII)

Cervical branch (CN VII)

Masseter

Frontal branch of superficial temporal artery

Frontal belly

Transverse facial artery

Supra-orbital nerve (CN V₁)

Temporal branch (CN VII)

Angular vein and artery

Lateral nasal artery

Infra-orbital nerve (CN V₂)

Zygomatic branch (CN VII)

Superior labial artery

Parotid duct

Inferior labial artery

Mental nerve

Marginal mandibular branch (CN VII)

Facial vein and artery

Parotid gland

FIGURE 7.18. Vasculature and nerves of face, relationship to parotid gland.

connective tissue in which they are embedded, limiting their ability to constrict when cut. Consequently, bleeding from scalp wounds is profuse. The arterial supply is from the *external carotid arteries* through the **occipital, posterior auricular,** and **superficial temporal arteries** and from the *internal carotid arteries* by way of the **supratrochlear** and **supra-orbital arteries** (Fig. 7.17*B*; Table 7.5). Arteries of the scalp supply little blood to the cranium, which is supplied primarily by the middle meningeal artery.

The **facial vein** provides the primary superficial venous drainage of the face (Figs. 7.18 and 7.19*A,B*). It begins at the medial angle of the eye as the **angular vein.** Among the tributaries of the facial vein is the **deep facial vein,** which drains the *pterygoid venous plexus* of the infratemporal fossa (Fig. 7.19*B*). Inferior to the margin of the mandible, the facial vein is joined by the anterior branch of the retromandibular vein. The facial vein drains directly or indirectly into the **internal jugular vein** (Fig. 7.19*A*). At the medial angle of the eye, the facial vein communicates with the *superior ophthalmic vein,* which drains into the *cavernous sinus.*

The **superficial temporal vein** drains the forehead and scalp and receives tributaries from the veins of the temple and face. Near the auricle, the superficial temporal vein enters the parotid gland (Fig. 7.18). The **retromandibular vein,** formed by the union of the superficial temporal vein and the maxillary vein, is a deep vein that

Pulses of Arteries of Face

The pulses of the superficial temporal and facial arteries can be used for taking the pulse. For example, anesthesiologists at the head of the operating table often take the *temporal pulse* anterior to the auricle as the artery crosses the zygomatic arch to supply the scalp. The *facial pulse* can be palpated where the facial artery crosses the inferior border of the mandible immediately anterior to the masseter.

Compression of Facial Artery

The facial artery can be occluded by pressure against the mandible where the vessel crosses it. Because of the numerous anastomoses between the branches of the facial artery and other arteries of the face, compression of the facial artery on one side does not stop all bleeding from a lacerated facial artery or one of its branches. In lacerations of the lip, pressure must be applied on both sides of the cut to stop the bleeding. In general, facial wounds bleed freely but heal quickly.

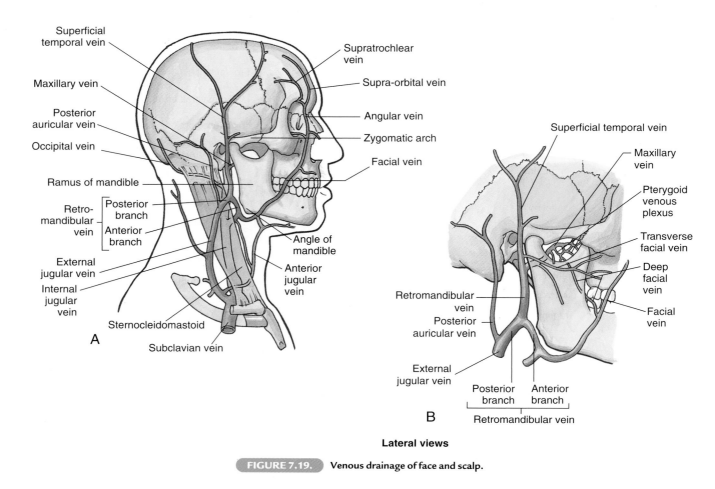

FIGURE 7.19. Venous drainage of face and scalp.

descends within the parotid gland, superficial to the external carotid artery and deep to the facial nerve (Fig. 7.19A,B). The retromandibular vein divides into an anterior branch, which unites with the facial vein, and a posterior branch, which joins the **posterior auricular vein** to form the **external jugular vein** (EJV). The EJV crosses the superficial surface of the sternocleidomastoid muscle to enter the subclavian vein in the root of the neck.

Venous drainage of the superficial parts of the scalp is through the accompanying veins of the scalp arteries, the **supra-orbital** and **supratrochlear veins,** which descend to unite at the medial angle of the eye to form the **angular vein,** which becomes the **facial vein** at the inferior margin of the orbit. The **superficial temporal veins** and **posterior auricular veins** drain the scalp anterior and posterior to the auricles, respectively. The **occipital veins** drain the occipital region of the scalp. Venous drainage of deep parts of the scalp in the temporal region is through **deep temporal veins,** which are tributaries of the pterygoid venous plexus.

There are no lymph nodes in the scalp or face except for the parotid/buccal region. Lymph from the scalp, face, and neck drains into the *superficial ring (pericervical collar) of*

lymph nodes—the submental, submandibular, parotid, mastoid, and *occipital*—located at the junction of the head and neck (Fig. 7.20). Lymph from the superficial ring of nodes drains into the **deep cervical lymph nodes** along the IJV. Lymph from these nodes passes to the jugular lymphatic trunk, which joins the thoracic duct on the left side and the IJV or brachiocephalic vein on the right side. A summary of the lymphatic drainage of the face follows:

- Lymph from the lateral part of the face and scalp drains to the superficial **parotid lymph nodes.**
- Lymph from the deep parotid nodes drains to the **deep cervical lymph nodes.**
- Lymph from the upper lip and lateral parts of the lower lip drains into the **submandibular lymph nodes.**
- Lymph from the chin and central part of the lower lip drains into the **submental lymph nodes.**

Parotid Gland

The parotid gland is the largest of three paired salivary glands. It is enclosed within a tough fascial capsule, the **parotid sheath,** derived from the investing layer of deep

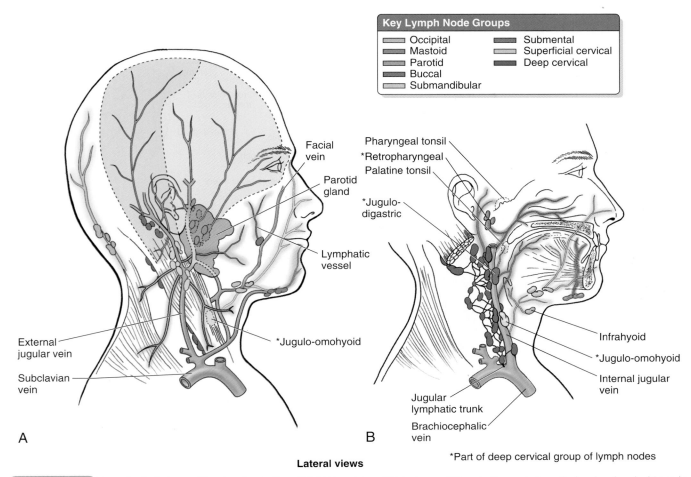

Key Lymph Node Groups

Occipital	Submental
Mastoid	Superficial cervical
Parotid	Deep cervical
Buccal	
Submandibular	

Facial vein

Parotid gland

Lymphatic vessel

External jugular vein

Subclavian vein

*Jugulo-omohyoid

A

Pharyngeal tonsil

*Retropharyngeal

Palatine tonsil

*Jugulo-digastric

Infrahyoid

*Jugulo-omohyoid

Internal jugular vein

Jugular lymphatic trunk

Brachiocephalic vein

B

Lateral views

*Part of deep cervical group of lymph nodes

FIGURE 7.20.   **Lymphatic drainage of head and neck.** Superficial (**A**) and deep (**B**) drainage. All lymphatic vessels from the head and neck ultimately drain into the deep cervical nodes, either directly or indirectly.

cervical fascia. The parotid gland has an irregular shape because the area it occupies, the **parotid bed,** is antero-inferior to the external acoustic meatus, where it is wedged between the ramus of the mandible and the mastoid process (Fig. 7.21). The apex of the parotid gland is posterior to the angle of the mandible, and its base is related to the zygomatic arch. The **parotid duct** passes horizontally from the anterior edge of the gland. At the anterior border of the masseter, the duct turns medially, pierces the buccinator, and enters the oral cavity through a small orifice opposite the second maxillary molar tooth. Embedded within the substance of the parotid gland, from superficial to deep, are the

Squamous Cell Carcinoma of Lip

Squamous cell carcinoma (cancer) of the lip usually involves the lower lip (Fig. B7.6). Overexposure to sunshine and irritation from pipe smoking over many years are contributing factors. Cancer cells from the central part of the lower lip, the floor of the mouth, and apex of the tongue spread to the submental lymph nodes, whereas cancer cells from lateral parts of the lower lip drain to the submandibular lymph nodes.

FIGURE B7.6.

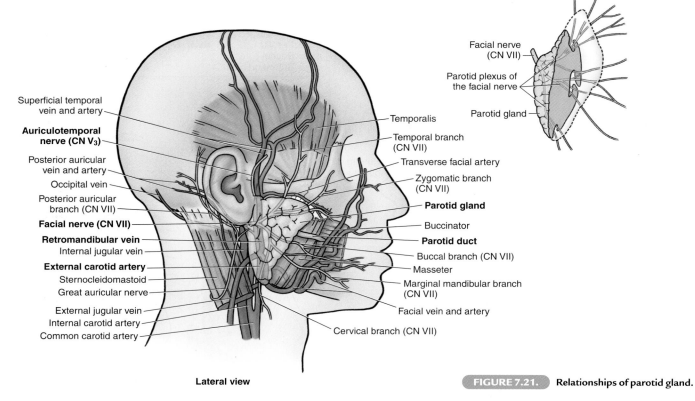

Superficial temporal
vein and artery

**Auriculotemporal
nerve (CN V₃)**

Posterior auricular
vein and artery

Occipital vein

Posterior auricular
branch (CN VII)

Facial nerve (CN VII)

Retromandibular vein

Internal jugular vein

External carotid artery

Sternocleidomastoid

Great auricular nerve

External jugular vein

Internal carotid artery

Common carotid artery

Temporalis

Temporal branch
(CN VII)

Transverse facial artery

Zygomatic branch
(CN VII)

Parotid gland

Buccinator

Parotid duct

Buccal branch (CN VII)

Masseter

Marginal mandibular branch
(CN VII)

Facial vein and artery

Cervical branch (CN VII)

Facial nerve
(CN VII)

Parotid plexus of
the facial nerve

Parotid gland

Lateral view

FIGURE 7.21. Relationships of parotid gland.

parotid plexus of the facial nerve (CN VII) and its branches, the *retromandibular vein*, and the *external carotid artery*. On the parotid sheath and within the gland are *parotid lymph nodes*.

The **great auricular nerve** (C2 and C3), a branch of the cervical plexus, provides sensory innervation to the parotid sheath, gland, and overlying skin (Fig. 7.16B; Table 7.4). The **auriculotemporal nerve,** a branch of CN V₃, also provides sensory innervation to the parotid gland and then passes superior to it with the superficial temporal vessels (Fig. 7.18). The parasympathetic component of the **glossopharyngeal nerve** (CN IX) supplies secretory fibers to the parotid gland; the postsynaptic fibers are conveyed from the *otic ganglion* to the gland by the auriculotemporal nerve.

Parotidectomy

About 80% of salivary gland tumors occur in the parotid glands. Surgical excision of the parotid gland (*parotidectomy*) is often performed as part of the treatment. Because the parotid plexus of CN VII is embedded in the parotid gland, the plexus and its branches are in jeopardy during surgery. An important step in parotidectomy is the identification and preservation of the facial nerve.

Infection of Parotid Gland

The parotid gland may become infected by infectious agents that pass through the bloodstream, as occurs in *mumps,* an acute communicable viral disease. Infection of the gland causes inflammation (*parotiditis*) of the gland. Severe pain occurs because the parotid sheath limits swelling. Often the pain is worse during chewing because the enlarged gland is wrapped around the posterior border of the ramus of the mandible and is compressed against the mastoid process when the mouth is opened. The mumps virus also may cause *inflammation of the parotid duct,* producing redness of the *parotid papilla,* where the parotid duct opens into the mouth opposite the second maxillary molar tooth. Because the pain produced by mumps may be confused with a toothache, redness of the papilla is often an early sign that the disease involves the gland and not a tooth.

Parotid gland disease often causes pain in the auricle, external acoustic meatus, temporal region, and TMJ because the auriculotemporal nerve, from which the parotid gland receives sensory fibers, also supplies sensory fibers to the skin over the temporal fossa and auricle.

Stimulation of the parasympathetic fibers produces a thin watery saliva. Sympathetic fibers are derived from the cervical ganglia through the **external carotid nerve plexus** on the external carotid artery (Fig. 7.21). The vasomotor activity of these fibers may reduce secretion from the parotid gland. Sensory nerve fibers pass to the gland and its sheath through the great auricular and auriculotemporal nerves.

ORBITS

The orbits are pyramidal, bony cavities in the facial skeleton with their bases (*orbital openings*) directed anterolaterally and their apices, posteromedially (Fig. 7.22). The orbits contain and protect the *eyeballs* and their muscles, nerves, and vessels, together with most of the lacrimal apparatus. All space in the orbits not occupied by structures is filled with **orbital fat.**

The orbit has a base, four walls, and an apex:

* The **superior wall** (roof) is approximately horizontal and is formed mainly by the **orbital part of the frontal bone,** which separates the orbital cavity from the anterior cranial fossa. Near the apex of the orbit, the superior wall is formed by the lesser wing of the sphenoid. Anterolaterally the lacrimal gland occupies the **fossa for the lacrimal gland** (lacrimal fossa) in the orbital part of the frontal bone.
* The **medial wall** is formed by the **ethmoid bone,** along with contributions from the frontal, lacrimal, and sphenoid bones. Anteriorly, the medial wall is indented by the **lacrimal groove** and **fossa for the lacrimal sac.** The

bone forming the medial wall is paper-thin, and the ethmoid air cells are often visible through the bone of a dried cranium.

* The **lateral wall** is formed by the **frontal process of the zygomatic bone** and the **greater wing of the sphenoid.** This is the strongest and thickest wall, which is important because it is most exposed and vulnerable to direct trauma. Its posterior part separates the orbit from the temporal lobes of the brain and middle cranial fossae.
* The **inferior wall** (floor) is formed mainly by the **maxilla** and partly by the **zygomatic** and **palatine bones.** The thin inferior wall is shared by the orbit superiorly and the maxillary sinus inferiorly. It slants inferiorly from the apex to the inferior orbital margin. The inferior wall is demarcated from the lateral wall by the **inferior orbital fissure.**
* The **apex** of the orbit is at the **optic canal** in the lesser wing of the sphenoid, just medial to the **superior orbital fissure.**

The bones forming the orbit are lined with **periorbita** (periosteum). The periorbita is continuous with:

* The periosteal layer of dura mater at the optic canal and superior orbital fissure.
* The periosteum covering the external surface of the cranium (pericranium) at the orbital margins and through the inferior orbital fissure.
* The orbital septa at the orbital margins.
* The fascial sheaths of the extra-ocular muscles.
* The orbital fascia that forms the fascial sheath of the eyeball.

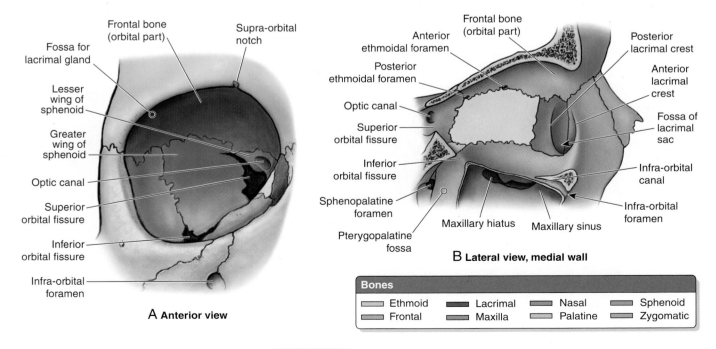

A Anterior view

B **Lateral view, medial wall**

Bones			
Ethmoid	Lacrimal	Nasal	Sphenoid
Frontal	Maxilla	Palatine	Zygomatic

FIGURE 7.22.   **Bones of right orbit.**

Fractures of Orbit

When the blows are powerful enough and the impact is directly on the bony rim, the resulting fractures usually occur at the sutures between the bones forming the orbital margin. Because of the thinness of the medial and inferior walls of the orbit, a blow to the eye may fracture the orbital walls while the margin remains intact. Indirect traumatic injury that displaces the orbital walls is called a "blowout" fracture. Fractures of the medial wall may involve the ethmoidal and sphenoidal sinuses, whereas fractures in the inferior wall may involve the maxillary sinus. Although the superior wall is stronger than the medial and inferior walls, it is thin enough to be translucent and may be readily penetrated. Thus a sharp object may pass through it into the frontal lobe of the brain. Orbital fractures often result in intra-orbital bleeding, which exerts pressure on the eyeball, causing *exophthalmos* (protrusion of the eyeball).

Orbital Tumors

Because of the closeness of the optic nerve to the sphenoidal and posterior ethmoidal sinuses, a malignant tumor in these sinuses may erode the thin bony walls of the orbit and compress the optic nerve and orbital contents. Tumors in the orbit produce exophthalmos. A tumor in the middle cranial fossa may enter the orbital cavity through the superior orbital fissure.

Eyelids and Lacrimal Apparatus

The eyelids and lacrimal fluid, secreted by the lacrimal glands, protect the cornea and eyeball from injury and irritation.

EYELIDS

When closed, the **eyelids** (L. *palpebrae*) cover the eyeball anteriorly, thereby protecting it from injury and excessive light (Fig. 7.24*B*). They also keep the cornea moist by spreading the lacrimal fluid. The eyelids are movable folds that are covered externally by thin skin and internally by a transparent mucous membrane, the **palpebral conjunctiva**. The palpebral conjunctiva is reflected onto the eyeball, where it is continuous with the **bulbar conjunctiva** (Figs. 7.23*A*,*B* and 7.24*B*). The bulbar conjunctiva is loose and wrinkled over the sclera and contains small blood vessels. The bulbar conjunctiva is adherent to the periphery of the cornea. The lines of reflection of the palpebral conjunctiva onto the eyeball form deep recesses, the **superior** and **inferior conjunctival fornices.** The **conjunctival sac** is the space bound by the palpebral and bulbar conjunctivae. The conjunctival sac is a specialized form of mucosal "bursa" that enables the eyelids to move freely over the surface of the eyeball as they open and close.

A Anterior view

B Lateral view

FIGURE 7.23. Surface anatomy of eyeballs and eyelids.

Levator palpebrae superioris

Orbicularis oculi (palpebral part)

Superior tarsal muscle

Superior tarsus — Skin

Tarsal glands

Palpebral conjunctiva

Ciliary glands

Eyelash

A **Sagittal MRI, lateral view**

Orbicularis oculi (1)

Levator palpebrae superioris

Superior rectus (8)

Orbital (intraconal) fat (7)

Superior conjunctival fornix

Superior tarsal muscle
Sclera

Bulbar and palpebral conjunctiva

Superior tarsus (tarsal plate)

Eyeball (2)

Palpebral fissure

Optic nerve (CN II)

Cornea
Inferior conjunctival sac
Inferior conjunctival fornix
Orbital septum
Inferior check ligament

Dural sheath (6)
Subarachnoid space (6)

Inferior rectus (5)

Fascial sheath of eyeball

Inferior oblique (3)
Orbital (extraconal) fat (4)

B **Sagittal section**

Superior tarsus

Levator palpebrae superioris

Medial palpebral ligament

Orbital part (O)

Orbicularis oculi

Palpebral part (P)

Lateral palpebral ligament

Medial angle

Inferior tarsus

Orbital septum

C **Anterior view, right side**

D **Anterior view, left side**

FIGURE 7.24.   **Orbit, eyeball, and eyelids. A.** The numbers are identified in part **B**. *S*, superior ophthalmic vein. *Circle,* optic canal. **B.** Contents of the orbit. *Inset,* details of superior eyelid. **C.** Parts of orbicularis oculi. **D.** Skeleton of eyelids and orbital septum.

The superior (upper) and inferior (lower) eyelids are strengthened by dense bands of connective tissue, the **superior** and **inferior tarsi** (singular **tarsus**; Fig. 7.24B,D). Fibers of the palpebral portion of the **orbicularis oculi** muscle are in the subcutaneous tissue superficial to these tarsi and deep to the skin of the eyelid (Fig 7.24B,C). Embedded in the tarsal plates are **tarsal glands,** the lipid secretion of which lubricates the edges of the eyelids and prevents them

from sticking together when they close (Fig. 7.24A). This secretion also forms a barrier that lacrimal fluid does not cross when produced in normal amounts. When production is excessive, it spills over the barrier onto the cheeks as tears.

The **eyelashes** (L. *cilia*) are in the margins of the eyelids. The large sebaceous glands associated with the eyelashes are the **ciliary glands.** The junctions of the superior and inferior eyelids make up the **medial** and **lateral palpebral**

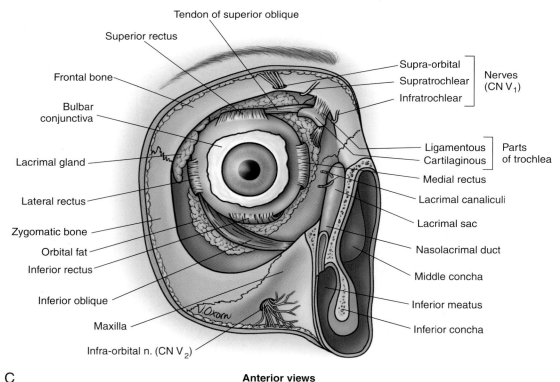

Anterior views

FIGURE 7.25. **Lacrimal apparatus. A.** Surface anatomy of the lacrimal apparatus. **B.** Surface anatomy of the eye, with the inferior eyelid retracted. **C.** Dissection of the anterior orbit and nose.

commissures, defining the **angles of the eyes** (Fig. 7.23). Thus each eye has medial and lateral angles, or *canthi.*

In the **medial angle of the eye,** a reddish shallow reservoir of tears, the **lacrimal lake,** can be observed. Within the lake is the **lacrimal caruncle,** a small mound of moist modified skin (Figs. 7.23*A* and 7.25*A,B*). Lateral to the caruncle is a **semilunar conjunctival fold,** which slightly overlaps the eyeball. When the edges of the eyelids are everted, a small pit the **lacrimal punctum** is visible at its medial end on the summit of a small elevation, the **lacrimal papilla** (Fig. 7.25*B*).

Between the nose and the medial angle of the eye is the **medial palpebral ligament,** which connects the tarsi to the medial margin of the orbit. The orbicularis oculi originates and inserts onto this ligament (Fig. 7.24*C*). A similar **lateral palpebral ligament** attaches the tarsi to the lateral margin of the orbit (Fig. 7.24*D*). The **orbital septum** is a weak membrane that spans from the tarsi to the margins of the orbit, where it becomes continuous with the periosteum. It keeps the orbital fat contained and can limit the spread of infection to and from the orbit.

LACRIMAL APPARATUS

The lacrimal apparatus consists of the following (Fig. 7.25):

- **Lacrimal glands** secrete lacrimal fluid (tears).
- **Lacrimal ducts** convey lacrimal fluid from the lacrimal glands to the conjunctival sac.
- **Lacrimal canaliculi** (L. small canals), each commencing at a *lacrimal punctum* (opening) on the *lacrimal papilla* near the medial angle of the eye, convey the lacrimal fluid from the *lacrimal lake* to the *lacrimal sac,* the dilated superior part of the nasolacrimal duct (Fig. 7.25*A,C*).
- **Nasolacrimal duct** conveys the lacrimal fluid to the nasal cavity.

The almond-shaped **lacrimal gland** lies in the *fossa for the lacrimal gland* in the superolateral part of each orbit. The production of lacrimal fluid is stimulated by parasympathetic impulses from CN VII. It is secreted through 8 to 12 **excretory ducts,** which open into the *superior conjunctival fornix* of the conjunctival sac. The fluid flows inferiorly within the sac under the influence of gravity. When the cornea becomes dry, the eyelid blinks. The eyelids come together in a lateral to medial sequence, pushing a film of fluid medially over the cornea. The lacrimal fluid containing foreign material such as dust is pushed toward the medial angle of the eye, accumulating in the *lacrimal lake* from which it drains by capillary action through the *lacrimal puncta* and *lacrimal canaliculi* to the *lacrimal sac.* From this sac, the lacrimal fluid passes to the nasal cavity through the *nasolacrimal duct* (Fig. 7.25*C*). Here the fluid flows posteriorly to the nasopharynx and is swallowed.

The **nerve supply of the lacrimal gland** is both sympathetic and parasympathetic. The presynaptic parasympathetic secretomotor fibers are conveyed from the facial nerve by the *greater petrosal nerve* and then by the *nerve of the pterygoid canal* to the *pterygopalatine ganglion,* where they synapse with the cell body of the postsynaptic fiber (Fig. 7.64*D*). Vasoconstrictive, postsynaptic sympathetic fibers—brought from the *superior cervical ganglion* by the *internal carotid plexus* and deep petrosal nerve—join the parasympathetic fibers to form the nerve of the pterygoid canal and traverse the pterygopalatine ganglion (Fig. 7.64*E*). Branches of the *zygomatic nerve* (from the maxillary nerve) then bring both types of fibers to the lacrimal branch of the ophthalmic nerve (CN V₁), by which they enter the gland.

Eyeball

The **eyeball** contains the optical apparatus of the visual system. It occupies most of the anterior portion of the orbit, suspended by six extrinsic muscles that control its movements, and a fascial *suspensory apparatus.* It measures approximately 25 mm in diameter. All anatomical structures

Injury to Nerves Supplying Eyelids

Because it supplies the levator palpebrae superioris, a lesion of the oculomotor nerve (CN III) causes paralysis of the muscle, and the superior eyelid droops (*ptosis*). Damage to the facial nerve (CN VII) involves paralysis of the orbicularis oculi, preventing the eyelids from closing fully. Normal rapid protective blinking of the eye is also lost. The loss of tonus of the muscle in the lower eyelid causes the lid to fall away (evert) from the surface of the eye. This leads to drying of the cornea and leaves it unprotected from dust and small particles.

Thus irritation of the unprotected eyeball results in excessive but inefficient lacrimation (tear formation).

Inflammation of Palpebral Glands

Any of the glands in the eyelid may become inflamed and swollen from infection or obstruction of their ducts. If the ducts of the ciliary glands become obstructed, a painful red suppurative (pus-producing) swelling, a *sty,* develops on the eyelid. Cysts of the sebaceous glands of the eyelids, called *chalazia,* may also form.

within the eyeball have a circular or spherical arrangement. The *eyeball proper* has three layers; however, there is an additional connective tissue layer that surrounds the eyeball, supporting it within the orbit. The connective tissue layer is composed posteriorly of the **fascial sheath of the eyeball** (bulbar fascia or Tenon capsule)**,** which forms the actual socket for the eyeball, and anteriorly of bulbar conjunctiva (Fig. 7.24*B*).

The fascial sheath is the most substantial portion of the suspensory apparatus. A very loose connective tissue layer, the **episcleral space** (a potential space), lies between the fascial sheath and the outer layer of the eyeball, facilitating movements of the eyeball within the fascial sheath. The three layers of the eyeball are the (Fig. 7.26):

1. *Fibrous layer* (outer coat), consisting of the *sclera* and *cornea*.
2. *Vascular layer* (middle coat), consisting of the *choroid*, *ciliary body*, and *iris*.
3. *Inner layer* (inner coat), consisting of the *retina*, which has both *optic* and *non-visual parts*.

FIBROUS LAYER OF EYEBALL

The **fibrous layer of the eyeball** is the external fibrous skeleton of the eyeball, providing shape and resistance. The **sclera** is the tough opaque part of the fibrous layer (coat) of the eyeball, covering the posterior five sixths of the eyeball (Figs. 7.26*A*) and providing attachment for both the extrinsic (extra-ocular) and the intrinsic muscles of the eye. The anterior part of the sclera is visible through the transparent bulbar conjunctiva as "the white of the eye" (Fig. 7.24*B*).

The **cornea** is the transparent part of the fibrous layer covering the anterior one sixth of the eyeball. The convexity of the cornea is greater than that of the sclera, and so it appears to protrude from the eyeball when viewed laterally.

The two parts of the fibrous coat differ primarily in terms of the regularity of the arrangement of the collagen fibers of which they are composed and the degree of hydration of each. While the sclera is relatively avascular, the cornea is completely avascular, receiving its nourishment from capillary beds around its periphery and fluids on its external and internal surfaces, the *lacrimal fluid* and *aqueous humor*, respectively (Fig. 7.27). Lacrimal fluid also provides oxygen absorbed from the air.

The cornea is highly sensitive to touch; its innervation is provided by the ophthalmic nerve (CN V$_1$). Even very small foreign bodies (e.g., dust particles) elicit blinking, flow of tears, and sometimes severe pain. Drying of the corneal surface may cause ulceration.

The **limbus** of the cornea is the angle formed by the intersecting curvatures of sclera and cornea at the **corneoscleral junction** (Figs 7.26*A* and 7.27*A*). The junction is a 1-mm-wide, gray, and translucent circle including numerous capillary loops involved in nourishing the avascular cornea.

VASCULAR LAYER OF EYEBALL

The **vascular layer of the eyeball** (also called the **uvea** or uveal tract) consists of the choroid, ciliary body, and iris (Fig. 7.26*B*).

The **choroid,** a dark reddish-brown layer between the sclera and the retina, forms the largest part of the vascular layer of the eyeball and lines most of the sclera (Fig. 7.27*A*). Within this pigmented and dense vascular bed, larger vessels are located externally (near the sclera). The finest vessels (the **capillary lamina of the choroid** or *choriocapillaris*, an extensive capillary bed) are innermost, adjacent to the avascular light-sensitive layer of the retina, which it supplies with oxygen and nutrients. Engorged with blood in life (it has the highest perfusion rate per gram of tissue of all vascular beds of the body), this layer is responsible for the "red eye"

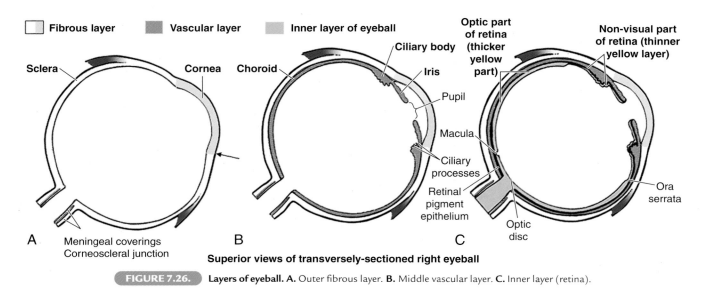

Superior views of transversely-sectioned right eyeball

FIGURE 7.26.   **Layers of eyeball. A.** Outer fibrous layer. **B.** Middle vascular layer. **C.** Inner layer (retina).

Pupil

Iridocorneal angle

Lens

Bulbar conjunctiva

Superior rectus muscle

Vorticose vein

Long posterior ciliary artery

Cornea
Site of aqueous humor
Iris
Scleral venous sinus
Corneoscleral junction
Ciliary process
Zonular fibers of suspensory ligament of lens
Medial rectus muscle
Ora serrata

Vitreous body occupying postremal chamber (posterior segment)

Optic part of retina
Choroid
Sclera
Macula of retina (macula lutea)
Optic disc

Sclera
Dura mater
Arachnoid mater
Subarachnoid space with cerebrospinal fluid (CSF)
Pia mater

Dural sheath of optic nerve
Optic nerve (CN II)
Central artery and vein of retina

A

Cornea
Limbal plexus
Anterior chamber (site of aqueous humor)
Scleral venous sinus
Iris
Sphincter pupillae
Pupil
Dilator pupillae
Posterior chamber
Lens
Ciliary muscle
Capsule of lens
Ciliary process
Zonular fibers of suspensory ligament of lens
Vitreous body (containing vitreous humor)

B

To anterior ciliary veins

Ciliary body
Corneoscleral junction (limbus of cornea)
Anterior ciliary arteries
To vorticose veins
Ora serrata
Muscular branches of ophthalmic artery

FIGURE 7.27. **Eyeball with quarter section removed. A.** Structure of eyeball. The inner aspect of the optic part of the retina is supplied by the central artery of the retina, whereas the outer, light-sensitive aspect is nourished by the capillary lamina of the choroid. The branches of the central artery are end arteries that do not anastomose with each other or any other vessel. **B.** Structures of ciliary region. The ciliary body is both muscular and vascular, as is the iris, the latter including two muscles: the sphincter pupillae and dilator pupillae. Venous blood from this region and the aqueous humor in the anterior chamber drain into the scleral venous sinus.

reflection that occurs in flash photography. The choroid attaches firmly to the pigment layer of the retina, but it can easily be stripped from the sclera. The choroid is continuous anteriorly with the ciliary body.

The **ciliary body** is a ring-like thickening of the layer posterior to the corneoscleral junction that is muscular as well as vascular (Figs. 7.26B and 7.27B). It connects the choroid with the circumference of the iris. The ciliary body provides attachment for the lens. The contraction and relaxation of the circularly arranged smooth muscle of the ciliary body controls thickness, and therefore the focus, of the lens. Folds on the internal surface of the ciliary body, the **ciliary processes,** secrete *aqueous humor.* Aqueous humor fills the **anterior segment of the eyeball**, the interior of the eyeball anterior to the lens, suspensory ligament, and ciliary body (Fig. 7.27B).

The **iris,** which literally lies on the anterior surface of the lens, is a thin contractile diaphragm with a central aperture, the **pupil,** for transmitting light (Figs. 7.26B, 7.27, and 7.28A). When a person is awake, the size of the pupil varies continually to regulate the amount of light entering the eye (Fig. 7.28B). Two involuntary muscles control the size of the pupil: the parasympathetically stimulated, circularly arranged **sphincter pupillae** decreases its diameter (constrict or contracts the pupil, *pupillary miosis*), and the sympathetically stimulated, radially arranged **dilator pupillae** increases its diameter (dilates the pupil). The nature of the pupillary responses is paradoxical: sympathetic responses usually occur immediately, yet it may take up to 20 minutes for the pupil to dilate in response to low lighting, as in a darkened theater. Parasympathetic responses are typically slower than sympathetic responses, yet parasympathetically stimulated papillary constriction is normally instantaneous. Abnormal sustained pupillary dilation (*mydriasis*) may occur in certain diseases or as a result of trauma or the use of certain drugs.

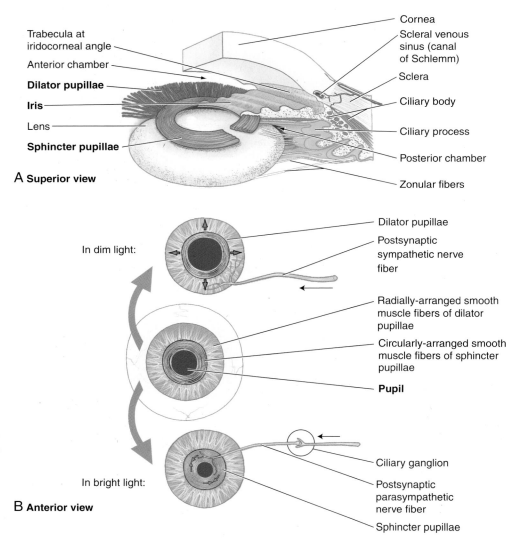

FIGURE 7.28. **Structure and function of the iris. A.** Iris dissected in situ. The iris separates the anterior and posterior chambers of the anterior segment of the eyeball as it bounds the pupil. **B.** Dilation and constriction of pupil. In dim light, sympathetic fibers stimulate dilation of the pupil. In bright light, parasympathetic fibers stimulate constriction of the pupil.

INNER LAYER OF EYEBALL

The inner, layer of the eyeball is the **retina** (Fig. 7.26C and 7.27). It consists grossly of two functional parts with distinct locations: the optic and non-visual parts. The **optic part of the retina** is sensitive to visual light rays and has two layers: a neural layer and pigmented layer. The **neural layer** is light receptive. The **pigmented layer** consists of a single layer of cells that reinforces the light-absorbing property of the choroid in reducing the scattering of light in the eyeball. The **non-visual retina** is an anterior continuation of the pigmented layer and a layer of supporting cells. The non-visual retina extends over the ciliary body (**ciliary part** of the retina) and the posterior surface of the iris (**iridial part** of the retina) to the pupillary margin.

Clinically, the internal aspect of the posterior part of the eyeball, where light entering the eyeball is focused, is referred to as the **fundus of the eyeball** (ocular fundus). The retina of the fundus includes a distinctive circular area called the **optic disc** (optic papilla) where the sensory fibers and vessels conveyed by the optic nerve (CN II) enter the eyeball (Figs. 7.26C, 7.27A, and 7.29). Because it contains no photoreceptors, the optic disc is insensitive to light. Consequently, this part of the retina is commonly called the *blind spot*.

Just lateral to the optic disc is the **macula of the retina** or **macula lutea** (L. yellow spot). The yellow color of the macula is apparent only when the retina is examined with red-free light. The macula lutea is a small oval area of the retina with special photoreceptor cones that is specialized for acuity of vision. It is not normally observed with an *ophthalmoscope* (a device for viewing the interior of the eyeball through the pupil). At the center of the macula of the retina is a depression, the **fovea centralis** (L. central pit), the area of most acute vision. The fovea is approximately 1.5 mm in diameter; its center, the **foveola**, does not have the capillary network visible elsewhere deep to the retina.

The optic part of the retina terminates anteriorly along the **ora serrata** (L. serrated edge), the irregular posterior border of the ciliary body (Figs. 7.26C and 7.27A). Except for the cones and rods of the neural layer, the retina is supplied by the **central artery of the retina,** a branch of the ophthalmic artery. The cones and rods of the outer neural layer receive nutrients from the *capillary lamina of the choroid,* or choriocapillaris (discussed in "Vasculature of Orbit," later in this chapter). It has the finest vessels of the inner surface of the choroid, against which the retina is pressed. A corresponding system of retinal veins unites to form the **central vein of the retina** (Fig. 7.28A).

REFRACTIVE MEDIA AND COMPARTMENTS OF EYEBALL

On their way to the retina, light waves pass through the refractive media of the eyeball: cornea, aqueous humor, lens, and vitreous humor (Fig. 7.27A). The *cornea* is the primary refractory medium of the eyeball—that is, it bends light to the greatest degree, focusing an inverted image on the light-sensitive retina of the *optic fundus*.

The **aqueous humor** (often shortened clinically to "aqueous") occupies the *anterior segment of the eyeball* (Figs. 7.27B and 7.28A). The anterior segment is subdivided by the iris and pupil. The **anterior chamber of the eye** is the space between the cornea anteriorly and the iris/pupil posteriorly. The **posterior chamber of the eye** is between the iris/pupil anteriorly and the lens and ciliary body posteriorly. Aqueous humor is produced in the posterior chamber by the **ciliary processes** of the ciliary body. This clear watery solution provides nutrients for the avascular cornea and lens. After passing through the pupil into the anterior chamber, the aqueous humor drains through a trabecular meshwork at the **iridocorneal angle** into the **scleral venous sinus** (L. *sinus venosus sclerae,* canal of Schlemm) (Fig. 7.28A). The humor is removed by the **limbal plexus,** a network of scleral veins close to the limbus, which drain in turn into both tributaries of the *vorticose* and the *anterior ciliary veins* (Fig. 7.27B). Intra-ocular pressure (IOP) is a balance between production and outflow of aqueous humor.

The **lens** is posterior to the iris and anterior to the vitreous humor of the vitreous body (Figs. 7.27 and 7.28A). It is a transparent, biconvex structure enclosed in a capsule. The highly elastic **capsule of the lens** is anchored by **zonular fibers** (collectively constituting the **suspensory ligament**

Branches of retinal vessels
(arterioles and venules)
Macula of retina
Optic disc

Ophthalmoscopic view

FIGURE 7.29.   **Right ocular fundus.** Retinal venules (wider) and retinal arterioles (narrower) radiate from the center of the oval optic disc. The dark area lateral to the disc is the macula. Branches of retinal vessels extend toward this area but do not reach its center, the fovea centralis—the area of most acute vision.

In the absence of nerve stimulation, the ciliary muscle is relaxed

Zonular fibers under tension

Lens is stretched thin to refract light for distant vision

A

Parasympathetic stimulation causes ciliary muscle to contract

Zonular fibers relax

In the absence of stretching, internal tension causes lens to become more spherical (thicker) to refract light for near vision

B

FIGURE 7.30. **Changing lens shape for distant and near vision (accommodation). A.** Distant vision. **B.** Near vision.

of the lens) to the encircling ciliary processes. Although most refraction is produced by the cornea, the convexity of the lens, particularly its anterior surface, constantly varies to fine-tune the focus of near or distant objects on the retina (Fig. 7.30). The isolated unattached lens assumes a nearly spherical shape. In other words, in the absence of external attachment and stretching, it becomes nearly round. The **ciliary muscle** of the ciliary body changes the shape of the lens. In the absence of nerve stimulation, the diameter of the relaxed muscular ring is larger. The lens suspended within the ring is under tension as its periphery is stretched, causing it to be thinner (less convex). The less convex lens brings more distant objects into focus (far vision). Parasympathetic stimulation via the oculomotor nerve (CN III) causes sphincter-like contraction of the ciliary muscle. The ring becomes smaller, and tension on the lens is reduced. The relaxed lens thickens (becomes more convex), bringing near objects into focus (near vision). The active process of changing the shape of the lens for near vision is called **accommodation**. The thickness of the lens increases with aging so that the ability to accommodate typically becomes restricted after age 40.

The **vitreous humor** is a watery fluid enclosed in the meshes of the **vitreous body,** a transparent jelly-like substance in the posterior four fifths of the eyeball posterior to the lens (**posterior segment of the eyeball**, also called the *postremal* or *vitreous chamber*) (Fig. 7.27A). In addition to transmitting light, the vitreous humor holds the retina in place and supports the lens.

Ophthalmoscopy

Physicians view the fundus (posterior part) of the eye with an *ophthalmoscope*. The retinal arteries and veins radiate over the fundus from the optic disc. The pale, oval optic disc appears on the medial side, with retinal vessels radiating from its center in the ophthalmoscopic view of the retina (Fig. 7.29). Pulsation of the retinal arteries is usually visible. Centrally, at the posterior pole of the eyeball, the macula of retina (macula lutea) appears darker than the reddish hue of surrounding areas of the retina.

Detachment of Retina

The layers of the developing retina are separated in the embryo by an intraretinal space. During the early fetal period, the embryonic layers fuse, obliterating this space. Although the pigment cell layer becomes firmly fixed to the choroid, its attachment to the neural layer is not firm. Consequently, detachment of the retina may follow a blow to the eye. A *detached retina* usually results from seepage of fluid between the neural and pigmented layers of the retina,

perhaps days or even weeks after trauma to the eye (Fig. B7.7). People with a retinal detachment may complain of flashes of light or specks floating in front of their eye.

Ophthalmoscopic view (*arrows*, wrinkles in detached retina)

FIGURE B7.7.

Papilledema

 An increase in CSF pressure slows venous return from the retina, causing *edema of the retina* (fluid accumulation). The edema is viewed during ophthalmoscopy as swelling of the optic disc, a condition called *papilledema*.

Presbyopia and Cataracts

 As people age, their lenses become harder and more flattened. These changes gradually reduce the focusing power of the lenses, a condition known as *presbyopia* (G. *presbyos,* old). Some people also experience a loss of transparency (cloudiness) of the lens from areas of opaqueness *(cataracts)*. *Cataract extraction* combined with an *intra-ocular lens implant* has become a common operation. An extracapsular cataract extraction involves removing the lens but leaving the capsule of the lens intact to receive a synthetic intra-ocular lens (Fig. B7.8*A,B*). Intracapsular lens extraction involves removing the lens and lens capsule and implanting a synthetic intra-ocular lens in the anterior chamber (Fig. B7.8*C*).

FIGURE B7.8.

Glaucoma

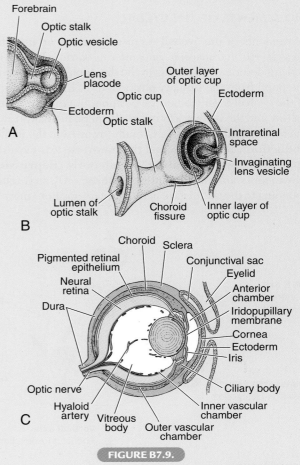 Outflow of aqueous humor through the scleral venous sinus into the blood circulation must occur at the same rate at which the aqueous is produced. If the outflow decreases significantly because the outflow pathway is blocked, pressure builds up in the anterior and posterior chambers of the eye, a condition called *glaucoma*. Blindness can result from compression of the inner layer of the eyeball (retina) and the retinal arteries if aqueous humor production is not reduced to maintain normal intraocular pressure.

Corneal Ulcers and Transplants

 Damage to the sensory innervation of the cornea from CN V$_1$ leaves the cornea vulnerable to injury by foreign particles. People with scarred or opaque corneas may receive *corneal transplants* from donors. Corneal implants of non-reactive plastic material are also used.

Development of Retina

 The retina and optic nerve develop from the **optic cup,** an outgrowth of the embryonic forebrain, the **optic vesicle** (Fig. B7.9*A*). As it evaginates from the forebrain (Fig. B7.9*B*), the optic vesicle carries the developing meninges with it. Hence the optic nerve is invested with cranial meninges and an extension of the subarachnoid space (Fig. B7.9*C*). The central artery and vein of the retina cross the subarachnoid space and run within the distal part of the optic nerve. The pigment cell layer of the retina develops from the outer layer of the optic cup, and the neural layer develops from the inner layer of the cup.

FIGURE B7.9.

Extra-ocular Muscles of Orbit

The **extra-ocular muscles of the orbit** are the *levator palpebrae superioris*, four *recti* (*superior, inferior, medial,* and *lateral*), and two *obliques* (*superior* and *inferior*). These muscles work together to move the superior eyelids and eyeballs (Figs. 7.31–7.33 and Table 7.7).

LEVATOR PALPEBRAE SUPERIORIS

The **levator palpebrae superioris** broadens into a wide bilaminar aponeurosis as it approaches its distal attachments. The superficial lamina attaches to the skin of the superior eyelid and the deep lamina to the superior tarsus (Fig. 7.24*B*). This muscle is opposed most of the time by gravity and is the antagonist of the superior half of the orbicularis oculi, the sphincter of the palpebral fissure. The deep lamina of the distal (palpebral) part of the muscle includes smooth muscle fibers, the **superior tarsal muscle,** that produce additional widening of the palpebral fissure, especially during a sympathetic response (e.g., fright). However, they seem to function continuously (in the absence of a sympathetic response) since an interruption of the sympathetic supply produces a constant *ptosis*—drooping of the upper eyelid.

MOVEMENTS OF THE EYEBALL

Movements of the eyeball occur as rotations around three *axes—vertical, transverse,* and *anteroposterior* (Fig. 7.31)—and are described according to the direction of movement of the pupil from the primary position, or of the superior pole of the eyeball from the neutral position. Rotation of the eyeball around the vertical axis moves the pupil medially (toward the midline, **adduction**) or laterally (away from the midline, **abduction**). Rotation around the transverse axis moves the pupil superiorly (**elevation**) or inferiorly (**depression**). Movements around the anteroposterior (AP) axis (corresponding to the axis of gaze in the primary position) move the

superior pole of the eyeball medially (**medial rotation**, or intorsion) or laterally (**lateral rotation**, or extorsion). These rotational movements accommodate changes in the tilt of the head. Absence of these movements resulting from nerve lesions contributes to double vision.

Movements may occur around the three axes simultaneously, requiring three terms to describe the direction of movement from the primarily position (e.g., the pupil is elevated, adducted, and medially rotated).

RECTI AND OBLIQUE MUSCLES

The four **recti muscles** (L. *rectus,* straight) run anteriorly to the eyeball, arising from a fibrous cuff, the **common tendinous ring,** that surrounds the optic canal and part of the superior orbital fissure at the apex of the orbit (Figs. 7.32 and 7.33*A,B*; Table 7.7). Structures that enter the orbit through this canal and the adjacent part of the fissure lie initially within the cone of recti. The four recti are named for their individual positions relative to the eyeball. Because they mainly run anteriorly to attach to the superior, inferior, medial, and lateral aspects of the eyeball anterior to its equator, the primary actions of the four recti in producing elevation, depression, adduction, and abduction are relatively intuitive.

Several factors make the actions of the obliques and the secondary actions of the superior and inferior recti more challenging to understand:

• The *apex of the orbit* is medially placed relative to the orbit, so that the *axis of the orbit* does not coincide with the *optical axis* (Figs. 7.33*D*). Therefore, *when the eye is in the primary position,* the superior rectus (SR) and inferior rectus (IR) muscles also approach the eyeball from its medial side, their line of pull passing medial to the vertical axis (Fig.7.32*A*, left side). This gives both muscles a secondary action of *adduction.* The SR and IR also extend laterally, passing superior and inferior to the AP axis, respectively, giving the SR a secondary action of

A-P axis
Lateral-Medial
Rotation

Transverse axis
Elevation-Depression

Vertical axis
Abduction-Adduction

FIGURE 7.31.   Axes around which movements of eyeball occur.

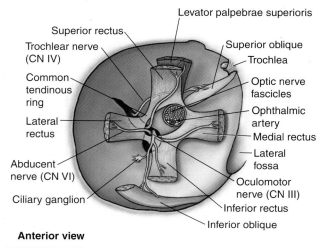

Superior rectus

Trochlear nerve
(CN IV)

Common
tendinous
ring

Lateral
rectus

Abducent
nerve (CN VI)

Ciliary ganglion

Levator palpebrae superioris

Superior oblique

Trochlea

Optic nerve
fascicles

Ophthalmic
artery

Medial rectus

Lateral
fossa

Oculomotor
nerve (CN III)

Inferior rectus

Inferior oblique

Anterior view

FIGURE 7.32.   Common tendinous ring, structural relationships.

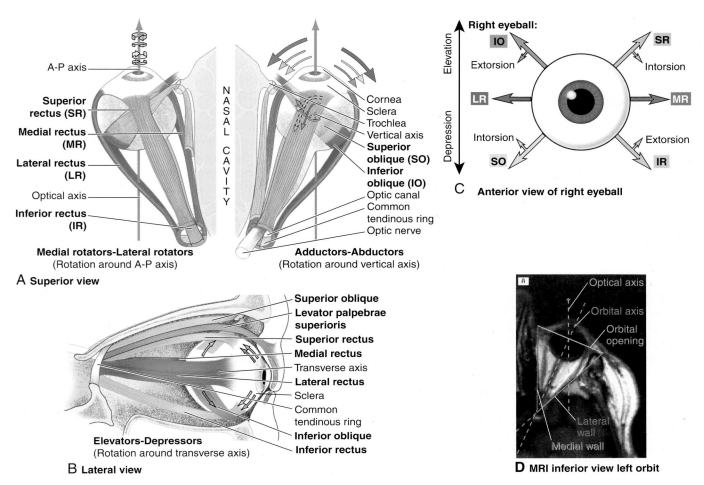

FIGURE 7.33. **Extra-ocular muscles and their movements. A.** Medial-lateral rotators (left eye) and adductors-abductors (right eye). *Arrows* indicate movements of the eyeball around the AP axis on the left, and around the vertical axis on the right. **B.** Elevator-depressors. *Arrows* indicate movements of the eyeball around the transverse axis. **C.** Unilateral diagram of extra-ocular muscle actions, starting from the primary position. For movements in any of the six cardinal directions (*large arrows*), the indicated muscle is the prime mover. Movements in directions between large arrows require synergistic actions by the adjacent muscles. *Small arrows* indicate muscles producing rotational movements around the AP axis. **D.** Orbital and optical axes.

TABLE 7.6 MUSCLES OF ORBIT

Muscle	Origin	Insertion	Innervation	Main Action(s)[a]
Levator palpebrae superioris	Lesser wing of sphenoid bone, superior and anterior to optic canal	Superior tarsus and skin of superior eyelid	Oculomotor nerve; deep layer (superior tarsal muscle) supplied by sympathetic fibers	Elevates superior eyelid
Superior oblique (SO)	Body of sphenoid bone	Tendon passes through trochlea to insert into sclera, deep to SR	Trochlear nerve (CN IV)	Abducts, depresses, and rotates eyeball medially (intorsion)
Inferior oblique (IO)	Anterior part of floor of orbit	Sclera deep to lateral rectus muscle	Oculomotor nerve (CN III)	Abducts, elevates, and rotates eyeball laterally (extorsion)
Superior rectus (SR)	Common tendinous ring	Sclera just posterior to corneoscleral junction	Oculomotor nerve (CN III)	Elevates, adducts, and rotates eyeball medially (intorsion)
Inferior rectus (IR)				Depresses, adducts, and rotates eyeball laterally (extorsion)
Medial rectus (MR)				Adducts eyeball
Lateral rectus (LR)			Abducent nerve (CN VI)	Abducts eyeball

[a]It is essential to appreciate that all muscles are continuously involved in eyeball movements; thus the individual actions are not usually tested clinically.

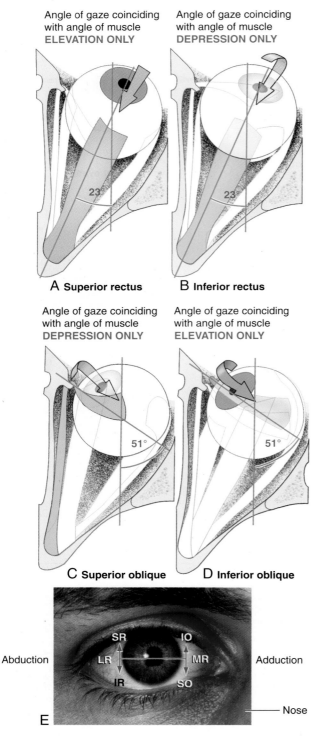

Angle of gaze coinciding with angle of muscle **ELEVATION ONLY**

Angle of gaze coinciding with angle of muscle **DEPRESSION ONLY**

23°

23°

A Superior rectus

B Inferior rectus

Angle of gaze coinciding with angle of muscle **DEPRESSION ONLY**

Angle of gaze coinciding with angle of muscle **ELEVATION ONLY**

51°

51°

C Superior oblique

D Inferior oblique

Abduction   SR   IO   Adduction
LR   MR
IR   SO
Nose
E

FIGURE 7.34. **Clinical testing of extra-ocular muscles.** Right eye is shown. **A** and **B.** When the eye is abducted by LR, only the rectus muscles can produce elevation and depression. However, when the eye is adducted by MR (**C** and **D**), only the oblique muscles can produce these movements. **E.** Following movements of the examiner's finger, the pupil is moved in an extended H pattern to isolate and test individual extra-ocular muscles and the integrity of their nerves.

medial rotation, and the IR a secondary action of *lateral rotation* (Fig.7.32A, right side).

- *If the gaze is first directed laterally* (abducted by the lateral rectus [LR]) so that the line of gaze coincides with plane of the IR and SR, *the SR produces elevation only* (and is solely responsible for the movement) (Fig. 7.34A), and *the IR produces depression only* (and is likewise solely responsible) (Fig. 7.34B). During a physical examination, the physician directs the patient to follow his or her finger laterally (testing the LR and abducent nerve [CN VI]), then superiorly and inferiorly to isolate and test the function of the SR and IR, and the integrity of the oculomotor nerve (CN III) that supplies both (Fig. 7.34E)

- The inferior oblique (IO) is the only muscle to originate from the anterior part of the orbit (immediately lateral to the lacrimal fossa) (Fig. 7.32). The superior oblique (SO) originates from the apex region like the rectus muscles (but superomedial to the common tendinous ring); however, its tendon traverses the *trochlea* just inside the superomedial orbital rim, redirecting its line of pull (Figs. 7.33A). Thus the inserting tendons of the oblique muscles lie in the same oblique vertical plane. When the inserting tendons are viewed anteriorly (Fig. 7.25C) or superiorly (Fig. 7.33A) with the eyeball in the primary position, it can be seen that the tendons of the oblique muscles pass mainly laterally to insert on the lateral half of the eyeball, posterior to its equator. Because they pass inferior and superior to the AP axis as they pass laterally, the IO is the primary lateral rotator, and the SO the primary medial rotator, of the eye.

- However, in the primary position the obliques also pass posteriorly across the transverse axis (Fig. 7.33B), and posterior to the vertical axis (Fig. 7.33A), giving the SO a secondary function as a depressor, the IO a secondary function as an elevator, and both muscles a secondary function as abductors.

- If the gaze is first directed medially (adducted by the medial rectus [MR]) so that the line of gaze coincides with plane of the inserting tendons of the SO and IO, the SO produces depression only (and is solely responsible for the movement) (Fig. 7.34C), and the IO produces elevation only (and is likewise solely responsible) (Fig. 7.34D). During a physical examination, the physician directs the patient to follow his/her finger medially (testing the MR and oculomotor nerve), then inferiorly and superiorly to isolate and test the functions of the SO and IO, and the integrity of the trochlear nerve (CN III) supplying the SO and of the inferior division of the oculomotor nerve (CN III) supplying the IO (Figs. 7.34E and 7.35). In practice the main action of the:

- SO is depression of the pupil in the adducted position (e.g., directing the gaze down the page when the

Elevation

| Inferior oblique | Superior rectus | | Superior rectus Inferior oblique | | Superior rectus | Inferior oblique |

| Lateral rectus | Medial rectus | | PRIMARY POSITION | | Medial rectus | Lateral rectus |

| Superior oblique | Inferior rectus | | Superior oblique Inferior rectus | | Inferior rectus | Superior oblique |

Depression

Right Abduction - Left Adduction   Left Abduction - Right Adduction

▭ Oculomotor nerve (CN III)   ▬ Trochlear nerve (CN IV)   ▬ Abducent nerve (CN VI)

FIGURE 7.35. **Binocular movements and muscles producing them.** All movements start from the primary position.

gaze of both eyes is directed medially [*converged*] for reading).

- IO is elevation of the pupil in the adducted position (e.g., directing the gaze up the page during **convergence** for reading).

Although the actions produced by the extra-ocular muscles have been considered individually, all motions require the action of several muscles in the same eye, assisting each other as synergists or opposing each other as antagonists. Muscles that are synergistic for one action may be antagonistic for another. For example, no single muscle can act to elevate the pupil directly from the primary position (Fig. 7.33C). The two elevators (SR and IO) act as synergists to do so (Fig. 7.35). However, these muscles are antagonistic as rotators, and so neutralize each other so that no rotation occurs as they work together to elevate the pupil.

Similarly, no single muscle can act to depress the pupil directly from the primary position. The two depressors, the SO and IR, both produce depression when acting alone, and also produce opposing actions in terms of adduction-abduction and medial-lateral rotation. However, when the SO and IR act simultaneously, their synergistic actions depress the

pupil as their antagonistic actions neutralize each other; therefore, pure depression results.

To direct the gaze, coordination of both eyes must be accomplished by the paired action of contralateral *yoke muscles.* For example, in directing the gaze to the right, the right lateral rectus and left medial rectus act as yoke muscles.

SUPPORTING APPARATUS OF EYEBALL

The *fascial sheath of the eyeball* envelops the eyeball, extending posteriorly from the conjunctival fornices to the optic nerve, forming the actual socket for the eyeball (Fig. 7.36A). The cup-like fascial sheath is pierced by the tendons of the extra-ocular muscles and is reflected onto each of them as a tubular *muscle sheath.* The muscle sheaths of the levator palpebrae superioris and superior rectus muscles are fused; thus, when the gaze is directed superiorly, the superior eyelid is further elevated out of the line of vision.

Triangular expansions from the sheaths of the medial and lateral rectus muscles, called the **medial** and **lateral check ligaments,** are attached to the lacrimal and zygomatic bones, respectively. These ligaments limit abduction and adduction. A blending of the check ligaments with the fascia

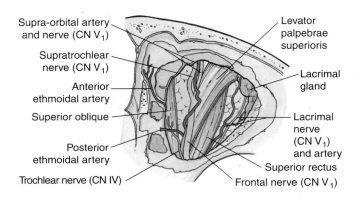

Supra-orbital artery and nerve (CN V₁)

Supratrochlear nerve (CN V₁)

Anterior ethmoidal artery

Superior oblique

Posterior ethmoidal artery

Trochlear nerve (CN IV)

Levator palpebrae superioris

Lacrimal gland

Lacrimal nerve (CN V₁) and artery

Superior rectus

Frontal nerve (CN V₁)

A Superior view

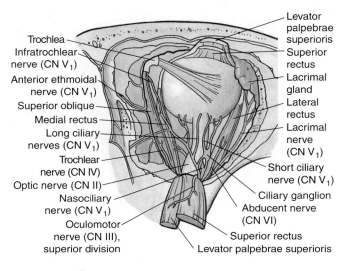

Trochlea

Infratrochlear nerve (CN V₁)

Anterior ethmoidal nerve (CN V₁)

Superior oblique

Medial rectus

Long ciliary nerves (CN V₁)

Trochlear nerve (CN IV)

Optic nerve (CN II)

Nasociliary nerve (CN V₁)

Oculomotor nerve (CN III), superior division

Levator palpebrae superioris

Superior rectus

Lacrimal gland

Lateral rectus

Lacrimal nerve (CN V₁)

Short ciliary nerve (CN V₁)

Ciliary ganglion

Abducent nerve (CN VI)

Superior rectus

Levator palpebrae superioris

B Superior view

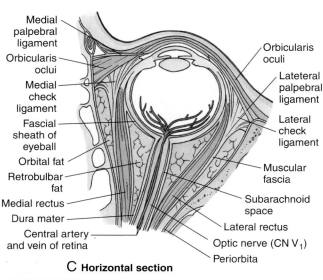

Medial palpebral ligament

Orbicularis oclui

Medial check ligament

Fascial sheath of eyeball

Orbital fat

Retrobulbar fat

Medial rectus

Dura mater

Central artery and vein of retina

Orbicularis oculi

Lateteral palpebral ligament

Lateral check ligament

Muscular fascia

Subarachnoid space

Lateral rectus

Optic nerve (CN V₁)

Periorbita

C Horizontal section

FIGURE 7.36.   **Dissections of right orbit. A.** Superficial. **B.** Deep. **C.** Fascial sheath of eyeball and check ligaments.

of the inferior rectus and inferior oblique muscles forms a hammock-like sling, the *suspensory ligament of the eyeball.* A similar check ligament from the fascial sheath of the inferior rectus retracts the inferior eyelid when the gaze is directed downward. Collectively, the check ligaments act with the oblique muscles and the **retrobulbar fat** to resist the posterior pull on the eyeball produced by the rectus muscles. In starvation or diseases that reduce the retrobulbar fat, the eyeball is retracted into the orbit (*inophthalmos*).

Nerves of Orbit

The large optic nerves (CN II) are purely sensory nerves that transmit impulses generated by optical stimuli and develop as paired anterior extensions of the forebrain. Throughout their course in the orbit the optic nerves are surrounded by extensions of the *cranial meninges* and *subarachnoid space*, the latter occupied by a thin layer of CSF (Fig. 7.38A, inset). The intra-orbital extensions of the cranial dura and arachnoid mater constitute the **optic sheath**, which becomes continuous anteriorly with the fascial sheath of the eyeball and the sclera. A layer of pia mater covers the surface of the optic nerve within the sheath. They exit the orbits via the optic canals.

In addition to the optic nerves, the nerves of the orbit include those that enter through the *superior orbital fissure* and supply the ocular muscles (Figs. 7.35 and 7.37A): **oculomotor** (CN III), **trochlear** (CN IV), and **abducent** (CN VI) nerves. A memory device for the innervation of the extraocular muscles moving the eyeball is similar to a chemical formula: $LR_6SO_4AO_3$ (**l**ateral **r**ectus, CN **VI**; **s**uperior **o**blique, CN **IV**; **a**ll **o**thers, CN **III**). The trochlear and abducent nerves pass directly to the single muscle supplied by each nerve. The oculomotor nerve divides into a superior branch supplying superior rectus and levator palpebrae superioris and an inferior branch supplying the medial and inferior rectus and inferior oblique, and carrying presynaptic parasympathetic fibers to the ciliary ganglion.

Three branches of the *ophthalmic nerve* (CN V₁) that pass through the superior orbital fissure and supply structures in the orbit are:

- The **lacrimal nerve,** which arises in the lateral wall of the cavernous sinus and passes to the lacrimal gland, giving sensory branches to the conjunctiva and skin of the superior eyelid; its distal part also carries secretomotor fibers conveyed to it from the zygomatic nerve (CN V₂).
- The **frontal nerve,** which enters the orbit through the superior orbital fissure and divides into the supra-orbital and supratrochlear nerves, providing sensory innervation to the superior eyelid, scalp, and forehead.
- The **nasociliary nerve,** the sensory nerve to the eyeball, which also supplies several branches to the orbit, face, paranasal sinuses, nasal cavity, and anterior cranial fossa. The **infratrochlear nerve,** a terminal branch of the nasociliary nerve, supplies the eyelids, conjunctiva, skin of

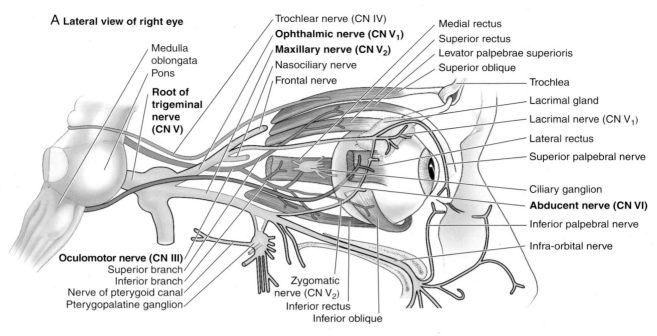

A Lateral view of right eye

Medulla oblongata
Pons
Root of trigeminal nerve (CN V)

Trochlear nerve (CN IV)
Ophthalmic nerve (CN V₁)
Maxillary nerve (CN V₂)
Nasociliary nerve
Frontal nerve

Medial rectus
Superior rectus
Levator palpebrae superioris
Superior oblique
Trochlea
Lacrimal gland
Lacrimal nerve (CN V₁)
Lateral rectus
Superior palpebral nerve
Ciliary ganglion
Abducent nerve (CN VI)
Inferior palpebral nerve
Infra-orbital nerve

Oculomotor nerve (CN III)
Superior branch
Inferior branch
Nerve of pterygoid canal
Pterygopalatine ganglion

Zygomatic nerve (CN V₂)
Inferior rectus
Inferior oblique

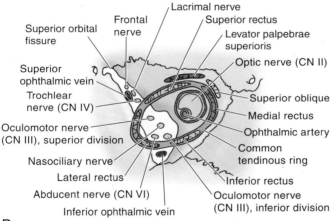

Lacrimal nerve
Frontal nerve
Superior rectus
Levator palpebrae superioris
Superior orbital fissure
Optic nerve (CN II)
Superior ophthalmic vein
Trochlear nerve (CN IV)
Superior oblique
Medial rectus
Oculomotor nerve (CN III), superior division
Ophthalmic artery
Nasociliary nerve
Common tendinous ring
Lateral rectus
Inferior rectus
Abducent nerve (CN VI)
Oculomotor nerve (CN III), inferior division
Inferior ophthalmic vein

B Anterior view

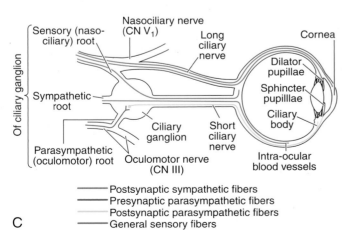

Of ciliary ganglion

Sensory (naso-ciliary) root
Nasociliary nerve (CN V₁)
Long ciliary nerve
Cornea
Dilator pupillae
Sphincter pupilliae
Ciliary body
Sympathetic root
Ciliary ganglion
Short ciliary nerve
Parasympathetic (oculomotor) root
Oculomotor nerve (CN III)
Intra-ocular blood vessels

⎯⎯ Postsynaptic sympathetic fibers
⎯⎯ Presynaptic parasympathetic fibers
⎯⎯ Postsynaptic parasympathetic fibers
⎯⎯ General sensory fibers

C

FIGURE 7.37. **Nerves of orbit. A.** Overview. **B.** Relationships at apex of orbit. **C.** Distribution of nerve fibers to ciliary ganglion and eyeball.

the nose, and lacrimal sac. The anterior and posterior **ethmoidal nerves,** also branches of the nasociliary nerve, supply the mucous membrane of the sphenoidal and ethmoidal sinuses and the nasal cavities and dura mater of the anterior cranial fossa. The **long ciliary nerves** are branches of the nasociliary nerve (CN V₁). The **short ciliary nerves** are branches of the ciliary ganglion (Fig. 7.36B).

The **ciliary ganglion** is a small group of postsynaptic parasympathetic nerve cell bodies associated with CN V₁. It is located between the optic nerve (CN I) and the lateral rectus toward the posterior limit of the orbit. The ganglion receives nerve fibers from three sources (Fig.7.37C):

- Sensory fibers from CN V₁ via the nasociliary nerve.
- Presynaptic parasympathetic fibers from CN III.
- Postsynaptic sympathetic fibers from the internal carotid plexus.

The *short ciliary nerves* arise from the ciliary ganglion and consist of postsynaptic parasympathetic fibers originating in the ciliary ganglion, afferent fibers from the nasociliary nerve, and postsynaptic sympathetic fibers that pass through the ganglion to the iris and cornea. The *long ciliary nerves,* which pass to the eyeball, bypassing the ciliary ganglion, convey postsynaptic sympathetic fibers to the dilator pupillae and afferent fibers from the iris and cornea.

Vasculature of Orbit

The **arteries of the orbit** are mainly from the **ophthalmic artery,** a branch of the internal carotid artery (Fig. 7.38A and

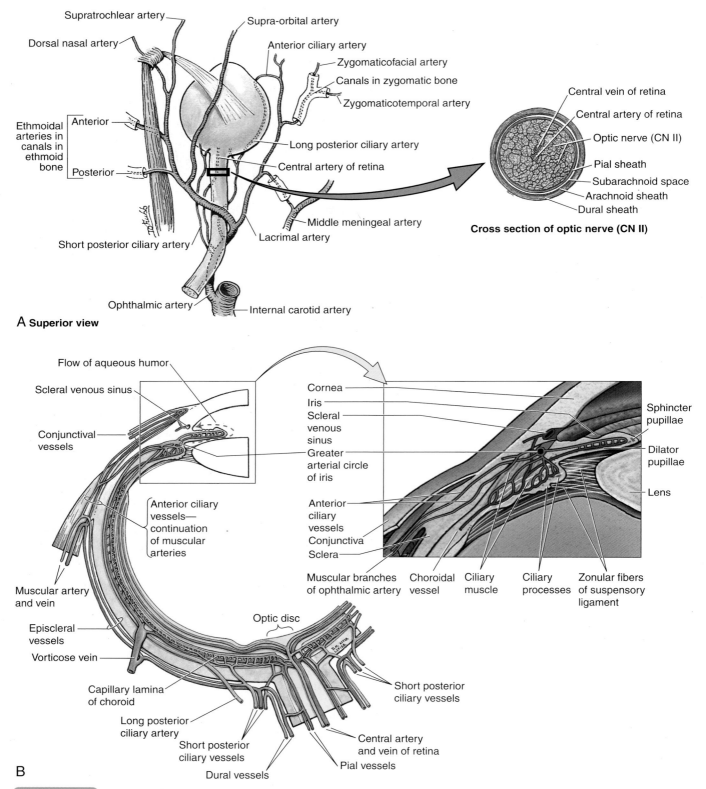

Supratrochlear artery

Dorsal nasal artery

Supra-orbital artery

Anterior ciliary artery

Zygomaticofacial artery

Canals in zygomatic bone

Zygomaticotemporal artery

Ethmoidal arteries in canals in ethmoid bone
Anterior
Posterior

Long posterior ciliary artery

Central artery of retina

Middle meningeal artery

Lacrimal artery

Short posterior ciliary artery

Ophthalmic artery

Internal carotid artery

A Superior view

Central vein of retina

Central artery of retina

Optic nerve (CN II)

Pial sheath

Subarachnoid space

Arachnoid sheath

Dural sheath

Cross section of optic nerve (CN II)

Flow of aqueous humor

Scleral venous sinus

Conjunctival vessels

Anterior ciliary vessels— continuation of muscular arteries

Muscular artery and vein

Episcleral vessels

Vorticose vein

Capillary lamina of choroid

Long posterior ciliary artery

Short posterior ciliary vessels

Dural vessels

Cornea

Iris

Scleral venous sinus

Greater arterial circle of iris

Anterior ciliary vessels

Conjunctiva

Sclera

Muscular branches of ophthalmic artery

Choroidal vessel

Ciliary muscle

Ciliary processes

Zonular fibers of suspensory ligament

Sphincter pupillae

Dilator pupillae

Lens

Optic disc

Short posterior ciliary vessels

Central artery and vein of retina

Pial vessels

B

FIGURE 7.38. **Arteries of orbit and eyeball. A.** Branches of ophthalmic artery. *Inset,* cross-section of optic nerve (CN II). **B. Partial horizontal section of right eyeball.** The artery supplying the inner part the retina (central retinal artery) and the choroid, which in turn nourishes the outer non-vascular layer of the retina, are shown. The vorticose vein (one of four or five) drains venous blood from the choroid into the posterior ciliary and ophthalmic veins. The scleral venous sinus returns the aqueous humor, secreted into the anterior chamber by the ciliary processes, to the venous circulation.

TABLE 7.7 **ARTERIES OF ORBIT**

Artery	Origin	Course and Distribution
Ophthalmic	Internal carotid artery	Traverses optic canal to reach orbital cavity
Central artery of retina	Ophthalmic artery	Pierces dural sheath and runs in optic nerve to eyeball; branches in center of optic disc; supplies optic retina (except cones and rods)
Supra-orbital		Passes superiorly and posteriorly from supra-orbital foramen to supply forehead and scalp
Supratrochlear		Passes from supra-orbital margin to forehead and scalp
Lacrimal		Passes along superior border of lateral rectus muscle to supply lacrimal gland, conjunctiva, and eyelids
Dorsal nasal		Courses along dorsal aspect of nose and supplies its surface
Short posterior ciliaries		Pierces sclera at periphery of optic nerve to supply choroid, which in turn supplies cones and rods of optic retina
Long posterior ciliaries		Pierces sclera to supply ciliary body and iris
Posterior ethmoidal		Passes through posterior ethmoidal foramen to posterior ethmoidal cells
Anterior ethmoidal		Passes through anterior ethmoidal foramen to supply anterior and middle ethmoidal cells, frontal sinus, nasal cavity, and skin on dorsum of nose
Anterior ciliary	Muscular branches of ophthalmic artery	Pierces sclera at attachments of rectus muscles and forms network in iris and ciliary body
Infra-orbital	Third part of maxillary artery	Passes along infra-orbital groove and foramen to face

Table 7.7). The **infra-orbital artery,** from the external carotid artery, also contributes to the supply of this region. The **central retinal artery,** a branch of the ophthalmic artery arising inferior to the optic nerve, pierces the dural sheath of the optic nerve and runs within the nerve to the eyeball, emerging at the optic disc (Fig. 7.36A and 7.38B). Branches of this artery spread over the internal surface of the retina. The terminal branches of the central retinal artery are *end arteries,* which provide the only blood supply to the internal aspect of the retina.

The external aspect of the retina is also supplied by the **capillary lamina of the choroid** (Fig. 7.38B). Of the eight or so posterior ciliary arteries (also branches of the ophthalmic artery), six **short posterior ciliary arteries** directly supply the choroid, which nourishes the outer nonvascular layer of the retina. Two **long posterior ciliary arteries,** one on each side of the eyeball, pass between the sclera and the choroid to anastomose with the **anterior ciliary arteries** (continuations of the **muscular branches of the ophthalmic artery** to the rectus muscles) to supply the ciliary plexus.

Venous drainage of the orbit is through the **superior** and **inferior ophthalmic veins,** which pass through the superior orbital fissure and enter the cavernous sinus (Fig. 7.39). The inferior ophthalmic vein also drains to the pterygoid venous plexus. The **central vein of the retina** usually enters the cavernous sinus directly, but it may join one of the

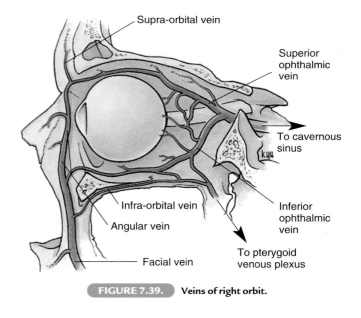

FIGURE 7.39. Veins of right orbit.

ophthalmic veins (Fig. 7.36C). The **vorticose veins** from the vascular layer of the eyeball drain into the inferior ophthalmic vein (Fig. 7.38B). The **scleral venous sinus** is a vascular structure encircling the anterior chamber of the eyeball through which the aqueous humor is returned to the blood circulation.

Blockage of Central Retinal Artery

 Because terminal branches of the central retinal artery are end arteries, obstruction of them by an embolus results in instant and total blindness. Blockage of the artery is usually unilateral and occurs in older people.

Blockage of Central Retinal Vein

 Because the central retinal vein enters the cavernous sinus, *thrombophlebitis* of this sinus may result in passage of a thrombus to the central retinal vein and produce a blockage in one of the small retinal veins. Occlusion of a branch of the central retinal vein usually results in slow, painless loss of vision.

Pupillary Light Reflex

 The **pupillary light reflex** is tested using a penlight during a neurological examination. This reflex, involving CN II (afferent limb) and CN III (efferent limb), is the rapid constriction of the pupil in response to light. When light enters one eye, both pupils constrict because each retina sends fibers into the optic tracts of both sides. The sphincter pupillae muscle is innervated by parasympathetic fibers; consequently, interruption of these fibers causes dilation of the pupil because of the unopposed action of the sympathetically innervated dilator pupillae muscle. The first sign of *compression of the oculomotor nerve* is ipsilateral slowness of the pupillary response to light.

Corneal Reflex

 During a neurological examination, the examiner touches the cornea with a wisp of cotton. A normal (positive) response is a blink. Absence of a blink response suggests a lesion of CN V₁; a lesion of CN VII (the motor nerve to the orbicularis oculi) may also impair this reflex. The examiner must be certain to touch the cornea (not just the sclera) to evoke the reflex. The presence of a contact lens may hamper or abolish the ability to evoke this reflex.

Paralysis of Extra-ocular Muscles/Palsies of Orbital Nerves

 One or more extra-ocular muscles may be paralyzed by disease in the brainstem or by a head injury, resulting in *diplopia* (double vision). Paralysis of a muscle is apparent by the limitation of movement of the eyeball in the field of action of the muscle and by the production of two images when one attempts to use the muscle.

Oculomotor Nerve (CN III) Palsy

 Complete oculomotor nerve palsy affects most of the ocular muscles, the levator palpebrae superioris, and the sphincter pupillae. The superior eyelid droops and cannot be raised voluntarily because of the unopposed activity of the orbicularis oculi (supplied by the facial nerve) (Fig. B7.10A). The pupil is also fully dilated and non-reactive because of the unopposed dilator pupillae. The pupil is fully abducted and depressed ("down and out") because of the unopposed activity of the lateral rectus and superior oblique, respectively.

Abducent Nerve (CN VI) Palsy

 When the abducent nerve (CN VI) supplying only the lateral rectus is paralyzed, the individual cannot abduct the pupil on the affected side (Fig. B7.10B). The pupil is fully adducted by the unopposed pull of the medial rectus.

Right eye   **Left eye:** Downward and outward gaze, dilated pupil, eyelid drooping (ptosis)

A **Left oculomotor (CN III) nerve paralysis**

Right eye: Does not abduct   **Left eye**
⟵ Direction of gaze

B **Right abducent (CN VI) nerve paralysis**

FIGURE B7.10.

TEMPORAL REGION

The **temporal region** includes the temporal and infratemporal fossae—superior and inferior to the zygomatic arch, respectively (Fig. 7.40).

Temporal Fossa

The **temporal fossa** (Fig. 7.40A,B), in which most of the temporalis muscle is located, is bounded:

- Posteriorly and superiorly by the superior and inferior temporal lines.
- Anteriorly by the frontal and zygomatic bones.
- Laterally by the zygomatic arch.
- Inferiorly by the infratemporal crest.

The *floor of the temporal fossa* is formed by parts of the four bones (frontal, parietal, temporal, and greater wing of the sphenoid) that form the **pterion**. The fan-shaped **temporalis muscle** arises from the bony floor and the overlying

A Lateral view

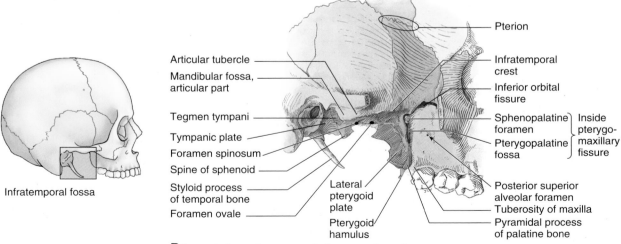

B Lateral view, after removal of zygomatic arch and ramus of mandible

FIGURE 7.40. **Bony boundaries of temporal and infratemporal fossae. A.** The lateral wall of the infratemporal fossa is formed by the ramus of the mandible. The space is deep to the zygomatic arch and is traversed by the temporal muscle and the deep temporal nerves and vessels. Through this interval, the temporal fossa communicates with the infratemporal fossa. **B.** Infratemporal fossa. This fossa communicates with the pterygopalatine fossa through the pterygomaxillary fissure.

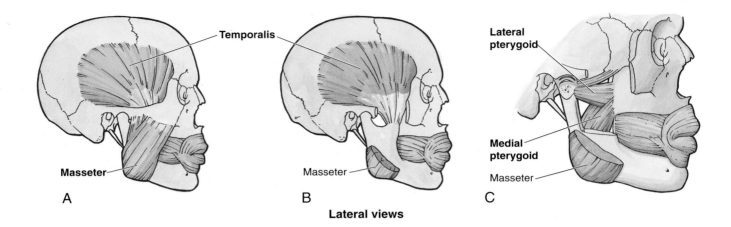

Lateral views

FIGURE 7.41. **Muscles of mastication. A.** Temporalis and masseter muscles. **B.** Temporalis muscle. **C.** Lateral and medial pterygoid muscles.

TABLE 7.8 MUSCLES OF MASTICATION ACTING ON THE MANDIBLE/TEMPOROMANDIBULAR JOINT (TMJ)

Muscle	Proximal Attachment	Distal Attachment	Innervation		Action on Mandible
Temporalis	Triangular muscle with broad attachment to floor of temporal fossa and deep surface of temporalis fascia	Narrow attachment to tip and medial surface of coronoid process and anterior border of ramus of mandible	Anterior trunk of mandibular nerve (CN V₃)	Via deep temporal nerves	Elevates mandible, closing jaws; posterior, more horizontal fibers are retractors of mandible
Masseter	Quadrate muscle attaching to inferior border and medial surface of maxillary process of zygomatic bone and the zygomatic arch	Angle and lateral surface of ramus of mandible		Via masseteric nerve	Elevates mandible; superficial fibers make limited contribution to protrusion of mandible
Lateral pterygoid	Triangular two-headed muscle from (a) infratemporal surface and crest of greater wing of sphenoid and (b) lateral surface of lateral pterygoid plate	Superior head attaches primarily to joint capsule and articular disc of TMJ; inferior head attaches primarily to pterygoid fovea on anteromedial aspect of neck of condyloid process of mandible		Via nerves to lateral pterygoid	Acting bilaterally, protracts mandible and depresses chin; acting unilaterally, swings jaw toward contralateral side; alternate unilateral contraction produces larger lateral chewing movements
Medial pterygoid	Quadrangular two-headed muscle from (a) medial surface of lateral pterygoid plate and pyramidal process of palatine bone and (b) tuberosity of maxilla	Medial surface of ramus of mandible, inferior to mandibular foramen; in essence, a "mirror image" of the ipsilateral masseter, the two muscles flanking the ramus		Via nerve to medial pterygoid	Acts synergistically with masseter to elevate mandible; contributes to protrusion; alternate unilateral activity produces smaller grinding movements

temporalis fascia, which makes up the *roof of the temporal fossa* (Fig. 7.41; Table 7.8). The temporalis fascia extends from the *superior temporal line* to the zygomatic arch. When the powerful masseter, attached to the inferior border of the arch, contracts and exerts a strong downward pull on the arch, the temporalis fascia provides resistance.

Infratemporal Fossa

The **infratemporal fossa** is an irregularly shaped space deep and inferior to the zygomatic arch, deep to the ramus

of the mandible, and posterior to the maxilla. The *boundaries of the fossa* are (Fig. 7.40B):

- Laterally: ramus of the mandible.
- Medially: lateral pterygoid plate.
- Anteriorly: posterior aspect of the maxilla.
- Posteriorly: tympanic plate and the mastoid and styloid processes of the temporal bone.
- Superiorly: inferior surface of the greater wing of the sphenoid bone.
- Inferiorly: where the medial pterygoid muscle attaches to the mandible near its angle (Table 7.8).

A Lateral view

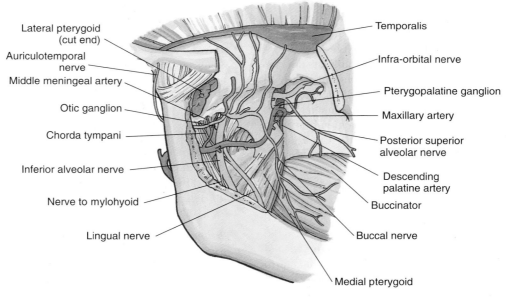

B Lateral view

FIGURE 7.42.   **Dissections of right infratemporal region. A.** Superficial **B.** Deep.

The *contents of the infratemporal fossa* are (Fig. 7.42):

- Inferior part of the temporalis muscle.
- Lateral and medial pterygoid muscles.
- Maxillary artery.
- Pterygoid venous plexus.
- Mandibular, inferior alveolar, lingual, buccal, and chorda tympani nerves, and the otic ganglion.

The **temporalis muscle** has a broad proximal attachment to the floor of the temporal fossa and is attached distally to the tip and medial surface of the coronoid process and anterior border of the ramus of the mandible (Fig. 7.41 A,B; Table 7.8). It elevates the mandible (closes the lower jaw); its posterior fibers retrude (retract) the protruded mandible.

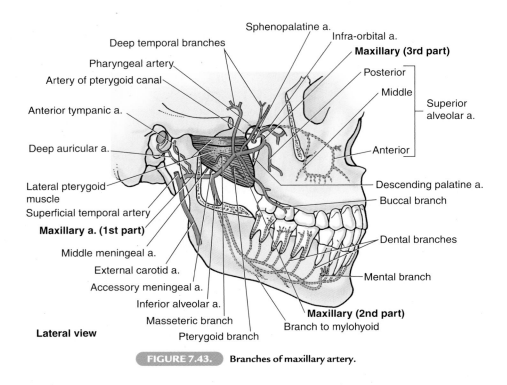

Deep temporal branches

Pharyngeal artery

Artery of pterygoid canal

Anterior tympanic a.

Deep auricular a.

Lateral pterygoid muscle

Superficial temporal artery

Maxillary a. (1st part)

Middle meningeal a.

External carotid a.

Accessory meningeal a.

Inferior alveolar a.

Masseteric branch

Pterygoid branch

Lateral view

Sphenopalatine a.

Infra-orbital a.

Maxillary (3rd part)

Posterior

Middle

Superior alveolar a.

Anterior

Descending palatine a.

Buccal branch

Dental branches

Mental branch

Maxillary (2nd part)

Branch to mylohyoid

FIGURE 7.43. Branches of maxillary artery.

The two-headed **lateral pterygoid muscle** passes posteriorly. Its superior head attaches to the joint capsule and disc of the TMJ, and the inferior head attaches primarily to the pterygoid fovea at the condylar process of the mandible.

The **medial pterygoid muscle** lies on the medial aspect of the ramus of the mandible. Its two heads embrace the inferior head of the lateral pterygoid and then unite (Fig. 7.42*A*). The medial pterygoid passes inferoposteriorly and attaches to the medial surface of the mandible near its angle. The attachments, nerve supply, and actions of the pterygoid muscles are described in Table 7.8.

The **maxillary artery,** the larger of the two terminal branches of the external carotid artery, arises posterior to the neck of the mandible, courses anteriorly deep to the neck of the mandibular condyle, and then passes superficial or deep to the lateral pterygoid (Figs. 7.43 and 7.44*A*). The artery passes medially from the infratemporal fossa through the **pterygomaxillary fissure** to enter the **pterygopalatine fossa** (Fig. 7.40*B*). The maxillary artery is thus divided into three parts by its relation to the lateral pterygoid muscle (Fig. 7.43).

Branches of the first, or retromandibular, part of the maxillary artery are the:

- *Deep auricular artery,* supplying the external acoustic meatus.
- *Anterior tympanic artery,* supplying the tympanic membrane.
- *Middle meningeal artery,* supplying the dura mater and calvaria.
- *Accessory meningeal arteries,* supplying the cranial cavity.

- *Inferior alveolar artery,* which supplies the mandible, gingivae (gums), teeth, and floor of the mouth.

Branches of the second, or pterygoid part, of the maxillary artery are the:

- *Deep temporal arteries,* anterior and posterior, which ascend to supply the temporalis muscle.
- *Pterygoid arteries,* which supply the pterygoid muscles.
- *Masseteric artery,* which passes laterally through the mandibular notch to supply the masseter muscle.
- *Buccal artery,* which supplies the buccinator muscle and mucosa of the cheek.

Branches of the third, or pterygopalatine, part of the maxillary artery are the:

- *Posterior superior alveolar artery,* supplying the maxillary molar and premolar teeth, the buccal gingiva, and the lining of the maxillary sinus.
- *Infra-orbital artery,* supplying the inferior eyelid, lacrimal sac, infra-orbital region of the face, side of the nose, and the upper lip.
- *Descending palatine artery,* supplying the mucous membrane and glands of the palate (roof of the mouth) and palatine gingiva.
- *Artery of pterygoid canal,* supplying the superior part of the pharynx, the pharyngotympanic (auditory) tube, and the tympanic cavity.
- *Pharyngeal artery,* supplying the roof of the pharynx, the sphenoidal sinus, and the inferior part of the pharyngotympanic tube.

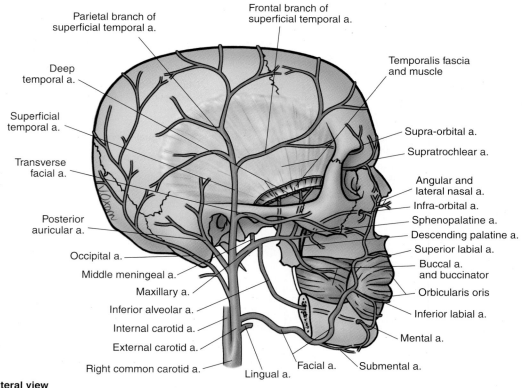

Parietal branch of
superficial temporal a.

Frontal branch of
superficial temporal a.

Deep
temporal a.

Temporalis fascia
and muscle

Superficial
temporal a.

Supra-orbital a.

Supratrochlear a.

Transverse
facial a.

Angular and
lateral nasal a.

Infra-orbital a.

Sphenopalatine a.

Posterior
auricular a.

Descending palatine a.

Superior labial a.

Occipital a.

Buccal a.
and buccinator

Middle meningeal a.

Orbicularis oris

Maxillary a.

Inferior alveolar a.

Inferior labial a.

Internal carotid a.

Mental a.

External carotid a.

Right common carotid a.

Lingual a.

Facial a.

Submental a.

A **Lateral view**

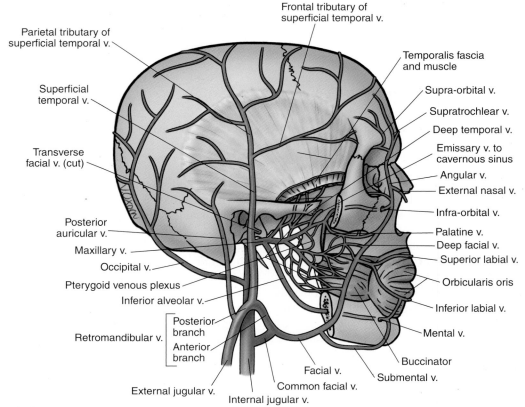

Parietal tributary of
superficial temporal v.

Frontal tributary of
superficial temporal v.

Superficial
temporal v.

Temporalis fascia
and muscle

Supra-orbital v.

Supratrochlear v.

Deep temporal v.

Transverse
facial v. (cut)

Emissary v. to
cavernous sinus

Angular v.

External nasal v.

Infra-orbital v.

Posterior
auricular v.

Palatine v.

Maxillary v.

Deep facial v.

Superior labial v.

Occipital v.

Pterygoid venous plexus

Orbicularis oris

Inferior alveolar v.

Inferior labial v.

Posterior
branch

Mental v.

Retromandibular v.

Anterior
branch

Buccinator

External jugular v.

Facial v.

Common facial v.

Submental v.

Internal jugular v.

B **Lateral view**

FIGURE 7.44.   **Vasculature of head. A.** Branches of external carotid artery. **B.** Venous drainage of face, scalp, and infratemporal fossa.

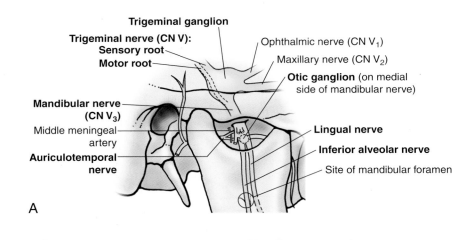

Trigeminal ganglion
Trigeminal nerve (CN V):
Sensory root
Motor root

Ophthalmic nerve (CN V₁)
Maxillary nerve (CN V₂)
Otic ganglion (on medial side of mandibular nerve)

Mandibular nerve (CN V₃)
Middle meningeal artery
Auriculotemporal nerve

Lingual nerve
Inferior alveolar nerve
Site of mandibular foramen

A

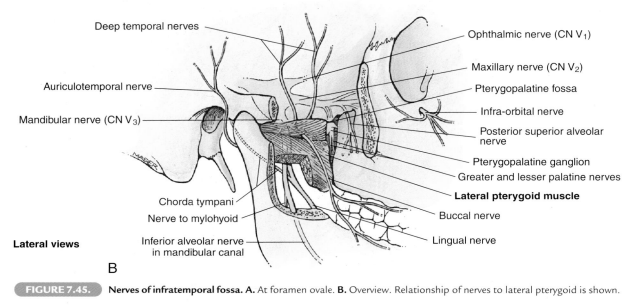

Deep temporal nerves

Auriculotemporal nerve

Mandibular nerve (CN V₃)

Chorda tympani
Nerve to mylohyoid
Inferior alveolar nerve in mandibular canal

Lateral views

B

Ophthalmic nerve (CN V₁)
Maxillary nerve (CN V₂)
Pterygopalatine fossa
Infra-orbital nerve
Posterior superior alveolar nerve
Pterygopalatine ganglion
Greater and lesser palatine nerves
Lateral pterygoid muscle
Buccal nerve
Lingual nerve

FIGURE 7.45. **Nerves of infratemporal fossa. A.** At foramen ovale. **B.** Overview. Relationship of nerves to lateral pterygoid is shown.

• *Sphenopalatine artery,* the termination of the maxillary artery, which supplies the lateral nasal wall, the nasal septum, and the adjacent paranasal sinuses.

The **pterygoid venous plexus** occupies most of the infratemporal fossa (Fig. 7.44B). It is located partly between the temporalis and pterygoid muscles. The plexus drains anteriorly to the facial vein via the deep facial vein but mainly drains posteriorly via the maxillary and then the retromandibular veins.

The **mandibular nerve** (CN V₃) receives the motor root of the trigeminal nerve (CN V) and descends through the foramen ovale to enter the infratemporal fossa, dividing into anterior and posterior trunks. The branches of the large posterior trunk are the auriculotemporal, inferior alveolar, and lingual nerves (Figs. 7.42 and 7.45A). The smaller anterior division gives rise to the **buccal nerve** (Fig. 7.45B) and branches to the four muscles of mastication (temporalis,

masseter, and medial and lateral pterygoids) but not the buccinator, which is supplied by the facial nerve (CN VII).

The **otic ganglion** (parasympathetic) is in the infratemporal fossa (Fig. 7.45A), just inferior to the foramen ovale, medial to the mandibular nerve, and posterior to the lateral pterygoid muscle. Presynaptic parasympathetic fibers, derived mainly from the glossopharyngeal nerve (CN IX), synapse in the otic ganglion. Postsynaptic parasympathetic fibers, which are secretory to the parotid gland, pass from the ganglion to this gland through the auriculotemporal nerve.

The **auriculotemporal nerve** arises via two roots that encircle the middle meningeal artery and then unite into a single trunk (Figs. 7.42 and 7.45). The trunk divides into numerous branches, the largest of which passes posteriorly, medial to the neck of the mandible and supplies sensory fibers to the auricle and temporal region. The auriculotemporal nerve also sends articular fibers to the TMJ and parasympathetic secretomotor fibers to the parotid gland.

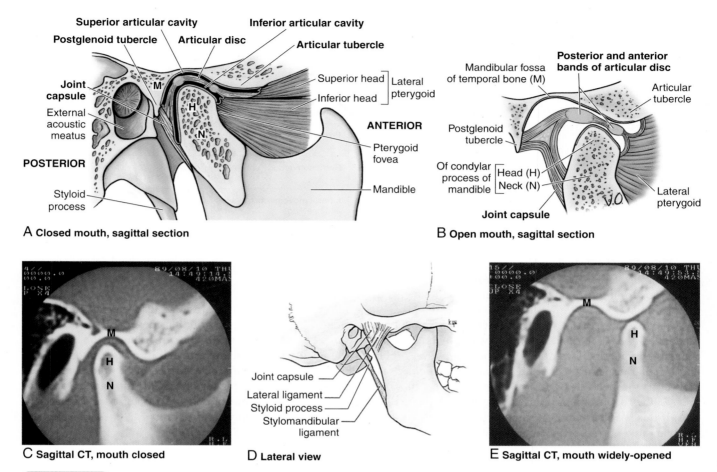

A Closed mouth, sagittal section

B Open mouth, sagittal section

C Sagittal CT, mouth closed   **D** Lateral view   **E** Sagittal CT, mouth widely-opened

FIGURE 7.46. **Temporomandibular joint (TMJ).** Anatomical and CT images of the TMJ in the closed-mouth (**A** and **C**) and open-mouth (**B** and **E**) positions. **D.** Lateral ligament.

The **inferior alveolar nerve** enters the mandibular foramen and passes through the mandibular canal, forming the **inferior dental plexus,** which sends branches to all mandibular teeth on that side. The *nerve to mylohyoid,* a small branch of the inferior alveolar nerve, is given off just before the nerve enters the mandibular foramen (Fig. 7.45B). A branch of the inferior dental plexus, the **mental nerve,** passes through the mental foramen and supplies the skin and mucous membrane of the lower lip, the skin of the chin, and the vestibular gingiva of the mandibular incisor teeth (see Fig. 7.52A).

The **lingual nerve** lies anterior to the inferior alveolar nerve (Figs. 7.42 and 7.52). It is sensory to the anterior two thirds of the tongue, the floor of the mouth, and the lingual gingivae. It enters the mouth between the medial pterygoid and the ramus of the mandible and passes anteriorly under cover of the oral mucosa, just medial and inferior to the third molar tooth.

The **chorda tympani nerve,** a branch of CN VII (Fig. 7.45B), carries taste fibers from the anterior two thirds of the tongue and presynaptic parasympathetic secretomotor fibers for the submandibular and sublingual salivary glands. The chorda tympani joins the lingual nerve in the infratemporal fossa.

TEMPOROMANDIBULAR JOINT

The **temporomandibular joint (TMJ)** is a modified hinge type of synovial joint, permitting movement in three planes. The articular surfaces involved are the **head of the mandible,** the **articular tubercle** of the temporal bone, and the **mandibular fossa** (Fig. 7.46A–C). The articular surfaces of the TMJ are covered by fibrocartilage rather than hyaline cartilage as in a typical synovial joint. An **articular disc** divides the joint cavity into two separate synovial compartments. The **joint capsule** of the TMJ is loose. The fibrous layer of the capsule attaches to the margins of the articular area on the temporal bone and around the neck of the mandible. The thick part of the joint capsule forms the intrinsic **lateral ligament** (temporomandibular ligament), which strengthens the TMJ laterally and, with the **postglenoid tubercle,** acts to prevent posterior dislocation of the joint (Fig. 7.46D).

Two extrinsic ligaments and the lateral ligament connect the mandible to the cranium. The **stylomandibular ligament,** a thickening of the fibrous capsule of the parotid gland, runs from the styloid process to the angle of the

FIGURE 7.47. Sphenomandibular and stylomandibular ligaments.

Labels: Spine of sphenoid; Styloid process; **Sphenomandibular ligament**; Lingula; **Stylomandibular ligament**; Angle of mandible

TABLE 7.9 MOVEMENTS AT THE TEMPOROMANDIBULAR JOINT

Movements of Mandible	Muscles
Elevation (close mouth)	Temporalis, masseter, and medial pterygoid
Depression (open mouth)	Lateral pterygoid and suprahyoid and infrahyoid muscles[a]
Protrusion (protrude chin)	Lateral pterygoid, masseter, and medial pterygoid[b]
Retrusion (retrude chin)	Temporalis (posterior oblique and near horizontal fibers) and masseter
Lateral movements (grinding and chewing)	Temporalis of same side, pterygoids of opposite side, and masseter

[a]The prime mover is normally gravity; these muscles are mainly active against resistance.

[b]The lateral pterygoid is the prime mover here, with minor secondary roles played by the masseter and medial pterygoid.

mandible (Fig. 7.46). It does not contribute significantly to the strength of the TMJ. The **sphenomandibular ligament** runs from the spine of the sphenoid to the lingula of the mandible (Fig. 7.47).

To enable more than a small amount of depression of the mandible—that is, to open the mouth wider than just separating the upper and lower teeth, the head of the mandible and articular disc must move anteriorly on the articular surface until the head lies inferior to the articular tubercle (Fig. 7.46E), a movement referred to as *translation* by dentists. If this anterior gliding occurs unilaterally, the head of the mandible on the retracted side rotates (pivots) on the inferior surface of the articular disc, permitting simple side-to-side chewing or grinding movements over a small range. During protrusion and retrusion of the mandible, the mandibular head and articular disc slide anteriorly and posteriorly on the articular surface of the temporal bone, with both sides moving together. TMJ movements are produced chiefly by the muscles of mastication. The attachments, nerve supply, and actions of these muscles are described in Tables 7.8 and 7.9.

Mandibular Nerve Block

 To perform a mandibular nerve block, an anesthetic agent is injected near the mandibular nerve where it enters the infratemporal fossa. This block usually anesthetizes the auriculotemporal, inferior alveolar, lingual, and buccal branches of the mandibular nerve.

Inferior Alveolar Nerve Block

An alveolar nerve block—commonly used by dentists when repairing mandibular teeth—anesthetizes the inferior alveolar nerve, a branch of CN V_3. The anesthetic agent is injected around the mandibular foramen, the opening into the **mandibular canal** on the medial aspect of the ramus of the mandible. This canal gives passage to the inferior alveolar nerve, artery, and vein. When this nerve block is successful, all mandibular teeth are anesthetized to the median plane. The skin and mucous membrane of the lower lip, the labial alveolar mucosa and gingiva, and the skin of the chin are also anesthetized because they are supplied by the mental branch of this nerve.

Dislocation of TMJ

Sometimes during yawning or taking a large bite, excessive contraction of the lateral pterygoids may cause the heads of the mandibles to dislocate anteriorly, by passing anterior to the articular tubercles (Fig. B7.11). In this

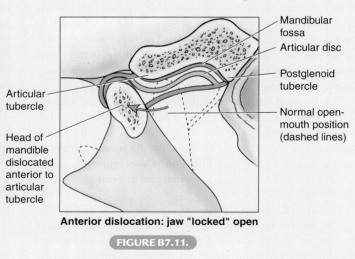

Labels: Mandibular fossa; Articular disc; Postglenoid tubercle; Normal open-mouth position (dashed lines); Articular tubercle; Head of mandible dislocated anterior to articular tubercle

Anterior dislocation: jaw "locked" open

FIGURE B7.11.

position, the mandible remains depressed and the person may not be able to close the mouth. Most commonly, a sideways blow to the chin when the mouth is open dislocates the TMJ on the side that received the blow. *Fracture(s) of the mandible* may be accompanied by dislocation of the TMJ. Because of the close relationship of the facial and auriculotemporal nerves to the TMJ, care must be taken during surgical procedures to preserve both the branches of the facial nerve overlying it and the articular branches of the auriculotemporal nerve that enter the posterior part of the joint. Injury to articular branches of the auriculotemporal nerve supplying the TMJ—associated with traumatic dislocation and rupture of the joint capsule and lateral ligament—leads to laxity and instability of the TMJ.

Arthritis of TMJ

 The TMJ may become inflamed from degenerative arthritis, for example. Abnormal function of the TMJ may result in structural problems such as dental occlusion and joint clicking (*crepitus*). The clicking is thought to result from delayed anterior disc movements during mandibular depression and elevation.

ORAL REGION

The **oral region** includes the oral cavity (mouth), teeth, gingivae (gums), tongue, palate, and the region of the palatine tonsils. The oral cavity is where food is ingested and prepared for digestion in the stomach and small intestine. When food is chewed, the teeth and saliva from the salivary glands facilitate the formation of a manageable *food bolus* (L. lump).

Oral Cavity

The **oral cavity** (mouth) consists of two parts: the *oral vestibule* and the *oral cavity proper* (Fig. 7.48). The oral vestibule communicates with the exterior through the mouth. The size of the **oral fissure** (opening) is controlled by muscles such as the orbicularis oris (the sphincter of the oral fissure). The **oral cavity proper** is the space posterior and medial to the upper and lower **dental arches.** It is limited laterally and anteriorly by the maxillary and mandibular alveolar arches housing the teeth. The **roof of the oral cavity proper** is formed by the palate. Posteriorly, the oral cavity communicates with the **oropharynx,** the oral part of the pharynx. When the mouth is closed and at rest, the oral cavity is fully occupied by the tongue.

Oral Vestibule

The **oral vestibule** is the slit-like space between the lips and cheeks superficially and the teeth and gingivae deeply. The **lips,** the mobile, fleshy muscular folds surrounding the mouth, contain the orbicularis oris and superior and inferior labial muscles, vessels, and nerves. They are covered externally by skin and internally by mucous membrane. The upper lip has a vertical groove, the **philtrum** (Fig. 7.49). As the skin of the lips approaches the mouth, it changes color abruptly to red; this red margin of the lips is the **vermillion border,** a transitional zone between the skin and mucous membrane. The skin of the **transitional zone** is hairless and so thin that it appears red because of the

FIGURE 7.48. Oral cavity.

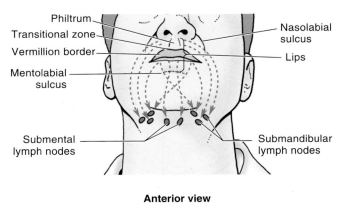

Anterior view

FIGURE 7.49. Surface anatomy and lymphatic drainage of cheeks, lips, and chin.

underlying capillary bed. The upper lip is supplied by superior labial branches of the **facial** and **infra-orbital arteries.** The lower lip is supplied by inferior labial branches of the **facial** and **mental arteries.** The upper lip is supplied by the superior labial branches of the **infra-orbital nerves** (CN V$_2$), and the lower lip is supplied by the inferior labial branches of the mental nerves (CN V$_3$) (Fig. 7.52*A*).

Lymph from the upper lip and lateral parts of the lower lip passes primarily to the **submandibular lymph nodes** (Fig. 7.49), whereas lymph from the medial part of the lower lip passes initially to the **submental lymph nodes.**

The **cheeks** (L. *buccae*) include the lateral distensible walls of the oral cavity and the facial prominences over the zygomatic bones. The cheeks have essentially the same structure as the lips, with which they are continuous. The principal muscles of the cheeks are the **buccinators** (Fig. 7.48). The lips and cheeks function as an oral sphincter that pushes food from the oral vestibule into the oral cavity proper. The tongue and buccinators work together to keep the food between the occlusal surfaces of the molar teeth during chewing. The **labial** and **buccal glands** are small mucous glands between the mucous membrane and the underlying orbicularis oris and buccinator muscles (Fig. 7.48).

Teeth and Gingivae

The **teeth** are hard conical structures set in the **dental alveoli** (tooth sockets) of the upper and lower jaws and are used in mastication (chewing) and assisting in articulation. Children have 20 **deciduous (primary) teeth**. The first tooth usually erupts at 6 to 8 months of age and the last tooth by 20 to 24 months of age. Eruption of the **permanent (secondary) teeth**, normally 16 in each jaw (3 molars, 2 premolars, 1 canine, and 2 incisors on each side), usually is complete by the midteens (Fig. 7.50), except for the third molars ("wisdom teeth"), which usually erupt during the late teens or early 20s.

A tooth has a crown, neck, and root. Each type of tooth has a characteristic appearance (Figs. 7.51 and 7.52). The **crown** projects from the gingiva. The **neck** is the part of the tooth between the crown and the root. The **root** is fixed in the

Superior view
Mandibular (lower) dental arcade

FIGURE 7.50.   **Adult mandibular dentition.**

B Lateral radiograph

1 Enamel   **2** Dentine   **3** Pulp cavity
4 Root canal   **5** Buccal cusp   **6** Root apex
7 Interalveolar septa (alveolar bone)
8 Interradicular septum (alveolar bone)

FIGURE 7.51.   **Parts of a tooth. A.** An incisor and molar tooth. **B.** Bite-wing radiograph of maxillary premolar and molar teeth.

alveolus (tooth socket) by the fibrous *periodontium* (periodontal membrane). Most of the tooth is composed of **dentine** (L. *dentinium*), which is covered by **enamel** over the crown and **cement** (L. *cementum*) over the root. The **pulp cavity** contains connective tissue, blood vessels, and nerves. The **root canal** (pulp canal) transmits the nerves and vessels to and from the pulp cavity through the **apical foramen.**

The **superior** and **inferior alveolar arteries,** branches of the **maxillary artery,** supply the maxillary (upper) and the mandibular (lower) teeth, respectively (Figs. 7.43 and 7.44*A*). **Veins** with the same names and distribution accompany the arteries (Fig. 7.44*B*). **Lymphatic vessels** from the teeth and gingivae pass mainly to the **submandibular lymph nodes** (Fig. 7.49). The superior and inferior **alveolar nerves,** branches of CN V$_2$ and CN V$_3$, respectively, form superior and inferior **dental plexuses** that supply the maxillary and mandibular teeth (Fig. 7.52*A*).

The **gingivae** (gums) are composed of fibrous tissue covered with mucous membrane, which is firmly attached to the alveolar processes of the mandible and maxilla and the necks of the teeth. The **buccal gingivae** of the mandibular molar

(A) Lateral view

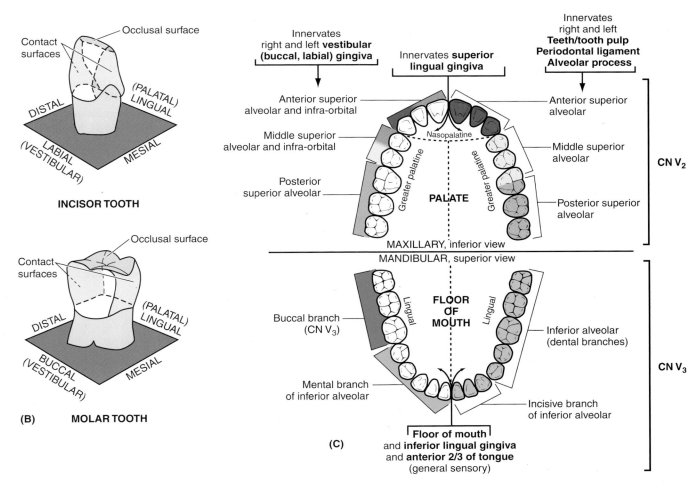

Dental Caries, Pulpitis, and Toothache

 Decay of the hard tissues of a tooth results in the formation of *dental caries* (cavities). Invasion of the pulp of the tooth by a carious lesion (cavity) results in infection and irritation of the tissues in the pulp cavity. This condition causes an inflammatory process (*pulpitis*). Because the pulp cavity is a rigid space, the swollen pulpal tissues cause pain (*toothache*).

Gingivitis and Periodontitis

Improper oral hygiene results in food deposits in tooth and gingival crevices, which may cause inflammation of the gingivae (*gingivitis*). If untreated, the disease spreads to other supporting structures (including the alveolar bone), producing *periodontitis*. Periodontitis results in inflammation of the gingivae and may result in absorption of alveolar bone and gingival recession. Gingival recession exposes the sensitive cement of the teeth.

teeth (Fig. 7.48) are supplied by the **buccal nerve,** a branch of the mandibular nerve (Fig. 7.52*C*). The **lingual gingivae** of all mandibular teeth are supplied by the **lingual nerve.** The **palatine gingivae** of the maxillary premolar and molar teeth are supplied by the **greater palatine nerve;** and the palatine gingivae of the incisors, by the **nasopalatine nerve**. The labial and buccal aspects of the maxillary gingivae are supplied by the anterior, middle, and posterior **superior alveolar nerves** (Fig. 7.52*A*).

Palate

The **palate** forms the arched roof of the oral cavity proper and the floor of the nasal cavities (Fig. 7.53). The palate consists of hard and soft parts: the hard palate anteriorly and the soft palate posteriorly. The hard palate separates the anterior part of the oral cavity from the nasal cavities, and the soft palate separates the posterior part of the oral cavity from the nasopharynx superior to it.

The **hard palate** is the anterior vaulted (concave) part; this space is filled with the tongue when it is at rest. The hard palate (covered by a mucous membrane) is formed by the palatine processes of the maxillae and the horizontal plates of the palatine bones (Fig. 7.54*A*). Three foramina open on the oral aspect of the hard palate: the incisive fossa and the greater and lesser palatine foramina. The **incisive fossa** is a slight depression posterior to the central incisor teeth. The **nasopalatine nerves** pass from the nose through a variable number of incisive canals and foramina that open into the incisive fossa (Fig. 7.54*B*). Medial to the

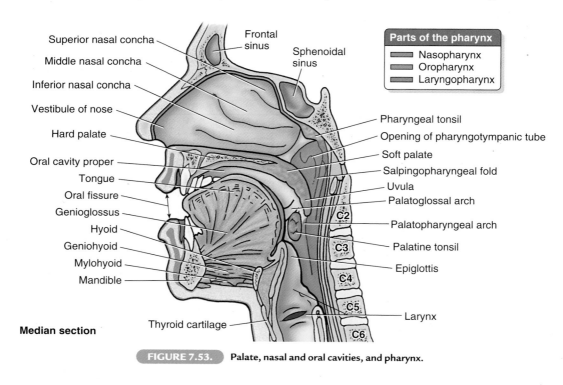

Median section

Parts of the pharynx
- Nasopharynx
- Oropharynx
- Laryngopharynx

Superior nasal concha
Middle nasal concha
Inferior nasal concha
Vestibule of nose
Hard palate
Oral cavity proper
Tongue
Oral fissure
Genioglossus
Hyoid
Geniohyoid
Mylohyoid
Mandible
Thyroid cartilage

Frontal sinus
Sphenoidal sinus
Pharyngeal tonsil
Opening of pharyngotympanic tube
Soft palate
Salpingopharyngeal fold
Uvula
Palatoglossal arch
Palatopharyngeal arch
Palatine tonsil
Epiglottis
Larynx

C2
C3
C4
C5
C6

FIGURE 7.53. Palate, nasal and oral cavities, and pharynx.

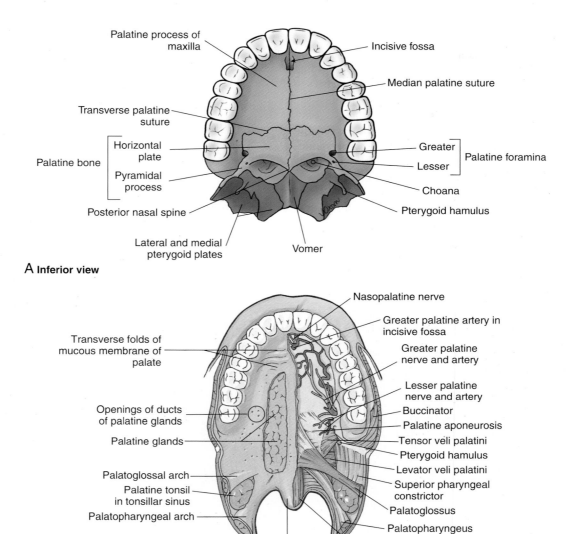

FIGURE 7.54. **Palate. A.** The bones forming the hard palate. **B.** Part of the right side has been dissected to show the palatine glands. The left side has been dissected to show the muscles of the soft palate and palatine arteries and nerves.

third molar tooth, the **greater palatine foramen** pierces the lateral border of the bony palate. The *greater palatine vessels and nerve* emerge from this foramen and run anteriorly on the palate. The **lesser palatine foramina** transmit the *lesser palatine nerves and vessels* to the soft palate and adjacent structures.

The **soft palate** is the movable third of the palate, which is suspended from the posterior border of the hard palate (Figs. 7.54B and 7.55). The soft palate extends postero-inferiorly as a curved free margin from which hangs a conical process, the **uvula**. The soft palate is strengthened by the **palatine aponeurosis,** formed by the expanded tendon of the **tensor veli palatini**. The aponeurosis, attached to the posterior margin of the hard palate, is thick anteriorly and thin posteriorly. The anterior part of the soft palate is formed

mainly by the palatine aponeurosis, whereas its posterior part is muscular.

When a person swallows, the soft palate is initially tensed to allow the tongue to press against it, squeezing the bolus of food to the back of the oral cavity proper. The soft palate is then elevated posteriorly and superiorly against the wall of the pharynx, thereby preventing passage of food into the nasal cavity. Laterally, the soft palate is continuous with the wall of the pharynx and is joined to the tongue and pharynx by the **palatoglossal** and **palatopharyngeal arches** (Figs. 7.54B and 7.55A), respectively. The **palatine tonsils,** often referred to as "the tonsils," are masses of lymphoid tissue, one on each side of the oropharynx (Fig. 7.55B). Each tonsil lies in a *tonsillar sinus* (fossa), bounded by the palatoglossal and palatopharyngeal arches and the tongue.

VASCULATURE AND INNERVATION OF PALATE

The palate has a rich blood supply, chiefly from the right and left **greater palatine arteries,** branches of the descending palatine arteries (Fig. 7.54B). The **lesser palatine artery,** a smaller branch of the descending palatine artery, enters the palate through the **lesser palatine foramen** and anastomoses with the ascending palatine artery, a branch of the facial artery. **Venous drainage of the palate,** corresponding to and accompanying the branches of the maxillary artery, involves tributaries of the **pterygoid venous plexus** (Fig. 7.44B).

The *sensory nerves of the palate* pass through the **pterygopalatine ganglion** and are considered branches of the maxillary nerve. The **greater palatine nerve** supplies the gingivae, mucous membrane, and glands of most of the hard palate (Fig. 7.54B). The **nasopalatine nerve** supplies the mucous membrane of the anterior part of the hard palate. The **lesser palatine nerves** supply the soft palate. The palatine nerves accompany the arteries through the greater and lesser palatine foramina, respectively. Except for the tensor veli palatini supplied by CN V$_3$, all muscles of the soft palate are supplied through the *pharyngeal plexus of nerves* (see Chapter 8), derived from pharyngeal branches of the vagus nerve (CN X).

MUSCLES OF SOFT PALATE

The **muscles of the soft palate** arise from the cranial base and descend to the palate (Figs. 7.54B and 7.55B). The soft palate may be elevated so that it is in contact with the posterior wall of the pharynx, sealing off the oral passage from the

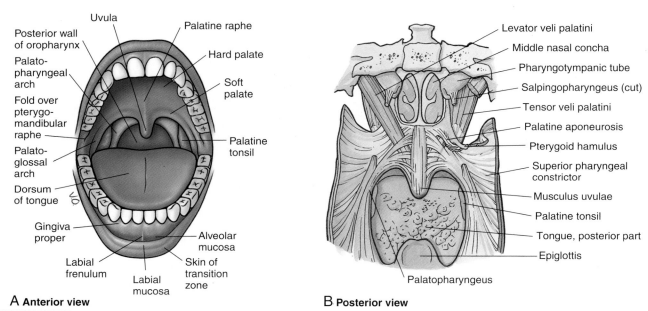

A Anterior view   **B** Posterior view

FIGURE 7.55. **Soft palate A.** Surface anatomy of oral cavity and soft palate. **B.** Dissection of the soft palate shows the muscles and their relationship to the posterior part of the tongue.

TABLE 7.10 MUSCLES OF SOFT PALATE

Muscle	Origin	Insertion	Innervation	Main Action(s)
Tensor veli palatini	Scaphoid fossa at root of posterior border of medial pterygoid plate, spine of sphenoid bone, and cartilage of pharyngo-tympanic tube	Palatine aponeurosis (Fig. 7.54B)	Nerve to medial pterygoid (a branch of CN V3) via otic ganglion	Tenses soft palate and opens mouth of pharyngotympanic tube during swallowing and yawning
Levator veli palatini	Cartilage of pharyngotympanic tube and petrous part of temporal bone		Pharyngeal branch of CN X via pharyngeal plexus	Elevates soft palate during swallowing and yawning
Palatoglossus	Palatine aponeurosis	Side of tongue		Elevates posterior part of tongue and draws soft palate onto tongue
Palatopharyngeus	Hard palate and palatine aponeurosis	Lateral wall of pharynx		Tenses soft palate and pulls walls of pharynx superiorly, anteriorly, and medially during swallowing
Musculus uvulae	Posterior nasal spine and palatine aponeurosis	Mucosa of uvula		Shortens uvula and pulls it superiorly

nasopharynx (e.g., when swallowing or breathing through the mouth). The soft palate can also be drawn inferiorly so that it is in contact with the posterior part of the tongue, sealing off the oral cavity from the nasal passage (e.g., when breathing exclusively through the nose, even with the mouth open). For attachments, nerve supply, and actions of the five muscles of the soft palate, see Fig. 7.55*B* and Table 7.10.

- The **levator veli palatini** (lifter of the soft palate) is a cylindrical muscle that runs infero-anteriorly, spreading out in the soft palate where it attaches to the superior surface of the palatine aponeurosis.
- The **tensor veli palatini** (tensor of the soft palate) is a muscle with a triangular belly that passes inferiorly; the tendon formed at its apex hooks around the **pterygoid hamulus**—the hook-shaped inferior projection of the medial pterygoid plate—before spreading out as the palatine aponeurosis.
- The **palatoglossus** is a slender slip of muscle that is covered with a mucous membrane; it forms the *palatoglossal arch*. Unlike the other muscles ending in *-glossus*, the palatoglossus is a palatine muscle (in function and innervation) rather than a tongue muscle.
- The **palatopharyngeus** is a thin, flat muscle also covered with a mucous membrane; it forms the *palatopharyngeal arch* and blends inferiorly with the longitudinal muscle of the pharynx.
- The **musculus uvulae** inserts into the mucosa of the uvula.

Tongue

The **tongue** (L. *lingua;* G. *glossa*) is a mobile muscular organ that can assume a variety of shapes and positions. The tongue is partly in the oral cavity proper and partly in the oropharynx (Fig. 7.53). At rest, it occupies essentially all the oral cavity proper. The tongue—mainly composed of muscles and covered by mucous membrane—assists with mastication (chewing), taste, deglutition (swallowing), articulation (speech), and oral cleansing. The tongue has a root, a body, an apex, a curved dorsal surface (dorsum), and an inferior surface (Fig. 7.56*A*). A V-shaped groove, the **terminal sulcus** (L. *sulcus terminalis*) of the tongue (Fig. 7.56*B*), marks the separation between the *anterior (presulcal) part* and the *posterior (postsulcal) part.*

The **root of the tongue** is the posterior third that rests on the floor of the mouth. The anterior two thirds of the tongue form the **body of the tongue.** The pointed anterior part of the body is the **apex (tip) of the tongue.** The body and apex are extremely mobile. The **dorsum (dorsal surface) of the tongue** is the posterosuperior surface of the tongue, which includes the **terminal sulcus.** At the apex of this groove is the **foramen cecum,** a small pit that is the non-functional remnant of the proximal part of the embryonic thyroglossal duct from which the thyroid gland developed. The mucous membrane on the anterior part of the tongue is rough because of the presence of numerous **lingual papillae** (Fig. 7.56*B*):

- **Vallate papillae** are large and flat-topped; they lie directly anterior to the terminal sulcus and are surrounded by deep moat-like trenches, the walls of which are studded by *taste buds;* the ducts of serous *lingual glands* (of von Ebner) open into these trenches.
- **Foliate papillae** are small lateral folds of lingual mucosa; they are poorly developed in humans.
- **Filiform papillae** are long, numerous, thread-like, and scaly; they contain afferent nerve endings that are sensitive to touch.

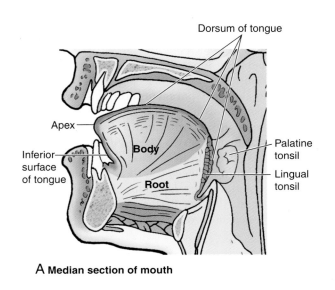

A Median section of mouth

Dorsum of tongue

Apex

Inferior surface of tongue

Body

Root

Palatine tonsil

Lingual tonsil

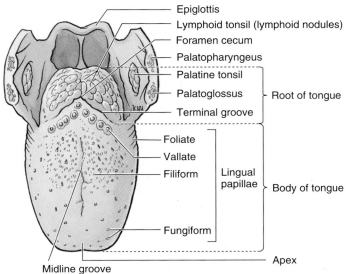

Epiglottis

Lymphoid tonsil (lymphoid nodules)

Foramen cecum

Palatopharyngeus

Palatine tonsil

Palatoglossus

Terminal groove

Root of tongue

Foliate

Vallate

Filiform

Lingual papillae

Body of tongue

Fungiform

Apex

Midline groove

B Superior view of dorsum of tongue

FIGURE 7.56. **Tongue. A.** Parts. **B.** Features of dorsum of tongue.

- **Fungiform papillae** are mushroom-shaped and appear as pink or red spots; they are scattered among the filiform papillae but are most numerous at the apex and sides (margins) of the tongue.

The vallate, foliate, and most of the fungiform papillae contain taste receptors in the **taste buds.** A few taste buds are also in the epithelium covering the oral surface of the soft palate, the posterior wall of the oropharynx, and the epiglottis.

The mucous membrane of the dorsum of the tongue is thin over the anterior part of the tongue and is closely attached to the underlying muscle (Fig. 7.56A). A depression on the dorsal surface, the **midline groove of the tongue** (median sulcus of tongue), divides the tongue into right and left halves (Fig. 7.56B). It also indicates the site of fusion of the embryonic distal tongue buds.

The **root** of the tongue lies within the oropharynx, posterior to the *terminal sulcus* and the *palatoglossal arches* (Fig. 7.56B). Its mucous membrane is thick and freely movable. It has no lingual papillae, but the underlying **lymphoid nodules,** known collectively as the lingual tonsil, give this part of the tongue its cobblestone appearance.

The **inferior surface of the tongue** is covered with a thin, transparent mucous membrane through which one can see the underlying **deep lingual veins.** With the tongue raised, the **lingual frenulum** (Fig. 7.57), a large midline fold of mucosa that passes from the gingiva covering the lingual aspect of the anterior alveolar ridge to the posteroinferior surface of the tongue, can be seen. The frenulum connects the tongue to the floor of the mouth while allowing the anterior part of the tongue to move freely. At the base of the frenulum are the *openings of the submandibular ducts* from the submandibular salivary glands.

MUSCLES OF TONGUE

The tongue is essentially a mass of muscles that is mostly covered by mucous membrane. Although it is traditional to

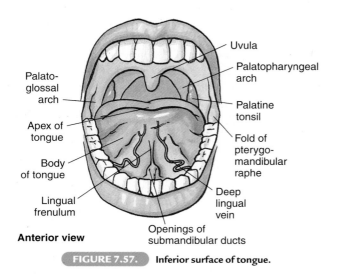

Palato-glossal arch

Apex of tongue

Body of tongue

Lingual frenulum

Uvula

Palatopharyngeal arch

Palatine tonsil

Fold of pterygo-mandibular raphe

Deep lingual vein

Openings of submandibular ducts

Anterior view

FIGURE 7.57.   **Inferior surface of tongue.**

do so, providing descriptions of the actions of tongue muscles by ascribing a single action to a specific muscle greatly oversimplifies the actions of the tongue and is misleading. The muscles of the tongue do not act in isolation, and some muscles perform multiple actions with parts of one muscle capable of acting independently, producing different—even antagonistic—actions. *In general, however, extrinsic muscles alter the position of the tongue and intrinsic muscles alter its shape* (Fig. 7.58 and Table 7.11).

The four intrinsic and four extrinsic muscles in each half of the tongue are separated by the fibrous **lingual septum,** which extends vertically from the midline groove of the tongue (Fig. 7.58C). The **intrinsic muscles of the tongue** (superior and inferior longitudinal, transverse, and vertical) are confined to the tongue and are not attached to bone. The **extrinsic muscles of the tongue** (genioglossus, hyoglossus, styloglossus, and palatoglossus) originate outside the tongue and attach to it.

INNERVATION OF TONGUE

All the muscles of the tongue are supplied by CN XII, the **hypoglossal nerve** (Fig. 7.59A), except for the palatoglossus (actually a palatine muscle supplied by the *pharyngeal plexus,* the plexus of nerves that includes motor branches of CN X). For general sensation (touch and temperature), the mucosa of the anterior two thirds of the tongue is supplied by the **lingual nerve,** a branch of CN V₃. For special sensation (taste), this part of the tongue, except for the vallate papillae, is supplied through the **chorda tympani nerve,** a branch of CN VII. The chorda tympani joins the lingual nerve and runs anteriorly in its sheath (Fig. 7.59B).

The mucous membrane of the posterior third of the tongue and the vallate papillae are supplied by the lingual branch of the **glossopharyngeal nerve** (CN IX) for both general and special sensation (taste). Twigs of the **internal laryngeal nerve,** a branch of the vagus nerve (CN X), supply mostly general but some special sensation to a small area of the tongue just anterior to the epiglottis. These mostly sensory nerves also carry **parasympathetic secretomotor fibers** to serous glands in the tongue. These nerve fibers probably synapse in the **submandibular ganglion** suspended from the lingual nerve (Fig. 7.59B).

There are four basic taste sensations: sweet, salty, sour, and bitter. Sweetness is detected at the apex, saltiness at the lateral margin, and sourness and bitterness at the posterior part of the tongue. All other "tastes" expressed by gourmets are olfactory (smell and aroma).

VASCULATURE OF TONGUE

The **arteries of the tongue** derive from the **lingual artery,** which arises from the *external carotid artery* (Fig. 7.60A). On entering the tongue, the lingual artery passes deep to the

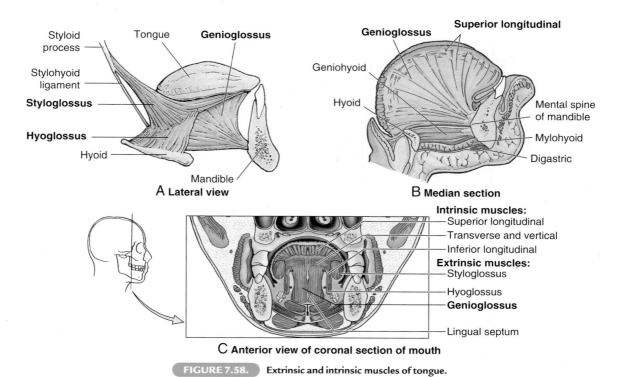

A Lateral view

B Median section

C Anterior view of coronal section of mouth

FIGURE 7.58. Extrinsic and intrinsic muscles of tongue.

TABLE 7.11 MUSCLES OF TONGUE

Muscle	Shape and Position	Proximal Attachment	Distal Attachment	Main Action(s)
Extrinsic muscles of tongue				
Genioglossus	Fan-shaped muscle; constitutes bulk of tongue	Via a short tendon from superior part of mental spine of mandible	Entire dorsum of tongue; inferior most and posterior most fibers attach to body of hyoid	Bilateral activity depresses tongue, especially central part, creating a longitudinal furrow; posterior part pulls tongue anteriorly for protrusion[a]; most anterior part retracts apex of protruded tongue; unilateral contraction deviates ("wags") tongue to contralateral side
Hyoglossus	Thin, quadrilateral muscle	Body and greater horn of hyoid	Inferior aspects of lateral part of tongue	Depresses tongue, especially pulling its sides inferiorly; helps shorten (retrude) tongue
Styloglossus	Short triangular muscle	Anterior border of distal styloid process; stylohyoid ligament	Margins of tongue posteriorly, interdigitating with hyoglossus	Retrudes tongue and curls (elevates) its sides, working with genioglossus to form a central trough during swallowing
Palatoglossus	Narrow crescent-shaped palatine muscle; forms posterior column of isthmus of fauces	Palatine aponeurosis of soft palate	Enters posterolateral tongue transversely, blending with intrinsic transverse muscles	Capable of elevating posterior tongue or depressing soft palate; most commonly acts to constrict isthmus of fauces (L. the throat)
Intrinsic muscles of tongue				
Superior longitudinal	Thin layer deep to mucous membrane of dorsum of tongue	Submucosal fibrous layer and median fibrous septum	Margins of tongue and mucous membrane	Curls tongue longitudinally upward, elevating apex and sides of tongue; shortens (retrudes) tongue
Inferior longitudinal	Narrow band close to inferior surface of tongue	Root of tongue and body of hyoid	Apex of tongue	Curls tongue longitudinally downward, depressing apex; shortens (retrudes) tongue
Transverse	Deep to superior longitudinal muscle	Median fibrous septum	Fibrous tissue at lateral lingual margins	Narrows and elongates (protrudes) tongue[a]
Vertical	Fibers intersect transverse muscle	Submucosal fibrous layer of dorsum of tongue	Inferior surface of borders of tongue	Flattens and broadens tongue[a]

[a]Act simultaneously to protrude tongue.

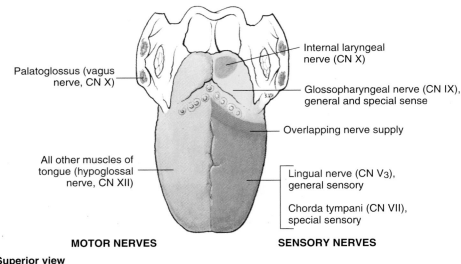

Internal laryngeal
nerve (CN X)

Palatoglossus (vagus
nerve, CN X)

Glossopharyngeal nerve (CN IX),
general and special sense

Overlapping nerve supply

All other muscles of
tongue (hypoglossal
nerve, CN XII)

Lingual nerve (CN V₃),
general sensory

Chorda tympani (CN VII),
special sensory

MOTOR NERVES   SENSORY NERVES

A Superior view

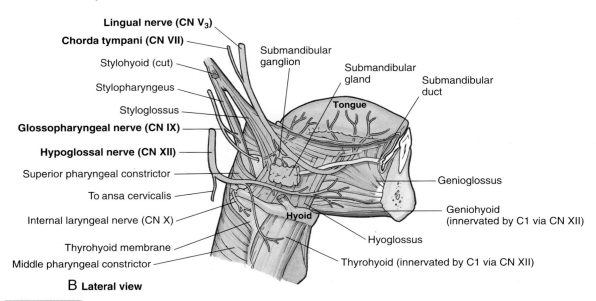

Lingual nerve (CN V₃)
Chorda tympani (CN VII)
Stylohyoid (cut)
Stylopharyngeus
Styloglossus
Glossopharyngeal nerve (CN IX)
Hypoglossal nerve (CN XII)
Superior pharyngeal constrictor
To ansa cervicalis
Internal laryngeal nerve (CN X)
Thyrohyoid membrane
Middle pharyngeal constrictor

Submandibular
ganglion

Submandibular
gland

Submandibular
duct

Tongue

Genioglossus

Geniohyoid
(innervated by C1 via CN XII)

Hyoid

Hyoglossus

Thyrohyoid (innervated by C1 via CN XII)

B Lateral view

FIGURE 7.59.   **Innervation of tongue. A.** Overview of sensory and motor innervation. **B.** Course of lingual and hypoglossal nerves.

hyoglossus muscle. The *main branches of the lingual artery* are the:

- **Dorsal lingual arteries,** which supply the posterior part, the root of the tongue, and send a tonsillar branch to the palatine tonsil.
- **Deep lingual artery,** which supplies the anterior part of the tongue; the dorsal and deep arteries communicate with each other near the apex of the tongue.
- **Sublingual artery,** which supplies the sublingual gland and the floor of the mouth.

The **veins of the tongue** are the:

- *Dorsal lingual veins,* which accompany the lingual artery.

- *Deep lingual veins* (Fig. 7.57), which begin at the apex of the tongue and run posteriorly beside the lingual frenulum to join the *sublingual vein.*

All lingual veins terminate, directly or indirectly, in the IJV.

Lymphatic drainage of the tongue takes the following routes (Fig. 7.60B,C):

- Lymph from the posterior third drains to the *superior deep cervical lymph nodes* on both sides.
- Lymph from the *medial part of the anterior two thirds* drains to the *inferior deep cervical lymph nodes.*
- Lymph from *lateral parts of the anterior two thirds* drains to the *submandibular lymph nodes.*

A Lateral view

B Superior view

C Lateral view

FIGURE 7.60.   **Blood supply and lymphatic drainage of tongue. A.** Arterial supply. **B and C.** Lymphatic drainage.

- Lymph from the *apex of the tongue and frenulum* drains to the *submental lymph nodes.*
- Lymph from the *posterior third* and the area near the midline groove drains bilaterally.

Salivary Glands

The **salivary glands** include the parotid, submandibular, and sublingual glands (Fig. 7.61A). Saliva, the clear, tasteless, odorless viscid fluid secreted by these glands and the mucous glands of the oral cavity:

- Keeps the mucous membrane of the mouth moist.
- Lubricates the food during mastication.

- Begins digestion of starches.
- Serves as an intrinsic "mouthwash."
- Plays a significant role in the prevention of tooth decay and in the ability to taste.

In addition to the three major salivary glands, small *accessory salivary glands* are scattered over the palate, lips, cheeks, tonsils, and tongue.

The **parotid glands** are the largest of the major salivary glands (Fig.7.61A). Each parotid gland has an irregular shape because it occupies the gap between the ramus of the mandible and the styloid and mastoid processes of the temporal bone. The purely serous secretion of the gland

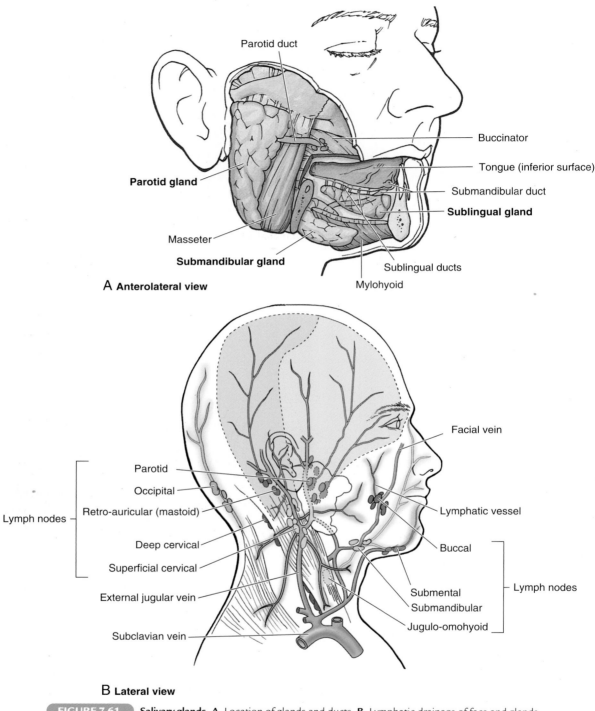

A Anterolateral view

Parotid duct

Buccinator

Tongue (inferior surface)

Submandibular duct

Sublingual gland

Parotid gland

Masseter

Submandibular gland

Sublingual ducts

Mylohyoid

B Lateral view

Facial vein

Lymphatic vessel

Buccal

Submental

Submandibular

Jugulo-omohyoid

Lymph nodes

Parotid

Occipital

Retro-auricular (mastoid)

Deep cervical

Superficial cervical

External jugular vein

Subclavian vein

Lymph nodes

FIGURE 7.61.   **Salivary glands. A.** Location of glands and ducts. **B.** Lymphatic drainage of face and glands.

passes through the **parotid duct** and empties into the vestibule of the oral cavity opposite the second maxillary molar tooth. In addition to its digestive function, it washes food particles into the mouth proper. The **arterial supply** of the parotid gland and duct is from branches of the *external carotid* and *superficial temporal arteries* (Fig. 7.44A). The **veins** from the parotid gland drain into the *retromandibular veins* (Fig. 7.44B). The **lymphatic vessels** from the parotid gland end in the **superficial and deep cervical lymph nodes** (Fig. 7.61B). The parotid gland was discussed earlier in this chapter, when its innervation was described.

The **submandibular glands** lie along the body of the mandible, partly superior and partly inferior to the posterior half of the mandible and partly superficial and partly deep to the mylohyoid muscle (Fig. 7.61A). The **submandibular duct** arises from the part of the gland that lies between the mylohyoid and the hyoglossus. Passing from lateral to medial, the **lingual nerve** loops under the submandibular duct as it runs anteriorly to open via one to three orifices on a small, fleshy *sublingual papilla* on each side of the lingual frenulum (Figs. 7.57 and 7.61A). The orifices of the submandibular ducts are visible, and saliva often sprays from it when the tongue is elevated and retracted.

The **arterial supply of the submandibular glands** is from the **submental arteries** (Fig. 7.44A). The **veins** accompany the arteries. The submandibular gland is supplied by presynaptic parasympathetic secretomotor fibers conveyed from the facial nerve to the lingual nerve by the *chorda tympani nerve* (Fig. 7.59B), which synapse with postsynaptic neurons in the *submandibular ganglion*. The latter fibers accompany arteries to reach the gland, along with vasoconstrictive postsynaptic sympathetic fibers from the superior cervical ganglion. The **lymphatic vessels** of the submandibular gland drain into the *deep cervical lymph nodes,* particularly the *jugulo-omohyoid lymph node* (Fig. 7.61B).

The **sublingual glands** are the smallest and most deeply situated (Fig. 7.61A). Each almond-shaped gland lies in the floor of the mouth between the mandible and the genioglossus muscle. The glands from each side unite to form a horseshoe-shaped mass around the lingual frenulum. Numerous small **sublingual ducts** open into the floor of the mouth alongside the lingual folds.

The **arterial supply of the sublingual glands** is from the *sublingual* and *submental arteries*—branches of the lingual and facial arteries, respectively (Figs. 7.44A and 7.60A). The **innervation** of the sublingual glands is the same as that described for the submandibular gland.

Sialography

The parotid and submandibular salivary glands may be examined radiographically after the injection of a contrast medium into their ducts. This special type of radiograph (*sialogram*) demonstrates the salivary ducts and some secretory units. Because of the small size and number of sublingual ducts of the sublingual glands, one cannot usually inject contrast medium into them.

Gag Reflex

One may touch the anterior part of the tongue without feeling discomfort; however, when the posterior part is touched, one usually gags. CN IX and CN X are responsible for the muscular contraction of each side of the pharynx. Glossopharyngeal branches (CN IX) provide the afferent limb of the gag reflex.

Paralysis of Genioglossus

When the genioglossus is paralyzed, the tongue mass has a tendency to shift posteriorly, obstructing the airway and presenting the risk of suffocation. Total relaxation of the genioglossus muscles occurs during general anesthesia; therefore, the tongue of an anesthetized patient must be prevented from relapsing by inserting an airway.

Injury to Hypoglossal Nerve

Trauma, such as a fractured mandible, may injure the hypoglossal nerve (CN XII), resulting in paralysis and eventual atrophy of one side of the tongue. The tongue deviates to the paralyzed side during protrusion because of the action of the unaffected genioglossus on the other side.

Sublingual Absorption of Drugs

For quick transmucosal absorption of a drug—for instance, when nitroglycerin is used as a vasodilator in angina pectoris (chest pain)—the pill (or spray) is put under the tongue, where the thin mucosa allows the absorbed drug to enter the deep lingual veins in less than a minute.

Lingual Carcinoma

Malignant tumors in the posterior part of the tongue metastasize to the superior deep cervical lymph nodes on both sides. In contrast, tumors in the apex and anterolateral parts usually do not metastasize to the inferior deep cervical nodes until late in the disease. Because the deep nodes are closely related to the IJVs, metastases from the carcinoma may spread to the submental and submandibular regions and along the IJVs into the neck.

A **Inferolateral and slightly posterior view, looking into infratemporal and pterygopalatine fossae**

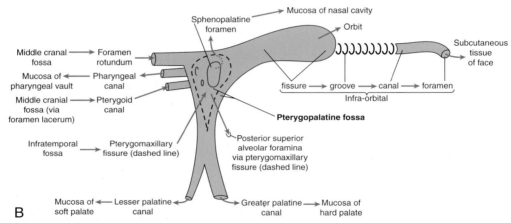

FIGURE 7.62. **Pterygopalatine fossa—location and communications.** The pterygopalatine fossa communicates with most compartments of the deep face via many passages (foramina, fissures, and canals). **A.** Photograph. **B.** Schematic illustration.

PTERYGOPALATINE FOSSA

The **pterygopalatine fossa** is a small pyramidal space inferior to the apex of the orbit. It lies between the pterygoid process of the sphenoid and the posterior aspect of the maxilla anteriorly (Fig. 7.62A). The fragile perpendicular plate of the palatine bone forms its medial wall. The incomplete *roof of the pterygopalatine fossa* is formed by the *greater wing of the sphenoid*. The *floor of the pterygopalatine fossa* is formed by the *pyramidal process of the palatine bone*. Its superior, larger end opens into the *inferior orbital fissure;* its inferior end is closed except for the palatine foramina. The pterygopalatine fossa communicates (Fig. 7.62B):

- Laterally with the *infratemporal fossa* through the *pterygomaxillary fissure.*
- Medially with the *nasal cavity* through the *sphenopalatine foramen.*

- Anterosuperiorly with the *orbit* through the *inferior orbital fissure.*
- Posterosuperiorly with the *middle cranial fossa* through the *foramen rotundum* and *pterygoid canal.*

The contents of the pterygopalatine fossa are the:

- Maxillary nerve (CN V_2), with which are associated the nerve of the pterygoid canal and the pterygopalatine ganglion (Figs. 7.63 and 7.64A).
- Terminal (third) part of the maxillary artery and its branches (Figs. 7.43 and 7.64B).

The **maxillary nerve** (CN V_2) enters the pterygopalatine fossa posterosuperiorly through the foramen rotundum and runs anterolaterally in the fossa (Figs. 7.63 and 7.64). Within the fossa, the maxillary nerve gives off the *zygomatic nerve,* which divides into the *zygomaticofacial* and *zygomaticotemporal nerves* (Fig. 7.63A). These nerves emerge from the

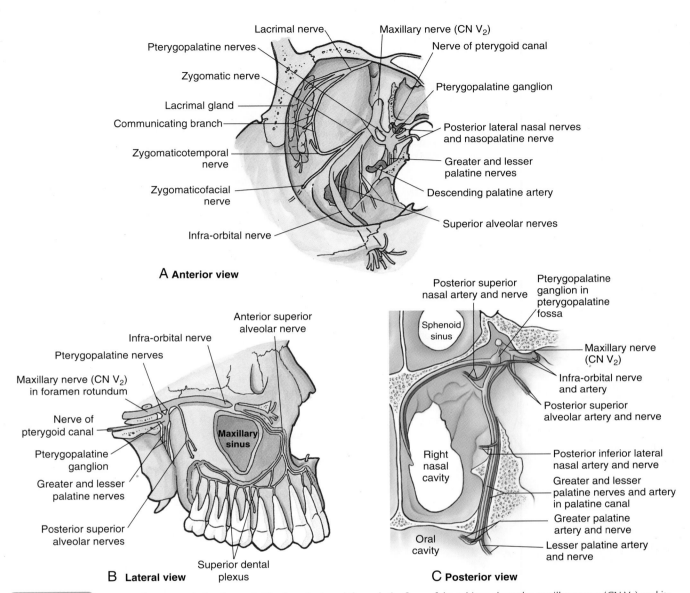

A Anterior view

Lacrimal nerve
Maxillary nerve (CN V₂)
Pterygopalatine nerves
Nerve of pterygoid canal
Zygomatic nerve
Pterygopalatine ganglion
Lacrimal gland
Communicating branch
Posterior lateral nasal nerves and nasopalatine nerve
Zygomaticotemporal nerve
Greater and lesser palatine nerves
Zygomaticofacial nerve
Descending palatine artery
Infra-orbital nerve
Superior alveolar nerves

B Lateral view

Anterior superior alveolar nerve
Infra-orbital nerve
Pterygopalatine nerves
Maxillary nerve (CN V₂) in foramen rotundum
Nerve of pterygoid canal
Pterygopalatine ganglion
Greater and lesser palatine nerves
Posterior superior alveolar nerves
Maxillary sinus
Superior dental plexus

C Posterior view

Posterior superior nasal artery and nerve
Pterygopalatine ganglion in pterygopalatine fossa
Sphenoid sinus
Maxillary nerve (CN V₂)
Infra-orbital nerve and artery
Posterior superior alveolar artery and nerve
Right nasal cavity
Posterior inferior lateral nasal artery and nerve
Greater and lesser palatine nerves and artery in palatine canal
Greater palatine artery and nerve
Oral cavity
Lesser palatine artery and nerve

FIGURE 7.63. Nerves of pterygopalatine fossa. **A.** The fossa is viewed through the floor of the orbit to show the maxillary nerve (CN V₂) and its branches. **B.** The fossa is viewed laterally. Part of the lateral wall of the maxillary sinus has been removed. **C.** In this coronal section, the nasopalatine and greater and lesser palatine nerves can be seen.

zygomatic bone through the cranial foramina of the same name and supply the lateral region of the cheek and the temple. The *zygomaticotemporal nerve* also gives rise to a communicating branch, which conveys parasympathetic secretomotor fibers to the lacrimal gland by way of the lacrimal nerve from CN V₁.

While in the pterygopalatine fossa, the maxillary nerve also gives off the two *pterygopalatine nerves,* which suspend the parasympathetic *pterygopalatine ganglion* in the superior part of the pterygopalatine fossa (Figs. 7.63A,B). The pterygopalatine nerves convey general sensory fibers of the maxillary nerve, which pass through the pterygopalatine ganglion without synapsing and supply the nose,

palate, tonsil, and gingivae (Figs. 7.64A,E). The maxillary nerve leaves the pterygopalatine fossa through the inferior orbital fissure, after which it is known as the *infra-orbital nerve.*

The **parasympathetic fibers to the pterygopalatine ganglion** come from the facial nerve by way of its first branch, the *greater petrosal nerve* (Fig. 7.64C). This nerve joins the *deep petrosal nerve* as it passes through the foramen lacerum to form the **nerve of the pterygoid canal.** This nerve passes anteriorly through the pterygoid canal to the **pterygopalatine fossa.** The parasympathetic fibers of the greater petrosal nerve synapse in the pterygopalatine ganglion (Fig. 7.64D).

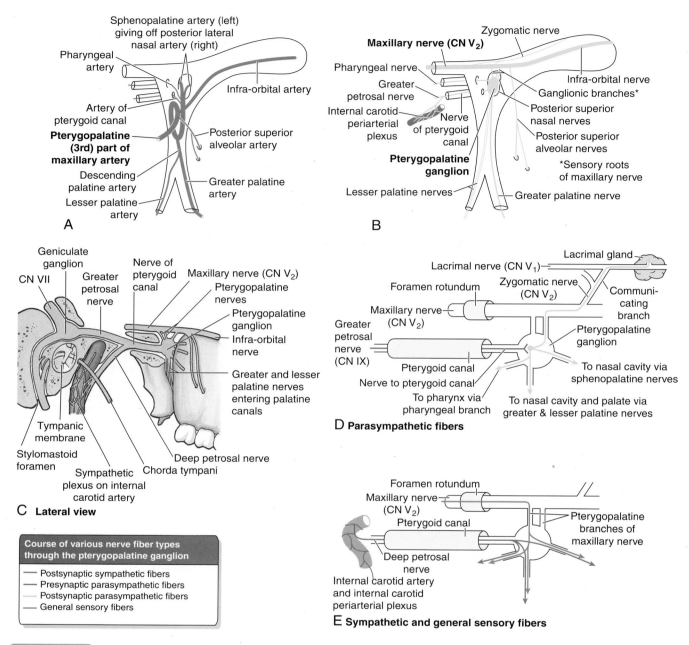

A. Pterygopalatine part of the maxillary nerve.

Sphenopalatine artery (left) giving off posterior lateral nasal artery (right)
Pharyngeal artery
Artery of pterygoid canal
Pterygopalatine (3rd) part of maxillary artery
Descending palatine artery
Lesser palatine artery
Infra-orbital artery
Posterior superior alveolar artery
Greater palatine artery

A

Zygomatic nerve
Maxillary nerve (CN V₂)
Pharyngeal nerve
Greater petrosal nerve
Internal carotid periarterial plexus
Nerve of pterygoid canal
Pterygopalatine ganglion
Lesser palatine nerves
Infra-orbital nerve
Ganglionic branches*
Posterior superior nasal nerves
Posterior superior alveolar nerves
*Sensory roots of maxillary nerve
Greater palatine nerve

B

Geniculate ganglion
CN VII
Greater petrosal nerve
Nerve of pterygoid canal
Maxillary nerve (CN V₂)
Pterygopalatine nerves
Pterygopalatine ganglion
Infra-orbital nerve
Greater and lesser palatine nerves entering palatine canals
Tympanic membrane
Stylomastoid foramen
Sympathetic plexus on internal carotid artery
Chorda tympani
Deep petrosal nerve

C Lateral view

Lacrimal gland
Lacrimal nerve (CN V₁)
Foramen rotundum
Zygomatic nerve (CN V₂)
Maxillary nerve (CN V₂)
Greater petrosal nerve (CN IX)
Pterygoid canal
Nerve to pterygoid canal
To pharynx via pharyngeal branch
Communicating branch
Pterygopalatine ganglion
To nasal cavity via sphenopalatine nerves
To nasal cavity and palate via greater & lesser palatine nerves

D Parasympathetic fibers

Course of various nerve fiber types through the pterygopalatine ganglion
— Postsynaptic sympathetic fibers
— Presynaptic parasympathetic fibers
— Postsynaptic parasympathetic fibers
— General sensory fibers

Foramen rotundum
Maxillary nerve (CN V₂)
Pterygoid canal
Deep petrosal nerve
Internal carotid artery and internal carotid periarterial plexus
Pterygopalatine branches of maxillary nerve

E Sympathetic and general sensory fibers

FIGURE 7.64. Schematic illustrations of arteries and nerves of pterygopalatine fossa. **A.** Pterygopalatine part of the maxillary nerve. **B.** Pterygopalatine part of the maxillary artery. **C.** Pterygopalatine ganglion in situ. **D.** Course of parasympathetic fibers. **E.** Course of sympathetic fibers.

The **deep petrosal nerve** is a sympathetic nerve arising from the *sympathetic plexus on the internal carotid artery* (Figs. 7.64C,E). It conveys postsynaptic fibers from nerve cell bodies in the superior cervical sympathetic ganglion. Thus these fibers do not synapse in the pterygopalatine ganglion but pass directly to join the branches of the ganglion (maxillary nerve). The postsynaptic parasympathetic and sympathetic fibers pass to the lacrimal gland and the glands of the nasal cavity, palate, and superior pharynx (Fig. 7.63C).

The **maxillary artery,** a terminal branch of the external carotid artery, passes anteriorly and traverses the infratemporal fossa. It passes over the lateral pterygoid muscle and enters the pterygopalatine fossa. The **pterygopalatine part of the maxillary artery,** its third part, passes through the *pterygomaxillary fissure* and enters the pterygopalatine fossa (Fig. 7.64*B*). The artery gives rise to branches that accompany all nerves in the fossa with the same names. The *branches of the third, or pterygopalatine, part of the maxillary artery* are the (Fig. 7.64*B*):

- Posterior superior alveolar artery.
- Descending palatine artery, which divides into greater and lesser palatine arteries.
- Artery of the pterygoid canal.
- Sphenopalatine artery, which divides into posterior lateral nasal branches to the lateral wall of the nasal cavity and its associated paranasal sinuses, and the posterior septal branches (Fig. 7.63*C*).
- Infra-orbital artery, which gives rise to the anterior superior alveolar artery and terminates as branches to the inferior eyelid, nose, and upper lip.

NOSE

The **nose** is the part of the respiratory tract superior to the hard palate and contains the peripheral organ of smell. It includes the external nose and nasal cavities, which are divided into right and left cavities by the *nasal septum* (Fig. 7.65*A*). Each nasal cavity is divisible into an *olfactory area* and a *respiratory area*. The functions of the nose and nasal cavities are:

- Olfaction (smelling).
- Respiration (breathing).
- Filtration of dust.
- Humidification of inspired air.
- Reception and elimination of secretions from the nasal mucosa, paranasal sinuses, and nasolacrimal ducts.

External Nose

The **external nose** varies considerably in size and shape, mainly because of differences in the nasal cartilages. The **dorsum of the nose** extends from its superior angle, the **root** (Fig. 7.65*A*), to the **apex** (tip) of the nose. The inferior surface of the nose is pierced by two piriform (L. pear-shaped) openings, the **nares** (nostrils, anterior nasal apertures), which are bound laterally by the **alae** (wings) of the nose and separated from each other by the **nasal septum.** The external nose consists of bony and cartilaginous parts (Fig. 7.65*B*).

The **bony part of the nose** consists of the:

- Nasal bones.
- Frontal processes of the maxillae.
- Nasal part of the frontal bone and its nasal spine.
- Bony part of the nasal septum.

The **cartilaginous part of the nose** consists of five main cartilages: two **lateral cartilages,** two **alar cartilages,** and a **septal cartilage.** The U-shaped alar cartilages are free and movable; they dilate or constrict the nares when the muscles acting on the nose contract.

A Lateral view

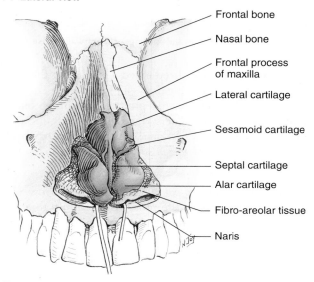

B Anterior view

FIGURE 7.65. **External nose. A.** Surface anatomy of nose. **B.** Nasal bones and cartilages (pulled inferiorly).

Nasal Cavities

The nasal cavities, entered through the nares (Fig. 7.65*A*), open posteriorly into the nasopharynx through the *choanae.* Mucosa lines the nasal cavities, except the *vestibule of the nose,* which is lined with skin (Fig. 7.66). The **nasal mucosa** is firmly bound to the periosteum and perichondrium of the supporting bones and cartilages of the nose (Fig. 7.67*A*). The mucosa is continuous with the lining of all the chambers with which the nasal cavities communicate: the nasopharynx posteriorly, the paranasal sinuses superiorly and laterally, and the lacrimal sac and conjunctiva superiorly. The inferior two thirds of the nasal mucosa is the **respiratory area,** and the superior one third is the **olfactory area** (Fig. 7.67*B*). Air passing over the respiratory area is warmed and moistened before it passes through the rest of the upper respiratory tract to the lungs. The

Frontal sinus

Openings of posterior ethmoidal sinus

Spheno-ethmoidal recess

Superior concha

Sphenoidal sinus

Rod from frontal sinus to middle meatus through frontonasal duct and ethmoidal infundibulum

Ethmoidal bulla

Semilunar hiatus

Vestibule of nose

Opening of nasolacrimal duct

Opening of middle ethmoidal sinus

Opening of pharyngo-tympanic tube

Opening of maxillary sinus (maxillary ostium)

Inferior concha

Medial view

FIGURE 7.66. **Features and openings of lateral wall of nose.** Parts of the conchae have been removed to show the openings of sinuses and other structures.

olfactory area is specialized mucosa containing the peripheral organ of smell; sniffing draws air to the area. The central processes of the olfactory receptor neurons in the olfactory epithelium unite to form nerve bundles that pass through the cribriform plate (Fig. 7.67A) and enter the **olfactory bulb.**

The *boundaries of the nasal cavity* (Fig. 7.67A) are as follows:

- The *roof of the nasal cavity* is curved and narrow, except at the posterior end; the roof is divided into three parts (frontonasal, ethmoidal, and sphenoidal), which are named from the bones that form each part.
- The *floor of the nasal cavity* is wider than the roof and is formed by the *palatine process of the maxilla* and the *horizontal plate of the palatine bone.*
- The *medial wall of the nasal cavity* is formed by the nasal septum, the main components of which are the *perpendicular plate of the ethmoid, vomer, septal cartilage,* and the *nasal crests of the maxillary and palatine bones.*
- The *lateral wall of the nasal cavity* is uneven because of the **nasal conchae (superior, middle,** and **inferior),** three elevations that project inferiorly like scrolls. The conchae curve inferomedially, each forming a roof for a **meatus,** or recess.

The **nasal conchae** (L. *shells*) divide the nasal cavity into four passages (Figs. 7.66 and 7.67A): spheno-ethmoidal recess, superior nasal meatus, middle nasal meatus, and inferior nasal meatus. The **spheno-ethmoidal recess,** lying superoposterior to the superior concha, receives the *opening of the sphenoidal sinus.* The **superior nasal meatus** is a narrow passage between the superior and the middle nasal conchae (parts of the ethmoid bone) into which the posterior ethmoidal sinuses open by one or more orifices. The **middle nasal meatus** is longer and deeper than the superior one. The anterosuperior part of this passage leads into the

ethmoidal infundibulum, an opening through which it communicates with the frontal sinus, via the **frontonasal duct.** The **semilunar hiatus** (L. *hiatus semilunaris*) is a semicircular groove into which the frontonasal duct opens. The **ethmoidal bulla** (L. bubble), a rounded elevation located superior to the semilunar hiatus, is visible when the middle concha is removed. The bulla is formed by *middle ethmoidal cells,* which constitute the *ethmoidal sinuses* (Fig. 7.68). The **maxillary sinus** also opens into the posterior end of the semilunar hiatus. The **inferior nasal meatus** is a horizontal passage, inferolateral to the inferior nasal concha (an independent, paired bone). The **nasolacrimal duct** from the lacrimal sac opens into the anterior part of this meatus.

The *arterial supply of the medial and lateral walls of the nasal cavity* is from branches of the **sphenopalatine artery, anterior and posterior ethmoidal arteries, greater palatine artery, superior labial artery,** and the **lateral nasal branches of the facial artery** (Figs. 7.63C and 7.67C). On the anterior part of the nasal septum is an area rich in capillaries (Kiesselbach area) where all five arteries supplying the septum anastomose. This area is often where profuse bleeding from the nose occurs. A rich *plexus of veins* drains deep to the nasal mucosa into the sphenopalatine, facial, and ophthalmic veins.

The *nerve supply of the posteroinferior half to two thirds of the nasal mucosa* is chiefly from CN V$_2$ by way of the **nasopalatine nerve** to the nasal septum and posterior lateral nasal branches of the **greater palatine nerve** to the lateral wall (Fig. 7.67B). The anterosuperior part of the nasal mucosa (both the septum and lateral wall) is supplied by the **anterior ethmoidal nerves,** branches of CN V$_1$.

Paranasal Sinuses

The **paranasal sinuses** are air-filled extensions of the respiratory part of the nasal cavity into the following cranial bones:

Lateral wall of nasal cavity

Nasal septum

Cribriform plate of ethmoid bone
Sphenopalatine foramen
Frontal bone
Superior concha
Superior meatus
Middle concha
Frontal process
Lacrimal bone
Middle meatus
Inferior concha
Inferior meatus
Medial pterygoid plate
Horizontal plate of palatine bone
Palatine process of maxilla
Pterygoid hamulus

A

Crista galli
Crest of sphenoid bone
Perpendicular plate of ethmoid bone
Nasal bone
Nasal spine of frontal bone
Septal cartilage
Vomer
Vomeronasal cartilage
Nasal crest of palatine bone
Nasal crest of maxilla

Anterior ethmoidal nerve
Olfactory bulb
Pterygopalatine ganglion
Nasal branch of anterior superior alveolar nerve
Maxillary nerve
Internal nasal branch of infraorbital nerve
Nerve of pterygoid canal
Nasopalatine nerve
Greater palatine nerve
Lesser palatine nerve
Pharyngeal nerve

B

Olfactory nerves in olfactory epithelium
Anterior ethmoidal nerve
Olfactory area (purple)
Respiratory area (pink)
Internal nasal branch of infraorbital nerve
CN V₁
CN V₂
Lesser palatine nerve
Greater palatine nerve
Nasopalatine nerve

Anterior ethmoidal arteries
Posterior ethmoidal arteries
Sphenopalatine artery traversing sphenopalatine foramen
Lateral nasal branches of facial artery
Greater palatine artery
Branches of sphenopalatine artery

C

Branch of sphenopalatine artery
Posterior ethmoidal arteries
Anterior ethmoidal arteries
Kiesselbach area (orange)
Incisive canal
Septal branch of superior labial artery
Greater palatine artery

Open-book views

FIGURE 7.67. Bones, arteries and nerves of lateral wall of nose and nasal septum.

Key

	Ethmoid sinus (E)
	Frontal sinus (F)
	Maxillary sinus (M)
	Sphenoid sinus (S)
HP	Hard plate
P	Pharynx

A **Medial view**

B **Left lateral radiograph**

C **Coronal CT**

Crista galli
Ethmoidal sinus
Maxillary ostium
Maxillary sinus
Nasal septum

Medial rectus
Eyeball
Middle concha
Middle meatus
Inferior concha
Inferior meatus

HP

FIGURE 7.68.   **Paranasal sinuses. A.** Location. **B.** Lateral radiograph. **C.** Coronal CT scan.

frontal, ethmoid, sphenoid, and maxilla (Fig. 7.68). They are named according to the bones in which they are located.

The **frontal sinuses** are between the outer and the inner tables of the frontal bone, posterior to the superciliary arches and the root of the nose. Each sinus drains through a **frontonasal duct** into the *ethmoidal infundibulum,* which opens into the *semilunar hiatus* of the middle meatus (Fig. 7.66). The frontal sinuses are innervated by branches of the *supraorbital nerves* (CN V$_1$).

The **ethmoidal cells (sinuses)** include several cavities that are located in the lateral mass of the ethmoid bone between the nasal cavity and the orbit. The **anterior ethmoidal cells** drain directly or indirectly into the middle meatus through the infundibulum (Fig. 7.66). The **middle ethmoidal cells** open directly into the middle meatus. The **posterior ethmoidal cells,** which form the **ethmoidal bulla,** open directly into the superior meatus. The ethmoidal sinuses are supplied by the anterior and posterior ethmoidal branches of the *nasociliary nerves* (CN V$_1$).

The **sphenoidal sinuses,** unevenly divided and separated by a bony septum, occupy the body of the sphenoid bone; they may extend into the wings of this bone in the elderly. Because of these sinuses, the body of the sphenoid is fragile. Only thin plates of bone separate the sinuses from

several important structures: the optic nerves and optic chiasm, the pituitary gland, the internal carotid arteries, and the cavernous sinuses. The *posterior ethmoidal artery* and *nerve* supply the sphenoidal sinuses.

The **maxillary sinuses** are the largest of the paranasal sinuses (Fig. 7.68). These large pyramidal cavities occupy the bodies of the maxillae. The **apex** of the maxillary sinus extends toward and often into the zygomatic bone. The **base** of the maxillary sinus forms the inferior part of the lateral wall of the nasal cavity. The **roof** of the maxillary sinus is formed by the floor of the orbit. The **floor** of the maxillary sinus is formed by the alveolar part of the maxilla. The roots of the maxillary teeth, particularly the first two molars, often produce conical elevations in the floor of the maxillary sinus. Each sinus drains by an opening, the **maxillary ostium** (Figs. 7.66 and 7.68), into the middle meatus of the nasal cavity by way of the semilunar hiatus. Because of the superior location of this opening, it is impossible for the sinus to drain when the head is erect until the sinus is full. The *arterial supply of the maxillary sinus* is mainly from superior alveolar branches of the *maxillary artery;* however, branches of the *greater palatine artery* supply the floor of the sinus. *Innervation of the maxillary sinus* is from the anterior, middle, and posterior *superior alveolar nerves* (Fig. 7.52A), branches of CN V$_2$.

Nasal Fractures

Because of the prominence of the nose, fractures of the nasal bones are common facial fractures in automobile accidents and sports (unless face guards are worn). Fractures usually result in deformation of the nose, particularly when a lateral force is applied by someone's elbow, for example. *Epistaxis* (nosebleed) usually occurs. In severe fractures, disruption of the bones and cartilages results in displacement of the nose. When the injury results from a direct blow, the cribriform plate of the ethmoid bone may also fracture, often accompanied by CSF rhinorrhea.

Deviation of Nasal Septum

The nasal septum is usually deviated to one side or the other (Fig. B7.12). This could be the result of a birth injury, but more often the deviation results during adolescence and adulthood from trauma (e.g., during a fist fight). Sometimes the deviation is so severe that the nasal septum is in contact with the lateral wall of the nasal cavity and often obstructs breathing or exacerbates snoring. The deviation can be corrected surgically.

Nasal septum deviated to left side

FIGURE B7.12.

Rhinitis

The nasal mucosa becomes swollen and inflamed (*rhinitis*) during severe upper respiratory infections and allergic reactions (e.g., hay fever). Swelling of the mucosa occurs readily because of its vascularity. Infections of the nasal cavities may spread to the:

- Anterior cranial fossa through the cribriform plate.
- Nasopharynx and retropharyngeal soft tissues.
- Middle ear through the *pharyngotympanic tube* (auditory tube), which connects the tympanic cavity and nasopharynx.
- Paranasal sinuses.
- Lacrimal apparatus and conjunctiva.

Epistaxis

Epistaxis (nosebleed) is relatively common because of the rich blood supply to the nasal mucosa (Fig. 7.67C). In most cases, the cause is trauma and the bleeding is from an area in the anterior third of the nose (Kiesselbach area). Epistaxis is also associated with infections and hypertension. Spurting of blood from the nose results from rupture of arteries. Mild epistaxis may also result from nose picking, which tears veins in the vestibule of the nose.

Sinusitis

Because the paranasal sinuses are continuous with the nasal cavities through apertures that open into them, infection may spread from the nasal cavities, producing inflammation and swelling of the mucosa of the sinuses (*sinusitis*) and local pain. Sometimes several sinuses are inflamed (*pansinusitis*), and the swelling of the mucosa may block one or more openings of the sinuses into the nasal cavities.

Infection of Ethmoidal Cells

If nasal drainage is blocked, infections of the ethmoidal cells may break through the fragile medial wall of the orbit. Severe infections from this source may cause blindness because some posterior ethmoidal cells lie close to the optic canal, which gives passage to the optic nerve and ophthalmic artery. Spread of infection from these cells could also affect the dural nerve sheath of the optic nerve, causing *optic neuritis*.

Infection of Maxillary Sinuses

The maxillary sinuses are the most commonly infected, probably because their ostia are commonly small and are located high on their superomedial walls. When the mucous membrane of the sinus is congested, the maxillary ostia are often obstructed. Because of the high location of the ostia, when the head is erect it is impossible for the sinuses to drain until they are full. Because the ostia of the right and left sinuses lie on the medial sides (i.e., are directed toward each other), when lying on one's side only the upper sinus (e.g., the right sinus if lying on the left side) drains. A cold or allergy involving both sinuses can result in nights of rolling from side-to-side in an attempt to keep the sinuses drained. A maxillary sinus can be cannulated and drained by passing a cannula from the nares through the maxillary ostium into the sinus.

Relationship of Teeth to Maxillary Sinus

The close proximity of the three maxillary molar teeth to the floor of the maxillary sinus poses potentially serious problems. During removal of a molar tooth, a fracture of a root may occur. If proper retrieval methods are not used, a piece of the root may be driven superiorly into the maxillary sinus. A communication may be created between the oral cavity and the maxillary sinus as a result, and an infection may occur.

EAR

The **ear** is divided into *external, middle,* and *internal parts* (Fig. 7.69A). The external and middle parts are mainly concerned with the transference of sound to the internal ear, which contains the organ for equilibrium (the condition of being evenly balanced) as well as for hearing. The *tympanic membrane* (eardrum) separates the external ear from the middle ear (Fig. 7.69B). The *pharyngotympanic (auditory) tube* joins the middle ear to the nasopharynx.

External Ear

The **external ear** is composed of the *auricle* (pinna), which collects sound, and the *external acoustic meatus (canal)*, which conducts sound to the tympanic membrane (Fig. 7.69B).

- External ear
- Middle ear
- Internal ear

A Coronal section

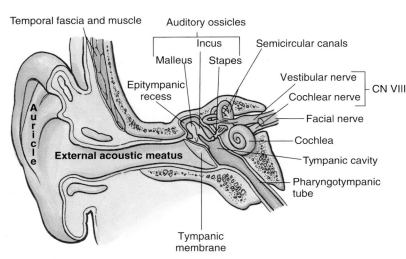

Temporal fascia and muscle

Auditory ossicles

Incus

Malleus   Stapes

Semicircular canals

Epitympanic recess

Vestibular nerve

Cochlear nerve

CN VIII

Facial nerve

Auricle

External acoustic meatus

Cochlea

Tympanic cavity

Pharyngotympanic tube

Tympanic membrane

B Coronal section

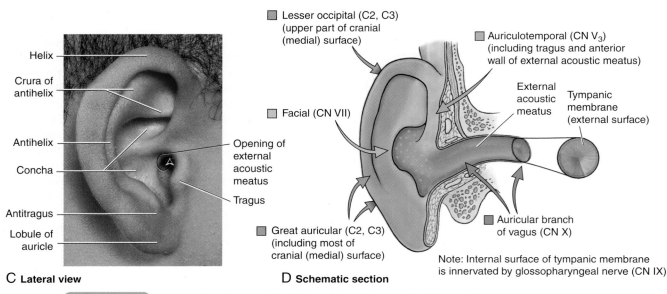

Helix

Crura of antihelix

Antihelix

Concha

Antitragus

Lobule of auricle

Opening of external acoustic meatus

Tragus

C Lateral view

- Lesser occipital (C2, C3) (upper part of cranial (medial) surface)

- Facial (CN VII)

- Great auricular (C2, C3) (including most of cranial (medial) surface)

- Auriculotemporal (CN V₃) (including tragus and anterior wall of external acoustic meatus)

External acoustic meatus

Tympanic membrane (external surface)

- Auricular branch of vagus (CN X)

Note: Internal surface of tympanic membrane is innervated by glossopharyngeal nerve (CN IX)

D Schematic section

FIGURE 7.69.   **Ear. A and B.** The external, middle, and internal ear are detailed. **C.** Surface anatomy. **D.** Innervation.

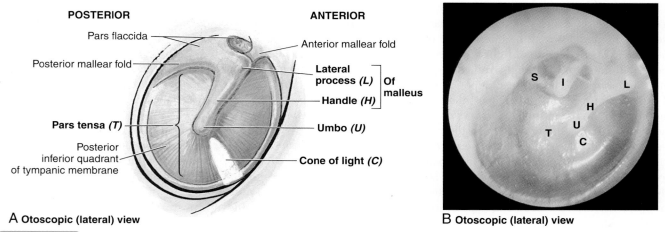

POSTERIOR   **ANTERIOR**

Pars flaccida — ...... — Anterior mallear fold

Posterior mallear fold — **Lateral process (L)** ⎤ **Of**
                                                 malleus
                                    Handle (H) ⎦

Pars tensa (T) — — **Umbo (U)**

Posterior inferior quadrant of tympanic membrane — **Cone of light (C)**

A Otoscopic (lateral) view

B Otoscopic (lateral) view

FIGURE 7.70. **Tympanic membrane and lateral approach to tympanic cavity. A.** Otoscopic view of the right tympanic membrane. The *cone of light* is a reflection of the light of the otoscope. **B.** The tympanic membrane has been rendered semitransparent and the lateral wall of the epitympanic recess has been removed to demonstrate the ossicles of the ear in situ. *I*, long limb of stapes; *S*, posterior limb if stapes.

The **auricle** (L. *auricula*) is composed of elastic cartilage covered by thin skin. The auricle has several depressions and elevations. The **concha** is the deepest depression, and the elevated margin of the auricle is the **helix** (Fig. 7.69C). The non-cartilaginous **lobule** (earlobe) consists of fibrous tissue, fat, and blood vessels. It is easily pierced for taking small blood samples and inserting earrings. The **tragus** is a tongue-like projection overlapping the opening of the external acoustic meatus. The **arterial supply** to the auricle is derived mainly from the *posterior auricular* and *superficial temporal arteries* (Fig. 7.71). The main **nerves to the skin of the auricle** are the *great auricular* and *auriculotemporal nerves* (Fig. 7.69D), with minor contributions from the facial (CN VII) and vagus (CN X) nerves.

Lymphatic drainage from the lateral surface of the superior half of the auricle is to the *superficial parotid lymph nodes*. Lymph from the cranial surface of the superior half of the auricle drains to the *mastoid* and *deep cervical lymph nodes* (Fig. 7.72). Lymph from the remainder of the auricle, including the lobule, drains to the *superficial cervical lymph nodes*.

The **external acoustic meatus** is a canal that leads inward through the tympanic part of the temporal bone from the auricle to the tympanic membrane, a distance of 2 to 3 cm in adults (Fig. 7.69B). The lateral third of this slightly S-shaped canal is cartilaginous and lined with skin, which is continuous with the skin of the auricle. Its medial two thirds is bony and lined with thin skin that is continuous with the external layer of the tympanic membrane. The ceruminous and sebaceous glands produce *cerumen* (earwax).

The **tympanic membrane,** approximately 1 cm in diameter, is a thin, oval, semitransparent membrane at the medial end of the external acoustic meatus (Fig. 7.70). It forms a partition between the meatus and the *tympanic cavity* of the middle ear. The tympanic membrane is covered with thin skin externally and the mucous membrane of the middle ear internally.

Viewed through an otoscope (an instrument used for examining the tympanic membrane), the tympanic membrane is normally translucent and pearly gray. It has a concavity toward the external acoustic meatus with a shallow, cone-like central depression, the peak of which is the **umbo**

Posterior auricular artery

Occipital artery

Superficial temporal artery

Maxillary artery

External carotid artery

Lateral view

FIGURE 7.71. **Arterial supply of auricle.**

Lymph node groups	
▨	Mastoid
▨	Parotid
▨	Superficial cervical
▨	Deep cervical

External jugular vein

FIGURE 7.72. **Lymphatic drainage of auricle.**

(Fig. 7.70). The handle of the malleus (one of the small ear bones, or auditory ossicles, of the middle ear) is usually visible near the umbo. From the inferior end of the handle of the malleus, a bright **cone of light** is reflected from the otoscope's illuminator. This light reflex is visible, radiating antero-inferiorly in a healthy ear. Superior to the attachment of the lateral process of the malleus, the membrane is thin and is called the **flaccid part** (L. *pars flaccida*). It lacks the radial and circular fibers present in the remainder of the tympanic membrane, called the **tense part** (L. *pars tensa*).

The tympanic membrane moves in response to air vibrations that pass to it through the external acoustic meatus. Movements of the membrane are transmitted by the **auditory ossicles** (malleus, incus, and stapes) through the middle ear to the internal ear (Fig. 7.73). The external surface of the tympanic membrane is supplied mainly by the *auriculotemporal nerve,* a branch of CN V$_3$ (Fig. 7.69D). Some innervation is supplied by a small *auricular branch of the vagus nerve* (CN X). The internal surface of the tympanic membrane is supplied by the *glossopharyngeal nerve* (CN IX).

Middle Ear

The **cavity of the middle ear**, or **tympanic cavity,** is the narrow air-filled chamber in the petrous part of the temporal bone. The cavity has two parts: the **tympanic cavity proper,** the space directly internal to the tympanic membrane, and the **epitympanic recess,** the space superior to the membrane (Fig. 7.73A,B). The tympanic cavity is connected anteromedially with the nasopharynx by the **pharyngotympanic tube** and posterosuperiorly with the **mastoid antrum.** The tympanic cavity is lined with mucous membrane, which is continuous with the lining of the pharyngotympanic tube, mastoid cells, and mastoid antrum.

The contents of the middle ear are the:

- Auditory ossicles: malleus, incus, and stapes.
- Stapedius and tensor tympani muscles.
- Chorda tympani nerve, a branch of CN VII.
- Tympanic plexus of nerves.

WALLS OF TYMPANIC CAVITY

The middle ear, shaped like a narrow box with concave sides, has six walls (Figs. 7.73 and 7.74):

- The **tegmental wall (roof)** is formed by a thin plate of temporal bone, the *tegmen tympani,* which separates the tympanic cavity from the dura mater on the floor of the middle cranial fossa.
- The **jugular wall (floor)** is formed by a layer of bone that separates the tympanic cavity from the superior bulb of the IJV.
- The **membranous wall (lateral wall)** is formed almost entirely by the peaked convexity of the *tympanic membrane;* superiorly, it is formed by the lateral bony wall of

the **epitympanic recess.** The handle of the malleus is attached to the tympanic membrane, and its head extends into the epitympanic recess.

- The **labyrinthine wall (medial wall)** separates the tympanic cavity from the internal ear. It also features the *promontory of the labyrinthine wall,* formed by the initial part (basal turn) of the cochlea, and the *oval* and *round windows.*
- The **carotid wall (anterior wall)** separates the tympanic cavity from the carotid canal, which contains the internal carotid artery; superiorly it has the **opening of the pharyngotympanic tube** and the **canal for the tensor tympani muscle.**
- The **mastoid wall (posterior wall)** has an opening in its superior part, the **aditus** (L. access) **to the mastoid antrum,** connecting the tympanic cavity to the mastoid cells; the canal for the facial nerve descends between the posterior wall and the antrum, medial to the aditus. The tendon of the **stapedius muscle** emerges from the apex of the **pyramidal eminence,** a hollow, bony cone enclosing the stapedius muscle.

The **mastoid antrum** is a cavity in the mastoid process of the temporal bone (Fig. 7.74). The mastoid antrum is separated from the middle cranial fossa by the thin plate of temporal bone called the **tegmen tympani.** The tegmen tympani forms part of the *tegmental wall* of the tympanic cavity and part of the floor of the middle cranial fossa lateral. The mastoid antrum is the common cavity into which the mastoid cells open. The antrum and mastoid cells are lined by mucous membrane, which is continuous with the lining of the middle ear. Antero-inferiorly, the mastoid antrum is related to the canal for the facial nerve.

AUDITORY OSSICLES

The **auditory ossicles** (malleus, incus, and stapes) form a mobile chain of small bones across the tympanic cavity from the tympanic membrane to the **oval window** (L. *fenestra vestibuli*), an oval opening on the labyrinthine wall of the tympanic cavity leading to the vestibule of the bony labyrinth (Fig. 7.73B). The ossicles are covered with the mucous membrane lining the tympanic cavity, but unlike other bones of the body, they are not directly covered with a layer of periosteum.

The **malleus** (L. hammer) is attached to the tympanic membrane (Fig. 7.73C). The rounded superior **head** of the malleus lies in the epitympanic recess. The **neck** lies against the flaccid part of the tympanic membrane, and the **handle** is embedded in the tympanic membrane with its tip at the umbo. The head of the malleus articulates with the incus; the tendon of the tensor tympani inserts into the handle of the malleus. The *chorda tympani nerve* crosses the medial surface of the neck of the malleus.

The **incus** (L. anvil) is located between the malleus and the stapes and articulates with them (Fig. 7.73B,D). The

A Anterior view

Epitympanic recess

Malleus
Incus
Stapes

Chorda tympani nerve

Tensor tympani

Tympanic membrane

1

3

5

2

Lesser petrosal nerve

Prominence of lateral semicircular canal

Facial nerve

Aditus to mastoid antrum (forming posterior wall)

Prominence of canal for facial nerve

Tympanic plexus on promontory of labyrinthine wall

Stapedius
Pyramidal eminence

Tympanic nerve (from CN IX)

Key

1.	Tegmental wall (roof)
2.	Jugular wall (floor)
3.	Membranous (lateral) wall
4.	Labyrinthine (medial) wall
5.	Mastoid (posterior) wall
	Carotid (anterior) wall was removed to provide this view

B Coronal section, anterior view

Incus

Epitympanic recess

Malleus

External acoustic meatus

Tympanic membrane

Base of stapes

Oval window

Stapes

Tympanic cavity

Pharyngotympanic tube

C Posteromedial view

Head

Neck

Lateral process

Handle

D Posterior view

Body

Short limb

Long limb

Lenticular process

E Superolateral view

Neck

Anterior limb

Head

Posterior limb

Base (footplate)

FIGURE 7.73. **Auditory ossicles. A.** Walls of the right tympanic cavity. **B.** Ossicles in situ. Features of: **C.** Malleus. **D.** Incus. **E.** Stapes.

body of the incus lies in the epitympanic recess where it articulates with the head of the malleus. The **long limb** lies parallel to the handle of the malleus, and its inferior end articulates with the stapes by way of the **lenticular process.** The **short limb** is connected by a ligament to the posterior wall of the tympanic cavity. The **base of the stapes** fits into the oval window on the medial wall of the tympanic cavity.

The **stapes** (L. a stirrup) is the smallest ossicle (Fig. 7.73E). The **base** (footplate) of the stapes is attached to the margins of the oval window. The base is considerably smaller than the tympanic membrane; as a result, the vibratory force of the stapes is increased approximately 10 times over that of the tympanic membrane. Consequently, the auditory ossicles increase the force but decrease the amplitude of the vibrations transmitted from the tympanic membrane.

Two muscles dampen or resist movements of the auditory ossicles; one also dampens movements (vibrations) of the tympanic membrane. The **tensor tympani** is a short muscle that arises from the superior surface of the cartilaginous part of the pharyngotympanic tube, the greater wing of the sphenoid, and the petrous part of temporal bone (Figs. 7.73A and 7.74). The tensor tympani inserts into the handle of the malleus. The tensor tympani, supplied by CN V_3, pulls the handle of the malleus medially, tensing the tympanic membrane and reducing the amplitude of its oscillations. This action tends to prevent damage to the internal ear when one is exposed to loud sounds. The **stapedius** is a tiny muscle inside the **pyramidal eminence** (pyramid), a hollow, cone-shaped prominence on the posterior wall of the tympanic cavity (Fig. 7.73A). Its tendon enters the

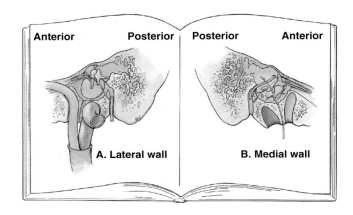

Anterior Posterior | Posterior Anterior

A. Lateral wall **B. Medial wall**

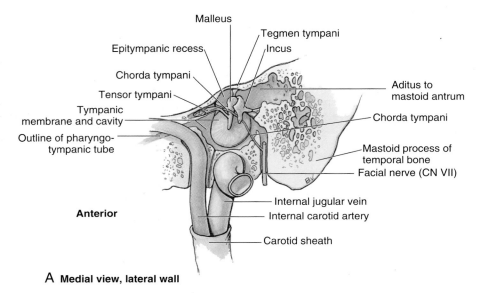

Malleus

Tegmen tympani

Epitympanic recess

Incus

Chorda tympani

Aditus to mastoid antrum

Tensor tympani

Tympanic membrane and cavity

Chorda tympani

Outline of pharyngo-tympanic tube

Mastoid process of temporal bone

Facial nerve (CN VII)

Internal jugular vein

Anterior

Internal carotid artery

Carotid sheath

A **Medial view, lateral wall**

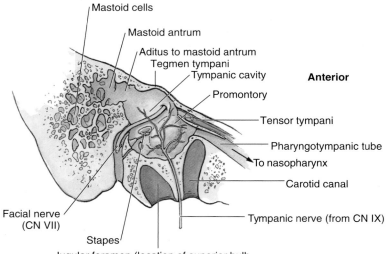

Mastoid cells

Mastoid antrum

Aditus to mastoid antrum

Tegmen tympani

Tympanic cavity

Anterior

Promontory

Tensor tympani

Pharyngotympanic tube

To nasopharynx

Carotid canal

Facial nerve (CN VII)

Tympanic nerve (from CN IX)

Stapes

Jugular foramen (location of superior bulb of internal jugular vein)

B **Lateral view, medial wall**

FIGURE 7.74. Dissections of right middle ear.

tympanic cavity by emerging from a small foramen in the apex of the pyramidal eminence and inserts on the neck of the stapes. The nerve to the stapedius arises from CN VII. The stapedius pulls the stapes posteriorly and tilts its base in the *oval window*, thereby tightening the anular ligament and reducing the oscillatory range. It also prevents excessive movement of the stapes.

PHARYNGOTYMPANIC TUBE

The **pharyngotympanic tube** connects the tympanic cavity to the nasopharynx (Figs. 7.74*B* and 7.75), where it opens posterior to the inferior nasal meatus. The posterolateral third of the tube is bony and the remainder is cartilaginous. The pharyngotympanic tube is lined by mucous membrane, which is continuous posteriorly with the lining of the tympanic cavity and anteriorly with the lining of the nasopharynx. The function of the pharyngotympanic tube is to equalize pressure in the middle ear with the atmospheric pressure, thereby allowing free movement of the tympanic membrane. By allowing air to enter and leave the tympanic cavity, this tube balances the pressure on both sides of the membrane. Because the walls of the cartilaginous part of the tube are normally in apposition, the tube must be actively opened. The tube is opened by the expanding girth of the belly of the *levator veli palatini* as it contracts longitudinally, pushing against one wall while the *tensor veli palatini* pulls on the

other (Fig. 7.75). Because these are muscles of the soft palate, equalizing pressure "popping the eardrums" is commonly associated with activities such as yawning and swallowing.

The **arteries** of the pharyngotympanic tube are derived from the *ascending pharyngeal artery*, a branch of the external carotid artery, the *middle meningeal artery*, and the *artery of the pterygoid canal*, branches of the maxillary artery (Fig. 7.43). The **veins** of the pharyngotympanic tube drain into the *pterygoid venous plexus*. The **nerves** of the pharyngotympanic tube arise from the *tympanic plexus* (Fig. 7.73), which is formed by fibers of CN IX. The anterior part of the tube also receives nerve fibers from the *pterygopalatine ganglion*.

Internal Ear

The **internal ear** contains the **vestibulocochlear organ** concerned with the reception of sound and the maintenance of balance. Buried in the petrous part of the temporal bone (Figs. 7.76 and 7.77*A*), the internal ear consists of the sacs and ducts of the membranous labyrinth. The *membranous labyrinth*, containing *endolymph*, is suspended within the perilymph-filled *bony labyrinth*, either by delicate filaments similar to the filaments of the arachnoid mater that traverse the subarachnoid space or by the spiral ligament. These fluids are involved in stimulating the end organs for balance and hearing, respectively.

BONY LABYRINTH

The **bony labyrinth** is a series of cavities (cochlea, vestibule, and semicircular canals) contained within the otic capsule of the petrous part of the temporal bone (Figs. 7.76 and 7.77*B*). The **otic capsule** is made of bone that is denser than the remainder of the petrous temporal bone and can be isolated from it using a dental drill. The otic capsule is often erroneously illustrated and identified as being the bony labyrinth. However, the bony labyrinth is the *fluid-filled space* that is surrounded by the otic capsule; it is most accurately represented by a cast of the otic capsule after removal of the surrounding bone (Fig. 7.77*C*).

The **cochlea** is the shell-shaped part of the bony labyrinth that contains the **cochlear duct,** the part of the internal ear concerned with hearing (Figs. 7.76 and 7.77*B*). The **spiral canal** of the cochlea begins at the vestibule and makes 2.5 turns around a bony core, the **modiolus** (Fig. 7.78). The modiolus contains canals for blood vessels and for the distribution of the branches of the cochlear nerve (Fig. 7.76). The large basal turn of the cochlea produces the *promontory of the labyrinthine wall* of the tympanic cavity. At the basal turn, the bony labyrinth communicates with the subarachnoid space superior to the jugular foramen through the **cochlear aqueduct** (Fig. 7.76). It also features the **round window,** closed by the **secondary tympanic membrane.**

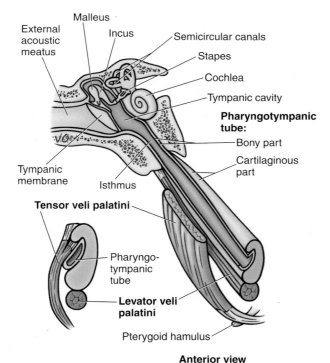

Anterior view

FIGURE 7.75. **Right pharyngotympanic tube.** The tube is open throughout its length by removing its membranous wall and the lateral part of its bony wall.

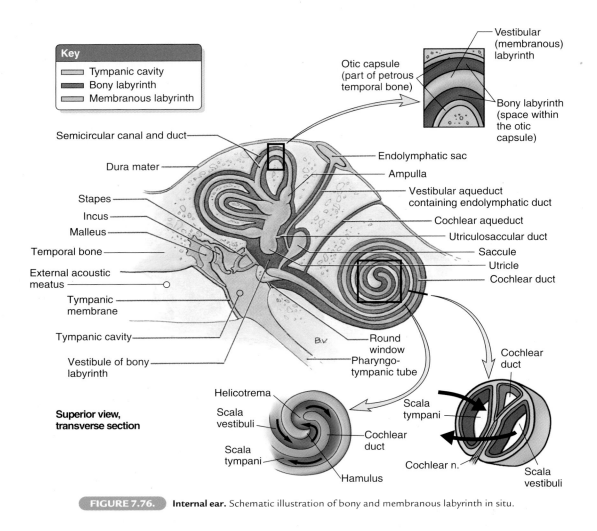

Key
- Tympanic cavity
- Bony labyrinth
- Membranous labyrinth

Semicircular canal and duct

Dura mater

Stapes

Incus

Malleus

Temporal bone

External acoustic meatus

Tympanic membrane

Tympanic cavity

Vestibule of bony labyrinth

Superior view, transverse section

Otic capsule (part of petrous temporal bone)

Vestibular (membranous) labyrinth

Bony labyrinth (space within the otic capsule)

Endolymphatic sac

Ampulla

Vestibular aqueduct containing endolymphatic duct

Cochlear aqueduct

Utriculosaccular duct

Saccule

Utricle

Cochlear duct

B.V.

Round window

Pharyngo-tympanic tube

Cochlear duct

Helicotrema

Scala vestibuli

Scala tympani

Cochlear duct

Hamulus

Scala tympani

Cochlear n.

Scala vestibuli

FIGURE 7.76.   **Internal ear.** Schematic illustration of bony and membranous labyrinth in situ.

The **vestibule of the bony labyrinth** is a small oval chamber (approximately 5 mm long) that contains the **utricle** and **saccule** and parts of the balancing apparatus (vestibular labyrinth) (Fig. 7.76). The vestibule features the *oval window* on its lateral wall, occupied by the base of the stapes. The vestibule is continuous with the bony cochlea anteriorly, the semicircular canals posteriorly, and the posterior cranial fossa by the **vestibular aqueduct.** The aqueduct extends to the posterior surface of the petrous part of the temporal bone, where it opens posterolateral to the *internal acoustic meatus.* The vestibular aqueduct transmits the **endolymphatic duct** and two small blood vessels.

The **semicircular canals** (anterior, posterior, and lateral) communicate with the vestibule of the bony labyrinth. The canals lie posterosuperior to the vestibule into which they open and are set at right angles to each other. They occupy three planes in space (Figs. 7.76 and 7.77*B*). Each semicircular canal forms about two thirds of a circle and is about 1.5 mm in diameter, except at one end where there is a swelling, the **bony ampulla.** The canals have only five openings into the

vestibule because the anterior and posterior canals share a common limb to both. Lodged within the canals are the *semicircular ducts* of the membranous labyrinth (Fig. 7.77*C,D*).

MEMBRANOUS LABYRINTH

The **membranous labyrinth** consists of a series of communicating sacs and ducts that are suspended in the bony labyrinth (Figs. 7.76 and 7.77*C,D*). The membranous labyrinth contains **endolymph,** a watery fluid similar in composition to intracellular fluid, thus differing in composition from the surrounding **perilymph** (which is like extracellular fluid), which fills the remainder of the bony labyrinth. The membranous labyrinth is composed of two divisions, the *vestibular labyrinth* and the *cochlear labyrinth,* and consists of more parts than does the bony labyrinth:

- **Vestibular labyrinth**—utricle and saccule, two small communicating sacs in the vestibule of the bony labyrinth.
- Three **semicircular ducts** in the semicircular canals.
- **Cochlear labyrinth**—cochlear duct in the cochlea.

The **spiral ligament**, a spiral thickening of the periosteal lining of the cochlear canal, secures the cochlear duct to the spiral canal of the cochlea (Fig. 7.78).

The **semicircular ducts** open into the *utricle* through five openings, reflecting the way the surrounding semicircular canals open into the vestibule. The utricle communicates with the saccule through the **utriculosaccular duct,** from which the *endolymphatic duct* arises (Fig. 7.76). The *saccule* is continuous with the cochlear duct through the **ductus reunions,** a uniting duct (Fig. 7.77*B*). The utricle and saccule have specialized areas of sensory epithelium called *maculae*. The **macula of the utricle** (L. *macula utriculi*) is in the floor of the utricle, parallel to the base of the cranium (Fig. 7.77*D*), whereas the **macula of the saccule** (L. *macula sacculi*) is vertically placed on the medial wall of the saccule. The **hair cells in the maculae** are innervated by fibers of the **vestibular division of the vestibulocochlear nerve** (CN VIII). The cell bodies of the sensory neurons are in the **vestibular ganglia,** which are in the internal acoustic meatus (Fig. 7.79).

The *endolymphatic duct* traverses the vestibular aqueduct and emerges through the bone of the posterior cranial fossa, where it expands into a blind pouch called the **endolymphatic sac.** It is located under the dura on the posterior surface of the petrous part of the temporal bone (Fig. 7.77*A,D*). The endolymphatic sac is a storage reservoir for excess endolymph formed by the blood capillaries in the membranous labyrinth.

Each **semicircular duct** has an **ampulla** at one end containing a sensory area, the **ampullary** crest (L. *crista ampullaris*) (Figs. 7.77 and 7.79). The crests are sensors for recording movements of the endolymph in the ampulla, resulting from rotation of the head in the plane of the duct. The hair cells of the crest, like those of the maculae, stimulate primary sensory neurons whose cell bodies are in the *vestibular ganglia.*

The **cochlear duct** is a spiral, blind tube, closed at one end and triangular in cross-section (Fig. 7.76). The duct is firmly suspended across the cochlear canal between the *spiral ligament* on the external wall of the cochlear canal and the **osseous spiral lamina** of the modiolus (Fig. 7.78). Spanning the spiral canal in this manner, the endolymph-filled cochlear duct divides the perilymph-filled spiral canal into two channels that communicate at the apex of the cochlea at the **helicotrema** (Fig. 7.76).

Waves of hydraulic pressure created in the perilymph of the vestibule by the vibrations of the base of the stapes ascend to the apex of the cochlea by one channel, the **scala vestibuli** (Fig. 7.80). The pressure waves then pass through the helicotrema and then descend back to the basal turn of the cochlea by the other channel, the **scala tympani.** There the pressure waves again become vibrations, this time of the *secondary tympanic membrane*, which occupies the round window. Here the energy initially received by the (primary) tympanic membrane is finally dissipated into the air of the tympanic cavity.

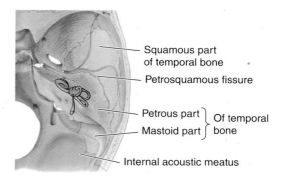

A Superior view of internal surface of cranial base

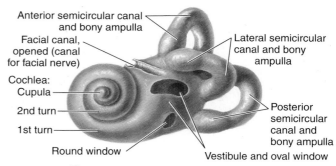

B Anterolateral view of left otic capsule

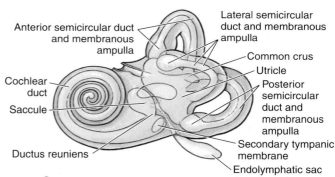

C Anterolateral view of left membranous labyrinth (through transparent otic capsule)

D Anterolateral view of left membranous labyrinth

FIGURE 7.77. Bony and membranous labyrinth of internal ear.

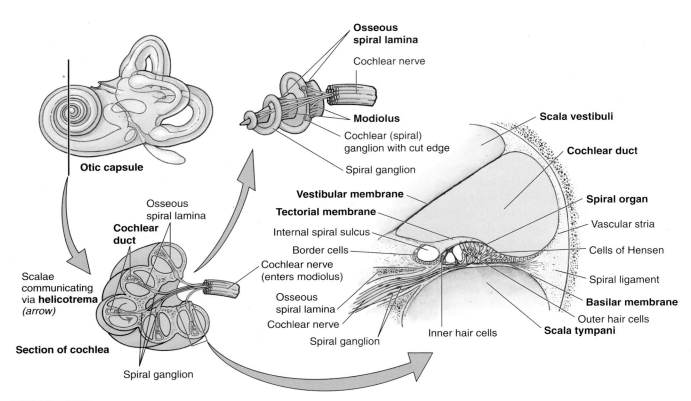

FIGURE 7.78. **Structure of cochlea.** The cochlea has been sectioned along the axis about which the cochlea winds (see the orientation figure in the upper left). An isolated, cone-like, bony core of the cochlea, the modiolus, is shown after the turns of the cochlea are removed, leaving only the spiral lamina winding around it like the thread of a screw. Details of the area enclosed in the rectangle are also shown.

The roof of the cochlear duct is formed by the **vestibular membrane** (Fig. 7.78). The floor of the duct is formed by part of the duct, the **basilar membrane,** plus the outer edge of the osseous spiral lamina. The receptor of auditory stimuli is the **spiral organ** (of Corti), situated on the basilar membrane. It is overlaid by the gelatinous **tectorial membrane.** The spiral organ contains hair cells, the tips of which are embedded in the tectorial membrane. The spiral organ is stimulated to respond by deformation of the cochlear duct induced by hydraulic pressure waves in the perilymph, which ascend and descend in the surrounding scala vestibuli and tympani (Fig. 7.80).

INTERNAL ACOUSTIC MEATUS

The **internal acoustic meatus** is a narrow canal that runs laterally for approximately 1 cm within the petrous part of the temporal bone (Fig. 7.77A). The **internal acoustic**

FIGURE 7.79. **Vestibulocochlear nerve (CN VIII).**

FIGURE 7.80. **Sound transmission through the ear.** The cochlea is depicted schematically as if consisting of a single coil to demonstrate the transmission of sound stimuli through the ear. 1. Sound waves entering the external ear strike the tympanic membrane, causing it to vibrate. 2. Vibrations initiated at the tympanic membrane are transmitted through the ossicles of the middle ear and their articulations. 3. The base of the stapes vibrates with increased strength and decreased amplitude in the oval window. 4. Vibrations of the base of the stapes create pressure waves in the perilymph of the scala vestibuli. 5. Pressure waves in the scala vestibuli cause displacement of the basilar membrane of the cochlear duct. Short waves (high pitch) cause displacement near the oval window; longer waves (low pitch) cause more distant displacement, nearer the helicotrema at the apex of the cochlea. Movement of the basilar membrane bends the hair cells of the spiral organ. Neurotransmitter is released, stimulating action potentials conveyed by the cochlear nerve to the brain. 6. Vibrations are transferred across the cochlear duct to the perilymph of the scala tympani. 7. Pressure waves in the perilymph are dissipated (dampened) by the secondary tympanic membrane at the round window into the air of the tympanic cavity.

opening of the meatus is in the posteromedial part of this bone, in line with the external acoustic meatus. The internal acoustic meatus is closed laterally by a thin, perforated plate of bone that separates it from the internal ear. The facial nerve (CN VII), the vestibulocochlear nerve (CN VIII), and

blood vessels pass through this plate of bone. The vestibulocochlear nerve divides near the lateral end of the internal acoustic meatus into two parts: a **cochlear nerve** and a **vestibular nerve** (Fig. 7.79). Sound transmission through the ear is summarized in Figure 7.80.

External Ear Injury

 Bleeding within the auricle resulting from trauma may produce an *auricular hematoma*. A localized collection of blood forms between the perichondrium and the auricular cartilage, causing distortion of the contours of the auricle. As the hematoma enlarges, it compromises the blood supply to the cartilage. If untreated (e.g., by aspiration of blood), fibrosis (formation of fibrous tissue) develops in the overlying skin, forming a deformed auricle (e.g., the cauliflower or boxer's ear of some professional fighters).

Otoscopic Examination

Examination of the external acoustic meatus and tympanic membrane begins by straightening the meatus. In adults, the helix is

grasped and pulled posterosuperiorly (up, out, and back). These movements reduce the curvature of the external acoustic meatus, facilitating insertion of the *otoscope* (Fig. B7.13*A*).

The meatus is relatively short in infants; therefore, extra care must be exercised to prevent injury to the tympanic membrane. The meatus is straightened in infants by pulling the auricle inferoposteriorly (down and back). The examination also provides a clue to tenderness, which can indicate inflammation of the auricle and/or the meatus.

The tympanic membrane is normally translucent and pearly gray (Fig. B7.13*B*). The handle of the malleus is usually visible near the center of the membrane (the umbo). From the inferior end of the handle, a bright *cone of light* is reflected from the otoscope's illuminator. This *light reflex* is visible radiating antero-inferiorly in the healthy ear.

FIGURE B7.13. *1*, cone of light; *2*, handle of malleus; *3*, umbo; *4*, long limb of fincus; *5*, posterior limb of stapes.

Acute Otitis Externa

Otitis externa is an inflammation of the external acoustic meatus. The infection often develops in swimmers who do not dry their meatus after swimming and/or use ear drops, but it may also be the result of a bacterial infection of the skin lining the meatus. The affected individual complains of itching and pain in the external ear. Pulling the auricle or applying pressure on the tragus increases the pain.

Otitis Media

An earache and a bulging red tympanic membrane may indicate pus or fluid in the middle ear, a sign of *otitis media* (Fig. B7.14*A*). Infection of the middle ear is often secondary to upper respiratory infections.

Inflammation and swelling of the mucous membrane lining the tympanic cavity may cause partial or complete blockage of the pharyngotympanic tube. The tympanic membrane becomes red and bulges, and the person may complain of "ear popping." An amber-colored bloody fluid may be observed through the tympanic membrane. If untreated, otitis media may produce impaired hearing

as the result of scarring of the auditory ossicles, limiting their ability to move in response to sound.

Perforation of Tympanic Membrane

Perforation of the tympanic membrane ("ruptured eardrum") may result from otitis media and is one of several causes of middle ear deafness. Perforation may also result from foreign bodies in the external acoustic meatus, trauma, or excessive pressure (e.g., during scuba diving).

Minor ruptures of the tympanic membrane often heal spontaneously. Large ruptures usually require surgical repair. Because the superior half of the tympanic membrane is much more vascular than the inferior half, incisions to release pus from a middle ear abscess (*myringotomy*), for example, are made posteroinferiorly through the membrane (Fig. B7.14*B*). This incision also avoids injury to the chorda tympani nerve and auditory ossicles. In persons with chronic middle ear infections, myringotomy may be followed by insertion of *tympanostomy or pressure-equalization (PE) tubes* in the incision to enable drainage of effusion and ventilation of pressure (Fig. B7.14*C*).

A **Otitis media**

B **Myringotomy incision**

C **Tympanostomy tube inserted**

FIGURE B7.14. Manubrium of Malleus – handle of malleous.

Medical Imaging of Head

Radiography, although replaced by newer imaging modalities in many specific cases, is often used for cranial examinations. Because crania vary considerably in shape, one must examine radiographs carefully for abnormalities (Fig. 7.81A,B). To visualize the arteries of the brain, a radiopaque contrast medium is injected into the carotid or vertebral artery and radiographs are taken, producing *arteriograms* (Fig. 7.81C). This type of radiograph is used for detecting cerebral aneurysms and arteriovenous malformations.

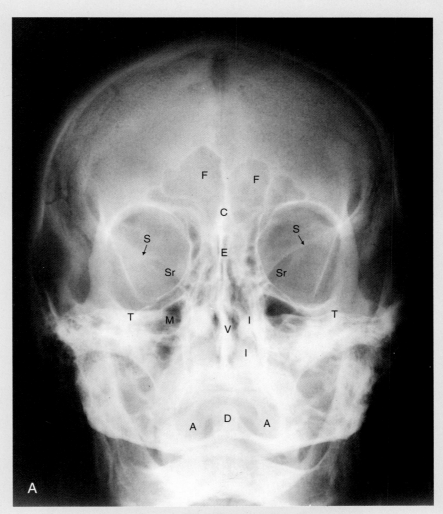

Anteroposterior view

FIGURE 7.81.   **Radiographs of cranium (skull). A.** The lateral masses of the atlas (*A*) and the dens of the axis (*D*) are superimposed on the facial skeleton (viscerocranium). Also identified are: crista galli (*C*), nasal septum formed by the perpendicular plate of the ethmoid (*E*) and the vomer (*V*); frontal sinus (*F*); inferior and middle conchae (*I*) of lateral wall of the nasal cavity; maxillary sinus (*M*); lesser wings of sphenoid (*S*); superior orbital fissure (*Sr*); and superior surface of petrous part of temporal bone (*T*).

Lateral radiograph

Lateral arteriogram

FIGURE 7.81. **Radiographs of cranium** *(Continued).* **B.** Identified are: anterior arch of the atlas (*A*); paranasal sinuses: ethmoidal (*E*), frontal (*F*), maxillary (*M*), sphenoidal (*S*), and mastoid cells (*Mc*); hypophysial fossa (*H*) for the pituitary gland; bony grooves for the branches of the middle meningeal vessels (*Mn*); nasopharynx (*N*); and the petrous part of the temporal bone (*T*). The right and left orbital parts of the frontal bone are not superimposed; thus the floor of the anterior cranial fossa appears as two lines (*L*). (Courtesy of Dr. E. Becker, Associate Professor of Diagnostic Imaging, University of Toronto, Toronto, Ontario, Canada.) **C.** Vertebrobasilar arteriogram. Identified are: the anterior cerebral artery (*A*), internal carotid artery (*I*), middle cerebral artery (*M*), and ophthalmic artery (*O*).

MRI is slower (longer acquisition time) and more expensive than CT but shows much more detail in the soft tissues than does CT (Fig. 7.82). MRI is the gold standard for detecting and delineating intracranial and spinal lesions because it provides good soft tissue contrast of normal and pathological structures. It also permits multiplanar capability, which provides three-dimensional information and relationships that are not so readily available with CT. MRI can also demonstrate blood and CSF flow. Magnetic resonance angiography (MRA) is useful for determining the patency of vessels of the cerebral arterial circle.

Orientation drawing for A

A Coronal MRI

Frontal lobe
Superior rectus
Lacrimal gland
Eyeball
Medial rectus
Inferior rectus
Middle concha
Nasal septum
Inferior concha
Maxillary sinus
Tongue

Orientation drawing for B

B Sagittal MRI

Cerebral hemisphere
Corpus callosum
Thalamus
Hypothalamus and pituitary gland
Midbrain
Pons
Fourth ventricle
Cerebellum
Medulla oblongata
Spinal cord

FIGURE 7.82.   MRI studies of head.

C **Transverse section of cadaveric head**

D **Transverse (axial) MRI scan**

1	Nasal bones	7	Posterior ethmoidal air cell	13	Retrobulbar fat
2	Angular artery	8	Sphenoidal sinus	14	Anterior chamber
3	Frontal process of maxilla	9	Orbicularis oculi muscle	15	Lens
4	Nasal septum	10	Medial rectus muscle	16	Vitreous body
5	Anterior ethmoidal air cell	11	Lateral rectus muscle	17	Optic nerve
6	Middle ethmoidal air cell	12	Cornea	18	Optic chiasm

19	Optic tract
20	Temporalis muscle
21	Superficial temporal vessels
22	Greater wing of sphenoid
23	Squamous portion of temporal bone

E **Transverse section of cadaveric head**

F **Transverse (axial) MRI scan**

1	Orbicularis oris muscle	12	Ramus of mandible	23	Transverse ligament of atlas
2	Levator anguli oris muscle	13	Lateral pterygoid muscle	24	Spinal cord
3	Facial artery and vein	14	Parotid gland	25	Vertebral artery in foramina transversaria
4	Zygomaticus major muscle	15	Superficial temporal vessels	26	Longus colli muscle
5	Buccinator muscle	16	Region of pharyngeal tubercle	27	Longus capitis muscle
6	Maxilla	17	Sphenoid bone	28	Internal carotid artery
7	Alveolar process of maxilla	18	Stylohyoid ligament and muscle	29	Internal jugular vein
8	Dorsum of tongue	19	Posterior belly of digastric muscle	30	Interior portion of helix of auricle
9	Soft palate	20	Occipital artery	a	Hard palate
10	Masseter muscle	21	First cervical vertebra (Atlas)	b	Palatoglossus muscle
11	Retromandibular vein	22	Dens (Axis)	c	Palatopharyngeus muscle

FIGURE 7.82.   MRI studies of head. (*continued*)

 Go to http://thePoint.lww.com/ECA4e for helpful study tools, including USMLE-style questions, case studies, images, and more!

Neck

FASCIA OF NECK / 594
Cervical Subcutaneous Tissue and Platysma / 594
Deep Cervical Fascia / 594

SUPERFICIAL STRUCTURES OF NECK: CERVICAL REGIONS / 596
Sternocleidomastoid Region / 596
Posterior Cervical Region / 598
Lateral Cervical Region / 598
Anterior Cervical Region / 604
■ Surface Anatomy of Cervical Regions and Triangles of Neck / 611

DEEP STRUCTURES OF NECK / 613
Prevertebral Muscles / 613
Root of Neck / 613

VISCERA OF NECK / 619
Endocrine Layer of Cervical Viscera / 619
Respiratory Layer of Cervical Viscera / 623
■ Surface Anatomy of Larynx / 624
Alimentary Layer of Cervical Viscera / 631

LYMPHATICS IN NECK / 638
MEDICAL IMAGING OF NECK / 641

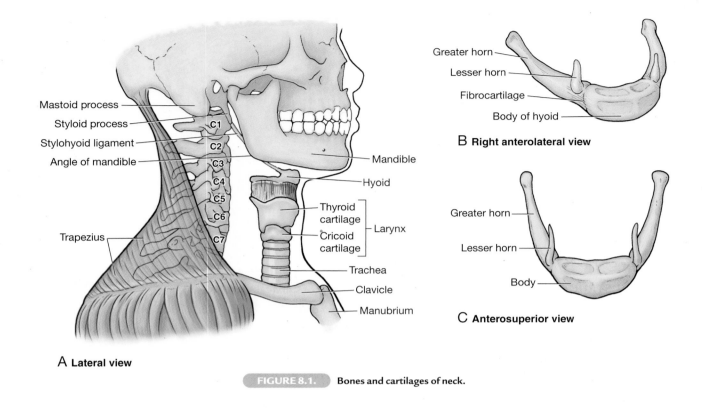

Mastoid process
Styloid process
Stylohyoid ligament
Angle of mandible

C1
C2
C3
C4
C5
C6
C7

Trapezius

Mandible

Hyoid

Thyroid cartilage
Cricoid cartilage
} Larynx

Trachea

Clavicle

Manubrium

A Lateral view

Greater horn
Lesser horn
Fibrocartilage
Body of hyoid

B Right anterolateral view

Greater horn

Lesser horn

Body

C Anterosuperior view

FIGURE 8.1. Bones and cartilages of neck.

The **neck** (L. *collum, cervix*) joins the head to the trunk and limbs and serves as a major conduit for structures passing between them. In addition, several important organs with unique functions are located here: the larynx, thyroid, and parathyroid glands, for example.

The *skeleton of the neck* is formed by the cervical vertebrae (C1–C7), **hyoid bone** (referred to as the *hyoid* in common usage), manubrium of the sternum, and clavicles (Fig. 8.1A). The mobile hyoid lies in the anterior part of the neck at the level of the C3 vertebra in the angle between the mandible and thyroid cartilage. The hyoid does not articulate with any other bone and functionally serves as an attachment for anterior neck muscles and a prop to keep the airway open (Fig. 8.1B, C).

FASCIA OF NECK

Structures in the neck are surrounded by a layer of fatty subcutaneous tissue (superficial fascia) and are compartmentalized by layers of deep cervical fascia. The fascial planes determine the direction in which an infection in the neck may spread.

Cervical Subcutaneous Tissue and Platysma

The **subcutaneous tissue of the neck** (superficial cervical fascia) is usually a thin layer of connective tissue that lies between the dermis of the skin and the investing layer of deep cervical fascia (Fig. 8.2B, C). It contains cutaneous nerves, blood and lymphatic vessels, superficial lymph nodes, and variable amounts of fat; anterolaterally, it contains the platysma.

The **platysma,** a muscle of facial expression, arises in subcutaneous tissue covering the superior parts of the deltoid and pectoralis major muscles and sweeps superomedially over the clavicle to the inferior border of the mandible (Fig. 8.2C).

Deep Cervical Fascia

The **deep cervical fascia** consists of three fascial layers (Fig. 8.2): *investing, pretracheal,* and *prevertebral.* These layers support the viscera (e.g., the thyroid gland), muscles, vessels, and deep lymph nodes. These fascial layers provide the slipperiness that allows structures in the neck to move and pass over one another without difficulty (e.g., when swallowing and turning the head and neck). These fascial

Buccopharyngeal fascia (part of pretracheal layer)

Pharynx

Mandible

Hyoid

Investing fascia

Larynx

Visceral part of tracheal layer

Isthmus of thyroid gland

Esophagus

Suprasternal space

Trachea

Manubrium of sternum

A Medial view

Occipital bone

Anterior longitudinal ligament

Body of vertebra

Buccopharyngeal fascia*

Intervertebral disc

Longus colli

Prevertebral fascia

Retropharyngeal space

Pharyngeal muscle

Pharynx

Plane of section for parts B and C

Isthmus of thyroid gland

B Anterosuperior view of part C

Nuchal ligament

Vertebral arch

Trapezius

Middle scalene

Anterior scalene

Longus colli

Esophagus

Omohyoid

Platysma

Sternothyroid

Sternohyoid

Posterior

Skin

Retropharyngeal space

Alar fascia

Lymph node

Carotid sheath

Vagus nerve

Internal jugular vein

Common carotid artery

Sternocleido-mastoid (SCM)

Thyroid gland

Trachea

Pretracheal layer

Anterior

C Superior view of transverse section (at level C7 vertebra)

Fascial layers

☐ Subcutaneous tissue of neck (superficial cervical fascia)

Layers of deep cervical fascia

▬ Investing layer

▬ Pretracheal layer *

▬ Prevertebral layer

▬ Alar fascia and carotid sheath

* Buccopharyngeal fascia is a component of the pretracheal layer

FIGURE 8.2. Cervical fascia. **A.** Fascia of the retropharyngeal region. **B.** Fascial compartments of the neck demonstrating an anterior midline approach to the thyroid gland. **C.** Cross-section of the neck passing through isthmus of the thyroid gland.

layers form *natural cleavage planes*, allowing separation of tissues during surgery.

INVESTING LAYER OF DEEP CERVICAL FASCIA

The **investing layer of deep cervical fascia,** the most superficial deep fascial layer, surrounds the entire neck deep to the skin and subcutaneous tissue (Fig. 8.2). At the "four corners" of the neck, the investing layer splits into superficial and deep layers of fascia to enclose (invest) the *sternocleidomastoid* (SCM) and *trapezius muscles.* Superiorly, the investing layer of fascia attaches to the superior nuchal line of the occipital bone, mastoid processes of the temporal bones, zygomatic arches, inferior border of the mandible, hyoid, and spinous processes of the cervical vertebrae. Just inferior to its attachment to the mandible, the investing layer of fascia splits to enclose the submandibular gland. Posterior to the mandible, it splits to form the fibrous capsule of the parotid gland.

Inferiorly, the investing layer of fascia attaches to the manubrium of the sternum, clavicles, acromions, and spines of the scapulae. The investing layer is continuous posteriorly with the periosteum covering the C7 spinous process and the nuchal ligament (L. *ligamentum nuchae*) (Fig. 8.2*B*). Just superior to the manubrium, the fascia remains divided into the two layers that enclose the SCM; one layer attaches to the anterior and the other to the posterior surface of the manubrium. A suprasternal space lies between these layers and encloses the inferior ends of the anterior jugular veins, the jugular venous arch, fat, and a few deep lymph nodes (Fig. 8.2*A*).

PRETRACHEAL LAYER OF DEEP CERVICAL FASCIA

The thin **pretracheal layer of deep cervical fascia** is limited to the anterior part of the neck (Fig. 8.2). It extends inferiorly from the hyoid into the thorax, where it blends with the fibrous pericardium covering the heart. The pretracheal layer includes a thin *muscular part*, which encloses the infrahyoid muscles, and a *visceral part*, which encloses the thyroid gland, trachea, and esophagus and is continuous posterosuperiorly with the *buccopharyngeal fascia*. The pretracheal layer blends laterally with the *carotid sheaths*.

The **carotid sheath** is a tubular fascial investment that extends from the cranial base to the root of the neck. This sheath blends anteriorly with the investing and pretracheal layers of fascia and posteriorly with the prevertebral layer of deep cervical fascia. The carotid sheath contains (Fig. 8.2*B, C*):

- The common and internal carotid arteries.
- The internal jugular vein (IJV).
- The vagus nerve (CN X).
- Some deep cervical lymph nodes.
- The carotid sinus nerve.
- Sympathetic nerve fibers (carotid periarterial plexuses).

The carotid sheath communicates with the mediastinum of the thorax inferiorly and the cranial cavity superiorly. These communications represent potential pathways for the spread of infection and extravasated blood.

PREVERTEBRAL LAYER OF DEEP CERVICAL FASCIA

The **prevertebral layer of deep cervical fascia** forms a tubular sheath for the vertebral column and the muscles associated with it, such as the *longus colli* and *longus capitis* anteriorly, the *scalenes* laterally, and the *deep cervical muscles* posteriorly (Fig. 8.2). This layer of fascia is fixed to the cranial base superiorly and inferiorly and fuses with the *anterior longitudinal ligament* centrally at approximately T3 vertebra. The prevertebral layer extends laterally as the *axillary sheath* (see Chapter 6), which surrounds the axillary vessels and brachial plexus.

RETROPHARYNGEAL SPACE

The **retropharyngeal space** is the largest and most clinically important interfascial space in the neck because it is the major pathway for the spread of infection (Fig. 8.2*A*). It is a potential space that consists of loose connective tissue between the visceral part of the prevertebral layer of deep cervical fascia and the *buccopharyngeal fascia*. Inferiorly, the buccopharyngeal fascia is continuous with the pretracheal layer of deep cervical fascia. The *alar fascia* crosses the retropharyngeal space. This thin layer is attached along the midline of the buccopharyngeal fascia from the cranium to the level of the C7 vertebra and extends laterally to blend with the carotid sheath. The retropharyngeal space is closed superiorly by the base of the cranium and on each side by the carotid sheath. This space permits movement of the pharynx, esophagus, larynx, and trachea relative to the vertebral column during swallowing.

SUPERFICIAL STRUCTURES OF NECK: CERVICAL REGIONS

To allow clear communications regarding the location of structures, injuries, or pathologies, the neck is divided into regions (Fig. 8.3). The four major regions are the (1) sternocleidomastoid region, (2) posterior cervical region, (3) lateral cervical region, and (4) anterior cervical region.

Sternocleidomastoid Region

The **sternocleidomastoid muscle** (SCM) visibly divides each side of the neck into *anterior* and *lateral cervical triangles*. The region between these triangular regions, corresponding to the area of this broad, strap-like muscle, is the **sternocleidomastoid region.** The SCM has two heads: the

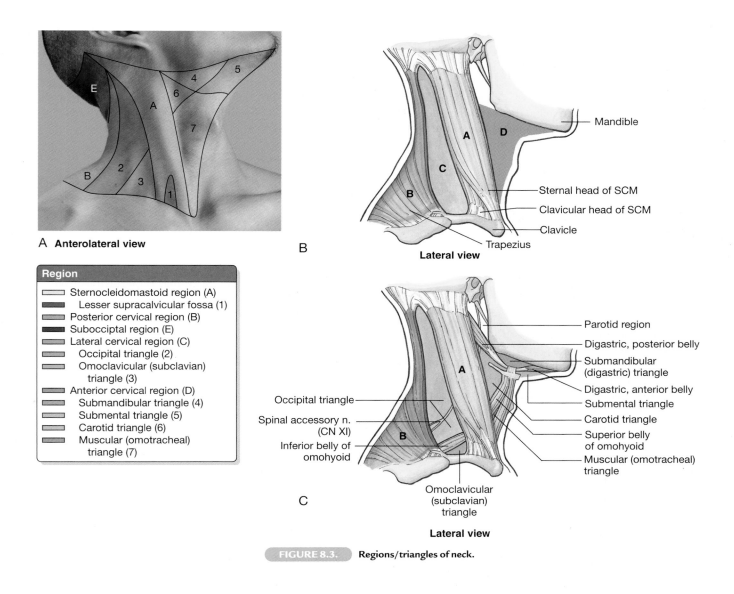

A Anterolateral view

B Lateral view

Mandible
Sternal head of SCM
Clavicular head of SCM
Clavicle
Trapezius

Region	
Sternocleidomastoid region (A)	
Lesser supraclavicular fossa (1)	
Posterior cervical region (B)	
Subocciptal region (E)	
Lateral cervical region (C)	
Occipital triangle (2)	
Omoclavicular (subclavian) triangle (3)	
Anterior cervical region (D)	
Submandibular triangle (4)	
Submental triangle (5)	
Carotid triangle (6)	
Muscular (omotracheal) triangle (7)	

Occipital triangle

Spinal accessory n. (CN XI)

Inferior belly of omohyoid

Omoclavicular (subclavian) triangle

Parotid region
Digastric, posterior belly
Submandibular (digastric) triangle
Digastric, anterior belly
Submental triangle
Carotid triangle
Superior belly of omohyoid
Muscular (omotracheal) triangle

C Lateral view

FIGURE 8.3.   Regions/triangles of neck.

Spread of Infection in Neck

The investing layer of deep cervical fascia helps prevent the spread of abscesses. If an infection occurs between the investing layer of deep cervical fascia and the muscular part of the pretracheal fascia surrounding the infrahyoid muscles, the infection usually does not spread beyond the superior edge of the manubrium. If, however, the infection occurs between the investing fascia and the visceral part of the pretracheal fascia, it can spread into the thoracic cavity anterior to the pericardium.

Pus from an abscess posterior to the prevertebral layer of deep cervical fascia may extend laterally in the neck and form a swelling posterior to the SCM. The pus may perforate the prevertebral layer of deep cervical fascia and enter the retropharyngeal space, producing a bulge in the pharynx (*retropharyngeal abscess*). This swelling may cause difficulty in swallowing (*dysphagia*) and speaking (*dysarthria*). Similarly, air from a ruptured trachea, bronchus, or esophagus (*pneumomediastinum*) can pass superiorly in the neck.

rounded tendon of the **sternal head** attaches to the manubrium, and the thick fleshy **clavicular head** attaches to the superior surface of the medial third of the clavicle. The two heads are separated inferiorly by a space, the **lesser supraclavicular fossa.** The heads join superiorly as they pass obliquely upward to attach to the mastoid process of the temporal bone and the superior nuchal line of the occipital bone. The attachments, innervation, and actions of the SCM are summarized in Table 8.1.

Posterior Cervical Region

The region posterior to the anterior border of the trapezius is the **posterior cervical region** (Fig. 8.3). The *suboccipital region* is deep to the superior part of this region.

Congenital Torticollis

Torticollis is a contraction of the cervical muscles that produces twisting of the neck and slanting of the head (Fig. B8.1). The most common type of *congenital torticollis* (wry neck) results from a fibrous tissue tumor (L. *fibromatosis colli*) that develops in the SCM before or shortly after birth. Occasionally, the SCM is injured when an infant's head is pulled excessively during a difficult birth, tearing its fibers (*muscular torticollis*). This tearing may result in a hematoma that may develop into a fibrous mass entrapping a branch of the spinal accessory nerve (CN XI), thus denervating part of the SCM. Surgical release of a partially fibrotic SCM from its distal attachments to the manubrium and clavicle may be necessary to enable the child to tilt and rotate the head normally.

Cervical dystonia (abnormal tonicity of the cervical muscles), commonly known as **spasmodic torticollis,** usually begins in adulthood. It may involve any bilateral combination of lateral neck muscles, especially the SCM and trapezius.

SCM

FIGURE B8.1.

The **trapezius** is a large, flat triangular muscle that covers the posterolateral aspect of the neck and thorax. It is a superficial muscle of the back, a muscle of the pectoral girdle, and a cervical muscle. The trapezius attaches the pectoral girdle to the cranium and vertebral column and assists in suspending it. Its attachments, nerve supply, and main actions are described in Table 8.1.

Lateral Cervical Region

The **lateral cervical region** (posterior triangle of the neck) is bounded (Fig. 8.3 and Table 8.1):

- Anteriorly by the posterior border of the SCM.
- Posteriorly by the anterior border of the trapezius.
- Inferiorly by the middle third of the clavicle between the trapezius and the SCM.
- By an *apex,* where the SCM and trapezius meet on the superior nuchal line of the occipital bone.
- By a *roof,* formed by the investing layer of deep cervical fascia.
- By a *floor,* formed by muscles covered by the prevertebral layer of deep cervical fascia.

The lateral cervical region wraps around the lateral surface of the neck like a spiral and is covered by skin and subcutaneous tissue containing the platysma.

MUSCLES IN LATERAL CERVICAL REGION

The floor of the lateral cervical region is usually formed by the prevertebral fascia overlying four muscles (Fig. 8.4): splenius capitis, levator scapulae, middle scalene (L. *scalenus medius*), and posterior scalene (L. *scalenus posterior*). Sometimes part of the inferior part of the anterior scalene (L. *scalenus anterior*) appears in the inferomedial angle of the lateral cervical region.

For more precise localization of structures, the lateral cervical region is divided into a larger occipital triangle superiorly and a small omoclavicular triangle inferiorly by the *inferior belly of the omohyoid* (Fig. 8.3). The important nerve crossing the **occipital triangle** is the *spinal accessory nerve* (CN XI). The small **omoclavicular (subclavian) triangle** is indicated on the superior surface of the neck by the *supraclavicular fossa.* The inferior part of the external jugular vein (EJV) crosses this triangle superficially (Fig. 8.4A); the *subclavian artery* lies deep in the triangle.

NERVES OF LATERAL CERVICAL REGION

The **spinal accessory nerve** passes deep to the SCM, supplying it before entering the lateral cervical region at or inferior to the junction of the superior and middle thirds of the posterior border of the SCM (Fig. 8.4B). It passes posteroinferiorly, within or deep to the investing layer of deep cervical fascia, running on the levator scapulae from which

TABLE 8.1 CUTANEOUS AND SUPERFICIAL MUSCLES OF NECK

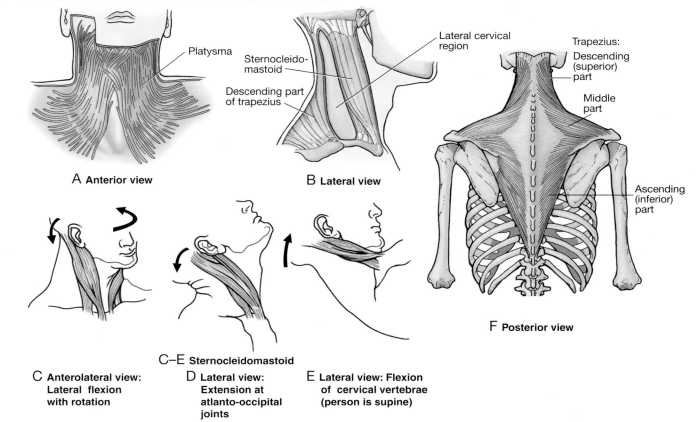

A Anterior view

B Lateral view

F Posterior view

C–E Sternocleidomastoid

C Anterolateral view:
Lateral flexion
with rotation

D Lateral view:
Extension at
atlanto-occipital
joints

E Lateral view: Flexion
of cervical vertebrae
(person is supine)

Muscle	Superior Attachment	Inferior Attachment	Innervation	Main Action(s)
Platysma (**A**)	Inferior border of mandible, skin, and subcutaneous tissues of lower face	Fascia covering superior parts of pectoralis major and deltoid muscles	Cervical branch of facial nerve (CN VII)	Draws corners of mouth inferiorly and widens it as in expressions of sadness and fright; draws skin of neck superiorly when teeth are clenched indicating tension
Sternocleidomastoid (**B–E**)	Lateral surface of mastoid process of temporal bone and lateral half of superior nuchal line	*Sternal head:* anterior surface of manubrium of sternum *Clavicular head:* superior surface of medial third of clavicle	Spinal accessory nerve (CN XI; motor); C2 and C3 nerves (pain and proprioception)	*Unilateral contraction:* tilts head to same side (i.e., laterally flexes neck) and rotates it so face is turned superiorly toward opposite side *Bilateral contraction:* (1) extends neck at atlanto-occipital joints, (2) flexes cervical vertebrae so that chin approaches manubrium, or (3) extends superior cervical vertebrae while flexing inferior vertebrae so chin is thrust forward with head kept level With cervical vertebrae fixed, may elevate manubrium and medial end of clavicles, assisting pump-handle action of deep respiration
Trapezius (**F**)	Medial third of superior nuchal line, external occipital protuberance, nuchal ligament, spinous processes of C7–T12 vertebrae	Lateral third of clavicle, acromion and spine of scapula	Spinal accessory nerve (CN XI; motor); C3 and C4 nerves (pain and proprioception)	Elevates, retracts, and rotates scapula *Descending (superior) part:* elevate pectoral girdle, maintain level of shoulders against gravity or resistance *Middle part:* retract scapula *Ascending (inferior) part:* depress shoulders *Descending and ascending parts:* rotate scapula upward With shoulders fixed, bilateral contraction extends neck; unilateral contraction produces lateral flexion to same side

Occipital vein

Posterior auricular vein

Splenius

Trapezius

Levator scapulae

Spinal accessory nerve (CN XI)

Middle and posterior scalene

Cervicodorsal vein

Omohyoid

Suprascapular vein

Superficial temporal vein

Maxillary vein

Retromandibular vein:
Posterior division
Anterior division

Facial vein

Common facial vein

Sternocleidomastoid

External jugular vein (EJV)

Communicating branch

Internal jugular vein (IJV)

Anterior jugular vein

Brachiocephalic vein

A Lateral view   Subclavian vein

FIGURE 8.4.   **Lateral cervical region. A.** Superficial veins of right side of neck.

it is separated by the prevertebral layer of fascia. CN XI then disappears deep to the anterior border of the trapezius at the junction of its superior two thirds with its inferior one third.

The **roots of brachial plexus** (anterior rami of C5–C8 and T1) appear between the anterior and the middle scalene muscles (Fig. 8.4). Five rami unite to form the *three trunks (superior, middle, and inferior) of the brachial plexus* (Fig. 8.4E), which descend inferolaterally through the lateral cervical region. The plexus then passes between the first rib, clavicle, and superior border of the scapula (the *cervicoaxillary canal*) to enter the axilla, providing innervation for most of the upper limb.

The **suprascapular nerve,** which arises from the superior trunk of the brachial plexus, runs across the lateral cervical region to supply the supraspinatus and infraspinatus muscles on the posterior aspect of the scapula. It also sends articular branches to the glenohumeral joint.

The anterior rami of C1–C4 make up the roots of the **cervical plexus,** which consists of nerve loops. The plexus lies anteromedial to the levator scapulae and middle scalene muscle and deep to the SCM. The superficial branches of the plexus that initially pass posteriorly are cutaneous branches (Fig. 8.4B, C). The deep branches passing anteromedially are motor branches, including the roots of the phrenic nerve and the **ansa cervicalis** (Fig. 8.5B).

Cutaneous branches of the cervical plexus emerge around the middle of the posterior border of the SCM, often called the **nerve point of the neck,** and supply the skin of the neck, superolateral thoracic wall, and the scalp between the auricle and the external occipital protuberance. Close to their origin, the roots of the cervical plexus receive communicating branches (L. *rami communicantes*), most of which descend from the *superior cervical ganglion* in the superior part of the neck.

The branches of the cervical plexus arising from the nerve loop between the anterior rami of C2 and C3 are the (Fig. 8.4A–C):

- **Lesser occipital nerve** (C2), supplying the skin of the neck and scalp posterosuperior to the auricle.
- **Great auricular nerve** (C2 and C3), ascending vertically across the SCM onto the parotid gland, where it divides and supplies skin over the gland, posterior aspect of the auricle, and the area of skin extending from the angle of the mandible to the mastoid process.
- **Transverse cervical nerve** (C2 and C3), supplying the skin covering the anterior cervical region; the nerve curves around the middle of the posterior border of the SCM and passes anteriorly and horizontally across it deep to the EJV and platysma.

Branches of the cervical plexus arising from the loop formed between the anterior rami of C3 and C4 are the

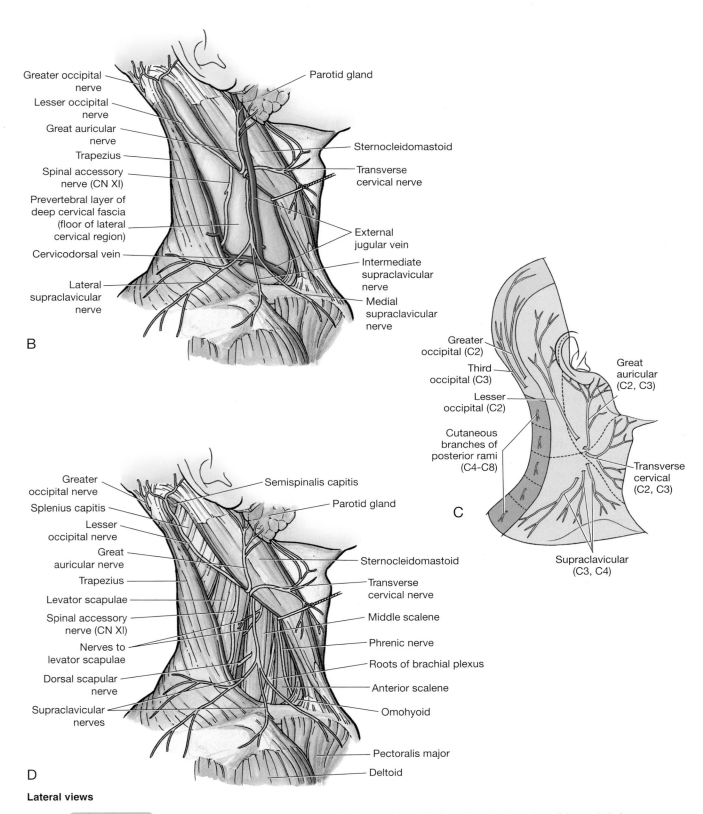

Greater occipital nerve

Lesser occipital nerve

Great auricular nerve

Trapezius

Spinal accessory nerve (CN XI)

Prevertebral layer of deep cervical fascia (floor of lateral cervical region)

Cervicodorsal vein

Lateral supraclavicular nerve

Parotid gland

Sternocleidomastoid

Transverse cervical nerve

External jugular vein

Intermediate supraclavicular nerve

Medial supraclavicular nerve

B

Greater occipital (C2)

Third occipital (C3)

Lesser occipital (C2)

Cutaneous branches of posterior rami (C4-C8)

Great auricular (C2, C3)

Transverse cervical (C2, C3)

Supraclavicular (C3, C4)

C

Greater occipital nerve

Splenius capitis

Lesser occipital nerve

Great auricular nerve

Trapezius

Levator scapulae

Spinal accessory nerve (CN XI)

Nerves to levator scapulae

Dorsal scapular nerve

Supraclavicular nerves

Semispinalis capitis

Parotid gland

Sternocleidomastoid

Transverse cervical nerve

Middle scalene

Phrenic nerve

Roots of brachial plexus

Anterior scalene

Omohyoid

Pectoralis major

Deltoid

D

Lateral views

FIGURE 8.4.   **Lateral cervical region** *(continued).* Superficial (**B**) and deep (**C**) dissections. **D.** Dissection of the cervical plexus.

E **Anterior view of right side**

FIGURE 8.4. *(continued)* **E.** A deeper dissection of the inferior part of the lateral cervical region.

supraclavicular nerves (C3 and C4), which emerge as a common trunk under cover of the SCM and send small branches to the skin of the neck and cross the clavicle to supply the skin over the shoulder (Fig. 8.4C). Deep motor branches include branches arising from the anterior rami of cervical nerves supplying the rhomboids—dorsal scapular nerve (C4 and C5), serratus anterior–long thoracic nerve (C5, C6, and C7) and nearby prevertebral muscles.

The **phrenic nerves** originate chiefly from the fourth cervical nerve (C4) but receive contributions from the C3 and C5 nerves. The phrenic nerves contain motor, sensory, and sympathetic nerve fibers. These nerves provide the sole motor supply to the diaphragm as well as sensation to its central part. In the thorax, the nerves supply the mediastinal pleura and the pericardium. Receiving variable communicating fibers in the neck and fibers from the cervical sympathetic ganglia or their branches, each phrenic nerve forms at the superior part of the lateral border of the anterior scalene muscle at the level of the superior border of the thyroid cartilage. The phrenic nerves descend obliquely with the IJVs across the anterior scalene, deep to the prevertebral layer of the deep cervical fascia and the cervicodorsal trunk and suprascapular artery (Fig. 8.4E).

On the left, the phrenic nerve crosses anterior to the first part of the subclavian artery; *on the right,* it lies anterior on the anterior scalene muscle and crosses anterior to the second part of the subclavian artery. On both sides, the phrenic nerve runs posterior to the subclavian vein and anterior to the internal thoracic artery as it enters the thorax. The contribution from C5 to the phrenic nerve may derive from an

accessory phrenic nerve, which is frequently a branch of the nerve to the subclavius. If present, the accessory phrenic nerve lies lateral to the main nerve and descends posterior and sometimes anterior to the subclavian vein. The accessory phrenic nerve joins the phrenic nerve either in the root of the neck or in the thorax.

VEINS IN LATERAL CERVICAL REGION

The **external jugular vein** begins near the angle of the mandible (just inferior to the auricle of the external ear) by the union of the posterior division of the *retromandibular vein* with the *posterior auricular vein* (Fig. 8.4A). The EJV crosses the SCM obliquely, deep to the platysma, and then pierces the investing layer of deep cervical fascia, which forms the roof of this region, at the posterior border of the SCM. The EJV descends to the inferior part of the lateral cervical region and terminates in the subclavian vein.

The major venous channel draining the upper limb, the **subclavian vein,** courses through the inferior part of the lateral cervical region, passing anterior to the anterior scalene muscle and phrenic nerve (Fig. 8.4E). The subclavian vein joins the IJV to form the **brachiocephalic vein** posterior to the medial end of the clavicle (Fig. 8.4A, E). Just superior to the clavicle, the EJV receives the cervicodorsal (*transverse cervical*), *suprascapular,* and *anterior jugular veins.*

ARTERIES IN LATERAL CERVICAL REGION

The arteries in the lateral cervical region are the cervicodorsal trunk (transverse cervical artery) and suprascapular artery, the third part of the subclavian artery, and part of the occipital artery (Fig. 8.4*E*).

The **cervicodorsal trunk** originates from the *thyrocervical trunk,* a branch of the subclavian artery, and divides into the superficial cervical and dorsal scapular arteries. The cervicodorsal trunk runs superficially and laterally across the phrenic nerve and anterior scalene muscle, 2 to 3 cm superior to the clavicle. It then crosses (passes through) the *trunks of the brachial plexus,* supplying branches to their *vasa nervorum* (blood vessels of nerves) and passing deep to the trapezius. The superficial cervical artery accompanies CN XI along the anterior (deep) surface of the trapezius. The dorsal scapular artery runs anterior to the rhomboid muscles, accompanying the dorsal scapular nerve. The dorsal scapular artery may arise independently, directly from the subclavian artery.

The **suprascapular artery,** from the cervicodorsal trunk, a branch of the thyrocervical trunk, or from the subclavian artery, passes inferolaterally across the anterior scalene muscle and phrenic nerve. It crosses the subclavian artery (third part) and the cords of the brachial plexus. It then passes posterior to the clavicle to supply muscles on the posterior aspect of the scapula. The suprascapular artery may arise directly from the subclavian artery.

The **occipital artery,** a branch of the external carotid artery (Fig. 8.5*A*), crosses the lateral cervical region at its apex and ascends to supply the posterior half of the scalp.

The **third part of the subclavian artery** supplies blood to the upper limb. It begins approximately a finger's breadth superior to the clavicle, opposite the lateral border of the anterior scalene muscle. It lies posterosuperior to the subclavian vein in the inferior part of the lateral cervical region (Fig. 8.4*E*). The pulsations of the artery can be felt

Lesions of Spinal Accessory Nerve (CN XI)

 Lesions of the CN XI are uncommon; however, the nerve may be damaged by penetrating trauma, surgical procedures, tumors, and fractures of the jugular foramen. A unilateral lesion usually does not produce an abnormal position of the head; however, weakness can occur in turning the head to one side against resistance.

Lesions of CN XI produce weakness and atrophy of the trapezius. *Drooping of the shoulder* is an obvious sign of injury to CN XI. *Unilateral paralysis of the trapezius* is evident by the patient's inability to elevate and retract the shoulder and by difficulty in elevating the arm superior to the horizontal level.

Subclavian Vein Puncture

 The right or left subclavian vein is often the point of entry to the venous system for *central line placement* (Fig. B8.2). Central lines are inserted to administer parenteral (venous nutritional) fluids and medications and to measure central venous pressure. The pleura and/or the subclavian artery are in danger of puncture during this procedure.

Prominence of External Jugular Vein

The EJV may serve as an "internal barometer." When venous pressure is in the normal range, the EJV is usually visible superior to the clavicle for only a short distance. However, when venous pressure rises (e.g., as in heart failure) the vein is prominent throughout its course along the side of the neck. Consequently, routine observation for distention of the EJVs during physical examinations may reveal diagnostic signs of heart failure, obstruction of the superior vena cava, enlarged supraclavicular lymph nodes, or increased intrathoracic pressure.

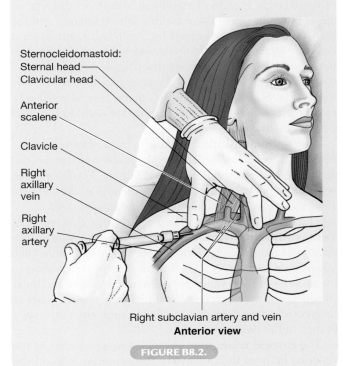

Sternocleidomastoid:
Sternal head
Clavicular head

Anterior scalene

Clavicle

Right axillary vein

Right axillary artery

Right subclavian artery and vein
Anterior view

FIGURE B8.2.

on deep pressure in the omoclavicular triangle just superior to the clavicle (Fig. 8.3). The artery is in contact with the first rib as it passes posterior to the anterior scalene muscle; consequently, compression of the artery against this rib can control bleeding in the upper limb.

Anterior Cervical Region

The **anterior cervical region** (anterior triangle of the neck) has a/an (Fig. 8.3*B*):

- *Anterior boundary:* formed by the median line of the neck.
- *Posterior boundary:* formed by the anterior border of the SCM.
- *Superior boundary:* formed by the inferior border of the mandible.
- *Apex:* located at the jugular notch in the manubrium of the sternum.
- *Roof:* formed by subcutaneous tissue containing the platysma.
- *Floor:* formed by the pharynx, larynx, and thyroid gland.

The anterior cervical region is subdivided into four smaller triangles (the unpaired submental triangle and three small paired triangles: submandibular, carotid, and muscular) by the digastric and omohyoid muscles (Fig. 8.3*C*).

The **submental triangle** is inferior to the chin. The apex of the triangle is at the mandibular symphysis, the site of union of the halves of the mandible during infancy, and the base of the triangle is formed by the hyoid. Laterally, it is bounded by the right and left anterior bellies of the digastric muscles. The floor of the submental triangle is formed by the two mylohyoid muscles, which meet in a median *fibrous raphe* (Fig. 8.5*D*). This triangle contains several small submental lymph nodes and small veins that unite to form the *anterior jugular vein* (Fig. 8.5*A*).

The **submandibular triangle** is a glandular area between the inferior border of the mandible and the anterior and posterior bellies of the digastric muscle. The floor of the submandibular triangle is formed by the mylohyoid and hyoglossus muscles, and the middle pharyngeal constrictor.

The **submandibular gland** nearly fills this triangle. **Submandibular lymph nodes** lie on each side of the gland and along the inferior border of the mandible. The *hypoglossal nerve* (CN XII) provides motor innervation to the muscles of the tongue. It passes into the submandibular triangle, as do the *nerve to the mylohyoid muscle,* parts of the *facial artery* and *vein,* and the *submental artery,* a branch of the facial artery (Fig. 8.5*B*).

The **carotid triangle** is a vascular area bounded by the superior belly of the omohyoid, the posterior belly of the

Severance of Phrenic Nerve and Phrenic Nerve Block

 Severance of a phrenic nerve results in paralysis of the corresponding half of the diaphragm. A phrenic nerve block produces a short period of paralysis of the diaphragm on one side (e.g., for a lung operation). The anesthetic agent is injected around the nerve where it lies on the anterior surface of the anterior scalene muscle.

Nerve Blocks in Lateral Cervical Region

 Regional anesthesia is often used for surgical procedures in the neck region or upper limb. In a **cervical plexus block,** an anesthetic agent is injected at several points along the posterior border of the SCM, mainly at the junction of its superior and middle thirds, the *nerve point of the neck* (Fig. B8.3). For anesthesia of the upper limb, the anesthetic agent in a *supraclavicular brachial plexus block* is injected around the supraclavicular part of the brachial plexus. The main injection site is superior to the midpoint of the clavicle.

Lateral view

FIGURE B8.3.

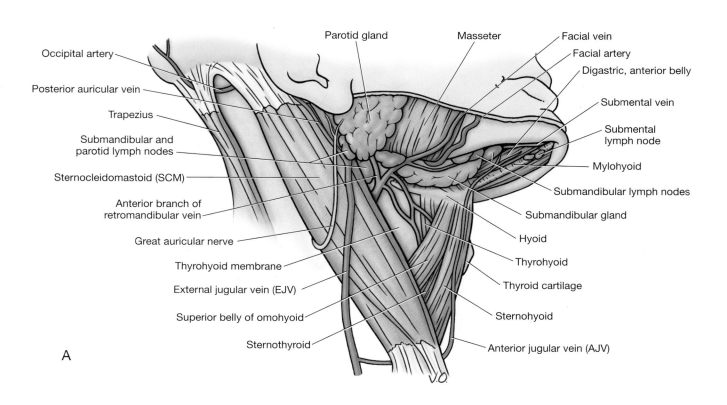

Occipital artery

Posterior auricular vein

Trapezius

Submandibular and parotid lymph nodes

Sternocleidomastoid (SCM)

Anterior branch of retromandibular vein

Great auricular nerve

Thyrohyoid membrane

External jugular vein (EJV)

Superior belly of omohyoid

Sternothyroid

Parotid gland

Masseter

Facial vein

Facial artery

Digastric, anterior belly

Submental vein

Submental lymph node

Mylohyoid

Submandibular lymph nodes

Submandibular gland

Hyoid

Thyrohyoid

Thyroid cartilage

Sternohyoid

Anterior jugular vein (AJV)

A

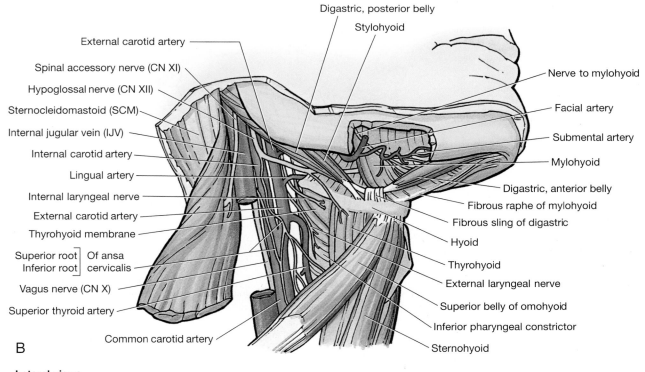

Digastric, posterior belly

Stylohyoid

External carotid artery

Spinal accessory nerve (CN XI)

Hypoglossal nerve (CN XII)

Sternocleidomastoid (SCM)

Internal jugular vein (IJV)

Internal carotid artery

Lingual artery

Internal laryngeal nerve

External carotid artery

Thyrohyoid membrane

Superior root ⌉ Of ansa
Inferior root ⌋ cervicalis

Vagus nerve (CN X)

Superior thyroid artery

Common carotid artery

Nerve to mylohyoid

Facial artery

Submental artery

Mylohyoid

Digastric, anterior belly

Fibrous raphe of mylohyoid

Fibrous sling of digastric

Hyoid

Thyrohyoid

External laryngeal nerve

Superior belly of omohyoid

Inferior pharyngeal constrictor

Sternohyoid

B

Lateral views

FIGURE 8.5. **Anterior cervical region and suprahyoid region.** Superficial (**A**) and deep (**B**) dissections are shown.

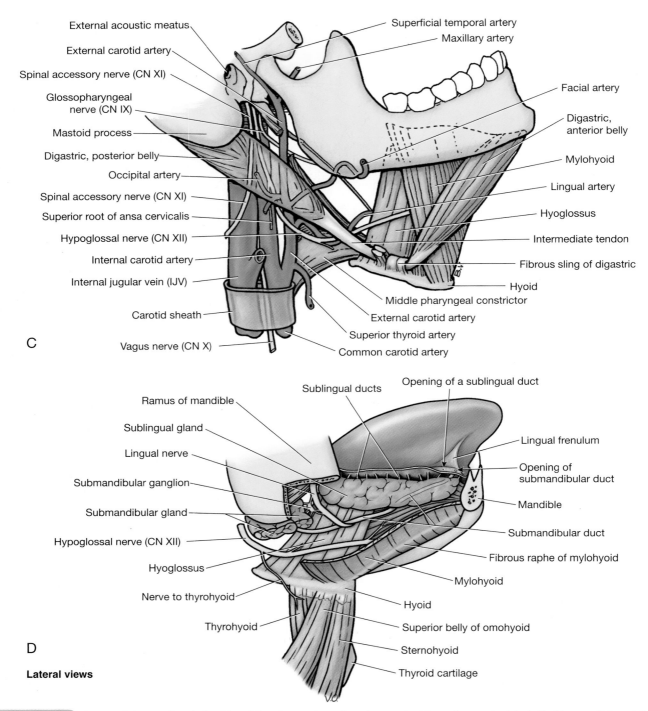

C

External acoustic meatus
External carotid artery
Spinal accessory nerve (CN XI)
Glossopharyngeal nerve (CN IX)
Mastoid process
Digastric, posterior belly
Occipital artery
Spinal accessory nerve (CN XI)
Superior root of ansa cervicalis
Hypoglossal nerve (CN XII)
Internal carotid artery
Internal jugular vein (IJV)
Carotid sheath
Vagus nerve (CN X)

Superficial temporal artery
Maxillary artery
Facial artery
Digastric, anterior belly
Mylohyoid
Lingual artery
Hyoglossus
Intermediate tendon
Fibrous sling of digastric
Hyoid
Middle pharyngeal constrictor
External carotid artery
Superior thyroid artery
Common carotid artery

D

Lateral views

Ramus of mandible
Sublingual gland
Lingual nerve
Submandibular ganglion
Submandibular gland
Hypoglossal nerve (CN XII)
Hyoglossus
Nerve to thyrohyoid
Thyrohyoid

Sublingual ducts
Opening of a sublingual duct
Lingual frenulum
Opening of submandibular duct
Mandible
Submandibular duct
Fibrous raphe of mylohyoid
Mylohyoid
Hyoid
Superior belly of omohyoid
Sternohyoid
Thyroid cartilage

FIGURE 8.5. *(continued)* **C.** Note the relationships of the nerves and vessels to the suprahyoid muscles. **D.** The right half of the mandible and the superior half of the mylohyoid muscle have been removed to show the suprahyoid region.

digastric, and the anterior border of the SCM (Fig. 8.5*A* and *B*). The **common carotid artery** ascends into the carotid triangle (Fig. 8.5*B* and *C*). Its pulse can be auscultated or palpated by compressing it lightly against the transverse processes of the cervical vertebrae.

At the level of the superior border of the thyroid cartilage (C4 vertebral level), the common carotid artery divides into the **internal** and **external carotid arteries** (Fig. 8.6*A*). At this bifurcation, there is a slight dilation of the proximal part of the internal carotid artery—the **carotid sinus** (Fig. 8.6*C*).

Innervated principally by the glossopharyngeal nerve (CN IX) through the **carotid sinus nerve,** as well as the vagus nerve, the carotid sinus is a *baroreceptor* (pressoreceptor) that reacts to changes in arterial blood pressure.

The **carotid body,** an ovoid mass of tissue, lies on the medial (deep) side of the bifurcation of the common carotid artery in close relation to the carotid sinus (Fig. 8.6*C*). Supplied mainly by the carotid sinus nerve (CN IX) and by CN X, the carotid body is a *chemoreceptor* that monitors the level of oxygen in the blood. It is stimulated by low levels of oxygen and initiates a reflex that increases the rate and depth of respiration, cardiac rate, and blood pressure.

The **muscular triangle** is bounded by the superior belly of the omohyoid muscle, the anterior border of SCM, and the median plane of the neck (Figs. 8.3*C* and 8.5*A*, *B*). This triangle contains the *infrahyoid muscles* and viscera, such as the thyroid and parathyroid glands.

MUSCLES IN ANTERIOR CERVICAL REGION

In the anterolateral part of the neck, the *hyoid* provides attachments for the suprahyoid muscles superior to it and the infrahyoid muscles inferior to it (Fig. 8.5). These **hyoid muscles** steady or move the hyoid bone and larynx. The attachments, innervation, and main actions of the suprahyoid and infrahyoid muscles are presented in Table 8.2.

The **suprahyoid muscles** are superior to the hyoid bone and connect it to the cranium. The suprahyoid muscle group includes the mylohyoid, geniohyoid, stylohyoid, and digastric muscles. As a group, these muscles constitute the substance of the floor of the mouth, supporting the hyoid in providing a base from which the tongue functions and in elevating the hyoid and larynx in relation to swallowing and tone production. Each **digastric muscle** has anterior and posterior bellies joined by an **intermediate tendon** that descends toward the hyoid. A **fibrous sling** allows the intermediate tendon to slide anteriorly and posteriorly as it connects this tendon to the body and greater horn of the hyoid bone (Fig. 8.5*B*, *C*).

The **infrahyoid muscles** (strap muscles) are inferior to the hyoid. These four muscles anchor the hyoid, sternum, clavicle, and scapula and depress the hyoid and larynx during swallowing and speaking (Table 8.2). They also work with the suprahyoid muscles to steady the hyoid, providing a firm base for the tongue. The infrahyoid group of muscles are arranged in two planes: a *superficial plane* made up of the sternohyoid and omohyoid, and a *deep plane* composed of the sternothyroid and thyrohyoid. The **omohyoid** has two bellies united by an intermediate tendon that is connected to the clavicle by a fascial sling. The **sternothyroid** is wider than the **sternohyoid,** under which it lies. The sternothyroid covers the lateral lobe of the thyroid gland, attaching to the oblique line of the lamina of the thyroid cartilage immediately superior to the gland. This muscle limits superior expansion of an enlarged thyroid gland. The **thyrohyoid,** running superiorly from the oblique line of the thyroid cartilage to the hyoid bone, appears to be a continuation of the sternothyroid muscle.

ARTERIES IN ANTERIOR CERVICAL REGION

The anterior cervical region contains the **carotid system of arteries,** consisting of the common carotid artery and its terminal branches, the internal and external carotid arteries (Figs. 8.5*C* and 8.6*C*). This region also contains the IJV and its tributaries and the anterior jugular veins (AJVs). The common carotid artery and one of its terminal branches, the *external carotid artery,* are the main arterial vessels in the carotid triangle.

Each **common carotid artery** ascends within the *carotid sheath* with the IJV and vagus nerve to the level of the superior border of the thyroid cartilage. Here, each common carotid artery terminates by dividing into the internal and external carotid arteries. The **right common carotid artery** begins at the bifurcation of the brachiocephalic trunk. In contrast, the **left common carotid artery** arises from the arch of the aorta and ascends in the neck.

The **internal carotid arteries,** the direct continuation of the common carotid arteries, have no branches in the neck. They enter the cranium through the carotid canals and become the main arteries of the brain and structures in the orbits.

The **external carotid arteries** supply most structures external to the cranium; the orbit and part of the forehead and scalp supplied by the supraorbital artery are the major exceptions (Figs. 8.5*B* and 8.6*C*). Each external carotid artery runs posterosuperiorly to the region between the neck of the mandible and the lobule of the auricle, where it is embedded in the parotid gland. Here it divides into two terminal branches: the *maxillary* and *superficial temporal arteries* (Fig. 8.6*C*). Before these terminal branches, six arteries arise from the external carotid artery (Figs. 8.5 and 8.6*C*):

- **Ascending pharyngeal artery** arises as the first or second branch of the external carotid artery and is its only medial branch; ascends on the pharynx and sends branches to the pharynx, prevertebral muscles, middle ear, and cranial meninges.
- **Occipital artery** arises from the posterior aspect of the external carotid artery, superior to the origin of the facial artery; passes posteriorly, immediately medial and parallel to the attachment of the posterior belly of the digastric muscle, ending in the posterior part of the scalp. During its course, it passes superficial to the internal carotid artery and CN IX–CN XI.
- **Posterior auricular artery,** a small posterior branch of the external carotid artery, ascends posteriorly between the external acoustic meatus and the mastoid process and contributes to the blood supply of adjacent muscles, parotid gland, facial nerve, structures in the temporal bone, auricle, and scalp.

TABLE 8.2 MUSCLES OF ANTERIOR CERVICAL REGION (EXTRINSIC MUSCLES OF LARYNX)

A Lateral view

B Anterior view

C Lateral view

D Superior view of hyoid

Muscle	Origin	Insertion	Innervation	Main Action(s)
Suprahyoid muscles				
Mylohyoid	Mylohyoid line of mandible	Mylohyoid raphe and body of hyoid	Nerve to mylohyoid, a branch of inferior alveolar nerve (from mandibular nerve, CN V₃)	Elevates hyoid, floor of mouth, and tongue during swallowing and speaking
Geniohyoid	Inferior mental spine of mandible	Body of hyoid	C1 via hypoglossal nerve (CN XII)	Pulls hyoid anterosuperiorly; shortens floor of mouth; widens pharynx
Stylohyoid	Styloid process of temporal bone		Stylohyoid branch of facial nerve (CN VII)	Elevates and retracts hyoid, thus elongating floor of mouth
Digastric	*Anterior belly*: digastric fossa of mandible *Posterior belly*: mastoid notch of temporal bone	Intermediate tendon to body and greater horn of hyoid	*Anterior belly:* nerve to mylohyoid, a branch of inferior alveolar nerve *Posterior belly:* digastric branch of facial nerve (CN VII)	Working with infrahyoid muscles, depresses mandible against resistance; elevates and steadies hyoid during swallowing and speaking
Infrahyoid muscles				
Sternohyoid	Manubrium of sternum and medial end of clavicle	Body of hyoid	C1–C3 by a branch of ansa cervicalis	Depresses hyoid after elevation during swallowing
Omohyoid	Superior border of scapula near suprascapular notch	Inferior border of hyoid		Depresses, retracts, and steadies hyoid
Sternothyroid	Posterior surface of manubrium of sternum	Oblique line of thyroid cartilage	C2 and C3 by a branch of ansa cervicalis	Depresses hyoid and larynx
Thyrohyoid	Oblique line of thyroid cartilage	Inferior border of body and greater horn of hyoid	C1 via hypoglossal nerve	Depresses hyoid and elevates larynx

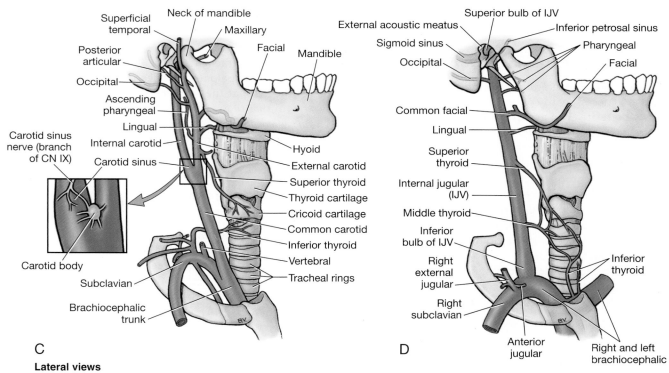

FIGURE 8.6. **Arteries and veins in neck. A.** Subclavian and carotid arteries. **B.** Internal jugular and subclavian veins. **C.** Branches of the subclavian and external carotid arteries. **D.** Internal jugular vein.

- **Superior thyroid artery,** the most inferior of the three anterior branches of the external carotid artery, runs anteroinferiorly deep to the infrahyoid muscles to reach the thyroid gland. In addition to supplying this gland, it gives off branches to the infrahyoid muscles and the SCM and gives rise to the superior laryngeal artery, supplying the larynx.
- **Lingual artery** arises from the anterior aspect of the external carotid artery, where it lies on the middle con-

stricter muscle of the pharynx; arches superoanteriorly and passes deep to CN XII, the stylohyoid muscle, and the posterior belly of the digastric muscle; and disappears deep to the hyoglossus muscle, giving branches to the posterior tongue. It then turns superiorly at the anterior border of this muscle, bifurcating into the deep lingual and sublingual arteries.
- **Facial artery** arises anteriorly from the external carotid artery, either in common with the lingual artery or

immediately superior to it; after giving rise to the *ascending palatine artery* and a *tonsillar branch,* passes superiorly under cover of the digastric and stylohyoid muscles and the angle of the mandible. It loops anteriorly and enters a deep groove in and supplies the submandibular gland and then gives rise to the submental artery to the floor of the mouth and hooks around the middle of the inferior border of the mandible to enter the face.

VEINS IN ANTERIOR CERVICAL REGION

Most veins in the anterior cervical region are tributaries of the **IJV,** usually the largest vein in the neck (Fig. 8.6*B, D*). The *IJV* drains blood from the brain, anterior face, cervical viscera, and deep muscles of the neck. The IJV commences at the jugular foramen in the posterior cranial fossa as the direct continuation of the sigmoid sinus (see Chapter 7). From the dilation at its origin, the **superior bulb of the IJV,** the vein runs inferiorly through the neck in the *carotid sheath* with the internal carotid artery superior to the carotid bifurcation and the common carotid artery and CN X inferiorly (Fig. 8.2*C*). The vein lies laterally within the sheath, with the nerve located posteriorly. The *cervical sympathetic trunk* lies posterior to the carotid sheath and is embedded in the prevertebral layer of deep cervical fascia. The IJV leaves the anterior cervical region by passing deep to the SCM.

Posterior to the sternal end of the clavicle, the IJV unites with the subclavian vein to form the *brachiocephalic vein.* The inferior end of the IJV dilates to form the **inferior bulb of the IJV** (Fig. 8.6*D*). This bulb has a bicuspid valve that permits blood to flow toward the heart while preventing backflow into the vein. The tributaries of the IJV are the inferior petrosal sinus and the facial, lingual, pharyngeal, and superior and middle thyroid veins. The **occipital vein** usually drains into the *suboccipital venous plexus,* drained by the deep cervical vein and the vertebral vein, but may drain into the IJV.

Ligation of External Carotid Artery

Sometimes *ligation of an external carotid artery* is necessary to control bleeding from one of its relatively inaccessible branches. This procedure decreases blood flow through the artery and its branches but does not eliminate it. Blood flows in a retrograde (backward) direction into the artery from the external carotid artery on the other side through communications between its branches (e.g., those in the face and scalp) and across the midline. When the external carotid or subclavian arteries are ligated, the descending branch of the occipital artery provides the main collateral circulation, anastomosing with the vertebral and deep cervical arteries.

Surgical Dissection of Carotid Triangle

The carotid triangle provides an important surgical approach to the carotid system of arteries, the IJV, the vagus and hypoglossal nerves, and the cervical sympathetic trunk. Damage or compression of the vagus and/or recurrent laryngeal nerves during surgical dissection of the triangle may produce an alteration in the voice because these nerves supply laryngeal muscles.

Carotid Pulse

The carotid pulse ("neck pulse") is easily felt by palpating the common carotid artery in the side of the neck, where it lies in a groove between the trachea and the infrahyoid muscles. It is usually easily palpated just deep to the anterior border of the SCM at the level of the superior border of the thyroid cartilage. It is routinely checked during *cardiopulmonary resuscitation* (CPR). Absence of a carotid pulse indicates cardiac arrest.

Carotid Occlusion and Endarterectomy

Atherosclerotic thickening of the intima of the internal carotid artery may obstruct blood flow. Symptoms resulting from this obstruction depend on the degree of obstruction and the amount of collateral blood flow to the brain from other arteries. A partial occlusion may cause a *transient ischemic attack* (TIA), a sudden focal loss of neurological function (e.g., dizziness and disorientation) that disappears within 24 hours. Arterial occlusion may also cause a *stroke.*

Carotid occlusion, causing stenosis (narrowing), can be relieved by opening the artery at its origin and stripping off the atherosclerotic plaque with the intima. This procedure is called *carotid endarterectomy.* Because of the relations of the internal carotid artery, there is risk of cranial nerve injury during the procedure involving one or more of the following nerves: CN IX, CN X (or its branch, the superior laryngeal nerve), CN XI, or CN XII.

Internal Jugular Pulse

Pulsations of the IJV can provide information about heart activity corresponding to electrocardiogram (ECG) recordings and right atrial pressure. The vein's pulsations are transmitted through the surrounding tissues and may be observed deep to the SCM superior to the medial end of the clavicle. Because there are no valves in the brachiocephalic vein or the superior vena cava, a wave of contraction passes up these vessels to the IJV. The pulsations are especially visible when the person's head is inferior to the feet (the *Trendelenburg position*). The internal jugular pulse increases considerably in conditions such as mitral valve disease, which increases pressure in the pulmonary circulation and the right side of the heart.

Internal Jugular Vein Puncture

A needle and catheter may be inserted into the IJV for diagnostic or therapeutic purposes. The right internal jugular vein is preferable because it is usually larger and straighter. During this procedure, the clinician palpates the common carotid artery and inserts the needle into the IJV just lateral to it

at a 30-degree angle, aiming at the apex of the triangle between the sternal and the clavicular heads of the SCM. The needle is then directed inferolaterally toward the ipsilateral nipple (Fig. B8.4).

Sternocleidomastoid

Internal jugular vein

Subclavian vein

Superior vena cava

Anterior view

FIGURE B8.4.

NERVES IN ANTERIOR CERVICAL REGION

The **transverse cervical nerve** (C2 and C3) supplies the skin covering the anterior cervical region (Fig. B8.3). The **hypoglossal nerve** (CN XII), the motor nerve of the tongue, enters the submandibular triangle deep to the posterior belly of the digastric muscle to supply the muscles of the tongue (Fig. 8.5*B–D*). Branches of the **glossopharyngeal** and **vagus nerves** are located in the submandibular and carotid triangles.

Surface Anatomy of Cervical Regions and Triangles of Neck

The cervical regions and triangles are outlined in Figure SA8.1*B*. Some of the important structures found in the regions and triangles are summarized in Table 8.3.

The **skin of the neck** is thin and pliable. The subcutaneous connective tissue contains the **platysma,** a thin sheet of striated muscle that ascends to the face (Fig. SA8.1*A*).

The **SCM** is the key muscular landmark of the neck. It defines the **sternocleidomastoid region** and divides the neck into anterior and lateral cervical regions (Fig. SA8.1*D*). This muscle is easy to observe and palpate throughout its length as it passes superolaterally from the clavicle and manubrium to the mastoid process of the temporal bone. The SCM can be made to stand out by asking the person to rotate the face toward the contralateral side and elevate the chin.

The **EJV** runs vertically across the SCM toward the angle of the mandible (Fig. SA8.1*D*). This vein may be prominent, especially if distended, and can be visualized by asking the person to take a deep breath (*Valsalva maneuver*). The **jugular notch** in the manubrium is the fossa between the sternal heads of the SCM. The lesser supraclavicular fossa, between the sternal and clavicular heads of the SCM, overlies the inferior end of the IJV. Deep to the superior half of the SCM is the cervical plexus, and deep to the inferior half of the SCM are the IJV, common carotid artery, and vagus nerve in the carotid sheath.

The anterior border of the **trapezius** defines the posterior cervical region. It may be observed and palpated when the shoulders are shrugged against resistance (Fig. SA8.1*C*).

A Anterior view

B Anterolateral view

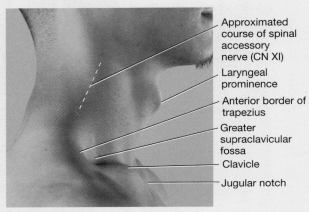

Approximated course of spinal accessory nerve (CN XI)

Laryngeal prominence

Anterior border of trapezius

Greater supraclavicular fossa

Clavicle

Jugular notch

C Lateral view

Key for B

A Sternocleidomastoid (SCM) region
B Lateral cervical region
C Anterior cervical region
D Posterior cervical region
E Suboccipital region
1 Lesser supraclavicular fossa
2 Occipital triangle
3 Omoclavicular triangle
4 Submental triangle
5 Submandibular triangle
6 Carotid triangle
7 Muscular triangle
X Carotid bifurcation
(take pulse inferior to this point)

Angle of mandible

External jugular vein

Laryngeal prominence

Trapezius

Clavicular ⎫
            ⎬ Heads of SCM
Sternal   ⎭

Jugular notch

Lesser   ⎫
          ⎬ Supraclavicular fossae
Greater   ⎭

D Anterolateral view

E Palpation of submandibular lymph nodes

FIGURE SA8.1.

Just inferior to the belly of the omohyoid is the greater supraclavicular fossa (Fig. SA8.1D), the depression overlying the omoclavicular triangle. The subclavian arterial pulsations can be palpated here in most people.

The **occipital triangle** contains the **spinal accessory nerve** (CN XI). Because of its vulnerability and frequency of iatrogenic injury (damage resulting from medical treatment), it is important to be able to estimate the location of the nerve (Fig. SA8.1*C*). Its course can be approximated by a line that intersects the junction of the superior and middle thirds of the posterior border of the SCM and the junction of the middle and lower thirds of the anterior border of the trapezius.

The **submandibular gland** nearly fills the submandibular triangle. It is palpable as a soft mass inferior to the body of the mandible, especially when the tongue is pushed against the maxillary incisor teeth. The **submandibular lymph nodes** lie superficial to the gland and, if enlarged, can be palpated by moving the fingers from the angle of the mandible along its inferior border (Fig. SA8.1*E*). If this is

continued until the examiner's fingers meet under the chin, enlarged **submental lymph nodes** can be palpated in the **submental triangle.**

The carotid arterial system is located in the **carotid triangle.** The **carotid sheath** can be mapped out by a line joining the sternoclavicular joint to a point midway between the mastoid process and the angle of the mandible (Fig. SA8.1*B*). The **carotid pulse** can be palpated by placing the index and third fingers on the thyroid cartilage and pointing them posterolaterally between the trachea and SCM. The pulse is palpable just medial to the SCM.

TABLE 8.3 SUMMARY OF CONTENTS OF REGIONS/TRIANGLES OF NECK

Region	Main Contents and Underlying Structures
Sternocleidomastoid region (**A**)	Sternocleidomastoid (SCM) muscle; superior part of the external jugular vein; greater auricular nerve; transverse cervical nerve
Lesser supraclavicular fossa (*1*)	Inferior part of internal jugular vein
Posterior cervical region (**D**)	Trapezius muscle; cutaneous branches of posterior rami of cervical spinal nerves; suboccipital region or triangle (**E**) lies deep to superior part of this region
Lateral cervical region (posterior triangle of neck) (**B**) Occipital triangle (*2*)	Part of external jugular vein; posterior branches of cervical plexus of nerves; spinal accessory nerve; trunks of brachial plexus; cervicodorsal trunk; cervical lymph nodes
Omoclavicular (subclavian) triangle (*3*)	Subclavian artery (third part); part of subclavian vein (sometimes); suprascapular artery; supraclavicular lymph nodes
Anterior cervical region (anterior triangle of neck) (**C**) Submandibular (digastric) triangle (*4*)	Submandibular gland almost fills triangle; submandibular lymph nodes; hypoglossal nerve; mylohyoid nerve; parts of facial artery and vein
Submental triangle (*5*)	Submental lymph nodes and small veins that unite to form anterior jugular vein
Carotid triangle (*6*)	Common carotid artery and its branches; internal jugular vein and its tributaries; vagus nerve; external carotid artery and some of its branches; hypoglossal nerve and superior root of ansa cervicalis; spinal accessory nerve; thyroid gland, larynx; pharynx; deep cervical lymph nodes; branches of cervical plexus
Muscular (omotracheal) triangle (*7*)	Sternothyroid and sternohyoid muscles; thyroid and parathyroid glands

DEEP STRUCTURES OF NECK

The **deep structures of the neck** are the prevertebral muscles, located posterior to the cervical viscera and anterolateral to the vertebral column, and structures located on the cervical side of the superior thoracic aperture, the root of the neck.

Prevertebral Muscles

The **anterior** and **lateral vertebral muscles** or **prevertebral muscles,** consisting of the longus colli and capitis and rectus capitis anterior and the anterior scalene muscles, lie directly posterior to the retropharyngeal space (Fig. 8.2). The **lateral vertebral muscles,** consisting of the rectus capitis lateralis, splenius capitis, levator scapulae, and

middle and posterior scalene muscles, lie posterior to the neurovascular plane of the cervical and brachial plexuses and subclavian artery, except the rectus capitis lateralis, which lies in the floor of the lateral cervical region. The muscles are illustrated and described in Table 8.4.

Root of Neck

The **root of the neck** is the junctional area between the thorax and the neck (Fig. 8.7*B*). The inferior boundary of the root of the neck is formed laterally by the first pair of ribs and their costal cartilages, anteriorly by the manubrium of the sternum, and posteriorly by the body of the T1 vertebra. Only the neurovascular elements of the root of the neck are described here; the visceral structures are discussed later in this chapter.

TABLE 8.4 PREVERTEBRAL MUSCLES

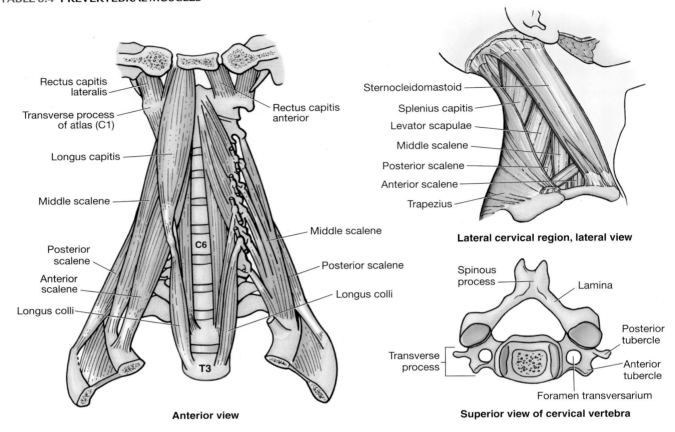

Rectus capitis lateralis

Transverse process of atlas (C1)

Longus capitis

Middle scalene

Posterior scalene

Anterior scalene

Longus colli

Rectus capitis anterior

Middle scalene

Posterior scalene

Longus colli

C6

T3

Anterior view

Sternocleidomastoid

Splenius capitis

Levator scapulae

Middle scalene

Posterior scalene

Anterior scalene

Trapezius

Lateral cervical region, lateral view

Spinous process

Lamina

Posterior tubercle

Anterior tubercle

Transverse process

Foramen transversarium

Superior view of cervical vertebra

Muscle	Superior Attachment	Inferior Attachment	Innervation	Main Action(s)
Anterior vertebral muscles				
Longus colli	Anterior tubercle of C1 vertebra (atlas); bodies of C1–C3 and transverse processes of C3–C6 vertebrae	Bodies of C5–T3 vertebrae; transverse processes of C3–C5 vertebrae	Anterior rami of C2–C6 spinal nerves	Flexes neck (anterior [or lateral] bending of cervical vertebrae C2–C7)
Longus capitis	Basilar part of occipital bone	Anterior tubercles of C3–C6 transverse processes	Anterior rami of C1–C3 spinal nerves	Flexion of head on neck (anterior [or lateral] bending of the head relative to the vertebral column at the atlanto-occipital joints)
Rectus capitis anterior	Base of cranium, just anterior to occipital condyle	Anterior surface of lateral mass of atlas (C1 vertebra)	Branches from loop between C1 and C2 spinal nerves	
Anterior scalene	Anterior tubercles of transverse processes of C3–C6 vertebrae	1st rib	Cervical spinal nerves C4–C6	Flexes neck laterally; elevates 1st rib during forced inspiration[a]

TABLE 8.4 PREVERTEBRAL MUSCLES (*continued*)

Muscle	Superior Attachment	Inferior Attachment	Innervation	Main Action(s)
Lateral vertebral muscles				
Rectus capitis lateralis	Jugular process of occipital bone	Transverse process of atlas (C1 vertebra)	Branches from loop between C1 and C2 spinal nerves	Flexes head and helps stabilize it[b]
Splenius capitis	Inferior half of nuchal ligament and spinous processes of superior six thoracic vertebrae	Lateral aspect of mastoid process and lateral third of superior nuchal line	Posterior rami of middle cervical spinal nerves	Laterally flexes and rotates head and neck to same side; acting bilaterally, extends head and neck[c]
Levator scapulae	Posterior tubercles of transverse processes of C1–C4 vertebrae	Superior part of medial border of scapula	Dorsal scapular nerve C5 and cervical spinal nerves C3 and C4	Elevates scapula and tilts its glenoid cavity inferiorly by rotating scapula
Middle scalene	Posterior tubercles of transverse processes of C4–C7 vertebrae	Superior surface of 1st rib; posterior groove for subclavian artery	Anterior rami of cervical spinal nerves	Flexes neck laterally; elevates 1st rib during forced inspiration[a]
Posterior scalene	Posterior tubercles of transverse processes of C4–C6 vertebrae	External border of 2nd rib	Anterior rami of cervical spinal nerves C7 and C8	Flexes neck laterally; elevates 2nd rib during forced inspiration[a]

[a]Flexion of neck = anterior (or lateral) bending of cervical vertebrae C2–C7.

[b]Flexion of head = anterior (or lateral) bending of the head relative to the vertebral column at the atlanto-occipital joints.

[c]Rotation of the head occurs at the atlanto-axial joints.

ARTERIES IN ROOT OF NECK

The **brachiocephalic trunk,** covered anteriorly by the sternohyoid and sternothyroid muscles, is the largest branch of the arch of the aorta. It arises in the midline, posterior to the manubrium, and passes superolaterally to the right. It divides into the right common carotid and right subclavian arteries posterior to the right sternoclavicular (SC) joint (Fig. 8.7*A*).

The **subclavian arteries** supply the upper limbs and send branches to the neck and brain. The **right subclavian artery** arises from the brachiocephalic trunk, and the **left subclavian artery** arises from the arch of the aorta (Figs. 8.6*A* and 8.7*A*). Their courses in the neck begin posterior to the respective SC joints as they ascend through the superior thoracic aperture. The arteries arch superolaterally, extending between their origin and the medial margin of the anterior scalene muscle. As the arteries begin to descend, they travel deep to the middle of the clavicles and cross the outer margin of the first ribs, where their name changes to the axillary arteries.

For purposes of description, the anterior scalene muscle divides each subclavian artery into three parts: the first part is medial to the muscle, the second is posterior to it, and the third is lateral to it (Fig. 8.7*D*). The cervical pleurae, covering the apices of the lungs, and sympathetic trunk lie posterior to the arteries (Fig. 8.7*B*). The **branches of the subclavian artery** are the (Fig. 8.7):

- *Vertebral artery, internal thoracic artery,* and *thyrocervical trunk* from the first part of the subclavian artery.

- *Costocervical trunk* from the second part of the subclavian artery.
- *Dorsal scapular artery*, often arising from the third part of the subclavian artery.

The **cervical part of the vertebral artery** arises from the first part of the subclavian artery and ascends in the pyramidal space formed between the scalene and the longus muscles (Fig. 8.7*A*). The artery then passes through the foramina of the transverse processes of vertebrae C1–C6. This **vertebral part of the vertebral artery** may enter a foramen more superior than the C6 vertebra. The **suboccipital part of the vertebral artery** courses in a groove on the posterior arch of the atlas before it enters the cranial cavity through the foramen magnum, demarcating the beginning of the **cranial part of the vertebral artery.**

The **internal thoracic artery** arises from the anteroinferior aspect of the subclavian artery and passes inferomedially into the thorax (Fig. 8.7*D*). The internal thoracic artery has no branches in the neck; its thoracic distribution is described in Chapter 1.

The **thyrocervical trunk** arises from the anterosuperior aspect of the first part of the subclavian artery, near the medial border of the anterior scalene muscle. It has two lateral branches, the suprascapular artery, supplying muscles on the posterior scapula, and the cervicodorsal trunk (Fig. 8.7*A, D*). Arising from the **cervicodorsal trunk** are the *dorsal scapular* and *superficial cervical arteries*, sending branches to muscles in the lateral cervical region,

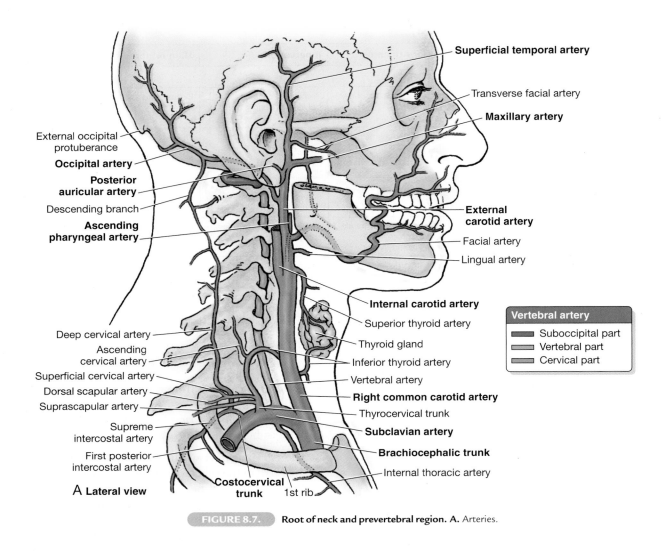

Superficial temporal artery

Transverse facial artery

Maxillary artery

External occipital protuberance

Occipital artery

Posterior auricular artery

Descending branch

Ascending pharyngeal artery

External carotid artery

Facial artery

Lingual artery

Internal carotid artery

Superior thyroid artery

Thyroid gland

Deep cervical artery

Inferior thyroid artery

Ascending cervical artery

Superficial cervical artery

Vertebral artery

Dorsal scapular artery

Right common carotid artery

Suprascapular artery

Thyrocervical trunk

Supreme intercostal artery

Subclavian artery

First posterior intercostal artery

Brachiocephalic trunk

Internal thoracic artery

A **Lateral view**   **Costocervical trunk**   1st rib

Vertebral artery	
	Suboccipital part
	Vertebral part
	Cervical part

FIGURE 8.7.   **Root of neck and prevertebral region. A.** Arteries.

the trapezius, and medial scapular muscles. The terminal branches of the thyrocervical trunk are the *inferior thyroid artery*, the primary visceral artery of the neck, and the ascending cervical artery, supplying lateral muscles of the upper neck.

The **costocervical trunk** arises posteriorly from the second part of the subclavian artery (posterior to the anterior scalene muscle on the right side and usually just medial to this muscle on the left side). The trunk passes posterosuperiorly and divides into the superior intercostal and deep cervical arteries, which supply the first two intercostal spaces and the posterior deep cervical muscles, respectively (Fig. 8.7*A, D*).

The **dorsal scapular artery** often arises from the cervicodorsal trunk, but it may be an independent branch of the second or third part of the subclavian artery. It runs deep to supply the levator scapulae and rhomboid muscles,

supplying both and participating in the arterial anastomoses around the scapula (see Chapter 6).

VEINS IN ROOT OF NECK

Two large veins terminate in the root of the neck: the **external jugular vein,** draining blood received mostly from the scalp and face, and the variable **anterior jugular vein** (Figs. 8.4 and 8.5*A*). The AJV typically arises near the hyoid bone from the confluence of superficial submandibular veins. At the root of the neck, the vein turns laterally, posterior to the SCM, and opens into the termination of the EJV or into the subclavian vein. Superior to the manubrium, the right and left AJVs commonly unite across the midline to form the **jugular venous arch** in the suprasternal space.

The *subclavian vein,* the continuation of the axillary vein, begins at the lateral border of the first rib and ends when it

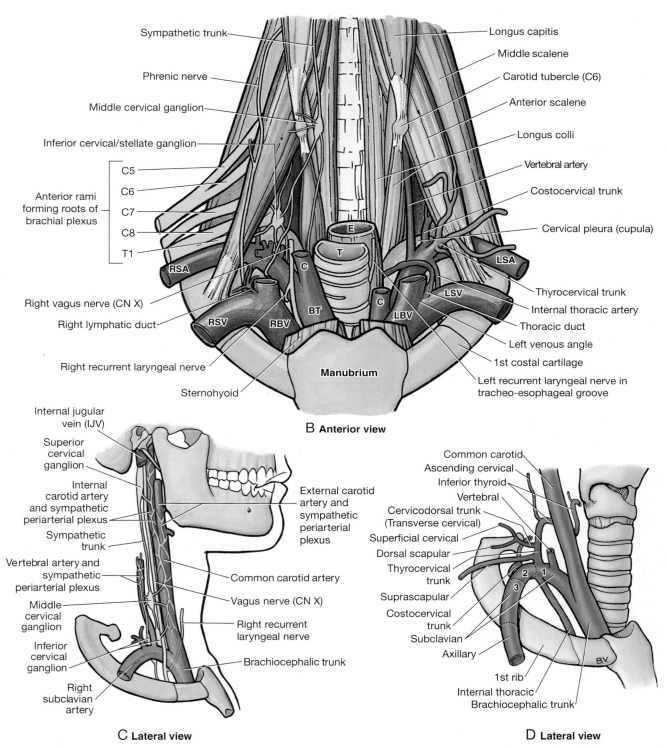

Sympathetic trunk

Phrenic nerve

Middle cervical ganglion

Inferior cervical/stellate ganglion

C5
C6
C7
C8
T1

Anterior rami forming roots of brachial plexus

Right vagus nerve (CN X)

Right lymphatic duct

Right recurrent laryngeal nerve

Sternohyoid

Longus capitis

Middle scalene

Carotid tubercle (C6)

Anterior scalene

Longus colli

Vertebral artery

Costocervical trunk

Cervical pleura (cupula)

Thyrocervical trunk

Internal thoracic artery

Thoracic duct

Left venous angle

1st costal cartilage

Left recurrent laryngeal nerve in tracheo-esophageal groove

E

T

C

BT

C

LSA

LSV

LBV

RSA

RSV   RBV

Manubrium

B **Anterior view**

Internal jugular vein (IJV)

Superior cervical ganglion

Internal carotid artery and sympathetic periarterial plexus

Sympathetic trunk

Vertebral artery and sympathetic periarterial plexus

Middle cervical ganglion

Inferior cervical ganglion

Right subclavian artery

External carotid artery and sympathetic periarterial plexus

Common carotid artery

Vagus nerve (CN X)

Right recurrent laryngeal nerve

Brachiocephalic trunk

C **Lateral view**

Common carotid

Ascending cervical

Inferior thyroid

Vertebral

Cervicodorsal trunk (Transverse cervical)

Superficial cervical

Dorsal scapular

Thyrocervical trunk

Suprascapular

Costocervical trunk

Subclavian

Axillary

2   1

3

1st rib

Internal thoracic

Brachiocephalic trunk

B.V.

D **Lateral view**

FIGURE 8.7. **Root of neck and prevertebral region** *(continued)*. **B.** Dissection of the root of the neck. *BT*, brachiocephalic trunk; *C*, left and right common carotid arteries; *E*, esophagus; *LBV*, left brachiocephalic vein; *LSA*, left subclavian artery; *LSV*, left subclavian vein; *RBV*, right brachiocephalic vein; *RSA*, right subclavian artery; *RSV*, right subclavian vein; *T*, trachea. **C.** Nerves. **D.** Branches of the subclavian artery.

unites with the IJV posterior to the medial end of the clavicle, to form the **brachiocephalic vein** (Fig. 8.7*B*). This union is commonly referred to as the **venous angle** and is the site where the *thoracic duct* (left side) and the *right lymphatic trunk* (right side) drain lymph collected throughout the body into the venous circulation. Throughout its course, the IJV is enclosed by the *carotid sheath* (Fig. 8.5*C*).

NERVES IN ROOT OF NECK

There are three pairs of major nerves in the root of the neck: (1) the vagus nerves, (2) the phrenic nerves, and (3) the sympathetic trunks (Fig. 8.7*B*).

Vagus Nerves (CN X). After their exit from the jugular foramen, each **vagus nerve** passes inferiorly in the neck within the posterior part of the **carotid sheath** in the angle between the IJV and the common carotid artery (Figs. 8.2*C* and 8.5*C*). The **right vagus nerve** passes anterior to the first part of the subclavian artery and posterior to the brachiocephalic vein and SC joint to enter the thorax (Fig. 8.7*B*). The **left vagus nerve** descends between the left common carotid and the left subclavian arteries and posterior to the SC joint to enter the thorax.

The **recurrent laryngeal nerves** arise from the vagus nerves in the inferior part of the neck. The nerves of the two sides have essentially the same distribution; however, they arise and recur (loop around) different structures and at different levels on the two sides. The **right recurrent laryngeal nerve** loops inferior to the right subclavian artery (Fig. 8.7*B*), and the **left recurrent laryngeal nerve** loops inferior to the arch of the aorta (Fig. 8.9*A, D*). After looping, both recurrent laryngeal nerves ascend superiorly to the posteromedial aspect of the thyroid gland, where they ascend in the **tracheo-esophageal groove,** supplying both the trachea and esophagus and all the intrinsic muscles of the larynx except the cricothyroid.

The **cardiac branches of CN X** originate in the neck as well as in the thorax and convey presynaptic parasympathetic and visceral afferent fibers to the cardiac plexus of nerves.

Phrenic Nerves. The **phrenic nerves** are formed at the lateral borders of the anterior scalene muscles (Fig. 8.7*B*), mainly from the C4 nerve with contributions from C3 and C5. The phrenic nerves descend anterior to the anterior scalene muscles under cover of the SCMs and IJVs. They pass deep to the prevertebral layer of deep cervical fascia, between the subclavian arteries and veins, and proceed through the thorax on each side of the mediastinum, supplying the diaphragm (see Chapter 1). In addition to their sensory distribution, they provide the sole motor supply to their own half of the diaphragm.

Sympathetic Trunks. The **cervical portion of the sympathetic trunks** lies anterolateral to the vertebral column, extending superiorly to the level of the C1 vertebra or the cranial base (Figs. 8.7*B, C*). The sympathetic trunks receive no white rami communicantes in the neck. The cervical portion of the trunks contains three **cervical sympathetic ganglia:** superior, middle, and inferior. These ganglia receive presynaptic fibers conveyed to the sympathetic trunk by the superior thoracic spinal nerves and their associated white rami communicantes, which then ascend through the sympathetic trunk to the ganglia. After synapsing with the postsynaptic neuron in the cervical sympathetic ganglia, postsynaptic neurons send fibers to the:

- Cervical spinal nerves via *gray* rami communicantes.
- Thoracic viscera via *cardiopulmonary splanchnic nerves.*
- Head and viscera of the neck via *cephalic arterial branches,* which accompany arteries (especially the vertebral and internal and external carotid arteries) as the *sympathetic periarterial plexuses.*

The **inferior cervical ganglion** usually fuses with the first thoracic ganglion to form the **cervicothoracic ganglion (stellate ganglion).** This star-shaped (L. *stella,* a star) ganglion lies anterior to the transverse process of the C7 vertebra, just superior to the neck of the first rib on each side and posterior to the origin of the vertebral artery. Some postsynaptic fibers from the ganglion pass via gray rami communicantes to the anterior rami of the C7 and C8 spinal nerves. Other fibers pass to the heart via the **inferior cervical cardiac nerve** (a cardiopulmonary splanchnic nerve), which passes along the trachea to the deep *cardiac plexus.* Other fibers pass via arterial branches to contribute to the sympathetic periarterial nerve plexus around the vertebral artery running into the cranial cavity.

The **middle cervical ganglion,** usually small and occasionally absent, lies on the anterior aspect of the inferior thyroid artery at the level of the cricoid cartilage and the transverse process of the C6 vertebra, just anterior to the vertebral artery. Postsynaptic fibers pass from the ganglion via gray rami communicantes to the anterior rami of the C5 and C6 spinal nerves, via a **middle cervical cardiac nerve** (cardiopulmonary splanchnic nerve) to the heart and via arterial branches to form periarterial plexuses to the thyroid gland.

The **superior cervical ganglion** is at the level of the C1 and C2 vertebrae. Because of its large size, it forms a good landmark for locating the sympathetic trunk. Postsynaptic fibers pass from it by means of cephalic arterial branches to form the internal carotid sympathetic plexus and enter the cranial cavity (Fig. 8.7*C*). This ganglion also sends arterial branches to the external carotid artery and gray rami communicantes to the anterior rami of the superior four cervical spinal nerves. Other postsynaptic fibers pass from it to the cardiac plexus of nerves via a **superior cervical cardiac nerve** (cardiopulmonary splanchnic nerve) (see Chapter 1).

Cervicothoracic Ganglion Block

Anesthetic injected around the cervicothoracic ganglion blocks transmission of stimuli through the cervical and superior thoracic ganglia. This ganglion block may relieve vascular spasms involving the brain and upper limb. It is also useful when deciding if surgical resection of the ganglion would be beneficial to a person with excess vasoconstriction of the ipsilateral limb.

Lesion of Cervical Sympathetic Trunk

A lesion of a sympathetic trunk in the neck results in a sympathetic disturbance called *Horner syndrome,* which is characterized by:

- Pupillary constriction, resulting from paralysis of the dilator pupillae muscle.
- Ptosis (drooping of the superior eyelid), resulting from paralysis of the smooth (tarsal) muscle intermingled with striated muscle of the levator palpebrae superioris.
- Sinking in of the eyeball (enophthalmos), possibly caused by paralysis of smooth (orbitalis) muscle in the floor of the orbit.
- Vasodilation and absence of sweating on the face and neck (anhydrosis), caused by a lack of sympathetic (vasoconstrictive) nerve supply to the blood vessels and sweat glands.

VISCERA OF NECK

The cervical viscera are organized in three layers, named for their primary function (Fig. 8.8). Superficial to deep, they are the *endocrine layer* (thyroid and parathyroid glands), the *respiratory layer* (larynx and trachea), and the *alimentary layer* (pharynx and esophagus).

Endocrine Layer of Cervical Viscera

The viscera of **the endocrine layer** are part of the body's endocrine system of ductless, hormone-secreting glands. The thyroid gland produces *thyroid hormone,* which controls the rate of metabolism, and *calcitonin,* a hormone controlling calcium metabolism. The parathyroid glands produce *parathormone* (PTH), which controls the metabolism of phosphorus and calcium in the blood.

THYROID GLAND

The **thyroid gland** is located anteriorly in the neck. It lies deep to the sternothyroid and sternohyoid muscles from the level of the C5–T1 vertebrae (Fig. 8.2*A*, *B*). It consists primarily of right and left **lobes,** anterolateral to the larynx and trachea. A relatively thin **isthmus** unites the lobes over the trachea, usually anterior to the second and third tracheal rings (Fig. 8.8*A*). The thyroid gland is surrounded by a thin **fibrous capsule,** which sends septa deeply into the gland. Dense connective tissue attaches the fibrous capsule to the cricoid cartilage and superior tracheal rings. External to the capsule is a loose *fascial sheath* formed by the visceral portion of the pretracheal layer of deep cervical fascia.

The rich blood supply of the thyroid gland is from the paired **superior** and **inferior thyroid arteries** (Fig. 8.9*A*, *B*). These vessels lie between the fibrous capsule and the loose fascial sheath. Usually, the first branches of the external carotid artery, the *superior thyroid arteries,* descend to the superior poles of the gland, pierce the pretracheal layer of deep cervical fascia, and divide into anterior and posterior branches. The *inferior thyroid arteries,* the largest branches of the thyrocervical trunks, arising from the subclavian arteries, run superomedially posterior to the carotid sheaths to reach the posterior aspect of the thyroid gland. The right and left superior and inferior thyroid arteries anastomose extensively within the gland, ensuring its supply while providing potential collateral circulation between the subclavian and the external carotid arteries.

In approximately 10% of people, a **thyroid ima artery** (L. *arteria thyroidea ima*) arises from the brachiocephalic trunk, the arch of the aorta, or from the right common carotid, subclavian, or internal thoracic arteries (Fig. 8.9*B*). This small artery ascends on the anterior surface of the trachea, which it supplies, and continues to the isthmus of the thyroid gland. The possible presence of this artery must be considered when performing procedures in the midline of the neck inferior to the isthmus because it is a potential source of bleeding.

Three pairs of thyroid veins usually drain the **thyroid plexus of veins** on the anterior surface of the thyroid gland and trachea (Fig. 8.9*A*, *C*). The **superior thyroid veins** accompany the superior thyroid arteries and drain the superior poles of the gland. The **middle thyroid veins** drain the middle of the lobes, and the **inferior thyroid veins** drain the inferior poles. The superior and middle thyroid veins drain into the IJVs, and the inferior thyroid veins drain into the brachiocephalic veins posterior to the manubrium.

The **lymphatic vessels of the thyroid gland** communicate with a capsular network of lymphatic vessels. From this network, the vessels pass initially to **prelaryngeal, pretracheal,** and **paratracheal lymph nodes,** which drain in turn to the **superior** and **inferior deep cervical nodes** (Fig. 8.10). Inferior to the thyroid gland, the lymphatic vessels pass directly to the **inferior deep cervical lymph nodes.** Some lymphatic vessels may drain into *brachiocephalic lymph nodes* or the *thoracic duct.*

The **nerves of the thyroid gland** are derived from the superior, middle, and inferior *cervical sympathetic ganglia*

Epiglottic cartilage

Lesser horn of hyoid

Lateral thyrohyoid ligament

Greater horn of hyoid

Thyrohyoid membrane

Triticeal cartilage

Thyroid cartilage

Superior thyroid notch

Cricothyroid ligament

Laryngeal prominence

Cricoid cartilage

Superior pole

Cricotracheal ligament

Left lobe

Right lobe

Inferior pole

Isthmus

Trachea

Esophagus

A Anterior view

Alimentary layer: Esophagus

Respiratory layer: Trachea

Endocrine layer: Parathyroid gland

Thyroid gland

Capsule and septa of thyroid gland

B Anterosuperior view

FIGURE 8.8.   Relationships of thyroid gland.

(Fig. 8.7C). They reach the gland through the *cardiac* and *superior and inferior thyroid periarterial plexuses* that accompany the thyroid arteries. These fibers are vasomotor, causing constriction of blood vessels. Endocrine secretion from the thyroid gland is hormonally regulated by the pituitary gland.

PARATHYROID GLANDS

The small flattened oval **parathyroid glands** lie external to the fibrous capsule on the medial half of the posterior surface of each lobe of the thyroid gland (Fig. 8.9D). Most people have four parathyroid glands. Approximately 5% of people have more; some have only two glands. The two **superior parathyroid glands** are usually at the level of the inferior border of the cricoid cartilage. The **inferior parathyroid glands** are usually near the inferior poles of the thyroid gland, but they may lie in a variety of positions.

The **inferior thyroid arteries** supply both the superior and the inferior parathyroid glands; however, these glands may also be supplied by branches from the superior thyroid arteries, the thyroid ima artery, or the laryngeal, tracheal, and esophageal arteries. The **parathyroid veins** drain into the *thyroid plexus of veins* of the thyroid gland and trachea (Fig. 8.9C). The **lymphatic vessels from the parathyroid glands** drain with those of the thyroid gland into the deep cervical and paratracheal lymph nodes (Fig. 8.10).

The **nerves of the parathyroid glands** are derived from *thyroid branches of the cervical sympathetic ganglia* (Fig. 8.9A). The nerves are vasomotor but not secretomotor because these glands are hormonally regulated.

Pyramidal Lobe of Thyroid Gland

Approximately 50% of thyroid glands have a small prominence, the *pyramidal lobe,* on the superior surface of the isthmus of the thyroid gland, usually to the left of the median plane. A band of connective tissue, often containing accessory thyroid tissue, may continue from the apex of the pyramidal lobe to the hyoid bone.

Thyroidectomy

During a thyroidectomy (e.g., excision of a malignant thyroid gland), the parathyroid glands are in danger of being inadvertently damaged or removed. These glands are safe during *subtotal thyroidectomy* because the most posterior part of the thyroid gland usually is preserved. Variability in the position of the parathyroid glands, especially the inferior ones, puts them in danger of being removed during surgery on the thyroid gland. If the parathyroid glands are inadvertently removed during surgery, the patient suffers from *tetany,* a severe convulsive disorder. The generalized convulsive muscle spasms result from a fall in blood calcium levels.

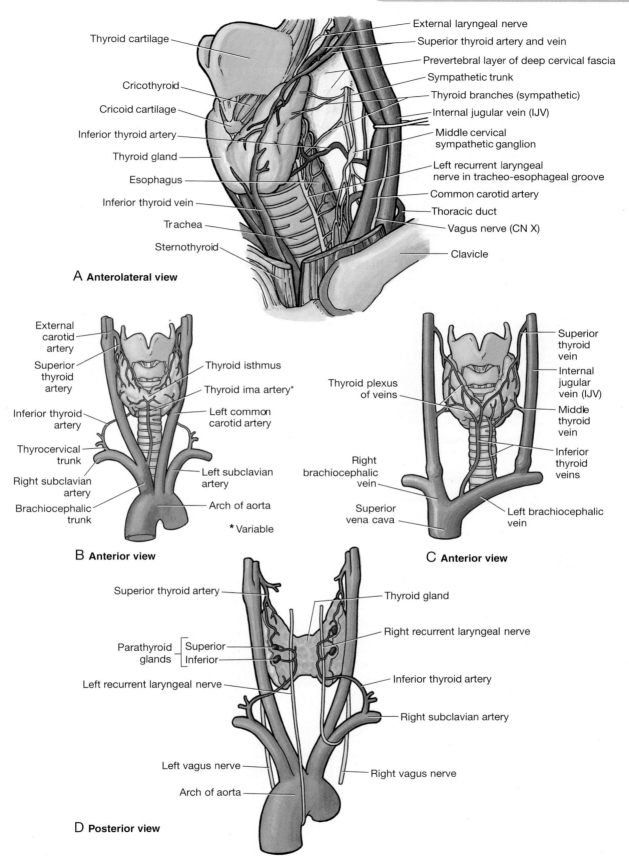

A Anterolateral view

- Thyroid cartilage
- Cricothyroid
- Cricoid cartilage
- Inferior thyroid artery
- Thyroid gland
- Esophagus
- Inferior thyroid vein
- Trachea
- Sternothyroid

- External laryngeal nerve
- Superior thyroid artery and vein
- Prevertebral layer of deep cervical fascia
- Sympathetic trunk
- Thyroid branches (sympathetic)
- Internal jugular vein (IJV)
- Middle cervical sympathetic ganglion
- Left recurrent laryngeal nerve in tracheo-esophageal groove
- Common carotid artery
- Thoracic duct
- Vagus nerve (CN X)
- Clavicle

B Anterior view

- External carotid artery
- Superior thyroid artery
- Inferior thyroid artery
- Thyrocervical trunk
- Right subclavian artery
- Brachiocephalic trunk

- Thyroid isthmus
- Thyroid ima artery*
- Left common carotid artery
- Left subclavian artery
- Arch of aorta
- *Variable

C Anterior view

- Thyroid plexus of veins
- Right brachiocephalic vein
- Superior vena cava

- Superior thyroid vein
- Internal jugular vein (IJV)
- Middle thyroid vein
- Inferior thyroid veins
- Left brachiocephalic vein

D Posterior view

- Superior thyroid artery
- Parathyroid glands { Superior / Inferior }
- Left recurrent laryngeal nerve
- Left vagus nerve
- Arch of aorta

- Thyroid gland
- Right recurrent laryngeal nerve
- Inferior thyroid artery
- Right subclavian artery
- Right vagus nerve

FIGURE 8.9. **Thyroid and parathyroid glands. A.** The vasculature and innervation of the root of the neck is shown. The arterial supply (**B**) and venous drainage (**C**) are detailed. **D.** The blood supply of the parathyroid glands is shown.

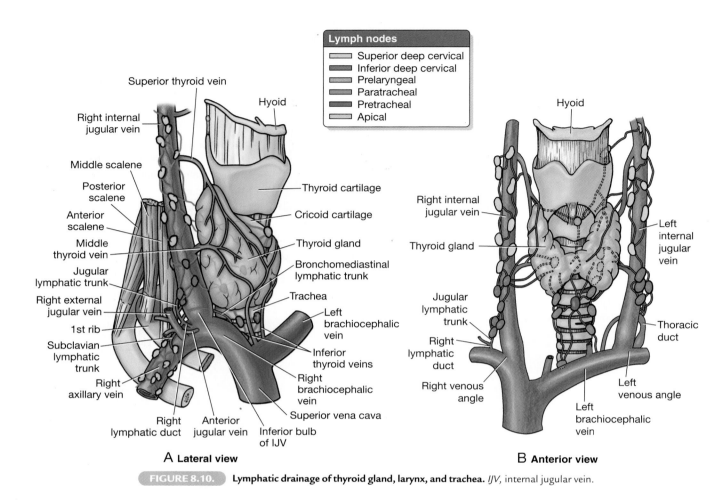

FIGURE 8.10. Lymphatic drainage of thyroid gland, larynx, and trachea. *IJV,* internal jugular vein.

Accessory Thyroid Tissue

Accessory thyroid tissue may develop in the neck lateral to the thyroid cartilage (Fig. B8.5); usually, the tissue lies on the thyrohyoid muscle. The pyramidal lobe and its connective tissue continuation may also contain thyroid tissue. Accessory thyroid tissue, like that of a pyramidal lobe, originates from remnants of the *thyroglossal duct*—a transitory endodermal tube extending from the posterior tongue region of the embryo carrying the thyroid-forming tissue at its descending distal end. Although the accessory tissue may be functional, it is usually too small to maintain normal function if the thyroid gland is removed.

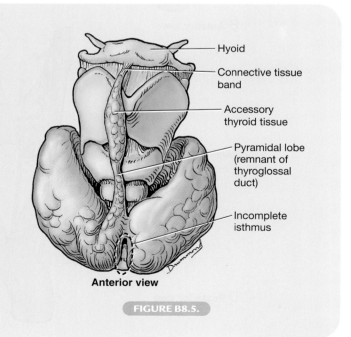

Anterior view

FIGURE B8.5.

Respiratory Layer of Cervical Viscera

The **viscera of the respiratory layer,** the larynx and trachea, contribute to the respiratory functions of the body (Fig. 8.8). The main functions of the respiratory viscera are:

- Routing air and food into the respiratory tract and esophagus, respectively.
- Providing a patent airway and a means of sealing it off temporarily.
- Producing voice.

LARYNX

The **larynx,** the complex organ of voice production, lies in the anterior part of the neck at the level of the bodies of the C3–C6 vertebrae (Fig. 8.1). It connects the inferior part of the pharynx (oropharynx) with the trachea. Although most commonly known for its role as the phonating mechanism for voice production, its most vital function is to guard the air passages, especially during swallowing, when it serves as a sphincter or valve of the lower respiratory tract, thus maintaining a patent airway.

Laryngeal Skeleton. The **laryngeal skeleton** consists of nine cartilages joined by ligaments and membranes (Fig. 8.11). Three cartilages are single (thyroid, cricoid, and epiglottic) and three are paired (arytenoid, corniculate, and cuneiform).

The **thyroid cartilage** is the largest of the cartilages. Its superior border lies opposite the C4 vertebra. The inferior two thirds of its two plate-like **laminae** are fused anteriorly

in the median plane to form the **laryngeal prominence** ("Adam's apple"). Superior to this prominence, the laminae diverge to form the V-shaped **superior thyroid notch** (Fig. 8.8A). The small **inferior thyroid notch** is a shallow indentation in the middle of the inferior border of the cartilage. The posterior border of each lamina projects superiorly as the **superior horn** and inferiorly as the **inferior horn** (Fig. 8.11A). The superior border and superior horns attach to the hyoid by the **thyrohyoid membrane.** The thick median part of this membrane is the **median thyrohyoid ligament,** and its lateral parts are the **lateral thyrohyoid ligaments.** The inferior horns of the thyroid cartilages articulate with the lateral surfaces of the cricoid cartilage at the **cricothyroid joints** (Fig. 8.11). The main movements at these joints are rotation and gliding of the thyroid cartilage, which result in changes in the length of the vocal folds.

The **cricoid cartilage** forms a complete ring around the airway, the only laryngeal cartilage to do so. It is shaped like a signet ring with its band facing anteriorly. The posterior (signet) part of the cricoid cartilage is the *lamina;* the anterior (band) part is the *arch.* The cricoid cartilage is smaller but thicker and stronger than the thyroid cartilage. The cricoid cartilage is attached to the inferior margin of the thyroid cartilage by the **median cricothyroid ligament** and to the first tracheal ring by the **cricotracheal ligament.** Where the larynx is closest to the skin and most accessible, the median cricothyroid ligament may be felt as a soft spot during palpation inferior to the thyroid cartilage.

A Lateral view

B Posterior view

FIGURE 8.11.   Skeleton of larynx and associated ligaments and membranes.

Surface Anatomy of Larynx

The U-shaped **hyoid bone** lies superior to the **thyroid cartilage** at the level of the C4 and C5 vertebrae (Fig. SA8.2). The **laryngeal prominence** is produced by the fused *laminae of the thyroid cartilage*, which meet in the median plane. The **cricoid cartilage** can be felt inferior to the laryngeal prominence. It lies at the level of the C6 vertebra. The cartilaginous **tracheal rings** are palpable in the inferior part of the neck. The second through fourth rings cannot be felt because the **isthmus** of the thyroid, connecting its right and left lobes, covers them. The first tracheal ring is just superior to the isthmus.

Anterior view

FIGURE SA8.2.

Key			
C	Cricoid cartilage	**RL**	Right lobe of thyroid gland
H	Hyoid	**S**	Isthmus
LL	Left lobe of thyroid gland	**T**	Thyroid cartilage
P	Laryngeal prominence	*****	Tracheal rings

The **arytenoid cartilages** are paired, three-sided pyramidal cartilages that articulate with lateral parts of the superior border of the cricoid cartilage lamina. Each cartilage has an apex superiorly, a vocal process anteriorly, and a large muscular process that projects laterally from its base (Fig. 8.11B). The **apex** of each arytenoid cartilage bears the corniculate cartilage and attaches to the aryepiglottic fold. The **vocal process** provides the posterior attachment for the vocal ligament, and the **muscular process** serves as a lever to which the posterior and lateral cricoarytenoid muscles are attached.

The **crico-arytenoid joints**, located between the bases of the arytenoid cartilages and the superolateral surfaces of the lamina of the cricoid cartilage, permit the arytenoid cartilages to slide toward or away from one another, to tilt anteriorly and posteriorly, and to rotate. These movements are important in approximating, tensing, and relaxing the vocal folds. The elastic **vocal ligaments** extend from the junction of the laminae of the thyroid cartilage anteriorly to the vocal process of the arytenoid cartilage posteriorly (Fig. 8.12C). The vocal ligaments form the submucosal skeleton of the vocal folds. The vocal ligaments are the thickened, free superior border of the **conus elasticus** or **cricovocal membrane** (Fig. 8.13A). The parts of the cricovocal membrane extending laterally between the vocal folds and the superior border of the cricoid are the **lateral cricothyroid ligaments.** The fibroelastic conus elasticus blends anteriorly with the *median cricothyroid ligament.* The **conus elasticus** and overlying mucosa close the tracheal inlet, except for the central **rima glottidis** (opening between the vocal folds).

The **epiglottic cartilage,** consisting of elastic cartilage, gives flexibility to the **epiglottis** (Figs. 8.11 and 8.12). It is a heart-shaped cartilage covered with mucous membrane. Situated posterior to the root of the tongue and the hyoid and anterior to the **laryngeal inlet,** the epiglottic cartilage forms the superior part of the anterior wall and the superior margin of the inlet. Its broad superior end is free; its tapered inferior end, the **stalk of the epiglottis,** is attached to the angle formed by the thyroid laminae and the **thyro-epiglottic ligament** (Fig. 8.13A).

The **hyo-epiglottic ligament** attaches the anterior surface of the epiglottic cartilage to the hyoid. A thin submucosal sheet of connective tissue, the **quadrangular**

membrane, extends between the lateral aspects of the ary- tenoid and epiglottic cartilages (Fig. 8.12*C*). Its free inferior margin constitutes the **vestibular ligament,** which is covered loosely by mucosa to form the **vestibular fold** (Fig. 8.12). This fold lies superior to the vocal fold and extends from the thyroid cartilage to the arytenoid cartilage. The free superior margin of the quadrangular membrane forms the **ary-epiglottic ligament,** which is covered with mucosa to form the **ary-epiglottic fold.**

The **corniculate and cuneiform cartilages** appear as small nodules in the posterior part of the ary-epiglottic folds (Figs. 8.11 and 8.12). The corniculate cartilages attach to the apices of the arytenoid cartilages; the cuneiform cartilages do not directly attach to other cartilages.

Interior of the Larynx. The **laryngeal cavity** extends from the *laryngeal inlet,* through which it communicates with the *laryngopharynx,* to the level of the inferior border of the cricoid cartilage. Here, the laryngeal cavity is continuous with the lumen of the trachea. The laryngeal cavity includes the (Fig. 8.12*A*):

- **Laryngeal vestibule,** between the laryngeal inlet and the vestibular folds.
- **Middle part of laryngeal cavity,** the central cavity (airway) between the vestibular and vocal folds.
- **Laryngeal ventricle,** recesses extending laterally from the middle part of the laryngeal cavity between vestibular and vocal folds. The **laryngeal saccule** is a blind pocket opening into each ventricle that is lined with mucosal glands.
- **Infraglottic cavity,** the inferior cavity of the larynx between the vocal folds and the inferior border of the cricoid cartilage, where it is continuous with the lumen of the trachea.

The **vocal folds** (true vocal cords) control sound production. The apex of each wedge-shaped fold projects medially into the laryngeal cavity (Figs. 8.12 and 8.13). Each fold contains a:

- *Vocal ligament,* consisting of thickened elastic tissue that is the medial free edge of the conus elasticus.
- *Vocalis muscle,* composed of exceptionally fine muscle fibers immediately lateral to and terminating at intervals relative to the length of the vocal ligaments (Table 8.5).

The **vocal folds** are the source of sounds (tone) that come from the larynx (Fig. 8.13). The vocal folds produce audible vibrations when their free margins are closely (but not tightly) apposed during phonation and air is forcibly expired intermittently. The vocal folds also serve as the main inspiratory sphincter of the larynx when they are tightly closed. Complete adduction of the folds forms an effective sphincter that prevents entry of air.

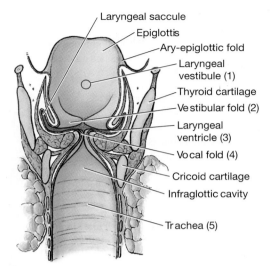

Laryngeal saccule
Epiglottis
Ary-epiglottic fold
Laryngeal vestibule (1)
Thyroid cartilage
Vestibular fold (2)
Laryngeal ventricle (3)
Vocal fold (4)
Cricoid cartilage
Infraglottic cavity
Trachea (5)

A Coronal section, posterior view

Pre-epiglottic fat   Tongue

B Coronal MRI

FIGURE 8.12.   **Interior and compartments of larynx.** **A.** Coronal section. **B.** Coronal MRI. Numbers in **B** refer to **A**.

The **glottis** (vocal apparatus of the larynx) makes up the vocal folds and processes, together with the **rima glottidis,** the aperture between the vocal folds. The shape of the rima (L. slit) varies according to the position of the vocal folds. During ordinary breathing, the rima is narrow and wedge-shaped (Fig. 8.13*B*); during forced respiration it is wide and kite-shaped. The rima glottidis is slit-like when the vocal folds are closely approximated during phonation (Fig. 8.13*C*). Variation in the tension and length of the vocal folds, in the width of the rima glottidis, and in the intensity of the expiratory effort produces changes in the pitch of the voice. The lower range of pitch of the voice of postpubertal males results from the greater length of the vocal folds.

The **vestibular folds** (false vocal cords), extending between the thyroid and the arytenoid cartilages (Fig. 8.12),

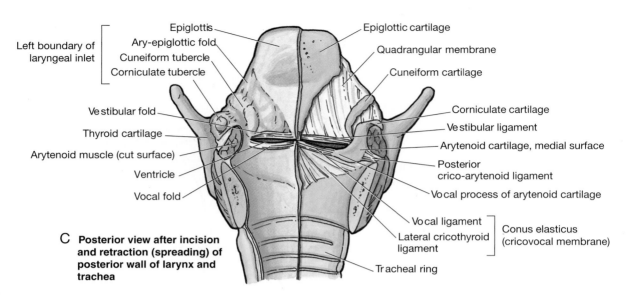

C **Posterior view after incision and retraction (spreading) of posterior wall of larynx and trachea**

FIGURE 8.12. **Interior and compartments of larynx** *(continued).* **C.** The posterior wall of the larynx is split in the median plane and the two sides are separated.

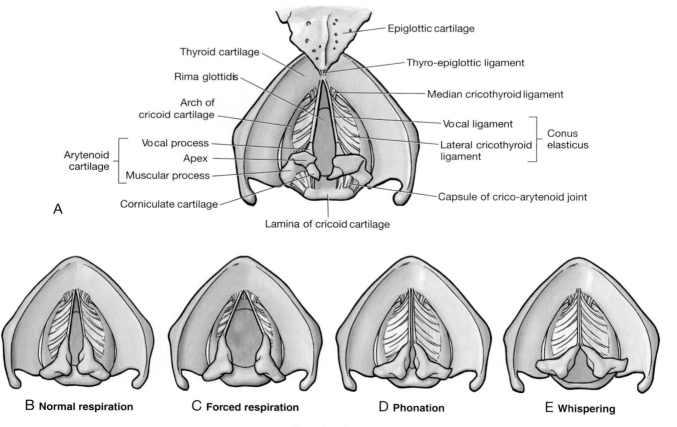

Superior views

FIGURE 8.13. **Rima glottidis. A.** Skeleton and ligaments of the larynx. **B–E.** Shape of the rima glottidis in relation to the position of the vocal folds.

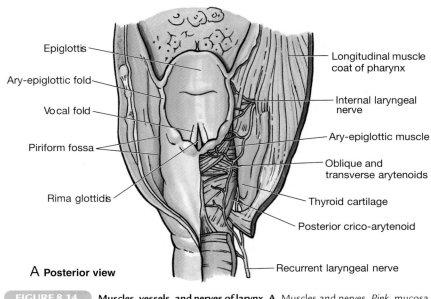

Epiglottis
Ary-epiglottic fold
Vocal fold
Piriform fossa
Rima glottidis

Longitudinal muscle coat of pharynx
Internal laryngeal nerve
Ary-epiglottic muscle
Oblique and transverse arytenoids
Thyroid cartilage
Posterior crico-arytenoid
Recurrent laryngeal nerve

A Posterior view

FIGURE 8.14. **Muscles, vessels, and nerves of larynx. A.** Muscles and nerves. *Pink,* mucosa.

play little or no part in voice production. They are protective in function. They consist of two thick folds of mucous membrane enclosing the *vestibular ligaments.* The space between these ligaments is the **rima vestibuli.** The lateral recesses between the vocal and the vestibular folds are the *laryngeal ventricles.*

Muscles of the Larynx. The laryngeal muscles are divided into extrinsic and intrinsic groups:

- The **extrinsic laryngeal muscles** move the larynx as a whole (Table 8.5). The *infrahyoid muscles* are depressors of the hyoid and larynx, whereas the *suprahyoid* and *stylopharyngeus muscles* are elevators of the hyoid and larynx.
- The **intrinsic laryngeal muscles** move the laryngeal parts, making alterations in the length and tension of the vocal folds and in the size and shape of the rima glottidis. All but one of the intrinsic muscles of the larynx are supplied by the *recurrent laryngeal nerve* (Fig. 8.14), a branch of CN X. The cricothyroid muscle is supplied by the external laryngeal nerve, one of the two terminal branches of the *superior laryngeal nerve.* The actions of the intrinsic laryngeal muscles are described in Table 8.5.

The **inferior laryngeal nerve,** the continuation of the recurrent laryngeal nerve (a branch of the vagus), supplies all intrinsic muscles of the larynx except the cricothyroid, which is supplied by the external laryngeal nerve. It also supplies sensory fibers to the mucosa of the infraglottic cavity. The inferior laryngeal nerve enters the larynx by passing deep to the inferior border of the inferior constrictor muscle of the pharynx. It divides into anterior and posterior branches that accompany the inferior laryngeal artery into the larynx.

Vessels of the Larynx. The laryngeal arteries, branches of the superior and inferior thyroid arteries, supply the larynx (Fig. 8.14B). The **superior laryngeal artery** accompanies the internal branch of the superior laryngeal nerve through the thyrohyoid membrane and branches to supply the internal surface of the larynx. The **inferior laryngeal artery,** a branch of the inferior thyroid artery, accompanies the *inferior laryngeal nerve* (terminal part of the recurrent laryngeal nerve) and supplies the mucous membrane and muscles in the inferior part of the larynx.

The laryngeal veins accompany the laryngeal arteries. The **superior laryngeal vein** usually joins the superior thyroid vein and through it drains into the IJV. The **inferior laryngeal vein** joins the inferior thyroid vein or the thyroid plexus of veins on the anterior aspect of the trachea, which empties into the left brachiocephalic vein.

The **lymphatic vessels of the larynx** superior to the vocal folds accompany the superior laryngeal artery through the thyrohyoid membrane and drain into the **superior deep cervical lymph nodes** (Fig. 8.10). The lymphatic vessels inferior to the vocal folds drain into the *pretracheal* or *paratracheal lymph nodes,* which drain into the **inferior deep cervical lymph nodes.**

Nerves of the Larynx. The nerves of the larynx are the superior and inferior laryngeal branches of the vagus nerve (Fig. 8.14). The **superior laryngeal nerve** arises from the **inferior vagal ganglion** and divides into two terminal branches within the carotid sheath: the internal laryngeal nerve (sensory and autonomic) and the external laryngeal nerve (motor).

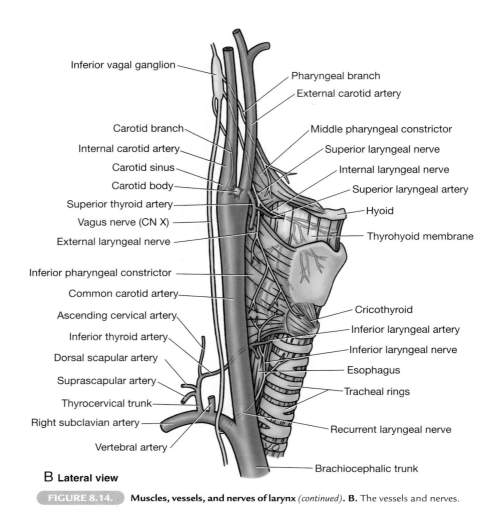

Inferior vagal ganglion

Carotid branch
Internal carotid artery
Carotid sinus
Carotid body
Superior thyroid artery
Vagus nerve (CN X)
External laryngeal nerve

Inferior pharyngeal constrictor
Common carotid artery
Ascending cervical artery
Inferior thyroid artery
Dorsal scapular artery
Suprascapular artery
Thyrocervical trunk
Right subclavian artery
Vertebral artery

Pharyngeal branch
External carotid artery
Middle pharyngeal constrictor
Superior laryngeal nerve
Internal laryngeal nerve
Superior laryngeal artery
Hyoid
Thyrohyoid membrane

Cricothyroid
Inferior laryngeal artery
Inferior laryngeal nerve
Esophagus
Tracheal rings

Recurrent laryngeal nerve

Brachiocephalic trunk

B **Literal view**

FIGURE 8.14.   **Muscles, vessels, and nerves of larynx** *(continued)*. **B.** The vessels and nerves.

The **internal laryngeal nerve,** the larger terminal branch of the superior laryngeal nerve, pierces the thyrohyoid membrane with the superior laryngeal artery, supplying sensory fibers to the laryngeal mucous membrane of the laryngeal vestibule and middle laryngeal cavity, including the superior surface of the vocal folds.

The **external laryngeal nerve** descends posterior to the sternothyroid muscle in company with the superior thyroid artery. At first the nerve lies on the inferior constrictor muscle of the pharynx; it then pierces the muscle, contributing to its innervation (with the pharyngeal plexus), and continues to supply the cricothyroid muscle.

TRACHEA

The **trachea,** extending from the inferior end of the larynx into the thorax, terminates at the sternal angle, where it divides into the right and left main bronchi (Fig. 8.9*A*). Deviation of the trachea from the midline often signals the presence of a pathological process. In adults, the trachea is approximately 2.5 cm in diameter, whereas in infants it is the diameter of a pencil.

The trachea is a fibrocartilaginous tube, supported by incomplete cartilaginous **tracheal rings.** They are deficient posteriorly where the trachea is adjacent to the esophagus (Fig. 8.8). The rings keep the trachea patent. The posterior gap in the tracheal rings is spanned by the involuntary **trachealis muscle,** smooth muscle connecting the ends of the tracheal rings.

Lateral to the trachea are the common carotid arteries and thyroid lobes (Fig. 8.14*B*). Inferior to the isthmus of the thyroid gland are the jugular venous arch and the inferior thyroid veins.

TABLE 8.5 MUSCLES OF THE LARYNX

Lateral view
Cricothyroid

Superior view
Posterior crico-arytenoid

Superior view
Transverse arytenoid

Superior view
Thyro-arytenoid

Superior view
Lateral crico-arytenoid

Superior view
Oblique arytenoid

Muscle	Origin	Insertion	Innervation	Main Action(s)
Cricothyroid	Anterolateral part of cricoid cartilage	Inferior margin and inferior horn of thyroid cartilage	External laryngeal nerve (from CN X)	Stretches and tenses vocal ligament
Thyro-arytenoid[a]	Lower half of posterior aspect of angle of thyroid laminae and cricothyroid ligament	Anterolateral arytenoid surface	Inferior laryngeal nerve (terminal part of recurrent laryngeal nerve, from CN X)	Relaxes vocal ligament
Posterior crico-arytenoid	Posterior surface of lamina of cricoid cartilage	Muscular process of arytenoid cartilage		Abducts vocal folds
Lateral crico-arytenoid	Arch of cricoid cartilage			Adducts vocal folds (interligamentous portion)
Transverse and oblique arytenoids[b]	One arytenoid cartilage	Contralateral arytenoid cartilage		Adduct arytenoid cartilages (adducting intercartilaginous portion of vocal folds, closing posterior rima glottidis)
Vocalis[c]	Lateral surface of vocal process of arytenoid cartilage	Ipsilateral vocal ligament		Relaxes posterior vocal ligament while maintaining (or increasing) tension of anterior part

[a]Superior fibers of the thyro-arytenoid muscles pass into the ary-epiglottic fold, and some of them reach the epiglottic cartilage; these fibers constitute the thyro-epiglottic muscle, which widens the laryngeal inlet.

[b]Some fibers of the oblique arytenoid muscles continue as ary-epiglottic muscles.

[c]This slender muscle slip lies medial to and is composed of fibers finer than those of the thyro-arytenoid muscle.

Injury to Laryngeal Nerves

The inferior laryngeal nerves are vulnerable to injury during thyroidectomy and other surgical operations in the anterior triangles of the neck. Because the inferior laryngeal nerve innervates the muscles moving the vocal fold, injury results in *paralysis of the vocal fold*. The voice is initially poor because the paralyzed fold cannot adduct to meet the normal vocal fold. When bilateral paralysis of the vocal folds occurs, the voice is almost absent because the vocal folds are motionless in a position that is slightly narrower than the usual neutral respiratory position. They cannot be adducted for phonation, nor can they be abducted for increased respiration, resulting in stridor (high-pitched, noisy respiration) often accompanied by anxiety. Injury to the external branch of the superior laryngeal nerve results in a voice that is monotonous in character because the paralyzed cricothyroid muscle supplied by it is unable to vary the length and tension of the vocal fold.

Hoarseness is the most common symptom of serious disorders of the larynx, such as carcinoma of the vocal folds.

Fractures of Laryngeal Skeleton

Laryngeal fractures may result from blows received in sports such as kick boxing and hockey or from compression by a shoulder strap during an automobile accident. Laryngeal fractures produce submucous hemorrhage and edema,

respiratory obstruction, hoarseness, and sometimes a temporary inability to speak. The thyroid, cricoid, and most of the arytenoid cartilages often ossify as age advances, commencing at approximately 25 years of age in the thyroid cartilage.

Laryngoscopy

Laryngoscopy is the procedure used to examine the interior of the larynx. The larynx may be examined visually by *indirect laryngoscopy* using a laryngeal mirror or it may be viewed by *direct laryngoscopy* using a tubular endoscopic instrument, a *laryngoscope*. The vestibular and vocal folds can be observed in Figure B8.6.

Aspiration of Foreign Bodies

A foreign object, such as a piece of steak, may accidentally *aspirate* through the laryngeal inlet into the vestibule of the larynx, where it becomes trapped superior to the vestibular folds. When a foreign object enters the vestibule, the laryngeal muscles go into spasm, tensing the vocal folds. The rima glottidis closes and no air enters the trachea. Asphyxiation occurs, and the person will die in approximately 5 minutes from lack of oxygen if the obstruction is not removed. Emergency therapy must be given to open the airway.

The procedure used depends on the condition of the patient, the facilities available, and the experience of the person giving first aid. Because the lungs still contain air, sudden compression of the abdomen (Heimlich maneuver) causes the diaphragm to elevate and compress the lungs, expelling air from the trachea into the larynx (Fig. B8.7). This maneuver usually dislodges the food or other material from the larynx.

Posterior wall of laryngopharynx
Piriform fossa
To esophagus
Mucosa over cricoid cartilage
Interarytenoid notch
Site of corniculate cartilages
Site of cuneiform cartilages
Ary-epiglottic fold
Rima glottidis
Vocal folds
Lateral walls of laryngeal vestibule (mucosa over quadrangular membrane)
Vestibular folds (medial edge)
Epiglottis
Median glosso-epiglottic fold
Right and left valleculae
Dorsum of tongue

Laryngoscopic examination

FIGURE B8.6.

Heimlich maneuver

FIGURE B8.7.

Tracheostomy

A transverse incision through the skin of the neck and anterior wall of the trachea (*tracheostomy*) establishes an airway in patients with upper airway obstruction or respiratory failure. The infrahyoid muscles are retracted laterally, and the isthmus of the thyroid gland is either divided or retracted superiorly. An opening is made in the trachea between the first and second tracheal rings or through the second through fourth rings. A *tracheostomy tube* is then inserted into the trachea and secured (Fig. B8.8). To avoid complications during a tracheostomy, the following anatomical relationships are important:

- The inferior thyroid veins arise from a venous plexus on the thyroid gland and descend anterior to the trachea.

- A small thyroid ima artery is present in approximately 10% of people; it ascends from the brachiocephalic trunk or the arch of the aorta to the isthmus of the thyroid gland.
- The left brachiocephalic vein, jugular venous arch, and pleurae may be encountered, particularly in infants and children.
- The thymus covers the inferior part of the trachea in infants and children.
- The trachea is small, mobile, and soft in infants, making it easy to cut through its posterior wall and damage the esophagus.

Skin incision for tracheostomy

Anterior views

Incision in trachea after retracting infrahyoid muscles and incising isthmus of thyroid gland

Tracheostomy tube inserted in tracheal opening

FIGURE B8.8.

Alimentary Layer of Cervical Viscera

The viscera of the alimentary layer take part in the digestive functions of the body. Although the pharynx conducts air to the larynx, trachea, and lungs, its constrictor muscles direct (and the epiglottis deflects) food to the esophagus. The esophagus, also involved in food propulsion, is the beginning of the *alimentary canal* (digestive tract).

PHARYNX

The **pharynx** is the superior expanded part of the alimentary system posterior to the nasal and oral cavities, extending inferiorly past the larynx (Fig. 8.16A). The pharynx extends from the cranial base to the inferior border of the cricoid cartilage anteriorly and the inferior border of C6 vertebra posteriorly. The pharynx is widest opposite the hyoid and narrowest at its inferior end, where it is continuous with the esophagus. The flat posterior wall of the pharynx lies against the prevertebral layer of deep cervical fascia (Fig. 8.2A).

Interior of the Pharynx. The pharynx is divided into three parts:

- *Nasopharynx*, posterior to the nose and superior to the soft palate.

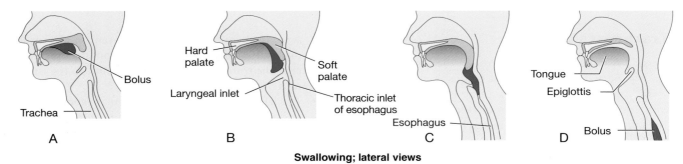

Swallowing; lateral views

FIGURE 8.15. Swallowing. **A.** The bolus of food is squeezed to the back of the oral cavity by pushing the tongue against the palate. **B.** The nasopharynx is sealed off and the larynx is elevated, enlarging the pharynx to receive food. **C.** The pharyngeal sphincters contract sequentially, squeezing food into the esophagus. **D.** The bolus of food moves down the esophagus by peristaltic contractions.

- *Oropharynx,* posterior to the mouth.
- *Laryngopharynx,* posterior to the larynx.

The **nasopharynx** has a respiratory function. It lies superior to the *soft palate* and is the posterior extension of the nasal cavities (Fig. 8.16A). The nose opens into the nasopharynx through two **choanae** (paired openings between the nasal cavity and nasopharynx). The roof and posterior wall of the nasopharynx form a continuous surface that lies inferior to the body of the sphenoid bone and the basilar part of the occipital bone.

The **lymphoid tissue** in the pharynx forms an incomplete *tonsillar ring* around the superior part of the pharynx. The lymphoid tissue is aggregated in certain regions to form masses called *tonsils.* The **pharyngeal tonsils** (commonly called adenoids when enlarged) are in the mucous membrane of the roof and posterior wall of the nasopharynx. Extending inferiorly from the medial end of the pharyngotympanic tube (auditory tube) is a vertical fold of mucous membrane, the **salpingopharyngeal fold.**

It covers the salpingopharyngeus muscle, which opens the pharyngeal orifice of the pharyngotympanic tube during swallowing. The collection of lymphoid tissue in the submucosa of the pharynx near the pharyngeal orifice of the pharyngotympanic tube is the **tubal tonsil.** Posterior to the **torus of the pharyngotympanic tube** and the salpingopharyngeal fold is a slit-like lateral extension of the pharynx, the **pharyngeal recess,** which extends laterally and posteriorly (Fig. 8.16B).

The **oropharynx** has a digestive function. It is bounded by the soft palate superiorly, the base of the tongue inferiorly, and the palatoglossal and palatopharyngeal arches laterally (Figs. 8.16 and 8.17). It extends from the soft palate to the superior border of the epiglottis.

Deglutition (swallowing) is the process that transfers a food bolus from the mouth through the pharynx and esophagus into the stomach. Solid food is masticated (chewed) and mixed with saliva to form a soft bolus (masticated morsel) that is easier to swallow. Deglutition occurs in three stages (Fig. 8.15):

- **Stage 1:** voluntary; the bolus is compressed against the palate and pushed from the mouth into the oropharynx, mainly by movements of the muscles of the tongue and soft palate.
- **Stage 2:** involuntary and rapid; the soft palate is elevated, sealing off the nasopharynx from the oropharynx and laryngopharynx. The pharynx widens and shortens to receive the bolus of food as the suprahyoid muscles and longitudinal pharyngeal muscles contract, elevating the larynx.
- **Stage 3:** involuntary; sequential contraction of all three pharyngeal constrictor muscles forces the food bolus inferiorly into the esophagus (Fig. 8.15D).

The **palatine tonsils** are collections of lymphoid tissue on each side of the oropharynx that lie in the **tonsillar sinus.** The sinus is between the **palatoglossal** and the **palatopharyngeal arches** (Fig. 8.17). The tonsillar bed is formed by the superior constrictor of the pharynx and the thin sheet of **pharyngobasilar fascia** (Fig. 8.18A). This fascia blends with the periosteum of the cranial base and defines the limits of the pharyngeal wall in its superior part.

The **laryngopharynx** (hypopharynx) lies posterior to the larynx, extending from the superior border of the epiglottis and the pharyngo-epiglottic folds to the inferior border of the cricoid cartilage, where it narrows and becomes continuous with the esophagus (Fig. 8.16). Posteriorly, the laryngopharynx is related to the bodies of the C4–C6 vertebrae. Its posterior and lateral walls are formed by the **middle** and **inferior pharyngeal constrictor muscles** (Fig. 8.18). Internally, the wall is formed by the *palatopharyngeus* and *stylopharyngeus muscles* (Fig. 8.17C). The laryngopharynx communicates with the larynx through the *laryngeal inlet* on its anterior wall (Fig. 8.12B).

The **piriform fossa** (recess) is a small depression of the laryngopharyngeal cavity on each side of the inlet (Fig. 8.16A).

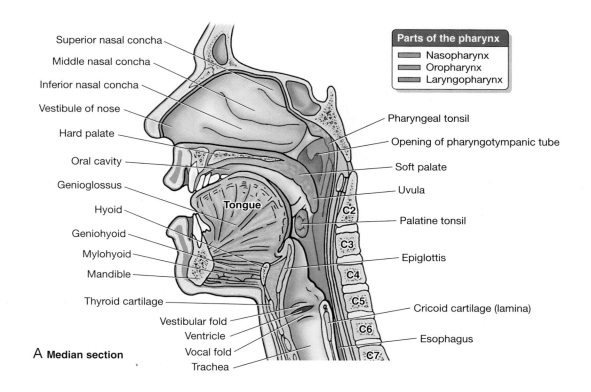

Parts of the pharynx
- Nasopharynx
- Oropharynx
- Laryngopharynx

Superior nasal concha
Middle nasal concha
Inferior nasal concha
Vestibule of nose
Hard palate
Oral cavity
Genioglossus
Hyoid
Geniohyoid
Mylohyoid
Mandible
Thyroid cartilage
Vestibular fold
Ventricle
Vocal fold
Trachea

Tongue

Pharyngeal tonsil
Opening of pharyngotympanic tube
Soft palate
Uvula
C2
Palatine tonsil
C3
Epiglottis
C4
C5
Cricoid cartilage (lamina)
C6
Esophagus
C7

A Median section

Pharyngobasilar fascia
Nasal septum

Levator veli palatini
Nasal conchae
Styloid process
Salpingopharyngeal fold
Stylopharyngeus
Palatine tonsil
Root of tongue and lingual tonsil
Epiglottis
Piriform fossa
Ary-epiglottic fold

Pharyngotympanic tube
Tensor veli palatini
Hamulus of medial pterygoid plate
Superior pharyngeal constrictor
Uvular muscle
Middle pharyngeal constrictor
Palatopharyngeus
Inferior pharyngeal constrictor
Oblique arytenoid
Transverse arytenoid
Posterior crico-arytenoid

B Posterior view

Esophagus

FIGURE 8.16.   **Nasopharynx, oropharynx, and laryngopharynx. A.** Structures of the head and neck. **B.** The posterior wall of the pharynx has been cut in the midline and reflected laterally, and the mucous membrane has been removed from the right side.

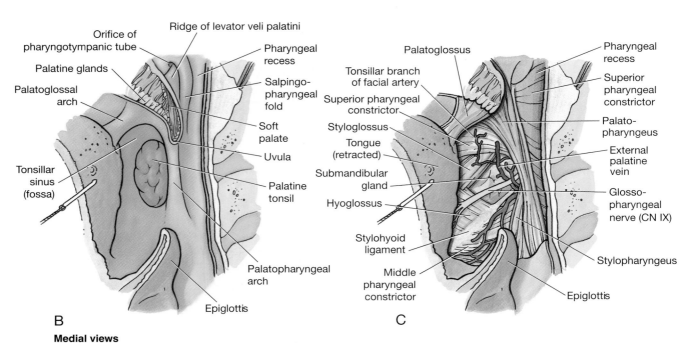

Medial views

FIGURE 8.17. **Oral cavity and tonsils. A.** Structures of the oral cavity in an adult male whose mouth is wide open with the tongue protruded. (Courtesy of Dr. B. Liebgott, Professor, Division of Anatomy, Department of Surgery, University of Toronto, Ontario, Canada.) **B.** Internal aspect of the lateral wall of the pharynx. **C.** Deep dissection of the tonsillar bed.

This mucosa-lined fossa is separated from the laryngeal inlet by the *ary-epiglottic fold.* Laterally, the piriform fossa is bounded by the medial surfaces of the thyroid cartilage and the *thyrohyoid membrane.* Branches of the internal laryngeal and recurrent laryngeal nerves lie deep to the mucous membrane of the piriform fossa.

Pharyngeal Muscles. The wall of the pharynx has a muscular layer composed entirely of voluntary muscle arranged mainly into an external circular and an internal longitudinal layer. In most of the **alimentary canal,** the muscular layer consists of smooth muscle. The external layer consists of three **pharyngeal constrictors: superior, middle,** and **inferior** (Figs. 8.15 and 8.18). The internal, mainly longitudinal, layer of muscles consists of the **palatopharyngeus,**

stylopharyngeus, and **salpingopharyngeus.** These muscles elevate the larynx and shorten the pharynx during swallowing and speaking. The attachments, nerve supply, and actions of the pharyngeal muscles are described in Table 8.6.

The pharyngeal constrictors have a strong internal fascial lining, the *pharyngobasilar fascia,* and a thin external fascial lining, the *buccopharyngeal fascia.* The pharyngeal constrictors contract involuntarily so that contraction takes place sequentially from the superior to the inferior end of the pharynx, propelling food into the esophagus. All three constrictors are supplied by the *pharyngeal plexus of nerves* that lies on the lateral wall of the pharynx, mainly on the middle constrictor (Fig. 8.18). The overlapping of the constrictor

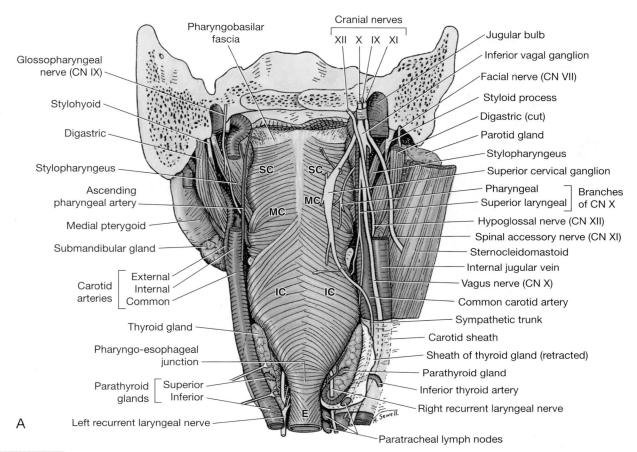

FIGURE 8.18. **Pharynx and related vasculature and nerves. A.** Overview. *SC*, superior pharyngeal constrictor; *MC*, middle pharyngeal constrictor; *IC*, inferior pharyngeal constrictor. A large wedge of occipital bone (including the foramen magnum) and the articulated cervical vertebrae have been separated from the remainder (anterior portion) of the head and cervical viscera at the retropharyngeal space and removed.

muscles leaves four gaps in the musculature for structures to enter or leave the pharynx (Fig. 8.18 and Table 8.6):

1. Superior to the superior constrictor, the levator veli palatini, pharyngotympanic tube, and ascending palatine artery pass through the *gap between the superior constrictor and the cranium.* It is here that the pharyngobasilar fascia blends with the buccopharyngeal fascia to form, with the mucous membrane, the thin wall of the pharyngeal recess (Fig. 8.20B).
2. A *gap between the superior and the middle pharyngeal constrictors* forms a passageway that allows the stylopharyngeus, glossopharyngeal nerve, and stylohyoid ligament to pass to the internal aspect of the pharyngeal wall.
3. A *gap between the middle and the inferior pharyngeal constrictors* allows the internal laryngeal nerve and superior laryngeal artery and vein to pass to the larynx.
4. A *gap inferior to the inferior pharyngeal constrictor* allows the recurrent laryngeal nerve and inferior laryngeal artery to pass superiorly into the larynx.

Vessels of the Pharynx. The **tonsillar artery,** a branch of the facial artery (Fig. 8.17C), passes through the superior constrictor muscle and enters the inferior pole of the tonsil. The tonsil also receives arterial twigs from the ascending palatine, lingual, descending palatine, and ascending pharyngeal arteries. The large **external palatine vein** (paratonsillar vein) descends from the soft palate and passes close to the lateral surface of the tonsil before it enters the pharyngeal venous plexus.

The **tonsillar lymphatic vessels** pass laterally and inferiorly to the lymph nodes near the angle of the mandible and the **jugulodigastric node** (Fig. 8.19). The jugulodigastric node is referred to as the *tonsillar node* because of its frequent enlargement when the tonsil is inflamed (*tonsillitis*). The palatine, lingual, and pharyngeal tonsils form the pharyngeal **tonsillar ring** (of Waldeyer), an incomplete circular band of lymphoid tissue around the superior part of the pharynx. The anteroinferior part of the ring is formed by the **lingual tonsil,** a collection of lymphoid tissue in the posterior part of the tongue (Fig. 8.15B). Lateral

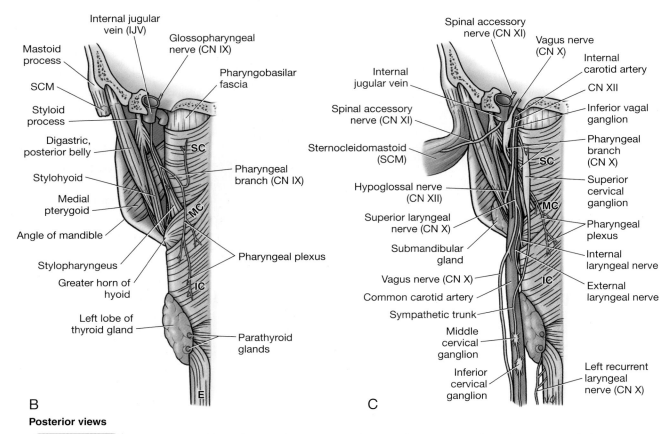

B

Posterior views

FIGURE 8.18. **Pharynx and related vasculature and nerves** *(continued)*. **B.** Muscles. **C.** Nerves and vessels. *SCM,* sternocleidomastoid.

parts of the ring are formed by the palatine and tubal tonsils, and posterior and superior parts are formed by the pharyngeal tonsil.

Pharyngeal Nerves. The **nerve supply to the pharynx** (motor and most of sensory) derives from the **pharyngeal plexus of nerves** (Fig. 8.18*B, C*). Motor fibers in the plexus are derived from the vagus nerve (CN X) via its pharyngeal branch(es). They supply all the muscles of the pharynx and soft palate, except the stylopharyngeus (supplied by CN IX) and the tensor veli palatini (supplied by CN V$_3$). The inferior pharyngeal constrictor also receives some motor fibers from the external and recurrent laryngeal branches of the vagus. Sensory fibers in the plexus are derived from CN IX. They supply most of the mucosa of all three parts of the pharynx. The sensory nerve supply of the mucous membrane of the anterior and superior nasopharynx is mainly from the maxillary nerve (CN V$_2$). The **tonsillar nerves** are derived from the *tonsillar plexus of nerves* formed by branches of CN IX and CN X and the pharyngeal plexus of nerves.

ESOPHAGUS

The **esophagus** is a muscular tube that extends from the laryngopharynx at the **pharyngo-esophageal junction** to the stomach at the cardial orifice. The esophagus consists of striated (voluntary) muscle in its upper third, smooth (involuntary) muscle in its lower third, and a mixture of striated and smooth muscle in between. Its first part, the **cervical esophagus,** begins at the inferior border of the cricoid cartilage (the level of the C6 vertebra) in the median plane.

Externally, the pharyngo-esophageal junction appears as a constriction produced by the **cricopharyngeal part of the inferior pharyngeal constrictor muscle** (the superior esophageal sphincter). The cervical esophagus lies between the trachea and the cervical vertebral bodies and is in contact with the cervical pleura at the root of the neck (Figs. 8.7*A* and 8.16*A*). The thoracic duct adheres to the left side of the esophagus and lies between the pleura and the esophagus.

The **arteries of the cervical esophagus** are branches of the *inferior thyroid arteries* (Fig. 8.14*B*). Each artery gives

TABLE 8.6 MUSCLES OF PHARYNX

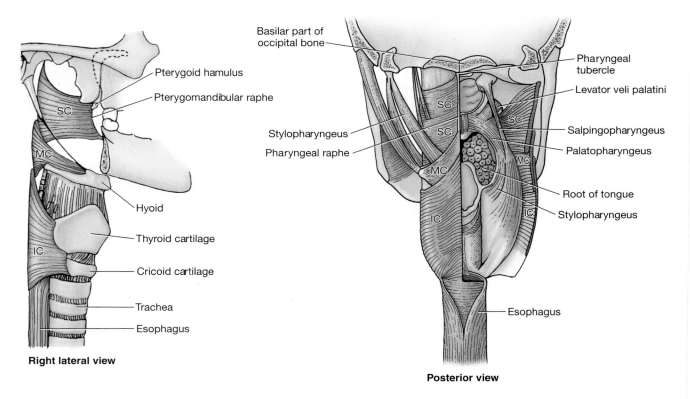

Right lateral view

Posterior view

Muscle	Origin	Insertion	Innervation	Main Action(s)
External layer				
Superior pharyngeal constrictor	Pterygoid hamulus, pterygo-mandibular raphe; posterior end of mylohyoid line of mandible and side of tongue	Pharyngeal tubercle on basilar part of occipital bone	Pharyngeal branch of vagus (CN X) and pharyngeal plexus	Constrict walls of pharynx during swallowing
Middle pharyngeal constrictor	Stylohyoid ligament and greater and lesser horns of hyoid	(Median) pharyngeal raphe	Pharyngeal branch of vagus (CN X) and pharyngeal plexus, plus branches of external and recurrent laryngeal nerves of vagus	
Inferior pharyngeal constrictor	Oblique line of thyroid cartilage and side of cricoid cartilage	Cricopharyngeal part encircles pharyngo-esophageal junction without forming a raphe.		
Internal layer				
Palatopharyngeus	Hard palate and palatine aponeurosis	Posterior border of lamina of thyroid cartilage and side of pharynx and esophagus	Pharyngeal branch of vagus (CN X) and pharyngeal plexus	Elevate (shorten and widen) pharynx and larynx during swallowing and speaking
Salpingopharyngeus	Cartilaginous part of pharyngotympanic tube	Blends with palatopharyngeus		
Stylopharyngeus	Styloid process of temporal bone	Posterior and superior borders of thyroid cartilage with palatopharyngeus	Glossopharyngeal nerve (CN IX)	

Lateral views

Lymph nodes and tonsils
- Occipital
- Retroauricular (mastoid)
- Parotid
- Buccal
- Submental
- Submandibular
- Jugulo-omohyoid
- Superficial cervical
- Deep cervical
- Retropharyngeal
- Jugulodigastric
- Infrahyoid
- A Pharyngeal tonsil
- P Palatine tonsil
- → Direction of flow of lymph

Jugular lymphatic trunk
Right internal jugular vein
Subclavian lymphatic trunk
Right lymphatic duct
Right subclavian vein
Right venous angle
Right brachiocephalic vein
Superior vena cava

Bronchomediastinal lymphatic trunk

Left internal jugular vein
Thoracic duct
Subclavian lymphatic trunk
Left venous angle
Left subclavian vein
Left brachiocephalic vein
Bronchomediastinal lymphatic trunk

C **Anterior view**

FIGURE 8.19. **Lymphatic drainage of head and neck. A.** Superficial lymph nodes. **B.** Deep lymph nodes. **C.** Termination of thoracic and right lymphatic ducts.

off ascending and descending branches that anastomose with each other and across the midline. The **veins** are tributaries of the *inferior thyroid veins*. **Lymphatic vessels** of the cervical esophagus drain into the *paratracheal lymph nodes* and *inferior deep cervical lymph nodes* (Fig. 8.10).

The **nerve supply** of the esophagus is somatic, motor, and sensory to the superior half and parasympathetic (vagal), sympathetic, and visceral sensory to the inferior half. The cervical esophagus receives the somatic fibers via branches from the *recurrent laryngeal nerves* and vasomotor fibers

from the *cervical sympathetic trunks* through the plexus around the inferior thyroid artery (Fig. 8.9A).

LYMPHATICS IN NECK

Most superficial tissues of the neck are drained by lymphatic vessels that enter the *superficial cervical lymph nodes*, which are located along the course of the EJV (Fig. 8.19A). Lymph from these nodes drains into *inferior deep cervical lymph nodes* (Figs. 8.10 and 8.19*B*). The specific group of inferior deep cervical nodes involved here descends across the lateral cervical region with the spinal accessory nerve (CN XI). Most lymph from the six to eight nodes then drains into the *supraclavicular lymph nodes,* which accompany the transverse cervical artery. The main group of deep cervical nodes forms a chain along the IJV, mostly under cover of the SCM.

Other deep cervical nodes include the prelaryngeal, pretracheal, paratracheal, and retropharyngeal nodes (Fig. 8.10). Efferent lymphatic vessels from the deep cervical nodes join to form the **jugular lymphatic trunks,** which usually join the thoracic duct on the left side. On the right side, the vessels enter the junction of the internal jugular and subclavian veins (*right venous angle*) directly or via a short right lymphatic duct (Fig. 8.19).

The *thoracic duct* passes through the superior thoracic aperture along the left border of the esophagus. It arches laterally in the root of the neck, posterior to the carotid sheath and anterior to the sympathetic trunk and vertebral and subclavian arteries (Fig. 8.7*A*). The thoracic duct enters the left brachiocephalic vein at the junction of the subclavian and IJVs (*left venous angle*) (Fig. 8.19*C*). The thoracic duct drains lymph from the entire body, except the right side of the head and neck, the right upper limb, and the right side of the thorax, which drain through the *right lymphatic duct.* The right jugular, subclavian, and bronchomediastinal lymphatic trunks unite to form this duct, which enters the right venous angle. Often, however, these lymphatic trunks enter the venous system independently in the region of the right venous angle.

Radical Neck Dissections

Radical neck dissections are performed when cancer invades the lymphatics. During the procedure, the deep cervical lymph nodes and the tissues around them are removed as completely as possible. Although major arteries, the brachial plexus, CN X, and the phrenic nerve are preserved, most cutaneous branches of the cervical plexus are removed. The aim of the dissection is to remove all tissue that contains lymph nodes in one piece. The deep cervical lymph nodes, particularly those located along the transverse cervical artery, may be involved in the spread of cancer from the thorax and abdomen. Because their enlargement may give the first clue to cancer in these regions, they are often referred to as the *cervical sentinel lymph nodes.*

Adenoiditis

Inflammation of the pharyngeal tonsils (adenoids) is called *adenoiditis.* This condition can obstruct the passage of air from the nasal cavities through the choanae into the nasopharynx, making mouth breathing necessary. Infection from the enlarged pharyngeal tonsils may also spread to the tubal tonsils, causing swelling and closure of the pharyngotympanic tubes. Impairment of hearing may result from nasal obstruction and blockage of the pharyngotympanic tubes. Infection spreading from the nasopharynx to the middle ear causes *otitis media* (middle ear infection), which may produce temporary or permanent hearing loss.

Foreign Bodies in Laryngopharynx

Foreign bodies entering the pharynx may become lodged in the piriform fossae. If the object (e.g., a chicken bone) is sharp, it may pierce the mucous membrane and injure the internal laryngeal nerve. The superior laryngeal nerve and its internal laryngeal branch are also vulnerable to injury if the instrument used to remove the foreign body accidentally pierces the mucous membrane. Injury to these nerves may result in anesthesia of the laryngeal mucous membrane as far inferiorly as the vocal folds. Young children swallow various objects, most of which reach the stomach and subsequently pass through the alimentary tract without difficulty. In some cases, the foreign body stops at the inferior end of the laryngopharynx, its narrowest part. A medical image such as a radiograph or a CT scan will reveal the presence of a radiopaque foreign body. Foreign bodies in the pharynx are often removed under direct vision through a pharyngoscope.

Tonsillectomy

Tonsillectomy (removal of the palatine tonsil) is performed by dissecting the tonsil from the tonsillar sinus or by a guillotine or snare operation. Each procedure involves removal of the tonsil and the fascial sheet covering the tonsillar sinus. Because of the rich blood supply of the tonsil, bleeding commonly arises from the large *external palatine vein* or less commonly from the tonsillar artery or other arterial twigs (Fig. 8.17C). The glossopharyngeal nerve accompanies the tonsillar artery on the lateral wall of the pharynx and is vulnerable to injury because this wall is thin. The internal carotid artery is especially vulnerable when it is tortuous as it lies directly lateral to the tonsil (Fig. B8.9).

Tensor veli palatini

Cartilage of pharyngotympanic tube

Levator veli palatini

Membranous lateral wall of pharyngotympanic tube

Salpingopharyngeus

Tonsillar branch of ascending palatine artery

Tonsillar branch of facial artery

Ligature retracting palatine tonsil

Medial view of right half of head

Tonsillectomy

FIGURE B8.9.

Zones of Penetrating Trauma

Three zones are common clinical guides to the seriousness of neck trauma (Fig. B8.10). The zones give physicians an understanding of structures that are at risk with penetrating neck injuries.

- **Zone I** includes the root of neck extending from the clavicles and manubrium to the inferior border of the cricoid cartilage. Structures at risk are the cervical pleurae, apices of lungs, thyroid and parathyroid glands, trachea, esophagus, common carotid arteries, jugular veins, and the cervical region of the vertebral column.
- **Zone II** extends from the cricoid cartilage to the angles of the mandible. Structures at risk are the superior poles of the thyroid gland, thyroid and cricoid cartilages, larynx, laryngopharynx, carotid arteries, jugular veins, esophagus, and cervical region of the vertebral column.
- **Zone III** occurs superiorly from the angles of the mandible. Structures at risk are the salivary glands, oral and nasal cavities, oropharynx, and nasopharynx.

Injuries in zones I and III obstruct the airway and have the greatest risk for **morbidity** (complications after surgical procedures and other treatments) and **mortality** (a fatal outcome) because injured structures are difficult to visualize and repair and vascular damage is difficult to control. Injuries in zone II are most common; however, morbidity and mortality are lower because physicians can control vascular damage by direct pressure and surgeons can visualize and treat injured structures more easily than they can in zones I and III.

Zone III

Zone II

Zone I

Angle of mandible

Cricoid cartilage

Trachea

Manubrium

FIGURE B8.10.

Medical Imaging of Neck

Radiographic examinations of the cervical vertebral column include anteroposterior (AP), lateral, and oblique projections. Lateral projections are common for evaluating severe neck injuries (Fig. 8.20). When a fracture is suspected, the lateral projection is examined before the person is moved for other projections. Observe the anterior and posterior margins of the vertebral bodies. Any deviation from the smooth curvature of these margins suggests a fracture and tearing of the associated ligaments. Observe that the intervertebral (IV) disc spaces are wider anteriorly than posteriorly. This difference exists because the IV discs are wedge-shaped. As the discs degenerate, the vertical height of the disc spaces decreases.

Transverse CT scans through the thyroid gland provide images of sections of the neck (Fig. 8.21A). They are oriented to show how a horizontal section of the person's neck appears to the physician standing at the foot of the bed. The superior edge of the CT image represents the anterior surface of the neck, and the right lateral edge of the image represents the left lateral surface. CT scans are used mainly as a diagnostic adjunct to conventional radiography. CT scans are superior to radiographs because they reveal radiodensity differences among and within soft tissues (e.g., in the thyroid gland).

MRI systems construct images of transverse, sagittal, and coronal sections of the neck and have the advantage of using no radiation (Fig. 8.21*B, C*). MRI studies of the neck are superior to CT studies for showing detail in soft tissues, but they provide little information about bones.

Ultrasonography is also a useful imaging technique for studying soft tissues of the neck. Ultrasound provides images of many abnormal conditions noninvasively, at relatively low cost, and with minimal discomfort. Ultrasound is useful for distinguishing solid from cystic masses, for example, which may be difficult to determine during physical examination. Vascular imaging of arteries and veins of the neck is possible using intravascular ultrasonography (Fig. 8.22). The images are produced by placing the transducer within the blood vessel. *Doppler ultrasound techniques* help evaluate blood flow through a vessel (e.g., for detecting stenosis [narrowing] of a carotid artery).

Angles of mandible

Intervertebral disc space

Body of C4 vertebra

Lamina of partly calcified cricoid cartilage

Intervertebral foramen

Body of C7 vertebra

Occipital bone

Posterior arch of atlas (C1)

Spinous process of axis (C2)

Zygapophysial joint

Spinous process of C7 vertebra

Lateral radiograph

FIGURE 8.20. Cervical region of vertebral column.

A   B

FIGURE 8.21. **Scans of neck through thyroid gland.** Transverse studies via CT (**A**) and MRI (**B**) revealing the structures of the neck. *1,* esophagus; *2,* trachea; *3,* lobes of thyroid gland; *4,* thyroid isthmus; *5,* SCM; *6,* sternohyoid; *7,* common carotid artery; *8,* IJV; *9,* vertebral artery; *10,* vertebral body; *11,* spinal cord in cerebrospinal fluid; *12,* deep muscles of the back; *13,* retropharyngeal space. (Courtesy of Dr. M. Keller, Assistant Professor of Medical Imaging, University of Toronto, Toronto, Ontario, Canada.) **C.** Median MRI study of the head and neck demonstrating that the air and food passages share the oropharynx. (Courtesy of Dr. W. Kucharczyk, Chair of Medical Imaging and Clinical Director, Tri-Hospital Resonance Centre, Toronto, Ontario, Canada.)

B Normal internal carotid artery

C Occluded carotid artery

A **Anterior View**

Key			
AR	Arch of aorta	LC	Left common carotid artery
BA	Basilar artery	LS	Left subclavian artery
BT	Brachiocephalic trunk	RC	Right common carotid artery
ECA	External carotid artery	RS	Right subclavian artery
ICA	Internal carotid artery	VA	Vertebral artery

FIGURE 8.22.   Normal Doppler color flow study of internal carotid artery.

Go to http://thePoint.lww.com/ECA4e for helpful study tools, including USMLE-style questions, case studies, images, and more!

Review of Cranial Nerves

OVERVIEW OF CRANIAL NERVES / 644

OLFACTORY NERVE (CN I) / 650

OPTIC NERVE (CN II) / 652

OCULOMOTOR NERVE (CN III) / 654

TROCHLEAR NERVE (CN IV) / 655

ABDUCENT NERVE (CN VI) / 656

TRIGEMINAL NERVE (CN V) / 659

FACIAL NERVE (CN VII) / 660
   Somatic (Branchial) Motor / 660
   Visceral (Parasympathetic) Motor / 660
   Somatic (General) Sensory / 660
   Special Sensory (Taste) / 660

VESTIBULOCOCHLEAR NERVE (CN VIII) / 663

GLOSSOPHARYNGEAL NERVE (CN IX) / 664
   Somatic (Branchial) Motor / 664
   Visceral (Parasympathetic) Motor / 664
   Somatic (General) Sensory / 664
   Special Sensory (Taste) / 665
   Visceral Sensory / 665

VAGUS NERVE (CN X) / 665
   Somatic (Branchial) Motor / 666
   Visceral (Parasympathetic) Motor / 666
   Somatic (General) Sensory / 668
   Sensory (Taste) / 668
   Visceral Sensory / 669

SPINAL ACCESSORY NERVE (CN XI) / 669

HYPOGLOSSAL NERVE (CN XII) / 671

The regional aspects of the cranial nerves are described in the preceding chapters, especially those for the head, neck, and thorax. This chapter summarizes the cranial nerves and the autonomic nervous system, using mainly figures and tables. Cranial nerve injuries, indicating the type or site of lesion and the abnormal findings, are also summarized.

OVERVIEW OF CRANIAL NERVES

Cranial nerves, like spinal nerves, contain sensory or motor fibers or a combination of these fibers (Figs. 9.1 and 9.2). Cranial nerves innervate muscles or glands or carry impulses from sensory receptors. They are called cranial nerves because they emerge from foramina or fissures in the cranium and are covered by tubular sheaths derived from the cranial meninges (Fig. 9.3). There are 12 pairs of cranial nerves, which are numbered I–XII, from rostral to caudal, according to their attachments to the brain (Fig. 9.1; Table 9.1). Their names reflect their general distribution or function.

Cranial nerves carry one or more of the following five main functional components (Fig. 9.2):

- **Motor (efferent) fibers**
  1. *Motor fibers innervating voluntary (striated) muscle:* Somatic motor (general somatic efferent) axons innervate the striated muscles in the orbit, tongue, and external muscles of the neck (sternocleidomastoid and trapezius) as well as striated muscles of the face, palate, pharynx, and larynx. The muscles of the face, palate, pharynx, and larynx are derived from the pharyngeal arches and their somatic motor innervation can be referred to more specifically as *branchial motor*.
  2. *Motor fibers involved in innervating glands and involuntary (smooth) muscle* (e.g., in viscera and blood vessels). These include *visceral motor* (general visceral efferent) axons that constitute the cranial outflow of the parasympathetic division of the autonomic nervous system. The presynaptic (preganglionic) fibers that emerge from the brain synapse outside the central nervous system in a parasympathetic ganglion. The postsynaptic (postganglionic) fibers continue to innervate glands and smooth muscle throughout the body.

- **Sensory (afferent) fibers**
  3. *Fibers conveying sensation from the viscera.* These include visceral sensory (general visceral afferent) fibers conveying information from the carotid body and sinus, pharynx, larynx, trachea, bronchi, lungs, heart, and gastrointestinal tract.
  4. *Fibers transmitting general sensation (e.g., touch, pressure, heat, cold) from the skin and mucous membranes.* These include *somatic (general) sensory* fibers, which are carried mainly by CN V but also by CN VII, CN IX, and CN X. *(Continued on page 000.)*

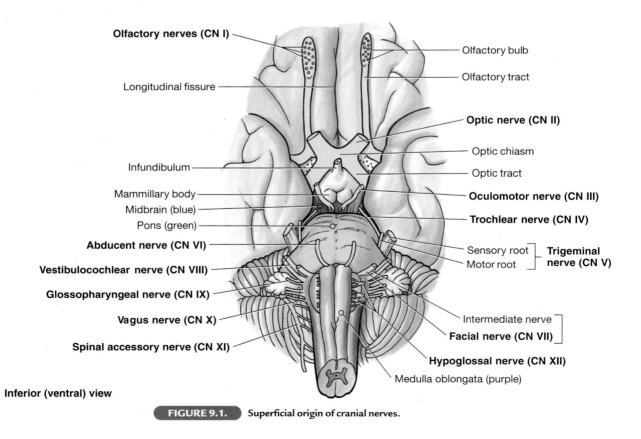

Olfactory nerves (CN I)
Olfactory bulb
Olfactory tract
Longitudinal fissure
Optic nerve (CN II)
Optic chiasm
Infundibulum
Optic tract
Mammillary body
Oculomotor nerve (CN III)
Midbrain (blue)
Pons (green)
Trochlear nerve (CN IV)
Abducent nerve (CN VI)
Sensory root ⎤ **Trigeminal**
Motor root ⎦ **nerve (CN V)**
Vestibulocochlear nerve (CN VIII)
Glossopharyngeal nerve (CN IX)
Intermediate nerve ⎤
Vagus nerve (CN X)
Facial nerve (CN VII) ⎦
Spinal accessory nerve (CN XI)
Hypoglossal nerve (CN XII)
Medulla oblongata (purple)
Inferior (ventral) view

FIGURE 9.1. Superficial origin of cranial nerves.

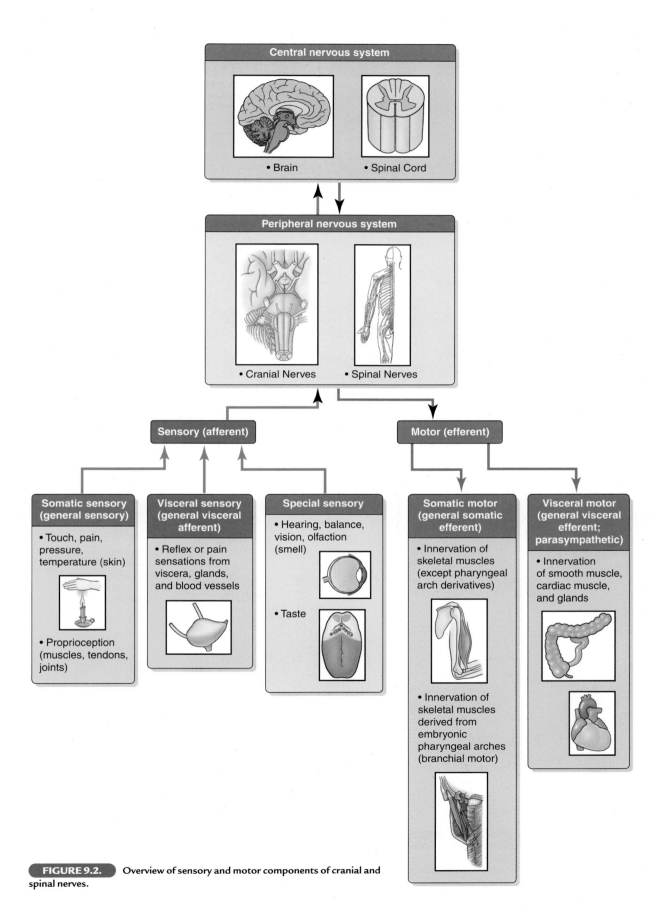

FIGURE 9.2. Overview of sensory and motor components of cranial and spinal nerves.

TABLE 9.1 SUMMARY OF CRANIAL NERVES

Trochlear—CN IV
Motor: superior oblique muscle of eye

Abducent—CN VI
Motor: lateral rectus muscle of eye

Oculomotor—CN III
Motor: ciliary muscles, sphincter pupillae, all extrinsic muscles of eye except those listed for CN IV and VI

Optic—CN II
Sensory: vision

Cranial nerve fibers
— Efferent (motor)
— Afferent (sensory)

Facial—CN VII
Primary root
Motor: muscles of facial expression

Olfactory—CN I
Sensory: smell

Trigeminal—CN V
Sensory root
Sensory: face, sinuses, teeth

Facial—CN VII
Intermediate nerve
Motor: submandibular, sublingual, lacrimal glands
Sensory: taste to anterior two thirds of tongue, soft palate

Trigeminal—CN V
Motor root
Motor: muscles of mastication

Vestibulocochlear—CN VIII
Vestibular nerve, sensory: orientation, motion
Cochlear nerve, sensory: hearing

Hypoglossal—CN XII
Motor: all intrinsic and extrinsic muscles of tongue (excluding palatoglossus—a palatine muscle)

Spinal accessory—CN XI
Motor: sternocleidomastoid and trapezius

Vagus—CN X
Motor: palate, pharynx, larynx, trachea, bronchial tree, heart, GI tract to left colic flexure
Sensory: pharynx, larynx; reflex sensory from tracheobronchial tree, lungs, heart, GI tract to left colic flexure

Glossopharyngeal—CN IX
Motor: stylopharyngeus, parotid gland
Sensory: taste: posterior third of tongue; general sensation: pharynx, tonsillar sinus, pharyngotympanic tube, middle ear cavity

CN I, CN II, CN III, CN IV, CN VI, CN V, CN V, CN VII, CN VII, CN VIII, CN IX, CN X, CN XI, CN XII

TABLE 9.1 SUMMARY OF CRANIAL NERVES

Nerve	Components	Location of Nerve Cell Bodies	Cranial Exit	Main Action(s)
Olfactory (CN I)	Special sensory (olfaction)	Olfactory epithelium (olfactory cells)	Foramina in cribriform plate of ethmoid bone	Smell from nasal mucosa of roof of each nasal cavity and superior sides of nasal septum and superior concha
Optic (CN II)	Special sensory (vision)	Retina (ganglion cells)	Optic canal	Vision from retina
Oculomotor (CN III)	Somatic motor	Midbrain (nucleus of oculomotor nerve)	Superior orbital fissure	Motor to superior rectus, inferior rectus, medial rectus, inferior oblique, and levator palpebrae superioris muscles; raises superior eyelid; turns eyeball superiorly, inferiorly, and medially
	Visceral motor	Presynaptic: midbrain (Edinger-Westphal nucleus) Postsynaptic: ciliary ganglion		Parasympathetic innervation to sphincter pupillae and ciliary muscle; constricts pupil and accommodates lens of eye
Trochlear (CN IV)	Somatic motor	Midbrain (nucleus of trochlear nerve)		Motor to superior oblique to assist in turning eye inferolaterally (or inferiorly when adducted)
Trigeminal (CN V)				
Ophthalmic (CN V$_1$)	Somatic (general) sensory	Trigeminal ganglion Synapse: sensory nucleus of trigeminal nerve	Superior orbital fissure	Sensation from cornea, skin of forehead, scalp, eyelids, nose, and mucosa of nasal cavity and paranasal sinuses
Maxillary (CN V$_2$)		Trigeminal ganglion Synapse: sensory nucleus of trigeminal nerve	Foramen rotundum	Sensation from skin of face over maxilla, including upper lip, maxillary teeth, mucosa of nose, maxillary sinuses, and palate
Mandibular (CN V$_3$)		Trigeminal ganglion Synapse: sensory nucleus of trigeminal nerve	Foramen ovale	Sensation from skin over mandible, including lower lip, side of head, mandibular teeth, temporomandibular joint, mucosa of mouth, and anterior two thirds of tongue
	Somatic (branchial) motor	Pons (motor nucleus of trigeminal nerve)		Motor to muscles of mastication, mylohyoid, anterior belly of digastric, tensor veli palatini, and tensor tympani
Abducent (CN VI)	Somatic motor	Pons (nucleus of abducent nerve)	Superior orbital fissure	Motor to lateral rectus to turn eye laterally
Facial (CN VII)	Somatic (branchial) motor	Pons (motor nucleus of facial nerve)	Internal acoustic meatus; facial canal; stylomastoid foramen	Motor to muscles of facial expression and scalp; also supplies stapedius of middle ear, stylohyoid, and posterior belly of digastric
	Special sensory (taste)	Geniculate ganglion Synapse: nuclei of solitary tract		Taste from anterior two thirds of tongue and palate
	Somatic (general) sensory	Geniculate ganglion Synapse: sensory nucleus of trigeminal nerve		Sensation from skin of external acoustic meatus
	Visceral motor	Presynaptic: pons (superior salivatory nucleus) Postsynaptic: pterygopalatine ganglion; submandibular ganglion		Parasympathetic innervation to submandibular and sublingual salivary glands, lacrimal gland, and glands of nose and palate
Vestibulocochlear (CN VIII)				
Vestibular	Special sensory (balance)	Vestibular ganglion Synapse: vestibular nuclei	Internal acoustic meatus	Vestibular sensation from semicircular ducts, utricle, and saccule related to position and movement of head
Cochlear	Special sensory (hearing)	Spiral ganglion Synapse: cochlear nuclei		Hearing from spiral organ
Glossopharyngeal (CN IX)	Somatic (branchial) motor	Medulla (nucleus ambiguus)	Jugular foramen	Motor to stylopharyngeus to assist with swallowing
	Visceral motor	Presynaptic: medulla (inferior salivatory nucleus) Postsynaptic: otic ganglion		Parasympathetic innervation to parotid gland
	Special sensory (taste)	Sensory ganglion (nuclei of solitary tract)		Taste from posterior third of tongue
	Somatic (general) sensory	Sensory ganglion Synapse: sensory nucleus of CN V		External ear, pharynx, middle ear
	Visceral sensory	Sensory ganglion (nuclei of solitary tract)		Carotid body and sinus

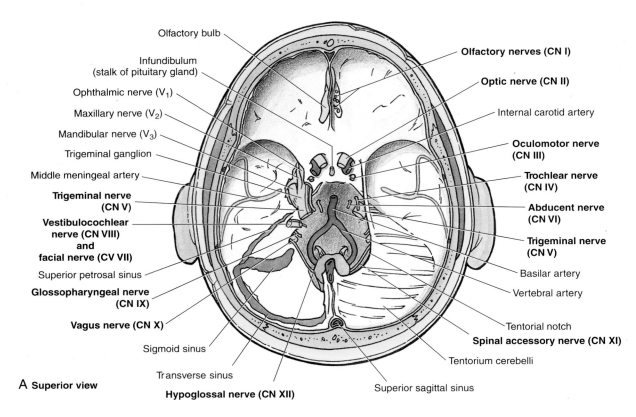

Olfactory bulb

Infundibulum
(stalk of pituitary gland)

Ophthalmic nerve (V₁)

Maxillary nerve (V₂)

Mandibular nerve (V₃)

Trigeminal ganglion

Middle meningeal artery

**Trigeminal nerve
(CN V)**

**Vestibulocochlear
nerve (CN VIII)
and
facial nerve (CV VII)**

Superior petrosal sinus

**Glossopharyngeal nerve
(CN IX)**

Vagus nerve (CN X)

Sigmoid sinus

Transverse sinus

Hypoglossal nerve (CN XII)

A Superior view

Olfactory nerves (CN I)

Optic nerve (CN II)

Internal carotid artery

**Oculomotor nerve
(CN III)**

**Trochlear nerve
(CN IV)**

**Abducent nerve
(CN VI)**

**Trigeminal nerve
(CN V)**

Basilar artery

Vertebral artery

Tentorial notch

Spinal accessory nerve (CN XI)

Tentorium cerebelli

Superior sagittal sinus

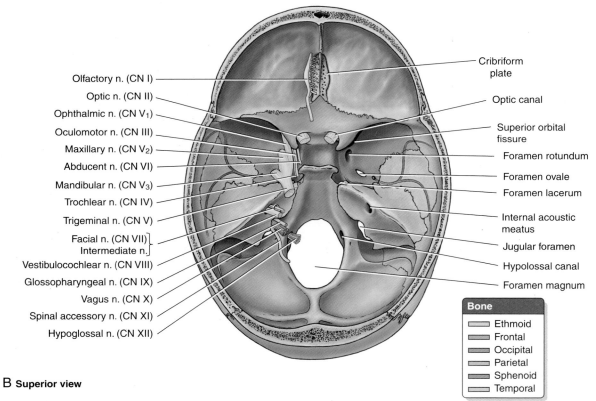

Olfactory n. (CN I)

Optic n. (CN II)

Ophthalmic n. (CN V₁)

Oculomotor n. (CN III)

Maxillary n. (CN V₂)

Abducent n. (CN VI)

Mandibular n. (CN V₃)

Trochlear n. (CN IV)

Trigeminal n. (CN V)

Facial n. (CN VII)
Intermediate n.

Vestibulocochlear n. (CN VIII)

Glossopharyngeal n. (CN IX)

Vagus n. (CN X)

Spinal accessory n. (CN XI)

Hypoglossal n. (CN XII)

Cribriform
plate

Optic canal

Superior orbital
fissure

Foramen rotundum

Foramen ovale

Foramen lacerum

Internal acoustic
meatus

Jugular foramen

Hypolossal canal

Foramen magnum

Bone

	Ethmoid
	Frontal
	Occipital
	Parietal
	Sphenoid
	Temporal

B Superior view

FIGURE 9.3. **Intracranial portions of cranial nerves. A.** Proximal parts of the cranial nerves, dura mater, and blood vessels.
B. Interior of base of cranium illustrating foramina and fissures and related cranial nerves.

TABLE 9.1 SUMMARY OF CRANIAL NERVES (*continued*)

Nerve	Components	Location of Nerve Cell Bodies	Cranial Exit	Main Action(s)
Vagus (CN X)	Somatic (branchial) motor	Medulla (nucleus ambiguus)	Jugular foramen	Motor to constrictor muscles of pharynx (except stylopharyngeus), intrinsic muscles of larynx, muscles of palate (except tensor veli palatini), and striated muscle in superior two thirds of esophagus
	Visceral motor	Presynaptic: medulla Postsynaptic: neurons in, on, or near viscera		Parasympathetic innervation to smooth muscle of trachea, bronchi, digestive tract, and cardiac muscle of heart
	Visceral sensory	Inferior ganglion Synapse: nuclei of solitary tract		Visceral sensation from base of tongue, pharynx, larynx, trachea, bronchi, heart, esophagus, stomach, and intestine
	Special sensory (taste)	Inferior ganglion Synapse: nuclei of solitary tract		Taste from epiglottis and palate
	Somatic (general) sensory	Superior ganglion Synapse: sensory nucleus of trigeminal nerve		Sensation from auricle, external acoustic meatus, and dura mater of posterior cranial fossa
Spinal accessory (CN XI)	Somatic motor	Spinal cord		Motor to sternocleidomastoid and trapezius
Hypoglossal (CN XII)	Somatic motor	Medulla	Hypoglossal canal	Motor to intrinsic and extrinsic muscles of tongue (except palatoglossus)

FIGURE 9.4. Cranial nerve nuclei. The motor nuclei are shown on the left side of the brainstem and the sensory nuclei on the right side. The sensory and motor nuclei are all paired—that is, located in both the right and left sides of the brainstem.

5. *Fibers transmitting unique sensations.* These include *special sensory* fibers conveying taste and smell and those serving the special senses of vision, hearing, and balance.

The fibers of cranial nerves connect centrally to **cranial nerve nuclei,** groups of neurons in which sensory or afferent fibers terminate and from which motor or efferent fibers originate (Fig. 9.4). Except for CN I and CN II, which are extensions of the forebrain, the nuclei of the cranial nerves are located in the brainstem. Nuclei of similar functional components are generally aligned into functional columns in the brainstem.

OLFACTORY NERVE (CN I)

The **olfactory nerves** (CN I) convey the sense of smell (Fig. 9.5). The cell bodies of the **olfactory receptor neurons** are located in the olfactory part of the nasal mucosa, or olfactory area, in the roof of the nasal cavity, and along the nasal septum and medial wall of the superior nasal concha (Fig. 9.5*B*). The central processes of the bipolar olfactory neurons are collected into bundles to form approximately 20 **olfactory nerves** on each side that collectively form the right or left olfactory nerve (Fig. 9.5*C*). The fibers pass through tiny foramina in the **cribriform plate** of the ethmoid bone, surrounded by sleeves of dura and arachnoid, and enter the **olfactory bulb** in the anterior cranial fossa. The olfactory nerve fibers synapse with **mitral cells** in the olfactory bulb. The axons of these cells form the **olfactory tract,** which conveys the impulses to the brain (Fig. 9.5*A* and *C*). The olfactory bulbs and tracts are technically anterior extensions of the forebrain.

Anosmia—Loss of Smell

Loss or decrease in olfaction usually occurs with aging. This may also occur due to excessive smoking and cocaine use. The chief complaint of most people with anosmia is the loss or alteration of taste; however, clinical studies reveal that in all but a few people, the dysfunction is in the olfactory system (Sweazey, 2002). Transitory olfactory impairment occurs as a result of viral or allergic rhinitis, inflammation of the nasal mucous membrane.

Injury to the nasal mucosa, olfactory nerve fibers, olfactory bulbs, or olfactory tracts may also impair smell. In severe head injuries, the olfactory bulbs may be torn away from the olfactory nerves, or some olfactory nerve fibers may be torn as they pass through a *fractured cribriform plate.* If all the nerve bundles on one side are torn, a complete loss of smell occurs on that side; consequently, anosmia may be a clue to a fracture of the cranial base and cerebrospinal fluid (CSF) rhinorrhea, a leakage of the fluid through the nose from the subarachnoid space. Olfaction disorders are also linked with psychiatric illnesses (e.g., schizophrenia) and epilepsy. These patients may experience distortion of smell (parosmia) or perceive an odor when there is none present (olfactory hallucination).

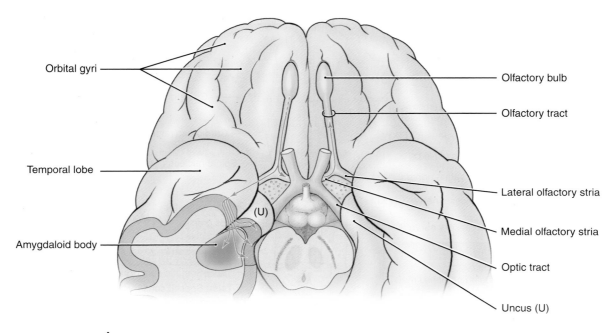

A Inferior view

FIGURE 9.5. **Olfactory system. A.** Olfactory bulbs, tracts, and medial and lateral striae.

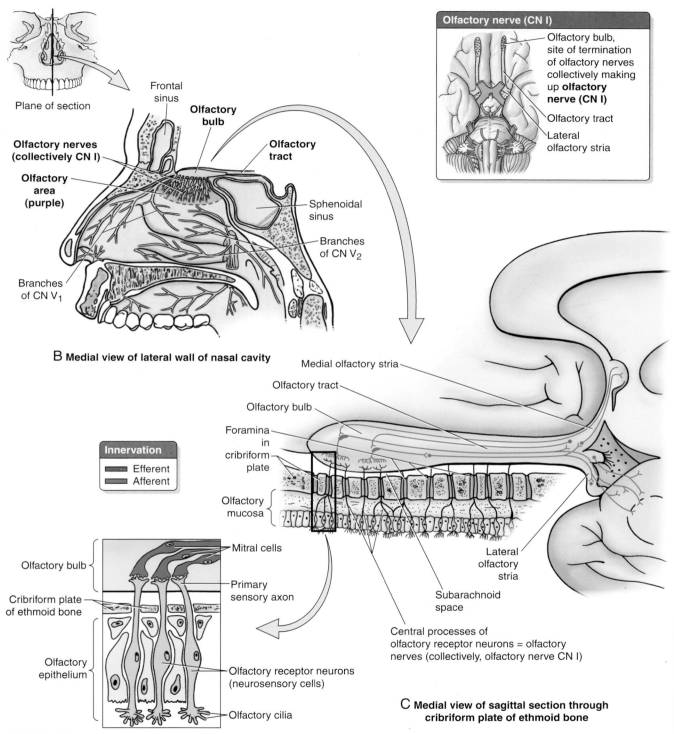

Plane of section

Frontal sinus

Olfactory bulb

Olfactory nerves (collectively CN I)

Olfactory tract

Olfactory area (purple)

Sphenoidal sinus

Branches of CN V₂

Branches of CN V₁

B **Medial view of lateral wall of nasal cavity**

Olfactory nerve (CN I)

Olfactory bulb, site of termination of olfactory nerves collectively making up **olfactory nerve (CN I)**

Olfactory tract

Lateral olfactory stria

Medial olfactory stria

Olfactory tract

Olfactory bulb

Foramina in cribriform plate

Innervation

- Efferent
- Afferent

Olfactory mucosa

Lateral olfactory stria

Subarachnoid space

Central processes of olfactory receptor neurons = olfactory nerves (collectively, olfactory nerve CN I)

Olfactory bulb

Mitral cells

Cribriform plate of ethmoid bone

Primary sensory axon

Olfactory epithelium

Olfactory receptor neurons (neurosensory cells)

Olfactory cilia

C **Medial view of sagittal section through cribriform plate of ethmoid bone**

FIGURE 9.5. **Olfactory system** *(continued)*. **B.** Sagittal section through the nasal cavity showing the relationship of the olfactory area to the olfactory bulb. **C.** Bodies of the olfactory receptor neurons are in the olfactory epithelium. These bundles of axons are collectively called the olfactory nerve (CN I).

Visual system. A. Right visual field representation on retinas, left lateral geniculate body, and left visual cortex. **B.** Overview of visual pathway.

OPTIC NERVE (CN II)

The **optic nerve** (CN II) conveys visual information. The optic nerves are paired, anterior extensions of the forebrain (diencephalon) and are, therefore, central nervous system (CNS) fiber tracts formed by axons of *retinal ganglion cells*. CN II is surrounded by extensions of the cranial meninges and subarachnoid space, which is filled with cerebrospinal fluid (CSF). CN II begins where the unmyelinated axons of the retinal ganglion cells pierce the sclera and become myelinated, deep to the **optic disc**. The nerve passes posteromedially in the orbit, exiting through the **optic canal** to enter the middle cranial fossa, where it forms the **optic chiasm** (Fig. 9.6). Here, fibers from the nasal (medial) half of each

retina decussate in the chiasm and join uncrossed fibers from the temporal (lateral) half of the retina to form the **optic tract.** The partial crossing of optic nerve fibers in the chiasm is a requirement for binocular vision, allowing depth-of-field perception (three-dimensional vision). Thus fibers from the right halves of both retinas form the right optic tract, and those from the left halves form the left optic tract. The decussation of nerve fibers in the chiasm results in the right optic tract conveying impulses from the left visual field and vice versa. The **visual field** is what is seen by a person with both eyes wide open and looking straight ahead. Most fibers in the optic tracts terminate in the **lateral geniculate bodies (nuclei)** of the thalamus. From these nuclei, axons are relayed to the visual cortices of the occipital lobes of the brain.

Visual Field Defects

Visual field defects may result from a large number of neurologic diseases. It is clinically important to be able to link the defect to a likely location of the lesion (Fig. B9.1).

Visual field defects of left eye

Temporal   Nasal

1

2

3

4

5

6

Visual field defects of right eye

Nasal   Temporal

1

2

3

4

5

6

1. Blindness of ipsilateral eye.
2. Bitemporal hemianopsia: loss of vision in the temporal fields of both eyes (tunnel vision).
3. Loss of vision in the temporal field of the ipsilateral eye.

4. Homonymous hemianopsia: visual loss is in same fields of each eye.
5. Homonymous hemianopsia.
6. Homonymous hemianopsia with macular sparing.

FIGURE B9.1.   Visual field defects.

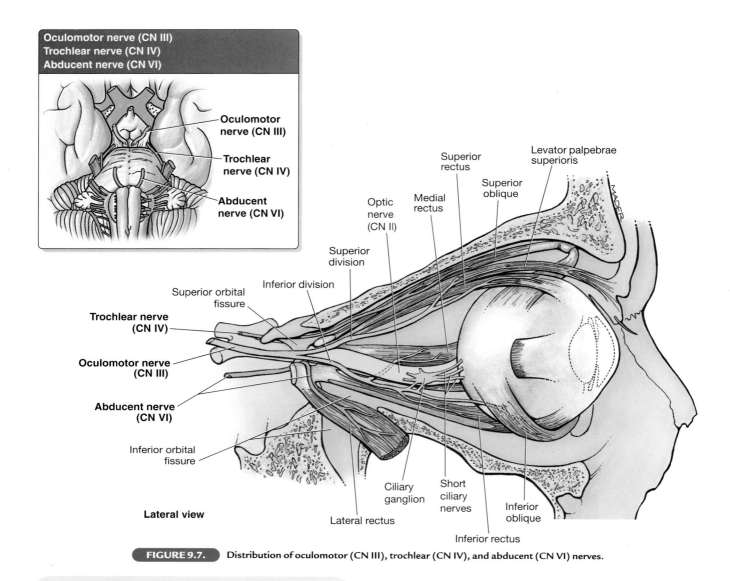

Oculomotor nerve (CN III)
Trochlear nerve (CN IV)
Abducent nerve (CN VI)

Oculomotor nerve (CN III)

Trochlear nerve (CN IV)

Abducent nerve (CN VI)

Superior rectus

Levator palpebrae superioris

Superior oblique

Optic nerve (CN II)

Medial rectus

Superior division

Inferior division

Superior orbital fissure

Trochlear nerve (CN IV)

Oculomotor nerve (CN III)

Abducent nerve (CN VI)

Inferior orbital fissure

Lateral view

Ciliary ganglion

Lateral rectus

Short ciliary nerves

Inferior oblique

Inferior rectus

FIGURE 9.7.   Distribution of oculomotor (CN III), trochlear (CN IV), and abducent (CN VI) nerves.

Demyelinating Diseases and the Optic Nerve

Because the optic nerves are actually CNS tracts, the myelin sheath that surrounds the fibers from the point at which they penetrate the sclera is formed by oligodendrocytes (glial cells) rather than by neurolemma (Schwann cells). Consequently, the optic nerves are susceptible to the effects of demyelinating diseases of the CNS, such as multiple sclerosis (MS).

OCULOMOTOR NERVE (CN III)

The **oculomotor nerve** (CN III) provides the following (Fig. 9.7):

- Somatic motor innervation to four of the six extra-ocular muscles (*superior, medial,* and *inferior rectus* and *inferior oblique*) and to the *levator palpebrae superioris*.
- Proprioceptive innervation to the previous muscles.
- Visceral (parasympathetic) innervation through the ciliary ganglion to the smooth muscle of the sphincter pupillae, which causes constriction of the pupil and ciliary muscle to produce accommodation (allowing the lens to become more rounded) for near vision (Fig. 9.8*B*).

CN III is the chief motor nerve to the ocular and extra-ocular muscles. It emerges from the midbrain, pierces the dura, and runs through the roof and lateral wall of the *cavernous sinus.* CN III leaves the cranial cavity and enters the orbit through the *superior orbital fissure*. Within this fissure, CN III divides into a **superior division,** which supplies the superior rectus and levator palpebrae superioris, and

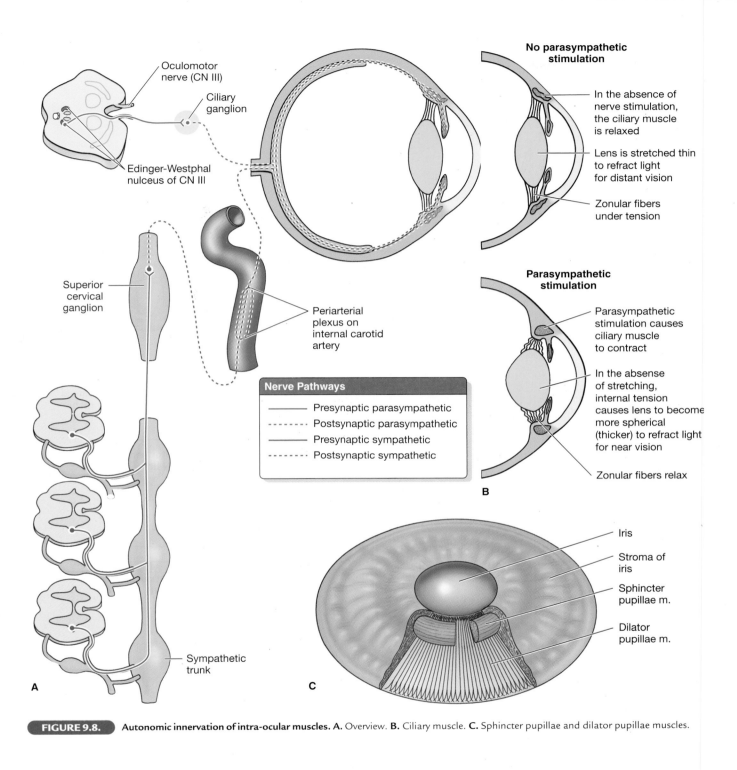

No parasympathetic stimulation

In the absence of nerve stimulation, the ciliary muscle is relaxed

Lens is stretched thin to refract light for distant vision

Zonular fibers under tension

Parasympathetic stimulation

Parasympathetic stimulation causes ciliary muscle to contract

In the absense of stretching, internal tension causes lens to become more spherical (thicker) to refract light for near vision

Zonular fibers relax

B

Oculomotor nerve (CN III)

Ciliary ganglion

Edinger-Westphal nulceus of CN III

Superior cervical ganglion

Periarterial plexus on internal carotid artery

Sympathetic trunk

A

Nerve Pathways

——— Presynaptic parasympathetic

- - - - Postsynaptic parasympathetic

——— Presynaptic sympathetic

- - - - Postsynaptic sympathetic

Iris

Stroma of iris

Sphincter pupillae m.

Dilator pupillae m.

C

FIGURE 9.8. Autonomic innervation of intra-ocular muscles. **A.** Overview. **B.** Ciliary muscle. **C.** Sphincter pupillae and dilator pupillae muscles.

an **inferior division,** which supplies the inferior and medial rectus and inferior oblique (Fig. 9.7). The inferior division also carries presynaptic parasympathetic (visceral efferent) fibers to the **ciliary ganglion,** where they synapse. Postsynaptic fibers from this ganglion pass to the eyeball in the *short ciliary nerves* to innervate the ciliary muscle and the sphincter pupillae.

TROCHLEAR NERVE (CN IV)

The **trochlear nerve** (CN IV) provides somatic motor and proprioceptive innervation to the contralateral **superior oblique**. The trochlear nerve, the smallest cranial nerve,

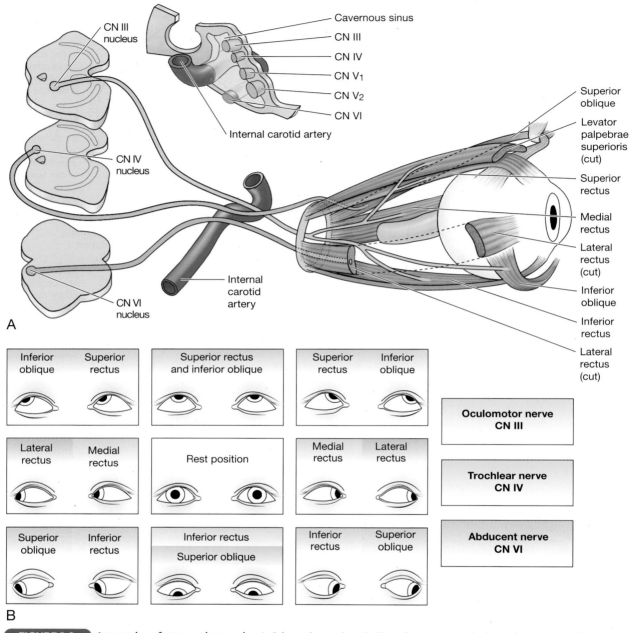

A

B

FIGURE 9.9. **Innervation of extra-ocular muscles. A.** Schematic overview. **B.** Binocular movements and muscles producing them. All movements start from the rest (primary) position.

arises from the nucleus of the trochlear nerve and crosses the midline prior to emerging inferior to the inferior colliculus of the posterior surface of the midbrain. It then passes anteriorly around the brainstem and pierces the dura mater at the margin of the tentorium cerebelli to course anteriorly in the lateral wall of the cavernous sinus. The nerve continues along the wall of the sinus to pass through the superior orbital fissure into the orbit, where it supplies the superior oblique (Fig. 9.7).

ABDUCENT NERVE (CN VI)

The **abducent nerve** (CN VI) provides somatic motor to and proprioceptive information from one extra-ocular muscle (**lateral rectus**). The abducent nerve emerges from the brainstem between the pons and the medulla and traverses the pontine cistern of the subarachnoid space. It then pierces the dura and runs the longest intracranial course within the cranial cavity of all the cranial nerves. During its intracranial course, it bends sharply over the crest of the petrous part of the temporal bone and then courses through the cavernous sinus, surrounded by venous blood like the internal carotid artery. CN VI then enters the orbit through the superior orbital fissure and runs anteriorly to supply the **lateral rectus,** which abducts the eye (Fig. 9.7).

The innervation and movements of the extra-ocular muscles from the primary position are summarized in Figure 9.9.

Ocular Palsies

The oculomotor (CN III), trochlear (CN IV), and abducent (CN VI) nerves may be compressed or completely paralyzed intra- and extracranially by neurologic diseases, tumors, aneurysms, etc.

Oculomotor Nerve (CN III)

Complete CN III Palsy

 Characteristic signs of a complete lesion of CN III are (Fig. B9.2):

- Ptosis (drooping) of the superior eyelid, caused by paralysis of the levator palpebrae superioris.
- Eyeball (pupil) abducted and directed slightly inferiorly (down and out) because of unopposed actions of the lateral rectus and superior oblique.
- No pupillary (light) reflex (constriction of the pupil in response to bright light) in the affected eye.
- Dilation of pupil, resulting from the interruption of parasympathetic fibers to the sphincter pupillae, leaving the dilator pupillae unopposed.
- No accommodation of the lens (adjustment to increase convexity for near vision) because of paralysis of the ciliary muscle.

Right eye: Downward and outward gaze, dilated pupil, eyelid manually elevated due to ptosis

Left: Normal

Right oculomotor (CN III) nerve palsy

FIGURE B9.2.

Partial CN III Palsy

Rapidly increasing intracranial pressure (e.g., resulting from an acute extradural or subdural hematoma) often compresses CN III against the petrous part of the temporal bone. Because the parasympathetic fibers in CN III are superficial, they are affected first (internal ophthalmoplegia). External ophthalmoplegia results from selective damage of the somatic motor fibers.

An aneurysm of a posterior cerebral or superior cerebellar artery may exert pressure on CN III as it passes between these vessels. Because CN III lies in the lateral wall of the cavernous sinus, injuries, infections, or tumors may also affect this nerve.

Trochlear Nerve (CN IV)

 CN IV is rarely paralyzed alone. The characteristic sign of trochlear nerve injury is *diplopia* (double vision) when looking down (e.g., when going down stairs). Diplopia occurs because the superior oblique normally assists the inferior rectus in depressing the pupil (directing the gaze downward) and is the only muscle to do so when the pupil is adducted.

Abducent Nerve (CN VI)

 Because CN VI has a long intracranial course, it is often stretched when intracranial pressure rises, partly because of the sharp bend it makes over the crest of the petrous part of the temporal bone after entering the dura. A space-occupying lesion such as a brain tumor may compress CN VI, causing paralysis of the lateral rectus muscle. Complete paralysis of CN VI causes medial deviation of the affected eye—that is, it is fully adducted at rest and does not fully abduct owing to the unopposed action of the medial rectus, leaving the person unable to abduct the eye (Fig. B9.3).

Right: Normal

Left eye: Does not abduct

Direction of gaze ———→

Left abducent (CN VI) nerve palsy

FIGURE B9.3.

Trigeminal nerve (CN V)

Sensory root ⎤
Motor root ⎦ Of CN V

A Lateral view

Sensory root

Trigeminal ganglion

Ophthalmic nerve (CN V₁)

Frontal nerve

Lacrimal nerve

Nasociliary nerve

Maxillary nerve (CN V₂)

Zygomatic nerve

Infra-orbital nerve

Anterior ⎤
Middle ⎬ Superior alveolar nerves
Posterior ⎦

Mandibular nerve (CN V₃)

Meningeal branch

Auriculotemporal nerve

Buccal nerve

Lingual nerve

Inferior alveolar nerve

B Lateral view

Trigeminal nerve (CN V) in A & B
- Ophthalmic nerve (CN V₁)
- Maxillary nerve (CN V₂)
- Mandibular nerve (CN V₃)

Lateral nasal wall

Olfactory mucosa

Pharyngeal nerve

CN V₁

CN V₂

Nasopalatine nerve

Greater palatine nerve

Lesser palatine nerve

Nasal septum

Anterior ethmoidal nerve

Olfactory mucosa

CN V₁

CN V₂

Lesser palatine nerve

Greater palatine nerve

Nasopalatine nerve

C Open-book view

FIGURE 9.10. **Distribution of trigeminal nerve (CN V). A.** Cutaneous (sensory) distribution of the three divisions of the trigeminal nerve. **B.** Branches of the ophthalmic (CN V₁), maxillary (CN V₂), and mandibular divisions (CN V₃). **C.** CN V₁ and CN V₂ innervation of the lateral wall and septum of the nasal cavity and palate.

TABLE 9.2 SUMMARY OF DIVISIONS OF TRIGEMINAL NERVE (CN V)

Divisions/Distributions	Branches

Ophthalmic nerve (CN V$_1$)
Somatic sensory only
Passes through superior orbital fissure
Supplies cornea, upper conjunctiva, mucosa of anterosuperior nasal cavity, frontal and ethmoidal sinuses, anterior and supratentorial dura mater, skin of dorsum of external nose, superior eyelid, forehead, and scalp
 	
	Tentorial nerve (a meningeal branch)
	Lacrimal nerve
	Communicating branch from zygomatic nerve
	Frontal nerve
	  Supra-orbital nerve
	  Supratrochlear nerve
	Nasociliary nerve
	  Sensory root of ciliary ganglion
	  Short ciliary nerves
	  Long ciliary nerves
	  Infratrochlear nerves
	  Anterior and posterior ethmoidal nerves

Maxillary nerve (CN V$_2$)
Somatic sensory only
Passes through foramen rotundum
Supplies dura mater of anterior part of middle cranial fossa; conjunctiva of inferior eyelid; mucosa of posteroinferior nasal cavity, maxillary sinus, palate and anterior part of superior oral vestibule; maxillary teeth; and skin of lateral external nose, inferior eyelid, anterior cheek, and upper lip
 	
	Meningeal branch
	Zygomatic nerve
	  Zygomaticofacial branch
	  Zygomaticotemporal branch
	  Communicating branch to lacrimal nerve
	Ganglionic branches to (sensory root of) pterygopalatine ganglion
	Posterior superior alveolar branches
	  Infra-orbital nerve
	  Anterior and middle superior alveolar branches
	  Superior labial branches
	  Inferior palpebral branches
	  External nasal branches
	Greater palatine nerves
	  Posterior inferior lateral nasal nerves
	Lesser palatine nerves
	Posterior superior lateral nasal branches
	Nasopalatine nerve
	Pharyngeal nerve

Mandibular nerve (CN V$_3$)
Somatic sensory and somatic (branchial) motor
Passes through the foramen ovale
Supplies sensory innervation to mucosa of anterior two thirds of tongue, floor of mouth, and posterior and anterior inferior oral vestibule; mandibular teeth; and skin of lower lip, buccal, parotid, and temporal regions of face; and external ear (auricle, upper external auditory meatus, and tympanic membrane)
Supplies motor innervation to muscles of mastication, mylohoid, anterior belly of digastric, tensor tympani, and tensor veli palatini
 	
	Somatic sensory branches
	  Meningeal branch (nervus spinosum)
	  Buccal nerve
	  Auriculotemporal nerve
	  Lingual nerve
	  Inferior alveolar nerve
	  Nerve to mylohyoid
	  Inferior dental plexus
	  Mental nerve
	Somatic (branchial) motor branches
	  Masseter
	  Temporal
	  Medial and lateral pterygoids
	  Mylohyoid
	  Anterior belly of digastric
	  Tensor tympani
	  Tensor veli palatini

TRIGEMINAL NERVE (CN V)

The **trigeminal nerve** (CN V) emerges from the lateral aspect of the pons by a large sensory root and a small motor root (Fig. 9.1). CN V is the principal general sensory nerve for the head (face, teeth, mouth, nasal cavity, and dura of the cranial cavity) (Fig. 9.10). The **sensory root of CN V** is composed mainly of the central processes of neurons in the **trigeminal ganglion** (Fig. 9.10B). The peripheral processes of the ganglionic neurons form three nerves or divisions: **ophthalmic nerve** (CN V₁), **maxillary nerve** (CN V₂), and sensory component of the **mandibular nerve** (CN V₃). For a summary of CN V, see Figure 9.10 and Table 9.2. The fibers of the **motor root of CN V** are distributed exclusively via the mandibular nerve (CN V₃) to the muscles of mastication, mylohyoid, anterior belly of the digastric, tensor veli palatini, and tensor tympani.

Injury to Trigeminal Nerve

CN V may be injured by trauma, tumors, aneurysms, or meningeal infections causing:
- Paralysis of the muscles of mastication with deviation of the mandible toward the side of the lesion.
- Loss of the ability to appreciate soft tactile, thermal, or painful sensations in the face.
- Loss of the corneal reflex (blinking in response to the cornea being touched) and the sneezing reflex.

Trigeminal neuralgia (tic douloureux), the principal disease affecting the sensory root of CN V, produces excruciating, episodic pain that is usually restricted to the areas supplied by the maxillary and/or mandibular divisions of CN V.

FACIAL NERVE (CN VII)

The **facial nerve** (CN VII) emerges from the junction of the pons and medulla as two divisions: the motor root and the intermediate nerve (L. *nervus intermedius*) (Fig. 9.1). The larger **motor root** (facial nerve proper) innervates the muscles of facial expression, and the smaller **intermediate nerve** carries taste, parasympathetic, and somatic sensory fibers (Fig. 9.11). During its course, CN VII traverses the posterior cranial fossa, internal acoustic meatus, facial canal, stylomastoid foramen of the temporal bone, and parotid gland. After traversing the internal acoustic meatus, the nerve proceeds a short distance anteriorly within the temporal bone and then turns abruptly posteriorly to course along the medial wall of the tympanic cavity. The sharp bend is the **geniculum of the facial nerve** (Fig. 9.11*A*) the site of the **geniculate ganglion** (sensory ganglion of CN VII). Within the facial canal, CN VII gives rise to the greater petrosal nerve, the nerve to the stapedius, and the chorda tympani nerve. After running the longest intraosseous course of any cranial nerve, CN VII emerges from the cranium via the *stylomastoid foramen;* gives off the posterior auricular branch; enters the parotid gland; and forms the **parotid plexus,** which gives rise to the following five terminal motor branches: temporal, zygomatic, buccal, marginal mandibular, and cervical.

Somatic (Branchial) Motor

As the nerve of the second pharyngeal arch, the facial nerve supplies the striated muscle derived from its mesoderm, mainly the muscles of facial expression and auricular muscles. It also supplies the posterior bellies of the digastric, stylohyoid, and stapedius muscles.

Visceral (Parasympathetic) Motor

The parasympathetic distribution of the facial nerve is detailed in Figure 9.12. CN VII provides presynaptic parasympathetic fibers to the **pterygopalatine ganglion** for innervation of the lacrimal, nasal, pharyngeal, and palatine glands and to the **submandibular ganglion** for innervation of the sublingual and submandibular salivary glands. The main features of parasympathetic ganglia associated with the facial nerve and other cranial nerves are summarized at the end of the chapter in Table 9.4. Parasympathetic fibers synapse in these ganglia, whereas sympathetic and other fibers pass through them.

Somatic (General) Sensory

Some fibers from the **geniculate ganglion** supply a small area of skin close to the external acoustic meatus (Fig. 9.11).

Special Sensory (Taste)

Fibers carried by the chorda tympani join the **lingual nerve** to convey taste sensation from the anterior two thirds of the tongue and soft palate (Fig. 9.11).

Injury to Facial Nerve

A *lesion of CN VII near its origin* or near the geniculate ganglion is accompanied by loss of motor, gustatory (taste), and autonomic functions. The motor paralysis of facial muscles involves upper and lower parts of the face on the ipsilateral (same) side (Bell palsy).

A *central lesion of CN VII* (lesion of the CNS) results in paralysis of muscles of the inferior face on the contralateral side. However, forehead wrinkling is not visibly impaired because it is innervated bilaterally. Lesions between the geniculate ganglion and the origin of the chorda tympani produce the same effects as that resulting from injury near the ganglion except that lacrimal secretion is not affected. Because it passes through the facial canal, CN VII is vulnerable to compression when a viral infection produces inflammation of the nerve (viral neuritis).

Facial nerve (CN VII)

Facial nerve (CN VII)

Geniculum of CN VII with geniculate ganglion

Tympanic membrane

Nerve to stapedius

Chorda tympani

Posterior auricular branch

Parotid plexus (branches to muscles of facial expression)

Greater petrosal nerve

CN V

Nerve of pterygoid canal

Pterygo-palatine ganglion

CN V₃:
Lingual nerve
Inferior alveolar nerve

A Lateral view

Facial nerve (CN VII)

Intermediate nerve

Somatic (branchial) motor

Muscles of facial expression

Facial nerve (CN VII)

Geniculate ganglion

Greater petrosal nerve

Carotid (sympathetic) plexus

Zygomatic nerve

Lacrimal nerve

Lacrimal gland

Maxillary nerve (CN V₂)

Nerve of pterygoid canal

Deep petrosal nerve

Nerve to stapedius

Internal carotid artery

Facial nerve

Chorda tympani

Mandibular nerve (CN V₃)

Lingual nerve

Pterygopalatine ganglion

Visceral (parasympathetic) motor

Lacrimal gland
Sublingual gland
Sub-mandibular gland

Special sensory (taste)

Taste

Sublingual gland

Submandibular ganglion

Submandibular gland

Temporal branch

Zygomatic branch

Buccal branch

Marginal mandibular branch

Posterior auricular branch

Cervical branch

B

Facial nerve fibers in B

■ Somatic (branchial) motor
□ Special sensory (taste)
■ Presynaptic parasympathetic (secretomotor) to pterygopalatine ganglion via greater petrosal nerve and to anterior tongue and submandibular ganglion via chorda tympani

FIGURE 9.11. **Distribution of facial nerve (CN VII). A.** Facial nerve in situ; intraosseous course and branches. **B.** Regional distribution of facial nerve.

A. Visceral (parasympathetic) motor to lacrimal gland

Greater petrosal nerve arises from CN VII at geniculate ganglion and emerges from superior surface of petrous part of temporal bone to enter middle cranial fossa.

Greater petrosal nerve joins deep petrosal nerve (sympathetic) at foramen lacerum to form nerve of pterygoid canal.

Nerve of pterygoid canal travels through pterygoid canal and enters pterygopalatine fossa.

Parasympathetic fibers from nerve of pterygoid canal in pterygopalatine fossa synapse in pterygopalatine ganglion.

Postsynaptic parasympathetic fibers from this ganglion innervate lacrimal gland via zygomatic branch of CN V_2 and lacrimal nerve (branch of CN V_1).

B. Visceral (parasympathetic) motor to submandibular and sublingual glands

The chorda tympani branch arises from CN VII just superior to stylomastoid foramen.

The chorda tympani crosses tympanic cavity medial to handle of malleus.

The chorda tympani passes through petrotympanic fissure between tympanic and petrous parts of the temporal bone to join the lingual nerve (CN V_3) in infratemporal fossa.

Parasympathetic fibers of chorda tympani synapse in submandibular ganglion; postsynaptic fibers follow arteries to glands.

FIGURE 9.12. Parasympathetic innervation involving facial nerve (CN VII).

Corneal Reflex

Loss of the corneal reflex may occur if either the ophthalmic nerve (CN V_1) or the facial nerve (CN VII) is lesioned. The corneal reflex is tested by touching the cornea with a cotton wisp. A bilateral blinking response should result. The afferent and efferent limbs of the corneal reflex are outlined in Fig. B9.4.

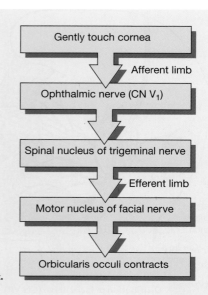

Gently touch cornea

Afferent limb

Ophthalmic nerve (CN V_1)

Spinal nucleus of trigeminal nerve

Efferent limb

Motor nucleus of facial nerve

Orbicularis occuli contracts

FIGURE B9.4. Corneal reflex.

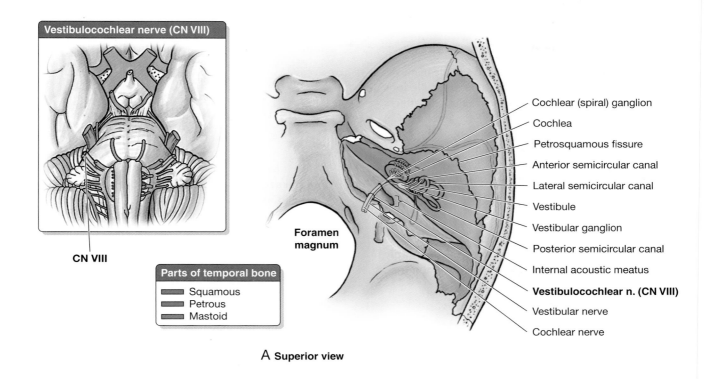

Vestibulocochlear nerve (CN VIII)

CN VIII

Parts of temporal bone
- Squamous
- Petrous
- Mastoid

Foramen magnum

Cochlear (spiral) ganglion
Cochlea
Petrosquamous fissure
Anterior semicircular canal
Lateral semicircular canal
Vestibule
Vestibular ganglion
Posterior semicircular canal
Internal acoustic meatus
Vestibulocochlear n. (CN VIII)
Vestibular nerve
Cochlear nerve

A **Superior view**

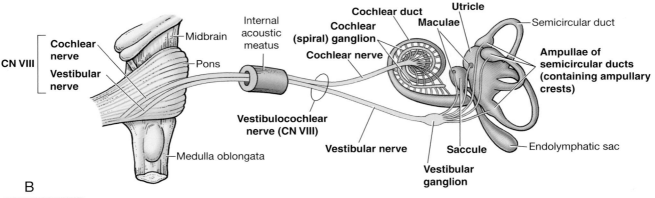

CN VIII

Cochlear nerve
Vestibular nerve

Midbrain
Pons
Medulla oblongata

Internal acoustic meatus

Vestibulocochlear nerve (CN VIII)

Cochlear (spiral) ganglion
Cochlear nerve

Cochlear duct
Maculae
Utricle
Semicircular duct

Ampullae of semicircular ducts (containing ampullary crests)

Vestibular nerve

Saccule

Vestibular ganglion

Endolymphatic sac

B

FIGURE 9.13. Distribution of vestibulocochlear nerve (CN VIII). **A.** Internal surface of cranial base showing the location of the bony labyrinth of the internal ear within the temporal bone and the internal acoustic meatus for CN VIII. **B.** Schematic overview.

VESTIBULOCOCHLEAR NERVE (CN VIII)

The **vestibulocochlear nerve** (CN VIII) is a special sensory nerve of hearing and equilibrium. The vestibulocochlear nerve emerges from the junction of the pons and medulla and enters the *internal acoustic meatus* (Fig. 9.1). Here, it separates into the vestibular and cochlear nerves (Fig. 9.13).

- The **vestibular nerve** is concerned with equilibrium. It is composed of the central processes of bipolar neurons in the **vestibular ganglion;** the peripheral processes of the neurons extend to the **maculae** of the utricle and saccule (sensitive to the linear acceleration relative to the position of the head) and to the **ampullae** of semicircular ducts (sensitive to rotational acceleration).
- The **cochlear nerve** is concerned with hearing. It is composed of the central processes of bipolar neurons in the **spiral ganglion;** the peripheral processes of the neurons extend to the spiral organ.

Injuries of Vestibulocochlear Nerve

Although the vestibular and cochlear nerves are essentially independent, peripheral lesions often produce concurrent clinical effects because of their close relationship. Hence lesions of CN VIII may cause *tinnitus* (ringing or buzzing of the ears), *vertigo* (dizziness, loss of balance), and impairment or loss of hearing. Central lesions may involve either the cochlear or vestibular divisions of CN VIII.

Deafness

There are two kinds of deafness: conductive deafness, involving the external or middle ear (e.g., otitis media, inflammation in the middle ear), and sensorineural deafness, which results from disease in the cochlea or in the pathway from the cochlea to the brain.

Acoustic Neuroma

Acoustic neuromas are benign tumors of the neurolemma of Schwann cells. The tumor begins in the vestibular nerve while it is in the internal acoustic meatus. The tumor is located at the cerebellopontine angle and presents initially with CN VIII dysfunction (i.e., hearing loss and ataxia). As the tumor grows it may involve CN VII and CN V, resulting in facial palsy and trigeminal sensory loss. Further progression of the tumor may compress CN IX, the cerebellum, and the brainstem.

GLOSSOPHARYNGEAL NERVE (CN IX)

The **glossopharyngeal nerve** (CN IX) emerges from the lateral aspect of the medulla and passes anterolaterally to leave the cranium through the *jugular foramen.* At this foramen are **superior** and **inferior ganglia,** which contain the cell bodies for the afferent (sensory) components of the nerve (Fig. 9.14). CN IX follows the stylopharyngeus, the only muscle the nerve supplies, and passes between the superior and the middle pharyngeal constrictor of the pharynx to reach the oropharynx and tongue. It contributes sensory fibers to the *pharyngeal plexus* of nerves. The glossopharyngeal nerve is afferent from the tongue and pharynx (hence its name) and efferent to the stylopharyngeus and parotid gland.

Somatic (Branchial) Motor

Motor fibers pass to one muscle, the stylopharyngeus, derived from the third pharyngeal arch.

Visceral (Parasympathetic) Motor

Following a circuitous route initially involving the tympanic nerve, presynaptic parasympathetic fibers are provided to the otic ganglion for innervation of the parotid gland (Fig. 9.15).

Somatic (General) Sensory

The *pharyngeal, tonsillar,* and *lingual branches* supply the mucosa of the oropharynx and isthmus of the fauces (*L.* throat), including the palatine tonsil, soft palate, and posterior third of the tongue. Stimuli determined to be unusual or unpleasant here may evoke the gag reflex or even vomiting. Via the tympanic plexus CN IX supplies the

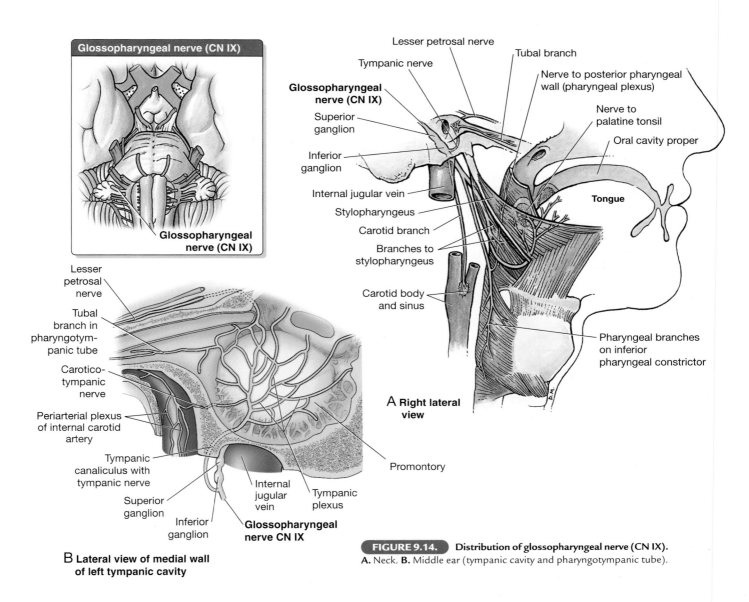

FIGURE 9.14. Distribution of glossopharyngeal nerve (CN IX). **A.** Neck. **B.** Middle ear (tympanic cavity and pharyngotympanic tube).

mucosa of the tympanic cavity, pharyngotympanic tube, and the internal surface of the tympanic membrane.

Special Sensory (Taste)

Taste fibers are conveyed from the posterior third of the tongue to the sensory ganglia.

Visceral Sensory

The *carotid sinus nerve* supplies the carotid sinus, a baro- (presso-) receptor sensitive to changes in blood pressure, and the carotid body, a chemoreceptor sensitive to blood gas (oxygen and carbon dioxide) levels.

VAGUS NERVE (CN X)

The vagus nerve arises by a series of rootlets from the lateral aspect of the medulla that merge and leave the cranium through the jugular foramen positioned between CN IX and CN XI (Fig. 9.16). What was formerly called "the cranial root of the accessory nerve" is actually a part of CN X (Fig. 9.1A). CN X has a **superior ganglion** in the jugular foramen that is mainly concerned with the general

Lesions of Glossopharyngeal Nerve

 Isolated lesions of CN IX or its nuclei are uncommon. Injuries of CN IX resulting from infection or tumors are usually accompanied by signs of involvement of adjacent nerves. Because CN IX, CN X, and CN XI pass through the jugular foramen, tumors in this region produce multiple cranial nerve palsies—the *jugular foramen syndrome.*

An isolated lesion would result in absence of taste on the posterior third of the tongue, changes in swallowing, absent gag reflex on the side of the lesion, and palatal deviation toward the unaffected side (Fig. B9.5). The afferent (sensory) limb of the gag reflex is via the glossopharyngeal nerve (CN IX) and the efferent (motor) limb is via the vagus nerve (CNX). The gag reflex is absent in about 37% of normal individuals (Davies, 1995).

Anterior view through widely opened mouth.

FIGURE B9.5. **Gag reflex.** In **B** note that the palate and posterior wall of the pharynx deviate to the left side when the gag reflex is elicited. This is due to a right CN IX/CN X lesion and is called the "curtain sign."

FIGURE 9.16. Relationship of structures traversing jugular foramen. CN IX, CN X, and CN XI are in numerical order, anterior to the internal jugular vein.

sensory component of the nerve. Inferior to the foramen is an **inferior ganglion** (nodose ganglion) concerned with the visceral sensory components of the nerve. In the region of the superior ganglion are connections to CN IX and the superior cervical (sympathetic) ganglion. CN X continues inferiorly in the carotid sheath to the root of the neck, supplying branches to the palate, pharynx, and larynx (Fig. 9.17; Table 9.3).

The course that CN X takes in the thorax differs on the two sides. CN X supplies branches to the heart, bronchi, and lungs. The vagi join the *esophageal plexus* surrounding the esophagus, which is formed by branches of the vagi and sympathetic trunks. This plexus follows the esophagus through the diaphragm into the abdomen, where the **anterior** and **posterior vagal trunks** break up into branches that innervate the esophagus, stomach, and intestinal tract as far as the left colic flexure (Fig. 9.17).

Somatic (Branchial) Motor

Fibers from the nucleus ambiguus supply:

- Pharyngeal muscles via the pharyngeal plexus with fibers of the glossopharyngeal nerve.
- Muscles of the soft palate.
- All muscles of the larynx.

Visceral (Parasympathetic) Motor

Fibers from the posterior (dorsal) nucleus of the vagus nerve supply the thoracic and abdominal viscera to the left colic (splenic) flexure.

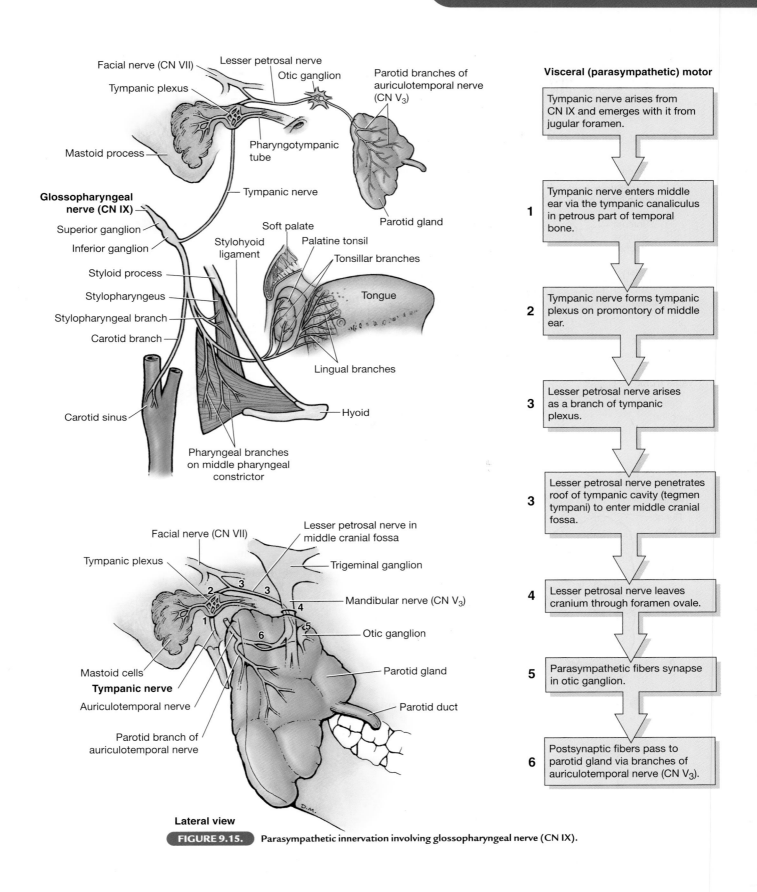

Visceral (parasympathetic) motor

Tympanic nerve arises from CN IX and emerges with it from jugular foramen.

1   Tympanic nerve enters middle ear via the tympanic canaliculus in petrous part of temporal bone.

2   Tympanic nerve forms tympanic plexus on promontory of middle ear.

3   Lesser petrosal nerve arises as a branch of tympanic plexus.

3   Lesser petrosal nerve penetrates roof of tympanic cavity (tegmen tympani) to enter middle cranial fossa.

4   Lesser petrosal nerve leaves cranium through foramen ovale.

5   Parasympathetic fibers synapse in otic ganglion.

6   Postsynaptic fibers pass to parotid gland via branches of auriculotemporal nerve (CN V₃).

Lateral view

FIGURE 9.15. Parasympathetic innervation involving glossopharyngeal nerve (CN IX).

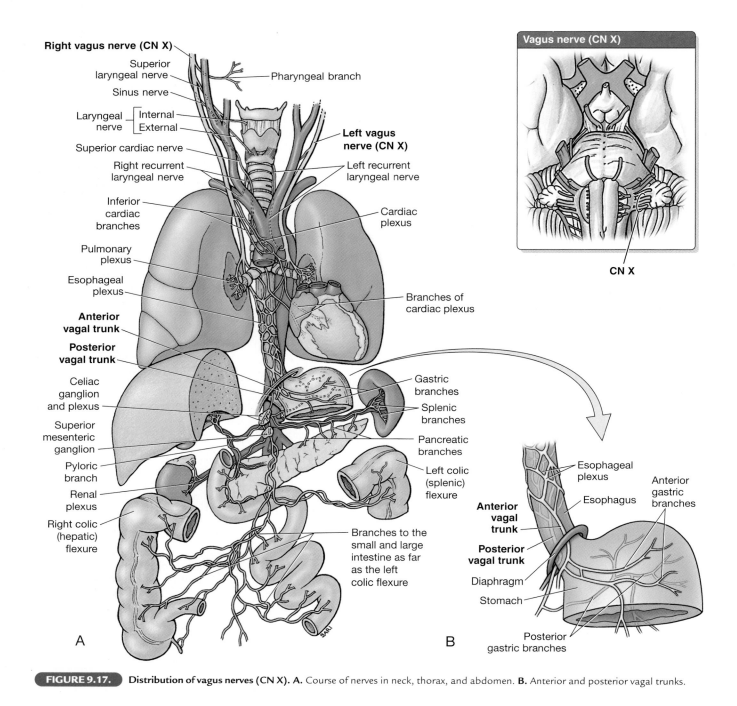

FIGURE 9.17.   **Distribution of vagus nerves (CN X). A.** Course of nerves in neck, thorax, and abdomen. **B.** Anterior and posterior vagal trunks.

Somatic (General) Sensory

Sensory from:

- Dura mater of posterior cranial fossa
- Skin posterior to the ear

- External auditory canal

Special Sensory (Taste)

Carry sense of taste from the root of the tongue and the taste buds on the epiglottis

Visceral Sensory

Convey sensory fibers from:

- Mucosa of the inferior pharynx at the esophageal junction, epiglottis, and ary-epiglottic folds

- Mucosa of larynx
- Baroreceptors in the aortic arch
- Chemoreceptors in the aortic bodies
- Thoracic and abdominal viscera

TABLE 9.3 SUMMARY OF VAGUS NERVE (CN X)

Divisions (Parts)	Branches
Cranial Vagi arise by a series of rootlets from medulla (includes traditional cranial root of CN XI)	Meningeal branch to dura mater (sensory; actually fibers of C2 spinal ganglion neurons that "hitch a ride" with vagus nerve) Auricular branch
Cervical Exit cranium/enter neck through jugular foramen; right and left vagus nerves enter carotid sheaths and continue to root of neck	Pharyngeal branches to pharyngeal plexus (motor) Cervical cardiac branches (parasympathetic, visceral afferent) Superior laryngeal nerve (mixed), internal (sensory), and external (motor) branches Right recurrent laryngeal nerve (mixed)
Thoracic Vagi enter thorax through superior thoracic aperture; left vagus contributes to anterior esophageal plexus; right vagus to posterior plexus; form anterior and posterior trunks	Left recurrent laryngeal nerve (mixed; all distal branches convey parasympathetic and visceral afferent fibers for reflex stimuli) Thoracic cardiac branches Pulmonary branches Esophageal plexus
Abdominal Anterior and posterior vagal trunks enter abdomen through esophageal hiatus in diaphragm	Esophageal branches Gastric branches Hepatic branches Celiac branches (from posterior trunk) Pyloric branch (from anterior trunk) Renal branches Intestinal branches (to left colic flexure)

Lesions of Vagus Nerve

Isolated lesions of CN X are uncommon. Injury to the pharyngeal branches of CN X results in *dysphagia* (difficulty in swallowing). Lesions of the superior laryngeal nerve produce anesthesia of the superior part of the larynx and paralysis of the cricothyroid muscle. The voice is weak and tires easily. Injury of a recurrent laryngeal nerve may be caused by aneurysms of the arch of the aorta and may occur during neck operations. Injury of the recurrent laryngeal nerve causes *hoarseness* and *dysphonia* (difficulty in speaking) because of paralysis of the vocal folds (cords). Paralysis of both recurrent laryngeal nerves causes *aphonia* (loss of voice) and *inspiratory stridor* (a harsh, high-pitched respiratory sound). Because of its longer course, lesions of the left recurrent laryngeal nerve are more common than those of the right. Proximal lesions of CN X also affect the pharyngeal and superior laryngeal nerves, causing difficulty in swallowing and speaking. Tachycardia and cardiac arrhythmia may occur.

SPINAL ACCESSORY NERVE (CN XI)

The spinal accessory nerve (CN XI) is somatic motor to the sternocleidomastoid (SCM) and trapezius muscles (Fig. 9.18). The traditional "cranial root" of CN XI is actually a part of CN X. CN XI emerges as a series of rootlets from the first five or six cervical segments of the spinal cord (Lachman et al., 2002). It joins CN X temporarily as they pass through the jugular foramen, separating again as they exit (Fig. 9.16). CN XI descends along the internal carotid

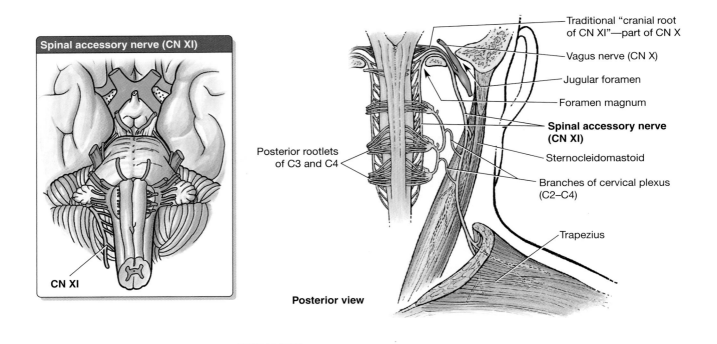

Spinal accessory nerve (CN XI)

CN XI

Traditional "cranial root of CN XI"—part of CN X

Vagus nerve (CN X)

Jugular foramen

Foramen magnum

Spinal accessory nerve (CN XI)

Sternocleidomastoid

Branches of cervical plexus (C2–C4)

Trapezius

Posterior rootlets of C3 and C4

Posterior view

FIGURE 9.18. Distribution of spinal accessory nerve (CN XI).

artery, penetrates and innervates the SCM, and emerges from the muscle near the middle of its posterior border. It crosses the posterior cervical region and passes deep to the superior border of the trapezius to innervate it. Branches of the cervical plexus conveying sensory fibers from spinal nerves C2–C4 join the spinal accessory nerve in the posterior cervical region, providing these muscles with pain and proprioceptive fibers.

Injury to Spinal Accessory Nerve

Because of its nearly subcutaneous passage through the posterior cervical region, CN XI is susceptible to injury during surgical procedures such as lymph node biopsy, cannulation of the internal jugular vein, and carotid endarterectomy.

Lesions of CN XI produce weakness (shrugging) and atrophy of the trapezius and impairment of rotary movements of the neck and chin to the opposite side as a result of weakness of the SCM (Fig. B9.6).

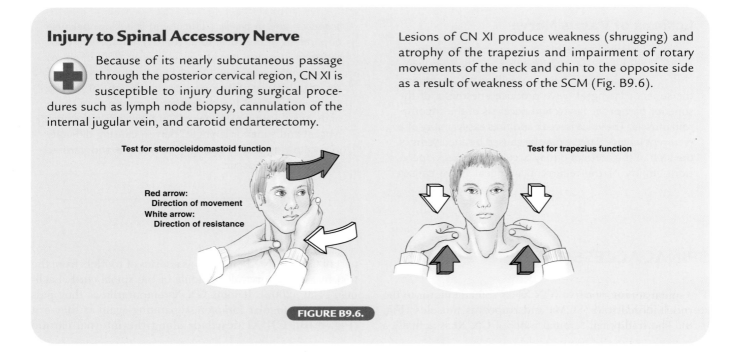

Test for sternocleidomastoid function

Red arrow:
Direction of movement
White arrow:
Direction of resistance

Test for trapezius function

FIGURE B9.6.

FIGURE 9.19. Distribution of hypoglossal nerve (CN XII).

Labels in figure: Hypoglossal nerve (CN XII); Intrinsic muscles of tongue; Styloglossus; CN XII; Anterior rami of cervical spinal nerves {C1, C2, C3}; Internal carotid artery; Hypoglossal nerve (CN XII); Ansa cervicalis {Inferior root, Superior root}; Genioglossus; Hyoglossus; Geniohyoid; Nerve to thyrohyoid; Thyrohyoid; Omohyoid; Sternohyoid; Sternothyroid; Lateral view

HYPOGLOSSAL NERVE (CN XII)

The **hypoglossal nerve** (CN XII) is somatic motor to intrinsic and extrinsic muscles of the tongue (styloglossus, hyoglossus, genioglossus). The hypoglossal nerve arises as a purely motor nerve by several rootlets from the medulla and leaves the cranium through the *hypoglossal canal* (Fig. 9.1). After exiting the cranial cavity, the nerve is joined by a branch or branches of the cervical plexus (Fig. 9.19), conveying general somatic motor fibers from C1 and C2 spinal nerves and general somatic sensory fibers from the spinal ganglion of C2. These spinal nerve fibers "hitch a ride" with CN XII to reach the hyoid muscles, with some of the sensory fibers passing retrograde along it to reach the dura mater of the posterior cranial fossa. CN XII passes inferiorly medial to the angle of the mandible and then curves anteriorly to enter the tongue.

CN XII ends in many branches that supply all the extrinsic muscles of the tongue, except the palatoglossus (which is actually a palatine muscle). CN XII has the following branches:

- A **meningeal branch** returns to the cranium through the hypoglossal canal and innervates the dura mater on the floor and posterior wall of the posterior cranial fossa. The nerve fibers conveyed are from the sensory spinal ganglion of spinal nerve C2, not from CN XII.
- The **superior root of the ansa cervicalis** branches from CN XII to supply the infrahyoid muscles (sternohyoid, sternothyroid, and omohyoid). This branch actually conveys only fibers from the cervical plexus (loop

between the anterior rami of C1 and C2) that joined the nerve outside the cranial cavity. Some fibers reach the thyrohyoid muscle.
- Terminal **lingual branches** supply the styloglossus, hyoglossus, genioglossus, and intrinsic muscles of the tongue.

Injury to Hypoglossal Nerve

Injury to CN XII paralyzes the ipsilateral half of the tongue. After some time, the tongue atrophies, making it appear shrunken and wrinkled. When the tongue is protruded, its apex deviates toward the paralyzed side because of the unopposed action of the genioglossus muscle on the normal side of the tongue (Fig. B9.7).

Right CN XII lesion

FIGURE B9.7.

TABLE 9.4 SUMMARY OF THE CRANIAL PARASYMPATHETIC GANGLIA

Ganglion	Location	Parasympathetic Root	Sympathetic Root	Main Distribution
Ciliary	Between optic nerve and lateral rectus, close to apex of orbit	Inferior branch of oculomotor nerve (CN III)	Branches from periarterial plexus on internal carotid artery in cavernous sinus	Parasympathetic postsynaptic fibers from ciliary ganglion pass to ciliary muscle and sphincter pupillae of iris; sympathetic postganglionic fibers from superior cervical ganglion pass to dilator pupillae and blood vessels of eye
Pterygopalatine	In pterygopalatine fossa, where it is suspended by ganglionic branches of maxillary nerve (sensory roots of pterygopalatine ganglion); just anterior to opening of pterygoid canal and inferior to CN V₂	Greater petrosal nerve from facial nerve (CN VII) via nerve of pterygoid canal	Deep petrosal nerve, a branch of periarterial plexus on internal carotid artery that is a continuation of postsynaptic fibers of cervical sympathetic trunk; fibers from superior cervical ganglion pass through pterygopalatine ganglion and enter branches of CN V₂	Parasympathetic postsynaptic (secretomotor) fibers from pterygopalatine ganglion innervate lacrimal gland via zygomatic branch of CN V₂; sympathetic postsynaptic fibers from superior cervical ganglion accompany branches of pterygopalatine nerve that are distributed to blood vessels of nasal cavity, palate, and superior parts of pharynx
Otic	Between tensor veli palatini and mandibular nerve (CN V₃); lies inferior to foramen ovale of sphenoid bone	Tympanic nerve from glossopharyngeal nerve (CN IX); from tympanic plexus tympanic nerve continues as lesser petrosal nerve	Fibers from superior cervical ganglion come from periarterial plexus on middle meningeal artery	Parasympathetic postsynaptic fibers from otic ganglion are distributed to parotid gland via auriculotemporal nerve (branch of CN V₃); sympathetic postsynaptic fibers from superior cervical ganglion pass to parotid gland and supply its blood vessels
Submandibular	Suspended from lingual nerve by two ganglionic branches (sensory roots); lies on surface of hyoglossus muscle inferior to submandibular duct	Parasympathetic fibers join facial nerve (CN VII) and leave it in its chorda tympani branch, which unites with lingual nerve	Sympathetic fibers from superior cervical ganglion via periarterial plexus on facial artery	Parasympathetic postsynaptic (secretomotor) fibers from submandibular ganglion are distributed to sublingual and submandibular glands; sympathetic fibers supply sublingual and submandibular glands and appear to be secretomotor

 Go to http://thePoint.lww.com/ECA4e for helpful study tools, including USMLE-style questions, case studies, images, and more!

References and Suggested Readings

Agur AMR, Dalley AF. *Grant's Atlas of Anatomy*, 12th ed. Baltimore: Lippincott Williams & Wilkins, 2009.

Brust JCM. Coma. *In* Rowland LP (ed), *Merritt's Textbook of Neurology*, 10th ed. Baltimore: Lippincott Williams & Wilkins, 2000.

Callen PW. *Ultrasonography in Obstetrics and Gynecology*, 4th ed. Philadelphia: WB Saunders, 2000.

Cormack DH. *Essential Histology*, 2nd ed. Baltimore: Lippincott Williams & Wilkins, 2001.

Cotran RS, Kumar V, Collins T. *Robbin's Pathologic Basis of Disease*, 6th ed. Philadelphia: WB Saunders, 1999.

Dean DX, Herbener TE. *Cross-Sectional Human Anatomy*. Baltimore: Lippincott Williams & Wilkins, 2002.

Federative Committee on Anatomical Terminology, 1998.

Foerster O. The dermatomes in man. *Brain* 56:1, 1933.

Gartner LP, Hiatt JL. *Color Textbook of Histology*, 5th ed. Philadelphia: Lippincott Williams & Wilkins, 2009.

Hardy SGP, Nafrel JP. Viscerosensory pathways. *In* Haines DE (ed), *Fundamental Neuroscience*, 2nd ed. New York: Churchill Livingstone, 2002.

Haines DE. *Neuroanatomy: An Atlas of Structures, Sections, and Systems*, 7th ed. Baltimore: Lippincott Williams & Wilkins, 2007.

Haines DE (ed). *Fundamental Neuroscience*, 2nd ed. New York: Churchill Livingstone, 2002.

Hutchins JB, Naftel JP, Ard MD. The cell biology of neurons and glia. *In* Haines DE (ed), *Fundamental Neuroscience*, 2nd ed. New York: Churchill Livingstone, 2002.

Keegan JJ, Garrett FD. The segmental distribution of the cutaneous nerves in the limbs of man. *Anat Rec* 102:409, 1948.

Kumar V, et al. Robbins & Cotran Pathologic Basis of Disease, 8th ed. Philadelphia: WB Saunders, 2009.

Lachman N, Acland RD, Rosse C. Anatomical evidence for the absence of a morphologically distinct cranial root of the accessory nerve in man. *Clin Anat* 15:4, 2002.

Mihailoff GA, Haines DE. Motor system II: Corticofugal systems and the control of movement. *In* Haines DE (ed), *Fundamental Neuroscience*, 2nd ed. New York: Churchill Livingstone, 2002.

Moore KL, Dalley AF. *Clinically Oriented Anatomy*, 6th ed. Baltimore: Lippincott Williams & Wilkins, 2010.

Moore KL, Persaud TVN. *The Developing Human: Clinically Oriented Embryology*, 8th ed. Philadelphia: WB Saunders, 2008.

Moore KL, Persaud TVN, Shiota K. *Color Atlas of Clinical Embryology*, 2nd ed. Philadelphia: WB Saunders, 2002.

Myers RP, Cahill DR, Devine RM, King BF. Anatomy of radical prostatectomy as defined by magnetic resonance imaging. *J Urol* 159:2148, 1998a.

Myers RP, King BF, Cahill DR. Deep perineal "space" as defined by magnetic resonance imaging. *Clin Anat* 11:132, 1998b.

Oelrich TM. The urethral sphincter in the male. *Am J Anat* 158:229, 1980.

Oelrich TM. The striated urogenital sphincter muscle in the female. *Anat Rec* 205:223, 1983.

Ross MH, Kaye G, Pawlina W. *Histology. A Text and Atlas*, 5th ed. Baltimore: Lippincott Williams & Wilkins, 2006.

Rowland LP (ed). *Merritt's Neurology*, 11th ed. Baltimore: Lippincott Williams & Wilkins, 2005.

Salter RB. *Textbook of Disorders and Injuries of the Musculoskeletal System*, 3rd ed. Baltimore: Lippincott Williams & Wilkins, 1999.

Swartz MH. *Textbook of Physical Diagnosis, History and Examination*, 6th ed. Philadelphia: WB Saunders, 2009.

Sweazy RD. Olfaction and taste. *In* Haines DE (ed), *Fundamental Neuroscience*, 2nd ed. New York: Churchill Livingstone, 2002.

Tank PW. *Grant's Dissector*, 14th ed. Baltimore: Lippincott Williams & Wilkins, 2009.

Torrent-Guasp F, Buckburg GD, Clemente C, Cox JL, Coghlan HC, Gharib M. The structure and function of the helical heart and its buttress wrapping. I. The normal macroscopic structure of the heart. *Semin Thoracic Cardiovasc Surg* 13:301–319, 2001.

Wendell-Smith C. Muscles and fasciae of the pelvis. *In* Williams PL, et al. (eds), *Gray's Anatomy. The Anatomical Basis of Medicine and Surgery*, 38th ed. New York: Churchill Livingstone, 1995.

Wilson-Pauwels L, Akesson EJ, Stuart PA, Spacey SO. *Cranial Nerves in Health and Disease*. Hamilton, ON, Canada: Decker, 2002.

Wilson-Pauwels L, Stuart PA, Akesson EJ. *Autonomic Nerves—Basic Science. Clinical Aspects, Case Studies*. Hamilton, ON, Canada: Decker, 1997.

Index

Note: Page numbers in *italics* indicate figures; those followed by t denote tables.

A

Abdomen, 116–203
  abdominal cavity, 117–135
  anterolateral wall of, 117–135. *See also*
    Abdominal wall
  diaphragm in, 185–191. *See also* Diaphragm
  inguinal region of, 127–135
  medical imaging of, 199, *199–203*, 203
  palpation of, 123
  peritoneum and peritoneal cavity, 135–140
  posterior wall of, 192–198. *See also*
    Abdominal wall
  protuberance of, 123
  quadrants of, *118*
  regions of, *118*
  sagittal section of, *122*
  surgical incisions of, 123
  transverse section of, *136*
  viscera of, 140–185. *See also* Abdominal
    viscera
    innervation of, summary, 180–185
Abdominal aorta, 195, *195–196*
  aneurysm of, 198, *198*
  and branches, 195–196, *195–196*
Abdominal cavity, 117–135. *See also* Abdominal
  viscera
Abdominal lymph nodes, 143, 145, 152, *157*
Abdominal ostium, 243
Abdominal pain, posterior, 198
Abdominal paracentesis, 141
Abdominal viscera, 140–185
  arteries of, *142*, 146t. *See also specific organ*
  bile ducts and gallbladder, 171–173
  embryologic development of, 155, *155*
  esophagus, 143
  jejunum and ileum, 152–154
  kidneys, ureters, suprarenal glands,
    174–180
  large intestine, 154–159
  liver, 165–171
  lymphatics and lymph nodes of, *147*. *See also*
    specific organ
  nerves and innervation of, 180–185, *183t,*
    184. *See also specific organ*
    autonomic innervation, 145–146
  pancreas, 162–164
  relationships of, 146, *149t, 150*
  small intestine, 146–154
  spleen, 161–162
  stomach, 143–146
  vasculature of, *151t, 152. See also specific*
    organ
Abdominal wall
  anterolateral, 117–135, *119*
    fascia of, 118, 122–123
    inguinal region of, 127–135

internal surface of, 121, *122*
  layers of, *129t*
  lymphatics of, 126, *126*
  muscles of, 119–121
  nerves of, 125–126, *125*, 125t
  palpation of, 123
  sagittal section of, *122*
  surface anatomy of, 124, *124*
  vasculature of, *125*, 126, 126t
  posterior, 192–198
    fascia of, 192, *192*
    lymphatics of, 196–197, *197*
    muscles of, 193, *193t, 304*
    nerves of, 193–195, *194*
    vasculature of, 195–196, *195–196*
Abdominopelvic cavity, 117, *117*, 205
Abdominopelvic splanchnic nerves, 39
Abducent nerve (CN VI), 544, *545*, 656–657
  distribution of, *654, 656*
  intracranial portion of, *648*
  nucleus of, *649*
  palsy of, 548, *548*, 657, *657*
  summary of, *646t–647t*
Abduction, *6*
Abductor digiti minimi, 373t, *374*, 462–463,
  463, 464t
Abductor hallucis, 373t, *374*
Abductor pollicis brevis, 462, *463*, 464t
Abductor pollicis longus, 451, *452*, 455t, *456*
Abrasions, 336
Accessory hemiazygos vein, 75, *76*, 111–112
Accessory ligaments, of intervertebral joints,
  289, *290*
Accessory pancreatic duct, 163, *164*
Accessory renal vessels, 181
Accomodation, of lens, 538
Acetabular fossa, 379, *380*
Acetabular labrum, *380*
Acetabular ligament, transverse, 379, *381*
Acetabulum, 205, *206*, 379, *380*
  lunate surface of, 379, *380*
Acetylcholine, 37
Acoustic meatus
  external, 497, *498*, 578, *578*, 587
  internal, *501*, 502, *585*, 586–587
Acoustic neuroma, 664
Acromial angle, 415–416
Acromioclavicular joint, *409*, 475–476, *476, 478*
  dislocation of, 480, *480*
  medical imaging of, *494*
  radiograph of, *478*
  surface anatomy of, 415
Acromioclavicular ligament, 476, *476*
Acromion, 407, *407*, 415
Acute respiratory distress, 79
Adamkiewicz, artery of, 299, 301, *302*
Adduction, *6*

Adductor brevis, 337, *338–339*, 339t
Adductor canal, *341*, 342
Adductor compartment, of palm, 461, *462*
Adductor group, of medial thigh, 337, *338–339*,
  339t
Adductor hallucis, 373t, *374*
Adductor hiatus, 339, 340, 342
Adductor longus, 337, *338–339*, 339t
Adductor magnus, 337, *338–339*, 339t, *350*
Adductor pollicis, 462, *463*, 464t
Adductor tubercle, 328
Adenoiditis, 639
Adhesions/adhesiotomy, 141
Adhesive capsulitis, 481
Aditus, 580, *581*
Adrenal glands. *See* Suprarenal glands
Alar cartilage, 573, *573*
Alar fascia, 595
Alar ligaments, *291*, 292
  rupture of, 293
Alimentary canal, 634
Alimentary (digestive) tract, 2–3, 140, *142*, 631.
  See also Abdominal viscera
  schematic overview of, *142*
  viscera of, 631–638
Alimentary layer, of cervical viscera, 620,
  631–638
Alveolar arch, of maxilla, 499, *500*
Alveolar ducts, 74, *74*
Alveolar nerves, superior and inferior, *658*
Alveolar process, 496, *497*, 499, *500*
Alveolar sacs, 74, *74*
Ampulla
  of duodenum, 150
  of rectum, 245, *246*
  of semicircular ducts, 585, *585–586*
Ampullary crest, 585, *585–586*
Anal canal, 259–260, *259*
  nerves and innervation of, *248, 259*, 260
  references to, 159, 203, 245, *246*
  vasculature and lymphatics of, 259–260, *259*
Anal columns, 245, 259
Anal sinuses, 245, 259
Anal sphincter
  external, 245, 251t, 259
  internal, 245, 259
Anal triangle, 250, 257–260
Anal valves, 245, 259
Anastomosis (anastomoses), 25
  arteriovenous, 28
  genicular, 356, 389
  periarticular arterial, 17, 486
  portacaval, 174, *174*
  portal-systemic, 173–174, *175*
  scapular arterial, 431
Anatomical planes, 3–4, *3*
Anatomical position, 2, *3*

Anatomical snuff box, 416, *452*, 456, 474
Anatomical variations, 7
Anatomicomedical terminology. *See also*
    Terminology
Anatomy
    clinical, 3
    individual variation in, 7
    regional and systemic, 2–3
Anconeus, *440*, *441t*, 443
Aneurysms, 112
    abdominal aortic, 198, *198*
    of ascending aorta, 112
    berry, 518, *518*
    popliteal, 357
    saccular, 511, 518
Angiography
    of cerebral arterial circle, 591
    of heart and great vessels, *115*
    left cardiac, 345
Angle of inclination/declination, of femur,
    322, *322*
Angular artery, *523t*, 524, *525*
Angular incisure, 144, *144*, 148
Angular vein, 525, *525–526*, 526
Ankle, 317, *317*
Ankle (jerk) reflex, 368
Ankle joint, 395–398
    arteries and nerves of, 397
    articular surfaces of, 395, *395*
    bones of, 323, *324*, 395
    coronal section of, 397
    dislocation of, 398, *398*
    injuries of, 397–398
    joint capsule, 395, *396*
    ligaments of, 396–397, *396*
    movements of, 397, 397t
    sprains of, 362, *397*
Anococcygeal body (ligament), 211, 257, 259
Anococcygeal nerves, 217, *218–219*
Anorectal flexure, *245*, 246
Anorectal junction, 259
Anosmia, 650
Ansa cervicalis, 600, *605*, 671
Anserine bursa, *390t*
Antagonistic muscle, 20
Antebrachial fascia, 417, *418*, 446
Antebrachial vein, median, 421, *421*
Anterior (ventral), definition of, *4t*
Anterior axillary line, 65, *65*
Anterior cardiac veins, *96*, 97
Anterior commissure
    of brain, *513*
    of labia, 268, *268*
Anterior cruciate ligament, 387, *387*
    injuries to, 393–394, *393*
    rupture of, 394
Anterior drawer sign, 394, *394*
Anterior (flexor) facial compartment, 417, *418*
Anterior horn, of spinal cord, 31, *33*
Anterior longitudinal ligament, 287, *288*, *289*
Anterior median (midsternal) line, 65, *65*
Anterior ramus (rami), of spinal nerve, *34*, 35
Anterior recesses, of ischioanal fossae, 257
Anterior root, of spinal nerve, *34*, 35

Anteroinferior pelvic wall, 211
Anterolateral abdominal wall. *See* Abdominal
    wall
Anular ligament, of radius, *482*, 483
Anulus fibrosus, 288, *289*
Anus, 250, *251*, *254*
Aorta, 103, *103–104*, 110t
    abdominal, 195–196, *195–196*
        aneurysm of, 198, *198*
        branches of, 142, *142*, 195–196,
            195–196
    arch of, 103, *103–104*, *109*, 110t
        variations of, 112–113, *113*
    ascending, 90
        aneurysm of, 112
    branches of, 103, *103–104*, 108, 110t
        abdominal, 195–196, *195–196*
        thoracic, 110, *110*
    coarctation of, 113, *113*
    in mediastinum, *106*
    thoracic, 103, *106*, 108, 110t
        branches of, 110, *110*
Aortic arch. *See* Aorta, arch of
Aortic hiatus, 108, *108–109*, 189
Aortic orifice, 90
Aortic sinuses, 90, *90*
Aortic valve, 90, *90*
    stenosis of, 92
Aortic vestibule, 90
Apex beat, 85, 92–94
Aphonia, 669
Apical foramen, of tooth root, 558, *558*
Aponeurosis, 17, 119
    bicipital, 440, *440*, 446
    epicranial, 503, *503*
    palatine, 561, *561*
    palmar, *418*, 461, *461*
    plantar, 371, *371*
Appendectomy, 160
Appendicitis, 160
Appendicular artery, *151t*, 156, *156*
Appendicular skeleton, 9, *9–10*
Appendix, 156–157, *156*
Aqueous humor, 535–536, 537
Arachnoid granulations, 505, *505*, *510*,
    514, *515*
Arachnoid mater, 31, 509–511, *510*
    cranial, 509–511, *510*
    spinal, 31, *33*, 297, *298*
Arachnoid trabeculae, *298*, 299, 509, *510*
Arches of foot, 400–402, *401*
    "fallen", 402, *402*
Arcuate artery, 376, *376*
Arcuate ligaments, medial and lateral, *188*,
    192, *192*
Arcuate line, 120, *121*, *122*
Arcuate popliteal ligaments, 387, *387*
Areola, 67, *67*
Arm, 406, *406*, 440–446
    arteries of, 440, 442–443, 443
    compartments of, transverse section, *443*
    cutaneous nerves of, 420, 421
    fascial compartments of, *418*
    medical imaging of, *492*

    muscles of, 440–443, *440*, *441t*, *442–443*. *See
        also* Forearm
    nerves of, 440, 442–443, 443–444
    surface anatomy of, 447, *447*
    veins of, 443, *443*
Arrector muscles, 7, 8, 20–22
Arterial arcades, 152–154
Arterial occlusion, five P signs of, 362
Arteries, 23–25, *26*. *See also vasculature of
        specific organs and regions*
    of abdominal viscera, *142*, 146t
    of abdominal wall
        anterolateral, *125*, 126, 126t
        posterior, 195–196, *195*
    of anal canal, 259–260, *259*
    of arm, 440, 442–443, 443
    articular, 17
    of bone, 12–13, *13*
    of brain, *516–517*, 517–519, 517t
    of breasts, 56, *57*
    of diaphragm, 189–190, 190t
    of duodenum, 150
    of dura mater, 508, *509*
    of ear, 579, *579*
    of esophagus, 108, 110t, 143, *143*
    of face, 522–524, *523t*, *525*
    of female pelvis/perineum, 237, *238*
    of foot, 357, *358*, 376, *376*
    of forearm, *452*, 456, *457*, 459t
    of gallbladder, 171–172, *173*
    of hand, *461*, 466–468, *467t*, *468*
    of heart, 94–96, 94t, *95*
    of hip joint, 383, *383*, 383t
    of intestines, *151t*, 156
    of knee joint, *355*, 389
    of larynx, 627, *628*
    of leg, 370t
    of liver, *145*, 146t, 168, *168*, 171
    of lungs and pleurae, 75, *75–76*, 108
    of nasal region, *523t*, 524, *525*
    of neck
        lateral region, 602–603, *602*
        root region, 615–616, *616*
    of orbit, 545–547, *546*, 547t
    of pancreas, *163*, 164
    of pelvis, 220–222, *221*, 222t
    of penis, 263, 263t, *264*, 267
    of pericardium, 82, *83*, 108, *110*, 110t
    of pharynx, 607, *616*, 635, *635*
    popliteal, *351*, 356, 370t
    pulmonary, 75, *75*
    of rectum, 259–260, *259*
    of scalp, *523*, 524–525
    of sciatic nerve, 349
    of scrotum, *131*, 132, 261, 263t
    of spermatic cord, *131*
    of spinal cord, 299, 301, *302*
    of spleen, *142*, *145*, 146t, 162
    of stomach, 144–145, *145*, 146t
    structure of, *24*
    of testes, 130, *130–131*
    of thigh, anteromedial, 343, *344t*
    of thoracic wall, *61*, 62–63, *63*, 64t
    of thymus, 102

of tongue, 564–566, 567
types of, 23–25, 24
of urethra, 228, 230, 232
of urinary bladder, 227, 228
of uterus, 241
of vertebral column, 294, 294
Arteriography. *See also* Angiography
abdominal, 203, 203
carotid artery, 590
Arterioles, 23, 24
Arteriosclerosis, 25, 312
Arteriovenous anastomoses, 28
Arthrodesis, 491
Arthroplasty, 394, 394
Articular arteries, 17
Articular cartilage, 10, 379
Articular disc, 555, 555
Articular process(es), 277, 278
Articular surface (facet), 277, 278
Articular system, 2
Articular veins, 17
Ary-epiglottic fold, 625, 625–627, 634
Ary-epiglottic ligament, 625
Ary-epiglottic muscle, 627
Arytenoid cartilages, 623, 624, 626
Arytenoid muscles, 626–627, 629t, 633
Ascending aorta, 90
Ascending colon, 157–158, 203
Ascitic fluid (ascites), 141
Aspiration, of foreign bodies, 78, 630
Asthma, 64
Atheromatous plaque, 25, 25
Atherosclerosis, 100
of coronary arteries, 100, 100
Atlanto-occipital joints, 291, 292
muscles producing movement of, 312t
Atlanto-occipital membranes, 291, 292
Atlantoaxial joints, 280, 291, 292
lateral and median, 291, 292
Atlantoaxial subluxation, 293
Atlas (C1 vertebra), 280t
Atria, of heart
left, 89–90, 89
right, 87, 87
Atrial septal defects, 91
Atrioventricular (AV) bundle, 97, 97
Atrioventricular (AV) nodal branch, coronary
artery, 95, 96
Atrioventricular (AV) node, 97
Atrioventricular orifice, right, 88, 89
Atrophy, bone, 12
Auditory ossicles, 580–583, 581
Auricle
of ear, 579, 579
right, of heart, 87, 87
Auricular artery(ies), posterior, 525, 525,
607, 609
Auricular nerve
great, 521, 522t
greater, 600, 601, 605
Auricular veins, posterior, 526, 526
Auriculotemporal nerve, 521, 522t, 528, 554, 554
Auscultation
of heart, 92, 93

of lungs/pleurae, 77, 78
Auscultatory areas, of chest, 92, 93
Autonomic innervation
of abdominal viscera, 183t, 184
of female pelvic viscera, 241, 241–242
of male pelvic viscera, 236, 236
of pelvic cavity, 219–220, 219
of smooth muscle, 22
of urinary bladder and urethra, 231
Autonomic nervous system (ANS), 31, 36–42
functions of, 37t
visceral afferent fibers of, 36, 36
visceral motor fibers of, 31, 36–37
AV bundle. *See* Atrioventricular (AV) bundle
AV node. *See* Atrioventricular (AV) node
AV shunts, 28
Avascular necrosis, 14, 414, 491
Avulsion, 318, 414, 438, 486
Axial line, 333
Axial skeleton, 9, 9–10
Axilla, 427–439
boundaries and contents of, 427–429, 429,
436–437
brachial plexus of, 433–439
lymphatics and lymph nodes of, 432–433, 432
vasculature of, 429–430, 430, 430t–431t
Axillary artery(ies), 63, 429, 430
compression of, 431
Axillary fascia, 417, 418
Axillary folds
anterior, 428, 429
posterior, 429
Axillary fossa, 65, 417, 418, 429
Axillary lymph nodes, 56, 421, 422, 432–433, 432
drainage pattern of, 56, 57
enlargement of, 58, 433
Axillary nerve, 413, 420, 434, 435t
injury to, 427
Axillary process, of breast, 56
Axillary sheath, 429, 437
Axillary tail, 58, 58
Axillary vein(s), 429–430, 432
injury to, 433
Axioappendicular muscles, 407
anterior, 422–423
posterior, 427–439
Axioappendicular skeleton, 9–10, 406–407
Axis (C2 vertebra), 280t
Axon, 30, 31
Azygos/hemiazygos venous system, 58–59, 111
Azygos lobe, of lung, 77
Azygos vein, 75, 76, 109, 111, 173

B

Back, 274–315
contents of, 275
curvatures of, 275–277, 276–277
medical imaging of, 314–315, 314–315
muscles of, 301–313
nerves and innervation of, 313, 313t
spinal cord and meninges of, 296–301
sprains and strains of, 313

surface anatomy of, 304, 304
vertebral column of, 275–295. *See also*
Vertebral column
Back muscles, 301–313
extrinsic, 303
intrinsic, 303–307
deep, 305, 307t, 308
intermediate, 303–304, 305t, 306
superficial, 303, 305t, 306
producing movements of atlanto-occipital
joints, 312t
producing movements of intervertebral
joints, 305–307, 309t–310t
suboccipital and deep neck, 311–312, 311
surface anatomy of, 304, 304
Back pain, 295
localized, 293
Back sprains and strains, 313
Ball and socket joints, 16t, 476
Bartholin (vestibular) glands, 269, 270
Baseball finger, 460, 460
Basilar artery, 516–517, 517t, 518
Basilar membrane, of cochlear duct, 586, 586
Basilic vein, 421, 421, 446
Basivertebral veins, 294, 295
Bell palsy, 524, 524
Benign hypertrophy of the prostate, 235
Berry aneurysm, 518, 518
Biceps brachii, 440, 440, 441t, 447
Biceps femoris, 349, 349t, 350
Biceps tendinitis, 444
Biceps tendon, 440, 440, 447
rupture of, 444, 444
Bicipital aponeurosis, 440, 440, 446
Bicipital groove(s), 410, 443, 447
Bicipital myotatic reflex, 444, 444
Bilateral, definition of, 5
Bile canaliculi, 171, 172
Bile duct, 162, 164, 171–173, 172
sphincter of, 171
Biliary colic, 173–174
Biliary ducts, 171, 171
Biliary system, 164
extrahepatic passages of, 172
Bipennate muscles, 17, 21
Bladder. *See* Urinary bladder
Blood pressure measurement, 445
Blood vessels. *See* Arteries; Veins; *specific
organ or system*
Bone, 9–10
dynamics of, 12
functions of, 9–10
grafts, 326
Bone(s), 11–14. *See also* Skeleton; *specific
structures*
accessory, 14
age of, assessment of, 14
classification of, 9, 11
development of, 12, 13
heterotopic, 11
markings of, 11–12
necrosis of, 14
types of, 11, 11
vasculature and innervation of, 12–14, 13

Bone marrow needle biopsy, 54
Bony ampulla, 584, *584*
Bony labyrinth, of internal ear, 583–584, *584–585*
  vestibule of, 584, *584*
Brachial artery(ies), *440*, *442–443*, 443, *446*
  compression of, 445, *445*
  deep (profunda brachii), *430*, 431t, *442*, 443
  occlusion or laceration of, 445
Brachial fascia, 417, *418*
Brachial plexus, 420, 433–439, *433–434*
  block, 439
  injuries of, 438–439, *439*
  nerves of, *434*, 434t–435t
  roots of, 433, *433–434*, 600, *617*
  supraclavicular and infraclavicular parts of,
    434t–435t, 438
  trunks and cords of, *434*, 438, *602*
  variations of, 438
Brachialis, 440, *440*, 441t, 447
Brachiocephalic trunk, 103, *103–104*, 609, 615,
  616
Brachiocephalic vein(s), 102–103, *103*, 600,
  602, *609*, 618
Brachioradialis, 454t
Brain, 31, *32*, 512–519
  injuries of, 512
  lobes of, 512
  parts of, 512, *513*
  vasculature of, *516–517*, *517–519*, 517t
  ventricular system of, 512–514, *515*
Brainstem, *513*
Breasts, 53–60
  carcinoma of, 58–59, *59*
  female, *56*
  lymphatic drainage of, 56–60, *57*
  mammography, 59, *59*
  nerves of, 60, *61*
  quadrants of, 58, *58*
  supernumerary, 58
  surface anatomy of, 67, *67*
  surgical procedures, 59, *59*
  vasculature of, 56, *57*
Breathing. *See* Respiration
Bregma, 499, *499*
Broad ligament, of uterus, 212t, 239, *240*
Bronchi, 71–74, *73–74*
  bronchial arteries, 75, *76*, 108
  bronchial tree, 72, *73–74*
  bronchial veins, 75, *76*
Bronchioles, terminal, 74, *74*
Bronchogenic carcinoma, 79
Bronchomediastinal lymphatic trunks, *638*
Bronchopulmonary lymph nodes, 76, *76*
Bronchopulmonary segment(s), 72–74, *73*
Bronchoscopy, 79, *79*
Buccal gingivae, 558–560, *559*
Buccal glands, *557*, 558
Buccal nerve, *521*, 522t, 554, *554*
Buccinator, 519, 520t, 528, *557*, 558
Buccopharyngeal fascia, 595, 634
Bulbar conjunctiva, 530, *530*
Bulbospongiosus, 237, *237*, 251, 251t, 261,
  267, *267*
Bulbourethral glands, 227, 235

Bundle branch block, 102
Bunions, 402, *402*
Burn injury, of skin, 8
Bursae
  of elbow joint, 483, *483*
  of glenohumeral joint, *478*, 479–480
  gluteal, 348, *348*
  of knee joint, 389, *390t*
  suprapatellar, 386, *386*, 389
Bursitis, 353, 486
Buttocks, 317

C

Calcaneal branches, of tibial and sural nerves,
  375t, 376
Calcaneal bursitis, 368
Calcaneal tendon, 363, *364*
Calcaneal tendon reflex, 368
Calcaneal tuberosity, 323, *324*
Calcaneocuboid joint, 398, *399*, 399t
Calcaneocuboid ligament, plantar, 398, *398*
Calcaneofibular ligament, 396, *396*
  injury to, 397
Calcaneonavicular ligament, plantar, 398, *398*
Calcaneus, *319*, 323, *324*
  fractures of, 327, *327*
  medial tubercle of, 329, *329*
Calices (calyces), major and minor, 177
Calvaria, 496, *497*, 498–499, *499*
Canal of Nuck, cysts or hernias of, 135
Capillaries, 23, *24*, 28
  lymphatic, 28, *29*
Capillary beds, 23, *24*, 28
Capitate, 411, *411–412*, *489*
Capitulum, of humerus, 410
Caput medusae, 174
Carbon particles, inhalation of, 79
Cardia, of stomach, 143, *144*
Cardiac cycle, 97, *98*, 99–100
Cardiac muscle, 17, *18t*
  characteristics of, 20
Cardiac nerves, cervical, 618
Cardiac notch, 71, *71*
Cardiac plexus, 76, 98, 105, 105t, *107*, 668
Cardiac referred pain, 102
Cardiac skeleton, 100
Cardiac tamponade, 84
Cardial notch, 143, *144*
Cardial orifice, 143, *144*, 148
Cardinal ligament, 215, *216*
Cardiomegaly, 84
Cardiopulmonary splanchnic nerves, 39
Cardiovascular system, 2, 23–28, *23*. *See also*
  Heart
  principal arteries, *26*
  principal veins, *27*
Carina, of bronchi, 79, *79*
Carotid artery(ies), 607, *609*
  arteriogram of, *590*
  bifurcation of, *612*
  common, 606, *606*, 609
  external, 528, *605*, 606, 607, *609*

branches of, *523t*, 525, *525*, *553*, 609
  ligation of, 610
internal, *505–506*, 506, *516–517*, *517–518*,
  517t, 607, 609
  and associated structures in
    cranium, *507*
  branches of, *523t*, 525
  Doppler color flow study of, *642*
left common, 103, *103*, 609
  occlusion of, 610
right common, 607, *609*
Carotid body, 607, *609*
Carotid canal, 499, *500*
Carotid nerve plexus, external, 528, *529*
Carotid pulse, 610, 613
Carotid sheath, 595, *596*, *606*, 613, 618
Carotid sinus, 606–607, *609*, 667
Carotid sinus nerve, 607, 665
Carotid triangle, 597, 604–606, *612*
  surgical dissection of, 610
Carotid tubercle, *617*
Carotid wall, of tympanic cavity, 580, *581*
Carpal bones, *489*
Carpal joints, 488, 488t, *489*
  structures limiting movements of, 486t, 491t
Carpal tunnel, *418*, *419*, 468
  medical imaging of, *493*
  release, 471
  syndrome, 460, 471, 491
Carpometacarpal joints, 488t, *489*, 491t
Carpus. *See* Wrist
Carrying angle, of elbow joint, 483, *483*
Cartilage, 9–10, *10–11*
  articular, 10, 379
  of nose, 573, *573*
Cartilagenous bone model, 12, *13*
Cartilagenous joints, 14, *15t*
  secondary, 288
Carvernous sinus, of cranial dura mater, 505
Cataracts, 539, *539*
Catheterization, urethral, 261, 270
Cauda equina, 289, 296, *297*
Caudal epidural block, 300, *301*
Caval opening, 188, *189*
Cavernous nerves, 265
Cavernous sinus, *505–506*, 506
Cecum, 140, 154–157, *156*
Celiac ganglia, 38, *147*, 668
Celiac lymph nodes, *147*, 152, 164, 172, *173*
Celiac plexus, *147*, 152, 162, 164, 171, 173,
  179, 185
Celiac trunk, 142, *142*, 145, 146t
Cell body, of neuron, 30, *31*
Cement, 558, *558*
Central artery, of retina, 546, *547*, 547t
  blockage of, 548
Central compartment, of palm, 461, *462*
Central lymph nodes, 432, 433
  superior, 154
Central nervous system (CNS), 31, *32*
  damage to, 31
Central tendon, of diaphragm, 187–188, *187*
Central vein, of retina, 547, *547*
  blockage of, 548

Cephalic arterial nerve branch, 39, *40*
Cephalic vein, 421, *421*, *446*
Cerebellar falx, 504, *505*
Cerebellar tentorium, 504, *505*
Cerebellomedullary cisterns, 512–514, *515*
Cerebellum, 512, *513*
Cerebral aqueduct, 512, *515*
Cerebral arterial circle, *517*, 519
Cerebral arteries, *516–517*, 517t, *518–519*
Cerebral falx, 504, *505*
Cerebral fissure, longitudinal, 504, *505*
Cerebral hemispheres, 512, *513*
  arterial supply of, 517t
Cerebral veins, 519
  great, 519
  occlusion of, 512, *513*
Cerebrospinal fluid (CSF)
  between cranial meninges, 31
  leakage of, 514
  between spinal meninges, 297, *300*
Cerebrovascular accident (CVA), 91
Cerebrum, 512, *513*
  injuries of, 512
Cervical arteries. *See* Cervical regions
Cervical canal, 236, *236*
Cervical cardiac nerves, inferior, middle,
    superior, 618
Cervical curvature, 275–276, 276, 277
Cervical enlargement, of spinal cord, 296–297,
  296
Cervical fascia, 594–596, *595*
Cervical ganglion (ganglia)
  inferior and middle, *617*, 618
  superior, 38, 39, *40*, 618, *655*
Cervical lordosis, *276*
Cervical lymph nodes
  deep, 526, 627
  deep, superior and inferior, 619, *622*, 627
Cervical lymph nodes, superficial and deep,
  568, *568*
Cervical nerve, transverse, 600, *601*, 611
Cervical pleura, 68, *69*
Cervical plexus, 420, 600, *601*
  block, 604, *604*
  cutaneous branches of, 600–602, *601*
Cervical regions, 596–613, *597*, 613t
  anterior, *597*, 604–611, *605–606*, 613t
    arteries in, *605*, 607–610, *609*
    innervation and nerves in, *606*
    muscles in, *605*, 607, *608t*
    nerves in, 611
    veins in, *609*, 610
  lateral, *597*, 598–604, *601–602*, 613t
    arteries in, 602–603, *602*
    muscles in, 598, *600*
    nerve blocks in, 604, *604*
    nerves in, 598–602, *601*
    veins in, *600*, 602
  posterior, *597*, 598, 613t
  root of neck, 613, *614*, *614–615t*. *See also*
    Neck, root of
  sternocleidomastoid, 596–598, *597*
  summary of, 613t
  surface anatomy of, 611–613, *612*

Cervical ribs, 54
Cervical sympathetic trunks, 618
  lesion of, 619
Cervical triangles, *597*, 611–613, *612*, 613t
Cervical vertebrae, *279t–280t*
Cervical viscera
  alimentary layer of, *620*, 631–638
  endocrine layer of, 619–622, *620*
  respiratory layer of, *620*, 623–631
Cervico-axillary canal, 427
Cervicodorsal trunk, *602*, 603, 615–616,
  616–617
Cervicothoracic ganglion, *76*, *617*, 618
  block, 619
Cervix, of uterus, 239, *239*
  cervical examination, 242, *242*
Chalazia, 533
Check ligaments, *531*, 543–544, *544*
Cheeks, 558
Chemoreceptor, 607
Chiasmatic cistern, 514, *515*
Childbirth, regional anesthesia for, 243, *243*
Choanae, 499, *500*, 632
Cholecystectomy, 174
Cholecystitis, 174
Chondroblasts, 12
Chorda tympani nerve, *554*, 555, 564, *566*, *581*,
  661
Chordae tendinae. *See* Tendinous cords
Choroid, 534, *534*
  capillary lamina of, 534–536, *546*, 547
Choroid plexuses, 514, *515*
Chylothorax, 77
Ciliary arteries, *546*, 547, 547t
Ciliary body, 534–535, 536
Ciliary ganglion, 545, *545*, *672t*
Ciliary glands, *531*, 532
Ciliary muscle, 537, *655*
Ciliary nerves, long and short, 545
Ciliary processes, 535, 536, 537
Ciliary veins, 537
Circular muscles, 19
Circulatory system, 2, 23–28, *23*
Circumcision, 266
Circumduction, 6
Circumflex branch, coronary artery, 94t, 96
Circumflex femoral arteries, 343, *344t*
  lateral and medial, 383, *383*
Circumflex humeral arteries, *430*, 431t
Circumflex iliac arteries, 126, 126t
Circumflex scapular arteries, *430*, 431t
Cirrhosis, of liver, 173
Cisterna chyli, *29*, 30, 110, 170, 197, *197*
Cisternal puncture, 514
Clavicle(s), 407, *407*
  fracture of, 412, *412*
  ossification of, 413
  surfaces and features of, 407, *407*
Clavicular notch, 49, 51, *51*
Clavipectoral fascia, 417, *418*
Clavipectoral triangle, 428
Claw hand, *438*, 439, 472, *472*
Clinical anatomy, 3
Clinoid processes, *501*, 502

Clitoris, 268, *268–269*
  body and root of, 268
  deep artery of, 263, 263t, *264*
  dorsal artery and nerve of, *219*
  frenulum and prepuce of, 268, *268*
  glans of, 268, *268–269*
Clivus, *501*, 502
Clunial nerves, inferior, middle, superior, 349,
  351, 352t
Coarctation of aorta, 113, *113*
Coccygeal plexus, 217–218, *218–219*, 218t
Coccygeal spinal nerves, 217, *218–219*
Coccygeus, 211, *213–214*, 213t, 252
  nerves to, 217, *219*
Coccyx, 205, *205*, *283t*
Cochlea, 583, *584–585*
  structure of, *586*
Cochlear aqueduct, 583, *584*
Cochlear duct, 583, *584–585*, 585, *586*
Cochlear labyrinth, 584
Cochlear nerve, *584*, 586–587, *587*, *646t–647t*,
  663
Colectomy, 160
Colic arteries, middle, right, left, *151t*, 158
Colic flexures, 158
Colic lymph nodes, 158
Colic veins, 174
Colitis, 160
Collar of callus, 12
Collateral circulation, 25, 431
Collateral ligaments
  of elbow, *482*, 483
  fibular, 358, 386–387, *387*
  of knee, 358, 386–387, *387*
  tibial, 387, *387*, 388
Colles fracture, 414, *414*, 491
Colon, 157–159, *157*, 203
Colonoscopy, 161
Colostomy, 161
Colostrum, 58
Comminuted fracture, 54
Common hepatic duct, 171, 172, *172*
Common tendinous ring, 540, *540*
Compact bone, 11, *11*
Comparison, terminology of, 4–5, *4t*
Compartment syndromes, of leg, 335
Compensatory hypertrophy, 23
Compressor urethrae, 232, 237, 251, 255, *255*
Computerized tomography (CT), 44, *45*
  of abdomen, *199*
  of arm and forearm, *492–493*
  of back, 314–315, *314–315*
  of neck/vertebral column, 641, *641–642*
  of thorax, *115*
Concentric contraction, 19
Concha, of auricle, *578*, 579
Conducting system, of heart, 97–98, *97*
  injury to, 102
Condylar canal, 500t
Condyle, *10*, 11
Condyloid joints, *16t*
Cone of light, 580, 587
Congenital diaphragmatic hernia (CDH), 191
Congenital torticollis, 598, *598*

Conjoint tendon, 128, *128*
Conjunctiva, 530, *530*
Conjunctival fornis (fornices), 530, *531*
Conjunctival sac, 530
Conoid ligament, 476, *476*
Constrictor muscles, of pharynx, 632, *633*, 634–635, *635*, *637t*
Contraction, skeletal muscle, 19–20
Contralateral, 5
Contusions, 340
Conus arteriosus, 88, *88*
Conus elasticus, 624, *626*
Conus medullaris, 296
Convergence, 543
Convergent muscles, 19
Coraco-acromial arch, 478, *479*
Coraco-acromial ligament, *478*, 479
Coracobrachialis, 440, *440*, *441t*
Coracoclavicular ligament, 476, *476*
Coracohumeral ligament, *478*, 479
Coracoid process, 410, *410*, 415, 428
Cornea, 534, *534*
Corneal reflex, 548, 662, *662*
Corneal ulcers and transplants, 539
Corneoscleral junction, 534, *534–535*
Corniculate cartilage, 625
Coronal suture, 499, *499*
Coronary angioplasty, 101, *101*
Coronary arteries, 94–96, 94t, *95*
    atherosclerosis of, 100, *100*
    circumflex branch of, 94t, 96
    imaging of, *114*
    lateral diagonal branch of, 96
    left, and branches, 94t, *95*, 96
    right, and branches, 94–96, 94t, *95*
    variations of, 101
Coronary arteriograms, *114*
Coronary artery disease (CAD), 100, *100*, 102
Coronary bypass graft, 101, *101*
Coronary ligaments, 388
Coronary sinus, 87, 96, *96*
    opening of, 87, *87*
Coronoid fossa, 410
Coronoid process, 410, *411*, *482*
Corpora cavernosa, 261, *262*, 267
Corpus callosum, *513*
Corpus spongiosum, 261, *262*, 267
Corrugator supercilii, *520*
Costal cartilages, 49, *50*, 54
Costal groove(s), 48, *50*, 62
Costal margins, 67
Costal notches, 51, *51*
Costocervical trunk, 616, *616*
Costochondral junction, dislocation of, 55
Costoclavicular ligament, 475, *476*
Costoclavicular syndrome, 55
Costocoracoid membrane, 417, *418*
Costodiaphragmatic recesses, 70, *70*, 161, *188*
Costomediastinal recesses, 70, *70*
Coxa valga, 325, *325*
Coxa vara, 325, *325*
Cranial fossae, anterior, middle, posterior, 500t, *501*, 502
Cranial meninges, 503–511, *504*

Cranial nerve nuclei, *649*
Cranial nerves, 32, 33–34, 643–672. *See also specific cranial nerve*
    emerging from brainstem, *513*, *644*
    ganglia, parasympathetic, *672t*
    intracranial portions of, *648*
    motor and sensory nerve fibers, *646t–647t*
    nuclei of, *649*
    overview of, 644–650, *645*
    sensory and motor components of, 644–650, *645–646*
    summary of, *646t–647t*
Cranial parasympathetic outflow, 42
Craniovertebral joints, *291*, *292*
Cranium, 496–502
    base of, 499, *499–500*, *500–501*
    facial aspect of, 496, *497*
    foramina and apertures of, 500t
    fractures of, 498, *498*
    lateral aspect of, 496–498, *497*
    medical imaging of, *589–590*
    meninges of, 503–511, *504*
    neuro- and viscerocranium, 496, *497*
    occipital aspect of, 498, *499*
    superior aspect of, 498–499, *499*
Cremasteric artery, 130, 132
Cremasteric fascia, 129, *129*
Cremaster muscle
Cremasteric reflex, 132
Crepitus, 557
Crest, bone, *10*, 11
Cribriform fascia, 330–331, *330*
Cribriform foramina, 500t
Cribriform plate, of ethmoid, *501*, 502, 575, 650
Crico-arytenoid joints, 623, *624*
Crico-arytenoid muscles, 627, 629t, *633*
Cricoid cartilage, 623, *623*, 624, *626*
Cricothyroid, 628, 629t
Cricothyroid joints, 623, *623*
Cricothyroid ligaments, 623, *623*, *626*
Cricotracheal ligament, 623, *623*
Cricovocal membrane, 624, *626*
Crista galli, *501*, 502, *575–576*
Crista terminalis, 87, *87*
Crown, of tooth, 558, *558*
Cruciate ligaments
    of atlantoaxial joint, *291*, *292*
    of knee joint, 387, *387–388*
Cruciform ligaments, of hand, 466
Crura
    of diaphragm, 188–189, *188*
    inguinal, 127
    of penis, 261, *262*, 267
Crural fascia, 330, 331
Crux, of heart, 96, *97*
CSF. *See* Cerebrospinal fluid
CT scan, 44, *45*. *See also* Computerized tomography (CT)
Cubital fossa, 446, *446*
    surface anatomy of, 447, *447*, 473
Cubital lymph nodes, *421*, 422
Cubital vein, *421*, 421, *446*, 446
Cuboid, *319*, 323, *324*, 329

Cuboid tuberosity, 323, *324*
Culdocentesis, 238
Cuneiform cartilage, 624, *626*
Cuneiforms, 319–320, 323–325, *324*, 329
Cuneonavicular joint, 399, *399t*
Cutaneous nerves/innervation
    of arm, *434*, 435t
    dermatomes and, 35, *35*
    of forearm, 440, 444, 446, *446*, *458*
    of hand, 469
    of lower limb, 132
    of thigh, 349, *351*, 352t
    of upper limb, 419–421, *419–420*
Cystic artery, *145*, 146t, 171, *172*
Cystic duct, 171, 172, *172*
Cystic lymph node, 172, *173*
Cystic veins, 172–173
Cystoscopy, 229, *229*
Cystotomy, suprapubic, 228

D

DAB (dorsal abduct) mnemonic, 372, 465–466
Dancer's fracture, 327, *327*
Dartos fascia, 131
Dartos muscle, 129, 131–132
Deafness, 664
Deep, definition of, *4t*
Deep circumflex iliac arteries, 195, *195*
Deep fascia, 7, 8, 329–330, *330*
Deep inguinal lymph nodes. *See also* Inguinal lymph nodes
Deep (internal) inguinal ring, 127, *128*
Deep lymphatic vessels, 29, 30, 126
Deep perineal pouch, 253–255, *254*
Deep veins
    of lower limb, 332, *333*
    of upper limb, *421*, 422
Deep venous thrombosis (DVT), 335–336
Deferentectomy (vasectomy), 132, 233
Deglutition, 632, *632*
Deltoid, 426t, *427*
    distal attachment of, 447, *447*
    surface anatomy of, 428, 447
Deltoid fascia, 417, *418*
Deltoid tuberosity, *408–409*, 410
Deltopectoral lymph nodes, *421*, 422
Deltopectoral triangle, *415*, 422, 428
Dendrites, 30, *31*
Dental arches, 557, *557*
Dental caries, 560
Dental plexuses, 558
Denticulate ligaments, 298, *299*
Dentine, 558, *558*
Dentition, adult mandibular, 558, *558*
Depression, 6
Dermatomes, 35, *35*
    dermatomally distributed skin lesion, 64
    of lower limb, 333, *334*
    maps of, 35, *35*
    of thorax, 62, *63*
    of upper limb, 419–420, *419*
Dermis, 7, 8

Descending colon, 158, *203*
Detrusor muscle, 226, *226–227*
Dialysis, intraperitoneal, 181
Diaphragm, 185–191
  actions during respiration, 187
  apertures of, *187–189*, 189
  congenital hernia of, 191, *191*
  crura of, 188–199, *188*
  domes of, 187, *187*
  innervation of, 105, *106–107*
  lymphatics of, 190, *190*
  paralysis of, 54, *54*, 191
  parts of, 188, *188*
  referred pain from, 191
  rupture of, 191
  stomach in relation to, 146, *149t*
  surfaces of, *187, 188*
  vasculature and nerves of, *187–188*, 189–190,
    190t
Diaphragma sellae, 504, *505*
Diaphysis, bone, 12, *13*
Diastole, *99*, 100
Diastolic blood pressure, 445
Diencephalon, 512, *513*
Digastric muscle type, 19, *21*
Digastric muscle(s), 607, *608t*
  anterior and posterior bellies, 597, 605
  intermediate tendon, and fibrous sling, 607,
    608t
Digestion, process of, 140
Digestive tract. *See* Alimentary (digestive) tract
Digital arteries, 376, *376, 461*, 467, *467t, 468*
Digital fibrous sheaths, of hand, 461, *461, 466,
    466*
Digital flexion creases, transverse, 474, *474*
Digital synovial sheaths, of hand, 466, *466*
Digits
  of foot, 317. *See also* Toes
  of hand, *406, 411*
    ischemia of, 470
    tenosynovitis of, 470–471, *471*
Dilator pupillae, 535–536, *536, 655*
Dinner fork deformity, 414, *414*
Diploë, *510*
Diploic vein, *510*
Diplopia, 657
Discs. *See* Intervertebral discs
Distal, definition of, *4t*, 5
Diverticulosis, 160
Doppler echocardiography, 101–102
Doppler ultrasound, 641, *642*
Dorsal artery
  of foot, 357, *358*
  of penis or clitoris, 263, *263t, 264, 267*
Dorsal horn. *See* Posterior horn
Dorsal interossei. *See* Interosseus muscles
Dorsal nerve of penis or clitoris, *219, 258, 259*
Dorsal pedis artery, 376, *376*
Dorsal ramus. *See* Posterior ramus
Dorsal root. *See* Posterior root
Dorsal scapular nerve, *434*, 434t
Dorsal venous arch, of foot, 25, *27*, 331–332,
    331–332
Dorsal venous network, of hand, 421, *421*

Dorsalis pedis artery, *370t*
Dorsalis pedis pulse, 362, *362*
Dorsiflexion, *6*, 397, 397t
Dorsum, *4t*, 5
  of foot, 317, *317*
Dorsum sellae, *501, 502*
Ductus deferens, 130, *130*, 131, 132, 233
  ampulla of, 233
  deferentectomy (vasectomy), 132, 233
  vasculature of, 233
Ductus deferens artery, 130, 222t, 233
Ductus reunions, 585, *585*
Duodenal ampulla, 150
Duodenal arteries, 150
Duodenal papilla(e), major and minor, 162,
    163, *164*, 171
Duodenal (peptic) ulcers, 160
Duodenojejunal flexure, 150
Duodenojejunal junction, 148, *149t*, 150, 152
Duodenum, 146–152
  arteries of, 150
  nerves and lymphatics of, *147*
  parts of, 148–150
  relationships of, *149t*, 150
  ulcers of, 160
  veins of, 150–152
Dupuytren contracture, 470, *470*
Dura-arachnoid interface, 297, *299*
Dura-arachnoid junction, 511
Dura-cranium interface, 511
Dura mater, 31, 504–509
  cranial, 504–509, *504, 510*
    headaches, origin from, 508–509
    infoldings or reflections of, 504, *505*
    vasculature and innervation of, 508, *509*
    venous sinuses, 504–508, *505–506*
  spinal, 31, *33*, 297, *298*
Dural root sheaths, 297, *298*
Dural sac, 297
Dural venous sinuses, 504–508, *505–506, 510*
  confluence of, 505, *505*
  metastasis of tumor cells to, 508
  occlusion of, 508
Dysarthria, 597
Dysphagia, 597, 669
Dyspnea, 64

E

Ear, 578–588, *578*
  auditory ossicles, 580–583, *581*
  external, 578, *578–580, 578*
    injury of, 587
  innervation and nerves of, *578, 663*
  internal, 583–587, *584–587*
  medical conditions of, 587–588
  middle, 580–583, *581*
  sound transmission through, 587
  surface anatomy of, *578*
  tympanic cavity, 580, *581–582*
  tympanic membrane, 579, *579*
  vasculature of, 579, *579*
Ear lobe (lobule), 578, *579*

Eccentric contraction, 19
Ecchymosis, 503
Echocardiography, 101–102
Ectopic tubal pregnancy, 249
Edinger-Westphal nucleus, *649, 655*
Efferent ductules, of epididymis, *130*, 131
Ejaculation, 265
Ejaculatory ducts, 233
Elbow bursitis, 486
Elbow joint, 482–483, *482–483*
  bursae of, 483, *483*
  carrying angle of, 483, *483*
  dislocation of, 486
  movements of, *410*
    structures limiting movements, 485t
  radiograph of, *482*
Elbow region, arterial anastomoses of, 443
Elbow tendinitis, 460
Electromyography, 22–23, 307
Elevation, *6*
Elevators of ribs. *See* Levator(es) costarum
Embolus/embolism, pulmonary, 79
Emissary veins, 503, 508, *510*
Emission, of semen, 265
Enamel, tooth, 558, *558*
Endarterectomy, 610
Endocardium, 84
Endochondral ossification, 12, 413
Endocrine layer, of cervical viscera, 619–622,
    620
Endocrine system, 3
Endolymph, 584
Endolymphatic duct, 584, *584–585*, 585
Endolymphatic sac, 585, *585*
Endometrium, 239, *239*
Endomysium, 20, *22*
Endoneurium, 31, 33, *33*
Endopelvic fascia, 215–217, *216*
Endoscopic surgery, 123
Endothoracic fascia, 68, *69*
Epicardium, 81–82, *81*, 84
Epicolic lymph nodes, 158
Epicondyles, *10*, 11
  of femur
    lateral, *319, 385*
    medial, *319, 385*
    surface anatomy of, *328*
  of humerus, *408–409*, 410, 416, *446*
    lateral, *408–409*, 410
    lateral epicondylitis, 460
    medial, *408–409*, 410
    surface anatomy of, *415*, 416
Epicranial aponeurosis, 503, *503*
Epidermis, 7, *7*
Epididymis, *129–130*, 131
  duct of, *130*, 131
  head, body, tail of, *130*, 131
Epidural anesthesia (block), 300, *301*
Epidural (extradural) hematoma, 511, *511*
Epidural space, 31, 297, *298*
Epidural venous plexus, 198, *294, 295*
Epigastric arteries, 126, 126t, 195, *195*
Epigastric fossa, 67
Epigastric veins, 174, 198

Epiglottic cartilage, 623, *623, 626*
Epiglottic stalk, 624
Epiglottis, *560, 627*
Epimysium, 20, *22*
Epineurium, *33, 33*
Epiphysial arteries, 13, *13*
Epiphysial line, 12–14, *13*
Epiphysial plates, 12, *13*
    fractures involving, 326, *326*
Epiphysial rim, *277, 278*
Epiphysis, 12, *13*, 14
Episcleral space, 534, *534*
Episiotomy, 253
Epistaxis, 577
Epitympanic recess, 580, *581*
Erb-Duchenne palsy, 438
Erectile dysfunction, 266
Erection, of penis, 265
Erector spinae muscles, 303–304, *306*
Esophageal arteries, 108, 110t, *145*
Esophageal hiatus, *109*, 110, 143, 189
Esophageal plexus, 105, 105t, *109*, 666
Esophageal sphincter, inferior, 143
Esophageal veins, 173
Esophagogastric junction, 143, *144*
Esophagus, 636–638
    arteries of, 108, 110t, *628*, 636–637
    lymphatics and lymph nodes of, *143*,
        638, *638*
    nerve supply of, 638
    references to, 108, *108*, 110, *142*, 143
Ethmoid bone
    cribriform plate of, *501, 502, 575*
    medial wall of, 529, *529*
Ethmoidal arteries, 574, *575*
Ethmoidal bulla, 574, *574*
Ethmoidal cells (sinuses), 576, *576*
    infection of, 577
Ethmoidal foramina, 500t
Ethmoidal nerves, 545
    anterior, 574, *575*
Extension, definition of, 5
Extensor carpi radialis brevis, 451, *452*, 454t
Extensor carpi radialis longus, 451, *452*, 454t
Extensor carpi ulnaris, 451, *452*, 454t
Extensor digiti minimi, 451, *452*, 454t
Extensor digitorum, 451, *452*, 454t
    tendinous sheath of, 453
Extensor digitorum brevis, *372, 373*
    contusion of, 379
Extensor digitorum longus, *358, 359t*
Extensor expansions, 453, *453, 455*
Extensor hallucis brevis, *372, 373*
Extensor hallucis longus, *358, 359t*
Extensor indicis, 451, *452*, 455t, *456*
    tendinous sheath of, 453
Extensor pollicis brevis, 451, *452*, 455t, *456*
Extensor pollicis longus, 451, *452*, 455t, *456*
Extensor retinacula (retinaculum)
    of ankle, *330*, 331
        superior and inferior, 357, *358*
    of wrist, 417–419, *418*, 451, *453*
Extensor tendons, and synovial sheaths, of
    wrist/hand, 451, *453*, 460

External acoustic meatus, *497, 498*, 578, *578, 587*
External carotid artery. *See* Carotid artery,
    external
External iliac lymph nodes, 223, *223*, 229t, 230t
External jugular vein, *600*, 602
    prominence of, 603
External oblique muscle, *21*, 119, *119*, 120t, 124
External occipital protuberance, 498, *499*
Exteroceptive sensation, 35
Extra-ocular muscles, 540–543, *540–541*, 540t
    clinical testing of, *542*
    innervation of, 656
    paralysis of, 548, *548*
Extradural (epidural) space, 297, *298, 300*
Extraperitoneal fat, 118, *118*
Extraperitoneal organs, 135, *136*
Eye. *See also* Eyeball; Orbit
    angles of, *530*, 533
    anterior and posterior chambers of, 537
    binocular movements of, *543*
    intra-ocular muscles, autonomic innervation
        of, *655*
Eyeball, *531*, 533–538, *534–535*
    arteries of, 545–547, *546*, 547t
    extra-ocular muscles, 540–543, *540–541*, 540t
    fascial sheath of, *531*, 534
    fibrous layer of, 534, *534*
    fundus of, *537, 537*
    horizontal section of, *546*
    inner layer of, *534–535, 537*
    movements of, 540, *540–541, 543*
    refractive media and compartments of,
        535–536, 537–538
    supporting apparatus of, 543–544, *544*
    surface anatomy of, *530*
    vascular layer of, 534–536, *534*
Eyelashes, *531, 532*
Eyelids, 530–533, *530–531*
    injury of nerves supplying, 533
    surface anatomy of, *530*

F

Face, 519–529
    arterial pulses in, 525
    injuries of, 519
    lymphatic drainage of, *568*
    muscles of, 519, 520t
    nerves and innervation of, 519–522
        cutaneous nerves, 521t–522t
        motor nerves, *520*, 522, *661*
    vasculature of, 522–526, 523t, *525, 553*
Facet, bone, *10*, 11
Facet joints. *See* Zygapophysial joints
Facial artery(ies), 522–524, 609–610, *609*
    branches of, 522–524, 523t, *525, 574*
    compression of, 525
    transverse, 523t, 524, *525*
Facial nerve (CN VII), 660–662, *661*
    chorda tympani branch of, *554, 555, 564,
        566, 581, 661*
    distribution/branches of, *520*, 522, 528,
        660, *661*

    injury to, 660
    intracranial portion of, *648*
    motor root and intermediate nerve of, 660,
        661
    nuclei of, *649*
    parasympathetic distribution, 660, *662*
    summary of, *646t–647t*
Facial pulse, 525
Facial vein, 525, *609*
    deep, 525, *525, 526*
    thrombophlebitis of, 508
Falciform ligament, *150*, 165, *166*
Falciform margin, 330, *330*
Fallopian tubes. *See* Uterine tubes
Falx cerebelli, 504, *505*
Falx cerebri, 504, *505*
Fascia
    of abdominal wall, 118, 122–123, 192, *192*
        clinical significance of, 122, *122*
    antebrachial, 417, *418, 446*
    of axilla, 417, *418*
    deep, 7, 8
    of eyeball, *531*, 534
    of female pelvis, *216, 240*
    of female perineum, 237
    of foot, 371–372, *371*
    of hand, 461–462, *461–462*
    investing, 595, *596*
    of kidneys, 176, *177*
    of lower limb, 329–331, *330*
    of male pelvis, 216
    of male perineum, 253–256, *254*
    of neck, 594–596, *595*
    of pelvis, 215–217, *216*
    of penis, 261, *262*
    of perineum, 227, 253, *254*
    of popliteal fossa, 355, *356*
    spermatic, 128–129, *128–129*
    superficial. *See* Subcutaneous tissue
    of thigh, 330, *331*
    of thoracic spine, 303, *304*
    of thorax, 68, *69*
    of upper limb, 417–419, *418*
    of urogenital triangle, 253–256, *254*
Fascia lata, 330, *330*
Fascial planes, 8
Fasciotomy, 335
Fat bodies, of ischioanal fossae, 257
Female breast, sagittal section of, *56*
Female external genitalia, 268–270, *268*
Female internal genital organs, 236–245
    infections of, 247
Female pelvis, *224, 227. See also* Pelvis;
    Perineum
    compared to male pelvis, 208t, 209
    fascia and ligaments of, *216, 240*
    floor of, *213*
        injury to, 217, *217*
    genital organs within, 236–245
    lymphatics and lymph nodes of, 229t
    medical imaging of, *244, 272–273*
    nerves and innervation of, 241, *241*
    osseoligamentous boundaries of, 250, *250*
    peritoneal reflections in, *212t*

supporting and compressive muscles of, 237
vasculature of, 238
Female perineum, 268–270, 268
external genitalia of, 268–270, 268
fascia and pouches of, 253–256, 254
lymphatics of, 229t
medical imaging of, 272–273
muscles of, 251–252, 252t
vasculature of, 263t, 264
Female urethra, 227, 230
dilation of, 270
innervation of, 230, 231
vasculature of, 229t, 230
Femoral artery, 341, 343, 344t
cannulation of, 345
Femoral canal, 343, 343
Femoral condyles, medial and lateral, 318,
319, 328
Femoral hernia, 345, 345
Femoral neck, fractures of, 384
Femoral nerve, 194, 194, 334, 341–343, 342
block, 336
Femoral pulse, 345, 345
Femoral ring, 343, 343
Femoral septum, 343, 343
Femoral sheath, 342–343, 343
Femoral triangle, 341–342, 341–342
Femoral vein, 331, 331–332, 341, 346
cannulation of, 345
Femoropatellar articulation, of knee joint, 385,
385, 389
Femorotibial articulations, of knee joint, 385,
385
Femur, 318–322, 319
angle of inclination of, 322, 322
changes in, 325, 325
condyles of, 318, 319, 328
fractures of, 325, 325
of femoral neck, 384
head of, 318, 319, 379, 380
artery to, 383, 383
ligament of, 318, 319, 380, 381
neck and shaft of, 319, 328
Q-angle, with tibia/fibula, 391, 392
torsion angle of, 322, 322
trochanters of, 318, 319, 327, 327–328
Fibroblasts, 12
Fibrous digital sheaths, 461, 461, 466, 466
Fibrous joints, 14, 15t
Fibrous layer, of joint capsules, 379, 381, 386,
386, 478, 482
Fibrous pericardium, 80–81, 81
Fibrous raphe, of mylohyoid, 604
Fibrous septa, of palm, 461, 462
Fibrous sling, for digastric tendon, 607, 608t
Fibula, 319, 322–323, 323
bone grafts from, 326
fractures of, 326, 326, 398, 398
surface anatomy of, 328–329, 328
Fibular artery, 361, 366, 370t
Fibular collateral ligament, 358, 386–387, 387, 393
Fibular nerves
common, 355, 357, 369t
injury to, 361

deep, 369t, 375t, 376
entrapment of, 362
superficial, 360, 360, 369t, 375t, 376
Fibular trochlea, 323, 324, 329
Fibularis brevis, 358, 359t, 360
Fibularis longus, 358, 359t, 360
Fibularis tertius, 358, 359t
Filiform papillae, 563, 563
Filum terminale, 296, 297
Fimbriae, of uterine tubes, 243
Fingers, 406, 406
Fissures, of brain, 512, 513
Fixator muscle, 20
Flail chest, 54
Flat bones, 9, 11
Flat feet, 402, 402
Flat muscles, 21
Flexion, definition of, 5
Flexor carpi radialis, 447, 449, 450t
tendon of, 473–474, 473
Flexor carpi ulnaris, 447, 449, 450t
Flexor digiti minimi brevis, 373t, 374, 462–463,
463, 464t
Flexor digitorum brevis, 373t, 374
Flexor digitorum longus, 364, 366, 366t
Flexor digitorum profundus, 449, 449–450,
451, 451t
muscle testing of, 460, 460
Flexor digitorum superficialis, 449, 449–450,
451, 451t
muscle testing of, 460, 460
Flexor hallucis brevis, 373t, 374
Flexor hallucis longus, 363, 364, 366t
Flexor pollicis brevis, 462, 463, 464t
Flexor pollicis longus, 449, 450, 451t
Flexor retinaculum (retinacula), 418, 419, 447
Flexor sheath, common, 463, 466
Flexor tendons
of forearm, 447
of hand, 463, 466, 466
Floating (free) ribs, 48, 49
Foliate papillae, 563, 563
Foot, 317, 317, 371–377. See also Sole of foot;
Toes
amputation of, 398
arches of, 400–402, 401
arteries of, 357, 358, 376, 376
ball of, 371, 400
bones of, 323–325, 324
fractures of, 327
surface anatomy of, 329, 329
deformities of, 402, 402
dorsal artery of, 370t, 376, 376
dorsal venous arch of, 331, 331–332
dorsum of, 317, 317, 371
fascia of, 371–372, 371
joints of, 398, 399, 399–400t
lymphatic drainage of, 377
movements, structures limiting, 400t
muscles of, 372–373, 373t, 374
dorsum, 358, 372–373, 372
PAD and DAB mnemonics, 372
plantar region, 372, 373t, 374
nerves of, 375t, 376

parts of, 371, 371
plantar region (sole) of, 317, 317, 371, 371
ligaments of, 398, 398
venous drainage of, 25, 27, 377
Foramen (in bone), 10, 11
Foramen cecum, 500t, 501, 502
of tongue, 563, 563
Foramen lacerum, 500t, 501, 502
Foramen magnum, 499, 500–501, 500t, 502
Foramen ovale, 500t, 501, 502, 570
Foramen rotundum, 500t, 501, 502, 572
Foramen spinosum, 500t, 501, 502
Forearm, 406, 406, 446–460
arteries of, 452, 456, 457, 459t
bones of, 446
cutaneous nerves of, 420, 421, 446, 446
fascial compartments of, 418
muscles of, 446–456
anterior compartment, 447–451, 448–450,
450t–451t
extensor, 451–453, 452–454, 454t–455t
flexor-pronator, 447–451, 449–450,
450t–451t, 473
posterior compartment, 448, 452, 454,
454t–455t
nerves of, 456, 457, 458t
motor and cutaneous innervation, 458
surface anatomy of, 473–474, 473–474
veins of, 457
Forefoot, 371, 371
Foreign bodies
aspiration of, 78, 630
in laryngopharynx, 639
Fossa, bone, 10, 11
Fourth ventricle, of brain, 512, 515
Fovea centralis, 537
Foveola, 537
Fractures, 12. See also specific structures
avulsion, 318
comminuted, 54, 414, 498
compound, 326, 326
depressed, 498, 498
Frenulum
of clitoris, 268, 268
of labia minora, 268
labial, 562
lingual, 564, 564, 606
of prepuce, 262
Frontal bone, 496, 497
foramen cecum of, 501, 502
orbital part of, 529, 529
orbital plates of, 501, 502
Frontal crest, 501, 502
Frontal nerve, 544, 545, 658
Frontal plane, 3–4, 3
Frontal sinus, 560, 576, 576
Frontonasal duct, 574, 576
Fundiform ligament, of penis, 263
Fundus
of bladder, 224, 226
of stomach, 143, 144, 148
of uterus, 239, 239
Fungiform papillae, 563, 564
Fusiform muscles, 17, 21

G

Gag reflex, 569, *666*
Gait cycle, 377–378
  fibular nerve injury and, 361, *362*
Gallbladder, *166, 171, 172*–173
  removal of, 174
  vasculature of, 171–172, *173*
Gallbladder fossa, 172
Gallstones, 173–174
Ganglion (ganglia), nerve, 33. *See also* Spinal
    ganglia; Sympathetic ganglia
Ganglion (synovial cyst), 460, *460*
Ganglion impar, 38, *39*, 219, *220*
Gastrectomy, 159
Gastric artery(ies), 145, *145*, 146t
  branches of, 143, *143, 145*
  right and left, 146t
Gastric canal, 144, *144*
Gastric folds, 144, *144*
Gastric lymph nodes, 145, *147*
Gastric veins
  left, 143, *145*
  right and left, 145, *145*
Gastro-omental artery(ies), 145, *145*, 146t
Gastro-omental lymph nodes, 145
Gastro-omental veins, 145, *145*
Gastrocnemius, *350*, 363, *364*, 365t
  strain, 367
Gastrocnemius bursa, 390t
Gastrocolic ligament, 137, *137*
Gastroduodenal artery, *145*, 171
Gastrophrenic ligament, 137, *137*
Gastrosplenic ligament, 137, *137*, 162
Gemellus (gemelli), superior and inferior, 347,
    347, 348t
General somatic (sensory) fibers, 34, *34*, 35
Genicular anastomosis, 356, 389
Genicular arteries, 355, *356*
Geniculate bodies, lateral, 652, *652*
Geniculate ganglion, 660, *661*
Geniculum, of facial nerve, 660, *661*
Genioglossus, *560*, 565t, *633*
  paralysis of, 569
Geniohyoid, 608t
Genital glands, auxiliary, 132
Genital organs
  female external, 268–270, *268*
  female internal, 236–245
  male external, 261–265, *262*
  male internal, *228*, 233–236
Genitofemoral nerve, 194, *194*
  genital branch of, 129, 130, *131*, 132
Genu valgum, 391, *392*
Genu varum, 391, *392*
Gingivae, 558–560, *559*
Gingivitis, 560
Glabella, 496, *497*
Glans
  of clitoris, 268, *268–269*
  of penis, 262, *263*, 266
Glaucoma, 539
Glenohumeral joint, *406*, 476–480, *478*

adhesive capsulitis of, 481
blood supply and innervation of, 479
bursae of, *478*, 479–480
capsule of, *478, 478*
dislocation of, 481, *481*
ligaments of, *478*, 479
medical imaging of, *494*
radiograph of, *478*
scapular movements and, *477*
Glenoid cavity, 410, *410*
Glenoid labrum, 478, *478*
Glial cells, 31
Glossopharyngeal nerve (CN IX), 664–665
  distribution of, *564, 566, 611*, 665
  intracranial portion of, *648*
  lesions of, *666, 666*
  nuclei of, *649*
  parasympathetic distribution, 664, *667*
  summary of, *646t–647t*
Glottis, 625
Gluteal arteries, superior and inferior, 222t,
    352, 353t
Gluteal bursae, 348, *348*
Gluteal fold, 327, *327*, 346, *346*
Gluteal lymph nodes, *351*, 353
Gluteal nerves, superior and inferior, 217, 218t,
    219, 349, *351*, 352t
  injury to, 354
Gluteal region, 317, *317*, 336–340, 346–355.
    See also Thigh
  intragluteal injections, 354, *354*
  muscles of, 347, *347*, 348t
  nerve injury in, 354
  nerves of, 349, *351*, 352t
  vasculature of, *351*, 352–353, *353t*
Gluteal veins, superior and inferior, 352, *353t*
Gluteofemoral bursa, 348, *348*
Gluteus maximus, 347, *347*, 348t
Gluteus medius, 347, *347*, 348t, 354
Gluteus minimus, 347, *347*, 348t
Gomphosis, 14, *15t*
Gonadal arteries, 222t
Gonads, relocation (descent) of, 133
Gracilis, 338–339, 339t, 340
  transplantation of, 340
Gray matter, 31, 33
Gray rami communicantes, 38, *40*, 194
Great cardiac vein, 96, *96*
Great cerebral vein, 519
Great vessels, of heart, 102–113, *103–104*
  in posterior mediastinum, 108, *110*
  in superior mediastinum, 102–105, *103*
  variations of, 112–113, *113*
Greater omentum, 137, *137–138*
  functions of, 141
Greater palatine nerve, 574, *575*
Greater pelvis, 207, *250*
Greater sac, of peritoneal cavity, 138,
    139–140
Greater trochanter, 318, *319*
Greater tubercle, of humerus, *408–409*,
    410, 416
Greater vestibular glands, 269
  inflammation of, 270

Groin pull, 340
Guarding, 123
Gyri, of brain, 512, *513*

H

Hair cells, of internal ear, 585, *586*
Hallux valgus, 402, *402*
Hamate, 411, *411–412, 489*
  fractures of, 414
Hamstring injuries, 354
Hamstrings, 349, 349t, *350*
Hand, 406, *406*, 461–474
  anesthesia of, 471
  arteries of, *461*, 466–468, *467t, 468*
  bones of, 411–412, *411*
    radiograph of, *489*
  claw hand, *438, 439*, 472, *472*
  compartments and spaces of, 461–462, *462*
  cutaneous innervation of, *469*
  dorsal venous network of, 468
  fascia of palm, 461–462, *461–462*
  fractures of, 414, *414*
  infections of, 470
  joints of, 488–491, *489*, 490t
    structures limiting movements of, 491t
  ligaments of, 461–462, *461–462, 489–490*
  movements of thumb, 462, *466*
  muscles of, 462–466, *463*, 464t–465t
    DAB and PAD mnemonics, 465–466
    extensor expansion and vinacula, *455*
    extensor tendons, 453
    extrinsic muscles tendons, *463*, 466, *466*
    hypothenar, 462–463, *463*, 464t
    long flexors of digits, 449, *449*, 451t
    short, 463–466, *463–465*, 465t
    thenar, 462, *463*, 464t
  nerves of, 468–469, *468*
  surface anatomy of, 473–474, *473–474*
  synovial sheaths and tendons of, *453, 463*,
    466, *466*
  thenar and hypothenar eminences, 461, *461*
  veins of, 468
Hard palate, 560–561, *560–561, 633*
Haustra, 154, *156*
Haversian systems, *13*
Head, 495–592
  brain, 512–519
  cranial meninges, 503–511
  cranium (skull), 496–502
  ear, 578–588
  face, 519–529
  injuries to, 511, *511*
  innervation of, posterior aspect, *313*, 313t
  lymphatics and lymph nodes of, 526, *527*,
    638
  medical imaging of, 589–592
  nose/nasal region, 573–578
  oral region, 557–569
  orbit and eye region, 529–548
  pterygopalatine fossa, 570–573
  scalp of, 502–503
  temporal region, 549–555

temporomandibular joint, 555–557
vasculature of, *553. See also specific region*
Headaches, 508–509
Heart, 84–102. *See also cardiac and cardiovascular entries;* Great vessels; Heart valves
  apex of, 85, *85–86*
    apex beat, 85, 92–94
  arteries of, 94–96, 94t, *95*
  atria of
    left, 89–90, *89*
    right, 87, *87*
  base of, 85, *85–86*
  borders of, 85, 87
  chambers of, *23,* 87–90
  circulatory cycle of, *23*
  collateral venous routes to, 112
  conducting system of, 97–98, *97,* 102
  development of, 82, *82*
  diseases of
    coronary artery disease, 100, *100*
    valvular heart disease, 91–92
  exterior of, *86*
  great vessels of, 102–105
  interior of, *88*
  layers of, 84
  lymphatic drainage of, 97
  medical conditions and procedures, 91–92, 100–102
  nerves and innervation of, 98–99
  orientation of, 84–87, *85*
  percussion of, 91
  referred pain and, 102
  skeleton of, 100
  surface anatomy of, 92–94, *92–93*
  surfaces of, 85–87, *86*
  valves of, 88, 89, *89,* 90, *90*
  veins of, 96–97, *96*
  ventricles of
    left, 90, *90*
    right, 88–89, *88*
Heart block, 102
Heart failure, dsypnea in, 64
Heart murmurs, 91
Heart valves, 88, 89, *89,* 90, *90*
  aortic, 90, *90*
    stenosis of, 92
  during diastole and systole, *99*
  mitral valve, *88,* 90, *90*
    prolapsed, 91–92
  pulmonary, 89, *89*
    stenosis of, 92
  tricuspid valve, 88, *88*
  valvular heart disease, 91–92
Heel region, of foot, 371, *371*
Heel strike, 377, *378t*
Heimlich maneuver, 630, *630*
Helicine arteries, 263
Helicobacter pylori, 159
Helicotrema, *584, 585, 586–587*
Helix, of auricle, *578, 579*
Hematocele, of testis, 132, *132*
Hematomas, 498, 511, *511*
  epidural, 511, *511*
Hemiazygos vein, *109,* 111

Hemopericardium, 84
Hemorrhoids, 260, *260*
Hemothorax, 77
Hepatic arteries, *145,* 146t, 168, *168,* 171, 172
Hepatic ducts, 171, 172, *172*
Hepatic lymph nodes, 164, 169, *170,* 172, 173
Hepatic nerve plexus, 171
Hepatic portal vein, 142–143, *142, 145,* 150, 162, 168–169, *168,* 173–174
  and portal-systemic anastomoses, 173–174, *175*
Hepatic portal venous system, *142,* 143, *145, 175*
Hepatoduodenal ligament, *137, 138,* 167, *168*
Hepatogastric ligament, *137, 138, 168*
Hepatopancreatic ampulla, 162, *164,* 171
Hepatopancreatic sphincter, 163, *164*
Hepatorenal recess, 165, *166*
Hernias
  of canal of Nuck, 135
  diaphragmatic, 191, *191*
  femoral, 345, *345*
  hiatal (hiatus), 159, *159,* 191
  incisional, 123
  inguinal, 134, *134t,* 135
  of viscera, 191
Herniated discs, 293, *293*
Herpes virus, 64
Herpes zoster (shingles), 64
Hesselbach triangles, 121
Hiatal (hiatus) hernia, 159, *159,* 191
Hindfoot, 371, *371*
Hinge joints, *16t*
Hip, 317, *317*
  contusions of, 340
Hip bone, 205, *206,* 318, *319, 321*
  fractures of, 318
  parts of, 318, *321*
Hip joint, 379–384, *380*
  arteries of, 383, *383,* 383t
  articular surfaces of, 379, *380*
  dislocation of, 384
  fibrous layer of capsule of, 379, *381*
  fractures of, 384
  joint capsule, 379–381, *381*
  ligaments of, 379–381, *381*
  movement restrictors of, 383t
  movements of, 382–383, *382*
  nerve supply of, 383
  orbicular zone of, 381, *381*
  surgical replacement of, 384, *384*
  synovial membrane of, *380,* 381
Hip prosthesis, 384, *384*
Hook of hamate, 411, *411,* 416
Horner syndrome, 619
Horns, in spinal cord, 31, *33*
Humeral axillary lymph nodes, *421,* 422
Humeral lymph nodes, *421,* 432, 433
Humerus, *408–409,* 410
  anatomical neck of, *408–409,* 410
  epicondyles of, *408–409,* 410, 416, *446*
  fractures of, 413, *413*
  shaft of, *408–409,* 410, 416
  surface anatomy of, 416
  surgical neck of, *408–409,* 410, 413

tubercles of, *408–409,* 410, 416
Hydrocele, in testis, 132, *132*
Hydrocephalus, 514, *514*
Hydrothorax, 77
Hymen, 269
Hymenal caruncles, *268,* 269
Hyo-epiglottic ligament, 624
Hyoglossus, 565t
Hyoid bone, 594, *594*
  surface anatomy of, 624, *624*
Hyoid muscles, *560,* 607, *608t*
Hypertension, 91
  portal, 174
Hypertrophy
  bone, 12
  of muscle, 23
Hypogastric nerves, 185, 219–220
Hypogastric plexus(es), 219, 220, 260
Hypogastric sheath, 215, *216*
Hypoglossal canal, 500t, *501,* 502
Hypoglossal nerve (CN XII), 671
  distribution of, *564, 566,* 611, *671*
  injury to, 569, 671, *671*
  intracranial portion of, *648*
  nucleus of, *649*
  summary of, *646t–647t*
Hypophysial fossa, *501,* 502
Hypothenar compartment, 461–462, *462*
Hypothenar eminence, 461, *461,* 474
Hypothenar muscles, 462–463, *463, 464t*
Hypothesia, of hand, 471
Hysterectomy, 242, *242*
Hysterosalpingography, 247–249, *247*
Hysteroscopy, 249

I

Ileal diverticulum, 160
Ileal orifice, 156, *156*
Ileocecal junction, 152
Ileocecal valve, 156, *156*
Ileocolic artery, *151t,* 156, *156,* 158
Ileocolic lymph nodes, 154, *157*
Ileocolic veins, 156, 158
Ileostomy, 160–161
Ileum, 152–154, *153*
  distinguishing characteristics of, 153t
Iliac arteries
  common, 195, *195–196*
  deep circumflex, 126, 126t, 195, *195*
  internal and external, 195, *195–196,* 220–222, *221,* 222t, 227
  superficial circumflex, 126, 126t
Iliac crest, 124, 205, *206,* 318, *321*
  surface anatomy of, 327, *327–328*
Iliac fossa, 205, *206*
Iliac lymph nodes, 179, 223, *223*
  common, 196, *197,* 223, *223*
  external, 223, *223*
  internal, 223, *223*
Iliac spine(s), 205, *206*
  anterior and posterior superior, 124, 205, *206*
  surface anatomy of, 327, *327–328*

Iliac vein(s), 222, 352, *353t*
Iliacus, 193, *193t*, 337t, *338*
Ilio-inguinal nerve, 125t, 132, 194, *194*
Ilio-inguinal nerve block, 270
Iliococcygeus, *213–214*, 215, *252*
Iliocostalis, 304, 305t, *306*
Iliofemoral ligament, 381, *381*
Iliohypogastric nerve, 125t, 194, *194*
Ilioinguinal nerve, 265
Iliolumbar artery, 222t
Iliolumbar ligaments, 209
Iliopsoas, 193, 198, 336, 337t, *338*
Iliopsoas test, 198
Iliopubic tract, 127, *127*
Iliotibial tract, 330, *330*
Ilium, 205, *206*, 318, *321*
Imaging, of body systems, 42–46. *See also*
      Medical imaging
Incisions, skin, 8
Incisive fossa, 499, *500*, 560, *561*
Incisor tooth, 558, *558*
Incontinence, stress, 217
Incus, 580–581, *581*, *587*
Infarction, 25
   pulmonary, 79
Inferior alveolar nerve, *554*, 555, 558, *559*
   block, 556
Inferior (caudal), definition of, *4t*
Inferior epigastric arteries, 126, 195, *195*
Inferior ganglion, 664, 666, *666*
Inferior gluteal nerve, 217, 218t, *219*
Inferior hypogastric plexuses, 185
Inferior longitudinal muscle, *565t*
Inferior mesenteric arteries, 142, *142*, *151t*,
      156, 158
Inferior mesenteric ganglion, 158
Inferior mesenteric lymph nodes, 196, *197*,
      229t, *230t*
Inferior mesenteric (nerve) plexus, 158, 182, 185
Inferior mesenteric vein, *145*, 158
Inferior oblique, *540–541*, 540t, *543*
Inferior pancreaticoduodenal artery(ies), 164
Inferior pharyngeal constrictor, *637t*
Inferior recess, 138
Inferior rectus, *531*, 540–543, *540–541*,
      540t, *543*
Inferior sagittal sinus, *505*, 505, *510*
Inferior vena cava. *See* Vena cava, inferior
Inferomedial, definition of, *4t*, *5*
Infra-orbital artery, *546*, 547, 547t, 558
Infra-orbital foramen, 496, *497*, 529
Infra-orbital nerve, *521t*
Infracolic compartment, 139, *139–140*
Infraglottic cavity, 625, *625*
Infrahyoid muscles, *312t*, 607, *608t*
Infrapatellar bursae, 389, *390t*
Infrapatellar bursitis, 394
Infrapatellar fat pad, 386, *386*
Infraspinatus, *426t*, 427
Infraspinous fossa, 407, *409–410*
Infrasternal angle, 67
Infratemporal fossa, *549*, 550–555
   contents of, *551*, 551
   nerves of, *554*

vasculature of, 553
Infratrochlear nerve, *521t*, 544–545, *545*
Infundibular pulmonary stenosis, 92
Infundibulum, of uterine tubes, *240*, 243
Inguinal canal, 128, *128*
Inguinal falx, 128, *128*
Inguinal fossae, 121, *122*
Inguinal hernias, 134, *134t*
   detection of, 135, *135*
Inguinal ligaments, 119, *119*, 124, 127, *127*
Inguinal lymph nodes, *229t*, *230t*, 260, 265,
      265, 332, 333
   enlarged, 336
Inguinal region, 127–135, *127*
   epididymis, *130*, 131
   ligaments of, 127, *127*
   relocation of gonads in, 133
   scrotum, 131–132, *131*
   spermatic cord, 128–130
   testes, 130–131, *130*
Inguinal ring(s), 127, *128*
   palpation of superficial, 135, *135*
Inguinal triangles, 121
Innervation. *See specific structures*
Insertion, of muscles, 19
Inspiratory stridor, 669
Integumentary system, 2, 7–8, *7*
Interatrial septum, 87, *87*
Intercarpal joints, *489*
Intercavernous sinuses, *505–506*, 506
Interclavicular ligament, *475*, 476
Intercostal arteries, 108, 110t, 126
Intercostal muscles, 61, *61*
Intercostal nerves, 61–62, *61*, *62*, 105t, 190
   atypical, 62
   nerve block, 64, *64*
Intercostal spaces, 48, *49*, 61
   contents of, *61*
Intercostal veins, 111
Intercostobrachial nerve, *420*, 421
Intercrural fibers, *127*, 128
Intergluteal cleft, 284, *285*, 346
Intermammary cleft, 67
Intermaxillary suture, 496, *497*
Intermediolateral cell columns, spinal cord, 38, *38*
Intermesenteric plexus, 182, 219
Intermetacarpal joints, *488t*
Intermetatarsal joints, *399*, *400t*
Intermuscular septa
   anterior and posterior, of lower limb, 331
   lateral, 330
   medial and lateral, 417, *418*
   transverse, of lower limb, *330*, 331
Internal acoustic meatus, *585*, 586–587
Internal carotid artery. *See* Carotid artery,
      internal
Internal ear, 583–587, *584–585*
Internal iliac artery(ies), 220–222, *221*, 222t
Internal iliac lymph nodes, 223, *223*, *229t*, *230t*
Internal jugular pulse, 611
Internal jugular vein puncture, 611, *611*
Internal jugular vein(s), *197*, 197
Internal oblique muscle, 119, *119*, 120t
Internal thoracic artery, 102, *430*, 430t

Interneuron, *34*
Interossei. *See* Interosseous muscles
Interosseous compartment, of foot, 372
Interosseous membrane
   of forearm, 446, *448*
   between tibia and fibula, 322, *323*
Interosseous muscles
   of foot (plantar), 372, 373t, *374*
   of hand, dorsal and palmar, 371, 372, 373t,
      374, 465–466, *465t*
Interosseous nerves, 452, 456, 457, *458t*
Interosseous sacro-iliac ligaments, 209, *210*
Interosseous talocalcaneal ligament, *398*, 398
Interosseous tibiofibular ligament, *391*, 391
Interpeduncular cistern, 514, *515*
Interphalangeal joints
   of foot, *399*, *400t*
   of hand, *490t*, 491t
Interpubic disc, 209
Interspinales, 305, 307t, *308*
Interspinous ligaments, 289, 290
Intertendinous connections, 453, *453*
Intertransversarii, 305, 307t, *308*
Intertransverse ligaments, 289, 290–292
Intertrochanteric crest, 318, *319*
Intertrochanteric line, 318, *319*
Interventricular branches, coronary artery, 95, 96
Interventricular foramina, 277, 278, 512, *515*
Interventricular septum, 88, *89*
Intervertebral discs, 287, *289*
   aging of, 290
   herniation of, 293, *293*
Intervertebral joints. *See also* Cranioverterbral
      joints
   accessory ligaments of, 289, 290
   lumbosacral, 209, *210*
   muscles producing movements of, 305–307,
      309t–310t
   thoracic, 51, *52*, 52t
Intervertebral veins, 294
Intestinal arteries, *151t*
Intestinal lymphatic trunks, 197, *197*
Intestines. *See* Large intestine; Small intestine
Intra-ocular muscles, autonomic innervation
      of, 655
Intragluteal injections, 354, *354*
Intramembranous ossification, 12, 413
Intraperitoneal injection, 181
Intraperitoneal organs, 135, *136*
Intrinsic back muscles. *See* Back muscles,
      intrinsic
Inversion, *6*
   injuries, 397, *398*
Investing fascia, 595, *596*
Involuntary muscle. *See* Smooth muscle
Ipsilateral, definition of, 5
Iridocorneal angle, 537
Iris, *534–536*, 536
Irregular bones, 9, 11
Ischemia, 25, 34, 42
Ischial bursa, 348, *348*
Ischial bursitis, 353
Ischial spine, 206, *206*
Ischial tuberosity, 206, *206*, 327

Ischio-anal abscesses, 258, *258*
Ischio-anal fossae, 257, *257*
Ischiocavernosus, *251*, 251t, 261, 267, *267*
Ischiococcygeus, 213t
Ischiofemoral ligament, 381, *381*
Ischiopubic ramus (rami), 318, *321*
Ischium, 206, *206*, 318, *321*
Isometric contraction, 19
Isotonic contraction, 19

J

Jejunum, 152–153
  characteristics of, distinguishing, 153t
Joints, 14–17. *See also specific joint*
  ankle, 395–398
  carpal (wrist), 488, 488t, *489*
  classification of, 14, *15t–16t*
  degenerative disease of, 17
  elbow, 482–483, *482–483*
  of foot, 398, *399*, 399–400t
  glenohumeral, *406*, 476–480, *478*
  of hand, 488–491, *489*, *490t*
  hip, 379–384
  intervertebral, 51, 52, 52t
  knee, 385–389
  of lower limb, 379–402
  of pectoral girdle, 406, *406*
  synovial, 14–17, *15t–16t*
  temporomandibular, 555–557, *555*
  of thoracic wall, 51, *52*, 52t
  tibiofibular, 389–391
  of upper limb, 475–492
  vasculature and innervation of, 17
  of vertebral bodies, 287, 288–290
  of vertebral column, 288–292, *289*
Joint capsule, 289, *289*
Jugular foramen, 499, *500*, 500t, *501*, 502
  structures traversing, *666*
Jugular foramen syndrome, 666
Jugular lymphatic trunks, 638, *639*
Jugular notch, *49*, 51, *51*, 415, 611
Jugular vein(s), *609*
  anterior, *609*, 616
  external, 526, *526*, 600, 602, 616
    prominence of, 603
  internal, *609*, 610
    pulse of, 611
    superior and inferior bulbs of, 610
    venipuncture of, 611, *611*
Jugular venous arch, 616
Jugular wall, of tympanic cavity, 580, *581*
Jugulodigastric lymph node, 527, 635, *636*, 638
Juxta-intestinal lymph nodes, 154

K

Kidney(s), 174–177, *176–177*. *See also renal
    entries*
  congenital anomalies of, 181–182
  fascia and fat of, 176, *177*
  hilum of, 176, *177*
  internal anatomic features of, 176–177,
    177, *178*
  lymphatics of, 179, *179*
  medical conditions related to, 181–182
  nerves of, 179–180, *179*
  suprarenal gland and, 177–179, *177*
  surface anatomy of, 180, *180*
  transplantation of, 181
  transverse tissue section of, *177*
  vasculature of, *178*, 179
Kidney stones, 181
Kiesselbach area, 575
Klumpke paralysis, 439, *439*
Knee, 317, *317*
Knee jerk reflex, 340
Knee joint, 385–389
  arteries and nerves of, 355, 389
  articular surfaces of, 385, *385*
  bones of, 385
  bursae of, 389, *390t*
  bursitis of, 394, *394*
  injuries and repair of, 393–394, *393–394*
  joint capsule, 385–386, *386*
  ligaments of, 386–388, *387*
  menisci of, 388, *388*
  movements of, 388–389, 389t
  replacement of, 394, *394*
Kyphosis, 276, *276*

L

Labia majora, 268, *268*
Labia minora, 268, *268*
Labial arteries, 263t
  inferior and superior, 522–524, *523t*
  superior, 574, 575
Labial glands, 557, *558*
Labial nerves, 270
Labyrinth
  bony, 583–584, *584–585*
  cochlear, 583
  membranous, 584–586, *584–585*
  vestibular, 584
Labyrinthine wall, of tympanic cavity, 580, *581*,
    581–582
Lacrimal apparatus, 532, *532*
Lacrimal artery, *546*, 547, 547t
Lacrimal canaliculi, 532, *533*
Lacrimal caruncle, *532*, 533
Lacrimal ducts, *532*, 533
Lacrimal gland, *532*, 533
  excretory ducts of, 533
Lacrimal gland(s)
  fossa for, 529, *529*
  nerve supply of, 533, 662
Lacrimal groove, 529
Lacrimal lake, *530*, 532, 533
Lacrimal nerve, *521t*, 544, *545*, 572
Lacrimal papilla, *531*, 533
Lacrimal punctum, *532*, 533
Lacrimal sac, fossa for, 529, *529*
Lacteals, 154
Lactiferous ducts, 56, *56*
Lactiferous sinuses, 56, *56*
Lacunar ligament, 127, *127*
Lambda, 498, *499*
Lambdoid suture, 499, *499*
Laminae, 277, *278*
  of laryngeal prominence, 623, *623*
Laminectomy, 278, *278*, 287
Laparoscopic appendectomy, 160
Laparoscopic examination, of pelvic viscera,
    249, *249*
Laparoscopic tubal ligation, 249
Laparotomy, 141
Large elastic arteries, 24, *25*
Large intestine, 140, 154–159
  arteries of, 156, *156*
  cecum and appendix of, 154–157
  colon of, 157–159
  lymphatics of, 156–157, *157*, 158
  nerves and innervation of, *157*, 158–159
  rectum and anal canal of, 159
  vasculature of, 151t
Laryngeal arteries, superior and inferior,
    627, *628*
Laryngeal cavity, 625, *625*
Laryngeal inlet, 624, 632
Laryngeal muscles, 627, 627–628, 629t
Laryngeal nerves
  external, 628, *628*
  inferior and superior, 627, *628*
  injury to, 630
  internal, 564, *566*, 627–628, *628*
  recurrent, 618, 627, *668*
    injury of, 112
    left, 103, *103*, 105t, *109*, 618, *621*
    right, *109*, *617*, 618
Laryngeal prominence, 623, *623*, 624
Laryngeal saccule, 625, *625*
Laryngeal skeleton, 623–625, *623*
  fracture of, 630
Laryngeal veins, superior and inferior, 627
Laryngeal ventricle, 625, *625*
Laryngeal vestibule, 625, *625*
Laryngopharynx, 560, 632–634, *633*
  foreign bodies in, 639
Laryngoscopy, 630, *630*
Larynx, 623–628, *623*
  interior of, 625–627, *625–626*
  lymphatic drainage of, 622, 627
  muscles of, 627, 627–628, 629t
  nerves of, 627–628, *628*
  skeleton of, 623–625, *623*
  surface anatomy of, 624, *624*
  vasculature of, 627, *628*
Lateral, definition of, *4t*
Lateral aperture, 512, *515*
Lateral cricoarytenoid, 629t
Lateral cutaneous nerve, *194*, 195
Lateral epicondyle
  of femur, *319*, 385
  of humerus, 408–409, *410*
Lateral epicondylitis, 460
Lateral geniculate bodies, 652, *652*
Lateral horns, of spinal gray matter, 38
Lateral inguinal fossae, 121, *122*

Lateral ligament, *555*
  of ankle, 396, *396*
  of urinary bladder, 215
Lateral malleolus, 322, *323*, 329
Lateral meniscus, 388, *388*
Lateral pelvic walls, 211
Lateral pterygoid, 550t, 552
  relationship of nerves to, *554*
Lateral rectus, *531*, 540–543, *540–541*, 540t, *543*
  innervation of, 656–657
Lateral rotation, *6*
Lateral umbilical folds, 121, *122*
Lateral ventricles, 512, *515*
Lateral wall, of tympanic cavity, 580, *581–582*
Laterality, terms of, *5*
Latissimus dorsi, 424, *425t*
  surface anatomy of, 429
Left atrium. *See* Atria, of heart
Left venous angle, 29, *30*
Left ventricle, 90, *90*
Leg, 357–370. *See also* Lower limb
  anterior compartment of, 357, *358–359*, *359t*
  compartment infections in, 361
  compartment syndromes in, 335
  fascia of, 330–331, *331*
  lateral compartment of, *359t*, 360, *360*
  leg region, 317, *317*
  medical imaging of, *404*
  muscles of
    anterior and lateral, 357, *358–359*, *359t*
    posterior deep, 363–366, *365*, 365t–366t, *366*
    posterior superficial, 363, *364*, 365t
  nerves of, *357*, *358*, 360, 366, *367*, 369t
  posterior compartment of, 363–370, *364*
  surface anatomy of
    anterior, *358*
    lateral, *360*
    posterior, *364*
  vasculature of, *370t*
Lens, 535–536, *537*
  changing, for distant and near vision, 538, *538*
Lenticular process, 581
Leptomeninx, 509
Lesser omentum, *137–138*, 138, 167, *168*
Lesser palatine nerves, 207–208
Lesser pelvis, 207–208, *250*
Lesser trochanter, 318, *319*
Lesser tubercle, of humerus, *408*, 410, 416
Lesser vestibular glands, 269–270
Levator ani, 211, *213–214*, 213t, 257
Levator palpebrae superioris, *531*, 540, *540–541*, 540t
Levator scapulae, 424–427, *425t*, 614, 615t
Levator veli palatini, 562t, *563*, 633
Levatores costarum, 305, 307t, *308*
Ligaments. *See also* Suspensory ligaments
  of abdominal viscera, 136–138, *137*
  accessory, *289*, 290
  of ankle joint, 396–397, *396*
  of cervical intervertebral joints, *291*, 292
  of Cooper, 56

of elbow, *482*, 483
of femoral head, 318, *319*, *380*, 381
of foot, 371–372, *371*
of glenohumeral joint, *478*, 479
of hand, 461–462, *461–462*, *489–490*
of hip joint, 379–381, *381*
of inguinal region, 127, *127*
of knee joint, 386–388, *387*
of laryngeal skeleton, 623, *623*
nuchal, *289*, 290, 596
of pelvis, *207*, 209–211, *210*
of plantar region, 398, *398*
pulmonary, 68
of radio-ulnar joints, *484*, 485
sternopericardial, 80
stylohyoid, *667*
tibiofibular, 389, *391*
umbilical, 121, *122*
of uterus, 239–240, *240*
of vertebral column, 288–292, *289*
Ligamenta flava, *289*, 290
Ligamentum arteriosum, 103, *103*, 105
Ligamentum venosum, 167
Light reflex, 587
Limbal plexus, 535–536, *537*
Limbus, of cornea, 534
Line, bone, *10*, 11
Linea alba, *119*, 120, 124, *124*
Linea aspera, 318, *319*, 339
Linea terminalis, 205
Lines of pleural reflection, 68
Lingual artery, 564, *567*, 605, 609, *609*
Lingual carcinoma, 569
Lingual frenulum, 564, *564*, 606
Lingual nerve, *554*, 555, 564, *566*, 569, 660, *661*
Lingual papillae, 563, *563*
Lingual septum, 564
Lingual tonsil, 633, 635
Lingual vein(s), 609
  deep, 564, *564*
Lingula, 71, *71*, 72
Lips, 557, *557*
  squamous cell carcinoma of, 527, *527*
  transition zone of, 557, *557*, 562
Lithotripsy, 225
Liver, 165–171, *166*. *See also hepatic entries*
  bare area of, *166*, 167
  biopsy of, 173
  borders of, 165, *166*
  cirrhosis of, 173
  lobectomies and segmentectomy, 173
  lobes and segments of, 167–169, *168–169*
  lymphatics of, 169–170, *170*
  peritoneal relations of, 165
  recesses of, 165, *166*
  rupture of, 173
  surface anatomy of, 167, *167*
  surfaces of, 165–167, *166*
  vasculature and nerves of, 168–171
  venous sinusoids of, 173
Lobar arteries, 75, *75*
Lobectomy
  hepatic, 173
  of lungs, 78

Lobes
  of liver, 167–169, *168–169*
  of lungs, 71, 72, *73*
Lobule, ear lobe, *578*, 579
Locomotion, 377, *378t*
Long bones, 9, 11
Long plantar ligament, 398, *398*
Long thoracic nerve, *434*, 434t
Longissimus, 304, 305t, *306*
Longissimus capitis, *306*
Longissimus thoracis, *306*
Longitudinal arch, of foot, 401, *401*
Longitudinal band ligaments, *291*, 292
Longitudinal muscles, of tongue, 565t
Longus capitis, *312t*, *614t*
Longus colli, *614t*, 617
Lordosis, 276, *276*
Lower limb, 316–404
  bones of, 318–329, *319–320*
    surface anatomy of, 327–329, *327–328*
  compartment syndromes of, 335
  cutaneous innervation of, 333–334, *334*, 335
  fascia of, 329–331, *330*
  joints of, 379–402
    ankle, 395–398
    hip, 379–384
    knee, 385–389
    tibiofibular, 389–391
  lymphatic drainage of, 332–333, *332*
  medical imaging of, *403–404*
  muscles of
    anterior thigh, 336–340
    foot, 372–373
    leg, 363–366
  nerves and innervation of. *See* Ankle; Foot; Gluteal nerves; Knee joint; Leg; Thigh
  overview of, 317, *317*
  regions of, *317*
    foot, 371–377
    leg, 357–370
    popliteal fossa, 356–357
    thigh and gluteal, 336–355
  subcutaneous tissue of, 329–331, *330*
  surface anatomy of, 327–329, *327–329*
  venous drainage of, 331–332, *331–332*
  walking and gait cycle, 377–378
Lumbar arteries, 195, *195–196*
  spinal and equatorial branches of, 294, *294*
Lumbar cistern, 296, 297, 298, 300
Lumbar curvature, 275–276, *276*, 277
Lumbar lymph nodes, 179, 196, *197*, 229t, *230t*
Lumbar lymph trunks, 196, *197*
Lumbar plexus, 194, *194*
Lumbar spinal cord, 296, 297
Lumbar spinal puncture, 300, *300*
Lumbar spinal stenosis, 286–287, *287*
Lumbar splanchnic nerves, *147*, 158, 182, *183t*, *184*, 241
Lumbar vertebrae, 277, 282t
  surface anatomy of, 284, *284*
Lumbocostal triangle, 191
Lumbosacral angle, 275
Lumbosacral enlargement, of spinal cord, 296, 297

Lumbosacral joints, 209, *210*
Lumbosacral trunk, 194, *194*, 217, *218–219*
Lumbricals, 373t, *374*, 463–466, *463*, 465t
Lunate, 411, *411–412*, 489
  anterior dislocation of, 491
Lung(s), *69*, *71*. *See also pulmonary entries*
  apex and hilum of, 71, *72*
  aspiration of foreign bodies into, 78
  auscultation and percussion of, 77, 78
  autonomic innervation of, 77
  blood clots in, 79
  borders of, 71, *71*, *72*
  bronchi of, 71–74, *73–74*
  collapse of, 77
  horizontal and oblique fissures, 71, *71*, 72
  internal structure of, 74, *74*
  lobes of, 71, 72, *73*
    variations in, 77
  lymphatics of, 75–76, *76*
  and pleurae, 68–79, *69*
    medical conditions involving, 77–79
    surface anatomy of, 70, *70*
    vasculature and nerves of, 75–79, *75–76*
  root of, 68
  surfaces of, 71, *72*
Lung cancer, 79
Lung resection, 78
Lymph, 28, 225
Lymph nodes, 29, *29*. *See also* Lymphoid system
  of abdominal viscera, 143, 145, *152*, 157
  anterior abdominal wall, 126, *126*
  axillary, *421*, 422, 432–433, *432*
  cancerous, 30
  cervical, deep, 526
  cubital, *421*, 422
  deltopectoral, *421*, 422
  of female pelvis and perineum, 229t
  gluteal, *351*, 353
  of head and neck, 527, 638
  inferior tracheobronchial, *76*, 97
  inguinal, *332*, 333
  laryngeal, 627
  lumbar, 132
  parotid, 526
  of pelvis, 223, *223*, 229t
  popliteal, *332*, 333, 356, *356*
  posterior mediastinum, 112
  pulmonary, 76, *76*
  submandibular, 526
  superficial inguinal, 126, *126*
Lymph vessels. *See* Lymphatic vessels
Lymphadenitis, 30
Lymphadenopathy, 336
Lymphangitis, 30
Lymphatic capillaries, 28, *29*
Lymphatic drainage/vessels. *See also specific*
    structures or organs drained
  of abdominal wall, anterolateral, 126, *126*
  of breast, 56–60, *57*
  of diaphragm, 190, *190*, 190t
  of posterior mediastinum, 111–112, *111*
  of scrotum, testis, and spermatic cord,
    131, *131*
  of thymus, *76*, 102

of urinary organs, 227–228
Lymphatic ducts, 30
  right, *29*, 30, 76, *76*, 103, *103*, 638
  thoracic duct, *29*, 30, 76, *76*, 103, *111*, 197,
    197, 649
Lymphatic plexus(es), 28, *29*
  deep, 76
  of diaphragm, 190, *190*
  of heart, 97
  in lungs, 75–76, *76*
  subareolar, 56, *57*
Lymphatic system. *See* Lymphoid system
Lymphatic trunks, *29*
  bronchomediastinal, *76*, 76
  descending thoracic, 197, *197*
  subclavian, 56, *57*
  thoracic duct and, *29*
Lymphatic vessels, 28–29, *29*. *See also* Lym-
    phoid system
Lymphedema, 30
Lymphocytes, 29
Lymphogenic metastasis, 58
Lymphoid nodules, of tongue, 564
Lymphoid organs, 30
Lymphoid system, 2, 28–31, *29*
  functions of, 28, 29–31

M

Macula
  of retina, 534–535, 537, *537*
  of utricle and saccule, 585, *585*
Macula lutea, 535, 537, *537*
Magnetic resonance imaging (MRI)
  of abdomen, 201–202
  angiogram of heart and great vessels, *115*
  of arm, *493*
  of glenohumeral and acromioclavicular
    joints, *494*
  of head, 591–592
  of lower limb, *403–404*
  of neck, 641, *642*
  of pelvis and perineum, 271–272
  of vertebral column, spinal cord, and CSF,
    314, 315
Main bronchus (bronchi), 44, *46*
Male genital organs
  external, 261–265, *262*
  internal, *228*, 233–236
  sterilization (vasectomy) and, 132, 233
Male gonads, relocation (descent) of, 133
Male pelvis, *224*, 227. *See also* Pelvis; Perineum
  compared to female pelvis, 208t, 209
  fascia and ligaments of, *216*
  genital organs within, *228*, 233–236
  innervation of, 236, *236*
  lymphatics and lymph nodes of, 230t
  medical imaging of, *271*
  peritoneal reflections in, 212t
  supporting and compressive muscles of, 232
Male perineum, 261–267
  distal urethra, 261
  fascia and pouches of, 253–256, *254*

innervation of, 265, *266*
lymphatics of, 230t, 265, *265*
medical imaging of, *271*
muscles of, *251–252*, 252t, 267, *267*
penis, 261–266
scrotum, 261, *262*
vasculature of, 263–265, 263t, *264*
Male urethra, 227, 231–232
  distal, 261
  innervation of, *231*, 232
  intermediate (membranous), 231, 232t, 261
  parts of, 232t
  rupture of, 256, *256*
  spongy, *226–227*, 231, 232t, 261
  vasculature of, 228, 232
Male urinary bladder, *226*
Male urogenital organs
  external, 261–265, *262*
  internal, *228*, 233–236
Malleolus, *10*, 12
Mallet finger, 460, *460*
Malleus, 580, *581*, 587
Mammary gland ligaments, 56
Mammary glands, 53, 56
Mammography, 59, *59*
Mandible, 496, *497*
  fractures of, 557
  head of, 555, *555*
Mandibular canal, 556
Mandibular fossa, 555, *555*
Mandibular nerve (CN V3), 554, *554*, 559
  block, 556
  cutaneous nerves from, 519, *521*, 522t
  distribution of, *658*
  motor innervation of face, 522
  summary of, *646t–647t*, 659t
Mandibular symphysis, 496, *497*
Manubrium, 49, 51, *51*
Marginal artery, 158
Marrow, bone
  in ribs, 48, *49*
  in sternum, 54
Masseter, *528*, 550t
Mastectomy, 59, *59*
Mastication, muscles of, 550t
Mastoid antrum, 580, *581*
Mastoid foramen, 500t
Mastoid process, 497, *498*, 499, *500*
Mastoid wall, of tympanic cavity, 580, *581*
Maxilla, 496, *497*
  frontal process of, 573, *573*
  palatine process of, *561*
Maxillary artery, 552, *552–553*
  branches of, 552–554, *552*, 558
  pterygopalatine part of, *572–573*, *572*
Maxillary nerve (CN V2), 559, *658*, 659t
  cutaneous nerves from, 519, *521t*
  in pterygopalatine fossa, 570–571, *571*
  summary of, *646t–647t*
Maxillary ostium, 576, *576*
Maxillary sinuses, 529, *529*, 574, 576, *576*
  apex, floor, base, and roof of, 576
  infection of, 577
  relationship of teeth to, 578

Maxillary teeth, 496, *497*
Medial, definition of, *4t*
Medial epicondyle, *319, 446*
　avulsion of, 486
　of femur, *319, 385*
　of humerus, *408–409, 410*
Medial inguinal fossae, 121, *122*
Medial ligament, of ankle, 396, *396*
Medial malleolus, 322, *323, 328*
Medial meniscus, 388, *388*
　tears in, and repair, 393–394, *393–394*
Medial pterygoid, *550t,* 552
Medial rectus, *531,* 540–543, *540–541,* 540t, *543*
Medial rotation, *6*
Medial wall, of tympanic cavity, 580, *581–582*
Median antebrachial vein, 421, *421*
Median aperture, 512, *515*
Median cubital vein, 421, *421,* 424
Median nerve, 456, *457, 458t*
　course of, *434,* 435t, *442–443,* 443
　in hand, 468, *468*
　recurrent branch of, *457*
　trauma to, 471–472, *472*
Median plane, 3, *3*
　of abdominal cavity, 117, *117*
Median sacral artery, 195, *196*
Median sternotomy, 54
Median umbilical fold, 121, *122*
Median umbilical ligament, 121, *122*
Mediastinal arteries, 108
Mediastinal lymph nodes, posterior, 170
Mediastinum, 80–84
　of testes, 130, *130*
　thoracic, 80–102, *80. See also* Thoracic
　　　mediastinum
　　anterior, 80, *80*
　　inferior, 80, *80*
　　levels of viscera in, 84, *84*
　　middle, 80–102, *80*
　　posterior, 80, 108–113, *109*
　　superior, 80, 102–108, *103–104*
Medical imaging, 42–46
　of abdomen, 199, *199–203*
　of back, 314–315, *314–315*
　of head, 589, *589–592,* 591
　of lower limb, *403–404*
　of pelvis and perineum, *271–273*
　of thorax, *114–115*
　of upper limb, *492–494*
Medium muscular arteries, 24, *25*
Medulla oblongata, 296, 512, *513*
Medullary arteries
　anterior and posterior, 299, 301, *302*
　great anterior segmental (of Adamkiewicz),
　　299, 301, *302*
Medullary cavity, of bone, 11, *11*
Membranous labyrinth, 584–586, *584–585*
Membranous wall, of tympanic cavity, 580,
　581–582
Meningeal artery, middle, 508, *509*
　hemorrhage of, 498
Meningeal branches
　of hypoglossal nerve, 671
　of spinal nerves, 294–295, *295*

of trigeminal nerve, *658*
of vagus nerve, 669t
Meningeal layer, of cranial dura mater, 504,
　505
Meninges
　cranial, 503–511, *504*
　　spaces associated with, 511
　herniation of, 285
　innervation of, *295*
　spinal, 31, *33, 297, 298*
　　spaces associated with, 299t
Meningocele, 285
Meningomyelocele, 285–286
Menisci, of knee joint, 388, *388*
Meniscofemoral ligament, posterior, *387,* 388
Mental artery, 558
Mental foramina, 496, *497*
Mental nerve, *521,* 522t, *554, 555*
Mental protuberance, 496, *497*
Mesenchyme, bone derivation from, 12, *13*
Mesenteric lymph nodes, *147,* 154
Mesentery(ies), 136, 152
　intestinal, 136, 138–139, *138–139*
　root of, 152
Mesoappendix, 156, *156*
Mesometrium, 239, *240*
Mesosalpinx, 239, *240*
Mesovarium, 239, *240,* 244
Metacarpal bones, 411, *411–412*
　bases and heads of, 411, *411,* 416, 474
Metacarpal ligament, superficial transverse,
　418, 419
Metacarpophalangeal joints, *490t*
Metaphysial arteries, 13, *13*
Metaphysis, bone, 12, *13*
Metastasis, 30
　of breast cancer, 58
Metatarsal arteries, dorsal and plantar, 376,
　376, 377
Metatarsal bones, *319–320, 324, 325*
　base, shaft, head of, *324, 325*
　fractures of, *327, 327*
　surface anatomy of, 329, *329*
　tuberosity of fifth, 329329
Metatarsophalangeal joints, 399, *400t*
Metatarsus, *324, 325*
Metopic suture, 496, *497*
Midaxillary line, 65, *66*
Midbrain, 512, *513*
Midclavicular lines, 65, *65*
Midclavicular planes, of abdominal cavity,
　117, *117*
Middle ear, 580–583, *581*
Middle mediastinum, 80–102, *80. See also*
　Heart; Pericardium
Middle pharyngeal constrictor, *637t*
Midfoot, 371, *371*
Midinguinal points, of abdominal cavity,
　117, *117*
Midpalmar space, 461, *462*
Mitral valve, *88, 90, 90*
　prolapsed, 92
Modiolus, 583, *586*
Molar tooth, 557–558, *558*

Mons pubis, 268, *268*
Motor (efferent) fibers, 34, *34,* 35–36, 644, *645*
Motor neuron, *30*
Motor nuclei, of cranial nerves, 649
Motor unit, 20, *22*
Movement, terminology of, 5, *5–6*
MRI scan. *See* Magnetic resonance imaging
Multifidus, 305, 307t, *308*
Mumps, 528
Murmurs, heart, 91
Muscle contraction, 19–20
Muscle fibers, *18, 22*
Muscle spindles, 307
Muscle testing, 22, 460, *460*
Muscle tone, 19
Muscles. *See also* Muscular system; *specific*
　　muscles and regions
　of abdominal wall
　　anterolateral, 119–121
　　posterior, 193, *193t*
　of arm, 440–443
　arrector, 7, *8,* 20–22
　atrophy of, 23
　of back, 301–313
　cardiac muscle, 17, *18t,* 20
　of face, 519, *520t*
　of female pelvis/perineum, 251–252, 252t
　of foot, 372–373, 373t, *374*
　of forearm, 446–456
　of gluteal region, 347, *347,* 348t
　of hand, 462–466
　hypertrophy of, 23
　intercostal, 61, *61*
　of leg, 357, 363–366
　of male pelvis/perineum, 251–252, 252t
　of mastication, *550t*
　muscle fiber, 20, *22*
　of neck. *See* Neck, muscles of
　of orbit, 540–543
　origin/insertion of, 19
　of pelvic walls and floor, 211–215
　of perineum, *251–252,* 252t
　shapes of (skeletal muscle), 18–19
　skeletal, 17–19, *18t,* 20
　smooth muscle, 17, *19t,* 20–22
　of thigh, 336–340
　of thoracic wall, 60–61, *60t*
　types of, 17, *18t–19t, 21*
Muscular (omotracheal) triangle, 597, 607, 613t
Muscular process, of arytenoid cartilage, 624, *626*
Muscular system, 2, 17–23. *See also* Muscles
Musculocutaneous nerve, *434,* 435t,
　　442–443, 444
　injury to, 445
Musculophrenic artery(ies), 126, 126t, *187*
Musculophrenic veins, *187*
Musculovenous pump, 28
Musculus uvulae, *562t,* 563
Mydriasis, 536
Myelin, 31
　demyelinating diseases, 654
Myelin sheath, *30, 31*
Myelinated nerves, 33
　neurolemma of, 31–33, *33*

Myelography, 314, *314*
Myeloid tissue, 30
Mylohyoid, *560*, *605–606*
  fibrous raphe of, 604
Myocardial infarction (MI), 23, 100
Myocardial necrosis, 23, 100
Myocardium, *18t*, 20, 84
Myometrium, 239, *239*
Myotomes, 35–36, *35*
  of thorax, 62, *63*
Myringotomy, 588, *588*

N

Nasal artery, *523t*, 524, *525*
Nasal cavity, 573–574, *574*
  section of, *560*
Nasal conchae, *496*, *497*, *560*, 574, *574–575*, *633*
Nasal fractures, 577
Nasal meatus, superior, middle, and inferior, 574, *575*
Nasal mucosa, 576
Nasal nerve, external, *521t*
Nasal region, 573–578
  bones and arteries of, *573*, *575*
Nasal septum, *496*, *497*, 499, *500*, 573, *573*, *633*
  bones, arteries and nerves of, *575*
  deviated, 577, *577*
  innervation of, *658*
Nasion, *496*, *497*
Nasociliary nerve, 544, *545*
Nasolacrimal duct, 532, *533*, 574
Nasopalatine nerves, *560*, *562*, 574, *575*
Nasopharynx, *560*, 631, *632*, *633*
Navicular, *319*, 323, *324*
Navicular tuberosity, 323, *329*
Neck, 593–642. *See also* Cervical regions; *cervical entries*
  bones and cartilages of, 594, *594*
  deep structures of, 613–619
  fascia of, 594–596, *595*
  infection, spread of, 597
  lymphatics and lymph nodes in, 638–639, *638*
  medical imaging of, 641, *641–642*
  muscles of
    anterior, 607, *608t*
    cutaneous and superficial, *599t*
    deep, 311–312, *311*
    laryngeal, 627, *627–628*, *629t*
    lateral, 598, *600*
    pharyngeal, 634–635, *635*
    prevertebral, 613, *614*, *614–615t*
  nerve point of, 600, 604, *604*
  nerves and innervation of
    lateral, 598–602, *601*
    root of, *621*
  radical dissection of, 639
  regions of, 596, *597*, 613t
    anterior, 604–611
    lateral, 598–604
    posterior, 598
    sternocleidomastoid, 596–598

summary of, 613t
root of, 613–618, *616–617*
  arteries of, 615–616, *616*
  nerves in, *617*, 618, *621*
  veins of, 616–618
skeleton of, 594, *594*
skin of, 611
subcutaneous tissue of, 594, *595*
superficial structures of, 596–613
surface anatomy of
  cervical regions and triangles, 611–613, *612*
  larynx, 624, *624*
  trauma, 640, *640*
  triangles of, 597, 611–613, *612*, 613t
  viscera of, 619–638
    alimentary layer of, *620*, 631–638
    endocrine layer of, 619–622, *620*
    respiratory layer of, *620*, 623–631
  zones of penetrating trauma, 640, *640*
Nerves. *See also* Nervous system; *specific structures and nerves*
  articular, 17
  cranial, *32*, 33–34, 643–672. *See also* Cranial Nerves
    overview of, 644–650, *645*
  ganglia of, 33. *See also* Parasympathetic ganglia; Spinal ganglia; Sympathetic ganglia
  myelinated, 33*33*
  peripheral, 31–33, *32*, *33*
  rami of, *34*, *35*
  spinal, *32*, 34–36. *See also* Spinal nerves
  vasomotor, 13
Nerve blocks. *See specific structure or nerve*
Nerve cell bodies, 30, *31*
Nerve ganglion (ganglia), 33. *See also* Spinal ganglia
Nerve point of neck, 600, 604, *604*
Nervous system, 2, 31–42. *See also* Nerves
  autonomic, 31, 36–42. *See also* Autonomic innervation; Autonomic nervous system
  central, 31, *32*. *See also* Brain; Spinal cord
  organization of, 31, *32*
  parasympathetic, 36, 42. *See also* Parasympathetic innervation
  peripheral, 31–34. *See also* Peripheral nerves
  somatic, 34–36
  spinal nerves of. *See also* Spinal nerves
  sympathetic, 36. *See also* Sympathetic innervation
Neurocranium, *496*, *497*
Neuroglia, 31
Neurolemma, *30*, 31–33
Neurons, 31
  motor, *30*
  myelinated and unmyelinated, 31–33, *33*
  presynaptic and postsynaptic, 36, *37*
  structure of, *30*, 31
Neurotransmittors, 31, 37
Nipples, 56, 67, *67*
  supernumerary, 58, *67*
Node of Ranvier, *33*

Norepinephrine, 37
Nose, 573–578, *575*
  bones and cartilages of, 573, *573*
  cavities of, 573–574
  external, 573, *573*
  fracture of, 577
  lateral wall, features and structures of, *574–575*
  paranasal sinuses, 574–576, *576*
  respiratory and olfactory areas of, 573–574, *575*
Notch, bone, *10*, 12
Nuchal ligament, 289, *290*, 596
Nuchal line(s), inferior and superior, 498, *499*
Nuck, canal of, 135
Nucleus, *31*, 32
Nucleus pulposus, 287, *288*, 289
  herniation of, 293, *293*
Nutrient artery
  of bone, 12–13, *13*
  of tibia, 367, *370*
Nutrient canal, 322
Nutrient foramina, 13, 322, *323*

O

Oblique arytenoid, *629t*, *633*
Oblique pericardial sinus, 81–82, *81–82*
Oblique popliteal ligament, 387, *387*
Obliquus capitis posterior, major and minor, 311, *311*
Obturator artery, *222t*, *344t*, 346
  replaced or accessory, 345
Obturator externus, 338–339, *339t*, *340*
Obturator fascia, 211, *213–214*
Obturator foramen, 206, *206*, 211
Obturator internus, 211, *213–214*, 214t, 347, *347*, 348t
  nerve to, *219*, 349, 351, 352t
Obturator nerve, 218, *219*, 346
  course of, 194, *194*, 211, *434*, 435t, *442–443*, 443
  injury to, 218
Occipital artery, 525, *525*, 603, *605*, *607*, *609*
Occipital bone, 499, *500*
Occipital condyles, 499, *500*
Occipital nerves
  lesser, *521*, 522t, 600, *601*
  lesser, greater, third, *521*, 522t
Occipital sinus, 505–506, *506*
Occipital triangle, 597, 598, *612*, 613t
Occipital vein, 526, *526*, *609*, 610
Occipitofrontalis, *520t*
Occiput, 498, *499*
Ocular palsies, 657, *657*
Oculomotor nerve (CN III), 544, *545*, 654–655, *654*
  distribution of, *654*, 656
  divisions of, 654–655, *654*
  intracranial portion of, *648*
  nucleus of, *649*
  palsy of, 548, *548*, 657, *657*
  summary of, *646t–647t*

Olecranon, 410, *411*, 416
Olecranon bursa, 483, *483*
Olecranon fossa, 410
Olfactory bulb, 650, *650*
Olfactory fibers, loss of (anosmia), 650
Olfactory nerve (CN I), 575, 650–651
  intracranial portion of, *648*
  summary of, *646t–647t*
Olfactory receptor neurons, 650
Olfactory system, 650–651
Olfactory tract, 650, *650*
Omental appendices, 154
Omental bursa, 138, *139–140*
  stomach in relation to, 146, *149t*
Omental foramen, *137*, 138–139
  lymph node of, 172
Omentum, 136–137
  greater, 137, *137–138*
  lesser, *137–138*, 138
Omoclavicular triangle, 597, 598, *612*, 613t
Omohyoid, 597, 605, 607, *608t*
Ophthalmic artery, 545–547, *546*, 547t
Ophthalmic nerve (CN V1), 658, 659t
  branches supplying orbit, 544, *545*
  cutaneous nerves from, 519, *521t*
Ophthalmic veins, 547, *547*
Ophthalmoscopy, 538, *538*
Opponens digiti minimi, 462–463, *463*, 464t
Opponens pollicis, 462, *463*, 464t
Optic canal, 496, *497*, 500t, *501*, 502, 529·
Optic chiasm, 652, *652*
Optic disc, 537, *537*, 652
Optic nerve (CN II), 652–654, *652*
  demyelinating disease of, 654
  entering the eyeball, *535*
  intracranial portion of, *648*
  summary of, *646t–647t*
Optic sheath, 544
Optic tract, 652, *652*
Ora serrata, *535*, 537
Oral cavity, 557, *557*
  median section of, *560*
  proper, 557, *557*
Oral fissure, 557, *557*
Oral region, 557–569
  lymphatics and lymph nodes of, 557, 558
Oral vestibule, 557–558, *557*
Orbicularis oculi, 519, *520t*, *531*, 532
Orbicularis oris, 519, *520t*
Orbit, 529–548, *529–532*
  apex of, 529, *545*
  bony features of, 529, *529*
  dissection of, superficial/deep, *544*
  extra-ocular muscles of, 540–543, *540–541*, 540t
    paralysis of, 548, *548*
  eyeball in, 533–538, *534–535*
  eyelids and lacrimal apparatus of, 530–533
  fascial sheath of, *544*
  fractures of, 530
  nerves of, 544–545, *545*
  tumors of, 530
  vasculature of, 545–547, *546*, 547t
Orbital fat, 529

Orbital fissure(s), 496, *497*
  superior, 529, *529*
Orbital plates, of frontal bone, *501*, 502
Orbital septum, *531*, 532
Orbitomeatal plane, 496
Origin, of muscles, 19
Oropharynx, 557, *560*, 632, *633*
Osgood-Schlatter disease, 326, *326*
Osseofibrous tunnels, 466, *466*
Osseus spiral lamina, 585, *586*
Ossification, 12, *13*
  of clavicle, 413
  endochondral, 12, 413
  intramembranous, 12, 413
Osteoarthritis, 17, 392
Osteons, *13*
Osteoporosis, 12
Otic capsule, 583, *584*, 586
Otic ganglion, 554, *554*, 667
  summary of, *672t*
Otitis externa, 588
Otitis media, 588, *588*
Otoscopic examination, 587, *588*
  of tympanic membrane, 579–580, *579*
Outcropping muscles, 456
Oval fossa, 87, *87*
Oval window, 580
Ovarian arteries, 222, 222t, 244
Ovarian fimbria, 243
Ovarian veins, 196, *196*, 244–245
Ovary(ies), *240*, 244–245
  fetal, relocation of, 133
  ligaments of, 239, *240*, 244
  vasculature and innervation of, *238*, 241–242, 244–245

P

P signs, of arterial occlusion, 362
Pacemaker, cardiac muscle as, 20
PAD (palmar adduct) mnemonic, 372, 465–466
Pain sensation, visceral referred, 186, *186*
Palate, 560–563, *560*
  bones of, *561*
  hard, 560–561, *560–561*
  soft, 560–562, 561
    muscles of, 562, *562*, 562t
  vasculature and innervation of, *561*, 562, 667
Palatine aponeurosis, 561, *561*
Palatine arteries, greater and lesser, 562, *562*, 574, 575
Palatine bone, 529, *529*
  horizontal plates of, 499, *500*
Palatine foramina, 499, *500*, 561, *561*, 562
Palatine gingivae, *559*, 560
Palatine nerves, greater and lesser, 560, 562, 574, 575
Palatine processes, of maxillae, 499, *500*
Palatine tonsils, 561, *562*, 632, *633*
Palatine vein, external, 635
Palatoglossal arches, 561, *561–562*, 632, *634*
Palatoglossus, *562t*, 563, *565t*
Palatopharyngeal arches, 561, *561–562*, 632,

634
Palatopharyngeus, 563, 632, *633*, 634, *635*, 637t
Palm, *4t*, 5. *See also* Hand
  arteries and nerves of, 466–469, *468–469*
  compartments and spaces of, 461–462, *462*
  fascia of, *418*, 419, 461–462, *461–462*
  skin creases of, 474, *474*
  wounds and surgical incisions of, 470
Palmar aponeurosis, *418*, 461, *461*
Palmar arch(es), 459t, 467–468, *467t*, *468*
  deep, *459*, 467, *467t*, *468*
  laceration of, 470
  superficial, 467, *467t*, *468*
Palmar carpal ligament, *418*, 447
Palmar digital arteries, *461*
Palmar fascia, *418*, 419, 461–462, *461–462*
  Dupuytren contracture of, 470, *470*
Palmar interosseous muscles, 371, *372*, 373t, *374*
Palmar ligament, 453
Palmaris brevis, *461*, 463
Palmaris longus, 447, *449*, 450t
  tendon of, 473–474, *473*
Palpation
  of abdomen, 123
  of dorsalis pedis pulse, 362, *362*
  of inguinal ring, 135, *135*
  of uterus, 243, *243*
Palpebral commissures, medial and lateral, 532–533
Palpebral conjunctiva, 530, *530*
Palpebral glands, inflammation of, 533
Palpebral ligaments, medial and lateral, *531*, 533
Pampiniform venous plexus, 130–131, *130*, 244
Pancreas, 162–164, *163*
  arteries of, *163*, 164
  head, body and tail of, 162
  neck of, 162
  nerves of, *163*
  relationships of, *149t*, 150
  rupture of, 165
  stomach in relation to, 146, *149t*
  surface anatomy of, 161, *161*
Pancreatic arteries, *163*, 164
Pancreatic cancer, 165
Pancreatic duct, 162–163, *164*, 171, *172*
  sphincter of, 162–163, *164*
Pancreatic veins, 164
Pancreaticoduodenal artery(ies), 146t, 171
  superior, *145*
  superior and inferior, 146t
Pancreaticoduodenal lymph nodes, 145, *147*, 152
Pancreaticoduodenal veins, *145*, 172
Pancreaticosplenic lymph nodes, 145, *147*, 162, 164
Pap smear, 242, *242*
Papillary muscles, of heart, 88, *88*, 90
Papilledema, 539
Paracentesis, 141
Paracolic gutters, 139–140, *140*, 158
Paracolic lymph nodes, 158

Paracolpium, *216*, 217
Paraesophageal hiatal hernia, 159
Parallel muscles, 19, *21*
Paranasal sinuses, 574–576, *576*, *577*
Paranephric fat, 176, *177*
Paraphimosis, 266
Pararectal fossae, *212t*
Pararectal lymph nodes, 223, *223*, *229t*, *230t*, 247, *247*
Parasympathetic fibers, 154
Parasympathetic ganglia, 77, *672t*
Parasympathetic innervation, 36–37, *36*, 37t.
    See also specific organs
    of abdomen, summary, *183t*, *184*, 185
    cranial and sacral nerves in, 42
    of heart, 99
    of intestines, 152, 154, *154*
    of intra-ocular muscles, *655*
    of pelvis, 220, *220*
    of stomach, 145–146, *147*
    visceral motor fibers in, 42, *43*
Parasympathetic secretomotor fibers, 564
Parathyroid glands, 620, *621*
Parathyroid veins, 620, *621*
Paratracheal lymph nodes, 619, *622*
Paraumbilical veins, 174
Paraurethral glands, 230, 269
Paravertebral sympathetic ganglia, 38, *39*, 77
Paravesical fossae, *212t*
Paresthesia, 336
    of hand, 471
Parietal eminences, 498, *499*
Parietal pelvic fascia, 215, *216*
Parietal peritoneum, 118, *118*, 135, *136*
    vessels and nerves of, 136
Parietal pleura, 68, *69*, 78
Parotid bed, 527
Parotid duct, 527, *528*, 568, *568*
    inflammation of, 528
Parotid gland, 526–529, *528*, 567–568, *568*
    infection and disease of, 528
    relationships with facial vasculature and
        nerves, *525*, 528
Parotid lymph nodes, 526
Parotid plexus, 660, *661*
Parotid sheath, 526–527
Parotidectomy, 528
Patella, *319*, 322, 328
    articular surfaces of, *319*, 322
    dislocation of, 392
Patellar ligament, 337, *338*, 386, *387*
Patellar retinacula, 337, *338*
Patellar tendon reflex, 340
Patellofemoral compartment, 392
Patellofemoral syndrome, 392
Peau d'orange sign, 58
Pecten pubis, 206
Pectinate line, *245*, 259, *259*
Pectineal ligament, 127, *127*
Pectineus, 336, 337t, *338*
Pectoral fascia, 417, *418*
Pectoral girdle, 406, *406*
    structures limiting movements of, 479t
Pectoral lymph nodes, 432, *432*

Pectoral muscles, 422, *422*, 423t
Pectoral nerves, medial and lateral, *434*, 435t
Pectoralis major, 422, *422*, 423t, 428
Pectoralis minor, 422, *422*, 423t
Pedicles, 277, 278
Pelvic arteries and veins, 220–222, *221*, 222t
Pelvic brim, 207
Pelvic cavity, 205, *205*
    walls and floor of, 211–215, *213t–214t*
Pelvic diaphragm, 211, *252*, 257
Pelvic examination, manual, 238
Pelvic fascia, 215–217, *216*
Pelvic floor, 211
    female, *213*
    injury to, 217
    muscles of, 211–215, *213t–214t*
Pelvic fractures, 209
Pelvic girdle, 205–209, 317
    joints and ligaments of, 209–211, *210*
    surface anatomy of, 327–328, *327–328*
Pelvic inlet, 205, *205*, 207
Pelvic ligaments, *207*, 209–211
    relaxation during pregnancy, 211
Pelvic muscles, 211–215, *213t–214t*
Pelvic nerves, 217–220, *218–219*, 218t
    autonomic, 219–220, *219*
    injury to, 218
Pelvic outlet, 205, *205*
Pelvic pain line, 220
Pelvic plexuses, *184*
Pelvic splanchnic nerves, 158, *183t*, 185, 218t, 220, 241
Pelvic venous plexuses, *221*, 222
Pelvic viscera, 223–269. *See also* Female pelvis;
        Male pelvis; Perineum
    female genital organs, 236–245
    laparoscopic examination of, 249, *249*
    lymphatic drainage of, *229t–230t*, 247
    male genital organs, 233–236
    nerves and innervation of, *231*, 248
    rectum, 245–249
    urinary organs, 223–232
Pelvirectal spaces, 217
Pelvis, 204–269. *See also* Pelvic girdle; Pelvic
        viscera
    bony, 205–209, *206*
        comparison of male and female,
            208t, 209
    boundaries of, 205, *205*
    fractures of, 209
    greater, 207, *250*
    lesser, 207–208, *250*
    ligaments of, *207*, 209–211
    lymph nodes of, 223, *223*
    male and female, *208t*, 209, *224*, *227*. *See
        also* Female pelvis; Male pelvis
    medical imaging of, 271–273, *271–273*
Penile raphe, *261*, 262
Penis, 261–266
    body of, 262–263, *262*
    crura of, 261, 262, *262*, 267
    deep arteries of, 263, 263t, *264*
    deep dorsal vein of, 263–265, *264*
    deep fascia of, 261, *262*

dorsal artery of, 263, 263t, *264*, 267
dorsal nerve of, *219*, 258, 259, 267
erectile cavernous tissue of, 261, *262*
erection, emission, ejaculation, and remis-
    sion, 265, 266
glans of, *262*, 263, 266
innervation of, 265, *266*
ligaments and muscles of, 262–263,
    267, *267*
lymphatic drainage of, 265, *265*
prepuce (foreskin) of, *262*, 263
    phimosis, paraphimosis, and circumcision
        of, 266
root of, 261–262, *262*
vasculature of, 263–265, 263t, *264*
Pennate muscles, 17, *21*
Peptic ulcers, 160
Percussion
    of heart, 91
    of lungs, 78
Percutaneous transluminal coronary angio-
        plasty, 101, *101*
Perforating arteries
    of foot, 377
    of thigh and gluteal region, 343, *344*
Perforating veins
    of lower limb, 332, *332*
    of upper limb, 421, *421*
Periarterial nerve plexus(es), 39, *40*, 154,
    158, 219
Periarticular arterial anastomoses, 17, 486
Pericardial cavity, 81, *81*
Pericardial effusion, 83
Pericardial friction rub, 83
Pericardial sac, 80, *81*, 83
Pericardial sinuses, 81–82, *82*
Pericardiocentesis, 84
Pericarditis, 83
Pericardium, 80–83, *81–83*
    arteries of, 82, 83, 108, *110*, 110t
    embryonic development of, 82, *82*
    epicardium, 81–82, *81*
    layers of, 81, *81*
    vasculature and innervation of, 82, 83
Perichondrium, 11
Pericranium, 503, *503*
Perilymph, 584, *585*, *587*
Perimetrium, 239, *239*
Perimysium, 20, *22*
Perineal artery, 258, 263t
    scrotal branches of, 132
Perineal body, 250, *251*, 257
    disruption of, 253
Perineal fascia, 227, 253, *254*
Perineal membrane, 250
Perineal muscles, 263, 267, *267*
Perineal nerves, deep and superficial,
    258–259, *258*
Perineal pouches
    deep, 253–255, *254*
    superficial, 253, *254*
Perineal raphe, *261*, 262
Perinephric abscess, 181
Perinephric fat, 176, *177*

Perineum, 250–270, *250. See also* Female perineum; Male perineum
  anal triangle, 257–260
  fascia and pouches of, 253–255, *254*
  female, 268–270, *268*
  male, 261–267
  medical imaging of, *271–273*
  muscles of, *251–252*, 252t
  subcutaneous tissue of, 253
Perineurium, 33, *33*
Periodontitis, 560
Periodontium, 558
Periorbita, 529, *529*
Periosteal arteries, 13, *13*
Periosteal bud, 12, *13*
Periosteal layer, of cranial dura mater, 504, *505*
Periosteal nerves, 13, *13*
Periosteum, 11, 13, *13*
Peripheral artery disease, 368
Peripheral nerve degeneration, 34
Peripheral nerves, 31–33, *32, 33*
  crushing injury of, 34
Peripheral nervous system (PNS), 31–34
Peristalsis, 22, 140. *See also* Abdominal viscera
Peritoneal adhesions, 141
Peritoneal cavity, 135, *136*
  closure of, in males *vs* females, 136
  subdivisions and compartments of, 138–140, *139–140*
Peritoneal dialysis, 181
Peritoneal fluid, 135–136
Peritoneal fold, *122*, 138
Peritoneal ligament, 136, *137*
Peritoneal recesses, 138
  clinical importance of, 142
Peritoneal reflections, *140*, 162
  in pelvis, male and female, 212t
Peritoneum, 135–140, *136*
  formations of, 136–138
  medical conditions involving, 141–142
  pelvic, 211, *212t*, 216
  surgical procedures of, 141
  vessels and nerves of, 136
Peritonitis, 141
Periureteric fascia, 176
Perivascular nerve plexus. *See* Periarterial nerve plexus
Pes planus (flatfeet), 402, *402*
Petrosal nerve
  deep, 572, *572*
  greater, 572
  lesser, 667
Petrosal sinuses, *505–506, 506–508*
Phagocytes, 79
Phalanx (phalanges)
  of foot, *319*, 324, 325
    proximal and distal, *319*, 325
  of hand, 411, *411–412*, 488
    bases and heads of, 411, *411*, 416
    fractures of, 414
Pharyngeal artery, ascending, 607, *616*, 635, *635*
Pharyngeal constrictor muscles, 632, *633*, 634–635, *635*, 637t
  cricopharyngeal part of, 636

Pharyngeal nerve, 575, *658*
Pharyngeal nerve plexus, 634, *635–636*, 636
Pharyngeal recess, 632, *633*
Pharyngeal tonsils, 560, 632, *633*
Pharyngo-esophageal junction, 636
Pharyngobasilar fascia, 632, 634, *635*
Pharyngotympanic tube, 580, 583, *583, 633*
  opening of, *560*, 580
Pharynx, *560*, 631–636, *633*
  interior of, 631–634, *633*
  muscles of, 632, *633*, 634–635, *635*
    gaps between, 635
  nerves of, *635–636*, 636
  parts of, *560*, 631–632, *633*
  swallowing and, 632, *632*
  vasculature of, *635–636*, 636
Phasic contraction, 19
Philtrum, 557, *557*
Phimosis, 266
Phrenic artery, *145, 188*
  left inferior, 143
  superior, 108, 110t
Phrenic lymph nodes, 170
Phrenic nerve(s), 105–106, 105t, *106–107*
  accessory, 602
  block of, 604
  diaphragmatic innervation by, 105–106, 105t, *187–188*
  injury of, and paralysis of diaphragm, 54, *54*
  left, 108, *187*, 190
  in neck region, *601–602*, 602, 618
  pericardial innervation by, 82, *83*
  right, 103, 105–106, 173, *187*, 190
  section of, 191
  severance of, 604
Phrenic vein, inferior, *188*
Phrenicolic ligament, 158
Pia mater, 31, 509–511, *510*
  cranial, 509–511, *510*
  spinal, 31, *33*, 298, *299*
Pineal body, *513*
Piriform aperture, 496, *497*
Piriform fossa, 627, 632–634, *633*
Piriformis, 211, *213–214*, 214t, 347, *347*, 348t
  innervation of, *219*
Piriformis syndrome, 354
Pisiform, 411, *411–412*, 416, *489*
  palpation of, *417*
Pisotriquetral joint, *489*
Pivot joints, *16t*
Plane joints, *16t*
Planes, of body, 3–4, *3*
Plantar aponeurosis, 371, *371*
Plantar arch, *353*, 376
  deep, 377
Plantar artery(ies), 367, 376, *376, 377*
Plantar calcaneocuboid ligament, 398, *398*
Plantar calcaneonavicular ligament, 398, *398*
Plantar fascia, 371, *371*
Plantar fasciitis, 377
Plantar ligaments, 398, *398*
Plantar muscles, 372, 373t, *374*
Plantar nerves, 373, *375t*, 376
  medial, entrapment of, 379

Plantar reflex, 379
Plantar region, of foot, 371, *371*
Plantarflexion, 6, 397, 397t
  absence of, 368
Plantaris, 363, *364*, 365t
Platysma, 520t, 594, 599t
  surface anatomy of, 611, *612*
Pleurae, 68–70, *69*
  injury and medical conditions, 77–79
  surface anatomy of, 70, *70*
  vasculature and nerves of, 75–79, *75–76*
Pleural cavity, 68, *69*
Pleural effusion, 77
Pleural reflection, lines of, 68
Pleural rub, 77
Pleural sleeve, 68, 71
Pleuritis, 77
Pneumomediastinum, 597
Pneumonectomy, 55, 78
Pneumothorax, 77
Polymastia, 58
Polythelia, 58
Pons, 512, *513*
Pontocerebellar cistern, 514, *515*
Popliteal aneurysm, 357
Popliteal artery, 351, 356, 370t
  aneurysm of, 357
  pulse of, 357
Popliteal bursa, 390t
Popliteal cysts, 392
Popliteal fossa, 355, 356–357
  fascia of, 355, 356
  nerves in, 355, 357
  vessels of, 355–356, 356
Popliteal ligaments, 350, 364, 386
Popliteal lymph nodes, 332, 333, 356, *356*
Popliteal pulse, 357
Popliteal vein, 356, *356*
Popliteus, 363, *364–365*, 365t
Porta hepatis, 167
Portacaval anastomosis, 174, *174*
Portal hypertension, 174
Portal-systemic anastomoses, 173–174, *175*
Portal triad, 167
Portal vein. *See* Hepatic portal vein
Portal venous system, *142*, 143, *145*, 173–174, *175*
Portosystemic shunts, 174, *174*
Positron emission tomography (PET), 46, *46*
Posterior (dorsal), definition of, *4t*
Posterior abdominal wall. *See* Abdominal wall
Posterior commissure, of labia, 268
Posterior cruciate ligament, 387–388, *387*
  injuries to, 393–394, *393*
Posterior drawer sign, 394, *394*
Posterior (extensor) facial compartment, 417, *418*
Posterior horn, of spinal cord, 31, *33*
Posterior intercostal arteries, 108, 110t, 126, 126t
Posterior longitudinal ligament, 287, 288–289, *289*
Posterior median furrow, 284, *285*
Posterior ramus (rami), of spinal nerves, 34, *35*

Posterior root, of spinal nerve, *34*, 35
Postganglionic neuron, *36*, 37
Postsynaptic parasympathetic fibers, 39, *41*
Postsynaptic (postganglionic) neuron, *36*, 37
Pott fracture-dislocation of ankle, *398*, *398*
Preaortic lymph nodes, 196–197, *197*
Prechiasmatic sulcus, *501*, 502
Preganglionic neuron, *36*, 37
Prelaryngeal lymph nodes, 619, *622*
Prepatellar bursitis, 394, *394*
Prepuce, *262*, 263, 266
Presbyopia, 539, *539*
Pressure sores, 353
Presynaptic (preganglionic) neuron, *36*, 37
Presynaptic sympathetic fibers, 38
Pretracheal layer, of deep cervical fascia, 595, 596
Prevertebral layer, of deep cervical fascia, 595, 596
Prevertebral neck muscles, 613, *614*, *614–615t*
Prevertebral sympathetic ganglia, 38, *39*
Primary cartilagenous joints, 14, *15t*
Primary curvature, of spine, 276–277, *276*
Primary ossification center, 12, *13*
Prime mover, 20
Princeps pollicis artery, 468
Process, bone, *10*, 12
Processus vaginalis, vestige of, 130
Profunda femoris artery, 343, *344t*
Pronation, *6*, 484, 485
Pronator quadratus, 449, *450*, 451, 451t
Pronator teres, 446, 447, *449–450*, 450t, 451
Proprioception, 17, 35
Prostate, 227, 233–235, *234*
    apex, base, isthmus of, 234, *234*
    autonomic innervation of, *236*
    cancer of, 235
    enlargement of, 235
    fibrous capsule of, 233–234
    lobes, lobules, and zones of, 234–235, *234*
    vasculature of, 235
Prostatectomy, 235
Prostatic ducts, 235, *235*
Prostatic sinuses, 235, *235*
Prostatic venous plexus, 227, 235
Protrusion (protraction), *6*
Protuberance, bone, *10*, 12
Proximal, definition of, *4t*, 5
Proximal radio-ulnar joint, *482*, 483–485, *484*
Psoas abscess, 198
Psoas fascia, 192, *192*
Psoas major, 193, *193t*
Pterion, *496*, 497, 549, *549*
    fracture of, 498
Pterygoid canal, nerve of, 571, *571*
Pterygoid hamulus, *561*, 563, 575, 633
Pterygoid muscles, lateral and medial, *550t*, 552
Pterygoid plates, 499, *500*, *561*, 570
Pterygoid processes, 499, *500*
Pterygoid venous plexus, 526, 553, 554, 562
Pterygomaxillary fissure, 552, *570*
Pterygopalatine fossa, 552, 570–573, *570*
    arteries of, 572–573, *572*
    location and communications, 570

nerves of, 570–572, *571–572*
Pterygopalatine ganglion, 562, 571, *571–572*, 575, 660
    summary of, *672t*
Ptosis, 533
Pubic arch, 206
Pubic crest, 206
Pubic ligaments, 209, *210*
Pubic symphysis, 209, *210*, 317, *317*
    references to, 124, *124*, 205, *205*
Pubic tubercles, 124, 206, *206*
Pubis, 206, *206*, 318, *321*
    body of, 318, *321*
    rami of, 318, *321*
Pubococcygeus, 211, *232*, 237, 252
Pubofemoral ligament, 381, *381*
Puboprostatic ligament, 215, 226
Puboprostaticus, 232
Puborectalis, 211, *219*, *232*, 237, *245*
Pubovaginalis, 237, *237*
Pubovesical ligament, 215, 226
Pubovesicalis, *232*, 237
Pudendal arteries
    deep external, scrotal branches of, 132
    external, 263, 263t, *264*
    internal, 222t, 352, *353t*
Pudendal canal, 258–259, *258*
Pudendal cleft, 268
Pudendal nerve block, 270
Pudendal nerves, *131*, 217, 218t, *219*, 258, 352t
    branches of, *131*, 132, 241, *258*
    to penis, 258, 265, *266*
    regions traversed by, *258*
Pudendal veins, internal, 352–353, *353t*
Pudendum, 268, *268*
Pulmonary alveolus, 74, *74*
Pulmonary artery(ies), 75, *75*
    left, *69*, *75*
    right, *69*, *75*
Pulmonary circulation, 23, 75, *75*
Pulmonary collapse, 77
Pulmonary embolism, 79
Pulmonary infarct, 79
Pulmonary ligament, 68
Pulmonary lymph nodes, 76, *76*
Pulmonary plexuses, *76*, 77, 105, 105t, *109*
Pulmonary sinuses, 89
Pulmonary thromboembolism, 336
Pulmonary trunk, 75, *75*
Pulmonary valve, 89, *89*
Pulmonary valve stenosis, 92
Pulmonary vein(s), 75, *75*, 89, *89*
    left, *75*, *83*
    right, *83*
Pulp cavity, of tooth, 558, *558*
Pulpitis, 560
Pupil, 535, *536*
Pupillary light reflex, 548
Push-off, in gait cycle, 377, *378t*
Pyloric antrum, 144, *144*
Pyloric canal, 144, *144*
Pyloric lymph nodes, 145, *147*, 152, 164
Pyloric orifice, 144, *144*
Pylorus, 144, *144*, 148

Pyramidal eminence, 580, 581, *581*
Pyramidalis muscle, *119*, 120

Q

Q-angle, 391, *392*
Quadrangular membrane, *623*, *624–625*, *626*
Quadratus femoris, 347, *347*, 348t, 385
    nerve to, 349, *351*, 352t
Quadratus lumborum, 193, *193t*
Quadratus plantae, 373t, *374*
Quadriceps femoris, 336, 337t, *338*
    paralysis of, 340
Quadriceps tendon, 337, *338*
Quadrigeminal cistern, 514, *515*
Quadriplegia, 293
Quervain tenosynovitis stenosans, 471, *471*

R

Radial artery, *446*, 456, 457, 459t, 467
    and branches, 467, 467t, *468*
Radial collateral ligament, *482*, 483
Radial epiphysis, fracture/separation of, *491*, 492
Radial fossa, *408*, 410
Radial groove, *409*, 410, 413
Radial head. *See* Radius, head of
Radial nerve, 456, 457, 458t
    course of, *434*, 435t, *442–443*, 444
    in hand, 469, *469*
    injury to, 445, 472
Radial notch, 410, *411*, 482
Radialis indicis artery, 467, *468*
Radiate ligament, *289*
Radical neck dissection, 639
Radicular arteries, anterior and posterior, 301, *302*
Radicular veins, anterior and posterior, 299, 301, *302*
Radio-ulnar joints
    distal, *484*, 485–486
    ligaments of, *484*, 485
    movements of, 485
        structures limiting movements, 485t
    proximal, *482*, 483–485, *484*
        radiograph of, *482*
Radiocarpal joint, 488t, *489*. *See also* Wrist joint
Radiography, 42–44, *44t*
    of back, 314, *314*
    of cranium (skull), 589–590
Radius, 408–409, 411, *411*
    fractures of, 414, *414*
    head of, *408*, 411, 416
        subluxation and dislocation of, *487*, 487
    styloid process of, *409*, 411, 416
Ramus (rami), 35
    communicantes, 62, *62*, 194, *194*
    of ischium, 318, *321*
    of pubis, 206, *206*, 318, *321*
    of spinal nerves, *34*, 35, 297, *298*

Raynaud syndrome, 470
Rectal arteries, 259–260, *259*
   inferior, *151t*, 263t, *264*
   middle and superior, *151t*, 222, 222t, 246, *246*
Rectal ligaments, lateral, *216*, 217
Rectal veins, 174, *259*, 260
Rectal venous plexus, 260
Recti muscles, extraocular, *531*, 540–543, *540–541*, 540t, *543*
Recto-uterine pouch, *212t*
Rectosigmoid junction, 245
Rectovesical pouch, *212t*
Rectovesical septum, 215, *216*, 246
Rectovesicalis, *232*, *237*
Rectum, 245–249, *245*
   ampulla and flexures of, *245*, *246*
   examination of, 249
   hemorrhoids of, 260, *260*
   innervation of, 247, *248*
   references to, *150*, 159, *203*
   resection of, 249
   vasculature and lymphatics of, *151t*, 246–247, *246–247*
Rectus abdominis, *119*, 120, 120t
Rectus capitis anterior, *312t*, *614t*
Rectus capitis lateralis, *614t*, 615t
Rectus capitis posterior, major and minor, 311, *311*
Rectus femoris, 336–337, 337t, *338*
Rectus muscles, extraocular, *531*, 540–543, *540–541*, 540t, *543*
Rectus sheath, 119–120, *119*, *121*
Recurrent Laryngeal nerves
   injury of, 112
   left, *103*, 103, 105t, *109*, *617*
   right, *109617*
Recurrent meningeal branches, of spinal nerves, 294–295, *295*
Referred pain
   in back, 295
   cardiac, 102
   diaphragmatic, 191
   visceral, 186, *186t*
Reflexive contraction, 19
Regional anatomy, 2
Regurgitation, heart valve, 91
Relationship, terminology of, 4–5, *4t*
Remission, of penis, 265
Renal arteries, 176, 179
Renal calculi, 181
Renal fascia, 176, *177*
Renal hilum, 176, *177*
Renal nerve plexus, 179
Renal papilla, 177
Renal pelvis, 176, *177*
Renal pyramid, 177
Renal sinuses, 176
Renal transplantation, 181
Renal veins, 176, 196, *196*
Reproductive system, 3
Respiration, thoracic wall movement in, 51–53, *53*
Respiratory bronchioles, 74, *74*
Respiratory layer, of cervical viscera, *620*, 623–631

Respiratory system, 3
Rete testis, 130, *130*, 131
Retina, *534–535*, 537
   central artery and vein of, *535*, 537, *546*, *547*, 547t
   detachment of, 538
   development of, 539, *539*
   optic, ciliary, and nonvisual parts of, 537
Retinacula
   extensor, of foot, *360*
   synovial folds, hip joint, *380*, 381
Retinacular arteries, 343, *344*, 381
Retinacular ligament, 453, *455*
Retrobulbar fat, 544
Retroinguinal space, 341
Retromandibular vein, 525, *526*, 528
Retropharyngeal abscess, 597
Retropharyngeal space, 595, *596*
Retropubic space, 215, *216*, 226, 234
Retrorectal space, 215, *216*
Retrusion (retraction), 6
Rhinitis, 577
Rhizolysis, percutaneous, 290
Rhomboid, major and minor, 425t, *427*
   surface anatomy of, 429
Ribs, 48–50, *50*, 67
   atypical, 48–50, *49*, *50*
   body, head, neck, tubercle of, 48, *50*
   dislocation of, 55
   false (vertebrochondral), 48, *49*
   floating (free), 48, *49*
   fracture of, 54
   supernumerary, 54
   true (vertebrocostal), 48, *49*
   typical, 48, *49*, *50*
Rider's bones, 11
Right atrium. *See* Atria, of heart
Right auricle, 87, *87*
Right lymphatic duct, 29, *30*, 76, *76*
Right venous angle, 29, *30*
Right ventricle, 88–89, *88*
Rima glottidis, 624, 625, *626–627*
Rima vestibuli, 627
Root canal, of tooth, 558, *558*
Root, of tooth, 558, *558*
Rotation, 6
Rotator cuff, 478
   injuries, 427, 480, *480*
   muscles, *426t*, 427, 478
Rotatores, 305, 307t, *308*
Round ligament
   of liver, *122*, *166*, 167
   of uterus, 239, *240*
Round window, 583, *584*

S

SA node. *See* Sinuatrial (SA) node
Sacciform recess
   of distal radioulnar joint, 485, *489*
   of proximal radioulnar joint, *484*, 485
Saccular aneurysm, 511, 518
Saccule, 584, *584*
   laryngeal, 625, *625*

Sacral arteries
   lateral and median, 222t
   median, 195, *196*, 222, 222t
Sacral cornua (horns), 283t
Sacral crest, 283t
Sacral curvature, 275–276, *277*
Sacral flexure, of rectum, 245–246
Sacral hiatus, 283t, 284, *285*, 297
Sacral lymph nodes, 229t, *230t*
Sacral parasympathetic outflow, 42
Sacral plexus, 217, *218–219*, 218t
Sacral promontory, 283t
Sacral sympathetic trunks, 219, *219*
Sacral triangle, 284, *285*
Sacro-iliac joints, 205, *206*, 209, *210*, 283t
Sacro-iliac ligaments, 209, *210*
Sacrococcygeal joint, *210*, 211
Sacrococcygeal ligaments, 211
Sacrospinalis, 303–304, *306*
Sacrospinous ligaments, 209, *210*, 218, 346, *346*
Sacrotuberous ligaments, 209, *210*, 346, *346*
Sacrum, 205, *206*, 283t
Saddle joints, *16t*
Sagittal plane, 3, *3*
Sagittal sinuses, 505, *505–506*, *510*
Sagittal suture, 499, *499*
Salivary glands, 567–569, *568*
Salpingopharyngeal fold, *560*, 632, *633*
Salpingopharyngeus, 634, *635*, 637t
Saphenous cutdown, 335
Saphenous nerve, 334, 342, *342–343*, 369t, *375t*, 376
   injury to, 335
Saphenous opening, of fascia lata, 330, *330*
Saphenous vein(s), 331, *331–332*, 332
Sarcolemma, 22
Sarcomere, 22
Sartorius, 336, 337t, *338*
Scala tympani, 585, *587*
Scala vestibuli, 585, *587*
Scalene muscles
   anterior, *614t*
   middle and posterior, *614t*, 615t
Scalene tubercle, 48, *50*
Scalp, 502–503, *503*
   arteries of, *523*, 524–525
   danger area of, 503
   injuries and infections of, 503
   lymphatic drainage of, 526, *527*
   muscles of, *520t*
   nerves and innervation of, *521t–522t*, *522*
Scaphoid, 411, *411–412*, 416, 489
   fractures of, 414, *414*, 491
Scaphoid tubercle, 411, *411*
Scapula, 407–410, *407–409*
   arterial anastomoses around, 431
   fracture of, 413
   movements of, *477*
   surface anatomy of, 416
   surfaces and features of, 407–409, *407–410*
   winged, 424, *424*
Scapular artery, dorsal, 616, *616*

Scapular lines, 66
Scapulohumeral muscles, *426t*, 427
Scapulothoracic joint, *477*
Schwann cells, *30*, 33. *See also* Neurolemma
Sciatic foramen, 346
Sciatic nerve, 217, 218t, *219*, 349, *351*, 352t
    artery to, 349
    injury to, 354
Sciatica, 293
Sclera, 534, *534–535*
Scleral venous sinus, *536*, 537, 547
Scoliosis, 277, *277*
Scrotal raphe, 261, *262*
Scrotal septum, 261
Scrotum, 131–132, *131*, 261, *262*
    cancer of, 132
    innervation of, *131*, 132, 261, *266*
    lymphatics of, *131*, 132
    vasculature of, 261, 263t, *264–265*
Secondary cartilagenous joints, 14, *15t*
Secondary curvature, of spine, 276–277, *276*
Secondary ossification center, 12, *13*
Segmental bronchi, 72, *73*
Segmentectomy, pulmonary, 78
Sella turcica, *501*, 502
Sellar diaphragm, 504, *505*
Semicircular canals, 584, *584*
Semicircular ducts, 584, *584*, 585
    ampullae of, 585, *585–586*
Semilunar hiatus, in nasal cavity, *574*
Semilunar lines, 124, *124*
Semimembranosus, 349, 349t, *350*
Semimembranosus bursa, *390t*
Seminal glands, 233, *236*
Seminiferous tubules, 130, *130*
Semispinalis, 305, *306*, 307t, *308*
Semispinalis capitis, 305, *306*, *308*
Semispinalis cervicis, 305, *308*
Semispinalis thoracis, 305, *308*
Semitendinosus, 349, 349t, *350*
Sensory (afferent) fibers, 36, *36*, 644–650, *645*
Sensory nuclei, of cranial nerves, *649*
Septal cartilage, 573, *573*
Septomarginal trabecula, *88*, 89, 97, *97*
Serous pericardium, 81, *81*
Serous pleural fluid, 68
Serratus anterior, 124, *422*, 423, *423t*
    paralysis of, 424
Serratus posterior, 303
Sesamoid bones, 9, 11
    of foot, 400, *401*
    of hand, 466
Sesamoid cartilage, *573*
Shin splints, 361
Shingles, 64
Short bones, 9, 11
Shoulder, 406, *406*
    rotator cuff muscles, *426t*, 427
Shoulder joint. *See* Glenohumeral joint
Sialography, 569
Sigmoid artery(ies), *151t*, 158
Sigmoid colon, 158, *203*
Sigmoid mesocolon, root of, 158
Sigmoid sinuses, *505–506*, 506
Sinuatrial (SA), nodal branch, coronary artery,

94, 94t, 95, *95*
Sinuatrial (SA) node, 97, *97*
Sinus venarum, 87, *87*
Sinuses, paranasal, 574–576, *576*
Sinusitis, 577
SITS muscles, *426t*, 427
Skeletal muscle, 17–19, *18t*, *20*
    characteristics of, 17
    contraction of, 19–20
    naming, 17
    origin and insertion of, 19
    shape and structure of, 17–19, *21*
    structural unit of, 20, *22*
Skeletal system, 2, 9–17, *9–10*
    anterior view, *9*
    bones of, 11–14
    cartilage of, 10–11
    joints of, 14–17
    posterior view, *10*
Skeleton, 9–17, *9–10*
    appendicular, 9, *9–10*
    axial, 9
    cranium, 496–502
    of foot, 323–325, *324*
    of hand, 411–412, *411*
    of heart, 100
    of larynx, 623–625, *623*
    nasal, 573, *573*
    of neck, 594, *594*
    of orbit, 529, *529*
    thoracic, 48–51, *49*
    vertebral column, 275–295
Skin, 7–8, *7*
    incisions and wounds, 8
    ligaments in, 7, 8
Skull. *See* Cranium
Sliding hiatal hernia, 159, *159*
Slipping rib syndrome, 55
Small arteries, *24*, 25
Small cardiac vein, 96, *96*
Small intestine, 140, 146–154. *See also*
        Duodenum; Ileum; Jejunum
    duodenum, 146–152
    jejunum and ileum of, 152–154
    mesentery of, *136*, *138*, 152
    nerves and innervation of, 154, *154*
    vasculature of, *151t*
Smoke, inhalation of, 79
Smoker's cough, 79
Smooth muscle, 17, *19t*
    characteristics of, 20–22
    innervation/"involuntary" nature of, 22
Soft palate, 560–562, *561*, 633
    muscles of, 562, *562t*
Sole of foot, 371, *371*
    arteries of, 376, *376*
    compartments of, 371–372, *372*
    definition of, *4t*, 5
    fascia and ligaments of, 371–372, *371*
    hemorrhaging wounds of, 377
    lateral and medial compartments of,
        371–372, *372*
    muscles of, 372, 373t, *374*
Soleus, 363, *364*, 365t
    tendinous arch of, 363, *364*

Somatic motor fibers, 34, *34*, 35–36, 63, *645*
Somatic nervous system (SNS), 31, 33–36
Somatic sensory fibers, 34, *34*, 35, 63, *645*
Spasmodic torticollis, 598
Special sensory fibers, *645*
Spermatic cord, 128–130, *131*
    constituents of, 130
    innervation, blood supply, and lymphatics of,
        131
    layers of, *129t*
Spermatic fascia, internal and external,
        128–129, *128–129*
Spheno-ethmoidal recess, 574, *574*
Sphenoid bone, 499, *500*
    crest of, *501*, 502, *575*
    greater wing of, 529, *529*
Sphenoidal sinuses, 576, *576*
Sphenomandibular ligament, 555, *556*
Sphenopalatine artery, 574, *575*
Sphenopalatine foramen, *570*, 575
Sphincter pupillae, *535–536*, 536
Spina bifida, 285–286, *286*
Spinal accessory nerve (CN XI), 669–670
    distribution of, 598–600, *601*, 670
    injury to, 670, *670*
    intracranial portion of, *648*
    lesions of, 603
    nucleus of, *649*
    summary of, *646t–647t*
Spinal arteries, 299, 301, *302*
Spinal cord, 31, *32*, 296–301
    compression of, 293
    herniation of, 285–286
    intermediolateral cell columns of, 38, *38*
    ischemia of, 303
    meninges of, 297–299, *298*
    nerves emanating from, 297, *298*
    segments of, 297
    vasculature of, 299, 301, *302*
    white matter and gray matter of, 31, *33*
Spinal dura mater, 31, *33*, 297, *298*
Spinal ganglia
    paravertebral, 38, *39*
    prevertebral, 38, *39*
    sympathetic, 38, *39*
Spinal meninges, 297–299, *298*
    spaces associated with, 299t
Spinal nerves, 32, 34–36, 297, *298*
    cervical, *521*, 522t
    coccygeal, 217
    lumbar, 193–194, *194*, 248
    meningeal branches of, 294–295, *295*
    overview of, 297, *298*
    pelvic, 217, 220, *231*, 248
    rami of, 297, *298*
    roots of, *34*, 35
        anterior (ventral), *34*, 35, 297, *298*
        posterior (dorsal), *34*, 35, 297, *298*
    sacral, 217, 243
    sensory and motor components of, *645*
    structure of, 34–36, *34*, 297, *298*
    thoracic, 125–126, 185
Spinal puncture, lumbar, 300, *300*
Spinal veins, 294, *294*
    anterior and posterior, 299, 301, *302*

Spinalis muscles, 304, 305t, *306*
Spine. *See also* Vertebral column
  of bone, *10*, 12
  vertebral column, 275–295
Spinous process, *277*, *278*
Spiral canal, 583, *584*
Spiral fold, *172*
Spiral ganglion, *586*
Spiral ligament, 585, *586*
Spiral organ, structure of, *586*
Splanchnic nerves, 39, *39–40*, 183t
  abdominopelvic, 39, 164, 179–180
    summary of, 182, *183t*, *184*
  cardiopulmonary, 39, *183t*
  greater and lesser, 152, 182, *183t184*
  least, *184*
  lower thoracic, 112, *147*, *157*, 182, *183t*
  lumbar, *147*, 158, 182, *183t*, *184*, 241
  pelvic, 158, *183t*, 185, 218t, 220, 241
  sacral, *183t*
Spleen, 30, 161–162, *162*
  nerves and arteries of, 162, *163*
  relationships of, *149t*
  rupture of, 165
  surface anatomy of, 161, *161*
Splenic artery, *142*, *145*, 146t, 162
Splenic vein, *145*, 162, 164
Splenius capitis, *306*, *614*, 615t
Splenius cervicis, *306*
Splenius muscles, 303, 305t, *306*
Splenomegaly, 165
Splenorenal ligament, 162
Spondylolisthesis, 286, *286*
Spongy bone, 11, *11*
Spongy urethra, *226–227*, 231, 261
Sprains
  of ankle, 362, 397
  of back, 313
Squamous cell carcinoma, 527, *527*
Stance phase, in gait cycle, 377, *378t*
Stapedius, 581, *581*
Stapedius muscle, 580
Stapes, 581, *581*, *587*
Stellate ganglion, *617*, 618
Stenosis
  aortic valve, of heart, 91
  pulmonary, 92
Sterilization
  female (tubal ligation), 249
  male (deferentectomy), 132, 233
Sternal angle, 51, *51*, 67
Sternal biopsy, 54
Sternoclavicular joint, *407*, 475–476, *475*
  capsule, 475
Sternoclavicular ligaments, *475*, 476
Sternocleidomastoid, *312t*, 596–598, *597*, *599t*
  sternal and clavicular heads of, *597*, *598*
  test for function, *670*
Sternocleidomastoid region of neck, 596–598, *597*, 613t
  surface anatomy of, 611, *612*
Sternocostal joint, dislocation of, 55
Sternocostal triangle (foramen), *188*, *189*
Sternohyoid muscle, *607*, 608t

Sternopericardial ligaments, 80
Sternothyroid muscle, *607*, *608t*
Sternum, *49*, *51*, *51*, 67
  fracture of, 54
  parts of, *49*, *51*, *51*
  surgical procedures involving, 54
Stomach, 140, 143–146. *See also gastric entries*
  body of, 144, *144*
  cancer and gastrectomy, 159
  interior of, 144, *144*
  parts and curvature of, 143–144, *144*, 148
  relations of, 146, *149t*
  surface anatomy of, 148, *148*
  ulcers of, 159–160
  vasculature and nerves of, 144–146, *145*, 146t
Stomach bed, 146, *149t*
Straight sinus, *505*, *505*, 519
Stretch marks, in skin, 8
Striated muscle. *See* Skeletal muscle
Strokes, 518
Styloglossus, *565t*
Stylohyoid ligament, *565*, *594*, *608*
Stylohyoid muscle, *566*, *592*, *605*, *607*, *608t*
Styloid process
  of radius, *409*, *411*
  of temporal bone, *497*, *498*, *555*, *633*
  of ulna, *408*, *410*, *411*
Stylomandibular ligament, 555–556, *555–556*
Stylomastoid foramen, *499*, *500*, *520*, *522*, 572
Stylopharyngeus, *632*, *633*, *634*, *635*, *637t*
Subacromial bursa, *478*, *480*
  inflammation and calcification of, 481
Subarachnoid cisterns, 512, *515*
Subarachnoid hemorrhage, 511, *511*
Subarachnoid space, 297–300, *300*, 509, *510*, 511
Subclavian artery(ies), *615*, *616*
  branches of, 62, *609*, 615, *616*
  left, 103–105, *103*, 197, *197*, *609*, 615, *616*
  right, *609*, 615, *616*
  third part of, *602*, 603–605
  variations of, 113
Subclavian lymphatic trunk, 56, *57*
Subclavian vein, 430, *600*, 602
Subclavian vein puncture, 603, *603*
Subclavius, 422–423, *422*, *423t*
  nerve to, *434*, 434t
Subcostal arteries, 108, 126t, 195, *195–196*
Subcostal nerves, 61, 105t, 125t, 190, 193
Subcostal plane, of abdominal cavity, 117, *117*
Subcutaneous infrapatellar bursa, *390t*
Subcutaneous prepatellar bursa, 389, *390t*
Subcutaneous tissue, 7, 8
  anterolateral abdominal, 118, *118*
  of lower limb, 329–331, *330*
  of neck, 594, *595*
  of perineum, 253
Subdural hematoma, 297, 511, *511*
Subinguinal space, 127, *128*
Sublingual absorption of drugs, 569
Sublingual artery, *567*
Sublingual glands, *568*, 569
Submandibular duct, 569

Submandibular ganglion, 564, *566*, 660
  summary of, *672t*
Submandibular glands, 569, *569*, 604, 613
Submandibular lymph nodes, 526, 557, 558, 604, *605*
Submandibular triangle, 597, 604, *612*, 613t
Submental arteries, 569
Submental lymph nodes, 526, 557, 558, 613
Submental triangle, 597, 604, *612*, 613, 613t
Suboccipital muscles, 311–312, *311*
Suboccipital nerve, 311, *311*
Suboccipital region, 311
  innervation of, *313*, 313t
Suboccipital triangle, 311, *311*
Subperitoneal endopelvic fascia, 215, *216*
Subphrenic abscesses, 167
Subphrenic recesses, 165, *166*
Subpubic angle, 206–207
Subscapular arteries, *430*, 431t
Subscapular bursa, *478*, 480
Subscapular fossa, *408*
Subscapular lymph nodes, 432, 433
Subscapular nerves, *434*, 435t
Subscapularis, 426t, 427
Subtalar joint, 398, *399*, *399t*
Subtendinous olecranon bursa, 441–443, *483*, *483*
Subtendinous olecranon bursitis, 486, *486*
Sulci, of brain, 512, *513*
Sulcus terminalis, 87, *87*
Superficial, definition of, *4t*
Superficial epigastric artery(ies), 126, 126t
Superficial fascia. *See* Subcutaneous tissue
Superficial fatty layer, anterolateral abdominal, 118, *118*
Superficial inguinal lymph nodes, 126, *126*
Superficial inguinal ring, 127, *128*
Superficial lymphatic vessels, 29, 30, 332–333
Superficial perineal pouch, 253, *254*
Superior (cranial), definition of, *4t*
Superior alveolar nerve, 558, 559, *559*
Superior cervical ganglion, 38, 39, *40*, 655
Superior costotransverse ligament, 289
Superior epigastric artery(ies), 126, 126t
Superior ganglion, 664
  of glossopharyngeal nerve, *666*
  of vagus nerve, 665–666, *666*
Superior gluteal nerve, 217, 218t, *219*
Superior hypogastric plexus, *157*, 182, 185, 219
Superior longitudinal muscle, *565t*
Superior mesenteric arteries, 142, *142*, *145*, 151t, *156*
Superior mesenteric lymph nodes, *147*, 152, 154, *157*, 158, 164
Superior mesenteric (nerve) plexus, *147*, 154, *157*, 158, 164, 185
Superior mesenteric vein, *145*
Superior oblique, 540–541, 540t
  innervation of, 655–656
Superior orbital fissure, *501*, 502
Superior pancreaticoduodenal artery(ies), 164, 171
Superior pharyngeal constrictor, *637t*
Superior phrenic arteries, 108, 110t

Superior recess, 138
Superior rectus, *531*, 540–543, *540–541*, 540t, *543*
Superior sagittal sinus, 505, *505–506*, 510
Superior thoracic artery, *430*, 431t
Superior vena cava. *See* Vena cava, superior
Supernumerary breasts, 58
Supernumerary nipples, 58, *67*
Supernumerary ribs, 54
Superolateral, *4t*, 5
Supination, *6*, *484*, 485
Supinator, *446*, *452*, 455t
Supinator fossa, 410, *411*
Supra-orbital artery, *523t*, 525, *525*, *546*, 547, 547t
Supra-orbital foramen, 496, *497*
Supra-orbital margin, 496, *497*
Supra-orbital nerve, *521t*
Supra-orbital notch, 496, *497*
Supra-orbital vein, 526, *526*
Supraclavicular fossa, lesser, 598, 613t
Supraclavicular lymph nodes, 639
Supraclavicular nerves, 420, *420*, *601*, 602
Supracolic compartment, 139, *139–140*
Suprahyoid muscles, 607, *608t*
Suprahyoid region, 605–606
Suprapatellar bursa, 386, *386*, 389, *390t*
Suprapatellar bursitis, 394, *394*
Suprapubic cystotomy, 228
Suprarenal arteries, 179
Suprarenal glands, *176–178*, *177–179*
   cortex and medulla of, 178, *178*, 184
   internal anatomy of, 178, *178*
   nerves of, 179–180, *179*
   sympathetic innervation of, 39, *39*
   vasculature and lymphatics of, 179, *179*
Suprarenal lymphatic vessels, 179, *179*
Suprarenal medulla, sympathetic innervation of, 184
Suprarenal veins, 179, *196*
Suprascapular artery, *430*, 430t, 602, *603*
Suprascapular nerve, *434*, 434t, 600, *601–602*
Suprascapular notch, 407, *408*
Supraspinatus, *426t*, 427
   injury of, 427
Supraspinatus tendinitis, calcific, 481
Supraspinous fossa, 407, *407*, *409*
Supraspinous ligaments, 289, *290*
Supratrochlear artery, *523t*, 525, *525*, *546*, 547, 547t
Supratrochlear nerve, *521t*
Supratrochlear vein, 526, *526*
Supraventricular crest, 88, *88*
Supravesical fossae, 121, *122*, 212t
Sural cutaneous nerve, medial, 355, *357*
Sural nerve, 366, *367*, 369t, 375t, 376
   grafts, 379
Suspensory ligaments
   of axilla, 417, *418*
   of breast, 56
   of eyeball, *535*, 537–538
   of ovary, 239, *240*
   of penis, 263
Suspensory muscle, of duodenum, 150

Sustentaculum tali, 323, *324*
Sutural bones, 14
Swallowing, 632, *632*
Swing phase, in gait cycle, 377, *378t*
Sympathetic ganglia, 39, 62
   cervical, 618
   intrinsic (enteric), 42
   paravertebral, 38, *39*, 77
   prevertebral, 38, *39*
Sympathetic ganglion cells, 77
Sympathetic innervation, 36–37, *36*, 37t
   of abdominal viscera, 182–185, *182–184*, 183t
   of heart, 98–99
   of pelvis, 220, *220*
   of viscera, 38–39, *40–41*, 145–146, *147*. *See also specific organs*
Sympathetic nerve fibers, 38–39, *39–41*, 154
   courses of, *40*
   postsynaptic, 38–39, *40*, 182
   presynaptic, 38, *40*, 182
Sympathetic trunks, 38, *41*
   cervical, *617*, 618
      lesion of, 619
   sacral, 219, *219*
   thoracic, 62, *62*, 82, 112, 143
Symphysis(es), 288
Synapse, *30*, 31
Syndesmosis, 14, *15t*
Synergistic muscle, 20
Synovial cyst, of wrist, *460*, 460
Synovial effusion, 392
Synovial folds, 380, *381*
Synovial joints, 14–17, *15t*
   degenerative disease of, 17
   types of, *16t*, 17
Synovial membrane
   of elbow joint, 482, *483*
   of glenohumeral joint, 478, *478*
   of hip joint, 379, *380*
Synovial sheaths, of hand, 451, *453*
Syntosis, of bone, 14
Systemic anatomy, 2
Systemic circulation, 23, *23*
Systole, *99*, 100
Systolic blood pressure, 445

T

Talar neck fractures, 327, *327*
Talocalcaneal joint ligaments, 396–397, *396*
Talocalcaneonavicular joint, 398, *399*, 399t
Talocrural articulation. *See* Ankle joint
Talocrural region, 317, *317*. *See also* Ankle
Talofibular ligaments, 396, *396*
   injury to, 397
Talus, *319*, 323, *324*, 329
   ankle joint articulation, 395, *395*
   neck of, fractures of, 327, *327*
   trochlea of, 395, *395*
Tarsal artery, lateral, 376, *376*
Tarsal glands, *531*, 532
Tarsal muscle, superior, 540, *540–541*, 540t

Tarsal tunnel syndrome, 397
Tarsometatarsal joint, 399, *399t*
Tarsus, 323–325, *324*
   superior and inferior, of orbits, *531*, 532
Taste, innervation of, 660, *661*, 665, *665*
Taste buds, 564
Tectorial membrane, *291*, 292
   of cochlear duct, 586, *586*
Teeth, 558–560, *558–559*
   deciduous and permanent, 558, *558*
   incisor and molar, *559*
   mandibular, *558*
   parts of, *558*
   relationship to maxillary sinus, 578
Tegmen tympani, 580
Tegmental wall, of tympanic cavity, 580, *581*
Temporal artery(ies), superficial, *523t*, 525, *525–526*, 609
Temporal bone
   articular tubercle of, 555, *555*
   petrous part and squamous part of, 499, *500*
Temporal fascia, 550
Temporal fossa, 496, *497*, 549–550, *549*
Temporal line(s), superior and inferior, 496, *497*
Temporal process, of zygomatic bone, 496, *497*
Temporal pulse, 525
Temporal region, 549–555
   infratemporal fossa, *549*, 550–555
   nerves of, 554–555, *554*
   temporal fossa, 549–550, *549*
   vasculature of, 552–555, *553*
Temporal vein
   deep, 526, *526*
   superficial, 525, *525–526*
Temporalis, *528*, 549–550, 550t, *551*
Temporalis fascia, 550
Temporomandibular joint (TMJ), 555–557, *555*
   arthritis of, 557
   dislocation of, 556–557, *556*
   movements at, 556t
   muscles acting on, *550t*
Tendinitis, 368
   degenerative, of rotator cuff, 480
Tendinous arch
   of levator ani, 211
   of pelvic fascia, 215
Tendinous cords, 88, *88*, 90, *90*
Tendinous intersections, *21*
   of rectus abdominis, *119*, 120, 124, *124*
Tendon, 17
Teniae coli, 154, *156*
Tennis elbow, 460
Tenosynovitis, 470–471, *471*
Tensor fasciae latae, *330*, 347, 348t
Tensor tympani muscle, 581, *581–582*
   canal of, 580
Tensor veli palatini, 561, *562t*, 563
Tentorium cerebelli, 504, *505*
Teres major, *426t*, 427, 429
Teres minor, *426t*, 427
Terminal arteries, 25
Terminal bronchioles, 74, *74*
Terminal groove, of tongue, 563, *563*

Terminal sulcus, of tongue, 563
Terminology, 3–6
    of anatomical planes, 3–4, *3*
    of anatomical position, *2*, 3
    of laterality, 5
    of movement, 5, *5, 6*
    of relationship or comparison, 4–5, *4t*
Testicular artery(ies), 130, *130–131*, 196, *196*
Testicular cancer, 132
Testicular veins, 130–131, *130–131*
Testis (testes), 130–131, *130*
    hydrocele of, 132
    innervation, blood supply, and lymphatics of,
        131, 236
    medical conditions of, 132
    relocation of, 133
Thenar compartment, 461, *462*
Thenar eminence, 416, 461, *461, 474*
    wasting of, 472, *472*
Thenar muscles, 462, *463, 464t*
Thenar space, 461–462, *462*
Thigh, 336–355
    anterior compartment of, 336
    fascial compartments of, 330, *331*
    gluteal region of, 346–355
    medical imaging of, *403*
    muscles of
        anterior, 336–337, *337t, 338*
        gluteal region, 347, *347, 348t*
        medial, 337–340, *338–339, 339t*
        medial and lateral rotators, *347*
        posterior, 349, *349t, 350*
    neurovascular structures and relationships in,
        341–346, *351*
    surface anatomy of, posterior and gluteal,
        346
    vasculature of
        anteromedial, 341–346
        posterior and gluteal, *351, 352–353, 353t*
Third ventricle, of brain, 512, *515*
Thoracic aorta, 103, *106,* 108, 110, *110t*
Thoracic aortic plexus, *107,* 108
Thoracic apertures, 48, *49*
Thoracic arteries, *430, 431t*
    internal, 615, *616*
    lateral and superior, *430, 431t*
Thoracic cavity and viscera, 68–113
    endothoracic fascia, 68, *69*
    heart and great vessels, 84–113. *See also*
        Great vessels; Heart
    lungs and pleurae, 68–79, *69. See also*
        Lung(s)
    mediastinum of, 80–84. *See also* Thoracic
        mediastinum
Thoracic curvature, 275–276, *276*
Thoracic duct, *29,* 30, 76, *76,* 103, 197, *197,*
    638, 649
    laceration of, 112
    and lymphatic trunks, 110–111, *111,*
        197, *197*
Thoracic interverte[   ] 51, 52, 52t
Thoracic kyphosi[
Thoracic media[   ]
    [   ]terior, 8[

esophagus in, 108, *108*
great vessels in, 102–113, *103*
heart and vasculature of, 84–102
inferior, 80, *80*
levels of viscera in, 84, *84*
lymphatics and lymph nodes in, 75–76, *76,*
    111–112, *111*
middle, 80–102, *80*
nerves and innervation of, 103, 105–108,
    105t
    posterior mediastinum, 112
    superior mediastinum, 105–108,
        107, 109
pericardium in, 80–83, *81–83*
posterior, 80, 108–113, *109*
superior, 80, 102–108, *103–104*
thymus in, 102
trachea and bronchi in, 71–74, *73–74,* 108
Thoracic muscles, of wall, 60–61, *60t*
Thoracic outlet, 48, *49*
Thoracic outlet syndrome, 55
Thoracic ribs, 48–50, *50*
Thoracic skeleton, 48–51, *49*
Thoracic splanchnic nerves, 112, *147, 157,* 182,
    183t
Thoracic vertebrae, 50, *50, 281t*
Thoracic wall, 48–67
    joints of, 51, 52, 52t
    movements of, 51–53, *53*
    muscles of, 60–61, *60t*
    nerves of, 61–62, *61, 62*
    skeleton of, 48–51, *49*
    surface anatomy of, 65–68, *65–68*
    vasculature of, 62–67
Thoraco-abdominal nerves, *125t*
Thoraco-acromial artery(ies), *430,* 431t
Thoracocentesis, 78
Thoracodorsal arteries, *430,* 431t
Thoracodorsal nerve, *434,* 435t
Thoracolumbar fascia, 192, *192,* 303, *304*
Thoracoscopy, 78–79, *79*
Thoracotomy, 55, *55*
Thorax, 47–115. *See also* Thoracic cavity and
        viscera; Thoracic wall
    medical imaging of, *114–115*
    surface anatomy of, 65–68, *65–68*
    thoracic cavity and viscera, 68–113
    thoracic wall, 48–67
Thrills, 91
Thromboembolism, pulmonary, 336
Thrombophlebitis, 336, 508
Thrombosis, deep venous, 335–336
Thrombus (thrombi), 508
Thumb
    median nerve injury and opposition of,
        472, *472*
    movements of, 462, *466*
Thymus, 102
    age changes in, 113
    as lymphoid organ, 30
Thyro-arytenoid, *629t*
Thyro-epiglottic ligament, 624, *626*
Thyrocervical trunk, 615, *616–617*
Thyrocervical trunk artery, *430,* 430t

Thyroglossal duct, 622, *622*
Thyrohyoid, *605*
Thyrohyoid ligaments, 623, *623*
Thyrohyoid membrane, *605,* 623, *623,* 634
Thyrohyoid muscle, 607, *608t*
Thyroid arteries
    inferior, 609, 619, *621*
        branches of, *628,* 636–638
    superior, 609, *609,* 619, *621*
Thyroid cartilage, *621, 623, 623,* 626
Thyroid gland, 619–620, *620*
    accessory tissue of, 622, *622*
    lobes, isthmus, capsule of, 619, *620,* 624
    lymphatics and lymph nodes of, 619, *622*
    medical imaging of, *642*
    nerves of, *617,* 619–620
    pyramidal lobe of, 620
Thyroid ima artery, 619, *621*
Thyroid notches, 623, *623*
Thyroid veins, superior, middle, inferior, 609,
    619, *621*
Thyroid venous plexus, 619, *621*
Thyroidectomy, 620
Tibia, 319, 322, *323*
    fractures of, 326, *326,* 398, *398*
    surface anatomy of, 328, *328*
Tibial arteries
    anterior, 357, *358,* 361, *370t,* 376, *376*
    posterior, 366, *367,* 370, 376, *376*
Tibial collateral ligament, 387, *387, 388, 393*
Tibial nerve, 355, 357, 365, 366, *369t*
    entrapment of, 397
    injury to, 368
Tibial pulse, posterior, 367–368, *368*
Tibial tuberosity, 337, *338*
Tibialis anterior, *358, 359t*
    strain (shin splints), 361
Tibialis posterior, *364,* 366, *366t*
Tibiofibular joints, 389–391, *391*
    superior, 389
Tibiofibular ligaments, 389–391, *391*
Tibiofibular syndesmosis, 389–391, *391*
Toes, 371
    great toe, 371
Tongue, 563–567, *563*
    carcinoma of, 569
    dorsum of, *563, 563*
    inferior surface of, 564, *564*
    innervation of, 564, *566*
    muscles of, 564, *565t*
    papillae and taste buds of, 563–564, *563*
    root, body, apex of, 563, *563–564, 564*
    vasculature and lymphatics of,
        564–567, *567*
Tonic contraction, 19
Tonsillar artery, *634, 635*
Tonsillar lymphatics, 635
Tonsillar nerves, 636
Tonsillar ring, 632, 635–636
Tonsillectomy, 640, *640*
Tonsils
    lingual, *633,* 635
    palatine, 561, *562,* 632, *633*
    pharyngeal, *560,* 632, *633*

Tooth. *See* Teeth
Toothache, 560
Torsion angle, of femur, 322, *322*
Torticollis, 598, *598*
Torus, of pharyngotympanic tube, 632
Trabeculae carneae, 88, *88*, 90
Trachea, 628–631
    bifurcation of, 71, *73–74*
    lymphatic drainage of, *622*
    references to, 72, *73*, 108, *109*
Tracheal layer of fascia, *595*
Tracheal rings, 624, 628
Trachealis muscle, 628
Tracheobronchial lymph nodes, 76, *76*
Tracheoesophageal groove, 618
Tracheostomy, 631, *631*
Tract, of nerve fibers, 31
Tragus, 578, *579*
Transient ischemic attacks (TIAs), 518, 610
Transitional zone, 557–558, *557*, *562*
Transtubercular plane, of abdominal cavity,
    117, *117*
Transumbilical plane, of abdominal cavity,
    117, *117*
Transversalis fascia, 118, *118*
Transverse acetabular ligament, 379, *381*
Transverse arch, of foot, 401–402, *401*
Transverse arytenoids, *629t*, 633
Transverse cervical nerve, 600, *601*, 611
Transverse colon, 158, *203*
Transverse facial artery, *523t*, 524, *525*
Transverse intermuscular septum, 331, *331*
Transverse ligaments
    of atlas, *291*, 292
        rupture of, 293
    humeral, *478*, 479
    of knee, 388, *388*
    of metacarpals, *418*, 419
    tibiofibular, 391, *391*
Transverse mesocolon, 139, *139–140*
Transverse muscle, of tongue, *565t*
Transverse pericardial sinus, 81, 82, *82*
Transverse perineal muscles, *251*, 251t
Transverse plane, *3*, 4
Transverse process(es), 277, *278*
Transverse sinuses, 505–506, *506*
Transverse tarsal joint, 398, *399*, *399t*
Transversospinal muscles, 305, *308*
Transversus abdominis muscle, 119, *119*, 120t
Trapezium, 411, *411–412*, 416, *489*
Trapezius, 598, *599t*
    references to, 303, 424, *425t*
    surface anatomy of, 429, 611, *612*
    test for function, *670*
Trapezoid, 411, *411–412*, *489*
Trapezoid ligament, 476, *476*
Trendelenburg position, 611
Trendelenburg sign, 384
Trendelenburg test, positive, 354, *354*
Triceps brachii, *440*, 441–443, *441t*, *442*, 447
Triceps surae, 363
Tricuspid orifice, 88, *88*
Tricuspid valve, 88, *88*
Trigeminal ganglion, 519, *658*, 659

Trigeminal nerve (CN V), 659–660
    distribution of, 519, 522, *658*
    divisions of, *658*, 659t
    injury to, 660
    intracranial portion of, *648*
    lesions of, 524
    nuclei of, *649*
    sensory and motor roots of, 659–660
    summary of, *646t–647t*
Trigeminal neuralgia, 524, 660
Trigone, of urinary bladder, 226, *227*
Triquetrum, 411, *411–412*, *489*
Trochanter
    bone, *10*, 12
    of femur, 318, *319*
Trochanteric bursa, 348, *348*
Trochanteric bursitis, 353
Trochlear nerve (CN IV), 544, *545*, 655–656
    distribution of, *654*, 656
    intracranial portion of, *648*
    nucleus of, *649*
    palsy of, 657
    summary of, *646t–647t*
Trochlear notch, 410, *411*, *482*
Tubal ligation, 249
Tubal pregnancy, ectopic, 249
Tubercle, of rib, 48, *50*
Tuberculum sellae, *501*, 502
Tuberosity, bone, *10*, 12
Tunica adventitia, 23, *24*
Tunica albuginea, 130, *130*, 261, *262*
Tunica intima, 23, *24*
Tunica media, 23, *24*
Tunica vaginalis, *129–130*, 130
Tympanic cavity, and walls, 580, *581–582*
Tympanic membrane, 579, *579*, *581*, 587
    flaccid and tense parts of, 580
    otoscopic viewing of, 579–580, *579*, 587
    perforation of, 588, *588*
    secondary, 583, *584*, *585*, 587
    tympanostomy (pressure-equilization) tubes,
        588, *588*
Tympanic nerve, 667

U

Ulcers, 159–160
Ulna, *408–409*, 410, *411*
    fractures of, 414, *414*
    styloid process of, *408*, 410, *411*
Ulnar artery, 456, *457*, *459t*, 466–467
    and branches, 466–467, *467t*, *468*
Ulnar canal, 468, *472*
Ulnar canal syndrome, 472, *472*
Ulnar collateral arteries, *430*, 431t
Ulnar collateral ligament, *482*, 483
    reconstruction of, 487, *487*
Ulnar nerve, 456, *457*, 458t
    course of, *434*, 435t, *442–443*, 443–444
    in hand, 468–469, *468*
    injury of, 472, *472*
Ultrasonography, 44, *45*
    of abdomen, *200*

of neck soft tissue, 641, *642*
    of pelvis, *273*
Umbilical artery, 222t
Umbilical folds, 121, *122*, *212*
Umbilical ligament, 121
Umbilicus, *119*
Umbo, 579–580, *579*
Uncinate process, 162
Uncovertebral joints, 288, *288*
Unilateral, definition of, 5
Unmyelinated nerves, 33, *33*
Upper limb, 405–494. *See also* Arm; Brachial
        plexus; Forearm; Hand; Shoulder
    bones of, 406–417, *406*, *408–409*
    brachial plexus of, 433–439, *434*,
        434t–435t
    compartments of, anterior and posterior,
        440, 446, *448*
    cutaneous nerves of, 419–421, *419–420*
    fascia of, 417–419, *418*
    joints of, 475–492. *See also* Elbow joint;
        Glenohumeral joint; Wrist joint
    lymphatics and lymph nodes of, *421*, 422
    medical imaging of, *492–494*
    muscles of
        anterior axioappendicular, 422–423, *422*,
            423t
        arm, 440–443
        forearm, 446–456
        hand, 462–466
        posterior axioappendicular, 423–427, *425t*
        scapulohumeral, *426t*, 427
    nerves and innervation of, 433–439,
        443–444, 456
    regions of, 406, *406*
        arm, 440–446
        axilla, 427–439
        cubital fossa, fossa, 446
        forearm, 446–460
        hand, 461–474
    surface anatomy of
        arm and cubital fossa, 447, *447*
        bones, 415–416, *415–417*
        pectoral and scapular regions, 428–429,
            429
    vasculature of. *See specific region*
    venous drainage of, 2, *421*, *421*
Ureteric calculi, 181, 225
Ureteric orifices, 226, *226*
Ureters, *176*, *177*, *178*, 223–225
    congenital anomalies of, 181–182
    nerves and innervation of, 179–180, *179*,
        225, *225*
    surface anatomy of, 180, *180*
    vasculature of, 179
Urethra. *See also* Female urethra; Male urethra
    catheterization of, 261
    female, 227, 230
    male, 227, 231–232
    vasculature and innervation of, *231*, 261
Urethral glands, 261
Urethral orifice
    external, 261, 269, *269*
    internal, 226, *226*

Urethral sphincter, 237
  external, 237, *251*, 251t, 255, *255*
  internal, 226, *226*, 232
Urethrovaginal sphincter, 237, *237*, *251*, 255, *255*
Urinary bladder, 226–228, *226*
  apex of, 226, *226*
  bed of, 226, *226*
  body and neck of, 226, *226*
  female and male, *227*
  fundus of, 226, *226*
  innervation of, 228, *231*
  male, *226*
  medical conditions and procedures, 228, 229
  rupture of, 228
  trigone of, 226, *227*
  uvula of, 226, *227*
  vasculature and lymphatics of, 227, *228*
Urinary organs, 223–232, *223*
  innervation of, 228, *231*
  lymphatics of, 227–228, 229t–230t
  vasculature of, *221–222*, 222t
Urinary stress incontinence, 217
Urinary system, 3
Urogenital organs, male. *See* Male urogenital
    organs
Urogenital triangle, 250
  fascia and pouches of, 253–256, *254*
Uterine artery(ies), 222t, 225, *225*, 241
Uterine tubes, *240*, 241–243
  ampullae and isthmus of, 243
  ectopic tubal pregnancy, 249
  infundibulum of, *240*, 243
  ligation of, 249
  patency of, 237–239
  vasculature and innervation of, *238*, *241*, *241–242*, *244–245*
Uterovaginal nerve plexus, 237, *241*
Uterus, 237–241, *239*
  body, body wall, isthmus of, 239, *239*
  cervix of, 239, *239*
  hysterectomy, 242, *242*
  innervation of, 241, *241–242*
  ligaments of, 239–240, *240*
  manual examination of, 243, *243*
  relationships of, 240–241
  smooth muscle during pregnancy, 23
  ultrasonography of, 273, *273*
  vasculature of, *238*, 240, *241*
Utricle, 584, *584*
Utriculosaccular duct, 585, *585*
Uvea, 534
Uvula, *560*, 562
  muscle of, 232, 562t, *563*, 633
  of urinary bladder, 226, *227*

V

Vagal ganglion, inferior, 627
Vagal trunks. *See* Vagus nerve
Vagina, 236–237, *236–237*
  distention and examination of, 238
  episiotomy and, 253

  innervation of, 241, *241–242*
  vasculature of, 237, *238*
  vestibule of, 236, *236*
Vaginal artery, 222t
Vaginal fornix, 236, *236*
Vaginal orifice, 269, *269*
Vaginal venous plexuses, 237
Vagus nerve (CN X), *36*, 105t, 665–669
  cardiac branches of, 618
  distribution of, 611, 618, *668*
    to abdominal viscera, *184*
    to ear, 578, *578*
    to intestines, 152, *157*
    intracranial portion of, *648*
    to lungs and pleurae, 76, *77*
    to pericardium, 82, *83*
    to stomach, 145
  left, 105, 618, *668*
  lesions of, 669
  nuclei of, *649*
  right, 105, 618
  summary of, 646t–647t, 669t
  trunks of, 143, *147*, 171, 666
    anterior, *185*, 666, *668*
    posterior, 154, *157*, *185*, 666, *668*
Vallate papillae, 563, *563*
Valves of heart. *See* Heart valves
Valvular heart disease, 91–92
Valvuloplasty, 91
Variations, anatomical, 7
Varicose veins, 28, 174, 335, *335*
Variocele, 132
Vasa nervorum, 36
Vasa recta, *153*, 154
Vasectomy, 132, 233
Vasomotor nerves, 13
Vastus intermedius, 337, 337t, *338*
Vastus lateralis, 337, 337t, *338*
Vastus medialis, 337, 337t, *338*
Veins, 25–28, *27*. *See also* Venous sinuses;
     specific organ or region
  abdominal, collateral routes, 198
  of abdominal wall, posterior, 196, *196*
  of anal canal, 259, *260*
  of arm, 443, *443*
  articular, 17
  of bone, 13, *13*
  of breasts, 56, *57*
  of diaphragm, 189–190, 190t
  of dura mater, 508, *510*
  of esophagus, 173
  of face and scalp, 553
  of female pelvis/perineum, 237, *238*
  of foot, 25, *27*, 377
  of hand, 468
  of heart, 96–97, *96*
  of intestines, *152*
  of large intestine and rectum, 151t
  of lungs and pleurae, 75, *75–76*
  of male pelvis/perineum, 235
  of neck, *600*, 602
    root of, 616–618
  of orbit, 547, *547*
  of pelvis, *221*, 222, 222t

  portal venous system, *142*, 143, *145*, 173–174, *175*
  pulmonary, 75, *75*, 89, *89*
  of spinal cord, 299, 301, *302*
  of stomach, pancreas, spleen, *152*
  structure of, *24*
  of temporal area, 525–526
  of testes, 130–131, *130–131*
  of thoracic wall, 63, *63*
  of thymus, 102
  of upper limb, 421, *421*
  of urinary organs, 227, *228*
  varicose, 28, 335
  vena cava. *See* Vena cava
  venae comitantes, 17
  of vertebral column, 294, *295*
Vena cava
  cardiac cycle flow through, *98*
  inferior, *86*, *136*, *169*
    azygous vein and, 111, *196*
    collateral venous routes, 112
    esophageal hiatus, passage through, *189*
    medical imaging of, *199–201*
    obstruction of, 112, 165
    opening of, 87, *87*
    relationships of, 149t
    schematic, with tributary veins, *196*
  superior, *86*, 86–87, *103–104*, 609
    obstruction of, and collateral venous
      routes, 112
    opening of, 87, *87*
Venae comitantes, 17
Venipuncture, 424
Venous angle, 618
Venous plexuses
  pelvic, *221*, 222
  prostatic, 227, *228*, 235
  rectal, 247
  uterine, *238*, 241
  vaginal, 237, *238*
Venous sinuses
  dural, 504–508, *505–506*
    occlusion of, 508
  scleral, *536*, 537, 547
Venous stasis, 335–336
Venous system, 25–28, *27*
  portal, 173–174, *175*
Venous valves, 28
Ventral horn. *See* Anterior horn
Ventral ramus. *See* Anterior ramus
Ventral root. *See* Anterior root
Ventricles
  of brain, 512–514, *515*
  of heart
    left, 90, *90*
    right, 88–89, *88*
  laryngeal, 625, *625*
Ventricular septal defects, 91
Venules, 25
Vermillion border, 557, *557*
Vertebrae. *See also* Vertebral column
  aging of, 290
  cervical, 279t–280t
  development of, hemivertebra, 277

dislocation of, 286
fractures of, 278
lumbar, 282t
medical conditions and procedures on, 278
regional characteristics of, 278–283
sacrum and coccyx, 283t
structure and function of, 277–278, 277
thoracic, 50, 50, 281t
Vertebral arch(es), 277, 278
joints of, 289–290, 289
Vertebral arteries, 312, 516–517, 517t, 518, 609, 617
cervical, vertebral, and suboccipital parts of, 615, 616
Vertebral body(ies), 277–278, 277
joints of, 287, 288–289
Vertebral canal, 277, 278, 296, 296
Vertebral column, 275–295. See also Vertebrae
curvatures of, 275–276, 276
abnormal, 276–277, 276–277
innervation of, 294–295, 295
joints and ligaments of, 288–292, 289
medical imaging of, 314–315, 314–315, 641
movements of, 292–294, 292
surface anatomy of, 284, 285–286
vasculature of, 294, 294–295
Vertebral foramen, 277, 278
stenotic, 286–287, 287
Vertebral joints, 288–292, 289
Vertebral muscles, anterior and lateral, 613, 614, 614–615t
Vertebral notches, 277, 278
Vertebral venous plexuses, 295, 299, 301
clinical significance of, 303
Vertebrochondral ribs, 48, 49
Vertebrocostal ribs, 48, 49
Vertex, 499, 499
Vertical muscle, of tongue, 565t
Vesical artery(ies), superior and inferior, 222t, 225, 225
Vesico-uterine pouch, 212t, 239, 240
Vestibular aqueduct, 584, 584
Vestibular folds, 625–627, 625–626
Vestibular ganglia, 585, 586

Vestibular glands, 269–270
inflammation of, 270
Vestibular labyrinth, 584
Vestibular ligament, 625, 625–626
Vestibular membrane, of cochlear duct, 586, 586
Vestibular nerve, 586, 587, 646t–647t, 663
Vestibule, 268–269, 269
of bony labyrinth, 584, 584
bulbs of, 269, 269
of vagina, 236, 236
Vestibulocochlear nerve (CN VIII), 663–664
distribution of, 585, 586, 663
injuries to, 664
intracranial portion of, 648
nuclei of, 649
summary of, 646t–647t
Vestibulocochlear organ, 583, 586–587
Vincula, 455
Visceral afferent (sensory) fibers, 36, 36, 220, 645
Visceral efferent (motor) fibers, 36–37, 36, 645
Visceral nervous system, 36, 36
Visceral pelvic fascia, 215, 216
Visceral peritoneum, 135, 136
vessels and nerves of, 136
Visceral pleura, 68, 69, 78
Visceral referred pain, 186, 186t
Visceral sensory fibers, 645
Viscerocranium, 496, 497
Visual field, 652, 652
defects in, 653
Visual system, 652
Vitreous body, 535, 538
Vitreous chamber, 535, 538
Vitreous humor, 538
Vocal folds, 625, 625–627
Vocal ligaments, 624, 625, 626
Vocal process, of arytenoid cartilage, 624, 626
Vocalis, 625, 629t
Voluntary muscle. See Skeletal muscle
Vomer, 499, 500, 561
Vorticose veins, 547, 547
Vulva, 268, 268–269, 270

W

Walking, and gait cycle, 377, 378t
White matter, 31, 33
White rami communicantes, 38, 40–41, 194
Winged scapula, 424, 424
Wormian bones, 14
Wounds, skin, 8
Wrist, 488, 488t, 489. See also Carpal tunnel
arteries of, 457, 459t
fractures and dislocations of, 491–492
ligaments of, 417–419, 418
skin creases of, 474, 474
synovial cyst of, 460, 460
Wrist-drop, 445, 445
Wrist joint, 488t, 489
structures limiting movements of, 486t

X

X-rays. See Radiography
Xiphisternal joint, 67
Xiphoid process, 51, 51, 124

Z

Z-line, 143, 144
Z movement, 466
Zonular fibers, 537
Zygapophysial joints, 289–290, 289
injury and disease of, 290
references to, 209, 210, 277, 278
Zygomatic arch, 496, 497
Zygomatic bone, 496, 497
frontal process of, 529, 529
Zygomatic nerve, 658
Zygomatic process, of temporal bone, 496, 497
Zygomaticofacial foramen, 496, 497
Zygomaticofacial nerve, 521t
Zygomaticotemporal nerve, 521t